W9-CRY-883

Chemical Carcinogens

Chemical Carcinogens

Second Edition, Revised and Expanded

Volume 1

Charles E. Searle, *Editor*
University of Birmingham, England

ACS Monograph 182

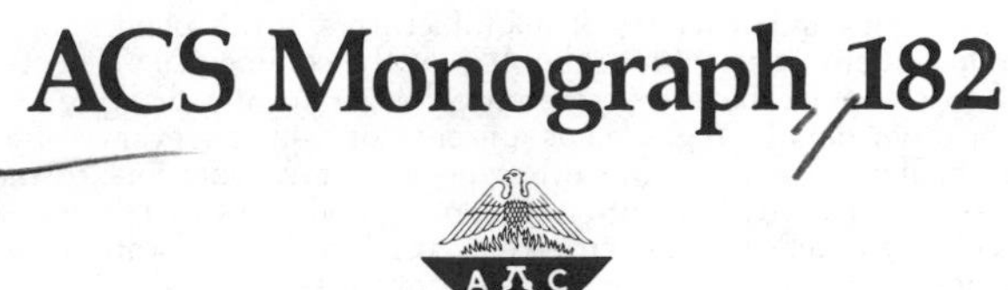

American Chemical Society
Washington, D.C. 1984

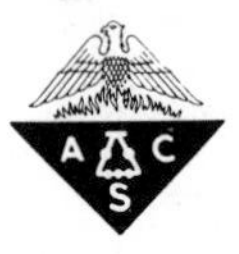

Library of Congress Cataloging in Publication Data

Chemical carcinogens.
(ACS monograph, ISSN 0065-7719; 182)

Includes bibliographies and indexes.

1. Carcinogens. 2. Carcinogenesis.
I. Searle, Charles E., 1922- . II. Series.
[DNLM: 1. Carcinogens. QZ 202 C517]

RC268.6.C48 1984 616.99'4071 84-20324
ISBN 0-8412-0869-7

PRINTED IN THE UNITED STATES OF AMERICA

FOREWORD

ACS MONOGRAPH SERIES was started by arrangement with the interallied Conference of Pure and Applied Chemistry, which met in London and Brussels in July 1919, when the American Chemical Society undertook the production and publication of Scientific and Technologic Monographs on chemical subjects. At the same time it was agreed that the National Research Council, in cooperation with the American Chemical Society and the American Physical Society, should undertake the production and publication of Critical Tables of Chemical and Physical Constants. The American Chemical Society and the National Research Council mutually agreed to care for these two fields of chemical progress.

The Council of the American Chemical Society, acting through its Committee on National Policy, appointed editors and associates to select authors of competent authority in their respective fields and to consider critically the manuscripts submitted. Since 1944 the Scientific and Technologic Monographs have been combined in the Series. The first Monograph appeared in 1921.

These Monographs are intended to serve two principal purposes: first to make available to chemists a thorough treatment of a selected area in form usable by persons working in more or less unrelated fields to the end that they may correlate their own work with a larger area of physical science; secondly, to stimulate further research in the specific field treated. To implement this purpose the authors of Monographs give extended references to the literature.

ABOUT THE EDITOR

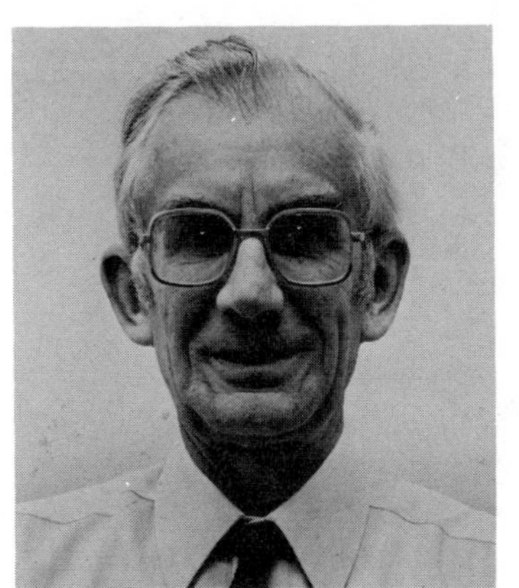

After receiving his B.Sc at University College of London, Charles E. Searle spent three years in industrial research. He then earned his doctorate in organic chemistry from the Battersea Polytechnic in London. From 1948 to 1956 he carried out thyroid research at University College Hospital Medical School and the Royal Free Hospital of Medicine. Currently, he is Senior Lecturer in the Department of Cancer Studies at the University of Birmingham where he has been involved in cancer research since 1956. He holds a D.Sc of the University of Birmingham and is a Fellow of the Royal Society of Chemistry and a member of the British Association for Cancer Research. His special interests are in chemical carcinogenesis and the prevention of cancer.

CONTENTS

Volume 1

Preface, **xv**

1. Cancer Epidemiology by R. A. Cartwright, **1**
   Background, **1**
   Sources of Data, **11**
   Methods in Epidemiology, **13**
   Natural History of Cancer, **18**
   Etiology of Cancer, **19**
   Occupation as a Cause of Cancer, **29**

2. Polynuclear Aromatic Carcinogens by Anthony Dipple, Robert C. Moschel, and C. Anita H. Bigger, **41**
   Nomenclature, **41**
   Introduction, **49**
   Chemical Structure and Carcinogenic Activity, **52**
   Chemistry of Polynuclear Carcinogens, **55**
   Biochemistry of Polynuclear Carcinogens, **66**
   Relationship Between Metabolism and Carcinogenic Action, **82**
   Tumorigenic Properties of Hydrocarbon Metabolites and Related Compounds, **99**
   Chemistry of Epoxides, Dihydrodiols, and Dihydrodiol Epoxides, **110**
   General Observations, **126**

3. Soots, Tars, and Oils as Causes of Occupational Cancer by M. D. Kipling and M. A. Cooke, **165**
   Early History, **165**
   Shale Oil, **167**
   Petroleum Oils, **167**
   Soots, **169**
   Pitch and Tar, **170**
   Lubricating and Cutting Oils, **170**
   Prognosis and Prevention, **172**

4. Carcinogenic Aromatic Amines and Related Compounds by R. C. Garner, C. N. Martin, and D. B. Clayson, **175**
   Mechanism of Action of Some Aromatic Amines, **178**

Structure–Activity Relationships, **201**
Conclusions, **263**

5. Epidemiology of Aromatic Amine Cancers by H. G. Parkes and A. E. J. Evans, **277**
Aromatic Amines of Industrial Importance, **279**
Epidemiology of Bladder Cancer, **286**
Industrial Bladder Cancer, **288**
Epidemiology of Industrial Bladder Cancer, **289**
The Work of R. A. M. Case, **290**
Screening, **294**
Compensation, **294**
Legal Liability, **295**
Legislation, **297**

6. Chemical Carcinogens as Laboratory Hazards by C. E. Searle, **303**
Epidemiological Studies of Chemists, **304**
Studies of Some Other Chemically Exposed Populations, **308**
Other Analytical Uses of Carcinogenic Amines, **312**
Possible Carcinogenicity of Some Other Reagents, **313**
Potency and Volatility of Chemical Carcinogens, **314**
Laboratory Precautions with Carcinogens, **314**
Carcinogens in Science Education, **319**

7. Carcinogenesis by Alkylating Agents by P. D. Lawley, **325**
Chemical Reactivity as a Factor Determining Carcinogenic Potency, **325**
Alkylation of DNA in Relation to Carcinogenic Potency of Alkylating Agents: Induction of Directly Miscoding Bases, **336**
In Vivo Dosimetry of Carcinogens Based on Alkylation of DNA, **368**
Dose–Response Relationships in Alkylation Carcinogenesis, **378**
Alkylating Agents and Cancer in Humans, **383**
Representative Oncogenesis Tests with Alkylating Agents, **400**
Oncogenesis Tests with Alkylating Agents in Relation to Their Chemical Structure and Reactivity, **404**
Summary and Conclusions, **460**

8. DNA Interactions of Reactive Intermediates Derived from Carcinogens by M. R. Osborne, **485**
Carcinogens that Alkylate DNA, **486**
Carcinogenicity and Reactivity, **501**
Position of Substitution, **501**
Regional Specificity, **503**
Spontaneous Loss of Alkyl Group, **507**
Depurination or Depyrimidination, **507**
Removal by Enzymes, **508**

DNA Breakage, **512**
Cross-linkage, **514**
Template Activity In Vitro, **514**

9. Carcinogenicity of Organic Halogenated Compounds by Helmut Greim and Thomas Wolff, **525**
Agents for Organic Synthesis, **526**
Fire Retardants, **534**
Solvents, **536**
Miscellaneous Agents, **544**
Polychlorinated Biphenyls (PCBs), **545**
Pesticides, **546**
Conclusion, **561**

10. Inorganic Carcinogenesis by John P. W. Gilman and Sabine H. H. Swierenga, **577**
Metals as Environmental and Occupational Carcinogens, **577**
Assessment of Carcinogenesis, **578**
Metal Carcinogens, **580**
Metal Cofactors in Carcinogenesis, **611**

11. Mineral Fiber Carcinogenesis by J. C. Wagner, **631**
Asbestos Minerals, **631**
Synthetic Mineral Fibers, **633**
Naturally Occurring Fibrous Minerals, **634**
Sequelae of Exposure to Asbestos Dust, **634**
Significance of Fiber Size, **637**
Effects of Other Fibers, **638**
Discussion, **639**

Author Index, **I1**

Subject Index, **I3**

Volume 2

12. N-Nitroso Carcinogens by R. Preussmann and B. W. Stewart, **643**
Chemistry: Recent Results, **644**
Biological Effects, **651**
Biotransformation, **682**
Mechanism of Carcinogenesis by N-*Nitroso Compounds*, **697**
Recent Developments, **728**

13. N-Nitroso Carcinogens in the Environment by R. Preussmann and G. Eisenbrand, **829**
Analytical Methodology, **831**

Preformed Environmental N-*Nitrosamines*, **832**
Occupational Exposure, **851**
In Vivo Nitrosation, **857**

14. Triazenes by G. F. Kolar, **869**
IUPAC Nomenclature and Classification, **870**
Historical Development, **870**
Use of Triazene Compounds, **872**
Chemistry of Triazenes, **872**
Biological Effects of Alkylaryltriazenes, **896**
Mechanism of Action and Metabolic Activation, **903**

15. Hydrazine Derivatives, Azo and Azoxy Compounds, and Methylazoxymethanol and Cycasin by Morris S. Zedeck, **915**
Background, **915**
Carcinogenesis Studies, **916**
Biochemical and Pathologic Alterations, **926**
Mutagenicity and Cell Transformation, **931**

16. Aflatoxins by William F. Busby, Jr. and Gerald N. Wogan, **945**
Historical Perspective, **946**
Chemistry, **947**
Mycology, **948**
Occurrence in Agricultural Commodities, **948**
Human Disease and Aflatoxin Exposure, **966**
Biological Activity, **970**
Metabolism, Excretion, and Tissue Distribution, **1029**
Biochemical Effects, **1076**
Structure–Activity Relationships, **1093**

17. Fusarial Mycotoxins and Cancer by R. Schoental, **1137**
Secondary Metabolites of Microfungi, **1138**
Epidemiological Considerations, **1140**
Esophageal Cancer, **1141**
T-2 Toxin, **1146**
Metabolism of T-2 Toxin, **1148**
Effects of T-2 Toxin and Related Trichothecenes on the Immune System, **1149**
Detection and Estimation of Trichothecenes Among Other Mycotoxins, **1150**
Estrogenic Agents, **1151**
Protection Against Fusarial Toxins, **1159**

18. Bracken Carcinogenicity by I. A. Evans, **1171**
Investigation of Biological Effects, **1171**
Chemical Studies, **1181**
Possible Environmental Hazard to Human Health, **1190**
General Conclusions, **1195**

19. Carcinogens in Food by Paul Grasso, **1205**
Species Responses to Carcinogens, **1206**
Genetic Factors, **1206**
The Statistical Approach, **1207**
Polycyclic Aromatic Hydrocarbons, **1209**
Nitrosamines, **1213**
Plant Sources, **1219**
Fungal Sources, **1220**
Metals, **1223**
Food Additives and Frying Oils, **1224**
Sweeteners, **1225**
Pesticides, **1226**
Diet and Cancer, **1227**
Conclusions, **1232**

20. Carcinogenicity of Medicines by T. A. Connors, **1241**
Agents Used in the Treatment of Cancer, **1241**
Medicines That are Converted to Carcinogens In Vivo, **1255**
Other Pharmaceutical Agents, **1266**
Estimation of Risk, **1272**

21. Inhibition of Chemical Carcinogenesis by Thomas J. Slaga and John DiGiovanni, **1279**
Inhibition of Tumor Initiation, **1282**
Inhibition of Tumor Promotion, **1298**
Summary, **1310**

22. Bioassay of Carcinogens: In Vitro and In Vivo Tests by J. H. Weisburger and G. M. Williams, **1323**
History of Carcinogen Bioassay, **1324**
Definition of Chemical Carcinogens, **1326**
The Carcinogenic Process, **1327**
Modifying Factors, **1328**
Mechanisms of Carcinogenesis, **1328**
Classes of Chemical Carcinogens, **1329**
Carcinogen Testing, **1332**
The Decision Point Approach, **1332**
Final Evaluation, **1356**
Health Risk Assessment, **1357**
Concluding Remarks, **1360**

Author Index, **I1**

Subject Index, **I3**

PREFACE

THE TERM CANCER COVERS A LARGE RANGE OF DISEASES for which a multiplicity of biological, physical, and chemical causes are known or suspected. Biological agents, predominantly viruses, cause a variety of cancers in animals, but their role in human cancer is much less certain. The evidence is strongest for the widespread Epstein-Barr virus, which normally causes glandular fever, but, under special circumstances, results in Burkitt lymphoma in African children or nasopharyngeal carcinoma in China. Viruses may also be involved in some other lymphomas, leukemias, and cancers of the liver, penis, and cervix.

Strict controls on exposure to ionizing radiation and radioactive substances arose from recognition of occupational cancers caused by careless use of these agents; meanwhile a great number of skin cancers are attributed to the UV component of sunlight. The study of chemical carcinogenic agents, important for identifying occupational and environmental causes of cancer and for cancer prevention, is the subject of this revised and expanded edition of Monograph 173.

Early knowledge of chemical carcinogens derived directly from cancers that occurred in industries where workers had daily contact with carcinogenic agents. Skin cancers caused by constituents of soots and mineral oils led to the first identification of pure chemical carcinogens, polycyclic aromatic hydrocarbons, around 1930. This discovery was followed by identification of the aromatic amines responsible for bladder cancer in the chemical and rubber industries. Later, various other occupational carcinogens such as vinyl chloride, certain alkylating agents, and some wood dusts were also identified. Some inorganic materials, such as dusts and fumes containing nickel and arsenic, have caused occupational cancers of the respiratory system. Some of these hazards have been removed by elimination of the carcinogenic agents or by major improvements in working conditions. However, asbestos remains a serious problem because of its widespread use, the difficulties in replacing it, and the huge amounts still remaining in buildings and ships.

Soon after the publication of the first edition of this monograph in 1976, the question of the percentage of cancer caused by chemicals in the workplace became a subject of heated controversy. A widely quoted document suggested that, at least in the United States, carcinogens in the workplace could be responsible for perhaps 20 or 30% of cancer cases; the expression "epidemic of cancer" is still heard. Currently, most epidemiologists and research workers believe that occupational cancers comprise at most 5 or 6% of all cancers in men and less in women. In recent decades the occurrence of lung cancer has increased dramatically, largely as a result of cigarette smoking, and the incidence of stomach cancer has declined, probably because of changes in eating habits. However, no major changes in other cancers have been observed; these cancers have been with us too long to be attributable to the great expansion in chemical usage after World War II. In their detailed review, "The Causes of Cancer: Quantitative Estimates of Avoidable Risks of Cancer in the United States Today," Doll and Peto estimated that approximately 4% of cancer deaths were attributable to occupational factors and 30% were due to tobacco (*J. Natl. Cancer Inst.* **1981,** *66,* 1191–1308; published separately by Oxford University Press, 1983).

However, this relatively low percentage of occupational cancers still represents a large number of people, and all reasonable steps must be taken to eliminate the causes. Apart from the continuing problems with asbestos and other materials, many questions still await answers. Is formaldehyde, which produces nasal cancer in rats with prolonged inhalation at high concentrations, a significant human hazard at the much lower levels widely encountered in many workplaces or through use of urea–formaldehyde foam insulation? Are some cases of lymphoma and brain cancer of occupational origin; and, if so, what are the causes? How should carcinogens be regulated? Are less stringent conditions adequate for agents believed to cause cancer only through nongenotoxic (epigenetic) mechanisms, such as tumor promoters and some hormones, or should they be treated similarly to carcinogens with a genotoxic action, such as the carcinogenic aromatic amines? Is it even sensible to regulate carcinogens separately from all other harmful chemicals?

In addition to exposing occupational cancers, studies of cancer epidemiology indicate possible causes of cancers in the general population. These studies reveal remarkably large differences in the incidence and mortality of cancers between different parts of the world and within individual countries. The incidence of some cancers can also change greatly with time, and changes found in migrant populations have been especially revealing. Frequently, the pattern of various cancers in a migrant population, such as the Japanese now residing in the United States, alters over a period of time from that characteristic of the country of origin toward one more like that of the country of adoption. Such changes in migrants were recently described as the most comforting news ever to come out of cancer research, because they convincingly demonstrate that much cancer is not inevitable but arises from environmental factors that differ from one location to another. Therefore, at least in theory, a major proportion of human cancer, not just occupational cancer, should be preventable.

The principal reasons for changes in cancers found in migrant populations, and the differences found between different localities, probably lie in dietary factors. Currently, much research seeks to elucidate the effects of specific types of diet on predisposition to certain forms of cancer. The identification of such associations and the discovery of plausible explanations for some of them are making it possible to give sound advice on diet and are raising real hopes of effecting significant reductions in some major cancers.

In many areas of the world, especially in the tropics, foods can become contaminated with toxic and carcinogenic products of plants and microorganisms. Together with nutritional deficiencies, this contamination can pose serious health problems in addition to those of infectious diseases. In technologically-advanced countries in the more temperate climates, known potent carcinogens of several classes are found also in foods, but generally only at concentrations of a few parts per billion. Although these concentrations are not necessarily insignificant, the actual proportions of the principal dietary constituents, especially very high intakes of fats and relatively low consumption of plant foods, are probably much more important.

In 1982, a committee of the U.S. National Research Council and National Academy of Sciences reviewed the relationship between diet and cancer in its report "Diet, Nutrition, and Cancer," and made recommendations for dietary modifications that offer hope of significantly reducing the incidence of several major cancers. The principal recommendations are the reduced consumption of fats and of foods preserved by smoking and salting, accompanied by increased regular consumption of whole-grain cereals, fruits, and vegetables. The study also noted the synergistic action of alcohol with smoking that causes cancers of the oral cavity, esophagus, and larynx.

Fortunately, these guidelines for reducing risks of cancer resemble earlier recommendations for reducing heart disease and other circulatory diseases such as those found in a 1977 U.S. Senate Committee report. This agreement is not very surprising because these and other diseases appear to be closely related to our present way of life, especially, but not exclusively, to our dietary and smoking habits. Although many recommendations are similar, differences of opinion exist about the relative merits and demerits of saturated and unsaturated fats.

The greatest unanimity is in the area of the prevention of smoking-related diseases. More than 30 years have passed since the first clear links were established between cigarette smoking and lung cancer. Since that discovery, we have seen lung cancer become by far the most important cause of cancer death in men; and, more recently, we have seen also rapid increases in the occurrence of lung cancer in women. Data from many countries indict smoking as a prime cause of lung and some other cancers and as a major precipitating factor in coronary heart diseases. Increasingly we are realizing that tobacco smoke harms not only the smoker but also the "passive smoker," from the fetus and young child to the nonsmoking spouses of smokers. Regrettably, most governments have remained unwilling to take serious steps to prevent the current epidemic of smoking-related diseases. They have shown even less willingness to curb the active exporting of smoking to developing countries that have crippling problems of poverty, malnutrition, and infectious disease.

Prevention of circulatory disease and prevention of cancer have unfortunately been treated as separate problems. Chances of success might be enhanced by greater cooperation between all groups involved in preventing these diseases. Thus governments and the public would be presented with sound and less confusing advice and perhaps would even be convinced that freedom from many serious diseases is possible and worth working for.

Chemicals now recognized as causing or modifying cancer now include a very extensive range of chemical classes, inorganic as well as organic. We have come a long way from the time when chemical carcinogen meant only a few polycyclic hydrocarbons and azo dyes and little else. This second edition of "Chemical Carcinogens" includes reviews of the nature, mode of action, and hazards of the major groups of chemical carcinogens.

Skin cancer caused by polycyclic aromatic contaminants of soots and mineral oils and bladder cancer resulting from exposure to a few identified aromatic amines have become less prominent problems of occupational medicine. On the other hand, research on the environmental aspects of *N*-nitroso carcinogens indicates some involvement by these compounds in human cancer. A new chapter is therefore devoted to this subject, and other chapters discuss carcinogenic triazenes, hydrazines, and related compounds.

Other important aspects of chemical carcinogenesis are now included: an introduction on cancer epidemiology to be used as a guide to recognizing carcinogens; accounts of carcinogenesis by halogenated solvents and pesticides; inhibition of carcinogenesis; carcinogenicity of drugs; and inorganic carcinogens other than asbestos. Carcinogenesis by asbestos is often regarded as an example of solid-state carcinogenesis, analogous to the development of cancer at the site of metal or plastic foils implanted inside animal tissues. Carcinogenesis of this type appears to depend on the dimensions and physical properties of the implant rather than on its chemical nature. Nevertheless, occupational and environmental carcinogenesis by asbestos is so important that a brief review is included again—with references to possible risks from other mineral fibers.

Unfortunately, we were unable to include certain areas of chemical carcinogenesis. Understanding the enhancement of carcinogenesis by tumor promoters and cocarcinogens is now regarded as very important for understanding the development of some human cancers. For discussions concerning tumor promoters and cocarcinogens, *see* Chapter 2 of the first edition and, for recent sources, *Environmental Health Perspectives,* Volume 50, U.S. Department of Health, Education, and Welfare, 1983. For discussions about occupational and environmental air pollution and smoking as causes of respiratory cancer, *see* Chapter 7 of the first edition; *Environmental Health Perspectives,* Volumes 47 and 52, 1983; "Smoking and Health: a Report of the Surgeon General," 1979, and "The Health Consequences of Smoking for Women; a Report of the Surgeon General," U.S. Department of Health, Education and Welfare, 1980. In addition the more modest report of the Royal College of Physicians of London "Health or Smoking," 1983, is recommended. (Perhaps the repeated use of the expression "smoking and health" rather than "smoking and disease" has been a psychological mistake.)

A comprehensive review of carcinogenesis testing systems presents extensive developments in short-term in vitro tests in the period since the first edition was published. Although potent carcinogens may be recognized easily by using small numbers of test animals, other chemicals give equivocal results even with full lifespan tests conducted on large numbers of animals that have been administered maximum tolerated doses. Apart from moral objections raised by such tests, they are also extremely expensive and quite unable to cope with the large numbers of chemicals that need to be evaluated.

Many unsuccessful attempts have been made to develop tests that might indicate carcinogenic activity rapidly and without the use of animals. The first test regarded as valuable was developed by Ames and colleagues. This test actually determines mutagenicity in special bacterial strains, and its use depends on the wide overlap between chemical mutagens and genotoxic carcinogens when allowance is made for metabolic activation. Various other short-term tests have been developed as a consequence of research on carcinogen–DNA interactions and the importance of DNA repair, but tests for agents acting by nongenotoxic mechanisms are still needed.

No short-term test alone is sufficient. However, a suitable battery of tests, which includes the Ames test and a test using mammalian cells, can give a great deal of valuable information on the likely carcinogenic hazards of chemicals and their mechanisms of action. Various logical and economical methods of short-term and animal testing are now being used to evaluate the nature and significance of potential carcinogenic hazards.

The problems inherent to chemical nomenclature still cause problems in chemical carcinogenesis. The use of 2-naphthylamine and β-naphthylamine for the same chemical is unlikely to cause confusion; but, nonchemists may not recognize 2-fluorenylacetamide as being the same carcinogen as 2-acetylaminofluorene, an obsolete name still used in chemical carcinogenesis literature. Polycyclic aromatic hydrocarbons have undergone various nomenclature changes; benzo[a]pyrene, for example, is found in older literature as both 3,4-benzpyrene and 1,2-benzpyrene. Nomenclature of these carcinogens is clarified at the start of Chapter 2. *N*-Nitroso derivatives of secondary amines, often still called dialkylnitrosamines, are more correctly termed *N*-nitrosodialkylamines as used in this volume. Nitrosamine is retained as a generic name, and acronyms are employed to avoid frequent repetition of cumbersome names, as in NDMA for *N*-nitrosodimethylamine (dimethylnitrosamine). I hope that the nomenclature in this volume is found reasonably consistent and free from avoidable confusion.

I regret to record the deaths of M. D. Kipling (1978) and W. H. S. George (1979), two authors who contributed to the first edition of this monograph. I express my thanks to other authors from the original edition who contributed to this second edition, to the new authors, who have also given most generously of their valuable time and expertise, and to my colleague Jennifer Teale for her advice and encouragement. Authoritative review of subjects as wide as chemical carcinogenesis makes multiauthor works virtually inevitable, but these tend to be criticized for their lack of balance and editorial control. However, many readers evidently found the first edition of considerable value despite such shortcomings. We hope this new edition will be useful in extending the understanding of the causes of cancer and in contributing to cancer prevention.

C. E. SEARLE
Birmingham, England

February 1984

1

Cancer Epidemiology

R. A. CARTWRIGHT

Yorkshire Regional Cancer Organisation, Cookridge Hospital, Leeds, LS16 6QB, England

THE ROLE OF OCCUPATION IN THE ETIOLOGY OF MALIGNANT DISEASE has been an important and debated issue; some scientists claim that well over 20% of all cancers are a result of occupational exposure (*1*), whereas others think only 3% are due to our work (*2, 3*). This topic has also been studied from a purely political point of view, and this approach has added to the difficulties of assessing how occupational cancers should be evaluated (*4, 5*). It is hoped this chapter will give a background to allow a critical analysis of broad generalizations and also to indicate that such a political approach to cancer etiology is facile (*6, 7*). This chapter is intended only to provide a framework for readers who wish to know more of the scope and applications of cancer epidemiology. It is not intended to be a comprehensive treatise, rather an introduction with emphasis on methods, in the hope that the readers will then be able to apply the principles themselves.

Background

Scope and Limitations. Cancer epidemiology can be broadly defined as the description of how malignant diseases influence human populations, together with the causes and natural history of the diseases. Etiologies vary with each type of cancer, as well as with the part of the world in which the descriptions are made and the particular year the observations are recorded.

The epidemiological approach has some advantages over other methods of analysis, but it also has quite a number of limitations (*8*).

The main advantage of epidemiology is that it measures events actually occurring in human populations rather than theoretical exposures inferred from an experimental approach. Furthermore, epidemiology allows insights into, and possibly confirmation of, mechanisms of carcinogenesis. A major disadvantage, however, is that epidemiology is a poor means to identify low levels of risk. Any risk that leads to an increase in cases of 40% or less cannot be determined with confidence by many epidemiological studies.

Another major weakness of epidemiology lies in the fact that cancer is a chronic disease with an undetectable starting point in an individual and a latent interval between exposure and diagnosis that extends up to and beyond 50 years.

0065-7719/84/0182-0001$08.75/1

Thus, details of exposure could be easily forgotten or records could be easily lost. Individuals can die of other causes before the malignancy becomes manifest. Exposure to only one possible hazard is unusual, and so distinguishing among various hazards and isolating their effects can be almost impossible.

A final difficulty is that the techniques of analysis that are used only allow an estimate of risk, together with confidence limits to be computed on the basis of known or putative hazards. If significant hazards concerned with the disease in question exist but are unknown, then the results of the supposed risk factors will be influenced accordingly. This situation can lead to spurious results; therefore, careful interpretation of the results of epidemiological studies is essential.

Historical Perspective. Epidemiological techniques have gradually emerged as a result of a series of clinical observations on populations with particular cancer problems. One early observation by Percivall Pott in 1775 (*9*) involved the occurrence of scrotal cancer among chimney sweeps. Since then, many hazardous substances that produce skin and scrotal cancer have been recognized. For example, in 1892, Butlin (*10*) demonstrated that Scottish shale oil workers were at risk, and in 1875, Volkmann (*11*) showed that tar and paraffin handlers were liable to such disorders. Mineral oils were shown to be responsible for Lancashire cotton mule spinners' cancers (*12*), and since then, mineral oil mists in the Birmingham area of England have led to a further epidemic of skin and scrotal cancer in lathe operators. This epidemic was first noted in 1950 (*13*) and has been studied extensively since then (*14*).

Other classical observations concerned the disease, first described as mala metallorum, that was found in excess in the Schneeberg miners in Germany in 1531, and it was finally identified as lung cancer in 1879 (*15*). Workers at the nearby uranium mines of Joachimstal (Jachymov) also had a long record of lung cancer, at times amounting to 43% of deaths among miners (*16*). In both mines, the concentrations of the radioactive gas radon and particulate respirable arsenic were very high.

Particular malignant diseases have been reliably reported to be linked with various occupations for more than a century. Epidemiological studies have gradually become more sophisticated. Early reports often described clinical observations of small case groups, such as the observations by Rehn from 1895 (*17*) of cases of bladder cancer in the aniline dye manufacturing industry. Later studies added information about the total workforce that was exposed to the hazard, and, more recently, a computation of "expected" rates for the malignancy was devised.

Epidemiological observations on types of cancer that are apparently not related to occupation have tended to lag behind these classical work-related clinical observations. For example, the two possible causes of the lung cancer epidemic, atmospheric pollution and cigarette smoking, were not investigated until the 1940s, because the epidemic nature of the increase of the disorder was not recognized prior to that date.

For all these historical and practical reasons, the emphasis in cancer epidemiological research might appear to be occupational. This emphasis some-

Table I

Distribution over Time of the Most Common Causes of Death in the United States Since 1950

	Death Rate[a]			
Cause	*1950*	*1960*	*1970*	*1977*
All causes	841.5	760.9	714.3	612.3
Heart disease	307.6	286.2	253.6	210.4
Neoplasms	125.4	125.8	129.9	133.0
Cerebrovascular disease	88.8	79.7	66.3	48.2
Accidents	57.5	49.9	53.7	43.8
Tuberculosis	21.7	5.4	2.2	1.0

[a]Death rates (deaths/100,000 population/year) are adjusted to the age structure of the population.

times leads to the incorrect assumption that occupational exposure is a major cause of malignant disease.

Cancer in the Modern World. More is known about the distribution of cancer throughout the world than any other group of diseases. This wealth of knowledge is partly due to the proliferation of cancer registries, from their origins in Europe to the rest of the world, and partly due to the fear, which is held by many nations, that when the infectious diseases are controlled, cancer will emerge as a major problem.

In the western world, cancer is a major disease entity. Table I shows the death rate attributable to malignant disease contrasted with other common causes of death in the United States (*18, 19*). Neoplasia is the second most common cause of all deaths; the most common cause, nowadays responsible for nearly half of all deaths, is disease of the arteries that leads to heart and cerebrovascular conditions.

Each year in England and Wales, 1 in 286 males and 1 in 317 females are newly diagnosed as having cancer. In other words, the chances of men who live to be 70 years old and of women who live to be 75 years old developing cancer are about one out of five. The differences that exist between the death (mortality) rates and the number of new cases (incidence) indicates that a proportion of cancer cases die of other disorders rather than the original cancer. This proportion is slowly increasing as treatment becomes more effective; indeed deaths from second malignancies in cases cured of one type of cancer will also increase.

Cancer Patterns. Cancer is a term that covers a loose aggregation of disorders, all of which are characterized by a clone of cells whose growth potential is uncontrolled. Terms such as tumor, new growth, and neoplasia refer to essentially the same phenomenon. Cancer tends to be defined by the site of the tumor, the specific type of cell of tumor origin (histopathology), and the degree of abnormality within the cells that make up the tumor (grade). The "stage" of a tumor is the degree to which it has spread from its point of origin into local or more distant tissues. Secondary growths can occur at some distance from the primary site but originate from it, and these secondary occurrences are called metastases. Tumors at certain sites are almost always of one particular histological type; for example, most bladder cancers are of a transitional cell type, and most skin tumors that are caused by industrial hazards are of squamous cell origin.

Malignancies arising in lymph glands (lymphomas) tend to be widespread in the body and difficult to define as arising from a particular site. The same is true of the various tumors of the blood-forming cells (leukemia), which are usually named by the origin of the putative cell, such as the lymphocytic leukemias.

Tumors commonly found in the United States are shown in Table II (*20*). In males, lung cancer accounts for 20% of the total malignancies. In females, 21% of all malignancies are breast cancer. Skin cancer is a common type of cancer but is not included in these figures.

Worldwide variation in tumor types is shown in Table III for the five most common tumors normally seen in males in the United States (*21, 22*). Skin cancer

Table II

Common Neoplasms Indicated in the Third National Cancer Survey from 1969 to 1971

	American Whites				*American Blacks*			
	Male		*Female*		*Male*		*Female*	
Site	N[a]	%[b]	N	%	N	%	N	%
Lung, trachea, and bronchus	17,010	21.0	4,313	5.3	2,096	23.8	405	5.6
Breast	174	0.2	22,487	27.5	18	0.2	1,673	23.0
Colon	7,753	9.6	9,125	11.2	600	6.8	740	10.2
Rectum	4,175	5.2	3,316	4.1	324	3.7	231	3.2
Stomach	3,299	4.1	2,129	2.6	484	5.5	240	3.3
Prostate	12,796	15.8	—	—	1,856	21.1	—	—
Bladder	5,478	6.8	1,920	2.3	261	3.0	110	1.5
Cervix uteri	—	—	4,419	5.4	—	—	1,012	13.9
Corpus uteri	—	—	6,207	7.6	—	—	329	4.5
Ovary	—	—	4,243	5.2	—	—	309	4.3
Esophagus	1,103	1.4	407	0.5	392	4.5	107	1.5
Pancreas	2,845	3.5	2,259	2.8	369	4.2	255	3.5
Brain	1,430	1.8	1,137	1.4	92	1.0	96	1.3
All lymphomas	3,036	3.7	2,462	3.0	235	2.7	147	2.0
All leukemias	3,100	3.8	2,315	2.8	250	2.8	176	1.4
All sites	81,006		81,713		8,793		7,266	

NOTE: Approximately 10% of all cases recorded were in the United States.
[a]Number of cases.
[b]Percentage distribution.
SOURCE: Ref. 20.

Table III

Worldwide Variation of New Cancer Cases in Sites Common in Western Societies for Males from 1960 to 1971

	Age-Standardized Occurrence Rate[a]				
Location	*Lung*	*Skin*	*Stomach*	*Prostate*	*Bladder*
Birmingham, England	100.2	37.3	29.9	22.3	21.6
Ibadan, Nigeria	0.4	0.6	2.4	1.8	0.9
Recife, Brazil	7.1	21.6	11.1	8.7	5.5
Cali, Colombia	8.2	19.4	20.3	7.8	3.1
Bombay, India	6.1	0.9	3.9	1.8	1.1
Texas, USA (whites)	38.7	122.0	14.8	37.2	16.1
Texas, USA (blacks)	34.9	4.5	27.9	59.3	9.4
Israel (Jews)	29.6	NA[b]	20.9	14.0	17.0
Miyagi, Japan	17.8	1.2	77.9	2.4	3.2
Shanghai, China[c]	24.4	NA	29.4	NA	2.0
Finland	78.0	24.4	36.9	21.0	8.6
Poland	64.3	10.8	36.4	14.7	10.7

[a]Occurrence rate is given in cases/100,000 population/year.
[b]NA = not available.
[c]Mortality data.

seems to increase in white populations with the quantity of UV light to which they are exposed. Stomach cancer is quite high in the Finns, but prodigiously so in the Japanese. Prostatic cancer is rare in Nigerians, but very common in American blacks. Lung cancer has its highest world incidence in Scotland (*22*). Cancer incidence in the five sites varies the least among the white populations of Europe, North America, Australia, and New Zealand. Undoubtedly regional and racial variations contain clues to the causes of the malignancies.

The cancers of the inhabitants of developing countries are quite different in their sites and histopathology. Table IV gives some distributional details of these tumors (*21*). Primary liver cell tumors are common in Southeast Asia and eastern Asia and are rare in America. Nasopharyngeal carcinoma, a rare disease in the West, is relatively common in the Chinese (*23*). Burkitt's lymphoma is virtually unknown in most of the world outside the central African malarial belt and parts of Southeast Asia.

The range in incidence worldwide for certain malignancies is enormous (*24*). Cancer of the esophagus is common in the Turkman tribes around the Caspian Sea and in certain regions of China. Particular tribes in Uganda have a high incidence of penile cancers, and many tribes of southern Africa are commonly affected by primary liver cancer. These observations must be indicative of the etiology of these tumors; unfortunately the investigations—for example of esophageal carcinoma in Iran and China—are proving to be far more complex than was originally envisaged.

Table IV

Worldwide Variation of New Cancer Cases in Sites Common in Some Developing Countries for Males from 1960 to 1971

	Age-Standardized Occurrence Rate[a]		
Location	*Primary Liver Cell Tumor*	*Nasopharyngeal Carcinoma*	*Esophageal Carcinoma*
Birmingham, England	1.2	0.5	6.4
Ibadan, Nigeria	4.9	0.3	0.3
Recife, Brazil	4.7	0.4	2.5
Cali, Colombia	1.1	0.1	1.2
Bombay, India	0.8	0.3	6.6
Texas, USA (whites)	2.9	0.8	3.8
Texas, USA (blacks)	5.6	1.2	10.3
Israel (Jews)	2.5	1.1	2.5
Miyagi, Japan	1.6	0.3	11.4
Shanghai, China[b]	22.7	17.5[c]	14.4
Finland	2.2	0.4	5.0
Warsaw, Poland	8.4	0.7	5.6

[a]Occurrence rate is given in cases/100,000 population/year
[b]Mortality data.
[c]Chung Shan, China.

Conversely, certain tumors vary little in their worldwide distribution, for example, female bladder cancer, myeloid leukemia, and nephroblastoma (Wilm's tumor) in children.

Not all cancers have equally common incidence rates in either sex within the same age range, or within the same social class. In developed countries, a few tumors are more common in females than in males, a few are equally distributed, and the rest tend to be more common in males (*20*). For example, gall bladder and thyroid cancers are more common in women, and bladder and larynx cancers are more common in men.

Age-specific incidence rates are strikingly different for each type of tumor (*20*). Table V gives some examples of the different rates at different ages for cases in the United States: some cancers in females, like cervical cancer, are common around the menopause. The usual situation, however, is that the incidence of malignancies increases with increasing age. Female breast cancer and Hodgkin's disease both have a bimodal distribution, with the antimode in the third or fourth decades. Testicular tumors are most commonly found in young men.

Social-class statistics are difficult to interpret on an international scale because each country has a distinct means of defining class. In the United Kingdom, however, such data have been available for over 60 years, and quite meaningful comparisons can be made between classes (*25*).

Table V

Cancer Incidence in Three Age Groups for All Races in the United States from 1969 to 1971

	Occurrence Rate[a]		
Site	*20–24 years old*	*50–54 years old*	*80–84 years old*
All sites (males)	29.7	414.6	2831.9
All sites (females)	30.1	507.7	1497.9
Prostate	0	18.2	847.6
Breast (females)	1.2	168.4	297.1
Hodgkin's (males)	5.4	4.8	10.7
Testis	6.2	2.9	2.4
Cervix	4.1	31.4	37.7

[a]Occurrence rates are given in cases/100,000 population/year.

Social class in England and Wales is exclusively based on occupation and has been criticized on a variety of counts (*26*). Social class varies from 1, the professional groups, to 5, the manual laborers (*26*). In general, cancer deaths occur most frequently in men of the "lower" social classes, i.e., manual workers of all description. This distribution is obtained partly because the total cancer deaths are weighted due to lung and stomach cancer deaths, and these cases are far more common among manual workers (*27*). In the United States and elsewhere, social-class statistics tend to be based on economic potential and are not readily comparable.

Secular Trends. Changes in the pattern of disease with time are of particular interest. In part, they help to predict the future health needs of a population and, in part, they highlight areas in which further etiological investigation of the disease is required.

Cancer as a cause of death has increased with respect to other causes of death and is still increasing slightly. Figure 1 shows the proportionate deaths caused by cancer of all types in 1923 and in 1973. In part, the overall proportionate increase in cancer deaths results from the advent of antibiotics and the general improvement of public health, which enables people to live longer and die of diseases other than infection; such diseases are often cancer. In addition, clearer diagnoses are now made with the increasingly scientific attitudes in clinical medicine, and the accuracy of the death-certificate recording has improved during this period. Changes in the lifestyle of the population also could have contributed to the general increase in cancer deaths, but the contribution is difficult to estimate quantitatively.

To make any comparison of secular trends, the results must be age-standardized in some way because of the ever-changing international age pattern of populations (*18*).

The increase of cancer in men and the recent increases in women partially

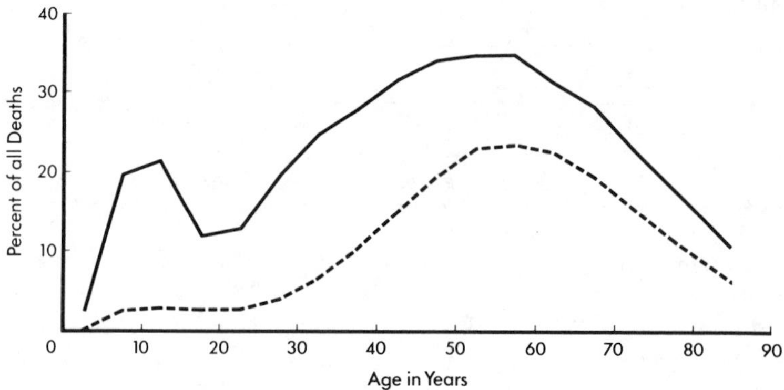

Figure 1. Proportion of all deaths attributed to neoplasms in England and Wales. vs. age. Key to year:—, 1973; and ----, 1923.

result from the influence of the enormous burden that the lung cancer statistics place on the total figures.

Secular trends for selected tumors for each sex are shown in semilogarithmic graphs in Figures 2 and 3. For some tumors, the overall resultant mortality rate has decreased; for other tumors, the rate has increased. The two major increases in mortality were due to lung cancer and leukemia in both sexes, although at different times. Pancreatic cancer deaths are almost certainly becoming more common. However, death certification in the United Kingdom is such that, even when a patient dies of an unrelated disorder, a past history of cancer could mean that the malignancy is placed on the certificate as one of the causes of death. This fact and possible changes in such practices have to be taken into account when secular changes in mortality are interpreted.

Despite many revisions in diagnostic techniques and treatment over the last 50 years, no marked change is seen in the number of female breast cancer mortalities. Carcinoma of the cervix had a declining mortality rate even before 1950, that is to say prior to the introduction of screening programs in Britain. The downward trend before 1950 has been among the factors that have made the value of screening for this disease difficult to assess.

More recently, several other malignancies have been shown to be on the increase, including malignant melanoma (*28*), non-Hodgkin's lymphoma (*29*), and multiple myeloma (*30*). Childhood lymphoblastic leukemia seems to have had a steep increase in incidence since 1970 in those populations that have been closely observed in the United States, United Kingdom, and Japan (*31*).

Childhood Tumors. The spectrum of tumors in children is very different from that in adults, in that very few tumors of the adult type are found in children, whereas an excess of tumors that originate from abnormal embryonic cells or tissues occurs (*32*). Close relationships exist between certain children's tumors and abnormalities in growth and development. For example, Wilm's tumor and congenital hemi-hypertrophy are occasionally linked. By inference, therefore, the causes of adult-

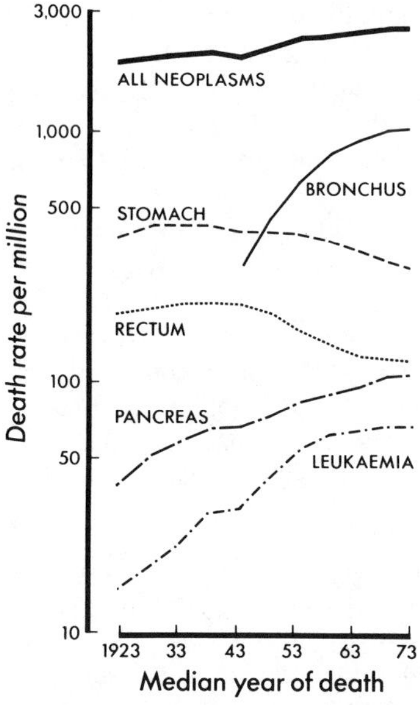

Figure 2. Secular trends in male cancer deaths 1921–75.

type tumors and childhood-type tumors are likely to be very different. The incidence of one type of eye tumor called retinoblastoma can be tracked in pedigrees and the inheritance pattern resembles that of a Mendelian dominant gene. This simple mode of inheritance is almost unique for cancer. These tumors are very rare: about four new cases per year for every 5 million of the total

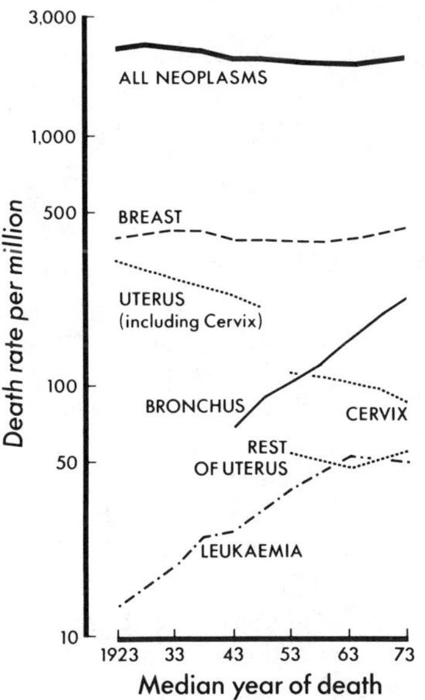

Figure 3. Secular trends in female cancer deaths 1921–75.

population (*33*). Other inherited syndromes cause childhood malignancies, but all of them are rarer than retinoblastomas.

Acute lymphoblastic leukemia has its peak incidence between 4 and 6 years of age and accounts for the childhood peak of cancer deaths shown in Figure 1. In Japan, the proportion of myeloid leukemia among children is much greater than in the western world (*34*).

Childhood malignancies do not appear to vary in incidence throughout the world except for some types of brain tumor, Ewing's sarcoma, and the lymphomas and leukemias (*35*).

Childhood leukemias tend to occur quite frequently in patients who have close contact. There are seasonal variations; leukemias occur more commonly in winter. Also, a greater incidence is seen in individuals born or living in a particular locality. These links in both time and space are known as clustering (*36, 37*). Clustering is often taken to indicate that an infective agent is associated with the etiology.

Natural History of Cancer. Some tumors grow rapidly, while other tumors grow so slowly that they are rarely truly responsible for deaths. This variation might be expected from different tumor types at different sites, but such variation also occurs in apparently identical tumors at the same site. Also in some tumors, survival is almost always the same irrespective of treatment. For example, 50% of women with breast cancer tend to survive about 5 years, whereas over 90% of people with lung and pancreatic cancers die within a few years. In contrast, death rarely results from basal cell cancers of the skin.

The major influence on most tumors, however, is whether or not they were treated and the exact mode of treatment. Nowadays, attempts are made to treat tumors either by surgery, radiotherapy, chemotherapy, or a combination of such measures. In many cases, except possibly the infirm, available treatments have had some success; survival rates have improved by 20–30% over the last few decades (*38*). Unfortunately little progress has been made in the treatment of some cancers, for example, pancreatic tumors.

The most remarkable advances have been made in the treatment of childhood malignancies. In the late 1950s, less than one in five children survived 5 years. Now well over half of all children treated at specialist centers survive, and almost all cases of certain specific tumor types survive.

Bladder cancer has a highly variable tumor incidence. It is more common in certain parts of the United Kingdom than in other parts. In the high-incidence areas, it has a worse prognosis and affects a greater percentage of women than elsewhere. Bladder cancer normally has a male:female ratio of 4:1, but in the high-incidence areas, this ratio is about 2:1 and the survival rate is perhaps 10% lower than elsewhere (*39*).

The reasons for such different behavior across populations for the same disease are not well understood. In part, the variance may be due to the different causes of the disease, but other factors such as the distinct genetic makeup of the individual affected might also be involved. The entire topic of disease natural history is quite new for modern chronic-disease epidemiologists to study. A malignancy can have many different causative factors, and these factors might influence the number of cases in a population and influence what happens to each case. In terms of cancer epidemiology, a malignancy can be either slow growing or rapidly invasive as part of its natural growth pattern. The normal aspects of cell surface variability, such as the ABO blood groups or the HLA types, also influence the natural history of a malignancy (*40*).

Sources of Data

Epidemiologists rely to a certain extent on the routine acquisition of information to uncover patterns in disease distributions and secular trends. Such data can be useful for a number of reasons: to determine the health needs for the community, to formulate hypotheses about cancer etiology, and to explain the peculiarities of cancer distribution.

Statistics on a national level are of prime importance to modern epidemiology as they provide data for contrast with a particular study population.

Early Mortality Records. Most industrialized countries had some sort of mortality surveillance system in operation by the latter half of the 19th century. This system was developed in England by William Farr (1807–83), the Compiler of Abstracts to the General Register Office. He is generally regarded as the founder of epidemiology (*41*). The annual reports of the Register Office for England and Wales are not specific to one disease but map out the overall pattern of changes in mortality. The value of such a system in any country is immeasurable for future public health concerns.

However, by the 1930s it was recognized that mortality from cancer and the occurrence of new cases could be different, and that it would be better to investigate the records of new cases—in particular, to follow the natural history of the diseases—and acquire more accurate morbidity information. This decision led to the development of cancer registries.

Cancer Registries. The cancer registry system has developed in two ways over the last 50 years, either as a hospital-based system or as a population-based system (*42*). The hospital cancer registry records details of all cases attending a certain center for treatment. Many cancer registries in America were of this type, as well as a few centers in Britain.

The Scandinavian countries and Britain have since developed a system of registries that are population-based; consequently, data on all cases, whether they are treated or not, are recorded. Cases are registered by the individual's address at the time of diagnosis rather than by treatment centers.

Certain registries in America are now population-based. One of the original registries is for Connecticut; although this registry was initiated in 1941, it recorded data retrospectively to 1935 (*43*).

The exact data that each registry collects tend to be unique in depth, scope, mode of collection, and overall accuracy. The minimal information required by many population- and hospital-based registries is divided into two categories:

1. Identification data—name, sex, date of birth (estimate if not known), address, and ethnic group.
2. Tumor data—topography, histology, anniversary date, basis of diagnosis, and source of information.

The anniversary date is the date a diagnosis is recorded by the best method available, for example, microscopic examination of the tumor, at best, or cause of death on a certificate, at worst. A good deal of variation is found between registries as to the definition of the date used to mark the onset of the tumor.

In the industrialized world, attempts are usually made to record follow-up information, date and causes of death, occupation, place of birth, and tumor stage. The accuracy of the data collected relies absolutely on the accuracy of the information available.

The registries that make use of the most varied sources of data are likely to be the most accurate because details can be cross-checked. One English registry (Yorkshire) makes use of many data sources and has an annual registration rate of 404 for males and 384 for females per 100,000 population from a total population of approximately 3.5 million persons. In other words, over 16,000 registrations are collected each year, but this figure includes duplicates, errors, and second malignancies, so the real number of cases is slightly less.

Cancer registries often deal with requests about particular problems within the areas they cover, and many of them publish routine reports about descriptive cancer epidemiology from time to time (*44*).

Other Data Sources. MORTALITY DATA. One of the major advantages of mortality data is that they have been available for a considerable period of time in many countries (*18*, *25*). Individual accuracy of death certification might be suspect, but the overall data are invaluable. Mortality data in the United Kingdom and elsewhere are routinely fed back to cancer registries as a final cross-check of registration. In England and Wales, some 8% of all primary registrations are made through death certificates.

SPECIALIZED REGISTRIES. Individual registries exist for very rare diseases, such as Burkitt's lymphoma in the United States (*38*), as well as bone and childhood tumors in England and Wales (*33*). These registries can be useful in that they often have specialized methods of data ascertainment and they can collect a considerable quantity of information about each case.

AT-RISK REGISTERS. A recent development has been the increase in numbers of registers that are being kept of selected groups of people who might have an increased risk of developing malignant disease. These registers include certain occupational groups, transplant patients, and those people with rare immunodeficiency disorders. The development of these registers is due in part to a greater appreciation of epidemiological methods. These methods allow a direct estimate of risk within the population of interest as opposed to local or national rates.

The main thrust in this field lies in the development of workforce registers that include records of all the possible hazards with which each individual has been in contact. This exercise has been started in some chemical companies in the United Kingdom in recent years in the hope of identifying any hazards related to specific chemicals or occupations. Thorough and updated files on possible hazards, occupations, and the composition of workforce will allow quick and efficient evaluation of safe uses or methods to the mutual benefit of the company and the workforce.

The medical and personnel departments of such industrial plants liaise to provide nominal lists that are continually updated with job or hazard descriptions and medical information. Such careful records that include data on all the workforce should be encouraged.

Methods in Epidemiology

Modern epidemiology plays two interlinking roles in studies on particular diseases. First, epidemiology tests hypotheses that are generated from outside epidemiology, and second, the results of epidemiological research tend to generate further hypotheses to be tested. Traditionally the hypotheses tested by epidemiologists arise from routinely collected general disease data, such as registry or mortality results.

A more modern approach to cancer epidemiology is to ascertain hypotheses on a multidisciplinary basis by using all possible data about the mechanisms that are involved in the disease process, as well as the clinical observations relevant to the disease in question. This approach often produces quite specific questions to be answered; for example: What is the role of saccharin in bladder cancer? Does a particular occupation lead to an excess of lung cancer deaths? The more the epidemiologist knows about the biology of the disease and its clinical course, the more likely the study will be able to answer the relevant question. The traditional sources of hypotheses tend to produce broad questions that are difficult to answer, whereas very specific lines of inquiry are more likely to be productive.

Methods Available. The techniques available for the epidemiological approach to disease are usually based on three levels of inquiry that can produce increasingly reliable results.

The simplest level is that of descriptive epidemiology that is essentially, although not always, based on routinely collected data, which is discussed in the preceding section. At an intermediate level, the cross-sectional approach to a population is of importance in acute disorders but is rarely used for chronic diseases such as cancer. At a more sophisticated level, analytical epidemiology has two more methods available to it: the case–control and the cohort study, two quite distinct ways of approaching a population under study. The type of study is of particular importance; each has advantages and disadvantages that can only be assessed on the basis of the questions to be answered and the techniques available in the analysis. A balanced view must be held, however, in that the strength of any study is its accuracy and ultimate reproducibility.

Descriptive Epidemiology. The descriptive epidemiology of cancer concentrates on such variables as site and histology of the cancers further categorized by age, sex, and places of residence of the patients. This approach has been a fertile field for epidemiologists who wish to study local disease patterns. In parts of West Yorkshire, England, for example, the mortality for men of working age with bladder cancer was over twice that of the population as a whole, and this information from descriptive work has led to a case–control study of this population group (*45*).

Table VI

Cancer Mortalities Grouped by Occupation for Men Aged 15–64 in England and Wales

Occupation	*Cancer Type*	*Standardized Mortality Ratios*
Farmers	Colon	120
Miners	Stomach	171
Furnace, forge, and foundry workers	Lung	155
Laborers	Stomach	150
	Larynx	186
	Lung	146
Sales workers	Colon	106
	Leukemia	111

One of the means of generating new hypotheses comes from the routine statistics that are available, especially on occupation and its possible influence on disease. However, the analysis of this type of routinely collected data has various disadvantages; in particular, the recorded occupation is often the current one held at the time of the disease event, death, or diagnosis and not necessarily the occupation held when the malignant process started. Also occupations on death certificates can often be grossly inaccurate or too general to be meaningful.

The interpretation of such data can only be of general value and lead to hypothesis testing. Table VI lists certain cancers and the occupational groups in whom an excess of deaths occurred in comparison with the national mortality rates (*25*). The standardized mortality ratio is set at 100 for the national experience; thus miners have a 71% excess of stomach cancer contrasted with the national data. Such leads need to be followed by higher levels of epidemiological inquiry that may demonstrate whether the relationship is real or spurious.

Descriptive cancer epidemiology continues because new descriptions of disease are continually required. For example, the lymphomas and leukemias have been reclassified many times in the last 30 years, and a lot of the older data are now meaningless (*46*). Some very rare diseases, such as soft tissue sarcomas, still need to be properly described (*47*). Finally, descriptive epidemiology is still lacking in many countries (*21, 42*).

Table VII lists some commonly used descriptive statistics used in this classical epidemiological approach with a brief description of each term (*48–50*).

Data in Analytical Epidemiology. Analytical epidemiology is only as reliable as the data collected, and thus a good deal of attention at the study-design stage is concerned with the way in which the data are acquired. The difficulty in cancer epidemiology is acquiring data about events at the putative time the malignant clone of cells was initiated; the initiation could have occurred 50 years before the study. Table VIII gives some indication of the reliability and quality of information. The judgments assume that the data sources are accurate and adequate, which may

Table VII

Statistics Commonly Used in Descriptive and Cross-sectional Cancer Epidemiology

Statistic	*Definition*
Crude incidence rate	Number of new cases per unit of observational time in the total population
Cumulative incidence rate	Cumulative proportion of a group who develop an illness over time
Incidence density	Rate at which new cases occur over a fixed time interval
Crude mortality rate	Number of deaths from the total population per unit of observational time
Standardized mortality ratio	Mortality experience standardized for the age/sex distribution of a population against a reference population
Prevalence rate	Existence of cases at a point in time
Case fatality rate	Proportion of all cases of illness that result in death over time
Survival rate	Total number of disease cases alive after a unit of time over the total number cases diagnosed (can be corrected against expected deaths)
Life table rate	Profile of deaths against time taking all cases into account

not always be the case with old records. The items of information in Table VIII are typical of the current general questions used in cancer epidemiology.

The ordinal scale of reliability indicates that the items marked 1 can be often obtained quite readily from two or more sources. The items marked 3 can only be obtained from one source, which normally cannot be checked. This source is usually the patient or the member of a cohort and depends on interview recall. The intermediate items may or may not be verifiable. Because of the aims of accuracy and reliability, studies in analytical epidemiology aim to achieve as much cross-checked data as possible. The basis of the data is usually an interview by a trained interviewer with a subject, either a case, a case-comparison subject, or a member of a cohort. This approach then allows all the checkable items to be identified and steps taken to verify the data. One interview can often initiate a dozen other lines of inquiry until ultimately a final data record is constructed.

Other forms of data acquisition exist: self-administered questionnaires or telephone interviews, for example. These are of low reliability and the cross-checkable data are far more vague and so the process to validate the data cannot always proceed.

When the poorer quality data are regarded as being of great importance for a particular study, the validity can be estimated by repeating the interview after some interval of time.

Table VIII

Types of Information Acquired in Analytical Epidemiology

Information	*Ability to Verify*	*Ordinal Scale of Degree of Reliability After Checking*
Names	Yes	1
Addresses	Not always	2
Date of birth	Yes	1
Sex	Yes	1
Hospital record No.	Yes	1
Current consumption of food	Yes with difficulty (weighed-intake study)	2
Past consumption of food	No	3
Current drinking habits	Not usually	2
Past drinking habits	No	3
Current and past intake of prescribed drugs	Yes	1
Current and past intake of self-administered medicines	No	3
Current tobacco consumption	Not always	2
Current occupation	Yes	1
Past occupation	Not always	2
Current and past medical history	Yes	1

Case–Control Studies. A "case–control" study, or a "case–case comparison" study is used as a means to test hypotheses. This type of study depends on the ability of the epidemiologist to identify cases of the disease in question and then to have access to them or their relatives for an interview or some other means of data acquisition.

The comparison or control group is usually ascertained on the basis of the demographic qualities of the cases. In cancer studies, the primary principle is that the controls should be selected as a group representative of the general population and with the same potential of having experienced the events (social, occupational, or other) that might be implicated in the hypotheses that are being tested by the study. For example, when a high incidence of bladder cancer is being examined, the control group should be of a similar age, sex, and locality as the case group so that the control group could have had similar occupations and experiences. Many case–control cancer studies chose controls matched for age, sex, locality, and occasionally for ethnic group.

Case–control studies are ideally suited for uncommon or rare disorders in which a range of possible hypotheses can be tested at the same time. Most studies collect incident cases over a period of time, often years. In some instances, both prevalent and subsequent incident cases can be incorporated if the hypotheses to be scrutinized are not influenced by the severity of the disease. A third alternative could be to take all new cases accruing for a fixed period prior to the start of the study and include the possibility of interviewing the relatives of dead cases.

These types of studies have the advantage of being relatively quick and cheap. They have the disadvantage that the disease or disease group must be known with some certainty as part of the hypotheses. Spurious results will be generated if crucial variables are not identified and incorporated into the hypotheses. For instance, in a study of asbestos exposure, if the protocol had not considered smoking habits, the results would have seemed to indicate a direct relationship between exposure to asbestos and lung cancer, whereas in fact, the risks to individuals are low unless they smoke cigarettes (*51*). Cohort studies should take such important factors into account; unfortunately it is often not possible to do so, because the required information on deceased members has often been lost.

Cohort Studies. A cohort is a group of people defined in a specific way. Classically a cohort was a group born during a similar period and thus having a lifetime experience of events quite similar to each other's and different from experiences of groups born earlier or later. To follow the disease experience of these types of cohort is essentially a descriptive exercise.

Analytical follow-up studies are of two broad types: those studies that collect the group to be studied retrospectively and those studies that start with a living population and note events that will occur in the future—the prospective cohort study. The distinction between the two types is quite important in that the study that uses retrospectively ascertained data is usually obliged to deal with major categories of death rather than the occurrence of specific diseases. Furthermore, the information about the individuals in the deceased cohort is limited; it must be extracted from routinely collected data, and not, for example, collected through specific inquiries about an individual's personal habits.

The cohort study differs fundamentally from the case–control approach. However ascertained, a cohort at its outset comprises a group of generally healthy people. A cohort can be defined partly or wholly as those people who are exposed for a certain minimum period to a putative hazard. This hazard could be associated with work or with personal lifestyle events, such as smoking habits or coffee consumption.

The aim of a cohort study is to follow the defined group over time and watch for the occurrence of major or definable events within the population. These events can be the diagnosis of a disease or death. Often the population has to be large and observations must continue for many years. These studies have various advantages over a case–control study. If a hazard is suspected but the disease or diseases that might result are not identified, then only a cohort study can be attempted. The cohort is often collected retrospectively to speed up the process, but prospectively ascertained cohorts have advantages: researchers can collect, without bias, data on all participants at the outset and can record diseases in a way that suits the study rather than relying on routinely collected mortality or morbidity data.

At the end of the study, the observations of events in the cohort can be contrasted with nationally collected data. Although this is routinely collected information, it has the advantage of being a very large data set in which errors are likely to be minimized. Routine data usually form the "expected" statistics if nationally available. If the data were quite unique then other parallel studies would be set up in groups representative of the general population to provide the relevant expected information. The ratio of expected to observed disease events forms the basis of the analyses as well as the confidence limits of the estimate.

An alternative approach is to use comparisons within the cohort; for example, one could contrast the previous experience of those who acquire a particular disease with that of other cohort members who do not.

Natural History of Cancer

In modern epidemiology, cancer studies must be linked in a meaningful fashion with clinical and basic laboratory work (*52*). In order to be an integral part of the team working on a problem, the epidemiologist must have a working knowledge of both the biological mechanisms involved and the clinical treatment.

Carcinogenesis. Chemicals that react with cells to produce malignant clones come from a wide variety of sources—including products of partial combustion, drugs, and foods—and are from a wide variety of chemical classes (*53*).

Many of the chemicals capable of producing malignant change can be metabolized to an electron pair-deficient state; this electrophilic molecule is then capable of very strong binding to nucleic acids.

The circumstances leading to the metabolic formation of an electrophile and its binding to DNA are known as initiation. Most frequently, the electrophile causes cell death or induces DNA damage, which is then repaired. An alternative and less likely path after binding is promotion, the next step in the carcinogenic process; a normal-looking but initiated cell becomes abnormal in appearance and becomes capable of clonal proliferation. Promoters include such substances as saccharin, viruses, and the phorbol esters. The abnormal cell is then capable of independently generating a malignant clone without further outside stimulation. On rare occasions when large quantities of initiating substances are present, promotion can be achieved by the initiators alone; for example, the extensive exposure of workmen to large quantities of 2-naphthylamine led to bladder cancers without additional promotional events (*54*).

Undoubtedly at every stage in the process, the individual genetic constitution of the host is of vital importance. The enzymic variation in the metabolic pathways dealing with initiation, the variation in the DNA repair mechanisms, and the presence of directly acting inhibitory substances all play a part (*55*). The variation of cell surface interactions might also alter promotional responses.

The whole process of carcinogenesis is complex and involves many interrelated steps. So far, attempts to isolate the responsible agent have uncovered further aberration. Most likely, several agents are acting in concert to form one type of malignancy, and any agent that metabolizes to electrophile reactants can potentially cause a variety of malignancies. In addition, different etiological agents can cause the same malignancy.

How do these concepts influence epidemiological studies; what are the etiological agents in cancer; what is the role of human variability; and what alters the natural history of the disease?

A careful regard for potential mechanisms adds to the difficulties of epidemiological inquiry. If there are at least two major steps in carcinogenesis, each caused by a variety of possible agents, then how can any study demonstrate the risk associated with one specific agent?

The studies quoted later in this chapter pay varying degrees of attention to these mechanisms and the problems they pose for epidemiology. Future studies should try to link laboratory work with epidemiology in a more direct fashion.

Human Variability. The aspects of human variability most pertinent to carcinogenesis have not been clearly defined (*56*). The mixed-function oxidases vary in their ability to induce malignant disease. Cell surface antigenic markers such as the ABO blood groups and the HLA system also vary a good deal, and certain subtypes have been implicated in the etiology and natural history of some cancers (*57*). An approach to these problems through a study of pharmacogenetics is indicated (*58*). A variety of syndromes are often associated with the subsequent development of malignant disease; for example, ataxia telangiectasia can lead to leukemia and lymphoma development and xeroderma pigmentes can predispose a person to skin cancers.

Cell surface markers appear to influence the way in which tumors behave in different individuals, and this aspect of the natural history of malignant disease might give useful information on the particular behavior of individual malignancies (*59*).

Etiology of Cancer

Cancer epidemiology has hitherto been based on the concept that one agent gives one cancer rather than the more accurate and complex picture just outlined. A number of studies in the following section adopted this simplistic approach partly because some of the tested agents are mixtures of numerous substances that include initiators as well as promoters; cigarette smoke, for example, contains well over 50 mutagenic or carcinogenic substances. As a result, the populations studied were usually limited to the most severely exposed groups.

Etiologic Agents and Public Health. One way of classifying etiological agents implicated in human carcinogenesis is by the circumstances surrounding exposure. The following categories best show the relationship to the social setting of the individual (*60, 62*). Habit-forming agents include, tobacco, alcohol, betel chewing, illegal drugs, and some physician-prescribed drugs. Non-habit-forming agents include over-the-counter drugs, drugs prescribed by physician for long-term therapy, diet, and trauma. Agents one could be exposed to in a work environment include radiation, chemicals, air pollution, and viruses. The final category, agents one could be exposed to in nonoccupational situations, includes radiation, chemicals, air pollution, and viruses from nonoccupational sources, as well as water pollution. The most difficult agents to withdraw as a preventative measure are those that are intrinsic to the individual's lifestyle and those that are habit forming; the easiest to eliminate are in the two more peripheral categories.

Table IX shows the major human cancer sites. Little is known of the etiological relationships in as many as 46% of all malignancies, intermediate knowledge in about 11%, and quite good knowledge only in cases of lung and skin cancer, which account for 28% of all malignancies.

Comparison of the exposure categories and Table IX shows that, from what little is known of cancer etiology, a substantial proportion of the major causes of cancer fall into the groups that are difficult, by their nature, to change acceptably. Occupation, in this very general sense, gets more than its fair share of attention, simply because it is relatively easy to alter exposure.

TOBACCO. Tobacco smoke is a potent source of initiators, mutagens, and promoters (*62*). All these substances are present in tiny amounts in each cigarette. A study

Table IX

Etiology of Common Tumors

Cancer Site	*Approximate Percentage of all Malignancies*	*Major Hypothesized Cause*
Esophagus	2	Smoking plus alcohol, diet, and burnt products
Stomach	7	Preservatives and other aspects of diet
Large intestine	7	Intestinal flora and diet
Rectum	5	Beer
Pancreas	3	Smoking
Lung	19	Smoking and occupation
Skin	9	UV radiation and occupation
Prostate	4	Endogenous hormones
Bladder	5	Occupation, diet, and smoking
Brain	2	Drugs
Lymphoma	2	Viruses, benzene, and irradiation
Leukemias	2	Viruses, benzene, and irradiation
Female breast	10	Radiation, hormones, and reproductive history
Uterine cervix	4	Viruses
Body of uterus	2	Exogenous hormones and reproductive history
Ovary	2	Reproductive history
TOTAL	85	

(*63*) showed that the urine of smokers becomes mutagenic after smoking cigarettes. Tobacco consumption is thus an ideal means of presenting many carcinogenic substances in small but regular doses.

Cigarette consumption over the years has been coupled with the observed increases in male and later in female lung cancer rates. Early studies (*64, 65*) have demonstrated a clear relationship between smoking and lung cancer in both men and women, with an overall risk ratio of 2.9 for men and 2.5 for women.

Since then numerous studies have confirmed this relationship. One study (*66*) followed 34,440 British male doctors between 1951 and 1971 who reduced their average tobacco consumption from about 10 cigarettes a day to about 4. A statistically significant decrease in lung cancer deaths, as well as a decrease in certain types of arterial disease was observed. The great mass of data from these types of studies suggests that the causes of many cancers and of arterial disease are very similar and clearly related to smoking.

The decrease in risk when a person stops smoking has been quantified. This decrease is complex and depends on previous consumption of cigarettes and the age at cessation. However, after 15 years of cessation, the risks for acquiring lung cancer become akin to risks for persons who never smoked.

Cigarette smoking confers other risks on an individual besides those of arterial disease and lung cancer. Perhaps 100,000 deaths a year are due to smoking-related diseases in the United Kingdom. The total risk for all cancers is increased, as well as for other malignancies associated with smoking. Vulnerable sites include oropharynx, larynx, bladder, and esophagus. The magnitude of the risks for these tumors is less than for lung cancer.

The introduction of low-tar cigarettes and the increased use of filters have been responsible for the decline in mortality from lung cancer and other smoking-related conditions in the younger cohorts. Detailed examination shows that this association is only valid if smoke inhalation and total cigarette consumption are not increased to compensate.

The risks relating cigarette smoking and lung cancer are so large in comparison with other risks that other causes of lung cancer are obscured. Increased cancer risk in the offspring of people who smoke has also been suggested (*67*), but epidemiological evidence is lacking at the present time.

ALCOHOL. Alcohol is related to the oral, laryngeal, pharyngeal, and esophageal malignancies seen in smokers and often causes multiplication of risks (*68*). A high incidence of carcinoma of the esophagus is observed in calvados drinkers in parts of Brittany and Normandy. Liver cancer may also be associated with alcohol consumption. The mechanism for this relationship is unclear (*69*). Beer has been associated with an increased risk of large bowel cancer in many studies, but it is not yet clear if this is an occupational or social hazard (*70*).

IONIZING RADIATION. Experiments showing that ionizing radiation can cause leukemia date back to 1906. The risks were quantified first for American radiologists and were found to be between 4.3 and 9.2 times the expected incidence in those employed before 1960. Since then these risks have declined and are negligible (*71*).

The atomic explosions in Japan led to an increase in leukemia cases; the increase was seen within 3 years of the explosions and rose to a peak between 5 and 7 years after the explosion (*72, 73*). Use of therapeutic low dose irradiation for nonmalignant disease has led to several studies into its consequences. The classic study by Court Brown and Doll (*74*) examined the fate of over 14,000 persons with ankylosing spondylitis who had had radiotherapy to the spine. Table X shows the excess risk experienced by this group in contracting leukemia, as well as the risk of other groups subjected to irradiation for nonmalignant conditions (*75–77*).

Although leukemia is perhaps the first and most easily recordable consequence of ionizing radiation, other tumors result from exposure. The dose received, the site irradiated, and the age at which irradiation occurred are all important variables.

Among the bomb survivors, exposed children suffered in excess from tumors of the salivary gland, brain, thyroid gland, and large bowel. External irradiation in adults seems to produce an excess of most tumors including breast, myeloma, large bowel, and lung (*78, 79*).

α-Emitters with long half-life can be ingested in occupational situations—as in the case of radium-dial painters and miners who inhaled radon gas or as a result of iatrogenic exposure—as with the use of thorotrast, which contains thorium dioxide as a contrast medium (*80–85*). The tumors induced are quite rare and the sites are quite specific—bone tumors in radium-dial painters and liver tumors in thorium-treated patients.

LOWER DOSES OF IONIZING RADIATION. Much attention is now given to the possible hazards of lower doses of ionizing radiation caused by low levels of fall-out, radioactive granite rocks, or diagnostic x-rays. The hazard of x-rays during pregnancy was demonstrated first by Alice Stewart (*86*). Her study indicates that x-irradiation of the fetus produced twice as many deaths due to childhood malignancy (mainly leukemia) as expected. The interpretation of this study is controversial, and it has been suggested that the results are confounded. The role that diagnostic x-rays might have in adult life has yet to be fully investigated, but Boice (*79*) has shown that the repeated fluorographs taken in some tuberculous patients led to an excess risk of breast cancer many years later.

Table X

Risk Estimates for Leukemia Subsequent to Irradiation

Medical History	*Population Size*	*Relative Risk*
A-bomb survivors (under 10 years old)	4,507	6.5
A-bomb survivors (aged 10 and over)	19,472	3.7
x-Rays to thymus	1,451	3.0
x-Rays for tinea capitis	2,043	4.4
x-Rays for menorrhagia	2,068	4.6
x-Ray treatment of spondylitics	14,554	9.5

Accidental exposure to radiation has to be put into perspective whether or not one accepts a lower threshold for the harmful effects of irradiation (*87–89*). Neutron emission is probably more harmful than γ-ray emission at low-dose levels in that a single neutron hit of DNA would cause a double-strand break while the same break would require two γ-ray hits. This gradation is partly substantiated by contrasting the results from Hiroshima and Nagasaki: the rates of leukemia in the low-dose groups were higher in the high neutron-exposed Hiroshima population (*72*).

The dosimetry data from Japan have since been questioned; the more recent view suggests that neutron exposures were identical in the two sites. In fact, more and more researchers question the fundamental assumption and the observations in these bomb-radiation studies. The cohort is, after all, a survivor population and is by no means a complete or evenly studied group.

The total background dose for all types of irradiation is about 100 mrem/year in the United Kingdom. The latest well-publicized leak from a nuclear reactor at Three Mile Island, Pa., produced a maximum dose of 80 mrem about 365 m away and vastly less in the local general population. The radiation came from iodine-131, a β-emitter, as well as a source of some γ-radiation with an 8-d half-life. The hazard of this type of leak to a local population is probably very slight, if there is any at all. However, even if a small risk is generated, epidemiologic techniques would probably not substantiate it because of the small numbers and very low doses involved. Nothing has emerged from studies of the Windscale disaster in the United Kingdom to suggest that these sorts of incidents are harmful (*90*). Modern therapeutic irradiation for malignant disease produces few additional malignancies in adults (*91*), in contrast to the widely used chemotherapeutic agents.

Nonionizing Radiation. Modern epidemiology is as much concerned with investigating possible hazards as with elucidating diseases that might result from a known hazard. Most nonionizing irradiation (e.g., magnetic fields, ultrasonic waves, and microwaves) does not appear to be a hazard. UV light, however, is one exception: exposure to UV light and paleness of the skin are related to skin malignancy. One study (*92*) suggests that sunspot activity is significant in the etiology of these skin cancers. The use of halocarbon compounds and the consequent potential loss of the ozone layer might be relevant, because depletion of the ozone layer would allow more UV-B light exposure, but this depletion has yet to be demonstrated. Even in the United Kingdom, a relationship between ambient UV light and melanoma incidence has been documented. Malignant melanoma is increasing in incidence in the United Kingdom, possibly as a result of changes in behavior patterns in relation to sunlight (i.e., greater desire to sunbathe) (*94*). Other skin tumors such as rodent ulcers or squamous cell tumors have also been associated with UV exposure. The hazard, if any, associated with the proliferation of sun beds has yet to be assessed, but would only be likely if exposure to UV-B light occurred.

The other types of nonionizing irradiation present a confused picture (*95, 96*). Sources of one main type of nonionizing radiation tend also to produce other types. There are no universally accepted measures of energy emission nor of absolute dose per mass of tissue. None of these types of irradiation are known to produce any malignancy, but some studies seem to suggest that ultrasonic waves at diagnostic energies disrupt the chromosomes' ability to divide normally. Similar claims have been made for magnetic (*97*) and electrical fields (*98*), although as many papers have claimed that such fields show no effects experimentally on cell nuclei in animals or in humans (*99*).

DRUGS AND IATROGENIC CANCER. Aside from drugs that emit radiation, two broad groups are capable of producing an increased risk of malignant disease: the immunosuppressants and the chemotherapeutic agents; cylophosphamide and chlornaphazine can both produce bladder cancer, for example. In addition a few specific agents are known to be hazardous; phenacetin induces renal tract tumors, for example. Epidemiological detection of iatrogenic cancer risk is very difficult and confused. Immunosuppressants, for example, are often given to patients with a pre-existing increased risk of malignant disease. The bias has been highlighted by two recent studies. One demonstrates that renal transplant patients on immunosuppressant therapy have a 60-fold excess of non-Hodgkins lymphoma (NHL) and of other malignancies, especially of the skin (*100*). Another smaller study has shown that cases with chronic renal failure on dialysis who do not receive immunosuppressive drugs also have an excess risk of NHL. The numbers are too small to quantify the risk reliably, perhaps about 30-fold (*101*). Similarly, even the cases who receive chemotherapeutic agents not known to cause further malignancies as part of their treatment for terminal diseases are intrinsically at risk of a second malignancy. In addition the topic is further confused because many cases die before they have time to develop second malignancies.

Long-term follow-up survivors is one means to assess the risks of these agents. Ovarian cancer is a tumor not prone to second malignancies (*43*). These reports indicate an enormous risk associated with alkylating agent chemotherapy for the subsequent development of acute leukemia, and virtually no risk at all for radical radiotherapeutic treatment when not combined with chemotherapy (*102*).

Many iatrogenic malignancies have never been investigated epidemiologically and the associations are based on case reports. Two exceptions are the studies of phenacetin abuse in Scandinavia and studies of transplacental carcinogenesis by diethylstilbestrol. The latter has been shown to be a transplacental carcinogen when used in early pregnancy; the very rare clear-cell adenocarcinoma of the cervix and vagina is seen in the female offspring (*103*).

Phenacetin abuse leads to transitional cell tumors of the upper urinary tract. The exact mechanism of action is still uncertain, but metabolic products of phenacetin are the suspect carcinogens (*104*).

Much controversy has surrounded the possible neoplastic sequelae of taking birth control pills, and recent studies have shown that birth control pills might induce certain cancers; possibly 117 women world-wide have had pill-associated liver tumors of various histologic types (*105*). Recent reports show no link between breast cancer and the consumption of oral contraceptives (*106*).

In addition, hormonal replacement therapy by an estrogen-containing compound taken to control the menopause has been suggested as a risk factor in cancer of the uterine body. Prolonged use of these compounds undoubtedly increases the risk of uterine cancer severalfold. Suggestions that a link exists between the menopausal use of these agents and breast cancer have not been supported by epidemiological studies.

TRAUMA AND INFLAMMATION. Continued chronic irritation of tissues can lead to the development of a malignancy. Such observations are always confounded by the possibilities that specific chemicals or specific physical agents are the real causative agent. Such malignancies are often of the skin and are almost always squamous cell carcinoma. The examples of such trauma tend to be rare, bizarre, and anthropologic rather than a common cause of malignancy. Short-stemmed clay pipes give lip and tongue cancer due to the repeated heat trauma to those sites. The migrating Turkman tribes of the Caspian littoral swallow the partly burnt remains of opium pipes and have a massive excess of esophageal cancer, possibly as a result (*107*), but now researchers suggest that the excess is due to the trauma from certain vegetable fibers in the diet. On the other hand, some of the Bantu tribes of Southern Africa also swallow partly burnt dross from their pipes and develop the same malignancy.

Some central American peasants smoke local cigars with the burning end inside their mouths giving themselves buccal and lingual cancers. South Asian populations commonly chew a mixture of tobacco and lime (betel), again leading to oropharyngeal malignancies in these populations (*108*).

Kangri, a bronze pot of burning embers carried around the abdomen and thigh by various populations in Asia and North Africa, leads to chronic scarring and carcinoma of the skin. Tropical ulcers produce a similar type of cancer.

In Western countries the chronic rubbing of reinforced corsets, the constant use of hair dyes, the rubbing of ill-fitting glass eyes or artificial limbs have all been reported to lead to squamous cell cancer at the site. Most of the reports describing these events have been clinical, and very little epidemiology has been attempted. We do know that the risk associated with hair dye use is minimal, if it exists at all. The significance of the other factors as a cause of disease in the various societies, however, is not yet understood.

Squamous cell carcinoma of the bladder results from chronic inflammation and occurs quite regularly as a result of bladder stones or more importantly with the parasitic infection schistosomiasis.

DIET. We consume many products that are carcinogenic initiators or promoters. Unfortunately the techniques of epidemiologic inquiry available for dietary studies are particularly limiting (*109*). The long latent periods and the diversity of even the simplest diets make a retrospective study unrewarding. Prospective studies are difficult to conduct due to great difficulties with even the most recent recall of food, and the weighed-intake technique is not suitable for large epidemiologically based studies.

The dietary associations that have been found are easy to criticize and tend to be the specific association of a readily acknowledged item of diet with a particular cancer. The relation between beer drinking and colorectal cancer is one example (*70*).

Two of the strongest relationships that exist between diet and cancer are (1) between the Japanese diet and stomach cancer and (2) between aflatoxins and liver cancer. Aflatoxin is a highly potent, liver-specific mutagen and it is produced by *Aspergillus flavus*—a fungus that grows on groundnuts, grain, and other foods when they are stored in damp conditions (*109*). Contaminated stores are found in Africa and the Far East and both these parts of the world have high rates for liver cancer (*110*).

Classic migrant studies showed how cancer incidence changes in different environments, for example, stomach and colon cancer in two generations of Japanese migrants in North America. In these two generations, stomach cancer rates have decreased and colon cancer rates have increased; both of these trends are towards the native American rates (*111*).

A large case–control study has shown that saccharin does not present a major bladder cancer risk, although it may account for some cases seen in non-coffee-drinking nonsmokers (*112*).

Fluoride has not been shown to increase the total cancer deaths in a population when due regard has been taken for the ethnic group, age, and sex of a population (*113, 114*).

More general dietary constituents have been implicated as risk factors through various types of correlation or follow-up studies. A putative association has been shown between excessive beef consumption and non-Hodgkins lymphoma. More convincing are the studies linking breast cancer with high-fat diets (*115*).

The relationship between diet and large-bowel cancer is more complex. Both the diet and the particular gut flora determine bile composition, which then affects the crucial factor of transit time. Pentose-containing fiber is one important dietary component that has been studied in relation to gut flora and transit time. Other dietary constituents have been linked to gall bladder disease, and high-fat and meat diets have been associated with colorectal cancer. Studies on these relationships have been summarized by Shottenfeld and Winawer (*116*).

Recently an increasing body of data has suggested that the lack of specific dietary supplements predisposes a person to epithelial cancers of various types. In particular, vitamin A deficiency has been associated in several studies with an increased risk of lung cancer (*117*).

ENVIRONMENTAL POLLUTION. There has never been a direct epidemiological study that clearly shows that noxious substances in the atmosphere or elsewhere in the common environment can produce cancers in humans.

In a sense, environmental pollution is an extension of occupational exposure. Many epidemiologic studies have shown that excess cancers have been caused by contact with particular chemicals at the workplace, and risks to the general population have been extrapolated from such studies. For example, on the basis of work that used benzo[*a*]pyrene levels as a general indicator of pollution (*118, 119*), Pike (*120*) concluded that air pollution has a modified additive effect that produces extra lung cancer cases at a rate of 1.4/100,000 persons/year/ng/m^3 of benzo[*a*]pyrene in the atmosphere for smokers and 0.4 for nonsmokers. This small but significant increase can never be directly tested by using epidemiologic techniques until the population's consumption of benzo[*a*]pyrene from cigarettes is drastically reduced.

Environmental levels of asbestos from numerous sources, of chromium salts, and of arsenic salts have all been measured in certain communities in amounts over the accepted threshold limit values. All these substances are known to have carcinogenic properties, but only a few of the contaminated populations have a demonstrated excess of malignancies as a result of these events; for instance, families of asbestos workers and those who were contaminated by strontium-90 fallout in Scotland during the 1950s.

Over the last two decades many other substances have been suggested as having a carcinogenic effect, as well as other deleterious effects, on humans. Such substances include the common pesticides such as dichlorodiphenyltrichloroethane (DDT), heptachlor, and *p*-dichlorobenzene; the polychlorinated biphenyls; the polybrominated biphenyls; dioxins; and the phthalic acid esters (*121*). Amitrole (aminotriazole) has been implicated as a weak carcinogen (*122*).

People argue that deleterious effects will surface only after many years. The Séveso incident in July 1976 was the result of a reaction tank explosion that sent approximately 1000 lb of trichlorophenol into the local environments. For miles the atmosphere was contaminated with dioxin (*123*). These and other similar at-risk populations are being carefully watched for possible sequelae. The dioxin-contaminated herbicides in Vietnam have been suggested as a cause of excess liver tumors among people in that area (*124*).

The role of environmental pollutants in human cancer incidence will remain unresolved until large and very long-term studies on well-monitored, nonsmoking populations are conducted.

VIRUSES. The role of viruses in human malignancy has been a contentious issue since virus-related malignancies were discovered in certain animals, for instance, a cat leukemia due to the feline leukemia virus and cattle tumors due to the bovine leukosis virus (*125*).

Much laboratory work suggests that viruses play a promotional role in carcinogenesis, and thus it would not be incompatible to link the viruses with other causes of cancer. Except in the most extreme situations, this link might actually cloud results and make the role of viruses even less clear.

The biology of viruses will not be discussed here except to say that virologists are now isolating human viruses that cause the human malignancy from which they were isolated (*126, 127*). In particular the human T cell lymphoma/leukemia virus (HTLV) causes a disease found in the Caribbean and in southern Japan, which is quite characteristic and distinct from other adult leukemias (*127*). A new reterovirus isolated from these cases is similar to the bovine leukosis virus (*128*).

The Epstein–Barr virus has been shown in cell cultures of the Burkitt's lymphoma. Also, cases of Burkitt's lymphoma (*129*), as well as cases of pharyngeal carcinoma (*130*), almost always show very high serum titers of antibodies to this virus, with an unexpected age distribution. The geographical distribution of these two tumors is rather peculiar. Burkitt's lymphoma, for example, is confined in Africa to a band where malaria is involved in the pathogenesis of the disease. It has also been suggested that immune depletion for any reason can lead to viral oncogenesis (*131*). On a similar level, a relationship exists among aflatoxins, chronic viral hepatitis, and primary liver cell cancer (*132*).

The *Herpes simplex* virus type II is similar to the very common oropharyngeal type I in many respects; therefore, serological distinction between the two types is difficult. Despite this difficulty some authorities claim, on the basis of epidemiological and laboratory studies, that there is clearly a risk associated with type II infections and carcinoma of the cervix, in situ carcinoma, and the cervical cellular dysplasias (*133, 134*). Since then studies have appeared that link carcinoma of the penis with that of the cervix. Carcinoma of the penis does arise often from large condylomata; therefore it is possible that genital warts should be implicated in the etiology of both conditions (*135*).

An outbreak of Kaposi's sarcoma in male homosexuals led to the discovery of a link between the cytomegalus virus and acute episodes of self-inflicted immune supression consequent to the use of amyl nitrite (*115*).

Another apparently confusing phenomenon that might link viruses with certain malignancies is that of time–space clustering. If viruses act in a truly promotional capacity, then a group of people within a population might easily be affected by a virus that is capable of creating a malignancy in those individuals' initiated cells under the proper conditions (i.e., if the local physiological environment is right and if the stem cells are cycling in the correct phase). In these malignancies that cluster, viruses might serve to start malignant clones. Malignancies that consistently occur as clusters in time and space are Burkitt's lymphoma, nasopharyngeal carcinoma, leukemia, Hodgkin's disease, non-Hodgkin's lymphoma, and penis and cervix cancers. A few reports indicate that testicular tumors and gastrointestinal tract cancers at all sites also form clusters in time and space. For 70 years childhood acute lymphoblastic leukemia has been reported to cluster sporadically, but all attempts to investigate the phenomenon have shown that a viral etiology is difficult to demonstrate epidemiologically—clustering is a variable phenomenon and there is little consensus about the statistical approaches to these problems (*136–39*). Similarly, Hodgkin's disease studies have shown that acquaintanceship networks exist among cases; for example, many cases were in the same class at school (*140*). Other studies have shown that on a case–control basis such networks are the norm and not peculiar to this particular disease group (*139*). If specific viruses were implicated, such studies might prove easier to conduct and interpret.

Studies on childhood cancers subsequent to maternal viral infections have produced unexpected results in a few instances; they do suggest that influenzal or chicken-pox infections in pregnancy might be related to leukemia and perhaps other tumors in the offspring (*141–43*). Clusters, however, tend to disappear. An early set of observations among Ugandans with Burkitt's lymphoma clearly showed time–space clustering when initially described, but then this phenomenon disappeared from all sites and has not been reported since (*144*).

Reproductive Factors. Reproductive factors have been studied intensively in many cancers but have only been particularly fruitful in malignancies of the reproductive system. Breast cancer is more common in women who have their first full-term delivery after the age of 35. Births before the mother's 20th year appear to afford some protection (*145*). Surgical menopause reduces the risk of post-menopausal breast cancer, while a naturally late onset of menopause increases the risk (*146*). Several contradictory studies have dealt with what role lactation might have in breast cancer, but the Tanka boat people from Hong Kong, who suckle children only with their right breasts, have breast cancer only of the left (*147*). This observation suggests that lactation has a protective effect.

Sexual activity has been associated with the occurrence of prostate cancer in a variety of studies. Past venereal disease, a greater number of sexual partners, more contraception use, and earlier age at first intercourse all suggest some etiological link, perhaps through endogenous hormones (*148*).

Ovarian cancer and uterine cancers are also associated with various reproductive factors; the factors that increase the risk of uterine cancer are similar to those for breast cancer, except for the risk of uterine body cancer associated with exogenous hormones.

Occupation as a Cause of Cancer

Occupation is the major opportunity an individual has for exposure to a highly select range of carcinogens. If individuals had a relatively carcinogen-free existence at home, then it would be easier to detect small occupational risks. In practice, however, any study is bound to contain a spectrum of home and work exposure. Studies on occupational topics have to be evaluated with these points in mind. Very few occupational studies contrast the health risks of the working lifestyle with those of the nonworking lifestyle, such as cigarette smoking or exposure to drugs.

Other difficulties peculiar to occupational epidemiology are centered on the problem of expectation: what would be the disease experience of the group of workers if they were not in their present occupation but were representative of the general population? This question is difficult to answer because the standard method in the follow-up study is to contrast the group with nationally collected statistics. In other words, a group of workers are contrasted with all other people including workers, the chronic physically handicapped, the mentally ill, and the unemployed. Consequently, the risk of disease in the total expected group is greater than that in the workforce and the result is the "healthy worker effect."

This spurious effect gives workers, even those at risk from an occupational hazard, the appearance of a better than expected chance of health. For example, the deaths from all cancers for talc miners, steel workers, and rubber workers are less than expected, which is clearly an underestimate (*144, 149, 150*). This phenomenon is particularly marked in the younger age groups, but it decreases with the length of time the cohort is studied, especially if workers have not been discriminated in their employment for the diseases under study.

This effect tends to be greater in the economically poorer subgroups of a community, for example, immigrant labor or minority group workers. The effect is certainly not the same for all causes of death: cases of rapid death following a silent onset would hardly be affected and some cancers come into this category. Many other local features modify this pattern: labor shortages make the healthy worker effect less marked and labor excesses make it worse.

Another factor to be evaluated in terms of occupational cancer epidemiology is the turnover of the workforce under study. High turnover leads to low average exposure per person and could be due to the unpleasant or hazardous nature of the job or the ill effects caused by the job. Obviously high turnover can occur for many other largely economic reasons, and this phenomenon will vary from country to country and from time to time. All these factors could influence the healthy worker effect. In addition, if people leave work because they are adversely affected by the working conditions—there is evidence this occurs, for example, in foundry workers—then the most severely affected will have the shortest exposure; this bias will distort any exposure–response relationship.

Workmen might also be exposed to a wide variety of noxious agents, not just one. Foundrymen, for example, are exposed to noise, carbon monoxide, heat, polycyclic hydrocarbons, metal fumes, and silica dust; thus, defining a specific hazard is often difficult. Also many industries until very recently have not provided quantitative exposure data to match local morbidity. The full cooperation of industry is essential for most of these studies.

One of the basic reasons for the continuing interest of epidemiologists in occupational matters is the constant search for chronic or long-term effects from unknown or new hazards. New chemicals are constantly being synthesized and many older products have never been fully tested for their carcinogenicity. Even if they have, a human carcinogen could very possibly turn up negative to short-term or animal tests. Short-term or acute effects present less of a problem in that a dose–response relationship could soon be calculated to determine the toxic dose. On the other hand, agents likely to cause cancer may have no threshold of effect. If this is true then low continuous exposure over a period of years is likely to be hazardous. The difficulties, therefore, surrounding the detection of chronic effects are of great importance. If one wished to know if very low levels of a known hazard were sufficient to produce, say, bladder cancer, then an extensive study would have to be undertaken. It would have to be very large and continue with environmental monitoring and epidemiological observations until sufficient man-years of exposure had elapsed to give a result that might reasonably be expected to differ from that of the general population if a hazard were present.

Studies such as those of the case–control type, which take cases as they arise, are dealing with historical events perhaps 25–40 years earlier, depending on the latent interval. On the other hand, case–control studies have fewer problems with the expected group and the analysis of confounding factors than follow-up studies. The working environment will undoubtedly have changed over the last 40 years, and the total relevance of the results for modern workers is always difficult to assess.

Occupations as Sources of Hazards. Table XI gives a list of hazards together with commonly associated malignancies and a few representative occupations where workers might be expected to come into contact with the hazard. Most epidemiological studies are obliged to assume the level of contact with the noxious agents, either because they lack environmentally monitored data or because the individual's exact occupation is not well understood.

As a result of the studies that led to the associations noted in Table XI, many substances such as benzidine and 2-naphthylamine were withdrawn from use in certain countries. The exposure regulations were tightened for other substances and low threshold limits set, as in the case of asbestos. The occupations that expose individuals to definable risks are listed in Table XI. They represent a largely historical group because of the nature of the studies.

In the future, new hazards, new types of occupational malignancy, and new occupations will be added to this list. The current concerns of all those working in industry are to know (a) whether the specified environmental threshold limit of

Table XI

Occupational Hazards and Malignancy

Agents	*Cancer Sites*	*Latent Intervals (years)*	*Occupations*
x-Rays	Bone marrow and skin	10–30	Medical and industrial (*151*)
Radon gas, radium, and uranium	Skin, lung, bone sarcoma, and bone marrow	10–30	Medical and industrial chemists, dial painters, and miners (*152*)
UV radiation	Skin	up to 70	Outdoor occupations (*153*)
Polycyclic hydrocarbons in soot, tar, oil, and resultant fumes and products of combustion	Lung, skin, larynx, bladder, and nasal cavity	10–40	Furnaces, and forges, and, foundaries, shale oil workers, gas workers and, retort men, chimney sweeps, lathe operators, textile workers, stokers, process workers, and many others (*154, 155*)
Benzene	Bone marrow and lymph nodes	5–15	Process workers, painters, textile workers, explosives workers (*156*)
1- and 2-Naphthylamine, auramine and magenta, 4-biphenylamine, and 4-nitrobiphenyl	Bladder	5–50	Dyestuffs makers, rubber workers and other chemical plant process workers, shoe workers, and printers (*157–61*)
Mustard gas	Bronchial tree, lung, and larynx	10–25	Production workers (*162*)
Isopropyl alcohol	Nasal cavity	over 10	Production workers (*154, 163*)
Vinyl chloride	Liver(angiosarcoma) and brain	5–40	Plastic manufacture (*164, 165*)
Chloroethers	Lung	at least 5	Chemical plant, process workers (*166*)
Chloroprene	Skin, lung, and liver	c10	Neoprene production (*167*)
Arsenic	Skin, lung, and liver	c10	Insecticide workers, miners and smelters, oil refiners (*168–70*)
Chromium	Lung, nasal cavity, and sinuses	10–25	Process and production workers, pigment workers (*171, 172*)
Cadmium	Lung, kidney, and prostate	10–20	Battery workers, smelters (*173*)
Nickel	Lung and nasal sinuses	5–30	Smelters and process workers (*174, 175*)
Asbestos and similar fibers	Lung, pleura and peritoneum, larynx, stomach, and large bowel	5–50	Miners, millers, manufacturers, users, and demolition workers (*171–73*)
Wood and leather particles	Nasal cavity	30–50	Wood and shoe workers (*179, 180*)
Unidentified organics	Lymph nodes	20–40	Chemists (*181*)

the known carcinogens is low enough to prevent an excess of cancers and (b) whether new cancers occur as a result of new manufacturing techniques or the production of new materials.

The answers to these questions are inevitably complex due to the multidisciplinary nature of the studies, and epidemiologists should take an initiatory and coordinating role.

Chemical Carcinogens. The International Agency for Research on Cancer has published a detailed evaluation of 514 chemicals (*182*). It showed that 19 chemicals or chemical processes were strongly associated with a carcinogenic risk and that many of these had current applications resulting in occupational exposure in some country. The paucity of true epidemiological data is striking—at least 100 chemicals with some evidence of carcinogenicity lack any such data. The risks associated with these chemicals are evaluated on the basis of all types of study and a list of proven and possible carcinogenic substances and processes can be derived (*see* list). For the majority of substances examined, however, there were insufficient data for evaluation.

The sources of chemical exposure in humans are often unknown. Those major groups that have had investigations are in industry or in pharmaceutical preparations. There is a marked and artificial deficit in chemicals associated with

Chemicals, Groups of Chemicals, or Industrial Processes That Are or May Be Carcinogenic for Humans

Proven	*Good Evidence (150)*	*Poor Evidence (150)*
Arsenic and arsenic compounds	Aflatoxins	Acrylonitrile
Asbestos	Cadmium and certain cadmium compounds	Aminotriazole (amitrole)
Auramine (manufacture)	Chlorambucil	Auramine
Benzene	Cyclophosphamide	Beryllium and certain beryllium compounds
Benzidine	Nickel and certain nickel compounds	Dimethylcarbamoyl chloride
4-Biphenylamine	Tris(1-aziridinyl) phosphine sulfide (thiotepa)	Dimethyl sulfate
N,N-Bis(2-chloroethyl-2-naphthylamine (chlornaphazine)		Ethylene oxide
Bis(chloromethyl) ether and technical grade chloromethyl methyl ether		Iron dextran
Chromium and certain chromium compounds		Oxymetholone
Diethylstilbestrol		Phenacetin
Conjugated estrogens		Polychlorinated biphenyls
Hematite mining (radon?)		Tetrachloromethane
2-Propanol manufacture (using strong acid process)		
Melphalan		
Mustard gas		
2-Naphthylamine		
Nickel refining		
Soots, tars, and oils		
Vinyl chloride		

the nonoccupational environment, because this area has yet to be fully explored. The chemicals studied so far represent a tiny fraction of all chemicals to which humans can be exposed.

Asbestos. Although it is not possible to describe in this chapter all examples of occupationally related malignancies, asbestos represents a good example of the interactions between the employees and industry in reaction to hazards and disease. The myriad uses of asbestos were exploited initially in the 1870s, and by 1900 the first disease, asbestosis, was noted. Another 30 years elapsed before it was associated with lung cancer, and it took yet another 20 years to implicate mesothelioma. Since then a wide range of industrial occupations are recognized to be at risk, and more diseases are likely to be asbestos-related (*183*). A study (*184*) on insulation workers in America has shown that bowel and stomach cancers also occur in excess, and since then laryngeal cancer has been added to the list.

More recently, other fibers have been shown to cause the same disease spectrum. Although there is no epidemiological confirmation, synthetic fibers with a diameter under 0.25 nm may be hazardous (*185*). Most interestingly, some isolated villages in central Anatolia, Karain and Tuzköy, have an exceedingly high death rate from mesothelioma, perhaps 1,000 times greater than elsewhere in the world (*186*). This part of Turkey does not contain asbestos, but the local zeolite rock is friable and is composed of fibers that have a very small mean diameter (*187*), and these are easily inhaled.

The carcinogenic action of asbestos is most likely limited to its physical and not its chemical properties, and therefore careful epidemiologic monitoring is required of artificial fibers that have similar dimensions to asbestos.

Is It Occupational? One final question concerns causal relationships and the multistage concepts of cancer. Most people have had more than one occupation. In a study of lifetime employment in Yorkshire, England, males had an average of 3.7 different occupations and 4.5 different employers (*26*). Very likely, individuals will have had more than one occupation associated with a malignancy risk. Who is to say which occupation is responsible for the disease, whether it was several, or whether it was a nonoccupational cause if the individual had smoked a great many cigarettes?

Epidemiologic methods can help to resolve these problems for a population, but one cannot extrapolate back to individual cases. One of the most helpful roles of epidemiology in this respect is to be able to contrast risks of smoking and risks of asbestos contact with respect to lung cancer. Unfortunately, assessing the respective roles of two occupations in relation to the same disease has not been done as frequently or as successfully. To date, most occupational epidemiological studies have been analyzed on the basis of one major occupation per case. The primary occupation is chosen in various ways, usually on the basis of length of employment in each occupation. Length of employment has little relevance in cancer epidemiology, though; even quite short exposure could ultimately lead to a malignancy.

When the results of the asbestos studies are carefully analyzed taking smoking into account, it is found that the risk of lung cancer in asbestos-exposed smokers is much higher than for smokers alone. The risk of lung cancer for nonsmoking asbestos workers is negligible (*188, 189*). As with smoking and alcohol, the effects of both factors are not equal, but one complements the other and multiplies the overall risks.

Acknowledgments

Many colleagues have contributed to the production of this chapter; in particular, I should like to mention the help of J. Birch, J. Cuzick, G. Draper, J. Miller, and J. Waterhouse. Thanks are also due to the Office of Population Censuses and Surveys in Britain (Figures 1–3 have been locally adapted from their data and figures), to The Yorkshire Cancer Registry and many other people in Yorkshire, and in particular to Fiona Landells on whom fell the burden of typing the various drafts. Finally, my wife's help in reading and commenting on this work has been invaluable.

Literature Cited

1. Bridbord, K. et al. "Estimates of the Fraction of Cancer in the United States related to Occupational Factors," statement by NCI, NIEHS, and NIOSH, September 15, 1978.
2. Wynder, E.L.; Gori, G.B. JNCI, J. Natl. Cancer Inst. **1977**, *58*, 825–32.
3. Doll, R. *Nature (London)* **1977**, *265*, 589–96.
4. "The Prevention of Occupational Cancer," ASTMS, London, 1980.
5. Epstein, S.S. "The Politics of Cancer"; Anchor: Los Angeles, 1980.
6. Higginson, J. *Science (Washington, D.C.)* **1979**, *205*, 1363–66.
7. Peto, R. *Nature (London)* **1980**, *284*, 297–300.
8. Hoover, R.N. *J. Med. Soc. N.J.* **1978**, *75*, 746–51.
9. Pott, P. "Chirurgical Observations Relative to the Cataract, the Polypus of the Nose, the Cancer of the Scrotum, the Different Kinds of Ruptures and the Mortification of Toes and Feet." L. Hawes: London, 1775.
10. Butlin, H.T. *Br. Med. J.* **1892**, *1*, 1341; *2*, 66.
11. Von Volkmann, R. *Beitr. Chirurg.* **1875**, 370.
12. Southam, A.H.; Wilson, S.R. *Br. Med. J.* **1922**, *2*, 971.
13. Cruickshank, C.N.D.; Squire, J.R. *Br. J. Ind. Med.* **1950**, *7*, 1.
14. Waterhouse, J. "Report on a Study of Occupational Skin Cancer"; Birmingham Univ.: Birmingham, England, 1975.
15. Haerting, F.H.; Hesse, W. *Wschr. Gerichtl. Med.* **1879**, *31*, 102.
16. Lorenz, E. *JNCI, J. Natl. Cancer Inst.* **1944**, *5*, 1.
17. Rehn, L. *Arch. Clin. Chir.* **1895**, *30*, 588.
18. "Trends in Mortality," Office of Population Censuses and Surveys, London, 1978.
19. "Mortality Surveillance 1968–1978," Office of Population Censuses and Surveys, Her Majesty's Stationery Office, London, 1980.
20. "Third National Cancer Survey," National Institutes of Health, NCI Publication No. 41, 1975.
21. "Cancer Incidence in Five Continents, Vol III," International Agency for Research on Cancer, WHO, Geneva, 1976.
22. Kaplan, H.S.; Tsuchitani, P.J. "Cancer in China"; Liss: New York, 1978.
23. Li, F.P.; Shiang, E.L. *JNCI, J. Natl. Cancer Inst.* **1980**, *65*, 217–21.
24. Segi, M. "Graphic Presentation of Cancer Incidence by Site and by Area and Population," Japan, 1977.

25. "Occupational Mortality 1970–1972," Office of Population Censuses and Surveys, Her Majesty's Stationery Office, London, 1978.
26. Cartwright, R.A. In "Human Ecology"; Clegg, E.J., Ed.; Taylor and Francis: London, 1980.
27. "Classification of Occupations," Office of Population Censuses and Surveys, Her Majesty's Stationery Office, London, 1970.
28. Swerdlow, A.J. *Br. Med. J.* **1979**, *2*, 1324–27.
29. Smith, P.G. In "Lymphoma," UICC Workshop, Geneva, 1978.
30. Cuzick, J., unpublished data.
31. Birch, J. *Lancet* **1979**, *2*, 854–55.
32. "Tumors in Children", 2nd Ed.; Marsden, H.B.; Steward, J.K., Eds.; Springer-Verlag: Berlin, 1976.
33. "Childhood Cancer in Britain 1953–1975," Office of Population Censuses and Surveys, Her Majesty's Stationery Office, London, 1981.
34. Miller, R.W. In "Genetics of Human Cancer"; Mulvihill, J.J.; Miller, R.W.; Fraumeni, J., Jr., Eds.; Raven: New York, 1977; pp. 1–41.
35. Muñoz, N. In "I Tumor Infantile"; Bucalossi, P. et al., Eds.; Casa Editrice Ambrosiana: Milan, 1976; pp. 5–15.
36. Glass, A.G.; Mantel, N.; Gunz, F.W.; Spears, G.F.S. *JNCI, J. Natl. Cancer Inst.* **1971**, *47*, 329–36.
37. Levine, P.H.; Connelly, R.R.; Berard, C.W.; O'Conor, G.T.; Dorfman, R.F.; Easton, J.M.; Devita, V.T. *Ann. Intern. Med.* **1975**, *83*, 31–36.
38. "Cancer Statistics—Survival," Office of Population Censuses and Surveys, Her Majesty's Stationery Office, London, 1980.
39. Cartwright, R.A., unpublished data, 1980.
40. Cohen, E.; Singal, D.P.; Khurana, U.; Gregory, S.G.; Cox, C.; Sinks, L.; Henderson, E.; Fitzpatrick, J.E.; Higby, D. In "HLA and Malignancy"; Murphy, G.P., Ed.; Allan Liss: New York, 1977; pp. 55–64.
41. Lilienfeld, D.E.; Lilienfeld, A.M. *Am. J. Epidemiol.* **1977**, *106*, 445–59.
42. Maclennan, R.; Muir, C.; Steinitz, R.; Winkler, A. "Cancer Registration and Its Techniques"; IARC: Lyon, 1978.
43. Schoenberg, B.S. "Multiple Primary Malignant Neoplasms"; Springer-Verlag: Berlin, 1977.
44. Waterhouse, J.A.H. "Cancer Handbook of Epidemiology and Prognosis"; Churchill Livingstone: Edinburgh, 1974.
45. Office of Population Censuses and Surveys, unpublished data, 1978.
46. Tulinius, H. In "Cancer Registry"; Grundmann, E.; Pedersen, E., Eds.; Springer-Verlag: Berlin, 1975; pp. 33–37.
47. Cartwright, R.A.; Cartwright, S.C. *J. Cancer Res. Clin. Oncol.* **1980**, in press.
48. Elandt-Johnson, R.C. *Am. J. Epidemiol.* **1975**, *102*, 267–71.
49. Barker, D.J.P.; Rose, G. "Epidemiology in Medical Practice", 2nd ed.; Churchill Livingstone: Edinburgh, 1979.
50. Meittinen, O.S. *Am. J. Epidemiol.* **1976**, *103*, 226–35.
51. Weiss, W.; Theodos, P.A. *J. Occup. Med.* **1978**, *20*, 341–45.
52. "Environmental Carcinogenesis"; Emmelot, P.; Kriek, E., Eds.; Elsevier: Amsterdam, 1979.
53. Brookes, P., Ed.; *Br. Med. Bull.* **1980**, *36*, 1–104.
54. Hicks, R.M. *Br. Med. Bull.* **1980**, *36*, 39–46.
55. Harris, C.C. *Ann. Intern. Med.* **1980**, *92*, 810–14.
56. Schmike, R.N. "Genetics and Cancer in Man"; Churchill Livingstone: Edinburgh, 1978.

57. Mourant, A.E.; Kopeć, A.C.; Domaniewska-Sobazak, K. "Blood Groups and Disease"; Oxford Univ.: Oxford, 1978.
58. Nebert, D.W. *JNCI, J. Natl. Cancer Inst.* **1980**, *64*, 1279–90.
59. Oliver, R.T.D. *Br. J. Hosp. Med.* **1977**, *18*, 449–55.
60. "Persons at High Risk of Cancer"; Fraumeni, J.F., Jr., Ed.; Academic: New York, 1975.
61. Mohr, U.; Schmähl, D.; Tomatis, L. "Air Pollution and Cancer in Man"; IARC: Lyon, 1977.
62. "Origins of Human Cancer"; Hiatt, H.H.; Watson, J.D.; Winsten, J.A., Eds.; Cold Spring Harbor, 1977.
63. Yamasaki, E.; Ames, B.N. *Proc. Natl. Acad. Sci. U.S.A.* **1977**, *74*, 3555–59.
64. Wynder, E.L.; Graham, E.A. *JAMA, J. Am. Med. Assoc.* **1950**, *143*, 329–36.
65. Doll, R.; Hill, A.B. *Br. Med. J.* **1952**, *2*, 1271–86.
66. Doll, R.; Peto, R. *Br. Med. J.* **1976**, *2*, 1525–36.
67. Bridges, B.A.; Clemmesen, J.; Sugimura, T. *Biol. Zentralbl.* **1979**, *98*, 338–40.
68. Tuyns, A.J.; Pequignot, G.; Jensen, O.M. *Bull. Cancer* **1977**, *64*, 45–60.
69. Wynder, C.L.; Covey, L.S.; Mabuchi, K.; Mushinaki, M. *Cancer* **1976**, 38.
70. Enstrom, J.E. *Br. J. Cancer* **1977**, *35*, 674–83.
71. Lewis, E.B. *Science (Washington, D.C.)* **1963**, *142*, 1492–94.
72. Ishimaru, T.; Otake, M.; Ichimaru, M. *Radiat. Res.* **1979**, *77*, 377–94.
73. "Sources and Effects of Ionizing Irradiation," UNSCEAR, United Nations: New York, 1977.
74. Court Brown, W.M.; Doll, R. *Br. Med. J.* **1965**, *2*, 1327–32.
75. Smith, P.G.; Doll, R. *Br. J. Radiol.* **1976**, *49*, 224–32.
76. Hempelmann, L.H.; Pifer, J.W.; Burke, G.J. *JNCI, J. Natl. Cancer Inst.* **1967**, *38*, 317–41.
77. Albert, E.R.; Omran, A.R. *Arch. Environ. Health* **1968**, *17*, 899–950.
78. Cuzick, J., unpublished data, 1980.
79. Boice, J.D. In "Advances in Medical Oncology, Research and Education," Vo. I; Pergamon: Oxford, 1979; pp. 147–56.
80. Polednak, A.P.; Stehney, A.F.; Rowland, R.E. *Am. J. Epidemiol.* **1978**, *107*, 179–85.
81. Sevc, J.; Kunz, E.; Placek, V. *Health Phys.* **1976**, *30*, 433–37.
82. Wagoner, J.K.; Archer, V.E.; Carroll, B.E. *JNCI, J. Natl. Cancer Inst.* **1964**, *32*, 787–801.
83. Farber, M. *Environ. Res.* **1979**, *18*, 37–43.
84. Speiss, H.; Gerspach, A.; Mays, C.W. *Health Phys.* **1978**, *35*, 61–81.
85. Mole, R.H. *Environ. Res.* **1979**, *18*, 192–215.
86. Stewart, A.M.; Barker, R. *Br. Med. Bull.* **1971**, *27*, 64–70.
87. "The Effect on Populations of Exposure to Low Levels of Ionizing Radiation"; Biological Effects of Ionizing Radiation Report III, National Acad. Sci.: Washington, 1981.
88. Gilbert, E.S.; Marks, S. *Radiat. Res.* **1979**, *79*, 122–48.
89. Anderson, T.W. *Health Phys.* **1978**, *35*, 743–50.
90. Dolphin, G.W., National Radiological Protection Board, NRPB–R.54, Her Majesty's Stationery Office, London, 1976.
91. Boice, J.D.; Hutchinson, G.B. *JNCI, J. Natl. Cancer Inst.* **1980**, *65*, 115–29.
92. Leading article, *Lancet* **1978**, *2*, 38.
93. Swerdlow, A.J. *Br. Med. J.* **1979**, *2*, 1324–27.
94. Elwood, J.M. *Int. J. Epidemiol.* **1974**, *3*, 325.
95. "Health Effects of Exposure to Electric and Magnetic Fields," World Health Organization, ICP/RCF, 801 (4), 1979.
96. "Health Implications of Exposure to Non-Ionizing Radiation,' World Health Organization, ICP/RCE, 801 (3), 1979.
97. Russner, P.; Mateika, M. *J. Hyg. Epidemiol. Microbiol. Immunol.* **1979**, *21*, 465–67.

98. Mitchell, J.T.; Marino, A.A.; Berger, T.J.; Becker, R.O. *Physiol. Chem. Phys.* **1978**, *10*, 79–85.
99. "Biological Effects of Static and Low-Frequency Electromagnetic Fields," Electrical Power Research Institute, EA-490-SR, 1977.
100. Kinlen, L.J.; Sheil, A.G.R.; Peto, J.; Doll, R. *Br. Med. J.* **1979**, *2*, 1461–166.
101. Kinlen, L.J.; Eastwood, J.B.; Derr, D.N.S.; Moorhead, J.F.; Oliver, D.O.; Robinson, B.H.B.; de Wardner, H.E.; Wing, A.J. *Br. Med. J.* **1980**, *1*, 1401–6.
102. Reimer, R.R.; Hoover, R.; Fraumeni, J.F., Jr.; Young, R.C. *New Engl. J. Med.* **1977**, *297*, 177–81.
103. Herbst, A.L.; Scully, R.E.; Robboy, S.J. *Natl. Cancer Inst. Monogr.* **1976**, *51*, 25–35.
104. Carro-Ciampi, G. *Toxicology* **1978**, *10*, 311–39.
105. Nissen, E.D.; Kent, F.; Kent, D.R. *Obstet. Gynecol. (N.Y.)* **1975**), *46*, 460–70.
106. Vessey, M.P.; Doll, R.; Jones, K.; McPherson, K.; Yeates, D. *Br. Med. J.* **1979**, *1*, 1755–58.
107. Knet, J.; Mahboubi, E. *Sciences (N.Y.)* **1972**, *175*, 846.
108. Hirayama, T. *Bull. W. H. O.* **1966**, *34*, 41.
109. Habs, M.; Schmähl, D. *J. Cancer Res. Clin. Oncol.* **1980**, *96*, 1–10.
110. Shank, R.C. In "Environmental Cancer"; Kraybill, H.F.; Mehlmann, M.A., Eds.; Wiley: New York, 1977.
111. Dunn, J.E. *Cancer Res.* **1975**, *35*, 3240–45.
112. Hoover, R.N.; Strasser, P.H. *Lancet* **1980**, *1*, 837–40.
113. Kinlen, L.J.; Clarke, C.A.; Doll, R. *Lancet* **1980**, *2*, 199.
114. Doll, R.; Kinlen, L.J. *Lancet* **1977**, *1*, 1300–1302.
115. Hymes, K.B.; Greene, J.B.; Marcus, A. *Lancet* **1981**, *2*, 598–600.
116. Armstrong, B.; Doll, R. *Int. J. Cancer* **1975**, *15*, 617–31.
117. Schottenfeld, D.; Winawer, S.J. In "Cancer Epidemiology and Prevention"; Schottenfeld, D.; Fraumeni, J.F., Eds.; Saunders: Philadelphia, 1982; pp. 703–27.
118. Doll, R.; Vessey, M.P.; Beasley, R.W.R. *Br. J. Ind. Med.* **1972**, *29*, 394–406.
119. Stocks, P. "Cancer in North Wales and Liverpool Regions," supplement to British Empire Campaign Report, 1957.
120. Pike, M.C.; Gordon, R.J.; Henderson, B.E.; Menck, H.R.; SooHoo, J. In "Persons at High Risk of Cancer"; Fraumeni, J.F., Jr., Ed.; Academic: New York, 1975; pp. 225–39.
121. Waldbott, G.L. "Health Effects of Environmental Pollutants," 2nd ed., Mosby: St. Louis, 1978.
122. Axelson, O.; Sucdell, L. *Work Environ. Health* **1974**, *11*, 21–28.
123. Lawther, P.J. *Proc. R. Soc. London Ser. B* **1979**, *205*, 63–75.
124. Tung, T.T. *Chirurgie* **1973**, *99*, 427–36.
125. Orth, G.; Breitburd, F.; Favre, M.; Croissant, O. In "Origins of Human Cancer"; Hiatt, H.H.; Watson, J.B.; Winsten, J.A., Eds.; Cold Spring Harbor Laboratory: Cold Spring Harbor, N.Y., 1977; pp. 1043–68.
126. Winters, W.D.; Neri, A.; Sykes, J.A.; O'Toole, C. *Prev. Detect. Cancer [Proc. Int. Symp.], 3rd* **1977**, *1*, 279–92.
127. Gallo, R.C.; Meyskens, F.L. *Semin. Hematol.* **1978**, *15*, 379–98.
128. Gallo, R.C.; Blattner, W.A.; Reitz, M.S.; Ito, Y. *Lancet* **1982**, *1*, 683.
129. de-Thé, G.; Geser, A.; Day, N.E.; Tukei, T.M.; Williams, E.H.; Ben, D.P.; Smith, P.G.; Dean, A.G.; Bornkamm, G.W.; Feerino, P.; Henle, W. *Nature (London)* **1978**, *274*, 756–61.
130. Ho, H.C.; Kwan, H.C.; Ng, M.H.; de-Thé, G. *Lancet* **1978**, *1*, 436.
131. Purtilo, D.T. *Lancet* **1980**, *1*, 300–303.
132. Blumberg, B.S.; Larouzé, B.; London, W.T.; Werner, B.; Hesser, J.E.; Millman, I.; Saimot, G.; Payet, M. *Am. J. Pathol.* **1975**, *81*, 669.
133. Kessler, I.I. *Cancer Res.* **1974**, *34*, 1091–110.

134. Kessler, I.I. *Prev. Detect. Cancer [Proc. Int. Symp.] 3rd* **1977**, *1*, 211–30.
135. Cocks, P.; Cartwright, R.A.; Adib, R. *Lancet* **1980**, *2*, 855–56.
136. Knox, E.G. *Appl. Stat.* **1964**, *13*, 25–29.
137. Pike, M.C.; Smith, P.G. *Biometrics* **1968**, *24*, 541–56.
138. Ohno, Y.; Aoki, N. *Int. J. Epidemiol.* **1979**, *3*, 273–81.
139. Smith, P.G.; Pike, M.C. *Cancer Res.* **1974**, *34*, 1156–60.
140. Vianna, N.J. *Cancer Res.* **1974**, *34*, 1149–55.
141. Austin, D.; Karp, S.; Divorsky, R. *Am. J. Epidemiol.* **1975**, *101*, 77–83.
142. Curnen, M.; Varma, A.; Christine, B. *JNCI, J. Natl. Cancer Inst.* **1974**, *53*, 943–7.
143. Vianna, N.J.; Polan, A.K. *Am. J. Epidemiol.* **1976**, *103*, 321–32.
144. Smith, P.G., unpublished data, 1979.
145. Bjelke, E. *Int. J. Cancer* **1975**, *15*, 561–165.
146. MacMahon, B.; Cole, P.; Lin, T.M. *Bull. W.H.O.* **1970**, *43*, 209–21.
147. Levin, M.L.; Sheehe, P.R.; Graham, S. *Am. J. Publ. Health* **1964**, *54*, 580–87.
148. Ing, R.; Ho, J.H.C.; Petrakis, N.L. *Lancet* **1977**, *2*, 124–27.
149. Ardjelkovich, D.; Taulbee, J.; Symons, M.; Williams, T. *J. Occup. Med.* **1977**, *19*, 397–405.
150. Boyd, J.T.; Doll, R.; Faulds, J.S. *Br. J. Ind. Med.* **1970**, *27*, 97–105.
151. Court Brown, W.M.; Doll, R. *Br. Med. J.* **1958**, 181–87.
152. Wagoner, J.K.; Archer, V.E.; Lundin, F.E. *New Engl. J. Med.* **1965**, *173*, 181–88.
153. Urbach, F. In "Biological Effects of Ultraviolet Irradiation"; Pergamon: Oxford, 1969.
154. Doll, R. *Br. J. Ind. Med.* **1959**, *16*, 181–90.
155. Lloyd, J.W. *J. Occup. Med.* **1971**, *13*, 53–68.
156. Aksoy, M.; Dinçol, K.; Erdem, S. *Am. J. Med.* **1972**, *52*, 160–66.
157. Case, R.A.M.; Hosker, M.E. *Br. J. Prev. Soc. Med.* **1954**, *8*, 39–80.
158. Case, R.A.M.; Hosker, M.E.; McDonald, D.B. *Br. J. Ind. Med.* **1954**, *11*, 75–104.
159. Case, R.A.M. *Ann. R. Coll. Surg. Engl.* **1966**, *39*, 213–35.
160. Cole, P.; Hoover, R.; Firedell, G.H. *Cancer* **1972**, *29*, 1250–60.
161. Koss, L.G.; Melamed, M.R.; Ricci, A. *New Engl. J. Med.* **1965**, *262*, 767–70.
162. Beebe, G.W. *JNCI, J. Natl. Cancer Inst.* **1960**, *25*, 1231–52.
163. Weil, C.S.; Smyth, H.F.; Nale, T.W. *Arch. Ind. Hyg.* **1952**, *5*, 535–47.
164. Monson, R.R.; Peters, J.M.; Johnson, M.N. *Lancet* **1974**, *2*, 297–98.
165. Tabershaw, I.R.; Gaffey, W. *New Engl. J. Med.* **1974**, *16*, 509–18.
166. Brown, S.M.; Selvin, S. *New Engl. J. Med.* **1973**, *289*, 693–94.
167. Khachatryan, E.A. *Probl. Oncol. (Engl. Transl.)* **1972**, *18*, 85.
168. Axelson, O.; Dahlgren, E.; Hansson, C.D.; Rehnlund, S.O. *Br. J. Ind. Med.* **1972**, *35*, 8–15.
169. Lee, A.M.; Fraumeni, J.F., Jr. *JNCI, J. Natl. Cancer Inst.* **1969**, *42*, 1045–52.
170. Yeh, S. *Hum. Pathol.* **1973**, *4*, 469–85.
171. Enterline, P.E. *J. Occup. Med.* **1974**, *16*, 523–26.
172. Ohsaki, Y.; Abe, S.; Kimura, K.; Tsuneta, Y.; Mikami, H.; Murao, M. *Thorax* **1978**, *33*, 372–74.
173. Lemen, R.A.; Lee, J.S.; Wagoner, J.K.; Blejer, H.P. *Ann. N. Y. Acad. Sci.* **1976**, *271*, 273.
174. Lessard, R.; Reed, D.; Maheux, B.; Lambert, J. *J. Occup Med.* **1978**, *20*, 815–17.
175. Pederson, E.; Hogetveit, A.; Anderson, A. *Int. J. Cancer* **1973**, *12*, 32–41.
176. Doll, R. *Br. J. Ind. Med.* **1955**, *12*, 81–86.
177. Selikoff, I.J.; Churg, J.; Hammond, E.C. *J. Am. Med. Ann.* **1964**, *188*, 22–26.
178. Wagner, J.C.; Sleggs, C.A.; Marchand, P. *Br. J. Ind. Med.* **1960**, *17*, 260–71.
179. Acheson, E.D.; Cowdell, R.H.; Hadfield, E. *Br. Med. J.* **1968**, *2*, 587–96.
180. Acheson, E.D.; Cowdell, R.H.; Jolles, B. *Br. Med. J.* **1970**, *1*, 385–93.
181. Olin, R.G. *Prev. Detect. Cancer [Proc. Int. Symp.] 3rd* **1977**, *1*, 847–55.

182. "Carcinogenic Risks. Strategies for Intervention," Report 25, WHO, IARC: Geneva, 1978.
183. Bogovski, P.; Gilson, J.C.; Timbrell, V.; Wagner, J.C. "Biological Effects of Asbestos," IARC: Lyon, 1973.
184. Selikoff, I.J.; Hammond, E.C.; Seidman, H. *Ann. N. Y. Acad. Sci.* **1979**, *330*, 91–116.
185. "Man-Made Mineral Fibers," Health and Safety Executive, Her Majesty's Stationery Office, London, 1979.
186. Artvinli, M.; Bariş, Y.I. *JNCI, J. Natl. Cancer Inst.* **1979**, *63*, 17–22.
187. Ataman, G. *C. R. Hebd. Seances Acad. Sci.* **1978**, *287*, 207–10.
188. Selikoff, I.J.; Hammond, E.C.; Churg, J. *JAMA J. Am. Med. Assoc.* **1968**, *204*, 106–12.
189. Selikoff, I.J.; Seidman, H.; Hammond, E.C. *JNCI, J. Natl. Cancer Inst.* **1980**, *65*, 507–13.

2

Polynuclear Aromatic Carcinogens

ANTHONY DIPPLE, ROBERT C. MOSCHEL, and C. ANITA H. BIGGER

National Cancer Institute, Frederick Cancer Research Facility, Chemical Carcinogenesis Program, Frederick, MD 21701

Nomenclature

Polynuclear Compounds. The nomenclature of polynuclear carcinogens has changed over the years, resulting in a certain degree of ambiguity in the literature. Even in recent years, several alternative systems for describing the stereochemistry of hydrocarbon derivatives have been employed and there is quite a potential for confusion in trying to follow the literature in this area. This brief outline on nomenclature is presented to eliminate some of this confusion as well as to define the nomenclature that will be used throughout this article.

Ambiguities in the naming of polynuclear carcinogens are exemplified in Structures IA–ID; using different nomenclature systems, the two isomeric benzpyrenes (IA and IB) have been assigned the same name, 1, 2-benzpyrene, because different peripheral numbering systems were used, as illustrated for pyrene (IC and ID). The system preferred by American scientists (IC) gave rise to the 3,4-benzpyrene (IA3) and 1,2-benzpyrene (IB3) nomenclature for the carcinogenic and noncarcinogenic benzpyrene isomers, respectively, while the system preferred by European workers (ID) led to the 1,2-benzpyrene (IA2) and 4,5-benzpyrene (IB2) nomenclature for these same compounds.

The currently accepted IUPAC rules give to pyrene the peripheral numbering illustrated by ID. This numbering is dictated by placing the polycyclic system so that (1) the maximum number of rings lies in a horizontal row; and (2) as many rings as possible are above and to the right of the horizontal row. If more than one orientation meets these requirements, the one with the minimum number of rings at the lower left is chosen. The system is then numbered in a clockwise direction starting with the carbon atom not engaged in ring fusion in the most counter-clockwise position of the uppermost ring or the uppermost ring that is farthest to the right. Atoms common to two or more rings are not numbered.

This numbering is applied throughout the hydrocarbon field, e.g., the isomeric benzpyrenes (IA and IB), picene (IIA), and chrysene (IIB), with the sole exceptions of phenanthrene, anthracene, and cyclopenta[*a*]phenanthrene, which are numbered as indicated in Structures IIIA–IIIC.

The peripheral numbering of heterocyclic aromatic compounds is dictated by the same principles but with the additional proviso that where a choice of

0065-7719/84/0182-0041$24.45/1

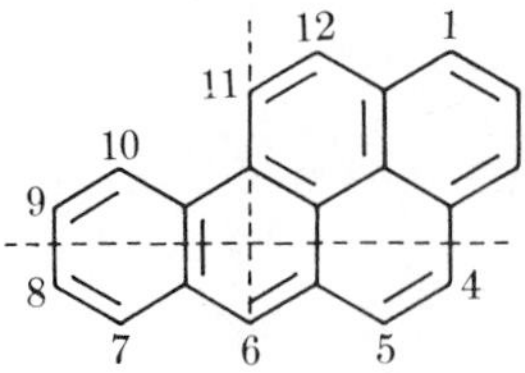

A. 1. Benzo[*a*]pyrene
2. 1, 2-Benzpyrene
3. 3, 4-Benzpyrene
(carcinogenic)

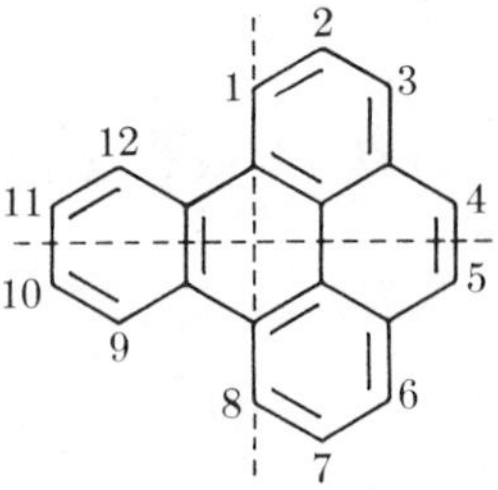

B. 1. Benzo[*e*]pyrene
2. 4, 5-Benzpyrene
3. 1, 2-Benzpyrene
(noncarcinogenic)

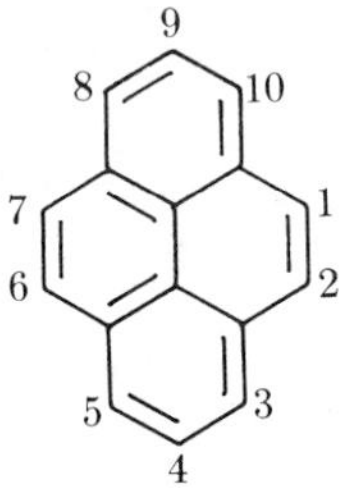

C. Pyrene

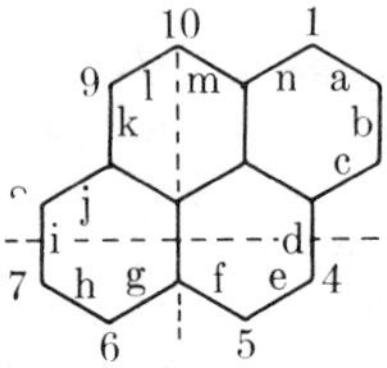

D. Pyrene

I

orientation is still available, low numbers are given to the hetero atoms. If a choice still remains, the lowest number is given to oxygen in preference to sulfur and to sulfur in preference to nitrogen. Exceptions to the systematic peripheral numbering system for heterocyclic compounds are the numbering for purine, carbazole (**IV**A), and acridine (**IVB**).

Thus, apart from a few exceptions, all the polycyclic hydrocarbons and heterocyclic compounds can be systematically numbered according to a few simple rules. The names of structures that have no trivial name are obtained by prefixing the name of a component ring system (the base component, which should contain as many rings as possible) with designations of the other component. Isomers are then distinguished by lettering the peripheral sides of the base component *a, b, c,* etc., beginning with *a* for the side 1,2; *b* for the side 2,3; etc., as illustrated earlier for pyrene (**I**D). With this system, the benzpyrene isomers are distinguished as benzo[*a*]pyrene (**I**A1) and benzo[*e*]pyrene (**I**B1), and the whole benzpyrene structure is then numbered according to the rules discussed.

Hydrocarbon Metabolites and Derivatives. In addition to the systematic descriptions, some trivial terms of wide usage are also worthy of mention and definition. The bond in a polycyclic aromatic hydrocarbon with the greatest double-bond character (i.e., lowest bond-localization energy), for example, the 5,6-bond in benz[*a*]anthracene (**V**), is described by the term "*K* region"; a region where electrons are relatively easily localized across *para*-positions (i.e., low *para*-locali-

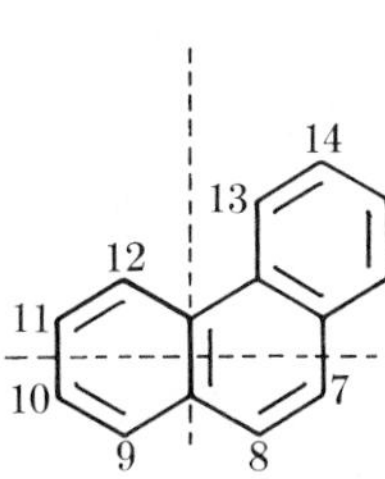

A. Picene

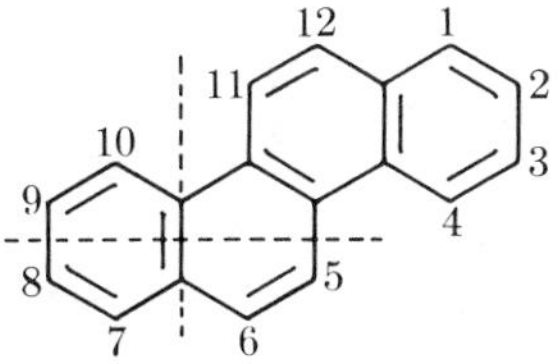

B. Chrysene

II

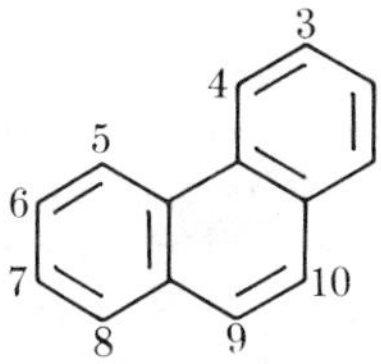

A. Phenanthrene

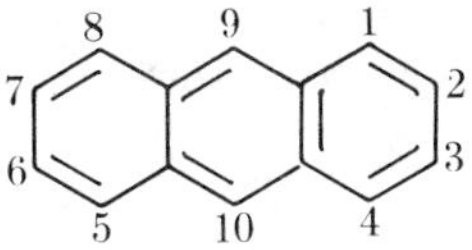

B. Anthracene

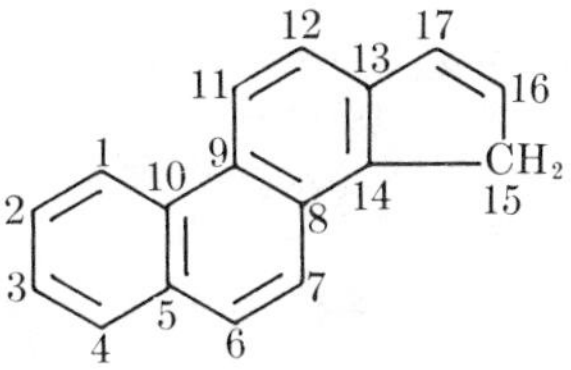

C. 15 *H*-Cyclopenta[*a*]phenanthrene

III

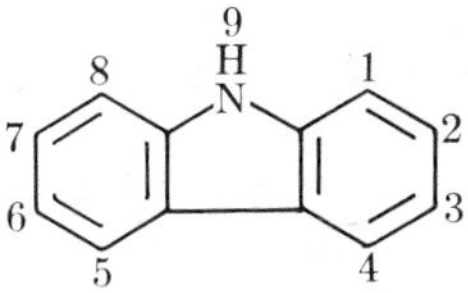

A. Carbazole

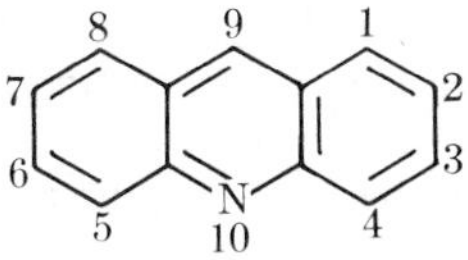

B. Acridine

IV

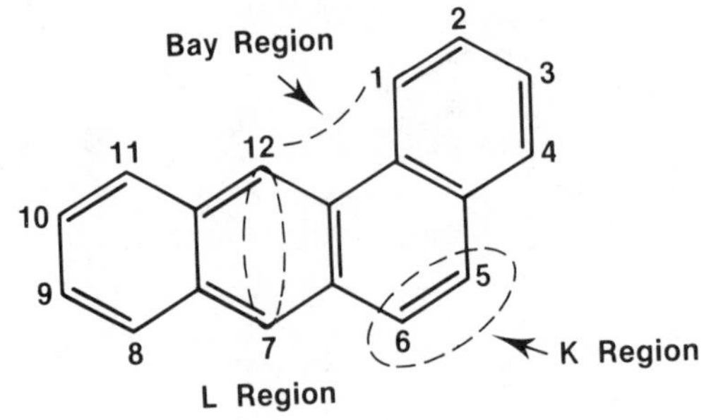

Bay Region
2
1
3
11
12
4
10
5
9
8
7
6
K Region
L Region

V

zation energy), for example, the region between the 7- and 12-positions in benz[*a*]anthracene, is described by the term "*L* region." The region generated by the angular addition of a benzene ring to a linear portion of an aromatic hydrocarbon, e.g., the region between the 1- and 12-positions in benz[*a*]anthracene, is termed a "bay region". Carcinogenic activity is frequently associated with the presence of a bay region, and this term is also used to distinguish between structural isomers of hydrocarbon dihydrodiol epoxides. Thus, only the benzo[*a*]pyrene dihydrodiol epoxide in which the epoxide ring involves a benzylic carbon that is part of the bay region would be referred to as a bay-region dihydrodiol epoxide; that is, Structure **VI**A but not **VI**B.

Nomenclature for the dihydrodiol epoxides is confusing for a variety of reasons, and no consensus on a particular nomenclature system has been reached. It apparently is correct either to utilize the prefix epoxy as in 7,8-dihydroxy-9,10-epoxy-7,8,9,10-tetrahydrobenzo[*a*]pyrene or to add on the word epoxide as in 7,8-dihydrobenzo[*a*]pyrene-7,8-diol 9,10-epoxide. However, the word epoxide is added to the name of an unsaturated system (e.g., ethylene epoxide), and the epoxy prefix precedes a description of the corresponding saturated system (e.g., 1,2-epoxyethane). Although the informal description of dihydrodiol metabolites of hydrocarbons has largely utilized the term dihydrodiol as in the benzo[*a*]pyrene dihydrodiols, for some reason the dihydro portion has mostly been dropped in informal reference to benzo[*a*]pyrene diol epoxides (**VI**A and **VI**B). This usage appears to be somewhat misleading because it might suggest that the diol refers to a catechol rather than a dihydrodiol; so we have opted to use the general terms benzo[*a*]pyrene dihydrodiol epoxide or just dihydrodiol epoxide in this chapter because we feel it is more consistent with the more formal nomenclature and the wide usage of dihydrodiol to describe the precursors of these metabolites. Also, a mixed usage of the words epoxide and oxide has been used to describe the oxirane rings in various hydrocarbon metabolites. Either of these terms is correct but epoxide is somewhat more specific, because it implies that the oxygen is connected to two atoms that are already linked in some way. We have decided to use the word epoxide in preference to oxide.

Hydrocarbon dihydrodiols and dihydrodiol epoxides contain asymmetric carbon centers, so that in addition to structural isomerism (**VI**A–**VI**B), stereoisomerism is also important. *Stereoisomers* are molecules that have the same constitution (i.e., the same sequential arrangement of atoms) but differ in the

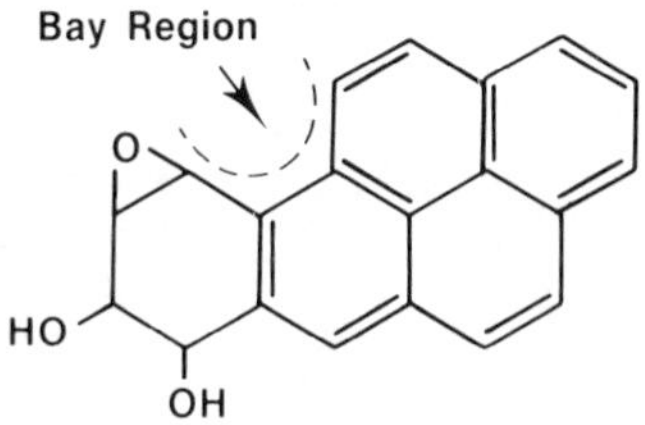

Bay Region

A. Bay-region dihydrodiol epoxide

(7,8-Dihydroxy-9,10-epoxy-7,8,9,10-tetrahydrobenzo[*a*]pyrene)

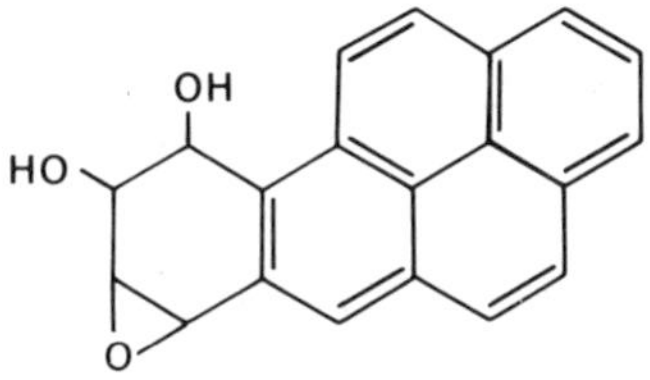

B. Non-bay-region dihydrodiol epoxide

(9,10-Dihydroxy-7,8-epoxy-7,8,9,10-tetrahydrobenzo[*a*]pyrene)

VI

spatial arrangement of their atoms. Two stereoisomers that are nonsuperimposable mirror images of each other are called *enantiomers,* and any two stereoisomers that are not related in this way are called *diastereomers.* These terms are mutually exclusive. Diastereomers may differ widely in physical and chemical properties, while enantiomers exhibit identical properties within a symmetrical environment. Enantiomers can be distinguished by their different responses in asymmetric environments or to asymmetric reagents. For example, the asymmetric character of plane-polarized light is frequently used to distinguish between enantiomers. Solutions of pure enantiomers will rotate the plane of plane-polarized light in opposite directions with the specific rotations for each enantiomer being of equal magnitude but of opposite sign.

An example of an enantiomeric pair from the hydrocarbon field, the (+)- and (−)-enantiomers of benzo[*a*]pyrene 4,5-epoxide, is illustrated by Structures **VII**A–**VII**C. Because the mirror-image relationship between the (+)- and (−)-enantiomers is not entirely obvious from the conventional structural representations of these molecules (**VII**A and **VII**C), the (−)-enantiomer is also depicted as **VII**B where its mirror-image relationship with the (+)-enantiomer (**VII**A) is clear. In all these representations, the dashed lines denote bonds that project below the plane of the paper, and the bold lines denote bonds that project out of the paper. Structures **VII**B and VIIC are the same [the (−)-enantiomer] viewed from either face of the molecule; Structure **VII**C has been drawn according to the rules for peripheral numbering outlined earlier. Throughout this chapter, such structures will be drawn according to these rules, and mirror-image relationships (e.g., between **VII**A and **VII**C) can be recognized by virtue of the fact that every bond that projects out of or into the paper in one enantiomer will project in the opposite direction in the other enantiomer. The pure enantiomers of benzo[*a*]pyrene 4,5-epoxide have been synthesized and their absolute stereochemistries have also been assigned (*1*), as indicated by the designation (4*S*,5*R*) in the name of the (+)-enantiomer (**VII**A).

This systematic notation of absolute configuration depends on assigning priorities to the four atoms attached to the carbon whose configuration is being described. Priority decreases with decreasing atomic number. When two of the attached atoms are the same, their relative priorities are determined by the

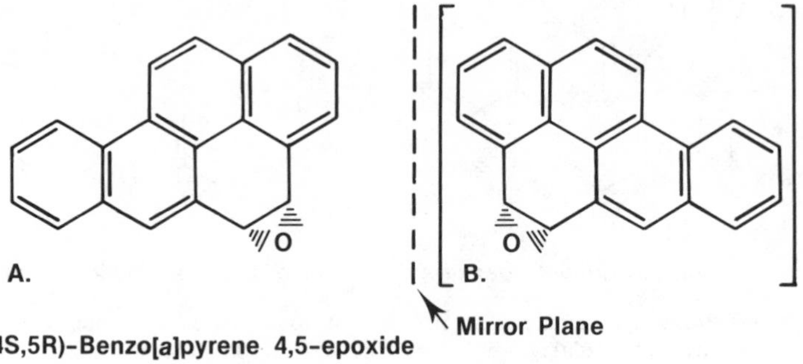

A.

B.

Mirror Plane

(+)-(4S,5R)-Benzo[*a*]pyrene 4,5-epoxide

C.

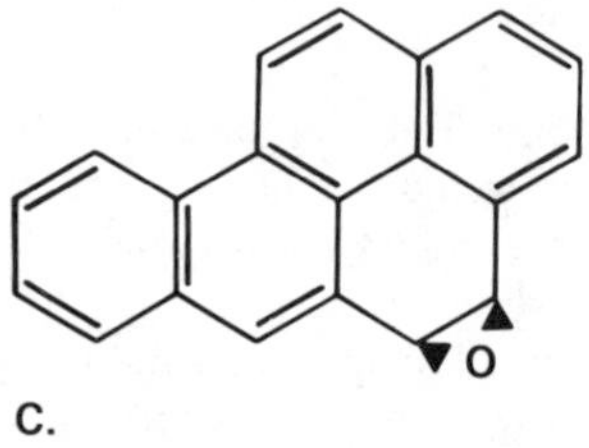

(-)-(4R,5S)-Benzo[*a*]pyrene 4,5-epoxide

VII

priorities of the atoms attached to them. The atom of lowest priority (frequently hydrogen) is then viewed *through* the triangle formed by the other three atoms. If priority decreases around this triangle in a clockwise direction, the configuration is specified as (*R*); if priority decreases in a counterclockwise direction, the configuration is specified as (*S*).

In addition to the arene epoxides, the vicinal *trans*-dihydrodiols, which are common metabolites of hydrocarbons, have two possible enantiomeric configurations, and in some cases, these enantiomers have been resolved. For example, Structures **VIII**A and **VIII**B illustrate the (−)- and (+)-enantiomers of *trans*-7,8-dihydroxy-7,8-dihydrobenzo[*a*]pyrene, respectively. Again, their absolute stereochemistry has been assigned (*2,3*).

The nomenclature for the arene epoxides and vicinal dihydrodiols is relatively straightforward, but the literature has become somewhat confusing with respect to the nomenclature for dihydrodiol epoxides. Each of the enantiomeric dihydrodiols (**VIII**A and **VIII**B) can give rise to two diastereomeric dihydrodiol epoxides depending on whether the epoxide oxygen is introduced above or below the plane of the polycyclic ring system. Thus, four stereoisomeric dihydrodiol epoxides are possible (**VIII**C and **VIII**E derived from **VIII**A, and **VIII**D and **VIII**F derived from **VIII**B). Of these, **VIII**C and **VIII**D represent one enantiomeric pair, and **VIII**E and **VIII**F represent another. The relationship between any other pairs of dihydrodiol epoxides (**VIII**C–**VIII**F) is diastereomeric. All the absolute configurations have

HO OH

Enantiomeric Relationship

HO OH

A. (−)(7R,8R)-*trans*-7,8-dihydroxy-7,8-dihydrobenzo[*a*]pyrene

B. (+)(7S,8S)-*trans*-7,8-dihydroxy-7,8-dihydrobenzo[*a*]pyrene

3. *r*-7,*t*-8-dihydroxy-*c*-9,10-epoxy-7,8,9,10-tetrahydrobenzo[*a*]pyrene
4. *cis* diol-epoxide
5. *syn* diol-epoxide
6. diol-epoxide-1
7. diol-epoxide II

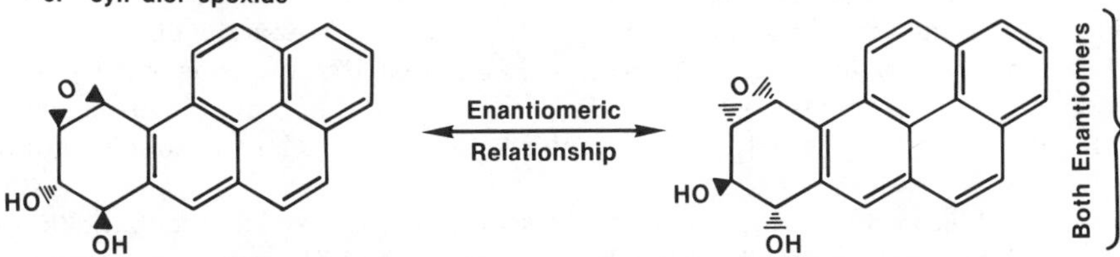

C. 1. (−)(7R,8S,9R,10S)-7,8-dihydroxy-9,10-epoxy-7,8,9,10-tetrahydrobenzo[*a*]pyrene

2. (−) 7β,8α-dihydroxy-9β,10β-epoxy-7,8,9,10-tetrahydrobenzo[*a*]pyrene

8. (−) *syn* 7,8-dihydrodiol 9,10-epoxide

D. 1. (+)(7S,8R,9S,10R)-7,8-dihydroxy-9,10-epoxy-7,8,9,10-tetrahydrobenzo[*a*]pyrene

2. (+) 7α,8β-dihydroxy-9α,10α-epoxy-7,8,9,10-tetrahydrobenzo[*a*]-pyrene

8. (+) *syn* 7,8-dihydrodiol 9,10-epoxide

Diastereomeric Relationships

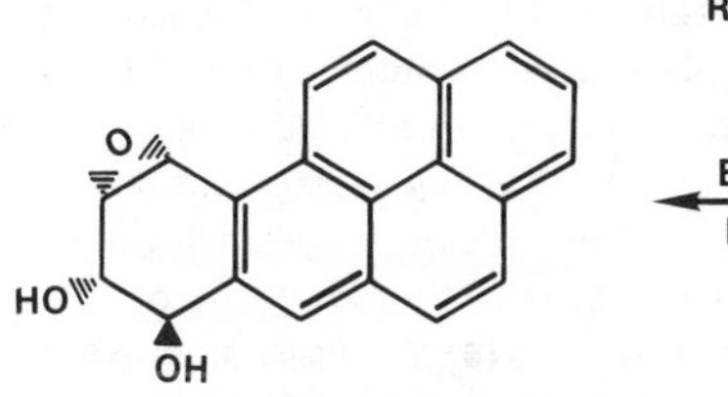

Enantiomeric Relationship

O HO OH

Both Enantiomers

E. 1. (+)(7R,8S,9S,10R)-7,8-dihydroxy-9,10-epoxy-7,8,9,10-tetrahydrobenzo[*a*]pyrene

2. (+) 7β,8α-dihydroxy-9α,10α-epoxy-7,8,9,10-tetrahydrobenzo[*a*]pyrene

8. (+) *anti* 7,8-dihydrodiol 9,10-epoxide

3. *r*-7,*t*-8-dihydroxy-*t*-9,10-epoxy-7,8,9,10-tetrahydrobenzo[*a*]pyrene
4. *trans* diol-epoxide
5. *anti* diol-epoxide

F. 1. (−)(7S,8R,9R,10S)-7,8-dihydroxy-9,10-epoxy-7,8,9,10-tetrahydrobenzo[*a*]pyrene

2. (−) 7α,8β-dihydroxy-9β,10β-epoxy-7,8,9,10-tetrahydrobenzo[*a*]pyrene

8. (−) *anti* 7,8-dihydrodiol 9,10-epoxide

6. diol-epoxide-2
7. diol-epoxide I

VIII

been assigned (reviewed in Ref. 4), but they have been described in the literature by using either the (*R*) and (*S*) system discussed earlier (i.e., **VIIIC**1, **VIIID**1, **VIIIE**1, and **VIIIF**1) or by using nomenclature borrowed from the steroid field. In the latter system, the structure is drawn according to the IUPAC rules discussed earlier, and substituents that project out of the plane of the paper are designated by the prefix β; those lying below this plane are designated by the prefix α. The names for the stereoisomeric dihydrodiol epoxides using this system are listed as **VIIIC**2, **VIIID**2, **VIIIE**2, and **VIIIF**2. In both of these systems for describing absolute configuration, the (+) or (−) preceding the name is not required to define the structure but it provides extra information about the direction in which these structures rotate the plane of plane-polarized light.

The nomenclature systems become somewhat clumsy in dealing with racemic mixtures. While each dihydrodiol-epoxide stereoisomer has an individual description using these systems, racemic mixtures are designated by prefixing one of these individual descriptions with (±), e.g., (±)-7α,8β-dihydroxy-9α,10α-epoxy-7,8,9,10-tetrahydrobenzo[*a*]pyrene, and this usage seems to be a contradiction in itself.

In addition to these systematic descriptions of absolute configuration, descriptions of relative configuration have also been used. The pair of enantiomers **VIIIC** and **VIIID** both have the 7-hydroxyl group and the epoxide ring on the same face of the 7,8,9,10-ring, while the pair of enantiomers **VIIIE** and **VIIIF** each have the 7-hydroxyl group and the epoxide ring on opposite faces of the 7,8,9,10-ring. These diastereomeric enantiomer pairs have been distinguished using the nomenclature listed as 3. In this system, the *r*-7 indicates that the 7-hydroxyl group is taken as a reference; the *t*-8 indicates that the 8-hydroxyl is *trans* to the reference group; and the *c*-9,10 or *t*-9,10 indicates that the 9,10-epoxy group is *cis* or *trans* to the reference group. Clearly, this nomenclature is the same for each member of an enantiomeric pair, but it does distinguish between diastereomers. If this nomenclature were preceded by either (+) or (−), then enantiomers would also be distinguished for convenient reference, but the names would not identify the absolute stereochemistry of each enantiomer. Other informal nomenclature has also been used to differentiate these structures. The pair of enantiomers with the 7-hydroxyl group and the epoxide ring on the same face of the 7,8,9,10-ring (i.e., **VIIIC** and **VIIID**) have been described as *cis*-diol epoxides (4), as *syn*-diol epoxides (5), as diol epoxide 1 (6), and as diol epoxide II (7). Correspondingly, the pair of enantiomers in which the 7-hydroxyl and the epoxide ring are on opposite sides of the 7,8,9,10-ring (i.e., **VIIIE** and **VIIIF**) have been identified as *trans*-diol epoxides, as *anti*-diol epoxides, as diol epoxide 2, and as diol epoxide I (4–7). Each of these nonsystematic approaches can identify any one of the four dihydrodiol-epoxides by preceding these trivial descriptions by (+) or (−) to distinguish enantiomers. The different choices of trivial nomenclature by different research laboratories make the literature in this area difficult to follow, but fully systematic nomenclature cannot be used on a routine basis because absolute stereochemistries for all dihydrodiol epoxides and dihydrodiols is not established; even when this information is known, the nomenclature is very cumbersome.

Of the trivial nomenclatures that have been used, we feel the least happy about using the diol epoxide 1 and 2 or the diol epoxide I and II systems because these names convey no structural information and the Arabic and Roman numerals could easily be confused. The *cis*- and *trans*-descriptions are potentially confusing because these terms are also used to describe the dihydrodiol function. A *cis*-dihydrodiol epoxide terminology might lead to confusion over whether the *cis* applies to the stereochemistry of the dihydrodiol or not. Although the *syn*- and *anti*-descriptions of the relative geometry of the hydroxyl group attached to the benzylic carbon and the epoxide ring are not ideal, they have been widely used and seem to offer fewer problems than the other informal nomenclatures; therefore, we have elected to use these terms throughout this chapter. The *syn*- and *anti*-descriptions distinguish between the diastereomer–enantiomer pairs of vicinal dihydrodiol epoxides with individual enantiomers being identified by the prefixes (+) or (−) where this distinction is appropriate. Thus, the four benzo[*a*]pyrene dihydrodiol epoxides of Structure **VIII** will be distinguished as listed under 8, i.e., as the (+)-*syn*-, (−)-*syn*-, (+)-*anti*-, or (−)-*anti*-benzo[*a*]pyrene 7,8-dihydrodiol 9,10-epoxides.

Introduction

The foundations for the scientific study of chemical carcinogenesis in general and hydrocarbon carcinogenesis in particular were laid by Percival Pott in 1775 (*5*) when he attributed the occurrence of scrotal cancer in chimney sweeps to their occupational exposure to soot. Subsequently, as new industries became established, other industrial carcinogens (coal tar, paraffin, and certain mineral oils) were recognized, again at the expense of much human tragedy. This painful and slow process of developing our knowledge of chemical carcinogens was finally curtailed (though unfortunately not concluded) in 1915 when Yamagiwa and Ichikawa (*6*) succeeded in inducing a carcinogenic response in the ears of rabbits through the persistent application of coal tar. Shortly thereafter, mouse skin was also found to be susceptible to the carcinogenic action of such tars (*7*), and this latter testing system is still in frequent use today. These findings created a first line of defense against environmental hazards and also provided an experimental tool with which the definition of chemical carcinogens could be refined.

In ensuing investigations into the identity of the carcinogenic constituent of coal tar, Bloch and Dreifuss (*8*) found that carcinogenic activity was concentrated in high-boiling fractions that were free from nitrogen, arsenic, and sulfur and that exhibited properties consistent with those of a complex polycyclic hydrocarbon. Kennaway (*9, 10*) subsequently showed that carcinogenic tars could be produced in the laboratory by various procedures and confirmed the conclusion that a hydrocarbon was responsible for the carcinogenic properties of coal tar. This confirmation was achieved by demonstrating carcinogenic activity in distillates from pyrolyses of hydrocarbons, such as isoprene and acetylene, in a hydrogen atmosphere.

In other attempts to synthesize carcinogenic materials in the laboratory, Kennaway investigated products from the reaction of tetralin with aluminum chloride at 30–40 °C. This reaction yielded more complex hydrocarbons (*11*). A number of carcinogenic distillates were obtained from such reactions, and a key property of these distillates was their fluorescence, which was obvious even in ordinary daylight. Mayneord (*12*) examined this fluorescence spectroscopically and by 1927 had shown that many carcinogenic mixtures and tars exhibited the same characteristic fluorescence spectrum. This discovery led to a search for an aromatic hydrocarbon that exhibited these spectral characteristics. Hieger observed that the spectrum of benz[*a*]anthracene was very similar to that of the carcinogenic fractions even though the compound fluoresced at a longer wavelength (*13*). Because of this similarity, Kennaway and Hieger (*14*) tested dibenz[*a,h*]anthracene for carcinogenic activity in mice shortly after Clar (*15*) had reported its synthesis. This hydrocarbon was found to be carcinogenic and the first chemical carcinogen of defined chemical constitution was recognized.

The fluorescence spectrum of dibenz[*a,h*]anthracene did not correspond exactly to that of the carcinogenic tars, and a large-scale isolation of the fluorescent carcinogenic constituent was undertaken starting with two tons of gas-works pitch. In 1930, a local gas, light, and coke company distilled this pitch, extracted the distillate with ethanol, and sent the extract to Kennaway's laboratory for further fractionation. By fractional distillation, differential extraction, and fractional crystallization and by following the fluorescence spectrum and carcinogenic activity of various fractions, Cook, Hewett, and Hieger obtained a small amount of a yellow material that exhibited the appropriate spectrum and was carcinogenic. Crystallization of the picrate from this material yielded three substances. One of these substances was perylene and the other two compounds were shown by structure-determining syntheses to be the hitherto unknown benzo[*a*]pyrene and benzo[*e*]pyrene isomers (**IA** and **IB**). Benzo[*a*]pyrene was carcinogenic and exhibited the fluorescence property of the carcinogenic tars, so that by 1933, the identity of the major carcinogenic constituent of coal tar had finally been established (*16*).

At this stage, the first phase of research into chemical carcinogenesis was complete. An animal test system was available for experimental investigations and for screening new compounds. Carcinogenic activity could be ascribed to defined chemical compounds. However, many important questions remained unanswered. Today, about 50 years later, many of these questions persist despite the considerable progress that has been made.

Can we assume, for example, that a compound that elicits a carcinogenic response in experimental animals is carcinogenic in humans, and more importantly, can we assume that a compound that does not elicit a carcinogenic response in experimental animals is not carcinogenic in humans? If we are to make the second assumption, how many different animal models are necessary to justify it? Is there a threshold phenomenon in the dose–response relationships for chemical carcinogens that would indicate safe levels of exposure for humans? Given the ever-increasing variety of chemical structures that can be associated with carcinogenic activity, can we assume that investigation of these questions with one type of chemical carcinogen is necessarily relevant to other types of carcinogens? Can we use tests other than long-term animal studies to help recognize carcinogenic hazards, and if so, how much confidence can we place in these tests?

These and other questions necessarily arise in trying to apply our knowledge of chemical carcinogens to the prevention of cancer in humans. They cannot be answered in any clear-cut, totally objective fashion, but at present require judgments that are based on an incomplete understanding of the carcinogenic process. This basic need for understanding of the mechanisms involved in the carcinogenic process has been the major motivation for much research in chemical carcinogenesis. However, carcinogenesis, wherein tumors appear in experimental animals many months after the initial exposure to a carcinogen, remains a poorly understood phenomenon.

It is well established that in mouse skin the process of carcinogenesis can be resolved into several stages. The first stage, *initiation*, is defined as a fairly rapid process whereby a carcinogen effects a permanent change within the cell population. The second stage, *promotion* (this has been further subdivided), requires a much longer time and can be effected by an agent, such as croton oil, that is not necessarily a carcinogen. Initiation is then the only stage that absolutely requires the presence of a carcinogen, and in appropriate experiments that use the two-stage mouse skin system, the measured carcinogenic potency of a carcinogen accurately reflects its capacity for tumor initiation. However, if a sufficiently large dose of carcinogen is administered to mouse skin, tumors will arise in the absence of any promotion. In this circumstance, carcinogenic potency need not necessarily reflect tumor-initiating capacity because the carcinogen may be effecting the necessary promotional stimulus, and it is not likely that all the polynuclear carcinogens would be equally effective promoters. However, because most of the approaches to mechanism involve structure–activity relationships to some extent, it is helpful to think of carcinogenic activity in terms of tumor-initiating capacity in the first instance, although the validity of the assumptions implicit in this approach remains a constant difficulty.

Two general types of mechanisms for chemical carcinogenesis have been conceived. First, the carcinogen may convert a normal cell into a tumor cell (the instructional theory), and second, the carcinogen may modify the environment of preexisting tumor cells so that they are permitted to grow (the selection theory) (*17*). The instructional theory encompasses several mechanisms through which the carcinogen may effect a heritable change within the cell. For example, the carcinogen may cause a mutational change in the DNA of the cell, may activate a latent oncogenic virus within the cell, or may alter the control systems of the cell in a way that leads to heritable change. Similarly, the selection theory accommodates mechanisms whereby the carcinogen interferes with the immune response and thus permits preexisting cancer cells to grow or whereby the carcinogen is simply toxic to normal cells and not to the preexisting cancer cells. A full discussion of the evidence relevant to these various views is outside the scope of this chapter. However, all these mechanisms require that the carcinogen enter some cell of the host and then interact with some cellular constituent; these two requisite conditions constitute the first step in the complex process of chemical carcinogenesis. The first event, tumor initiation, and the various factors that could conceivably modify the ability of a carcinogen to effect it are illustrated in Scheme I.

Examination of this scheme reveals that a simple relationship between chemical structure and tumor-initiating activity need not exist, even though the chemical structure of a carcinogen must ultimately determine its biological activity in a given system. Nonetheless it is the only approach available, and all studies of

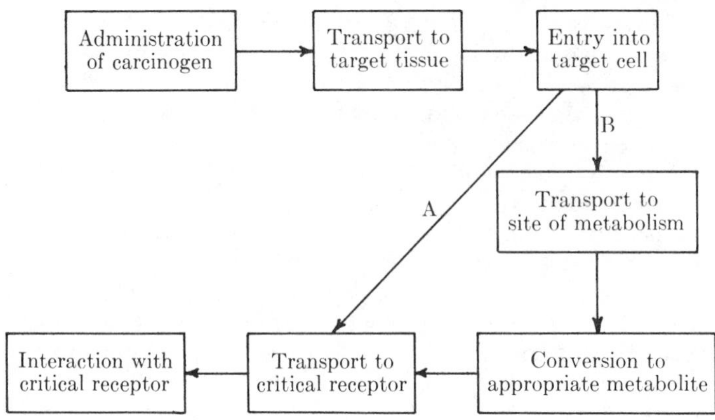

Scheme I. Possible factors involved in tumor initiation.

the mechanism of carcinogenesis by polynuclear carcinogens originate from attempts to correlate the various properties of these carcinogens with their carcinogenic activities.

Chemical Structure and Carcinogenic Activity

In the 1930s, a large-scale program aimed at defining those structural features of chemical compounds necessary for carcinogenic activity was begun. A large number of the compounds synthesized and subsequently screened for carcinogenic activity were polycyclic aromatic hydrocarbons and heterocyclics. All types of chemical carcinogens are covered in the literature (*18, 19*), and many authors have contributed excellent reviews of polynuclear carcinogens (*20–24*). Lacassagne et al. (*25*) dealt specifically with the angular benzacridines. The bibliography, "Survey of Compounds Which Have Been Tested for Carcinogenic Activity," (*26–30*) is invaluable.

The status of various polynuclear compounds with respect to carcinogenic activity is summarized in the appendix. Literature references are cited only in cases where they are not readily accessible through the sources listed in the previous paragraph. Unfortunately, many of these compounds are described in the literature by a variety of alternative names.

None of the various proposals for the expression of experimentally determined carcinogenic activities (*19, 20, 31–33*) has been generally accepted and applied. In Appendices B–G, therefore, carcinogenic activities are based upon the percentage of treated animals that developed tumors, i.e., up to 33%, slight activity; 33–66%, moderate activity; and above 66%, high activity. The compounds listed in these tables have not necessarily been tested under strictly comparable conditions, and the relative activities given must be regarded as crude approximations. For example, 7-methylbenz[*a*]anthracene and 7,12-dimethylbenz[*a*]anthracene are both listed under "high activity" (Appendices B and C), because either compound can elicit a carcinogenic response in over 90% of the animals exposed to them. Nevertheless, when the activities of the two compounds are compared at relatively low-dose levels, the dimethyl derivative is considerably more active than the monomethyl derivative (*28*).

Appendix A summarizes the carcinogenic activities of unsubstituted aromatic hydrocarbons comprised of six-membered rings, up to and including hexacyclic structures. Most of these compounds were tested in mice either by subcutaneous injections (giving rise to sarcomas) or by topical application to the skin (giving rise to benign papillomas and malignant epitheliomas). The most active carcinogens have been the subject of numerous studies, but in several cases the status of inactive compounds depends on surprisingly limited experimentation. The initiating activities of some compounds in this category were recently studied by Scribner (*34*), who found that considerable activity was associated with benz[*a*]anthracene, chrysene, benzo[*e*]pyrene, and dibenz[*a,c*]anthracene; phenanthrene, picene, and benzo[*b*]chrysene also showed some activity.

In addition to the compounds listed, a number of larger structures have been examined. No carcinogenic activity was demonstrated for pyranthrene (*35*), benzo[*a*]coronene, dibenzo[*a,l*]pentacene, phenanthro[9,10-*b*]triphenylene, benzo[*b*]naphtho[1,2-*k*]chrysene, dinaphtho[1,2-*b*:1,2-*k*]chrysene, or dinaphtho-[1,2-*b*:2,1-*n*]perylene. Coronene was inactive after subcutaneous injections in mice (*35*) but has produced skin papillomas after topical applications (*36*). Benzo[*a*]-naphtho[2,1,8-*hij*]naphthacene (*37*), benzo[*a*]naphtho[8,1,2-*cde*]naphthacene, and dibenzo[*cd,lm*]perylene exhibit slight carcinogenic activity, while tribenzo[*a,c,j*]-naphthacene is inactive at the injection site in mice but elicits leukemia and ovarian tumors (*23*). Dibenzo[*h,rst*]pentaphene, though not particularly potent, is perhaps the most active carcinogen among these large molecules (*38*).

Appendices B and C list the carcinogenic activities of the various substituted benz[*a*]anthracenes that have been examined; Appendices D and E cover derivatives of other aromatic hydrocarbons; and Appendix F lists the activities of some hydrocarbons that contain a five-membered ring. These appendices do not represent a comprehensive survey of the literature. Major omissions are the partially hydrogenated derivatives of the compounds in the appendices (*24, 44*), amino-substituted compounds (*see* Chapter 4), and several compounds containing five-membered rings, such as fluoranthene derivatives (*24, 47*), fluorene derivatives, acephenanthrene derivatives, and aceanthrene derivatives. The carcinogenic activities of hydrocarbon epoxides, dihydrodiols, and dihydrodiol epoxides are summarized elsewhere in this chapter.

The activities of some heterocyclic carcinogens are also listed in Appendix G. Although a number of derivatives of compounds in this appendix have been tested, the only compounds for which information on a substantial number of derivatives is available are the inactive benz[*a*]acridine and benz[*c*]acridine (Appendix H). The isochromeno derivatives in the appendix of heterocyclic carcinogens contain a lactone ring and should be regarded, perhaps, as carcinogenic alkylating agents rather than heterocyclic compounds.

Clearly, no obviously general structure–activity relationship, that would account for all the experimental data can be formulated. In view of the variety and complexity of the numerous compounds examined, it is conceivable that the limiting factor for the expression of carcinogenic activity (Scheme I) may be different for different groups of compounds; therefore, relationships that extend over only a limited series of compounds are still worthy of consideration and do represent valuable information even when the current lack of understanding of carcinogenesis precludes the direct interpretation and application of this information.

Derivatives of benz[*a*]anthracene constitute the most extensive series of polynuclear compounds for which structure–activity relationships have been examined (Appendices B and C). The carcinogenic activity of the parent hydrocarbon can be enhanced by substitution with either electron-donating or electron-withdrawing groups, and the magnitude of the effect depends on the position of substitution (Appendix B). In most cases, a methyl substituent effects a more pronounced increase in carcinogenic activity (relative to that of benz[*a*]anthracene) than higher alkyl substituents. Methyl substitution at positions 6, 7, 8, and 12 is particularly effective, but substitution at positions 1, 2, 3, and 4 on the angular benzene ring results in compounds that are inactive in the majority of the test systems. This latter finding is also reflected, to some extent, in the carcinogenic activities of the dimethylbenz[*a*]anthracenes (Appendix C). All such compounds with a methyl group on the angular ring, with the exception of 4,5-dimethylbenz[*a*]anthracene, are inactive. This guideline holds for the 1,2-; 1,12-; 4,7-; and 4,12-dimethyl compounds even though the 7-, and 12-monomethylbenz[*a*]anthracenes are both potent carcinogens. The simplest interpretation of these observations is that the unsubstituted angular ring is required for carcinogenic activity. Indeed, this relationship is consistent with our present understanding of the mechanism of action of hydrocarbons, but this simple and direct interpretation was not recognized until 1976, when Jerina and Daly (*76*) suggested that bay-region dihydrodiol epoxides (e.g., **VIA**) might be the active metabolites for most hydrocarbon carcinogens.

Examinations of structure–activity relationships have generated a number of more general observations. Carcinogenic activity may depend on the molecular size of polynuclear compounds (*22, 24*), or on their molecular thickness (*48, 54*). The relationship between steroid and polynuclear carcinogen structures has excited researchers for a number of years, largely because the steroids might be converted into polycyclic hydrocarbons in vivo, thereby accounting for the incidence of "spontaneous" tumors (*23, 66, 77*). Other studies tend to emphasize the alternative possibility that polynuclear carcinogens interfere with normal steroid hormone action. For example, Williams and Rabin (*78*) have shown that several carcinogens interfere with membrane–ribosome association. These authors suggest that the carcinogens produce this effect by occupying or destroying sites on the membrane that are normally available to steroid hormones. Similarly, Litwack et al. (*79*) have found that a corticosteroid-binding protein of rat liver, ligandin, also binds the polynuclear carcinogen 3-methylcholanthrene.

The most generally applicable structure–activity relationship for polynuclear carcinogens is that most of the carcinogenic hydrocarbons can be regarded as phenanthrene derivatives (*80*). This relationship again is consistent with current views of the structural features associated with carcinogenic activity. The notable exceptions not included in the appendices are 6,12-dimethylbenzo[*b*]thionaphtheno[3,2-*f*]thionaphthen and 6,12-dimethylbenzo[*b*]thionaphtheno[2,3-*f*]thionaphthen, which are both potent sarcomagens in mice (*81*), and the carcinogens, benzo[*j*]fluoranthene and benzo[*k*]fluoranthene (*82, 83*).

Although contributions to and modifications of our knowledge of the carcinogenic activities of polynuclear carcinogens are still being made today, much of the work over the last 25 years has been directed primarily at the mechanism of action of these compounds. This work can be somewhat arbitrarily classified into two main approaches. A great deal of work has been done on chemical carcinogens apart from any biological system. This approach largely involves the implicit assumption that the critical step in the carcinogenic process is the interaction of the unmodified carcinogen with some cellular receptor (e.g., path A in Scheme I). The other approach involves the properties of carcinogens within a biological system together with the attendant response of the biological system to the carcinogen. This strategy relates more closely, but not exclusively, to path B in Scheme I.

Considerable interaction between these two approaches has occurred over the years, and each one has undoubtedly stimulated further development of the other. Nevertheless, most of this work can be more conveniently examined in separate sections under the arbitrary headings of either chemistry or biochemistry of polynuclear carcinogens.

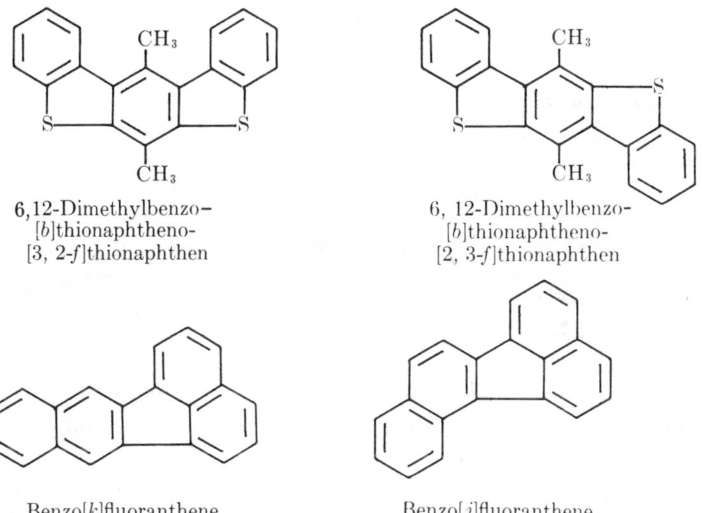

6,12-Dimethylbenzo-[*b*]thionaphtheno-[3, 2-*f*]thionaphthen

6, 12-Dimethylbenzo-[*b*]thionaphtheno-[2, 3-*f*]thionaphthen

Benzo[*k*]fluoranthene

Benzo[*j*]fluoranthene

Chemistry of Polynuclear Carcinogens

A comprehensive survey of the chemistry of polycyclic hydrocarbons can be found in the two volumes by Clar (*84*). However, a few points that are particularly relevant to the carcinogenic action of these compounds are outlined in this section.

Aromatic compounds cannot be accurately described by the conventional structural formulas given in Appendices A and G. These formulas represent only one of the possible Kékulé structures and erroneously suggest that aromatic compounds contain a framework of carbon atoms linked together by alternating single and double bonds. This interpretation would be totally inconsistent with the chemical properties of these compounds, and in fact, all the carbon–carbon bond lengths lie at various values between those of an isolated single bond and an isolated double bond. Furthermore, aromatic compounds exhibit a greater stability (i.e., a lower energy) than that which would be expected for the structure represented by the most stable canonical form. The difference between the energy of the actual compound and the energy of the most stable hypothetical Kékulé structure is defined as resonance energy. This difference may be computed from experimental values for heats of combustion, heats of hydrogenation, etc., or calculated by the application of quantum mechanics. Resonance energy has no absolute meaning, however, because it merely reflects an increase in the stability of an actual compound over that which would be expected for a hypothetical structure. This stability is not related to chemical reactivity, which is determined by the difference in free energy between the reactants and the transition states for specific chemical reactions. Thus, resonance energy increases along the series: benzene (36 kcal/mol), naphthalene (61 kcal/mol), and anthracene (84 kcal/mol). Chemical reactivity also increases along this series.

The inconsistencies between the properties of aromatic compounds and those expected from the structural representations of these compounds arise because the pi electrons of aromatic compounds are not localized in discrete bonds. Instead, the electrons are delocalized over the whole aromatic molecule, contrary to the tacit assumption made in drawing the conventional structural representations. The pi electron density distribution varies from compound to compound and is determined for any given aromatic hydrocarbon by the geometry of the carbon atom framework. This distribution primarily determines the chemical properties of aromatic hydrocarbons, and many methods of visualizing this distribution have been devised. The most useful of these methods is resonance theory, which describes the real structures of aromatic compounds as weighted averages of the possible conventional structures, with the greatest weights being given to the most stable conventional structures. More detailed descriptions can be obtained by the application of the valence-bond and molecular-orbital methods of quantum mechanics (*85*), and the localization theory of chemical reactions is of particular value for predicting chemical reactivity (*86*).

The chemical stability of benzene arises from the even distribution of the six pi electrons over the ring. Hexagonal symmetry is the result, and in the ground state, the length of each bond is 1.39 Å. For a Kékulé structure, alternating single bonds (1.54 Å) and double bonds (1.33 Å) would be expected. Benzene is not particularly reactive and appears to undergo substitution reactions (which preserve its aromatic character) more readily than addition reactions. The polycyclic aromatic hydrocarbons that most closely resemble benzene with respect to their chemical stability are triphenylene, dibenzo[*fg,op*]naphthacene, and phenanthro[9,10-*b*]-triphenylene. All of these compounds can be formulated as condensed polyphenyls, and their chemical properties clearly indicate that this formulation reasonably approximates their actual structures. These compounds are inactive in carcinogenesis experiments.

In general, the most reactive class of polycyclic aromatic hydrocarbons is the acenes: naphthalene, anthracene, naphthacene, and pentacene (Appendix A). Reactivity increases with increasing molecular weight, and heptacene is so unstable that it has been impossible to prepare this compound in a pure state. The most notable feature of acene reaction chemistry is the relative ease with which additions across *para*-positions can occur. Maleic anhydride adds across the 1,4-positions of naphthalene to only a very small extent, but an extensive 9,10-addition occurs with anthracene, and the reaction across the 5,12-positions of naphthacene and the 6,13-positions of pentacene occurs very readily. These chemical reactions of the acenes indicate that a pair of pi electrons can be localized across *para*-positions relatively easily. Again, no compound of this group has been shown to be carcinogenic.

In the phene series: phenanthrene, benz[*a*]anthracene, pentaphene, and benzo[*b*]pentaphene (Appendix A), general reactivity is usually lower than in the isomeric acene. In contrast to the acenes, addition reactions across a double bond occur fairly easily, e.g., across the 9,10-bond of phenanthrene (**III**A). This double bond in the central ring of phenanthrene exhibits properties that are similar to those of an isolated ethylenic double bond, and to a large extent, a pair of pi electrons is localized in this double bond. However, in addition to a reactive double bond, the higher phenes also contain reactive *para*-positions (e.g., the 7- and 12-positions of benz[*a*]anthracene) that will add reagents such as maleic anhydride. With the exception of benz[*a*]anthracene, none of the phenes mentioned has been reported to be carcinogenic, but many potent carcinogens can be found among substituted benz[*a*]anthracenes (Appendices B and C), and as noted earlier, many carcinogenic hydrocarbons can be considered to be phenanthrene derivatives.

Many of the more complex hydrocarbon carcinogens also contain a reactive double bond, such as the 4,5-bond in benzo[*a*]pyrene. None of the highly carcinogenic pyrene derivatives undergo facile *para*-addition reactions, although substitutions occur very readily in some cases (e.g., at the 6-position of benzo[*a*]pyrene).

From these observations, attention was directed toward a possible relationship between the chemical reactivity of a specific bond in a polycyclic hydrocarbon (i.e., a bond with high double-bond character, such as the 9,10-bond in phenanthrene) and carcinogenic activity. The early work on the application of theoretical chemistry to predicting chemical reactivity for polynuclear carcinogens has been reviewed by Coulson (*87*). Pullman (*88a, 88b, 89*) introduced the term *K* region to describe the bond in a polynuclear compound that has the greatest double-bond character; for example, the 9,10-bond in phenanthrene (**III**A) and the 5,6-bond in benz[*a*]anthracene (**V**). She later used the term *L* region to describe the region of a hydrocarbon that exhibits properties similar to the 9- and 10-positions of anthracene (*90*); for example, carbons 7 and 12 in benz[*a*]anthracene. Although it is chronologically incorrect, the use of this terminology simplifies the following discussion.

Schmidt (*91–93*) originated the attempts to relate the carcinogenic activities of polycyclic hydrocarbons to their pi electron density distributions. His methods

Table I

Properties of Some Benzacridines

Compound	*K Region*			
	Total Charge[a]		*Excess Charge*[b]	pK_a[c]
	A	*B*		
Benz[*a*]acridine	1.260	1.973	−0.039	3.95
10-Methylbenz[*a*]acridine			−0.039	4.22
Benz[*c*]acridine	1.270	1.984	−0.003	3.24
12-Methylbenz[*a*]acridine	1.273	1.989	−0.036	4.60
10-Methylbenz[*c*]acridine		1.998		3.68
8-Methylbenz[*c*]acridine		2.00		3.67
10,11-Dimethylbenz[*c*]acridine		2.008		3.74
8,9,12-Trimethylbenz[*a*]acridine		2.018		4.59
9,12-Dimethylbenz[*a*]acridine	1.284	2.002	−0.023	5.13
8,12-Dimethylbenz[*a*]acridine	1.286		−0.033	
7,11-Dimethylbenz[*c*]acridine	1.302	2.022	0.035	
8,10,12-Trimethylbenz[*a*]acridine	1.298		0.038	
7,10-Dimethylbenz[*c*]acridine	1.304	2.025	0.049	3.99
7,9-Dimethylbenz[*c*]acridine	1.304	2.024	0.039	4.26
7,9,11-Trimethylbenz[*c*]acridine	1.312		0.039	
7,8,9,11-Tetramethylbenz[*c*]acridine				3.98

[a]Values given under A are from Pullman (*89*) where total charge is defined as the sum of twice the mobile bond order plus the two free valence numbers. Values given under B are from Lacassagne et al. (*25*) and arise from the modified definition of total charge from Buu-Hoi et al. (*95*). Both sets of figures were obtained from the valence-bond method.

[b]Values are taken from Greenwood (*96*) and represent the sum of the charges (which arise on the introduction of a nitrogen atom or a methyl group into benz[*a*]anthracene) of the two atoms at the *K* region. These values were obtained from the molecular-orbital method.

[c]Values taken from Pagès-Flon et al. (*97*).

were crude and qualitative, but regions of high pi electron density (particularly at *L* regions) were indicated, and he related the presence of such regions to biological activity. Svartholm (*94*) developed this approach further by applying the ideas of resonance, but the major contributions came later (detailed documentation of individual contributions may be found in Ref. 87). This later work applied the more sophisticated quantum mechanical approaches of the valence-bond method (and later the molecular-orbital method) to studies of polynuclear compounds and calculated many molecular parameters. As a result, correlations between carcinogenic activity and electronic structure could be evaluated more precisely.

Pullman (*88a, 88b, 89*) showed that an index describing the electrical properties of the *K* region (i.e., the "total charge on the *K* region" which was defined as the sum of twice the mobile bond order plus the two free valence numbers) seemed to vary with carcinogenic potency for several methylbenz[*a*]anthracenes, methylbenzo[*c*]-phenanthrenes, methylbenz[*a*]acridines, and methylbenz[*c*]acridines. For example, Table I lists some benzacridines in roughly increasing order of carcinogenic potency (*see* Appendix H) along with experimentally determined pK_a values and some calculated indices for the pi electron distribution at the *K* region.

The relationship between the *K* region indices and carcinogenic activity is really quite convincing.

For many compounds, carcinogenic activity seemed to relate to a fairly high pi electron density at the *K* region, and this finding indicated that the interaction between the hydrocarbon and the cell that was responsible for initiating the carcinogenic process took the form of an addition reaction at the *K* region. There were, however, numerous exceptions to the original relationship, and most of these were unsubstituted polycyclic compounds (*see* Appendix A and Table II). The rate of osmium tetroxide addition to the *K* region of these unsubstituted hydrocarbons followed the theoretical predictions reasonably well (*21*) and the exceptions did not arise from any inadequacies in the theoretical predictions of chemical reactivity. Similarly, experimentally determined reaction rates of unsubstituted hydrocarbons with trichloromethyl radicals were correlated with the highest free valence numbers for these compounds (*106*). Kooyman and Heringa (*107*) then suggested that carcinogenic potency might depend on both the highest free valence number and the highest bond order for a given molecule.

Pullman (*90*) arrived at a similar conclusion, but she suggested that the presence in a polynuclear compound of an *L* region (*see* **V**), which always contains the two carbon atoms of highest free valence, could inactivate that compound, even though the properties of its *K* region were consistent with carcinogenic activity. This proposition (the *K*- and *L*-region theory), which was based on calculations related to the ground states of these polynuclear compounds, was then restated more explicitly in terms of the localization theory of chemical reactions (*86, 108*). Thus for a polynuclear compound to exhibit carcinogenic properties, it had to have a reactive *K* region (the sum of the bond-localization energy and the minimum carbon-localization energy had to be less than a certain value) and an unreactive *L* region (the sum of the *para*-localization energy and the minimum carbon-localization energy at the *para*-positions had to be greater than another fixed value). This theory accommodated the known carcinogenic activities of unsubstituted aromatic hydrocarbons tolerably well, and it was concluded that the critical reaction (or the rate-determining step in the reaction) between the carcinogen and the cell involved an addition at the *K* region. However, in cases where a reactive *L* region was present, an addition at this latter region would occur rendering the compound ineffective as a carcinogen (*86*). A number of theoreticians, some using different indices to describe chemical reactivity, have reexamined this structure–activity relationship, but all of them seem to confirm the general concept that a reactive *K* region and an unreactive *L* region are associated with carcinogenic activity (*109–16*). Several unsubstituted aromatic hydrocarbons, which for many years were regarded as inactive, are now known to be carcinogenic, e.g., naphtho[8,1,2-*cde*]naphthacene and dibenz[*a,c*]anthracene. These findings now make the *K*- and *L*-region theory seem somewhat less convincing (Table II).

The Pullman-complex indices for unsubstituted hydrocarbons are given in Table VIII, where the compounds are listed in increasing order of carcinogenic activity. Also given are the bond orders and the coefficients of the highest filled or lowest empty molecular orbitals. The molecular orbital coefficients describe the electron-donor and electron-acceptor properties of these molecules (*101*). The compounds with the lowest coefficients should be the most effective electron donors or electron acceptors. These properties are of interest because several workers have suggested that the critical molecular event in carcinogenesis might be the formation of a charge-transfer complex between the carcinogen and a cellular receptor (*117–20*). Pullman and Pullman (*101*) pointed out that for aromatic hydrocarbons there is no correlation between electron-donor or -acceptor properties and carcinogenicity when a large series of compounds is studied. This conclusion was also reached from experimental studies on charge-transfer complex formation (*121, 122*). Table II also lists the experimentally determined affinities

Table II

Properties of Some Unsubstituted Aromatic Hydrocarbons

	K Region			*L Region*
Compound[a]	*Bond*[b]	*Bond Order*[c]	*C.L.E.*$_{min}$ + *B.L.E.*[b]	*C.L.E.*$_{min}$ + *P.L.E.*[b]
Benzene	1,2	1.667	4.07	6.54
Naphthalene	1,2	1.725	3.56	5.98
Anthracene	1,2	1.738	3.53	5.38
Phenanthrene	9,10	1.775	3.36	—
Pyrene	4,5	1.777	3.33	—
Naphthacene	1,2	1.741	3.33	5.25
Triphenylene	1,2	1.690	3.81	—
Pentacene	1,2	1.742	3.27	5.03
Picene	5,6	1.758	3.37	—
Pentaphene	6,7	1.790	3.23	5.56
Dibenzo[*c,g*]phenanthrene	5,6		3.38	—
Benzo[*b*]chrysene	5,6		3.27	5.47
Dibenzo[*b,g*]phenanthrene	7,8		3.30	5.48
Dibenzo[*def,mno*]chrysene	4,5		3.20	—
Dibenzo[*b,k*]chrysene	6,7		3.24	5.44
Dibenzo[*a,j*]naphthacene	5,6		3.24	5.42
Chrysene	5,6	1.754	3.38	—
Benz[*a*]anthracene	5,6	1.783	3.29	5.53
Dibenz[*a,c*]anthracene	10,11	1.727	3.51	5.67
Dibenz[*a,j*]anthracene	5,6	1.780	3.31	5.66
Benzo[*c*]phenanthrene	5,6	1.762	3.41	—
Dibenz[*a,h*]anthracene	5,6	1.778	3.30	5.69
Benzo[*c*]chrysene	7,8	1.764	3.41	—
Naphtho[8,1,2-*cde*]naphthacene	4,5		3.14	5.30
Benzo[*a*]pyrene	4,5	1.787	3.23	—
Dibenzo[*b,def*]chrysene	5,6		3.17	—
Benzo[*rst*]pentaphene	6,7		3.16	—

[a] *See* Appendix A for structures and carcinogenic activities.

[b] Pullman and Pullman (*86*). C.L.E., B.L.E., and P.L.E. are carbon-localization energy, bond-localization energy, and *para*-localization energy, respectively. The Pullmans' requirements for carcinogenic activity were: C.L.E.$_{min}$ + B.L.E. should be equal to or smaller than 3.31 β and, if an *L*-region is present, C.L.E.$_{min}$ + P.L.E. should be equal to or greater than 5.66 β.

[c] By the molecular-orbital method (*98–100*).

of some polycyclic hydrocarbons (in the vapor phase) for thermal electrons (*105*) and lists Badger's relative rates of reaction between osmium tetroxide and the *K* regions of polycyclic compounds (*21*). The ionization potentials of these compounds should reflect the ease of their conversion to radical cations, but again no correlation with carcinogenic activity is seen (*102*).

The carcinogenic activities of the 12 isomeric monomethylbenz[*a*]anthracenes have been studied extensively (Appendix B), and these compounds can be arranged in order of carcinogenic potency with some confidence (Table III). The 2- and 3-methyl derivatives are totally inactive; the 6-, 8-, 12-, and 7-methyl

Coefficient of Highest Filled or Lowest Empty M.O.[d]	*Ionization Potentials*[e]	*Absorption Coefficient for Thermal Electrons*[f]	*Relative Rate of Reaction with* OsO_4[g]
1		0.01	
0.618	8.12	0.01	
0.414	7.23	12	
0.605	8.02	0.05	0.1
0.445	7.58	6.0	0.66
0.295	6.64	1.7	
0.684	8.13	0.015	
0.220	6.23		
0.501	7.62		
0.437	7.35		
0.535	—		
0.405	7.29		
0.419	7.11		
0.291	6.84		
0.348	—		
0.358	6.82		
0.520	7.72		slow
0.452	7.35	29	1.0
0.499	7.43		
0.492	7.42		
0.566	7.76	1.3	
0.473	7.42		1.3
0.550	7.71	1.2	slow
0.303	6.70		
0.371	7.15		2.0
0.342	6.75		
0.342	7.06		

[d] Values taken from Pullman and Pullman (*101*). The lower this coefficient, the greater are both the electron-donor and electron-acceptor properties of the molecule.
[e] Taken from Refs. 102–4.
[f] Lovelock et al. (*105*).
[g] Badger (*21*).

Table III

Properties of Monomethylbenz[*a*]anthracenes

	K Region			
Position of Methyl Group[a]	*Total Charge*[b]	*Excess Charge*[c]	*Rate of OsO_4 Attack*[d]	*Excitation Energy*[e]
2		0.036		0.9116
3		0.011		0.9154
1		0.001		0.9164
4		0.024		0.9134
11	1.292	−0.001		0.9059
10	1.294	0.013		0.9099
9	1.294	0.003	0.64	0.9120
5	1.298	−0.164	0.50	0.9067
6	1.298	−0.164		0.9061
8	1.296	0.009		0.9042
12	1.296	0.003	0.96	0.8984
7	1.306	0.039	0.91	0.8934

[a]*See* Appendix B for carcinogenic activities.
[b]Defined in footnote *a* to Table I and in text. Values from Pullman (*89*).
[c]Defined in footnote *b* to Table I. Values from Greenwood (*96*).
[d]Experimental values from Badger (*127*).
[e]Calculated energy change involved in promoting an electron from the highest occupied to the lowest unoccupied molecular orbital; Pullman et al. (*123*).

derivatives are all highly active carcinogens; the other isomers have all exhibited some slight activity in one system or another. The properties of the *K* regions of these molecules do not really distinguish the potent carcinogens from the weakly active or the inactive compounds as seen in Table III. However, reasonable relationships with carcinogenic activity exist (1) for the calculated excitation energies for these compounds (*123*); (2) for the conjugating ability of the carbon to which the methyl group is bound, as represented by the free valences for benz[*a*]anthracene (*21*); (3) for the bathochromic shift of the 287-nm band of the benz[*a*]anthracene spectrum as a result of methyl substitution (*124*); (4) for the nucleophilicities of these compounds for silver ion (*125*); and (5) for stabilities of arylmethyl cations derived from these compounds, as represented by decreasing values for the coefficient of the nonbonding molecular orbital at the positive carbon atom (*126*) (*see* Table III). The best correlation with biological activities appears to lie with the experimentally determined nucleophilicities. All the other properties are undoubtedly interrelated, and it is interesting from this viewpoint that 11-methylbenz[*a*]anthracene is an exception in all these cases.

Many polynuclear compounds exhibit the property of photodynamic action, which is the phenomenon whereby a combination of light energy and a chemical sensitizer produces effects that are not induced by either component alone. Studies with limited numbers of polynuclear compounds suggested a possible relationship between the photodynamic action of these compounds and their carcinogenic

Free Valence at Methylation Site[f]	NBMO Coefficient at Methyl Carbon[g]	Equilibrium Constant for Reaction with Ag^{+} [h]	Bathochromic Shift in nm[i]
0.357	0.693	1.23	
0.352	0.729	1.34	
0.388	0.703		0.5
0.399	0.676		
0.404	0.639	1.34	3.0
0.356	0.693	1.25	1.0
0.355	0.703	1.32	2.0
0.404	0.639	1.25	
0.403	0.639	1.35	1.5
0.406	0.631	1.41	2.0
0.484	0.583	1.64	3.5
0.467	0.561	1.66	4.5

[f]Values from Berthier et al. (*99*).
[g]Values from Dipple et al. (*126*).
[h]Equilibrium constant for the reaction: $Ar + Ag^{+} \rightleftharpoons ArAg^{+}$ (*125*).
[i]The bathochromic shift of the 287-nm band in the spectrum of benz[*a*]anthracene as a result of methyl substitution (*124*).

activities (*128, 129*). However, when a more extensive range of compounds was studied, no direct link between carcinogenic and photodynamic properties was established (*130*).

A similar conclusion has been reached from studies of the physical interactions between polycyclic hydrocarbons and cellular constituents. Aromatic hydrocarbons are more soluble in purine solutions (*131, 132*) or in DNA solutions (*133, 134*) than in water alone, and many researchers have studied the interactions involved in these phenomena. Most of the data presented appear to support the view that the interaction with DNA involves the insertion of the hydrocarbon molecule between base pairs of the DNA as was proposed for acridine dye–DNA complexes (*135*), although this may not be the only type of interaction involved (*136*). No conclusive proof of this intercalation model for hydrocarbons has been presented yet, but it does seem clear that physical interaction with DNA is related to the size of the hydrocarbons and bears no obvious relationship to their carcinogenic activities (*137*).

Occasional studies of the relationship between carcinogenic potency and various properties of polycyclic hydrocarbon carcinogens appear in the more recent literature (*138, 139*); but this approach, which involves the implicit assumption that the hydrocarbon itself directly initiates the carcinogenic process, has been largely superceded. The more popular approach is investigating the properties of various metabolites in relation to the carcinogenic properties of the

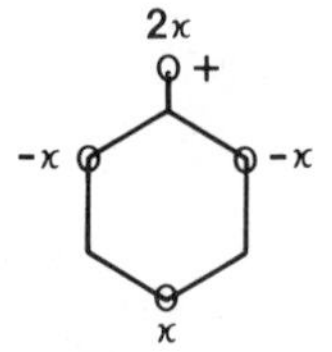

A. Benzyl Cation

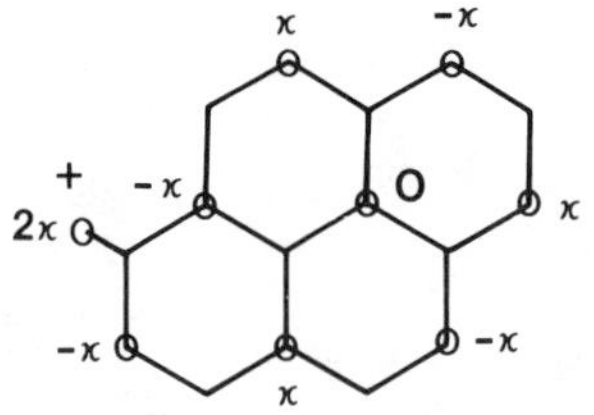

B. Pyrenyl-1-methyl Cation

IX

parent compounds. Following the Millers' demonstration of the role played by metabolic activation in the mechanism of action of the aromatic amine carcinogens (*140*), Dipple et al. (*126*) have made the first attempts to relate carcinogenic activity to the chemical reactivity of putative carcinogenic metabolites. These authors used a delocalization coefficient (1-a_{0r}) based on the readily calculable nonbonding molecular orbital (NBMO) coefficient, a_{0r}, at the site of carbonium ion formation to estimate the relative stabilities of putative reactive metabolites. Among other ideas arising from this investigation, it was suggested that the 9,10-bond in benzo[*a*]pyrene and analogous bonds in the dibenzpyrenes might be the sites of formation of the reactive carcinogenic metabolites for these hydrocarbons (*126*). Although this proposition is now believed to be the case, dihydrodiol epoxides were not known at that time; therefore, most studies of this type followed Sims' discovery of the dihydrodiol epoxide mechanism for activation of benzo[*a*]pyrene (*141*) and Jerina and Daly's concept that the active metabolites for most hydrocarbons might be bay-region dihydrodiol epoxides (**VI**A) (*76*).

Because several investigators have used indices related to the NBMO coefficients in their studies (*142*), the calculation of these coefficients (*143*) is briefly reviewed herein. For an odd alternant hydrocarbon cation, e.g., the benzyl cation (**IX**A) or the pyrenyl-1-methyl cation (**IX**B), the charge densities over the aromatic system are determined by coefficients of the NBMO. These coefficients have nonzero values only at every other carbon atom in these structures, i.e., those circled in **IX**A and **IX**B. Using the facts: (1) the sum of the coefficients for atoms attached to a noncircled atom is zero; and (2) the sum of the squares of all the coefficients is unity, the numerical values of these coefficients are readily obtained. This assignment can often be done by inspection, but in some cases a little algebra may be required. For the benzyl cation, if we assign a value of x for the coefficient at the 4-position, the coefficients for the *ortho*-positions must both be $-x$ and the coefficient for the benzylic carbon must then be $2x$, all from (1) above. Application of (2) then generates the relationship $7x^2 = 1$; so that $x = 1/\sqrt{7}$. The NBMO coefficient of the benzylic carbon is then $2/\sqrt{7}$. The squares of these coefficients indicate the charge density in the NBMO at that position in the molecule. Assigning coefficients of the NBMO in the pyrenylmethyl cation requires a little more effort because the coefficient for the central circled carbon in the pyrene system turns out to be zero. However, the process is still simple and the coefficient for the benzylic carbon is $2/\sqrt{11}$ in this case.

Jerina et al. (*144–46*) have calculated the ease of carbonium ion formation from various dihydrodiol epoxides using these kinds of calculations, in which an estimate of the increase in delocalization energy on going from an epoxide to a cation, ΔE_{deloc}, can be approximated to $2(1 - a_{0r})\beta$ where β is a resonance integral (*143*). Jerina has used the index $\Delta E_{deloc}/\beta$ to monitor the relative ease of carbonium ion formation, which is simply $2(1 - a_{0r})$ where a_{0r} is the NBMO coefficient for the atom carrying the positive charge (Scheme II). Because the saturated 7-, 8-, and 9-positions play no role in determining this, a_{0r} is actually calculated for the pyrenylmethyl cation (**IXB**), i.e., $a_{0r} = 2/\sqrt{11}$ and $\Delta E_{deloc}/\beta$ or $2(1 - a_{0r})$ is then 0.794. Overall, these calculations have indicated that a bay-region dihydrodiol epoxide should ionize to a cation more readily than a non-bay-region dihydrodiol epoxide from the same parent hydrocarbon, but comparisons of this index calculated for bay-region dihydrodiol epoxides from several different hydrocarbons do not show a good correlation with the carcinogenic activities of the parent hydrocarbons (*144–46*). While the discovery of dihydrodiol epoxides has directed interest away from the older *K*- and *L*-region concepts, some of the exceptions to the new correlations would be eliminated if the requirement for a nonreactive *L* region was conserved.

In a similar approach, Fu et al. (*147*) have calculated Dewar reactivity numbers, N_t, for the benzylic carbon of the epoxide in dihydrodiol epoxides. Because N_t is $2a_{0r}\beta$ when a_{0r} is the NBMO coefficient for the same atom as in Jerina's calculations (Scheme II), these calculations result in similar conclusions. Smith et al. (*148*) have examined several indices describing polycyclic hydrocarbons in relation to their carcinogenicity and have concluded that an index Q_b describing the net pi electron charge at the benzylic carbon of an ionized bay-region dihydrodiol epoxide represents the best correlation with Jerina's $\Delta E_{deloc}/\beta$ index. Because the perturbation approach would describe Q_b as a_{0r}^2, this observation again is not surprising. Osborne (*149*) has found that the sum of all the NBMO coefficients, without regard to sign, for bay-region dihydrodiol epoxides (e.g., $9/\sqrt{11}$ for the benzo[*a*]pyrene bay-region dihydrodiol epoxide (Structure **IXB** and Scheme II)) gives a better correlation with carcinogenicity of the parent hydrocarbons than the other indices discussed. Other types of calculations based on resonance theory (*150*) or involving more sophisticated methods that take account of sigma bonding as well as pi bonding (*151*) have led to similar conclusions.

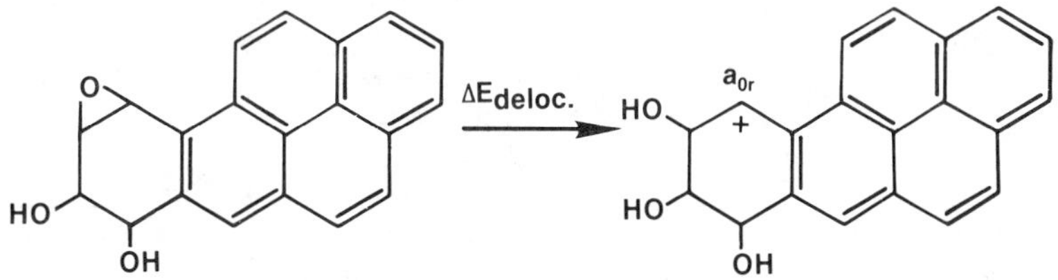

Scheme II. Estimate of energy change involved in ionization of a dihydrodiol epoxide. $\Delta E_{deloc} = 2(1\text{-}a_{0r})\beta$ (144–46).

Despite these extensive studies of the chemical and physical properties of polynuclear carcinogens, no single property of these compounds can be related quantitatively to their biological activities. This is not surprising in view of the many factors that could potentially modify biological activity (Scheme I). Because of this and the possibility that the process of carcinogenesis may be initiated through various mechanisms, not even the most limited correlation of carcinogenic activity with some chemical or physical property can be totally ignored. Nevertheless, the various relationships reported need to be evaluated. From this point of view, the relationships between the reactivities of dihydrodiol epoxides and carcinogenic activity are of the greatest interest at present. This priority does not stem from the predictive power of the correlations as much as from the experimental studies on these compounds. However, the facts that many of the potent carcinogens have low ionization potentials, are good electron donors, form charge-transfer complexes readily, and exhibit quite high photodynamic activities should not be completely forgotten, even though many noncarcinogens also exhibit these properties.

Biochemistry of Polynuclear Carcinogens

Enzymes Involved in Metabolism. The enzyme system primarily responsible for polycyclic hydrocarbon metabolism is the mixed-function oxidase system (*152*), which is membrane bound and requires NADH or NADPH and molecular oxygen to convert nonpolar hydrocarbons into more polar epoxy or hydroxy derivatives. The terminal oxidase is a family of hemoproteins called cytochromes P-450; the term is derived from the fact that the carbon monoxide complex of the reduced cytochrome exhibits an absorbance maximum at around 450 nm. The mixed-function oxidase activity of microsomal preparations has been solubilized and reconstituted, showing that cytochrome P-450, NADPH–cytochrome P-450 reductase, and phosphatidylcholine are required for activity, that substrate specificity is controlled by the cytochrome P-450, and that multiple cytochromes P-450 exist. Treatment of animals with various chemicals leads to the induction of different cytochromes P-450 and therefore leads to different metabolic fates for subsequently administered carcinogens. The different pathways should be particularly noted because many studies of the metabolism of hydrocarbons have utilized variously induced rat liver microsomal preparations, and one cannot assume that these findings are directly transferable to carcinogenesis studies in which the liver is not the target organ and inducers of microsomal enzymes are not routinely administered. In 1980, Lu and West (*153*) concluded that some 20 individual cytochromes P-450 had been described; five to seven of these have been isolated from rat liver microsomes. Nomenclature is inconsistent in the original literature. For example, the major cytochrome P-450 induced in rat liver by treatment with 3-methylcholanthrene has been named cytochrome P-450*c* (*154*), cytochrome P-448 (*155*), or cytochrome P_1-450 (*156*). The volume of work in this area is also very large, but many excellent reviews are available on the multiplicity of the cytochromes P-450 (*153, 157*), on the mechanisms of their catalytic action (*158, 159*), on the mechanism of oxygen activation in these systems (*160*), and on their genetic control (*161*). While these enzyme systems are primarily associated with microsomal preparations, hydrocarbon-metabolizing activity has been found also in preparations of nuclei (*162*). This observation has been pursued in several laboratories, because a major concern has been that the nuclear activity might arise from contamination with endoplasmic reticulum (reviewed in Refs. 163 and 164), but at present, the weight of evidence suggests that nuclei do contain such enzyme activities. Although still in a very early stage, attempts are being made (*165, 166*) to clone DNA sequences containing information for specific cytochromes P-450, and this new approach can be expected to lead to major advances in our concepts of the multiplicity and genetics of this fascinating enzyme system.

Hydrocarbon metabolites generated by the mixed-function oxidases are subject to further enzymic modification. Hydrocarbon epoxides, for example, may be substrates for the enzyme epoxide hydrolase, which hydrates these epoxides to yield vicinal *trans*-dihydrodiols. This enzyme is also referred to as epoxide hydrase or epoxide hydratase. Until relatively recently, only one form of this enzyme appeared to be in a given tissue and this enzyme, like the mixed-function oxidase, is a membrane-bound inducible microsomal enzyme (reviewed in Refs. 157, 167, and 168). Guengerich et al. (*169, 170*) have recently provided evidence for multiple forms of microsomal epoxide hydrolase within individual tissues, and Guenthner et al. (*171*) have demonstrated that a soluble epoxide hydrolase in rodent liver differs immunologically, as well as with respect to substrate specificity, from the microsomal enzyme. Epoxide hydrolase plays a key role in the metabolic formation of hydrocarbon dihydrodiol epoxides; it is required to convert an initially formed epoxide to a *trans*-dihydrodiol, and of equal importance may be the fact that bay-region dihydrodiol epoxides seem to be very poor substrates for this enzyme. Again, attempts are being made to clone the information for this enzyme (*172*).

Hydroxylated metabolites of hydrocarbons may be conjugated with glucuronic acid to give glucuronides. This reaction is catalyzed by microsomal UDP–glucuronyltransferases, which are inducible by various xenobiotics and which appear to exist in multiple forms (reviewed in Ref. 157). Other conjugations are catalyzed by cytosolic enzymes such as sulfotransferases and glutathione-*S*-transferases. Multiple forms of glutathione transferases have been purified, and these activities are also inducible (reviewed in Refs. 157 and 163). In general, the conjugation reactions convert hydrocarbon metabolites to anionic species that are more water-soluble and therefore more readily transported and excreted.

Metabolic Reactions at Various Sites on Hydrocarbons. The basis for the study of metabolism of polynuclear carcinogens is the idea that the actual initiator of the carcinogenic process is a metabolite of the carcinogen rather than the administered compound (path B in Scheme I). Evidence supportive of this idea was obtained some 20 years ago for the aromatic amines (*140, 173*) in the form of data showing that some metabolites are more carcinogenic than their parent compounds. For the polynuclear carcinogens, evidence of this nature has only been developed in recent years.

In the earliest of several reviews of the older literature (*18, 19, 174, 175*), Boyland postulated that because the dihydrodiol derivatives that resulted from metabolic attack at aromatic double bonds in naphthalene, anthracene, and phenanthrene were *trans*-diols, the initial metabolic product and the precursor of the diols was probably an epoxide. He also suggested that the reaction of such epoxides with tissue constituents could represent the critical event in the process of carcinogenesis by polycyclic hydrocarbons, and this possibility has been the subject of intensive study. Boyland's suggestion was supported when the urinary metabolite of naphthalene that was an acid-labile precursor of 1-naphthylmercapturic acid was identified by Boyland and Sims (*176*) as *N*-acetyl-*S*-(1,2-dihydro-2-hydroxy-1-naphthyl)-L-cysteine. These authors noted that the formation of this metabolite as well as the 1,2-dihydrodiol could both be accounted for by the proposed 1,2-naphthalene epoxide intermediate. In their subsequent extensive studies of aromatic hydrocarbon metabolism, these authors showed that most of the metabolic products that they identified could have arisen from intermediate epoxides (*177*).

The identification of this mercapturic acid precursor may have wrongly assigned the cysteine residue to the 1-position instead of the 2-position, though this error would not affect the argument about an epoxide precursor. The assigned structure was based on the dehydration of the mercapturic acid precursor to yield a 1-substituted naphthalene. However, the 1,2-naphthalene epoxide has now been shown to open primarily by nucleophilic attack at the 2-position (*178*), and the acid-catalyzed dehydration of *trans*-1-hydroxy-2-thioethyl-1,2-dihydronaphthalene has been shown to yield 1-thioethylnaphthalene as a result of the migration of the thioethyl group via a cyclic sulfonium intermediate (*179*) (Scheme III). A similar migration was also implicated in the dehydration of the analogous glutathione derivative.

The first synthesis of hydrocarbon epoxides was by Newman and Blum (*180*) in 1964, and thereafter it could be shown that metabolites obtained from polycyclic hydrocarbons also could be obtained from metabolism of the appropriate epoxide (*181, 182*). Conclusive proof that arene epoxides were transient metabolic intermediates was not provided, however, until Jerina et al. (*183*) used a radiotracer trapping technique to demonstrate the metabolic formation of 1,2-naphthalene epoxide from naphthalene in a microsomal system.

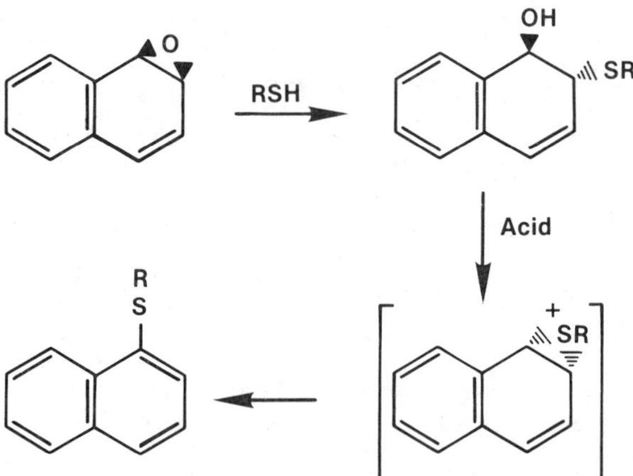

Scheme III. Migration of thioalkyl group during acid-catalyzed dehydration (179).

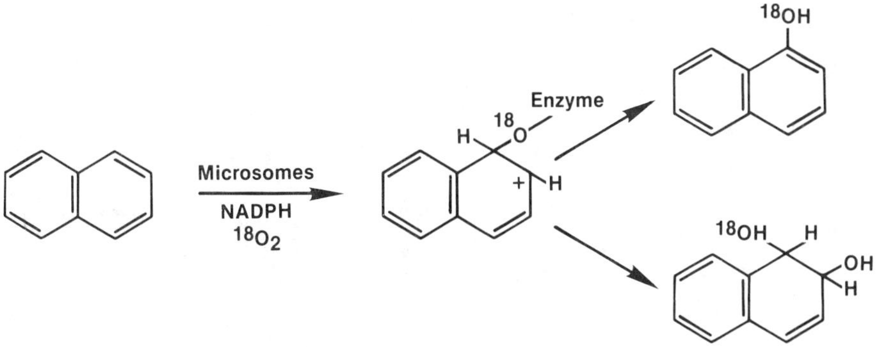

Scheme IV. Mechanism for microsomal metabolism of naphthalene based on $^{18}O_2$ *incorporation studies* (184).

Holtzman et al. (*184*) had previously examined the consequences of subjecting naphthalene to microsomal metabolism in the presence of an atmosphere of isotopic ^{18}O. They found that the 1-naphthol that was produced contained the heavy isotope and that the *trans*-1,2-dihydrodiol contained one atom of ^{18}O and one atom of ^{16}O, which presumably had originated from water. Furthermore, heating the diol in acid gave 95% 1-naphthol and 5% 2-naphthol; only the 1-naphthol contained ^{18}O. Thus, the diol contained ^{18}O exclusively in the 1-hydroxyl group. The mechanistic scheme that these authors postulated to accommodate their data was essentially that illustrated in Scheme IV, where the initially formed cationic species can be regarded as the immediate precursor of 1-naphthol (by loss of a proton from the 1-position) and as the immediate precursor of the dihydrodiol (arising by the attack of water at the 2-position).

This scheme accounted perfectly well for the then known facts, but when Vogel and Klärner (*185*) synthesized 1,2-naphthalene epoxide, they found that this compound readily rearranged to 1-naphthol but was not hydrated nonenzymically to a dihydrodiol. Furthermore, Jerina et al. (*186*) showed that 1,2-naphthalene epoxide in the presence of microsomes and $[^{18}O]H_2O$ was enzymically converted to the *trans*-dihydrodiol and that the ^{18}O was located primarily in the 2-hydroxyl group. Thus, their data were consistent with the data of Holtzman et al. (*184*) but showed that the epoxide was a suitable precursor for the dihydrodiol, because the specificity of the attack by water at the 2-position of the epoxide was enzymically directed. [Hanzlik et al. have shown that microsomal epoxide hydrolase selectively catalyzes attack by water at the least hindered epoxide carbon (*187*)]. In addition, 1,2-naphthalene epoxide reacted with glutathione (but not with *N*-acetylcysteine) both enzymically and nonenzymically to yield the same *S*-(1,2-dihydro-1-hydroxy-2-naphthyl)glutathione found as a naphthalene metabolite. At the time this work was published, the glutathione residue was thought to bind at the 1-position (*see* Scheme III and earlier discussion). These workers (*186*) showed that 1,2-naphthalene epoxide could give rise to all the end products of metabolism found for naphthalene in the microsomal system, i.e., 1-naphthol, *trans*-1,2-dihydro-1,2-dihydroxynaphthalene, and *S*-(1,2-dihydro-1-hydroxy-2-naphthyl)glutathione; the

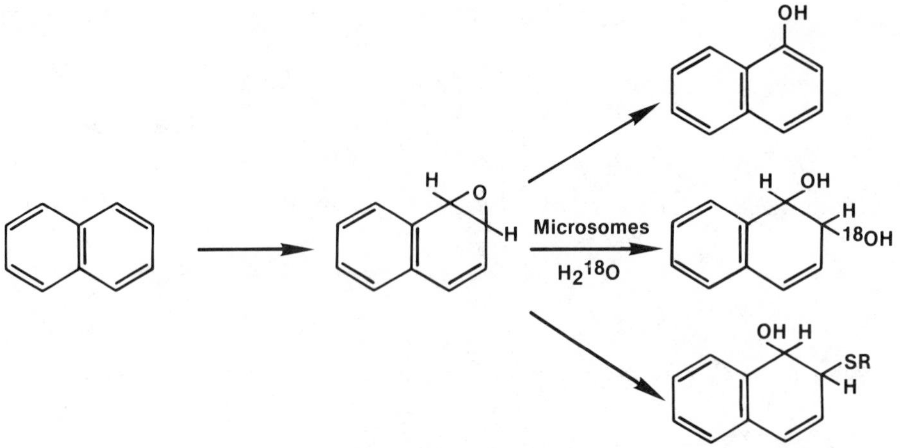

OH
H O
H Microsomes
$H_2{}^{18}O$
H OH
H
^{18}OH
OH H
SR
H

Scheme V. Modified mechanism accounting for [^{18}O]H_2O incorporation studies (186), *the failure of the epoxide to be converted to a dihydrodiol nonenzymically* (185), *and preferred nucleophilic attack on the 2-position of the intermediate epoxide* (178, 179).

last compound is only formed of course when a liver supernatant fraction and glutathione are added to the microsomal system. Moreover, the presence of styrene epoxide—a competitive substrate for epoxide hydrolase—during the microsomal metabolism of naphthalene decreased the dihydrodiol yield and concomitantly increased the naphthol yield. Increased concentrations of glutathione increased the yield of glutathione derivative at the expense of both dihydrodiol and phenol during the metabolism of naphthalene in the microsomes plus liver supernatant system. This finding strongly supported the view that all the metabolites arose from a common intermediate, namely 1,2-naphthalene epoxide (Scheme V).

One consequence of the discovery of the hydroxylation-induced migration of aromatic substituents (the NIH shift of Guroff et al. (*188*) was a further refinement of the mechanistic description of these metabolic reactions. Jerina et al. (*189*) had shown that the isomerization of [4-^{2}H]3,4-toluene epoxide to [3-^{2}H]4-hydroxytoluene exhibited a deuterium retention as great as that observed in the enzymic conversion of [4-^{2}H]toluene to [3-^{2}H]4-hydroxytoluene. Therefore, they suggested that arene epoxides were likely metabolic intermediates in the enzymic formation of phenols. Similar findings were obtained from a study of the microsomal conversion of naphthalene to 1-naphthol (*190*), where both [1-^{2}H]naphthalene or [2-^{2}H]naphthalene were converted to [2-^{2}H]1-naphthol with approximately 64% of the original deuterium retained in either case. Under the same conditions both [1-^{2}H]1,2-naphthalene epoxide and [2-^{2}H]1,2-naphthalene epoxide rearranged to [2-^{2}H]1-naphthol with approximately 72–75% deuterium retention. These results suggested the formation of a common intermediate during the metabolism of either deuterated naphthalene and the isomerization of either deuterated 1,2-naphthalene epoxide. The keto form of 1-naphthol, which arises by the migration of either hydrogen or deuterium from the 1- to the 2-position, was proposed as the

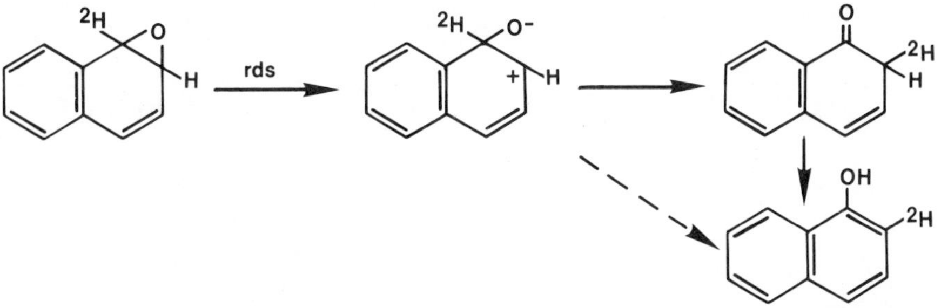

Scheme VI. Mechanism for isomerization of 1,2-naphthalene epoxide to 1-naphthol (190, 191).

common intermediate. Deuterium is retained depending on an isotope effect in the subsequent enolization.

Further investigation of the mechanism of isomerization of arene epoxides to phenols (*191*) indicated that for 1,2-naphthalene epoxide, a stepwise rather than a concerted mechanism is involved. This mechanism is described in Scheme VI. The deuterium retentions of 1,2-naphthalene epoxide under physiological conditions require that all the phenol should arise from its keto form. However, for other arene epoxides (or for 1,2-naphthalene epoxide in acid solution), some phenol arises from direct loss of a proton at the cation stage. Because the route to the phenol does involve a cation intermediate, the distinction between Schemes IV and V for naphthalene metabolism becomes less clear, i.e., is the epoxide a necessary intermediate en route from naphthalene to 1-naphthol? Similarly detailed mechanistic studies have not been carried out for the more complex carcinogenic hydrocarbons, although they are needed as a sound basis to interpret the findings on metabolism of these compounds.

The metabolism of aromatic hydrocarbons has been studied in systems ranging from the microsomal preparations discussed earlier to liver homogenates, liver slices, cultured cells, and whole animals. The metabolites that were found vary with the system used, because all the in vitro systems are metabolically deficient with respect to the whole animal; therefore, results of metabolic studies must be discussed in the context of the system used.

The metabolism in animals of a number of aromatic hydrocarbons has been studied, and in general, the findings with either rats or rabbits are comparable. Metabolic studies in whole animals are far more complex than in microsomal systems, because conjugations with sulfuric and glucuronic acids occur, and the conjugates can then give rise to other metabolites. However, most of the metabolites reported for naphthalene in animals can be seen to have arisen through one or the other of the primary routes indicated in Scheme V for the microsomal metabolism. Sims (*192*) pointed out that the naphthalene metabolites in rabbits appear to arise from three routes. The first involves the direct generation of 1-naphthol that is found in urine as either sulfuric acid or glucuronic acid conjugates and not as the phenol. The second route involves the primary production of the *trans*-1,2-dihydrodiol. This compound is then conjugated with either sulfuric acid or glucuronic acid, and these conjugates break down, as originally proposed by

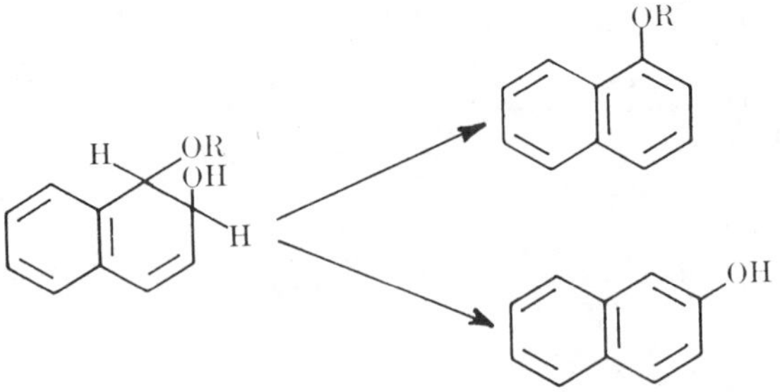

Scheme VII. Metabolic breakdown of sulfates or glucosiduronates of trans-*1,2-dihydro-1,2-dihydroxynaphthalene* (193). *R* = SO_3H *or* $C_6H_9O_6$.

Corner and Young (*193*), to yield 1-naphthyl sulfate, 1-naphthyl glucosiduronate, and the 2-naphthol that is found unconjugated in the urine (Scheme VII). The dehydrogenation of the dihydrodiol or its conjugates leads to another group of urinary metabolites: sulfuric acid conjugates and glucuronic acid conjugates of 1,2-dihydroxynaphthalene. The third primary metabolic route involves the formation of the glutathione derivative *S*-(1,2-dihydro-1-hydroxy-2-naphthyl)glutathione which appears to be the starting point for the formation of the urinary mercapturic acid *N*-acetyl-*S*-(1,2-dihydro-1-hydroxy-2-naphthyl)-L-cysteine. In rat bile, a series of amino acid conjugates of naphthalene was found, and from these conjugates the precursor–product relationship of the glutathione derivative and the mercapturic acid was established by Boyland et al. (*194*).

All the naphthalene metabolites arise from metabolic attack at the 1,2-bond, but when more complex molecules are examined, several sites of metabolic attack are detected. A comparison of the metabolism at a double bond in different hydrocarbons (e.g., the *K* region) is interesting when examining how products vary with the different electron densities at this bond. The compounds that have been studied in whole animals will be dealt with in order of increasing reactivity of their *K* regions as indicated by bond orders and complex indices listed in Table II.

The results of studies of the products of metabolic attack at the *K* region of anthracene (1,2-bond) in rats differ dramatically from those found for naphthalene in that neither 1- nor 2-hydroxyanthracene nor conjugates thereof are detected (*195*). On the other hand, *trans*-1,2-dihydro-1,2-dihydroxyanthracene and 1,2-dihydroxyanthracene are produced and excreted mainly as sulfuric acid and glucuronic acid conjugates. A mercapturic acid, *N*-acetyl-*S*-(1,2-dihydro-2-hydroxy-1-anthracenyl)cysteine, is also excreted in the urine. However, because characterization again depended on acid treatment, the cysteine residue may have been attached to the 2-position (*see* earlier discussion and Refs. 178 and 179).

A similar situation is found for the *K* region of phenanthrene (9,10-bond). No 9-hydroxyphenanthrene or conjugate thereof is present in the untreated urine of either rats or rabbits (*196*). The major metabolite is *trans*-9,10-dihydro-9,10-dihydroxyphenanthrene, which is also excreted as sulfuric acid and glucuronic acid conjugates (*177*). A sulfuric acid conjugate of 9,10-dihydroxyphenanthrene is found in the urine, as is *N*-acetyl-*S*-(9,10-dihydro-9-hydroxy-10-phenanthryl) cysteine (*197*).

For the *K* region of pyrene (4,5-bond), no evidence of phenol formation is found. The 4,5-dihydrodiol is detected in relatively small amounts, and no 4,5-dihydroxypyrene derivatives are found. The major metabolite appears to be the mercapturic acid *N*-acetyl-*S*-(4,5-dihydro-4-hydroxy-5-pyrenyl)-L-cysteine (*198*).

In the case of benz[*a*]anthracene (*199*), the major metabolite at the *K* region (5,6-bond) is again a mercapturic acid, *N*-acetyl-*S*-(5,6-dihydro-6-hydroxy-5-benz[*a*]anthracenyl)cysteine, and whereas the dihydrodiol at the *K* region of phenanthrene is the major metabolic product, the 5,6-dihydrodiol of benz[*a*]anthracene is only a minor metabolite. Phenols are not formed at the *K* region of benz[*a*]anthracene.

For both phenanthrene and benz[*a*]anthracene, Boyland and Sims (*177, 199*) estimate that the extent of metabolic attack at any given bond increases with increasing bond order, i.e., the most extensive metabolic attack occurs at the *K* region. As indicated by the previous discussion, the final products of metabolic attack at *K* regions vary with the bond order of this region. Thus for naphthalene, all the three primary metabolic routes (Scheme V) are followed, and phenol, dihydrodiol, and mercapturic acid are formed, but as the double-bond character of the *K* region increases on going to anthracene, the phenol route becomes inoperative. Similarly, as double-bond character increases further on going to pyrene and then to benz[*a*]anthracene, the dihydrodiol route appears to be less favored also, and the main metabolic route becomes mercapturic acid formation. These observations are interesting to consider with respect to the mechanisms outlined in Schemes IV, V, and VI. Apparently phenols are formed only at bonds where the energy required to localize a pair of electrons at that bond (bond-localization energy) is fairly high. This behavior is to be expected because the higher the bond-localization energy, the greater the gain in energy on reverting from the arene epoxide or cation intermediates in Schemes IV, V, and VI to the fully aromatic system. However, the rate-determining step in the formation of 1-naphthol from 1,2-naphthalene epoxide (Scheme VI) does not involve regeneration of the fully aromatic system (*191*); this only occurs during the enolization step. In fact, ketones are usually much more stable than their enolic forms, and 2-tetralone has been isolated (*200*) from an acid hydrolysis of a mercapturic acid metabolite of 1,2,3,4-tetrahydro-1,2-naphthalene oxide. This example is somewhat extreme because the bond-localization energy for the isolated double bond in a dihydronaphthalene would be very low, but it does illustrate the point that phenol formation could be interrupted at the enolization step of Scheme VI for compounds with relatively low bond-localization energies. Raha (*201*) isolated a compound presumed to be the keto form of a *K*-region phenol of benzo[*a*]pyrene; Pullman and Pullman (*202*) calculated that for the *K*-region double bond of this compound, the keto form of a phenol would be the most stable form, while at any other bond in the molecule, the enol form would be favored. Newman and Olson (*203*) isolated tautomeric mixtures of phenols and ketones in attempts to prepare the *K*-region phenols of 7,12-dimethylbenz[*a*]anthracene, while Harvey et al. (*204*) isolated a 5-oxo-5,6-dihydro derivative after reductive cleavage of 5-acetoxy-7,12-dimethylbenz[*a*]anthracene. Dipple et al. (*205*) obtained both the 5- and 6-oxo-5,6-

dihydro derivatives via acid-catalyzed dehydration of the *cis*-diol, but these ketones did not exhibit any carcinogenic activity in mice. Similar dehydrations of the *K*-region *cis*-diols of phenanthrene and benzo[*a*]pyrene gave no evidence of ketone formation, though the existence of the keto form of 9-phenanthrol at low temperature (77 K) is evident from IR spectra of UV-irradiated suspensions of the 9,10-epoxide in Nujol (*206*). For 7,12-dimethylbenz[*a*]anthracene at least, a *K*-region epoxide could possibly lead to *K*-region ketones through analogous steps to those in Scheme VI, but the generation of such ketones through metabolism has not been reported.

The preponderance of *K*-region dihydrodiols as metabolic products in animals also appears to decrease with decreasing bond-localization energies at the *K* region. Pandov and Sims (*207*) have shown that this is consistent with the behavior of the epoxide intermediates, because phenanthrene 9,10-epoxide is converted to a dihydrodiol by the enzyme epoxide hydrolase in rat liver homogenates or microsomes much more rapidly than is dibenz[*a,h*]anthracene 5,6-epoxide. Similarly, with liver preparations, a dihydrodiol is the major metabolic product at the 8,9-double bond in 7,12-dimethylbenz[*a*]anthracene, while at the *K* region (lower bond-localization energy), a glutathione conjugate is the major metabolic product (*208*). Also, with a system containing both epoxide hydrolase and glutathione transferase activities, benz[*a*]anthracene 5,6-epoxide is converted to a glutathione conjugate more rapidly than the 8,9-epoxide, while the 8,9-epoxide is converted to a dihydrodiol more rapidly than the 5,6-epoxide (*209*).

Although the metabolic products at double bonds in hydrocarbons have been discussed in terms of the bond-localization energies at these bonds, once an epoxide intermediate is formed, the fate of the epoxide will then be influenced by the residual aromatic system as discussed earlier (*126*). The temptation then is to think that where the aromatic system can effectively delocalize developing charge that results from the opening of the epoxide ring, the intermediate may be more sensitive to a softer nucleophile (*210*) like glutathione, and when charge delocalization is less effective, the harder nucleophile water is preferred even though these reactions are enzymically mediated. Where there is even less charge delocalization possible, isomerization to the phenol apparently becomes competitive with these other routes. A related phenomenon is the difference in chemistry between the mercapturic acid formed from naphthalene and from benz[*a*]anthracene. In the studies cited earlier, Boyland and Sims (*176*) found that the mercapturic acid from naphthalene was converted by acid into 1-naphthylmercapturic acid plus traces of 1-naphthol, 2-naphthol, and naphthalene. The mercapturic acid from benz[*a*]anthracene gave primarily benz[*a*]anthracene and *N,N'*-diacetylcystine along with a trace of the arylmercapturic acid (*199*).

Changes in the spectrum of metabolites produced along with changes in the chemistry of the bond attacked can also be seen in the metabolic reactions at bonds other than the *K* region, as in benz[*a*]anthracene, for example. Thus, 3,4-dihydro-3,4-dihydroxybenz[*a*]anthracene; 8,9-dihydro-8,9-dihydroxybenz[*a*]anthracene; and 3-, 4-, 8-, and 9-hydroxybenz[*a*]anthracenes were detected as metabolites in animals. Metabolic reactions at these bonds are therefore similar to those found at the 1,2-bond of naphthalene. Although 10,11-dihydro-10,11-dihydroxybenz[*a*]-anthracene was also detected, no 10- or 11-hydroxybenz[*a*]anthracene was found;

the metabolic reactions at this bond appear to relate more closely to those at the 1,2-bond of anthracene than to those at the 1,2-bond of naphthalene. Another pattern of products results from metabolic attack at the 1,2-bond of pyrene. In this case the only metabolite detected is 1-hydroxypyrene.

Some metabolic products resulting from attack at the *L* region of benz[*a*]-anthracene have been found and identified as 7-hydroxybenz[*a*]anthracene and possibly 7,12-dihydro-7,12-dihydroxybenz[*a*]anthracene. According to Boyland and Sims (*199*), these products could have arisen from an initial epoxidation across the 7- and 12-positions. Metabolism also occurs at the methyl groups of methylated hydrocarbons yielding hydroxymethyl derivatives and carboxylic acids (*211, 212*). The mechanism of the first step in these reactions involves the direct displacement of a proton by a positive oxygen species rather than the generation of an intermediate aralkyl cation. This conclusion follows because studies with $^{18}O_2$ have shown that in the microsomal conversion of ethylbenzene to methylphenyl carbinol, the oxygen atom in the carbinol originates from atmospheric oxygen rather than from water (*213*). A similar conclusion was reached by Grandjean and Cavalieri (*214*) who examined the microsomal metabolites produced from 7-methylbenz[*a*]anthracene and 7,12-dimethylbenz[*a*]anthracene in the presence of $[^{18}O]H_2O$ or $^{18}O_2$.

Most of the more recent studies of the metabolism of polycyclic hydrocarbons (which include studies of the more carcinogenic hydrocarbons: 7,12-dimethylbenz[*a*]anthracene, benzo[*a*]pyrene, dibenz[*a,h*]anthracene, and 3-methylcholanthrene) have used only the in vitro systems of rat liver slices, rat liver homogenates, cultured cells, and liver microsomal preparations. The results of these experiments are consistent with the generalizations made on the basis of the animal studies. In general, the metabolites found in the in vitro systems are also found in animal studies, but the animal studies yield additional metabolites not seen in the in vitro systems. Glutathione conjugates are not formed in the simple microsomal system because the necessary enzyme activity and glutathione are not present. However, liver homogenates are competent in this respect, and glutathione conjugates at the *K* regions of benz[*a*]anthracene, dibenz[*a,h*]anthracene (*181*), 3-methylcholanthrene (*182*), and 7,12-dimethylbenz[*a*]anthracene (*208*) are detected.

In summary, the primary metabolic fates that befall the polycyclic aromatic hydrocarbons can be classified according to the chemistry of the sites that are modified (Scheme VIII and Table IV):

1. Metabolic reactions occur at *L* regions, but because the presence of such regions of low *para*-localization energy is usually associated with an absence of carcinogenic activity, these metabolic reactions are probably not involved in the expression of carcinogenic activity.
2. Metabolic reaction also occurs on saturated carbon atoms in polycyclic aromatic hydrocarbons leading to the sequential formation of hydroxy compounds, ketones, and aldehydes (the aldehyde in Scheme VIII has not been found as a metabolite though it is presumably formed as an intermediate), and carboxylic acids. Some of these products, notably the aldehydes and ketones, have exhibited

Metabolism at L Regions (195)

H OH

HO H

air ?

OH

OH

O

O

Metabolism at Saturated Carbon Atom

CH₃ → CH₃ → [CH₃ CHO] → CH₃

CH₃ CH₂OH CHO COOH

20/20 [87 days]	4/16 [162 days]	15/15 [102 days]	Sarcoma in rats [mean latent period] *(215)*
10/10 [118 days]	17/18 [120 days]	19/19 [132 days]	Sarcoma in mice [mean latent period] *(216)*

Metabolism at (K Region) Double Bonds (see text for references and discussion)

Mercapturic acid

HCl

Phenols, Arylmercapturic acid
Parent
Hydrocarbon

Scheme VIII. Summary of metabolic modifications of polycyclic hydrocarbons.

Table IV

Summary of K-Region Metabolites Found in Studies on Whole Animals

K-Region Metabolites *Found in Studies on Whole Animals for*	*Phenol*	*Dihydrodiol*	*Glutathione Conjugates*	*Products of Acid Hydrolysis of Mercapturic Acids*		
				Phenols	*Arylmercap-turic Acid*	*Parent Hydrocarbon*
Naphthalene	found	found	found	minor	major	minor
Anthracene	absent	found	found	minor	major	minor
Phenanthrene	absent	major	found		minor	major
Pyrene	absent	minor	major		minor	major
Benz[a]anthracene	absent	minor	major		trace	major

high carcinogenic activities and could therefore be involved in the expression of the carcinogenic potential of the parent compounds.

3. Metabolic modification of "aromatic" double bonds is the most predominant and most extensively studied type of metabolic reaction. This modification yields a spectrum of metabolic products that could be involved in expressing carcinogenic activity. The relative abundance and the chemical properties of the products obtained vary with the bond-localization energy of the particular bond concerned as illustrated for the *K* regions of several hydrocarbons in Scheme VIII and Table IV.

Stereochemical Course of Metabolism. In some of the earliest studies of hydrocarbon metabolism, the reactions involved were recognized as highly stereoselective. Thus, Boyland and Levi (*217*) isolated (+)-*trans*-1,2-dihydro-1,2-dihydroxyanthracene from the urine of rabbits dosed with anthracene, but they isolated the (−)-enantiomer from similarly treated rats (*218*). Over the last decade, the emphasis has been on metabolic studies with in vitro systems rather than whole animals, and while this focus has dramatically increased our knowledge of the stereochemistry of metabolism, it should be remembered that in different tissues of different species, different stereochemistry may be involved.

A summary of some of the studies of metabolic reactions at the 4,5-bond in benzo[*a*]pyrene is presented in Scheme IX. Cytochrome P-450*c* has been shown to be highly selective in its oxidation of this bond in that more than 97% of the epoxide formed is the (+)-(4*S*,5*R*)-epoxide (*219*). This could be considered to represent selective attack on the bottom rather than the top face of the conventional representation of benzo[*a*]pyrene. Each enantiomeric benzo[*a*]pyrene 4,5-epoxide gives rise to two glutathione derivatives on chemical reaction with glutathione. These products result from a *trans* opening of the epoxide ring in which glutathione reacts equally effectively at either the 4-position or the 5-position (*219*). However, when reaction of the racemic epoxide with glutathione is catalyzed by rat liver cytosolic glutathione transferases, apparently the two (4*S*,5*S*)-positional isomers are preferentially formed and an even greater selectivity for these two isomers is exhibited when skate liver glutathione transferase 4 is used (*220*). Thus, while the chemical reaction occurs with attack at either the 4- or 5-position on either face of the molecule, the enzyme-mediated reactions occur at the 5-position on the top face or at the 4-position on the bottom face, i.e., at the carbons with (*R*)-absolute configuration. In contrast to the glutathione reactions, epoxide hydrolase-mediated hydration of each enantiomeric epoxide (Scheme IX) yields primarily the same (+)-(4*R*,5*R*)-dihydrodiol resulting from preferential attack at the 4-position of the (+)-epoxide and the 5-position of the (−)-epoxide, i.e., at the carbon atom with (*S*)-absolute configuration in each case (*221*). [The major dihydrodiol produced is described herein as the (+)-enantiomer following Kedzierski et al. (*1*) and Armstrong et al. (*221*), who report a value of $[\alpha]_D^{20}$ of +39° measured in tetrahydrofuran. However in methanol, the sign changes to minus, and in the earlier literature, this same dihydrodiol was referred to as the (−)-enantiomer (*222, 223*)].

Although these metabolic reactions at the 4,5-bond in benzo[*a*]pyrene demonstrate a high degree of stereoselectivity, this is not general for all such

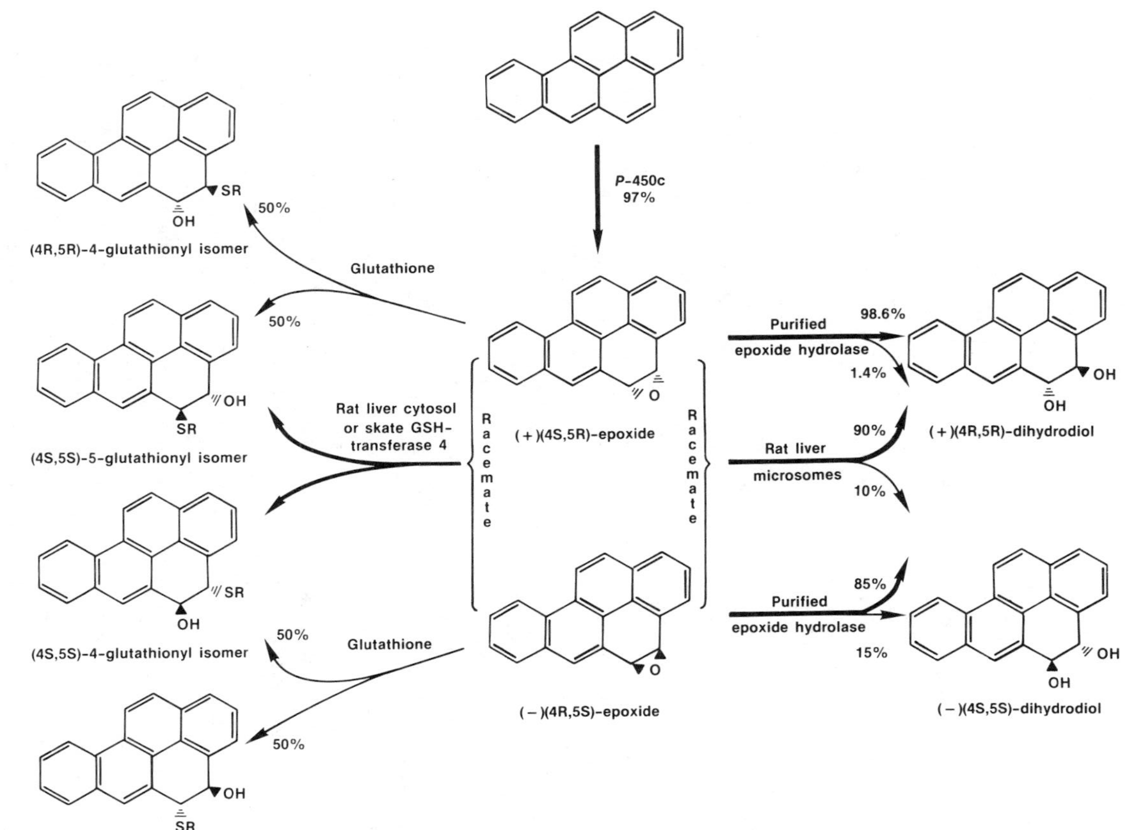

Scheme IX. Stereochemistry of metabolism at the 4,5-bond of benzo[a]pyrene (219–22).

reactions at *K* regions. For example, either purified epoxide hydrolase or microsomal preparations convert phenanthrene 9,10-epoxide or (−)-benz[*a*]-anthracene 5,6-epoxide into roughly 40:60 mixtures of (+)- and (−)-dihydrodiols respectively, while for (+)-benz[*a*]anthracene 5,6-epoxide, an 87:13 ratio is obtained (*221*). Similarly, with different substrates, the positional selectivity of the epoxide hydrolase-mediated reaction varies. While preferential attack at the epoxide carbon with (*S*)-absolute configuration was observed for benzo[*a*]pyrene 4,5-epoxide, water attacks both carbons of (*R*)- and (*S*)-absolute configuration in the case of phenanthrene 9,10-epoxide and (−)-benz[*a*]anthracene 5,6-epoxide, with a slight preference for attack at the carbon with (*R*)-absolute configuration in each case; attack at the carbon of (*S*)-absolute configuration is again preferred with (+)-benz[*a*]anthracene 5,6-epoxide as the substrate (*221*). The situation becomes more complex when the rates of various reactions are considered, and overall, no simple rule to predict the stereochemistry of these metabolic reactions has emerged. Nonetheless, this kind of information is being used to generate descriptions of the topology of the enzyme active site, and these descriptions may eventually lead to a predictive capability (*221, 224*).

The metabolic reactions that lead to bay-region dihydrodiol epoxides of benzo[*a*]pyrene again show a high degree of stereoselectivity or even stereospecificity in some cases (Scheme X). Liver microsomes from rats pretreated with 3-methylcholanthrene oxidize the 7,8-bond of benzo[*a*]pyrene with a very high degree of stereoselectivity to yield almost exclusively the (+)-(7*R*,8*S*)-epoxide (*4, 223, 225*). Each enantiomer of the 7,8-epoxide is stereospecifically converted by microsomal preparations (*4, 223, 225*) or by purified epoxide hydrolase (*221*), through attack of water at the 8-position in each case, to a single enantiomeric dihydrodiol. Rat liver epoxide hydrolase metabolizes the (−)-7,8-epoxide three to four times faster than the (+)-7,8-epoxide, but the enzyme has a higher affinity for the (+)-7,8-epoxide. Thus, hydration of the racemic 7,8-epoxide is rather complex, and this reaction appears to be more stereoselective at the initial stages of the reaction than at later stages (Scheme X) (*4*). As a result, apparently contradictory reports exist in the literature of both high (*223, 225*) and low (*222*) enantiomeric purity for the product of hydration of the racemic 7,8-epoxide. Further oxidation of benzo[*a*]pyrene-7,8-dihydrodiol to the vicinal dihydrodiol epoxide exhibits a high degree of stereoselectivity when liver microsomes from 3-methylcholanthrene-pretreated rats are used but a lower stereoselectivity when microsomal preparations from untreated or phenobarbital-treated rats are used (*225–27*). The ratios of products indicated in Scheme X are taken from Thakker et al. (*227*). With the microsomal system from 3-methylcholanthrene-pretreated rats, the 7,8-dihydrodiol formed from benzo[*a*]pyrene is almost exclusively the (−)-enantiomer. This isomer, in turn, is preferentially converted to the (+)-*anti*-7,8-dihydrodiol 9,10-epoxide which is the most carcinogenic of the four isomeric dihydrodiol epoxides in Scheme X. This situation may not obtain in other biological systems, and studies of the DNA-bound dihydrodiol epoxide metabolites of benzo[*a*]pyrene in mouse skin (*228*) or cell culture systems (*229*) indicate that while the (+)-*anti*-dihydrodiol epoxide probably predominates, it is not formed as selectively in these systems as in the microsomal system. Similarly, Deutsch et al. (*230*), who used a reconstituted system of various purified cytochromes P-450 from rabbit liver, have

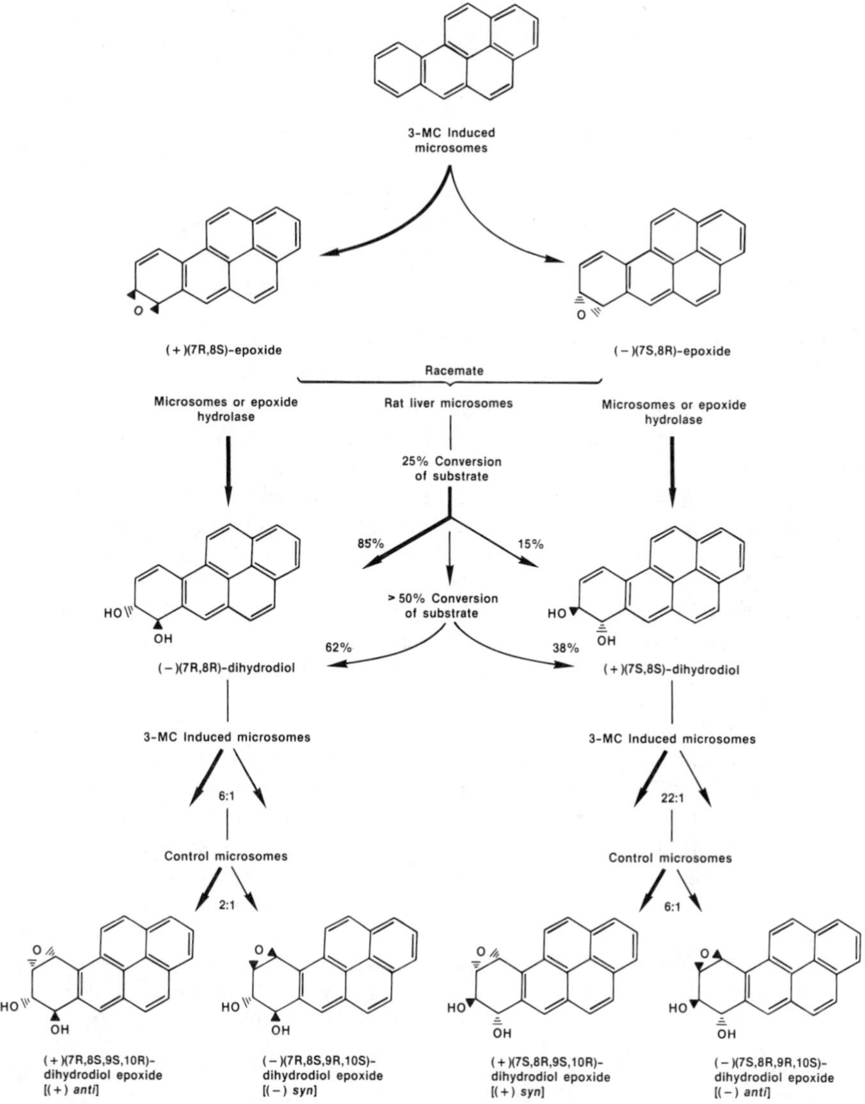

Scheme X. Stereochemistry of metabolism at the 7,8- and 9,10-bonds of benzo[a]pyrene (4, 221–23, 225–27).

shown that the conversion of the (−)-7,8-dihydrodiol of benzo[*a*]pyrene to a dihydrodiol epoxide ranges between a ratio of 11:1 to 1.8:1 in favor of the (+)-*anti*-isomer, according to which purified cytochrome P-450 is used, and that conversion of the (+)-7,8-dihydrodiol ranges from a (+)-*syn* to (−)-*anti* ratio of 0.4 to 3.0. By focusing on a single form of cytochrome P-450 (i.e., P-450*c*), Jerina et al. (*231*) have developed a model for the shape of the active site on this cytochrome that, so far, has permitted the stereochemistry of certain oxidations to be successfully predicted. The further development of this approach, perhaps involving other purified cytochromes P-450, may eventually account for much of the fascinating stereochemistry involved in these reactions.

Relationship Between Metabolism and Carcinogenic Action

Over the years, a direct mechanism of action for the hydrocarbon carcinogens, in which metabolism serves only a detoxification role, and an indirect mechanism of action, wherein a metabolite of the hydrocarbon is responsible for the initiation of carcinogenesis, have both been advocated strongly at various times. It was possible to support both these mutually exclusive hypotheses and a number of different ideas, in the case of the indirect mechanism, about which particular metabolite(s) might be responsible for carcinogenic activity, because there was a complete lack of any critical evidence which could exclude one possibility or another. In the last few years, this situation has changed considerably, and it is becoming increasingly clear that the carcinogenic action of the hydrocarbons is probably expressed through metabolites associated with the dihydrodiol epoxide pathway. This realization has been and continues to represent a very exciting development in hydrocarbon carcinogenesis, and it is of interest and significance that the discovery of this mechanism of metabolic activation did not arise through the "classical approach" of identifying metabolites that exhibited greater carcinogenic potency than the parent compound (*140, 173*). In fact, dihydrodiol epoxides were first identified as the hydrocarbon metabolites responsible for DNA binding in mammalian cells (*141*), and only subsequently were their carcinogenic activities investigated. For the purpose of the present chapter, we have considered it prudent to include a discussion of the background relating to the role of metabolism in the carcinogenic action of hydrocarbons and to discuss various putative mechanisms of metabolic activation that have been investigated, in addition to describing the development of the dihydrodiol epoxide mechanism of hydrocarbon activation.

Background. It has been known for many years that polynuclear carcinogens become covalently bound to certain tissue constituents of animals treated with these carcinogens. By exploiting the intense fluorescence of benzo[*a*]pyrene, Miller (*232*) showed that this carcinogen was covalently bound to epidermal proteins of mouse skin. Such covalent interactions do not occur in the absence of metabolic activity, and these findings required that the carcinogen be metabolized in vivo to a chemically reactive form that can react covalently with cellular macromolecules. Wiest and Heidelberger (*233*) applied radiotracer techniques to studies of hydrocarbon binding to cellular constituents, and Heidelberger and Moldenhauer (*234*) subsequently showed a positive correlation between carcinogenic activity and the extents to which seven out of eight radioactive polycyclic hydrocarbons were bound to soluble mouse skin proteins. The exception was dibenz[*a,c*]anthracene which was extensively bound and was believed to be noncarcinogenic. Next, binding to a specific electrophoretic fraction of the soluble proteins was compared with carcinogenic activity, and an excellent correlation with carcinogenic activity was found for the 12 compounds studied (*235*). This finding established a link between binding and carcinogenic activity, and consequently, a link between metabolism and carcinogenic activity. The binding of polynuclear carcinogens to other cellular macromolecules has also been reported. Heidelberger and Davenport (*236*) noted that covalent binding of hydrocarbons to nucleic acids occurred in mouse skin, but they experienced difficulty in confirming this observation (*237*). Brookes and Lawley (*238*) showed that firm binding of hydrocarbons to DNA, RNA, and proteins of mouse skin did occur and that the extent of binding to DNA was positively correlated with carcinogenic potency.

The respective correlations between carcinogenic potency and protein binding or carcinogenic potency and DNA binding have been used to support the protein deletion hypothesis of carcinogenesis (*239*) and the somatic mutation hypothesis of carcinogenesis (*240*), respectively, and both of these correlations support the concept that a chemically reactive metabolite may be involved in the process of chemical carcinogenesis. More direct evidence for the generation of chemically reactive metabolites came from the work of Grover and Sims (*241*) and of Gelboin (*242*) who independently demonstrated that a covalent interaction between aromatic hydrocarbons and DNA does occur in the presence of liver microsomal preparations.

Other suggestive evidence for the involvement of metabolism in the carcinogenic action of polynuclear carcinogens arises from various studies of the biological effects of aromatic hydrocarbons. Haddow (*243*) observed that primary tumors are more resistant to the growth-inhibitory properties of aromatic hydrocarbons than are normal cells, and several studies have subsequently confirmed the generality of this observation, which is subject to only a few exceptions (reviewed in Ref. 244). Diamond et al. (*245*) found that cells that are sensitive to the toxic action of 7,12-dimethylbenz[*a*]anthracene bind considerably more of the carcinogen to their nucleic acids and proteins than do resistant cells. Furthermore, Andrianov et al. (*246*) demonstrated directly that cells that resist the toxic effects of benzo[*a*]pyrene exhibit a considerably reduced capacity for metabolizing this carcinogen relative to that of cells that are sensitive. Similarly, Gelboin et al. (*247*) demonstrated that the levels of aryl hydrocarbon hydroxylase activity in various cell types are positively correlated with sensitivity to the toxic effects of benzo[*a*]pyrene. These workers also provided conclusive proof that the toxic effects of aromatic hydrocarbons require metabolic transformation of the hydrocarbon to a toxic metabolite when they showed that a benzo[*a*]pyrene metabolite, namely 3-hydroxybenzo[*a*]pyrene, is cytotoxic to cells irrespective of their capacities for metabolism of the parent hydrocarbon. Cells can metabolize hydrocarbons yet be resistant to toxic effects; for example, Iype et al. (*248*) recently found that hepatoma cells in culture were far more resistant to the toxic effects of 7,12-dimethylbenz[*a*]anthracene than were normal liver epithelial cells, and this resistance was attributed to the greater ability of the malignant cells to detoxify some cytotoxic metabolite.

7,8-Benzoflavone
(α-Naphthoflavone)

2,3,7,8-Tetrachlorodibenzo-p-dioxin
(TCDD)

5,6-Benzoflavone
(β-Naphthoflavone)

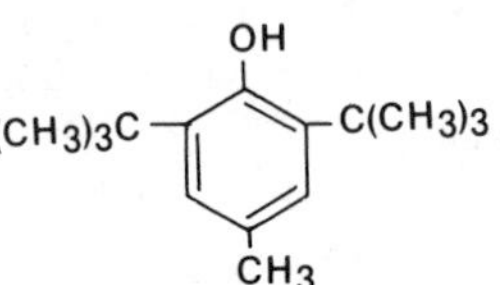

Butylated
Hydroxytoluene

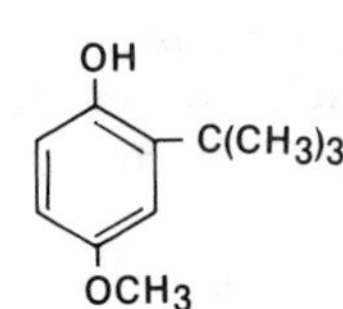

Butylated
Hydroxyanisole

3,3′,4′,5,7-Pentahydroxyflavone
(Quercetin)

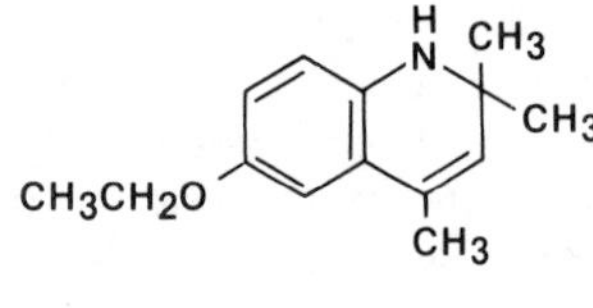

Ethoxyquin

A relationship between metabolism and toxicity of aromatic hydrocarbons is therefore firmly established, but toxicity and carcinogenicity need not necessarily be expressed through similar mechanisms. In fact, from studies analogous to those cited, a rather confusing picture of the relationship between metabolism and carcinogenic action emerges.

Many compounds capable of altering metabolism of polycyclic aromatic hydrocarbons also inhibit polycyclic hydrocarbon carcinogenesis (Table V, reviewed in Refs. 249–52). Thus, the yield of mammary tumors in rats in response to treatment with 7,12-dimethylbenz[*a*]anthracene is decreased by treatment of animals with various other polycyclic hydrocarbons (*261, 263*), as well as with compounds such as 5,6-benzoflavone (*253*), 1,1,1-trichloro-2,2-bis(*p*-chlorophenyl)ethane (DDT) (*266*), and certain antioxidants (*271, 275*). The carcinogenic action of 3-methylcholanthrene in mouse skin is inhibited by 7,8-benzoflavone

Table V

Inhibition of Polycyclic Hydrocarbon Carcinogenesis

Inhibitor	*Carcinogen*	*Species and Target Tissue*
Flavones		
5,6-Benzoflavone (β-Naphthoflavone)	7,12-Dimethylbenz[*a*]anthracene	Rat mammary gland (*253*), and mouse lung (*254*) and skin (*255*)
	Benzo[*a*]pyrene	Mouse lung and skin (*256*)
	3-Methylcholanthrene	Mouse skin (*255*)
7,8-Benzoflavone (α-Naphthoflavone)	7,12-Dimethylbenz[*a*]anthracene	Mouse lung (*254*) and skin (*255, 257–59*)
	Benzo[*a*]pyrene	Mouse skin (*250*)
	3-Methylcholanthrene	Mouse skin (*250*)
3,3′,4′,5,7-Pentahydroxy-flavone (Quercetin)	7,12-Dimethylbenz[*a*]anthracene	Mouse skin (*250, 260*)
	Benzo[*a*]pyrene	Mouse skin (*250*) and lung (*256*)
Polycyclic Hydrocarbons		
Benz[*a*]anthracene	7,12-Dimethylbenz[*a*]anthracene	Rat mammary gland (*261*) and mouse skin (*262*)
3-Methylcholanthrene	7,12-Dimethylbenz[*a*]anthracene	Rat mammary gland (*263*)
Benzo[*e*]pyrene or Dibenz[*a,c*]anthracene	7,12-Dimethylbenz[*a*]anthracene	Mouse skin (*250, 264, 265*)
Chrysene	7,12-Dimethylbenz[*a*]anthracene	Rat mammary gland (*261*)
	Benzo[*a*]pyrene	Mouse skin (*270*)
Halogenated Hydrocarbons		
1,1,1-Trichloro-2,2-bis-(*p*-chlorophenyl)ethane (DDT)	7,12-Dimethylbenz[*a*]anthracene	Rat mammary gland (*266*)
Aroclor 1254	7,12-Dimethylbenz[*a*]anthracene	Mouse skin (*267*)
2,3,7,8-Tetrachloro-dibenzo-*p*-dioxin (TCDD)	7,12-Dimethylbenz[*a*]anthracene	Mouse skin (*267, 268*)
	Benzo[*a*]pyrene	Mouse skin (*267, 268*)
	3-Methylcholanthrene	Mouse skin (*269*)
Antioxidants		
Butylated hydroxy-anisole	7,12-Dimethylbenz[*a*]anthracene	Mouse forestomach (*271*), skin (*272*), and lung (*273*), and rat mammary gland (*271*)
	Benzo[*a*]pyrene	Mouse forestomach (*271*) and lung (*273*)
	Dibenz[*a,h*]anthracene	Mouse lung (*273*)

Continued on next page

Table V Continued

Inhibitor	*Carcinogen*	*Species and Target Tissue*
Butylated hydroxy-toluene	7,12-Dimethylbenz[*a*]anthracene	Mouse skin (*272*) and rat mammary gland (*271*)
	Benzo[*a*]pyrene	Mouse forestomach (*271*)
Ethoxyquin	7,12-Dimethylbenz[*a*]anthracene	Mouse forestomach and rat mammary gland (*271*)
	Benzo[*a*]pyrene	Mouse forestomach (*271*)
Vitamin C or Vitamin E	7,12-Dimethylbenz[*a*]anthracene	Mouse skin (*272*)
Selenium (Na_2Se)	7,12-Dimethylbenz[*a*]anthracene	Mouse skin (*274*) and rat mammary gland (*275*)
	Benzo[*a*]pyrene	Mouse skin (*274*)
	3-Methylcholanthrene	Mouse skin (*274*)

(*250*), 2,3,7,8-tetrachlorodibenzo-*p*-dioxin (TCDD) (*269*), and selenium (*274*), and the carcinogenic activity of benzo[*a*]pyrene is inhibited by 5,6-benzoflavone (*256*), 7,8-benzoflavone (*250*), quercetin (*250*), chrysene (*270*), selenium (*274*), and TCDD (*267, 268*). Similar though not identical patterns of inhibition of carcinogenesis by polycyclic hydrocarbons are seen in other target tissues (*see* Table V).

Because many of these inhibitors of carcinogenesis are known to induce metabolism of the hydrocarbon carcinogens, a possible conclusion from consideration of these data is that metabolism is not involved in the carcinogenic action of polycyclic aromatic hydrocarbons. However, carcinogenesis by 2-acetylaminofluorene is known to be inhibited by dietary 3-methylcholanthrene (*276, 277*), yet this aromatic amine does express its carcinogenic potential via metabolic activation (*173, 278*). The explanation of this apparent inconsistency was provided by Miller et al. (*279*) who showed that dietary 3-methylcholanthrene enhanced the production of some of the noncarcinogenic urinary metabolites of 2-acetylaminofluorene at the expense of the carcinogenic metabolite *N*-hydroxy-2-acetylaminofluorene. Thus, induction or inhibition of specific enzymes by modifiers of carcinogenesis could shift the balance of metabolism into detoxification pathways or into activation pathways, and thereby inhibition or enhancement of carcinogenesis could result.

The inhibitors of carcinogenesis listed in Table V are known to affect hydrocarbon metabolism in different ways. Some of these compounds including polycyclic hydrocarbons (3-methylcholanthrene, benz[*a*]anthracene, and dibenz[*a,c*]anthracene), 5,6-benzoflavone, and halogenated hydrocarbons induce the microsomal enzymes involved in hydrocarbon oxidation in a variety of tissues and cell culture systems (*249, 250, 280–84*). Other compounds including 7,8-benzoflavone and benzo[*e*]pyrene can inhibit the enzymes involved in metabolism (*249–52*). The situation is complicated even more by the fact that some compounds that inhibit the carcinogenic action of one hydrocarbon actually enhance the carcinogenic potency of others. For example, 7,8-benzoflavone was found to enhance tumor initiation by dibenz[*a,h*]anthracene in mouse skin (*285*). Benzo[*e*]pyrene enhances tumor initiation by benzo[*a*]pyrene in mouse skin (*250, 264*), and under certain conditions, TCDD enhances the formation of 3-methylcholanthrene-induced subcutaneous fibrosarcomas (*286*).

These complexities are further exemplified by the different properties of the isomeric 5,6- and 7,8-benzoflavones (*254, 257–59, 287, 288*). Diamond and Gelboin (*287*) found that 7,8-benzoflavone inhibits hydrocarbon metabolism and hydrocarbon toxicity in hamster embryo cell cultures. Furthermore, this compound inhibits the aryl hydrocarbon hydroxylase activity (this activity refers to the rate of conversion of benzo[*a*]pyrene into 3-hydroxybenzo[*a*]pyrene) of hamster cell homogenates and rat liver microsomes only when these activities have been induced by prior treatments with benz[*a*]anthracene and 3-methylcholanthrene, respectively. No inhibition of aryl hydrocarbon hydroxylase activities in homogenates and microsomes from noninduced cells and rats is observed. More recently, Huang et al. (*289*), using a reconstituted system containing individual P-450 isozymes isolated from rabbit liver to examine the metabolism of benzo[*a*]pyrene, found that 7,8-benzoflavone was a potent inhibitor when P-450LM6 from TCDD-induced liver was used. They also found that 7,8-benzoflavone had smaller effects with three other isozymes (P-450LM2, P-450LM4, and P-450LM3*b*), and surprisingly, it had a stimulatory effect on metabolism when P-450LM3*c* from untreated liver was used. Both 5,6- and 7,8-benzoflavones are inducers of microsomal enzymes as well as inhibitors of the enzyme activity, and different studies have suggested that both the enzyme-inducing (*256*) and enzyme-inhibiting (*255*) activities of flavones can correlate with inhibitory effects on hydrocarbon carcinogenesis.

Somewhat surprising differences between these two flavones were found when their effects on hydrocarbon-initiated skin tumorigenesis were examined. Wattenberg and Leong (*256*) showed that topically applied 5,6-benzoflavone induces the aryl hydrocarbon hydroxylase present in the skin and inhibits skin carcinogenesis elicited by benzo[*a*]pyrene. No enzyme induction is observed after topical application of 7,8-benzoflavone, yet this treatment inhibits skin tumorigenesis initiated by a single dose of 7,12-dimethylbenz[*a*]anthracene by 55–80% (*257–59*) and inhibits covalent binding of this carcinogen to DNA, RNA, and protein in mouse skin by 50–70% (*258, 259*). Under these same conditions, 7,8-benzoflavone does not inhibit skin tumorigenesis that is initiated by a single dose of benzo[*a*]pyrene to any appreciable extent (*258*). It does, however, inhibit the covalent binding of benzo[*a*]pyrene to RNA and protein of skin by about 50% but inhibits covalent binding of this carcinogen to DNA by only 18% (*258*).

The mechanisms of carcinogenesis inhibition by other types of inhibitors are equally complex. For the antioxidants, the initial postulate was that, because they act as free-radical scavengers, inhibition might be through direct reaction with free-radical intermediates produced during polycyclic hydrocarbon metabolism. However, Sullivan et al. (*290*) showed that this was unlikely because antioxidants did not react with free radicals of benzo[*a*]pyrene. Butylated hydroxyanisole and butylated hydroxytoluene do not induce mouse skin aryl hydrocarbon hydroxylase, nor do they affect the activity of this enzyme when added directly to epidermal homogenate metabolizing systems (*272, 291*). However, Speier and

Wattenberg (*292*) have shown that liver microsomes from butylated hydroxyanisole-fed mice are not able to stimulate as much covalent binding of benzo[*a*]pyrene to DNA as control microsomes. The pattern of metabolism of benzo[*a*]pyrene by these microsomes is altered (*293*); activation of benzo[*a*]pyrene through epoxidation is decreased while yields of 3-hydroxybenzo[*a*]pyrene, a detoxification product, are increased. The activities of glutathione-*S*-transferase (*294*), UDP–glucuronyltransferase (*295*), and epoxide hydrolase (*294*) have been shown to increase in butylated hydroxyanisole-fed mice, and these changes could also modify the activation of the carcinogen. Anderson et al. (*296*) have found that the major benzo[*a*]pyrene–deoxyribonucleoside adduct formed in mouse lung following a carcinogenic dose of benzo[*a*]pyrene is decreased by 55% if the animal is treated with butylated hydroxyanisole. This decrease appears to correlate with the inhibition of pulmonary adenoma formation by butylated hydroxyanisole.

Similar types of data have been assembled on the inhibitory properties of halogenated hydrocarbons (reviewed in Refs. 250 and 252) and polycyclic hydrocarbons (reviewed in Refs. 249, 250, and 252). The halogenated hydrocarbon inhibitors and some of the polycyclic hydrocarbon inhibitors are potent inducers of microsomal enzymes. For the halogenated hydrocarbons, their ability to inhibit carcinogenesis correlates well with their ability to induce microsomal enzymes and with a decrease in binding of the carcinogen to DNA. On the other hand, the ability of polycyclic hydrocarbons to inhibit carcinogenesis does not correlate with their ability to induce enzymes. Instead, competition of the inhibitor polycyclic hydrocarbon with the carcinogen polycyclic hydrocarbon seems the most likely mechanism though in neither case is a mechanism firmly established. The inhibition of carcinogenesis by the flavones also could occur through several possible mechanisms.

Overall, the sensitivity of hydrocarbon carcinogenesis to the modifying effects of agents that influence hydrocarbon metabolism in some way suggests that metabolic transformations of these carcinogens are key steps in carcinogenesis, even though a detailed interpretation of the data is not available in all cases.

Proposed Mechanisms for Metabolic Activation. A variety of possible mechanisms through which polynuclear carcinogens might conceivably be converted in vivo to chemically reactive entities that can react with cellular receptors and thereby initiate the carcinogenic process have been considered. Numerous studies of covalent interactions occurring in vitro have been made in the belief that the in vivo covalent binding of polynuclear carcinogens to cellular macromolecules represents an important step in the carcinogenic action of these compounds.

The in vitro studies have involved two general approaches. In the first, various mechanisms through which the parent hydrocarbons themselves may become covalently linked to cellular macromolecules in vitro have been investigated. In the second, specific mechanisms of metabolic activation have been postulated; suitable chemically reactive hydrocarbon derivatives have been prepared; and the chemistry and carcinogenic activities of these derivatives have been investigated.

Benzo[*a*]pyrene is covalently bound to DNA or to DNA constituents after irradiation of mixtures or physical complexes of these components with light at or near the wavelength of the absorption bands of the hydrocarbon (*297, 298*). Covalent interactions similarly occur when hydrocarbon–DNA physical complexes are irradiated with X-rays (*299*), treated with hydrogen peroxide (*300, 301*), treated with iodine (*301, 302*), or exposed to the ascorbic acid model hydroxylating system of Udenfriend et al. (*303*), as described by Lesko et al. (*302*). More detailed studies of the iodine-induced reactions revealed that carcinogenic hydrocarbons are more extensively bound to DNA than are noncarcinogenic hydrocarbons and that iodine-induced binding of benzo[*a*]pyrene occurs more readily with polyguanylic acid than with other homopolyribonucleotides (*304*). Rice (*298*) and Antonello et al. (*305*) thought that the photochemical reaction between benzo[*a*]pyrene and pyrimidines involved the formation of a cyclobutane ring in which the 5,6-double bond of the pyrimidine is fused with a double bond of the hydrocarbon. However, by applying elemental analysis and IR, UV, and NMR spectroscopy, Cavalieri and Calvin (*306*) have shown that the photoproduct from benzo[*a*]pyrene and 1-methylcytosine is, in fact, 6-(1-methylcytos-5-yl)benzo[*a*]pyrene. An analogous structure has been assigned to the major photoproduct from thymine and benzo[*a*]pyrene, although it was thought to be contaminated with an isomeric product in which the thymine is linked to either the 1- or 12-position of the hydrocarbon (*307*). Hoffman and Müller (*308*) reported that one of the products formed by irradiation of benzo[*a*]pyrene and DNA involves the formation of a covalent bond between the 6-position of benzo[*a*]pyrene and the 8-position of guanine nucleotides.

The 6-position of benzo[*a*]pyrene is also involved in the iodine-induced reactions discussed. Benzo[*a*]pyrene forms a charge-transfer complex with iodine, which exhibits a strong electron spin resonance signal (*119, 121*). Furthermore, exposure of benzo[*a*]pyrene to iodine vapor generates the 6,12-, 3,6-, and 1,6-benzo[*a*]pyrene quinones together with benzo[*a*]pyrene dimers linked together through the 6-positions (*309*). The involvement of radical cation intermediates in these reactions was suggested, and in the presence of iodine, benzo[*a*]pyrene was subsequently shown to react covalently with pyridine to yield benzo[*a*]pyren-6-ylpyridinium salts (*310*). Evidence for similar covalent interactions with purines and pyrimidines has also been presented (*311*).

Because the metabolism of polycyclic hydrocarbons is an oxidative process, chemically reactive intermediates or potentially carcinogenic metabolites have been sought in in vitro oxidations of polycyclic hydrocarbons. The study by Jeftic and Adams (*312*) of the electrochemical oxidation of benzo[*a*]pyrene is particularly interesting with respect to the observations on the in vitro covalent interactions of this carcinogen. The initial step in the oxidation involves a one-electron process that yields the benzo[*a*]pyrene radical cation. The cation is consumed either by dimerization to 6,6′-dibenzo[*a*]pyrenyl followed by further oxidation or by reaction with water to form a neutral radical that is oxidized further to 6-hydroxybenzo[*a*]pyrene. The hydroxy compound is then oxidized to a neutral phenoxy radical that is ultimately transformed into a mixture of benzo[*a*]pyrene quinones. Thus, if cellular oxidations occur through analogous mechanisms, a number of reactive radical intermediates (both neutral and cationic) would be generated, and any one of these intermediates could be involved in carcinogenesis.

The one-electron-transfer oxidation of 7,12-dimethylbenz[*a*]anthracene effected by manganese dioxide, ferricyanide, or Ce(IV) has been described by Fried and Schumm (*313*). All the identified reaction products could be accounted for by the generation of the radical cation followed by attack of solvent at the 7- and 12-positions and at the methyl groups. This observation provides an interesting contrast to the iodine-induced reaction of 7,12-dimethylbenz[*a*]anthracene with pyridine, which was reported to yield a 7,12-dimethylbenz[*a*]anthracen-5-ylpyridinium salt (*310*). However, Cavalieri (*314*) reported that the iodine-induced reaction of 7,12-dimethylbenz[*a*]anthracene with pyridine yields a 12-methylbenz-[*a*]anthracenyl-7-methylpyridinium salt, which is more consistent with expectation based on the report of Fried and Schumm (*313*). The binding of hydrocarbons to DNA in the presence of horseradish peroxidase and hydrogen peroxide is thought to involve the intermediacy of one-electron-oxidation products (*315*), and it has been suggested that carcinogenesis in rat mammary gland, in particular, might involve radical cations (*316*).

Miller and Miller (*317*) suggested, by analogy with their findings on the metabolic activation of 2-acetylaminofluorene, that hydroxymethyl metabolites of methyl-substituted hydrocarbons might be esterified to reactive benzylic esters and that these esters could be the carcinogenic metabolites. However, the hydroxymethyl metabolites, like the arene epoxides, are now known to be less carcinogenic than the parent hydrocarbons; therefore, Dipple et al. (*126*) suggested that metabolic precursors of these metabolites might be responsible for the carcinogenic action of polycyclic hydrocarbons. The cationic species of Scheme VI were regarded as possible precursors of the *K*-region epoxides, and arylmethyl cations were regarded as possible precursors of the hydroxymethyl derivatives that are found as metabolites of methyl-substituted hydrocarbons. A good correlation between the calculated stabilities of such arylmethyl cations and carcinogenic potency for the 12 isomeric monomethylbenz[*a*]anthracenes was found (*see* Table III). Also, some experimental support for the postulated involvement of cationic species in the carcinogenic process was obtained when carcinogenic potency for five out of six 7-bromomethylbenz[*a*]anthracenes was found to increase with an increasing tendency to react through a kinetically first-order process (*49*). However, McMahon et al. (*213*) and Grandjean and Cavalieri (*214*) have shown that carbocations are not intermediates in the microsomal conversion of alkylhydrocarbons to alcohols.

The carcinogenic activities of several compounds that could be regarded as models for reactive esters of 7-hydroxymethylbenz[*a*]anthracenes have been studied. Several 7-bromomethylbenz[*a*]anthracenes are carcinogenic in a variety of animal tests (*49, 50, 56*) as are a number of derivatives of 7-hydroxymethyl-12-methylbenz[*a*]anthracene (*55*) (data are presented in Appendix C). Where comparable tests were made, none of these synthetic derivatives was more carcinogenic than the parent hydrocarbon, but Flesher and Sydnor (*318*) have shown that the effective dose of the modified hydrocarbon, in certain cases at least, can be considerably less than that of the parent compound because of differences in transport or diffusion of the two compounds.

The 7-bromomethylbenz[*a*]anthracenes are useful tools for investigating various aspects of chemical carcinogenesis (*319–22*), and the reaction chemistry of both 7-bromomethylbenz[*a*]anthracene and 7-bromomethyl-12-methylbenz[*a*]-anthracene with nucleic acids has been studied (*323, 324*). The reaction of 7-bromomethylbenz[*a*]anthracene with nucleosides in dimethylacetamide results in the aralkylation of ring nitrogens of purine and pyrimidine nucleosides, as is found in studies with most alkylating agents (*325*). However, when reactions with nucleosides or nucleic acids in aqueous solutions are examined, completely different and novel aralkylation products are found that result from substitutions on the amino groups of guanine, adenine, and cytosine residues. These products are also found in DNA of mouse skin that has been exposed to these bromo compounds (*321*), and they represent the first polycyclic hydrocarbon–nucleic acid products to be characterized. This novel chemistry is now known to apply also to the reactions of dihydrodiol epoxides with nucleic acids in aqueous solution and will be discussed later in this chapter.

If DNA is the critical target with which carcinogenic metabolites must react to initiate the carcinogenic process, then the final carcinogenic metabolite of 7-methylbenz[*a*]anthracene could not be an ester of 7-hydroxymethylbenz[*a*]-anthracene. This conclusion follows from the studies of Baird et al. (*326*) who showed that after enzymic conversion to deoxyribonucleosides, the reaction products of 7-bromomethylbenz[*a*]anthracene with DNA are chromatographically separable from analogous products obtained from the DNA of cell cultures that had been exposed to [^{3}H]7-methylbenz[*a*]anthracene.

Another possible mechanism for metabolic activation of polycyclic hydrocarbon carcinogens involves their conversion into free radicals. After stirring benzo[*a*]pyrene with mouse skin homogenates for several days, Nagata et al. (*327*) have observed that a free radical may be detected by electron spin resonance spectroscopy. Furthermore, a radical is similarly produced from another carcinogen, 3-methylcholanthrene, but not from pyrene, phenanthrene, and dibenz-[*a,c*]anthracene. The benzo[*a*]pyrene radical is also obtained after stirring with albumin solution, and the electron spin resonance spectrum of this radical is identical to that of the 6-phenoxy radical obtained by the oxidation of 6-hydroxybenzo[*a*]pyrene (*328*). Photoirradiation of benzo[*a*]pyrene in organic solvents can also yield the 6-phenoxy radical (*329*). This radical is also present in benzene solutions of 6-hydroxybenzo[*a*]pyrene and this benzo[*a*]pyrene metabolite will react covalently with DNA at room temperature (*330*). The chemistry of this interaction has not been elucidated (*331*), but 6-hydroxybenzo[*a*]pyrene does not exhibit carcinogenic activity (Appendix E).

HYDROCARBON *K*-REGION EPOXIDES. As discussed earlier, Boyland (*174*) had postulated that epoxides were intermediates in hydrocarbon metabolism and that their reaction with cellular constituents might be the initiating event in carcinogenesis. This postulate together with the early theoretical studies focusing attention on the *K* regions of hydrocarbons (*86*) and the discovery of the synthetic accessibility of *K*-region epoxides in 1964 (*180*) led to an upsurge in interest in the *K*-region epoxides (Structure **VII**) in the late 1960s and early 1970s.

Initial studies of the carcinogenicity of hydrocarbon *K*-region epoxides were disappointing in that these compounds did not exhibit the high carcinogenic potencies that would have been expected for the carcinogenic metabolites of the hydrocarbon carcinogens, and these epoxides overall were less carcinogenic than their parent hydrocarbons. The carcinogenic activities of 7-methylbenz[*a*]anthracene 5,6-epoxide and benz[*a*]anthracene 5,6-epoxide, which had been synthesized by Newman and Blum (*180*), were compared with the activities of the parent hydrocarbons by Miller and Miller (*317*). 7-Methylbenz[*a*]anthracene 5,6-epoxide was considerably less active than 7-methylbenz[*a*]anthracene after subcutaneous injections in either rats or mice, after repeated topical applications to mice, and in initiation–promotion experiments in mouse skin. In this last system, benz[*a*]-anthracene 5,6-epoxide was slightly more active than benz[*a*]anthracene itself, and this was the only test applied to these compounds. The arene epoxides examined by Boyland and Sims (*57, 216*) were tested only by subcutaneous injection into mice. 3-Methylcholanthrene 11,12-epoxide, dibenz[*a,h*]anthracene 5,6-epoxide, and benz[*a*]anthracene 5,6-epoxide were less active than their parent hydrocarbons while, at the dose levels used, 7-methylbenz[*a*]anthracene 5,6-epoxide and chrysene 5,6-epoxide evoked tumor incidences comparable with those of the parent hydrocarbons. However, the latent period was longer for the epoxides. Van Duuren et al. (*332*) showed that the *K*-region epoxides of phenanthrene, 7-methylbenz[*a*]anthracene, and dibenz[*a,h*]anthracene exhibit initiating activity in mouse skin but that this activity is rather feeble compared with that of dibenz[*a,h*]anthracene. These initial reports were published in 1967, and although the simple interpretation was that the hydrocarbons did not express their carcinogenic activities through metabolic conversion to *K*-region epoxides, it was possible that these reactive compounds were destroyed before reaching the appropriate receptors in the target tissues and that the simple interpretation of these data was incorrect. This possibility had to be weighed even more carefully after the later experimental demonstrations that (1) epoxides are intermediates in hydrocarbon metabolism (*183*); (2) *K*-region epoxides of several hydrocarbons are formed in microsomal systems (*333–36*); (3) *K*-region epoxides react with DNA, RNA, and histone in vitro (*337*) and bind to DNA, RNA, and proteins in cells in culture (*338, 339*); (4) several *K*-region epoxides are more effective than their parent hydrocarbons in effecting malignant transformation of cells in culture (*340–42*); and (5) several *K*-region epoxides evoke mutations in mammalian cells in culture (*343*), in bacteriophage (*344*), in bacteria (*345*), and in *Drosophila* (*346*). Many more recent studies have confirmed these earlier findings of the comparatively weak carcinogenic potency of *K*-region epoxides (*347–50*) and of their mutagenic activities in various systems (*351–56*), but the balance of evidence supporting their potential role as the carcinogenic metabolites of the hydrocarbons was drastically altered in a negative sense by developments in the investigation of hydrocarbon–DNA interactions.

In 1973, Baird et al. (*326*) were able to demonstrate that the products of interaction of the *K*-region epoxide of 7-methylbenz[*a*]anthracene with DNA in vitro were different from the DNA adducts that were formed when 7-methylbenz[*a*]anthracene was metabolically activated for DNA binding in cells in culture. Thus, if the interactions with DNA were responsible for initiation of carcinogenic action, then the *K*-region epoxide could not be the carcinogenic metabolite. Similar observations have since been reported for other hydrocarbons (*141, 357–60*), but most of these observations followed the discovery of the dihydrodiol epoxide route of activation of hydrocarbon carcinogens (*141*).

DIHYDRODIOL EPOXIDES: DNA-BINDING STUDIES. The synthesis and carcinogenic activities of dihydrodiols and vicinal dihydrodiol epoxides are discussed in subsequent sections of this chapter. This section will focus on the DNA binding studies that, for many hydrocarbons, provided the initial evidence for the existence of dihydrodiol epoxide metabolites.

Following the demonstration of a correlation between carcinogenic potency and extent of binding to DNA in mouse skin for a series of polycyclic hydrocarbons (*238*), Brookes et al. showed that rodent embryo cells in culture represent a convenient system for obtaining DNA that is modified by polycyclic hydrocarbons (*245, 361, 362*). They developed procedures for the enzymic degradation of such DNA and for the chromatographic analysis of the resulting hydrocarbon–nucleoside adducts (*326, 361, 363*). It was presumed that the DNA interaction was a key event in carcinogenesis and by identifying the metabolite responsible for DNA binding, the metabolite responsible for carcinogenic activity was also being identified. Using these methodologies, Baird et al. (*326*) in 1973 were able to demonstrate that the DNA-binding metabolite formed from 7-methylbenz[*a*]anthracene in mammalian cells was not the *K*-region epoxide.

In the same year, Borgen et al. (*364*) reported their findings on the microsome-catalyzed binding of benzo[*a*]pyrene and various *trans*-dihydrodiol metabolites of benzo[*a*]pyrene to DNA. The relative extents of binding were 3 for the 9,10-dihydrodiol, 5 for the 4,5-dihydrodiol, 11 for benzo[*a*]pyrene itself, and 168 for the 7,8-dihydrodiol. Because the binding to DNA was more than an order of magnitude greater for the 7,8-dihydrodiol than for benzo[*a*]pyrene itself, these authors concluded that the 7,8-dihydrodiol was an intermediate in the activation of benzo[*a*]pyrene for DNA binding and that this dihydrodiol must be further metabolized to yield an active alkylating agent. Based on this report, Sims and his colleagues (*141, 365*) conceived the idea that for the case of the 7,8-dihydrodiol of benzo[*a*]pyrene (and analogous derivatives of other hydrocarbons, such as the 8,9-dihydrodiol of benz[*a*]anthracene), a second microsomal oxidation occurred on the double bond adjacent to the dihydrodiol to yield a vicinal dihydrodiol epoxide (Scheme XI) that might be the species responsible for reaction with DNA and perhaps for carcinogenic activity. Using the chromatographic techniques developed in Brookes' laboratory (*363*) and an *m*-chloroperoxybenzoic acid oxidation of radioactive benzo[*a*]pyrene 7,8-dihydrodiol to generate a crude preparation of the benzo[*a*]pyrene dihydrodiol epoxide, Sims et al. (*141*) were able to show that the dihydrodiol epoxide reacted with DNA in vitro to yield products that were similar to or identical with those formed when rodent embryo cells were exposed to the parent hydrocarbon, benzo[*a*]pyrene. While this study did not address the question of which stereoisomers of the 7,8-dihydrodiol 9,10-epoxide (Structures **VIIIC–VIIIF** and Scheme X) were responsible for DNA binding, the conclusion (Scheme XI) that benzo[*a*]pyrene is metabolically activated for DNA binding by conversion to the *trans*-7,8-dihydrodiol, as suggested by Borgen et al. (*364*), followed by further conversion to a vicinal dihydrodiol epoxide, as suggested by Sims et al. (*141*), has proven to be correct (reviewed in Ref. 163).

Fluorescence spectroscopy, which played a key role in identifying benzo[*a*]-pyrene as a carcinogenic constituent of coal tar some 50 years ago, has very recently been a valuable aid in determining which metabolites of hydrocarbons become covalently bound to DNA in mammalian systems. Using a specially constructed photon-counting spectrophotofluorometer, Daudel et al. (*366*) were able to show that the fluorescence emission spectrum of hydrocarbon residues

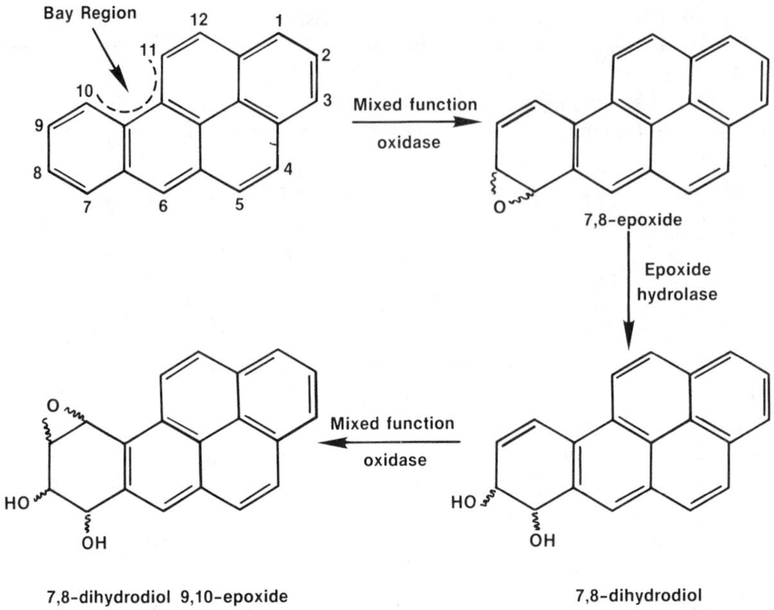

Bay Region 12 1 11 2 10 3 9 8 4 7 6 5 Mixed function oxidase 7,8-epoxide Epoxide hydrolase Mixed function oxidase 7,8-dihydrodiol 9,10-epoxide 7,8-dihydrodiol

*Scheme XI. The dihydrodiol epoxide route of metabolic activation of benzo[*a*]pyrene* (141, 364).

attached to DNA from mouse skin, which had been exposed in vivo to benzo[*a*]pyrene, was very similar to that for DNA reacted in vitro with the 7,8-dihydrodiol 9,10-epoxide. A similar result was subsequently reported by Ivanovic et al. (*367*), but these investigators demonstrated that commercially available fluorescence spectrophotometers were capable of detecting the low levels of hydrocarbons bound to DNA in cellular systems (~ 1 hydrocarbon per 10^5 nucleotides). While studies of this nature and further studies of the binding of dihydrodiols to DNA (*368*) were consistent with the 7,8-dihydrodiol 9,10-epoxide mechanism for DNA binding, the critical confirmatory information arose from the chemical synthesis and characterization of this dihydrodiol epoxide (*369–71*). In the reports from Jerina's laboratory (*370*) and Harvey's laboratory (*371*), both the *syn*- and the *anti*-7,8-dihydrodiol 9,10-epoxide stereoisomers were described. These well-characterized preparations were used to prepare markers through reactions with DNA in vitro, and benzo[*a*]pyrene–DNA binding was shown to occur primarily through the *anti*-7,8-dihydrodiol 9,10-epoxide in mammalian cells in culture (*372, 373*) or in mouse skin in vivo (*228*), although some products arose through the intermediacy of the *syn*-isomer. The *syn*-isomer can be a major contributor to DNA binding in hamster embryo cells at relatively short exposure times (4–6 h), but by 24 h, binding through the *anti*-isomer predominates (*229*). Some caution is needed, therefore, in making generalizations, but under the conditions of the following studies, the *anti*-isomer of benzo[*a*]pyrene-7,8-dihydrodiol 9,10-epoxide is responsible for the majority of benzo[*a*]pyrene–DNA or benzo[*a*]pyrene–RNA binding observed in such diverse systems as mouse skin in vivo (*228, 374*); rat skin in vivo

(*374*); mouse lung and liver in vivo (*296, 375, 376*); tracheobronchial tissues from mice, rats, hamsters, and cows (*377–79*); cultured human bronchial tissue (*378, 379*); cultured human esophagus (*380*), colon (*381*), and peripheral lung tissue (*382*); cultured rodent embryo cells (*229, 373, 383, 384*); rat hepatocytes (*385*); mouse cells (*386*); human alveolar tumor cells (*382*); and WI-38 human fibroblasts (*387*).

Although in intact mammalian cells, the vast majority of benzo[*a*]pyrene–DNA binding clearly arises through isomeric forms of the 7,8-dihydrodiol 9,10-epoxide, the active metabolites for other hydrocarbons are less clearly defined. Naturally, once the involvement of a dihydrodiol epoxide in benzo[*a*]pyrene metabolism was recognized, it was reasonable to anticipate the formation of such metabolites from other hydrocarbons. Booth and Sims described an 8,9-dihydrodiol 10,11-epoxide of benz[*a*]anthracene (*365*) at the same time that the benzo[*a*]pyrene work was reported. For benz[*a*]anthracene (*see* Structure **V** for numbering system) one could envisage three other vicinal dihydrodiol epoxides, i.e., the 10,11-dihydrodiol 8,9-epoxide, the 1,2-dihydrodiol 3,4-epoxide, and the 3,4-dihydrodiol 1,2-epoxide, but which of these might be most likely to be the key reactive intermediate was not immediately obvious.

A generalization described by Jerina and Daly (*76*) has been most helpful in this regard. They examined structure–mouse skin carcinogenicity data for hydrocarbons, particularly with respect to the effects of methyl and fluoro substitutions and observed that these structure–activity relationships would be expected if the vicinal dihydrodiol epoxide that was responsible for biological activity was formed in the angular ring, i.e., the 1,2,3,4-ring in the case of benz[*a*]anthracene. Furthermore, because the epoxide ring in the active metabolite of benzo[*a*]pyrene is immediately adjacent to a bay region, they suggested that such bay-region dihydrodiol epoxides (Structure **VI**A) may be the active metabolites of hydrocarbons in most cases. For benz[*a*]anthracene, this metabolite would be the 3,4-dihydrodiol 1,2-epoxide. Overall, this generalization has held remarkably well; the presently available evidence indicates that DNA binding usually occurs through a bay-region dihydrodiol epoxide and that the most carcinogenic metabolites for any given hydrocarbon seem to be the dihydrodiol precursors of the bay-region dihydrodiol epoxides and the epoxides themselves.

In the specific case of benz[*a*]anthracene, discordant reports appear in the literature. While the tumor initiating activities of the 3,4-dihydrodiol and the 3,4-dihydrodiol 1,2-epoxide are consistent with the bay-region dihydrodiol epoxide generalization (explained further in the next section), workers from Sims' laboratory have argued that DNA binding in mouse skin or in hamster embryo cell cultures occurs primarily through the 8,9-dihydrodiol 10,11-epoxide (*388–90*). In their studies, chromatographic comparisons were made between the benz[*a*]anthracene products formed in cellular systems and the products of reaction of 8,9,10,11-ring dihydrodiol epoxide with DNA in vitro. However, when these authors included a 3,4-dihydrodiol 1,2-epoxide-modified DNA marker in their studies (*391*), they found that these bay-region dihydrodiol epoxide products were not separable from the 8,9-dihydrodiol 10,11-epoxide adducts except by derivatization and further chromatography. It was then possible to observe that binding through both the bay-region and non-bay-region dihydrodiol epoxides was

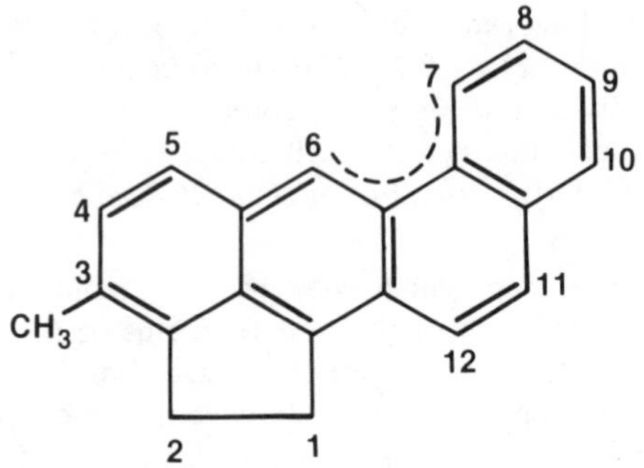

X

occurring for benz[*a*]anthracene (*391*) even though fluorescence studies (*389*) suggested that only an 8,9-dihydrodiol 10,11-epoxide was involved. Benz[*a*]anthracene is only a weak carcinogen, and this is reflected in low levels of binding to DNA (*238*). This low binding, in conjunction with the difficulties experienced in efficiently degrading this bound material to deoxyribonucleosides for chromatographic analysis (*388*), can complicate DNA analyses of this type, and further work may be needed to clarify the benz[*a*]anthracene–DNA interactions.

Several laboratories have investigated the nature of the products obtained when 3-methylcholanthrene (**X**) is bound to DNA in cells in culture or mouse tissues in vivo and all report data that are consistent with the proposal that bay region dihydrodiol epoxide (i.e., 9,10-dihydrodiol 7,8-epoxide) intermediates are responsible for DNA binding (*360, 375, 392–96*). Fluorescence spectra of DNA from mouse skin exposed to 3-methylcholanthrene (*392*), of 3-methylcholanthrene–deoxyribonucleoside adducts obtained from mouse skin DNA (*396*), and of mouse embryo cell DNA (*360*) all resemble the fluorescence of anthracene; this finding suggests that binding occurs through a dihydrodiol epoxide generated in the 7,8,9,10-ring. Two metabolites of 3-methylcholanthrene—tentatively identified as the 9,10-dihydrodiol—and the 9,10-dihydrodiol carrying a hydroxyl group on either the 1- or 2-position or on the 3-methyl substituent (*393*) can bind to DNA in the presence of a microsomal system to yield DNA adducts that seem, by chromatography, to be the same as those adducts formed from the parent hydrocarbon in cellular systems (*360*). Thus, both the bay-region dihydrodiol epoxide of 3-methylcholanthrene and of a hydroxylated metabolite of 3-methylcholanthrene have been implicated in DNA binding, but a more precise characterization of these DNA adducts probably will require the synthesis of the appropriate reactive intermediates.

The limited evidence for the structure of the 7-methylbenz[*a*]anthracene metabolite involved in DNA binding is again consistent with the bay-region dihydrodiol epoxide generalization. Fluorescence measurements on DNA, to which this hydrocarbon has been bound in cellular systems (*397*), or on 7-methylbenz[*a*]anthracene–deoxyribonucleoside adducts isolated from such DNA (*398*) indicate that an anthracene fluorophore is present, as would be expected if binding occurs through the bay-region 3,4-dihydrodiol 1,2-epoxide. In concert with these findings, both the 1,2-dihydrodiol and the 3,4-dihydrodiol, but not the

8,9-dihydrodiol, bind to the DNA of mouse skin in vivo (*399*). Also, the chromatographic properties of deoxyribonucleoside adducts obtained from treatment of DNA with the bay-region 3,4-dihydrodiol 1,2-epoxide resemble those of the metabolically generated 7-methylbenz[*a*]anthracene–deoxyribonucleoside adducts more closely than do those of the adducts derived from the 1,2-dihydrodiol 3,4-epoxide (*399*). However, the present evidence is again insufficient to constitute a proof that the bay-region dihydrodiol epoxide is the only metabolite involved in the binding of 7-methylbenz[*a*]anthracene to DNA in cellular systems.

7,12-Dimethylbenz[*a*]anthracene is perhaps the most potent of the hydrocarbon carcinogens, and it differs from the hydrocarbons discussed previously in that it carries a methyl substituent, the 12-methyl group, in the bay region. Nevertheless, the present weight of evidence suggests that the bay-region dihydrodiol epoxide is responsible for the metabolism-mediated binding of this carcinogen to DNA in cellular systems. The photosensitivity of 7,12-dimethylbenz-[*a*]anthracene–DNA adducts formed in hamster embryo cells provided the first clue that a bay-region dihydrodiol epoxide might be the active metabolite for this carcinogen (*400*). Moschel et al. were able to confirm that the 1,2,3,4-ring is saturated during the binding process by showing that the fluorescence spectra of 7,12-dimethylbenz[*a*]anthracene–deoxyribonucleoside adducts that were obtained from mouse embryo cells are derived from a dimethylanthracene fluorophore (*401*). The fluorescence of 7,12-dimethylbenz[*a*]anthracene-modified DNA from mouse skin (*392*) or from hamster embryo cells (*402*) is also consistent with this interpretation. The inhibition of DNA binding in mouse embryo cells by an inhibitor of epoxide hydrolase (*see* Scheme XI) suggests that a dihydrodiol epoxide is responsible for DNA binding (*403*). Evidence that the bay-region 3,4-dihydrodiol 1,2-epoxide is largely responsible for DNA binding, rather than a 1,2-dihydrodiol 3,4-epoxide, can be derived (1) from fluorescence data (*398*); (2) from the fact that microsome-catalyzed binding to DNA is higher for the *trans*-3,4-dihydrodiol than for 7,12-dimethylbenz[*a*]anthracene itself (*404*); and (3) from comparisons of the chromatographic (*405*) and fluorescence (*406*) properties of 7,12-dimethylbenz[*a*]anthracene–deoxyribonucleoside adducts with those of products generated from DNA and a crude preparation of the 3,4-dihydrodiol 1,2-epoxide. It has been suggested that oxidation at the 7-methyl group to yield a 7-hydroxymethyl metabolite might precede dihydrodiol epoxide formation in the activation of 7,12-dimethylbenz[*a*]anthracene (*402*). However this is not a major pathway in mouse skin or in mouse embryo cell cultures, because treatment with the hydroxymethyl derivative leads to products that are different from those obtained with the parent hydrocarbon (*407, 408*).

Another carcinogen with a methyl group in the bay region is 15, 16-dihydro-11-methylcyclopenta[*a*]phenanthren-13-one (*409*) (*see* Structure **III**C for numbering system). Abbott and Coombs (*410*) have shown that the major hydrocarbon–deoxyribonucleoside adduct formed in mouse skin is also formed with calf thymus DNA and a microsomal system. The ability to generate this adduct in subcellular systems allowed them to show that the 3,4-dihydrodiol was an intermediate in the formation of this adduct. Also, through application of pyrolysis–electron impact mass-analyzed ion kinetic energy spectrometry to calf thymus

DNA that was modified with the carcinogen in vitro, Wiebers et al. (*411*) were able to develop structural evidence suggesting that the major adduct that was formed resulted from reaction of the bay-region dihydrodiol epoxide (i.e., the 3,4-dihydrodiol 1,2-epoxide) on the amino group of guanine residues in DNA.

Binding of other polycyclic compounds to DNA has been reported in the literature, but there is little evidence so far relating to the structures of the metabolites responsible for binding. No radioactive hydrocarbon–deoxyribonucleoside adducts were detectable in DNA from mouse skin that was exposed to radioactive dibenz[*a,c*]anthracene (*412*), but some adducts were formed in hamster embryo cells (*413*). Products from DNA treated with the non-bay-region 10,11-dihydrodiol 12,13-epoxide in vitro elute in the same region of Sephadex LH-20 chromatograms as the hamster embryo cell adducts, but the elution profiles are not identical (*413*). Even less structural information is available on DNA adducts with other compounds, such as dibenz[*a,h*]anthracene (*412, 414*), dibenzo[*a,e*]fluoranthrene (*415, 416*), and benzo[*e*]pyrene (*417*).

The study of the DNA binding of polycyclic hydrocarbons, insofar as it has led to the recognition of dihydrodiol epoxide metabolites, has had a major impact on the direction of research in hydrocarbon carcinogenesis. Some DNA binding studies have not, however, produced substantial and definitive results. Several major technical difficulties are associated with such studies; for instance the relatively low levels of binding to DNA that occur in cellular systems. These levels depend on the hydrocarbon involved (*238, 362*). For 7,12-dimethylbenz[*a*]anthracene, which binds the most extensively to DNA, binding on the order of one hydrocarbon per 10^4 nucleotides can be obtained, but for other hydrocarbons, binding can be less than one hydrocarbon per 10^6 nucleotides. A second problem is that the radioactivity associated with DNA is not always efficiently converted by enzymic hydrolysis to products that behave like hydrocarbon–deoxyribonucleoside adducts; therefore, in some of the analyses discussed, the radioactive products studied by chromatography are not definitively proven to be representative of the total DNA binding. With the exception of work on the benzo[*a*]pyrene bay-region dihydrodiol epoxide, the dihydrodiol epoxides used in DNA studies often constitute solutions of a dihydrodiol incubated with *m*-chloroperoxybenzoic acid, rather than a dihydrodiol epoxide that has been isolated and fully characterized. The reason for using such solutions is, of course, the limited availability of the dihydrodiols in most cases.

Larger quantities of material can usually be obtained from microsomal incubations with exogenous DNA than from intact cellular systems. Such systems are useful in binding dihydrodiol metabolites to DNA, but microsomal incubations with the parent hydrocarbons usually result in the formation of products that differ qualitatively and/or quantitatively from those formed in intact tissues or cells (*358, 359, 410, 418*). Bigger et al. have found that, in contrast to cellular systems, the nature of the products formed in the microsomal systems varies with substrate concentration (*419–22*), and these limitations restrict the substitution of microsomal systems for cellular systems to specific cases (*410*). Of course, it is not absolutely certain that carcinogen–DNA interactions are a critical component of the carcinogenic process, despite the wealth of circumstantial evidence now supportive of this. Clearly, more than these interactions are required, because Phillips et al. (*395*) found that the different susceptibilities of different strains of mice to hydrocarbon carcinogenesis are not reflected in differences in DNA binding nor are the different susceptibilities of mouse and rat skin (*374*). Carcinogenesis is clearly complex, and different susceptibilities to the promotional stages of carcinogenesis could rationalize these findings with a mutational mechanism of carcinogenesis.

In summary, hydrocarbon–DNA interactions in cellular systems have been studied extensively, but technical limitations make the findings less definitive than can be considered ideal. Nevertheless, these studies provide strong indications that the bay-region dihydrodiol epoxide metabolites of several different hydrocarbons are responsible for most of the interactions with DNA in intact tissues or cellular systems. In the case of benz[*a*]anthracene, a non-bay-region dihydrodiol epoxide may also be involved, and in the case of benzo[*a*]pyrene, minor products have also been attributed to modification of DNA by the *K*-region epoxide (*423, 424*) and by the *K*-region epoxide of 9-hydroxybenzo[*a*]pyrene (*423–25*).

Tumorigenic Properties of Hydrocarbon Metabolites and Related Compounds

With the exception of the *K*-region epoxides of several hydrocarbons, few hydrocarbon metabolites had been subjected to evaluations of biological activity prior to 1976. This situation has changed dramatically in the past 6–7 years, and the benzo[*a*]pyrene derivatives, in particular, have been assayed for many different biological activities. The hydrocarbons are included in this volume because of their carcinogenicity, so we have focused on this specific biological activity. This selection of material from the literature is further justified by the fact that our present concept of the role played in the carcinogenic process by *K*-region epoxides of hydrocarbons is consistent with their carcinogenic properties, not, for example, with their mutagenic or cytotoxic properties (*see* earlier discussion). Nevertheless, some fascinating studies of the mutagenicity of hydrocarbon derivatives have been reported, and this literature can be located through several excellent reviews, such as that by Levin et al. (*426*). In collecting information on the tumorigenic properties of hydrocarbon derivatives, comparative studies of derivatives and the parent hydrocarbons have been selected, and in the following tables, the tumorigenic activities of derivatives related to the activity of the parent compounds tested under the same conditions are presented. This approach permits a ready evaluation of whether a given metabolite is more carcinogenic than the parent hydrocarbon. This has long been considered to be a property that should be exhibited by metabolites responsible for carcinogenic activity.

The majority of studies on the carcinogenic properties of benzo[*a*]pyrene derivatives have involved (1) repeated applications of the test compound to the skin of female mice (complete carcinogenesis in skin); or (2) initiation of the skin of female mice by a single dose of the test compound followed by promotion with 12-*O*-tetradecanoylphorbol 13-acetate (TPA); or (3) intraperitoneal injection of several doses of test compound in newborn mice. Data from these different assays are tabulated separately (Tables VI, VII, and VIII) but not every test or dose level reported has been included.

Of the benzo[*a*]pyrene epoxides tested in the complete carcinogenesis assay on mouse skin (Table VI), only benzo[*a*]pyrene 7,8-epoxide exhibits substantial activity relative to that of benzo[*a*]pyrene. Even this epoxide is less potent than benzo[*a*]pyrene itself. While the parent compound and the 7,8-epoxide both yield tumors in almost 100% of the mice at a dose of 0.4 μmol every 2 weeks, the incidence for the epoxide at a 0.15-μmol dose falls to 18%, but remains at 100% for the parent compound. Even a 0.1-μmol repetitive dose of benzo[*a*]pyrene yields tumors in 94% of the treated animals, while fewer than 10% of the animals develop tumors at this dose of the 7,8-epoxide.

In contrast to these findings, *trans*-7,8-dihydro-7,8-dihydroxybenzo[*a*]pyrene, which is the metabolic product of the action of epoxide hydrolase on the 7,8-epoxide, exhibits comparable carcinogenicity with that of benzo[*a*]pyrene at 0.15- and 0.1-μmol doses but clearly exceeds the activity of the parent hydrocarbon at a 0.025-μmol dose in this system. Moreover, tests of the pure enantiomeric 7,8-dihydrodiols indicate that the (−)-enantiomer is largely responsible for this biological activity. The 7,8,9,10-tetrahydro-7,8-diol is inactive as a carcinogen, and this finding indicates that the 9,10-double bond is necessary for the carcinogenic activity of the *trans*-7,8-dihydrodiol (*431*). In this system, the *trans*-7,8-dihydrodiol is the only benzo[*a*]pyrene metabolite with demonstrably greater carcinogenic potency than benzo[*a*]pyrene; tests of the *syn*-7,8-dihydrodiol 9,10-epoxide revealed no activity at all, and the stereoisomeric *anti*-dihydrodiol epoxide exhibited only weak activity.

In addition to the findings summarized in Table VI, all of the 12 hydroxybenzo[*a*]pyrenes (phenols) have been examined in this system (*429, 433*). At a 0.4-μmol repetitive dose, only two of the isomeric phenols, 11-hydroxybenzo[*a*]-pyrene and 2-hydroxybenzo[*a*]pyrene, induced any tumors at all. The 11-hydroxy compound yielded tumors in only 14% of the treated animals, but the 2-hydroxy isomer yielded a 100% tumor incidence at this dose as did benzo[*a*]pyrene itself (*429*). The parent compound also yielded an almost 100% tumor incidence at a 0.1-μmol repetitive dose (*427*); studies at lower dose levels of 2-hydroxybenzo[*a*]pyrene were not reported initially. Subsequently, doses of 0.1, 0.05, and 0.025 μmol of 2-hydroxybenzo[*a*]pyrene and benzo[*a*]pyrene were compared, and the carcinogenic activities of these two compounds were found to be similar through this dose range (*434*).

In summary, studies with the complete carcinogenesis system in mouse skin have demonstrated that (1) benzo[*a*]pyrene 7,8-epoxide exhibits substantial activity, but is less potent than benzo[*a*]pyrene; (2) 2-hydroxybenzo[*a*]pyrene is of comparable potency with that of benzo[*a*]pyrene itself; and (3) the activity of the racemic 7,8-dihydrodiol (attributed primarily to the (−)-enantiomer) demonstrably exceeds that of benzo[*a*]pyrene.

A very wide range of benzo[*a*]pyrene derivatives have been examined in the initiation–promotion system in mouse skin, and some of these findings are summarized in Table VII. As in the studies using repeated application to mouse skin, benzo[*a*]pyrene 7,8-epoxide is more potent than the other arene epoxides tested, though the other epoxides do exhibit some activity in this system. Somewhat surprisingly, the 4,5-dihydrodiol and 9,10-dihydrodiol have exhibited some activity in this system. As in the other skin system, the 7,8-dihydrodiol is the most active derivative tested to date with the (−)-enantiomer again demonstrating greater activity than the (+)-enantiomer and yielding an initiating potency comparable with that of benzo[*a*]pyrene itself. The racemic *syn*-7,8-dihydrodiol

Table VI

Carcinogenic Activity of Derivatives of Benzo[*a*]pyrene in the Skin of Female C57BL/7J Mice

		Activity of Derivative/ Activity of Parent Compound		
Benzo[a]pyrene Derivative	*Dose*[a] *(μmol)*	*Percent of Mice with Tumors*	*Total No. of Tumors*	*Ref.*
4,5-Epoxide	0.1	6/94	2/46	427
	0.4	3/100	1/44	427
7,8-Epoxide	0.1	9/94	3/46	427
	0.15	18/100	5/40	428
	0.4	94/100	52/44	427
9,10-Epoxide	0.1 or 0.4	0/100	0/44	427
11,12-Epoxide	0.1 or 0.4	0/100	0/34	429
(±)-9,10-Dihydrodiol	0.15	0/97	0/38	430
(±)-7,8-Dihydrodiol	0.025	22/7	7/2	431
	0.1	92/91	28/24	431
	0.15	100/100	39/40	428
(+)-7,8-Dihydrodiol	0.1	5/100	1/24	432
(−)-7,8-Dihydrodiol	0.1	100/100	24/24	432
(±)-*syn*-7,8-Dihydrodiol 9,10-epoxide	0.02, 0.1, or 0.4	0/100	0/40	431
(±)-*anti*-7,8-Dihydrodiol 9,10-epoxide	0.02	0/4	0/1	431
	0.1	7/50	2/15	431
	0.4	13/100	3/40	431

[a]Indicated dose was administered once every 2 weeks for 60 weeks.

9,10-epoxide has proved to be a weak initiator, as have the pure (+)- and (−)-enantiomers, and the activity of the racemic *anti*-7,8-dihydrodiol 9,10-epoxide seems to be attributable to the (+)-enantiomer. This (+)-enantiomer exhibits substantial activity that approaches but does not equal that of benzo[*a*]pyrene itself. The activity of the *anti*-dihydrodiol epoxide varies substantially with the solvent in which it is administered. Its activity was found to be almost twice as high when tetrahydrofuran was used as solvent instead of acetone (*438*), but even in tetrahydrofuran, its activity is less than that of the parent compound. The 12 isomeric phenols have also been tested in the initiation–promotion system (*441*). More of them demonstrated some activity than in the other skin assay, but again the 2- and 11-hydroxybenzo[*a*]pyrenes are the most active. With an initiating dose of 0.4 μmol, benzo[*a*]pyrene produced papillomas in 90% of surviving mice with an average of 8.4 papillomas per surviving mouse. For the 11-hydroxy compound, these values were 72% and 2.8, and for the 2-hydroxy compound, they were 78% and 8.5.

Table VII

Tumor-Initiating Activity of Benzo[*a*]pyrene Derivatives in Swiss CD-1 and Sencar Female Mice

			Activity of Derivative/Activity of Parent Compound[a]			
Benzo[a]pyrene Derivative	*Dose (μmol)*	*Micrograms of TPA (treatments per week)*	*Time (weeks)*	*Percent of Mice with Tumors*	*Papilloma per Mouse*	*Ref.*
4,5-Epoxide	0.2	10 (2)	23	0.21	0.04	435
4,5-Dihydrodiol	0.087	1 (3)	27	0.35	0.29	436
9,10-Epoxide	0.2	10 (2)	30	0.16	0.04	437
9,10-Dihydrodiol	0.087	1 (3)	27	0.17	0.35	436
	0.4	10 (2)	30	0.14	0.01	438
11,12-Epoxide	0.2	10 (2)	30	0.41	0.08	437
7,8-Epoxide	0.2	10 (2)	23	0.86	0.4	435
(±)-7,8-Dihydrodiol	0.2	10 (2)	23	0.95	0.96	435
	0.087	1 (3)	27	0.74	0.56	436
(+)-7,8-Dihydrodiol	0.1	10 (2)	21	0.30	0.17	439
(−)-7,8-Dihydrodiol	0.1	10 (2)	21	1.0	1.46	439
(±)-*syn*-7,8-Dihydrodiol 9,10-epoxide	0.2	10 (2)	30	0.08	0.01	437
(−)-*syn*-7,8-Dihydrodiol	0.1	10 (2)	24	0.15	0.05	440
9,10-epoxide	0.1	5 (2)**	24	0.15	0.05	440
(+)-*syn*-7,8-Dihydrodiol	0.1	10 (2)	24	0.25	0.08	440
9,10-epoxide	0.1	5 (2)**	24	0.12	0.04	440
(±)-*anti*-7,8-Dihydrodiol	0.2	10 (2)	23	0.23	0.08	435
9,10-epoxide	0.4	10 (2)	30	0.3	0.04	438
	0.2	10 (2)	30	0.75	0.28	437
(−)-*anti*-7,8-Dihydrodiol	0.1	10 (2)	24	0.09	0.03	440
9,10-epoxide	0.1	5 (2)**	24	0.03	0.01	440
(+)-*anti*-7,8-Dihydrodiol	0.1	10 (2)	24	0.69	0.52	440
9,10-epoxide	0.1	5 (2)**	24	0.87	0.71	440

NOTE: Most of these studies involved Swiss CD-1 mice. Those that involved Sencar mice are indicated by the presence of ** in the TPA column.
[a]The values for % of mice with tumors and papillomas/mouse for benzo[*a*]pyrene are: 94%, 4.8 (*435*); 77%, 3.4 (*436*); 92%, 5.3 (*437*); 90%, 7.5 (*438*); and 77%, 2.6 (*439*); CD-1 mice, 68%, 2.1, Sencar mice, 86%, 2.8 (*440*). These control values and the tabulated data above allow the experimental data to be readily generated.

To summarize the relative activities in this system, the (−)-enantiomer of *trans*-7,8-dihydro-7,8-dihydroxybenzo[*a*]pyrene apparently has the highest tumor-initiating activity of the derivatives tested and, at a 0.1-μmol dose, this activity is similar to that of the parent hydrocarbon benzo[*a*]pyrene (Table VII). At a higher dose of 0.4 μmol, 2-hydroxybenzo[*a*]pyrene also exhibits activity comparable with that of benzo[*a*]pyrene, but whether it has a comparable activity at a lower dose is not known. Although none of the bay-region dihydrodiol epoxides exhibits the same activity as benzo[*a*]pyrene or the 7,8-dihydrodiol, the (+)-enantiomer of the *anti*-stereoisomer is the most active compound in this class.

Table VIII

Lung Adenomas Induced by Benzo[*a*]pyrene Derivatives After Intraperitoneal Injection in Newborn Swiss–Webster Mice

			Activity of Derivative/ Activity of Parent Compound		
Benzo[a]pyrene Derivative	*Total Dose (μmol)*	*Time (weeks)*	*Percent of Mice with Adenoma*	*Adenomas per Mouse*	*Ref.*
4,5-Epoxide	1.4	24	2/85	0.02/9.92	442
9,10-Epoxide	1.4	24	0/85	0/9.92	442
11,12-Epoxide	1.4	24	12/85	0.24/9.92	442
7,8-Epoxide	1.4	24	64/85	2.0 /9.92	442
(±)-7,8-Dihydrodiol	0.028	28	57/7	1.64/0.11	443
	1.4	17	90/64	59 /4.03	444
(+)-7,8-Dihydrodiol	1.4	17	84/64	18.4 /4.03	444
(−)-7,8-Dihydrodiol	1.4	17	90/64[a]	4.9 /4.03[a]	444
(±)-*syn*-7,8-Dihydrodiol 9,10-epoxide	0.028	28	0/7	0/0.11	443
(−)-*syn*-7,8-Dihydrodiol 9,10-epoxide	0.014	34–37	11/4	0.13/0.03	445
(+)-*syn*-7,8-Dihydrodiol 9,10-epoxide	0.014	34–37	4/4	0.22/0.03	445
(±)-*anti*-7,8-Dihydrodiol 9,10-epoxide	0.028	28	74/7	4.29/0.11	443
(−)-*anti*-7,8-Dihydrodiol 9,10-epoxide	0.014	34–37	1/4	0.01/0.03	445
(+)-*anti*-7,8-Dihydrodiol 9,10-epoxide	0.014	34–37	89/4	7.55/0.03	445

NOTE: In this system, a spontaneous adenoma incidence ranging from 8 to 12% of surviving mice with adenomas and 0.08–0.13 adenomas/mouse is found. The appropriate control value has been subtracted from the data for each test compound to generate the numbers given in the table.

[a]Only two animals survived to 17 weeks. At lower doses of 0.7 and 0.14 μmol, 29 and 46 mice survived yielding corrected values of 90 and 88% of mice with adenomas and 32.1 and 9.18 adenomas/mouse, respectively. The (+)-enantiomer gave values of 44% (2.25) and 6% (0.06) at the 0.7 and 0.14-μmol doses. These data are not tabulated because benzo[*a*]pyrene was not tested at these doses.

Quite different conclusions result from consideration of data on lung adenomas induced by three intraperitoneal injections in newborn mice (Table VIII). Again, benzo[*a*]pyrene 7,8-epoxide is the most active of the arene epoxides tested, but in this system, the 11,12-epoxide is more effective than the 4,5-epoxide or the 9,10-epoxide, neither of which exhibit any demonstrable activity. Nevertheless, at a total dose of 1.4 μmol, benzo[*a*]pyrene is more active than the 7,8-epoxide. In these studies, control values for untreated mice ranged from 8 to 12% tumor incidences and from 0.08 to 0.13 adenomas per mouse. These control values have been subtracted from treated-group data to generate Table VIII.

From the available data, it appears that the activity of benzo[*a*]pyrene in this system is exceeded by the racemic 7,8-dihydrodiol and by either pure enantiomer of this dihydrodiol. The (−)-enantiomer, however, is far more potent than the (+)-enantiomer (*see* footnote *a* in Table VIII), as found in the other systems. In contrast to the other systems, the racemic *anti*-dihydrodiol epoxide is clearly more potent than benzo[*a*]pyrene, and this activity seems to reside in the (+)-enantiomer. The (−)-enantiomer has no significant activity. Although tested at a low dose, where benzo[*a*]pyrene itself was not significantly active, the data for the (−)-*syn*-dihydrodiol epoxide suggest that it may be active in this system, but tests at higher doses would be needed to demonstrate this. The 7,8-dihydrodiol at a 1.4-μmol dose also induces a significant number of malignant lymphomas (*446*), while these are not seen with benzo[*a*]pyrene itself. 2-Hydroxybenzo[*a*]pyrene is also a potent carcinogen in this system (*434*); it exceeds the activity of benzo[*a*]pyrene at a 1.4-μmol total dose, and exhibits an activity just slightly below that listed for the (+)-7,8-dihydrodiol at this dose (Table VIII). In summary, the newborn mouse system seems to be very sensitive to the benzo[*a*]pyrene metabolites, with 2-hydroxybenzo[*a*]pyrene, the racemic 7,8-dihydrodiol, the (+)-7,8-dihydrodiol, the (−)-7,8-dihydrodiol, and the racemic *anti*- and the (+)-*anti*-dihydrodiol epoxide all exhibiting greater activity than the parent compound.

In all of these tests, 2-hydroxybenzo[*a*]pyrene has proven to be a potent carcinogen. However, whether this phenol is metabolically formed from benzo[*a*]-pyrene is not established (*434*), so the significance of its biological activity with respect to the mechanism of action of benzo[*a*]pyrene remains unclear. With the exception of this phenol, all of the other benzo[*a*]pyrene derivatives that exhibit substantial activity are involved in the bay-region dihydrodiol epoxide pathway of benzo[*a*]pyrene metabolism (Scheme XI). This finding strongly supports the concept that carcinogenic activity, like DNA binding, is expressed through the metabolic conversion of benzo[*a*]pyrene to the bay-region dihydrodiol epoxide (*76, 141*). Moreover, these tumorigenicity assays indicate that the (−)-enantiomer of the 7,8-dihydrodiol and the (+)-enantiomer of the *anti*-dihydrodiol epoxide are more potent carcinogens than their isomers; therefore, a specific stereochemical course of metabolism (i.e., the left-hand route of Scheme X) is probably involved in the activation of benzo[*a*]pyrene.

In comparison with the carcinogenic activity of benzo[*a*]pyrene, however, the activities of these metabolites do not absolutely prove that the bay-region dihydrodiol epoxide metabolic activation pathway is a complete explanation for the metabolic activation of benzo[*a*]pyrene. The fact that the 7,8-epoxide is less active than benzo[*a*]pyrene in these carcinogenicity assays could be attributed to instability (rearrangement to a phenol) or to a less efficient uptake of the epoxide by target tissues, because the metabolic product from this epoxide, the 7,8-dihydrodiol, consistently demonstrates a carcinogenic activity that is greater than or equal to that of the parent compound. In contrast, the limited tumorigenic activities of the dihydrodiol epoxides in the mouse skin systems are difficult to reconcile with the view that the metabolic activation of benzo[*a*]pyrene merely requires its conversion to the bay-region dihydrodiol epoxide. This discord is particularly worrisome with regard to the initiation–promotion experiments (Table VII) in which the test compound is only required to initiate the carcinogenic process. Brookes (*447*) has found that equimolar doses of benzo[*a*]pyrene and the *anti*-7,8-dihydrodiol 9,10-epoxide applied to mouse skin result in roughly similar levels of binding to DNA. Because benzo[*a*]pyrene would not be quantitatively converted to the dihydrodiol epoxide, this finding demonstrates that the topically applied dihydrodiol epoxide is very inefficiently transferred to the skin DNA, but it also shows that the limited tumor-initiating activity of this metabolite cannot be attributed simply to its inability to reach the target tissue. Further investigations are clearly warranted. Conceivably, a second metabolite, which can be formed from the 7,8-dihydrodiol but not from the dihydrodiol epoxide, is required in addition to the dihydrodiol epoxide itself to initiate the carcinogenic process efficiently in mouse skin. The greater activity of the *anti*-dihydrodiol epoxide in the lung adenoma test in newborn mice compared with that of benzo[*a*]pyrene (Table VIII) could be considered to outweigh the mouse skin data. On the other hand, the substantial spontaneous tumor incidence in mouse lung tissue might be an indication that tumor initiation in this system is simpler than in mouse skin.

As part of a broadly based investigation of the role of such metabolites in carcinogenesis, a number of epoxides, dihydrodiols, and dihydrodiol epoxides that are derived from other polycyclic aromatic compounds have been subjected to testing for carcinogenic activity. Many hydrocarbon derivatives of this type have been obtained with difficulty and in limited quantities either by synthesis or, in some cases, by metabolic generation. As a result, most of the carcinogenicity assays reported have utilized the initiation–promotion protocol in mouse skin because it requires only small amounts of test compound. Representative information on the relative tumor initiation activities of these various derivatives has been collected together in Table IX.

Phenanthrene dihydrodiols do not exhibit significant tumor-initiating activity, nor does phenanthrene itself. Benzo[*e*]pyrene is also only feebly active as are most of its derivatives. The 9,10-dihydrodiol of benzo[*e*]pyrene exists preferentially in a quasi-diaxial conformation (as will be discussed later) and neither it, nor the bay-region dihydrodiol epoxide derived from it, is notably carcinogenic. The 9,10-dihydrobenzo[*e*]pyrene, which presumably could be metabolically converted to an 11,12-epoxide, is clearly the most tumorigenic of the benzo[*e*]pyrene derivatives listed in Table IX. Dibenz[*a,c*]anthracene is another feebly active tumor initiator and the non-bay-region 10,11-dihydrodiol 12,13-epoxide is even less active.

Chrysene, so far, appears to resemble benzo[*a*]pyrene in this tumor initiation assay in that the 1,2-dihydrodiol is more active than chrysene itself, but the bay-region *anti*-1,2-dihydrodiol 3,4-epoxide is clearly less active than chrysene and, incidentally, is less active than the 1,2,3,4-tetrahydrochrysene 3,4-epoxide. The large number of benz[*a*]anthracene derivatives that have been evaluated include all the possible *trans*-dihydrodiols and most of the stereoisomeric dihydrodiol epoxides. The 3,4-dihydrodiol is clearly the most active dihydrodiol, and its activity exceeds the weak activity of benz[*a*]anthracene itself. The (−)-enantiomer of this dihydrodiol is more active than the (+)-enantiomer, but neither of these compounds is as active as the bay-region *anti*-3,4-dihydrodiol 1,2-epoxide. As for the analogous benzo[*e*]pyrene derivative, 3,4-dihydrobenz[*a*]anthracene is the most active derivative of benz[*a*]anthracene listed in Table IX. Dibenz[*a,h*]-anthracene is more active than any of its derivatives. Benzo[*c*]phenanthrene,

Table IX

Tumor-Initiating Activities of Derivatives of Various Hydrocarbons in Female Mice

		Activity of Derivative/ Activity of Parent Compound				
Compound	*Dose (μmol)*	*Micrograms of TPA*[a] *(treatments per week)*	*Time (weeks)*	*Percent of Mice with Tumors*	*Papilloma per Mouse*	*Ref.*
Phenanthrene (**IIIA**)						
1,2-dihydrodiol (BR)	10	10(2)*	35	21/17[b]	0.21/0.28[b]	448
3,4-dihydrodiol	10	10(2)*	35	26/17[b]	0.41/0.28[b]	448
9,10-dihydrodiol	10	10(2)*	35	3/17[b,c]	0.03/0.28[b,c]	448
Benzo[e]pyrene (**IB**)						
4,5-dihydrodiol	6	10(2)*	35	12/14[d]	0.17/0.14[d]	449
	6	10(2)*	35	11/14[d]	0.11/0.14[d]	449
9,10-dihydrodiol (BR)	2	2(2)**	15	32/17[e]	0.6/0.2[e]	450
9,10,11,12-tetrahydro-9,10-diol	6	10(2)*	35	18/14[d]	0.25/0.14[d]	449
9,10-dihydro	2.5	10(2)*	35	67/11[d]	1.43/0.11[d]	449
anti-9,10-dihydrodiol 11,12-epoxide (BR)	2	2(2)**	15	6/17[e]	0.1/0.2[e]	450
Dibenz[a,c]anthracene						
10,11-dihydrodiol	2	2(2)**	15	10/27[e]	0.1/0.5[e]	450
anti-10,11-dihydrodiol 12,13-epoxide	2	2(2)**	15	10/27[e]	0.1/0.5[e]	450
Chrysene (**IIB**)						
1,2-dihydrodiol (BR)	1.25	10(2)*	25	60/43[d]	1.8/0.97[d]	451
3,4-dihydrodiol	1.25	10(2)*	25	13/43[d]	0.13/0.97[d]	451
5,6-dihydrodiol	1.25	10(2)*	25	0/43[d]	0.0/0.97[d]	451
1,2-dihydro	2	10(2)*	25	64/67[f]	2.21/1.7[f]	448
1,2,3,4-tetrahydro-3,4-epoxide	2	10(2)*	25	77/67[f]	1.5/1.7[f]	448
anti-3,4-dihydrodiol 1,2-epoxide	2	2(2)**	15	7/73	0.2/1.6	450
anti-1,2-dihydrodiol 3,4-epoxide (BR)	2	2(2)**	15	38/73	0.6/1.6	450
Benz[a]anthracene (**V**)						
1,2-dihydrodiol	0.4	10(2)*	20	4/14[f]	0.04/0.14	452
3,4-dihydrodiol (BR)	0.4	10(2)*	20	77/14[f]	2.4/0.14	452
5,6-dihydrodiol	0.4	10(2)*	20	7/14[f]	0.07/0.14	452
8,9-dihydrodiol	0.4	10(2)*	20	7/14[f]	0.1/0.14	452
10,11-dihydrodiol	0.4	10(2)*	20	13/14[f]	0.13/0.14	452
anti-10,11-dihydrodiol 8,9-epoxide	2	10(2)*	15	7/38	0.1/0.5	453
syn-8,9-dihydrodiol 10,11-epoxide	2	10(2)*	15	0/38	0/0.5	453
anti-8,9-dihydrodiol 10,11-epoxide	2	10(2)*	15	25/38	0.3/0.5	453

Table IX Continued

Compound	Dose (μmol)	Micrograms of TPA[a] (treatments per week)	Time (weeks)	Percent of Mice with Tumors	Papilloma per Mouse	Ref.
		Activity of Derivative/Activity of Parent Compound				
anti-1,2-dihydrodiol 3,4-epoxide	2	10(2)*	15	0/38	0/0.5	453
anti-3,4-dihydrodiol 1,2-epoxide (BR)	2	10(2)*	15	100/38	4.2/0.5	453
3,4-dihydro	0.4	10(2)*	20	86/7[f]	4.5/0.07[f]	454
(+)-3,4-dihydrodiol (BR)	0.4	10(2)*	20	45/7[f]	1.3/0.07[f]	454
(±)-3,4-dihydrodiol[g] (BR)	0.4	10(2)*	20	20/7[f]	0.4/0.07[f]	454
(−)-3,4-dihydrodiol[g] (BR)	0.4	10(2)*	20	50/7[f]	1.8/0.07[f]	454
syn-3,4-dihydrodiol 1,2-epoxide (BR)	0.4	10(2)*	20	43/7[f]	0.6/0.07[f]	454
anti-3,4-dihydrodiol 1,2-epoxide (BR)	0.4	10(2)*	20	70/7[f]	1.9/0.07[f]	454
Dibenz[a,h]anthracene						
1,2-dihydrodiol	0.04	10(2)*	25	7/53[e]	0.07/1.4[e]	455
3,4-dihydrodiol (BR)	0.04	10(2)*	25	50/53[e]	1.17/1.4[e]	455
5,6-dihydrodiol	0.04	10(2)*	25	14/53[e]	0.17/1.4[e]	455
3,4-dihydrodiol 1,2-epoxide (BR)	0.1	2(2)**	15	7/50	0.1/1.4	450
Benzo[c]phenanthrene						
1,2-dihydrodiol	0.4	10(2)*	20	3/17[h]	0.03/0.17	456
3,4-dihydrodiol (BR)	0.4	10(2)*	20	28/17[h]	0.41/0.17	456
5,6-dihydrodiol	0.4	10(2)*	20	7/17[h]	0.07/0.17	456
syn-3,4-dihydrodiol 1,2-epoxide (BR)	0.4	10(2)*	20	87/17[h]	6.47/0.17	456
anti-3,4-dihydrodiol 1,2-epoxide (BR)	0.4	10(2)*	20	80/17[h]	7.13/0.17	456
3-Methylcholanthrene (**X**)						
4,5-dihydrodiol	0.08	1(2)*	32	39/65[i]	0.47/1.7[i]	457
7,8-dihydrodiol	0.08	1(2)*	32	8/65[i]	0.08/1.7[i]	457
9,10-dihydrodiol (BR)	0.08	1(2)*	32	43/65[i]	1.0/1.7[i]	457
11,12-dihydrodiol	0.08	1(2)*	32	5/65[i]	0.05/1.7[i]	457
1-keto	0.03	10(2)*	30	3/59	0.03/2.1	458
1-hydroxy	0.03	10(2)*	30	21/59	0.34/2.1	458
1-hydroxy-9,10-dihydrodiol (BR)	0.03	10(2)*	30	68/59	1.44/2.1	458
2-keto	0.03	10(2)*	30	66/59	1.48/2.1	458
2-hydroxy	0.03	10(2)*	30	59/59	1.68/2.1	458
7-Methylbenz[a]anthracene (**V**)						
1,2-dihydrodiol	0.09	0.5(3[j])*	40	27/57[k]	0.3/0.8[k]	459
	0.09	0.5(3[j])*	40	73/57[k]	1.53/0.8[k]	459

Continued on next page

Table IX Continued

Compound	Dose (μmol)	Activity of Derivative/Activity of Parent Compound: Micrograms of TPA[a] (treatments per week	Time (week)	Percent of Mice with Tumors	Papilloma per Mouse	Ref.
3,4-dihydrodiol (BR)	0.4	2(2)**	15	100/83	6.8/3.8	450
5,6-dihydrodiol	0.09	0.5(3[j])*	40	7/57[k]	0.07/0.8[k]	459
8,9-dihydrodiol	0.09	0.5(3[j])*	40	23/57[k]	0.27/0.8[k]	459
anti-3,4-dihydrodiol 1,2-epoxide (BR)	0.4	2(2)**	15	22/83	0.3/3.8	450
5-Methylchrysene (**XI**)						
1,2-dihydrodiol (BR)	0.011(10)	2.5(3)***	20	95/75[l]	7.3/3[l]	460
7,8-dihydrodiol	0.011(10)	2.5(3)***	20	50/75[l]	1.1/3[l]	460
9,10-dihydrodiol	0.011(10)	2.5(3)***	20	0/75[l]	0/3[l]	460
8-Methylbenz[a]anthracene (**V**)						
3,4-dihydrodiol (BR)	0.1	10(2)*	31	73/40[m]	2.2/0.97[m]	461
5,6-dihydrodiol	0.1	10(2)*	31	0/40[n]	0/0.97[n]	461
8,9-dihydrodiol	0.1	10(2)*	31	23/40[m]	0.5/0.97[m]	461
7,12-Dimethylbenz[a]anthracene (**V**)						
3,4-dihydrodiol (BR)	0.003	10(2)*	23	92/76	9.8/2.9	462
	0.009	10(2)*	23	77/85	10.9/6.0	462
	0.1	2(2)**	15	100/100	22.8/10.2	463
5,6-dihydrodiol	0.009	10(2)*	23	0/85[o]	0/6.0[o]	462
8,9-dihydrodiol	0.009	10(2)*	23	4/85	0.07/6.0	462
10,11-dihydrodiol	0.009	10(2)*	23	7/85	0.11/6.0	462

NOTE: Dihydrodiols that are precursors of bay-region dihydrodiols are indicated by BR. The strain of mice used is indicated in the TPA column: *, Swiss CD-1; **, Sencar; and ***, Swiss–Webster.

[a]TPA represents 12-*O*-tetradecanoylphorbol-13-acetate.

[b]Vehicle-only control: 7% of mice with tumors; 0.1 papilloma/mouse.

[c]Less active than control.

[d]Vehicle-only control: 7% of mice with tumors; 0.07 papilloma/mouse.

[e]Vehicle-only control: 10% of mice with tumors; 0.1 papilloma/mouse.

[f]Vehicle-only control: 3% of mice with tumors; 0.03 papilloma/mouse.

[g]At the lower dose of 0.1 μmol, the (−)-enantiomer (43% of mice with tumors; 1 papilloma/mouse) is clearly more active than the (+)-enantiomer (3% of mice with tumors; 0.07 papilloma/mouse). This dose could not be tabulated because comparable data for benz[*a*]anthracene were not presented (*454*).

[h]No tumors in vehicle-control group.

[i]Initiating dose for 3-methylcholanthrene was 0.09 μmol.

[j]After 26 weeks, dose was changed to 1 μg applied 3 times each week.

[k]Initiating dose of 7-methylbenz[*a*]anthracene was 0.1 μmol.

[l]Initiating dose of 5-methylchrysene was 0.012 μmol applied 10 times.

[m]Vehicle-only control: 13% of mice with tumors, 0.23 papilloma/mouse.

[n]Only nine mice used in this group.

[o]The 5,6-dihydrodiol also had little activity in the studies of Slaga et al. (*463*), but Chouroulinkov et al. (*457*) reported activity comparable to the parent hydrocarbon.

however, is similar to benz[*a*]anthracene in that, for both of these hydrocarbons, tumorigenic activity increases along the series: hydrocarbon, dihydrodiol, and bay-region dihydrodiol epoxide. In addition to this distinction, benzo[*c*]phenanthrene is unique, at present, in that the *syn*- and *anti*-stereoisomeric bay-region dihydrodiol epoxides exhibit similar carcinogenic activities. In all other cases in which comparisons have been made, the *anti*-stereoisomer has proven to be more carcinogenic than the *syn*-isomer. Jerina and his colleagues (*464*) have pointed out that the hydroxyl groups in the *anti*-stereoisomers usually adopt the quasi-diequatorial conformation in contrast to the quasi-diaxial conformation of the *syn*-diastereomers. However both stereoisomers of the bay-region dihydrodiol epoxide of benzo[*c*]phenanthrene adopt the quasi-diequatorial conformation (*464*).

For 3-methylcholanthrene the 9,10-dihydrodiol precursor of the bay-region dihydrodiol epoxide is less tumorigenic than the parent hydrocarbon as is 1-hydroxy-3-methylcholanthrene. However, the 9,10-dihydrodiol derived from this hydroxy compound is, surprisingly, more active than either the dihydrodiol or the hydroxy compound. The activities of other derivatives of this hydrocarbon would be of interest. For 7-methylbenz[*a*]anthracene, 8-methylbenz[*a*]anthracene, and 7,12-dimethylbenz[*a*]anthracene, the 3,4-dihydrodiol is more tumorigenic than the parent hydrocarbon. The corresponding bay-region 3,4-dihydrodiol 1,2-epoxide has only been examined for 7-methylbenz[*a*]anthracene; it is less tumorigenic than the dihydrodiol or the parent hydrocarbon.

5-Methylchrysene (**XI**) is an interesting compound, because it has two bay regions, one of which is substituted with the 5-methyl group. The 1,2-dihydrodiol—which is the precursor for the bay-region dihydrodiol epoxide in which the bay region is substituted—is more active as a tumor initiator than the 7,8-dihydrodiol.

The tumor initiation data summarized in Table IX is sparse compared with extensive data available for benzo[*a*]pyrene and its derivatives. Nevertheless, the data can be subjected to a preliminary evaluation. Twelve hydrocarbons are listed in Table IX, and for 11 of these, comparisons between the parent hydrocarbon and the dihydrodiol precursor of the bay-region dihydrodiol epoxide have been reported; for 9 of these 11, the dihydrodiol is at least as active, and in most cases, is more active in this assay than the parent hydrocarbon. The activities of the bay-region dihydrodiol epoxides have been examined for only six of these hydrocarbons; for four of these six hydrocarbons, the dihydrodiol epoxide is less active than either the parent hydrocarbon or the dihydrodiol precursor. In the other two cases, benz[*a*]anthracene and benzo[*c*]phenanthrene, the dihydrodiol epoxide is more active than either the parent hydrocarbon or the dihydrodiol precursor.

These studies were initiated to determine whether metabolic activation to a bay-region dihydrodiol epoxide represents a general mechanism through which the hydrocarbon carcinogens express their carcinogenic activity. So far, the results of these studies have generally supported such a mechanism. However, the carcinogenic properties of the dihydrodiol epoxides themselves are not entirely consistent with the generalization. The inconsistencies may be because of the inherent difficulties associated with testing reactive compounds in animal systems or because the tumor initiation process requires more from a hydrocarbon than the generation of a reactive dihydrodiol epoxide metabolite.

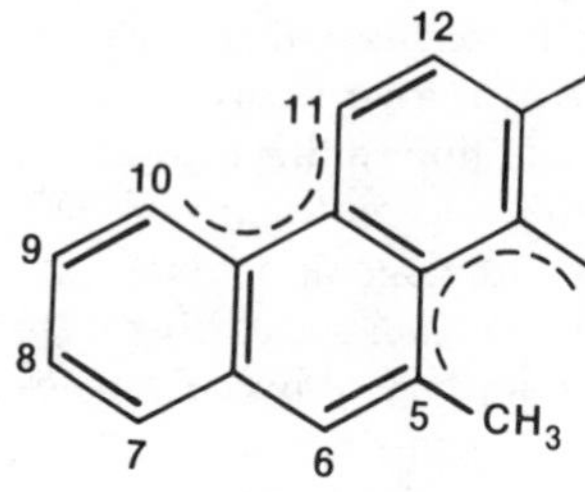

XI

Chemistry of Epoxides, Dihydrodiols, and Dihydrodiol Epoxides

Synthetic Chemistry. Considerable literature on the synthesis and properties of arene epoxides, dihydrodiols, and dihydrodiol epoxides of polycyclic aromatic hydrocarbon carcinogens has developed over the last decade (reviewed in Refs. 142 and 465–68). In this chapter, the salient features of the syntheses are surveyed to provide an overview of the chemical methods that have been applied to prepare useful amounts of well-characterized compounds. This summary excludes the preparation of hydrocarbon derivatives that use in vitro metabolic activation systems. Often, more than one synthetic route to a particular hydrocarbon derivative has been published, and the reader should consult the primary references for more detailed descriptions and discussions of the relative merits of any particular synthetic route.

K-Region Arene Epoxides and Dihydrodiols. Since the first synthesis of hydrocarbon *K*-region arene epoxides in 1964 (*180*), several synthetic methods have been described (*469–73*), and a general summary of all useful routes to *K*-region arene epoxides and dihydrodiols is given in Scheme XII. The key intermediate in most of these synthetic sequences is the *K*-region *cis*-dihydrodiol, which is readily available from the parent hydrocarbon through osmium tetroxide oxidation (*474*). Further oxidation of this material with sodium periodate provides the corresponding dialdehyde that may be cyclized to the epoxide with tris(dimethylamino)phosphine (*180*). Alternatively, oxidation of the *cis*-dihydrodiol with pyridine–sulfur trioxide reagent in dimethyl sulfoxide (DMSO) provides the *K*-region *o*-quinone (*469, 470*). Reduction of this compound with lithium aluminum hydride furnishes the *K*-region *trans*-dihydrodiol or a mixture of the *cis*- and *trans*-isomers. The *trans*-dihydrodiol may then be cyclized to the *K*-region arene epoxide with the dimethylacetal of dimethylformamide (*469, 470*). By another sequence, treatment of the *cis*-dihydrodiol with trimethyl orthoacetate produces a 2-methyl-2-methoxy-1,3-dioxolane derivative that forms a *trans*-chlorohydrin acetate ester on reaction with trimethylsilyl chloride. Subsequent cyclization of this ester with sodium methoxide yields the *K*-region arene epoxide (*471*).

More recent reports indicate that, for certain hydrocarbons, direct oxidation of the parent compound with *m*-chloroperoxybenzoic acid (*472*) or with sodium hypochlorite in the presence of a phase-transfer catalyst (*473*) leads to *K*-region arene epoxides. All of these sequences, which are outlined in Scheme XII, have

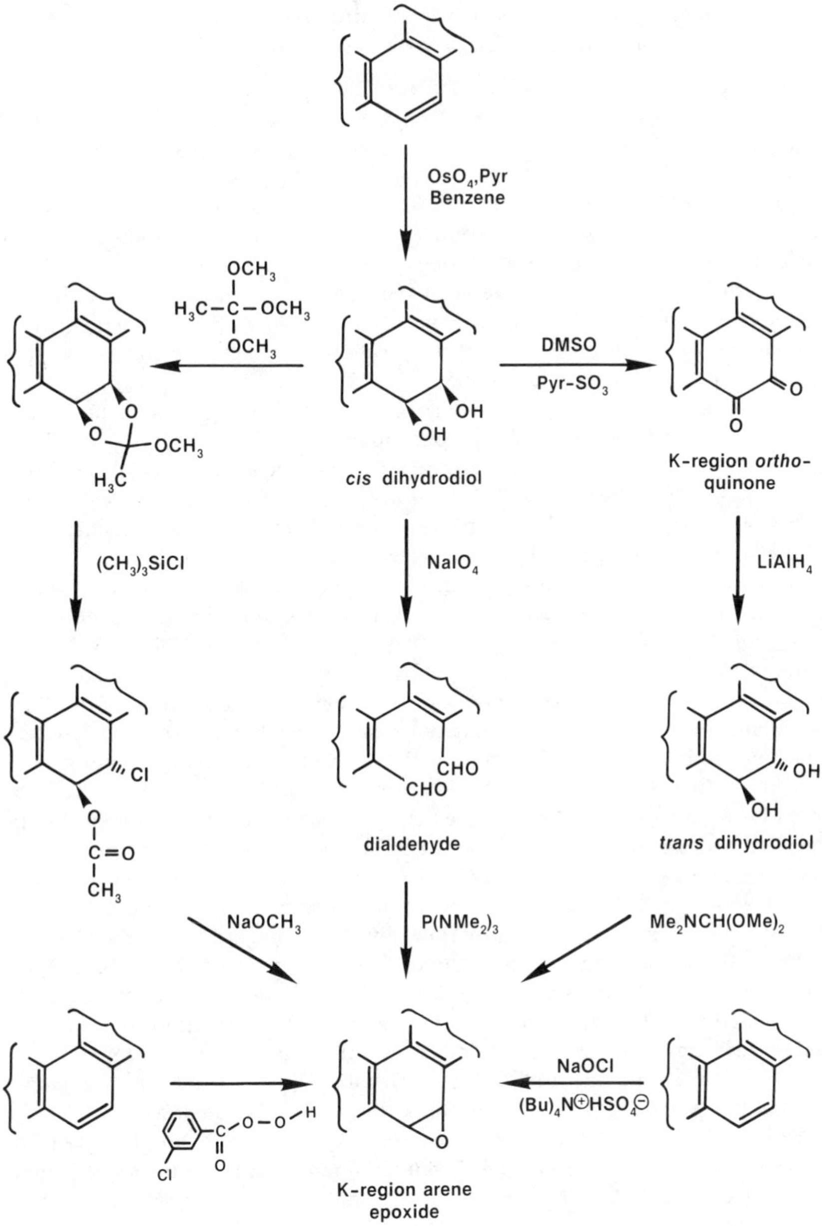

Scheme XII. Synthetic routes to K-region arene epoxides.

been employed to prepare the *K*-region dihydrodiols and arene epoxides of a wide variety of hydrocarbons and of some heterocyclic aromatics (*475, 476*).

NON-*K*-REGION ARENE EPOXIDES AND DIHYDRODIOLS. Synthetic access to non-*K*-region arene epoxides and dihydrodiols is considerably more complex than for the *K*-region analogs. Key intermediates are dihydroarenes (generalized structures **A** and **B** in Scheme XIII) that are generally available through a multistep sequence: (1) Friedel–Crafts succinoylation of an appropriate aromatic nucleus (*477*); (2) reduction to an arylbutyric acid; and (3) acid-catalyzed cyclization (*478*) to the cyclic ketone. Reduction of the ketone with either sodium borohydride or lithium aluminum hydride furnishes the corresponding alcohol that can be dehydrated under acid conditions to dihydroarenes such as **A** or **B** in Scheme XIII. The particular dihydroarene depends on the position of the ketone that is obtained as a result of the original succinoylation.

Scheme XIII also illustrates that intermediates **A** or **B** may be obtained sometimes through selective dehydrogenation of tetrahydroarenes (*479*) that are available, in some cases, through catalytic hydrogenation (*480*) or through dissolving-metal reduction (*467, 481*) of fully aromatic precursors.

Bromination of the dihydroarene intermediate (**A** or **B** in Scheme XIII) followed by magnesium carbonate-catalyzed hydrolysis of the benzylic bromide provides an intermediate bromohydrin that may be transformed into a non-*K*-region arene epoxide by either Route I or II in Scheme XIII. Earlier syntheses of such non-*K*-region arene epoxides (e.g., benzo[*a*]pyrene 7,8-epoxide (*482*), benzo[*a*]pyrene 9,10-epoxide (*482*), dibenz[*a,c*]anthracene 10,11-epoxide (*483*), benz[*a*]anthracene 8,9-epoxide (*484*), or naphthalene 1,2-epoxide (*185*)) followed essentially a sequence of steps outlined in Route I of Scheme XIII. By this route, the intermediate bromohydrin is treated with base to form a tetrahydro epoxide. The epoxide is then brominated with *N*-bromosuccinimide (NBS) to form a bromo epoxide intermediate that undergoes dehydrobromination to the non-*K*-region arene epoxide when treated with base. 1,5-Diazabicyclo[4.3.0]non-5-ene (*185*) was found to be a particularly effective base for the dehydrobromination reaction.

Overall yields for non-*K*-region arene epoxides from bromohydrin intermediates were substantially improved by Yagi and Jerina (*485, 486*) who introduced the modified reaction sequence outlined in Route II of Scheme XIII. By this route, bromohydrins are protected as bromohydrin esters that are further brominated to form a dibromo ester. Treatment of the latter dibromo compounds with base brings about cyclization and dehydrobromination in one step to the non-*K*-region arene epoxide thereby circumventing bromination of a preformed tetrahydro epoxide that is generally unstable under these conditions. Using the methods outlined in Scheme XIII, workers have prepared non-*K*-region arene epoxides of naphthalene (*185, 485, 486*), 1-methylnaphthalene (*487*), phenanthrene (*485, 486*), benzo[*a*]pyrene (*482, 486*), benz[*a*]anthracene (*484*), and dibenz[*a,c*]anthracene (*483*).

As indicated earlier, synthesis of non-*K*-region dihydrodiols also proceeds through dihydroarenes (**A** and **B** in Scheme XIII). These dihydroarenes are readily converted to *trans*-tetrahydro diesters by application of the Prévost reaction (Scheme XIV) (*488*). Treatment of the dihydroarene (**A** in Scheme XIV) with the silver salt of benzoic or acetic acid and iodine yields the *trans*-tetrahydro diester.

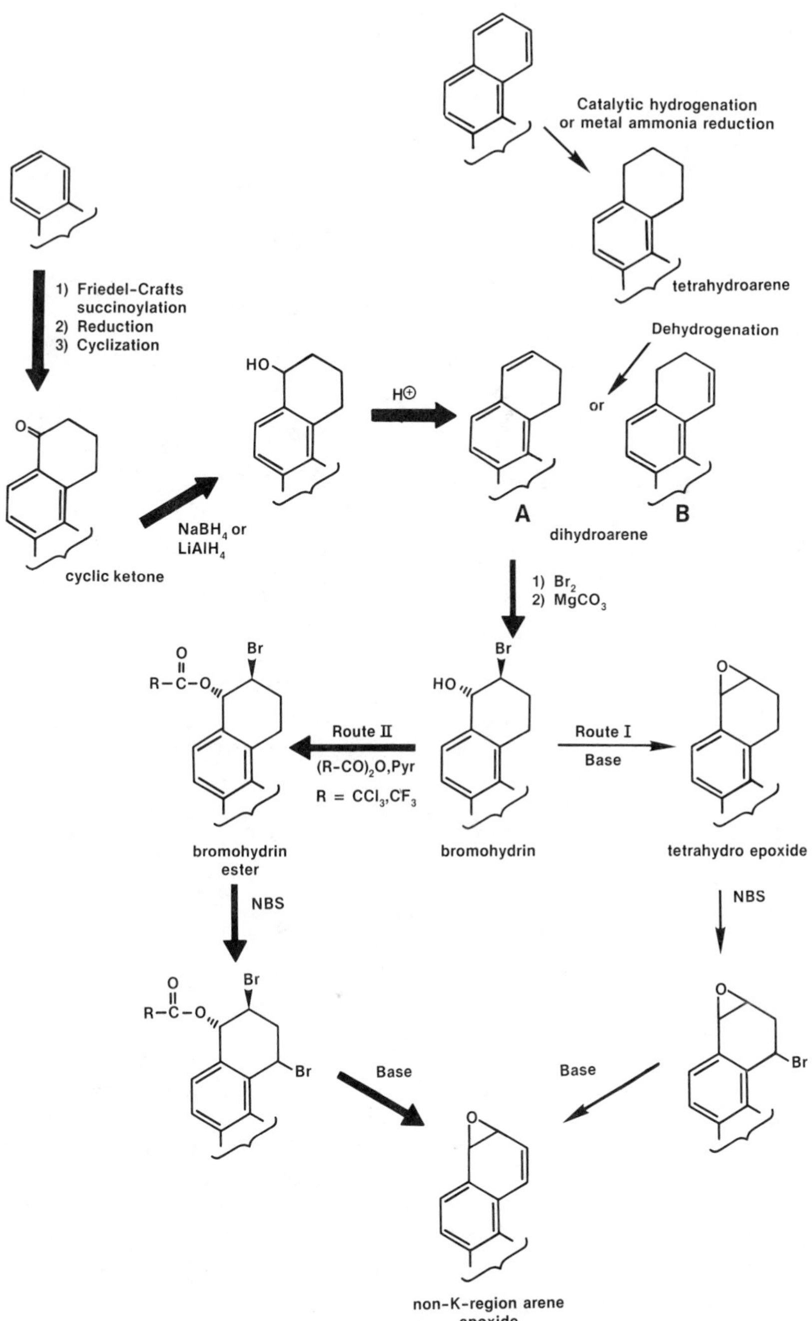

Scheme XIII. Synthetic routes to non-K-region arene epoxides.

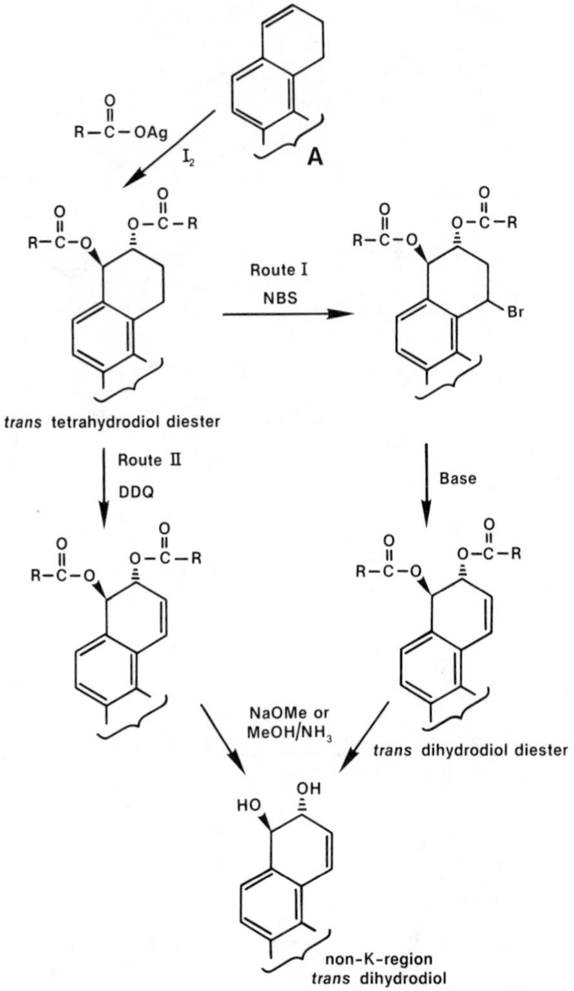

Scheme XIV. Synthetic routes to non-K-region dihydrodiols. NBS represents N-bromosuccinimide, and DDQ represents 2,3-dichloro-5,6-dicyano-1,4-benzoquinone.

This diester is then dehydrogenated by either Route I or II in Scheme XIV. By Route I, bromination of the *trans*-diester with *N*-bromosuccinimide (NBS) furnishes a bromo diester intermediate that, in a second step, undergoes base-catalyzed dehydrobromination to the dihydrodiol diester (*489*). By Route II, dehydrogenation of the tetrahydro diester with 2,3-dichloro-5,6-dicyano-1,4-benzoquinone (DDQ) furnishes the *trans*-dihydrodiol diester in one step (*467, 479, 490*). Finally, removal of the ester groups with base yields the corresponding non-*K*-region *trans*-dihydrodiol.

Through the sequences outlined in Schemes XIII and XIV, reliable routes to the non-*K*-region dihydrodiols of anthracene and phenanthrene (*489*), benz[*a*]-

anthracene (*467, 489, 491*), chrysene (*492, 493*), dibenz[*a,h*]anthracene (*492, 494*), benzo[*a*]pyrene (*369, 467, 490, 495*), benzo[*e*]pyrene (*496, 497*), triphenylene (*497*), dibenzo[*a,i*]pyrene and dibenzo[*a,h*]pyrene (*498*), benzo[*c*]phenanthrene (*499*), 7-methylbenz[*a*]anthracene (*490, 500*), 7,12-dimethylbenz[*a*]anthracene (*501*), dibenz[*a,c*]anthracene (*502*), dibenz[*c,h*]acridine (*503*), 7-methylbenzo[*a*]-pyrene (*504*), and benzo[*b*]fluoranthene, benzo[*j*]fluoranthene, and benzo[*k*]-fluoranthene (*505*) are now available.

Somewhat less satisfactory syntheses of non-*K*-region *trans*-dihydrodiols were carried out previously through lithium aluminum hydride reduction of non-*K*-region *o*-quinones (*506, 507*). As mentioned earlier, such reduction of *K*-region *o*-quinones provides the corresponding *trans*-dihydrodiols in good yield, but with the non-*K*-region *o*-quinones, complex mixtures of products, which may include the *cis*-dihydrodiol, tetrahydrodiols, and catechols (*507*), are frequently obtained. However, recent reports suggest that modified procedures for *o*-quinone reduction can provide improved yields of non-*K*-region dihydrodiols of both unsubstituted (*508, 509*) and methyl-substituted polycyclic hydrocarbons (*508, 510*). Finally, trace amounts of non-*K*-region dihydrodiols can be prepared through oxidation (ascorbic acid/ferrous sulfate/EDTA) of 7-methylbenz[*a*]anthracene (*511*), benz-[*a*]anthracene and 7,12-dimethylbenz[*a*]anthracene (*512*), 3-methylcholanthrene (*513*), 7-hydroxymethyl-12-methylbenz[*a*]anthracene (*514*), chrysene, dibenz-[*a,h*]anthracene, and dibenz[*a,c*]anthracene (*515*), and benzo[*c*]phenanthrene (*499*).

An important aspect of the structure of these dihydrodiols is the conformation of the vicinal *trans*-hydroxyl groups. This conformation is referred to as either quasi-diequatorial or quasi-diaxial. The term quasi indicates that this conformation only resembles and cannot be identical to the analogous conformation in, for example, *trans*-1,2-cyclohexane diol, because the arene dihydrodiols are conformationally more restrained. The conformation of the hydroxyl groups in a dihydrodiol is determined from the proton NMR spectrum. The quasi-diequatorial or quasi-diaxial conformation is assigned on the basis of the magnitude of the coupling constant for the adjacent carbon-bound (carbinol) protons of the dihydrodiol grouping. When the adjacent hydroxyl groups are oriented in a quasi-diequatorial conformation, coupling constants for the carbon-bound protons, which must be quasi-diaxial, are of the order of 10–12 Hz. When the hydroxyl groups assume the quasi-diaxial conformation, coupling constants for the carbinol hydrogens, which are quasi-diequatorial, are near 2 Hz. From such measurements, it has become clear that the quasi-diequatorial conformation is the preferred conformation for *trans*-dihydrodiols that are not in the bay region (*489, 507, 511, 516, 517*) or situated *peri* to a methyl substituent in methylated hydrocarbons (*511, 517*). For these latter cases, the quasi-diaxial conformation is observed.

VICINAL DIHYDRODIOL EPOXIDES. Epoxidation of the remaining double bond in the ring that bears the dihydrodiol grouping furnishes a vicinal dihydrodiol epoxide. The stereochemistry of the final product (i.e., whether it be the *syn, anti,* or a mixture of both diastereomeric dihydrodiol epoxides) depends on the reagent(s) employed to form the oxirane ring and the conformation of the *trans*-hydroxyl groups of the dihydrodiol precursor.

As shown in Scheme XV, epoxidation of a quasi-diequatorial *trans*-dihydrodiol with *m*-chloroperoxybenzoic acid introduces the epoxide ring *cis* to the non-benzylic hydroxyl group to provide stereoselective formation of an *anti*-dihydrodiol epoxide. Alternatively, treatment of the same quasi-diequatorial dihydrodiol with *N*-bromoacetamide (NBA) or *N*-bromosuccinimide (NBS) affords a bromohydrin intermediate with the bromine atom on the same face of the ring as the non-benzylic hydroxyl group. Cyclization of the bromohydrin with base then produces the *syn*-dihydrodiol epoxide. Thus, attack by both peracid and brominating agent occurs with high stereoselectivity on the diequatorial *trans*-dihydrodiols presumably as a consequence of a directive influence exerted by the quasi-equatorial non-benzylic hydroxyl group (*370, 516, 518*).

After initial preparations of the *trans*-7,8-dihydrodiol 9,10-epoxide of benzo[*a*]pyrene where stereochemistry was not specified (*141,369*), both the *syn*- and *anti*-diastereomers were fully characterized after stereoselective synthesis by the routes outlined in Scheme XV (*370, 371, 467, 519*). Additional vicinal *trans*-dihydrodiol epoxides prepared by these routes include the following compounds: *syn*- and *anti*-1,2-dihydrodiol 3,4-epoxide of phenanthrene (*520*), the *syn*-1,2-dihydrodiol 3,4-epoxide of chrysene (*520*), the *anti*-1,2-dihydrodiol 3,4-epoxide of chrysene (*493, 520*), *syn*- and *anti*-benz[*a*]anthracene-3,4-dihydrodiol 1,2-epoxide (*491, 521*), *syn*- and *anti*-benz[*a*]anthracene-1,2-dihydrodiol 3,4-epoxide (*491*), the *syn*-and *anti*-8,9-dihydrodiol 10,11-epoxide and the *syn*- and *anti*-10,11-dihydrodiol 8,9-epoxide of benz[*a*]anthracene (*521*), the *anti*-10,11-dihydrodiol 8,9-epoxide of 7-methylbenz[*a*]anthracene (*490*), the *anti*-3,4-dihydrodiol 1,2-epoxide of 7-methylbenz[*a*]anthracene (*500*), the *anti*-8,9-dihydrodiol 10,11-epoxide of 7,12-dimethylbenz[*a*]anthracene (*501*), the *anti*-10,11-dihydrodiol 12,13-epoxide of dibenz[*a,c*]anthracene (*502*), the *anti*-3,4-dihydrodiol 1,2-epoxide of dibenz[*a,h*]anthracene (*494*), the *syn*-9,10-dihydrodiol 11,12-epoxide of benzo[*e*]pyrene (*516*), the *anti*-9,10-dihydrodiol 11,12-epoxide of benzo[*e*]pyrene (*497, 516*), the *syn*-1,2-dihydrodiol 3,4-epoxide of triphenylene (*516*), the *anti*-1,2-dihydrodiol 3,4-epoxide of triphenylene (*497, 516*), the *anti*-3,4-dihydrodiol 1,2-epoxide of dibenzo[*a,i*]pyrene (*498*), the *anti*-1,2-dihydrodiol 3,4-epoxide of dibenzo[*a,h*]pyrene (*498*), and both the *syn*- and *anti*-3,4-dihydrodiol 1,2-epoxide of benzo[*c*] phenanthrene (*464*).

In contrast to the stereoselectivity observed in the peracid epoxidation of quasi-diequatorial *trans*-dihydrodiols, peracid epoxidation of *trans*-dihydrodiols whose hydroxyl groups assume a quasi-diaxial conformation—as is the case for dihydrodiols in the sterically crowded bay region—provides a mixture of both the *syn*- and *anti*-dihydrodiol epoxides (Scheme XV). Stereoselectivity is markedly reduced in these cases presumably because the axial non-benzylic hydroxyl group can no longer exert a directive influence on peracid attack. This lack of stereoselectivity is exemplified in the epoxidation of *trans*-dihydrodiols in the bay regions of benzo[*e*]pyrene (*516*), triphenylene (*516*), chrysene (*522*), dibenz[*a,h*]-anthracene (*494*), and benzo[*a*]pyrene (*430*). However, epoxidation of the *trans*-1,2-dihydrodiols of dibenz[*a,h*]anthracene (*494*) and 7-methylbenz[*a*]anthracene (*500*) appears to be exceptional, because the *syn*-1,2-dihydrodiol 3,4-epoxides are apparently formed predominantly (*523*).

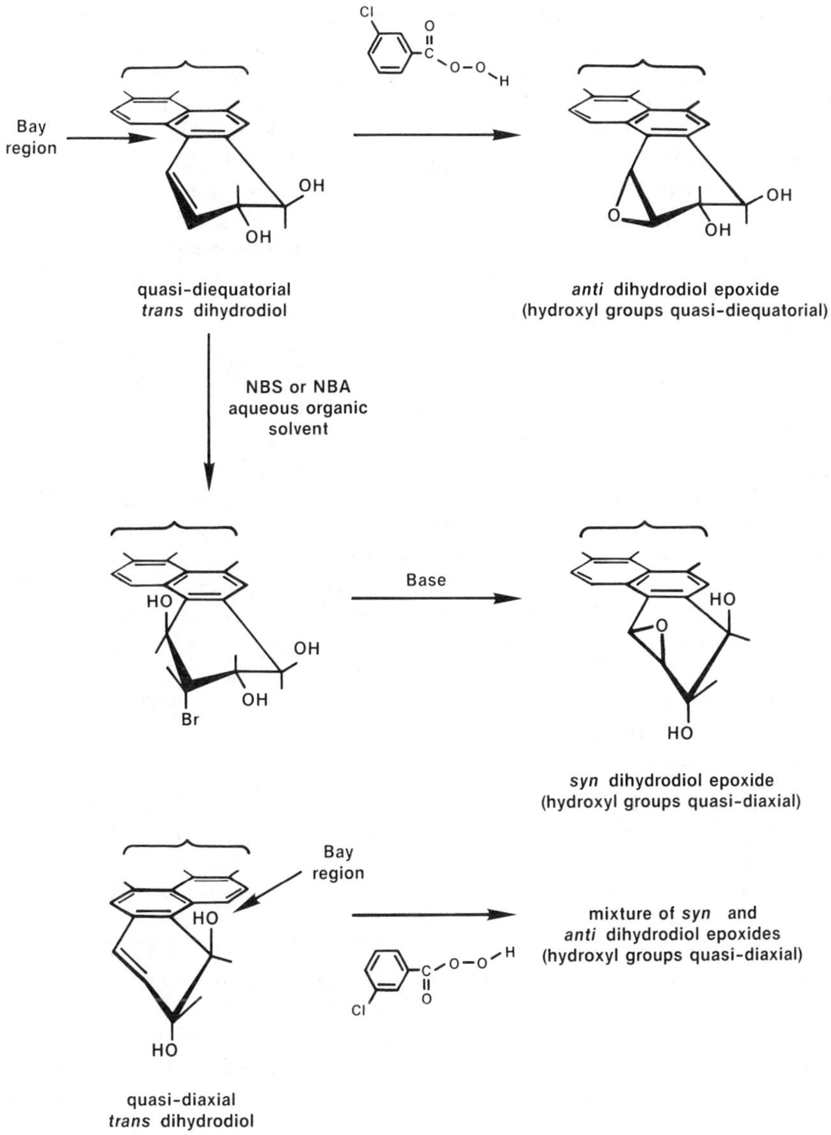

Cl
O
C
O–O
H

Bay region

OH
OH

OH
O
OH

quasi-diequatorial
trans dihydrodiol

anti dihydrodiol epoxide
(hydroxyl groups quasi-diequatorial)

NBS or NBA
aqueous organic
solvent

HO
OH
OH
Br

Base

HO
O
HO

syn dihydrodiol epoxide
(hydroxyl groups quasi-diaxial)

Bay region

HO
HO

C
O–O
H
O
Cl

mixture of *syn* and
anti dihydrodiol epoxides
(hydroxyl groups quasi-diaxial)

quasi-diaxial
trans dihydrodiol

Scheme XV. Synthesis and conformational considerations of vicinal dihydrodiol epoxides.

Scheme XV also illustrates that the preferred conformation of the *trans*-nydroxyl groups in an *anti*-dihydrodiol epoxide is quasi-diequatorial ($J \cong 9$ Hz), whereas for a *syn*-dihydrodiol epoxide, the quasi-diaxial conformation predominates ($J = 3$–6 Hz) (*520, 524*). The quasi-diaxial conformation is also observed for dihydrodiol epoxides whose hydroxyl groups are in a bay region (*516*). However, a notable exception to these generalizations is found for the 3,4-dihydrodiol 1,2-epoxides of benzo[*c*]phenanthrene where, in both the *syn*- and *anti*-diastereomers, the hydroxyl groups adopt the quasi-diequatorial conformation (*464*). This exception presumably results from a need to relieve unfavorable steric interactions that are brought about by having the oxirane ring in a highly congested bay region or "fjord region" (*464. 499*).

Reactivity. Arene Epoxides. A number of investigations of the hydrolysis and reactions with nucleophiles of arene epoxides have been reported (*525–30*), but the discoveries of the dihydrodiol epoxides have resulted in a shift of effort into the study of these latter compounds. The non-*K*-region arene epoxides rearrange in aqueous solution to yield phenols, and evidence from the product distributions obtained indicates that the epoxides open preferentially to form the vinylogous benzylic carbonium ion (*525, 528, 529*). Only strong nucleophiles can effectively compete with the rearrangement to phenols for the non-*K*-region arene epoxides (*526*), but the *K*-region epoxides yield both *cis*- and *trans*-dihydrodiols in addition to phenols (*527, 528*). The distribution of products is pH dependent, with a phenol as the major product from several epoxides in the acid range (*525, 527, 528*); the *trans*-dihydrodiol is extensively favored in the more alkaline range for phenanthrene 9,10-epoxide (*528*), as a result of nucleophilic attack of water or hydroxide ion on the epoxide. The *cis*-dihydrodiol is thought to arise below pH 7 through the trapping of the carbonium ion (*527, 528*).

Vicinal Dihydrodiol Epoxides. The published syntheses of both diastereomers of the *trans*-7,8-dihydrodiol 9,10-epoxide of benzo[*a*]pyrene were accompanied by accounts of their reactions with the sulfur nucleophiles (abbreviated as Nu: in Scheme XVI), the *t*-butylthiol anion in aqueous dioxane (*371*), and *p*-nitrophenylthiolate in *t*-butyl alcohol (*370*). For both diastereomers—i.e., the *syn*-dihydrodiol epoxide (generalized structure **A** in Scheme XVI) and the *anti*-dihydrodiol epoxide (generalized structure **F** in Scheme XVI)—the products obtained are the result of backside displacement at C-10 (represented by the benzylic carbon to which the oxirane ring is attached in **A** and **F** in Scheme XVI) of the dihydrodiol epoxide. This displacement results in the *trans*-stereospecific ring opening of the oxirane ring (as in generalized structures **B** and **G** in Scheme XVI). Similar *trans*-ring opening is also observed in the reaction of both dihydrodiol epoxides of benzo[*a*]pyrene with sodium methoxide and aniline as nucleophiles in non-aqueous media (*519*). Although detailed kinetic data for all these reactions are not available, the reaction of *p*-nitrophenylthiolate in *t*-butyl alcohol with the *syn*-dihydrodiol epoxide of benzo[*a*]pyrene is more than two orders of magnitude faster than with the *anti*-isomer (*370*).

Although reactions of the benzo[*a*]pyrene dihydrodiol epoxides with water in either mixed solvent (*531*) or largely aqueous media (*519,532*) also result in nucleophilic attack exclusively at C-10, the stereochemistry of the resulting tetrols

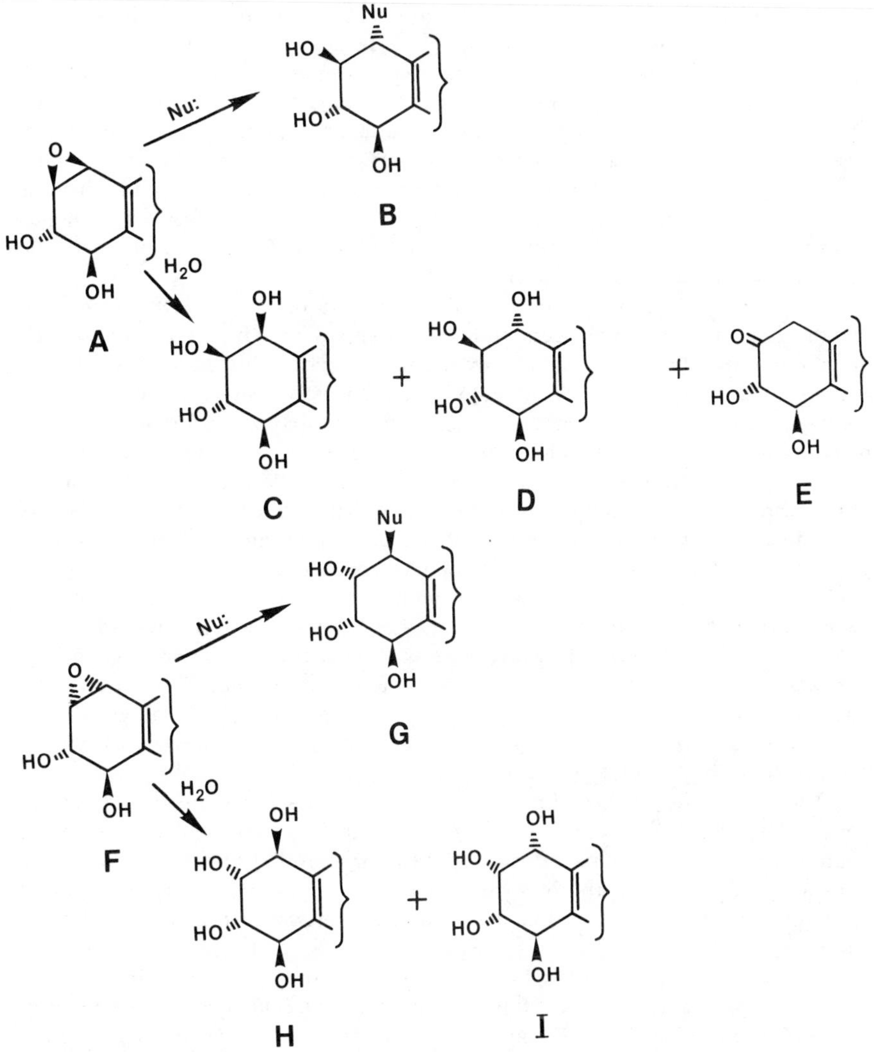

Scheme XVI. Reactions of vicinal dihydrodiol epoxides. Nu: represents a nucleophile.

indicates that, for the *anti*-isomer (**F** in Scheme XVI), both *trans*- and *cis*-addition to C-10 occurs to yield tetrols **H** and **I** (Scheme XVI), respectively. For the *syn*-isomer (**A** in Scheme XVI), *cis*-addition by water predominates yielding tetrol **C** (Scheme XVI) as the major product (*519, 531, 532*) accompanied by lesser amounts of the product of *trans*-addition (**D** in Scheme XVI) and a ketone [**E** in Scheme XVI, namely, *trans*-7,8-dihydroxy-9-keto-7,8,9,10-tetrahydrobenzo[*a*]pyrene (*519*)]. Yields for this ketone derivative are highest under neutral or alkaline conditions in less aqueous media (*519, 533*). The distribution of tetrols from the hydrolysis of the *syn*-dihydrodiol epoxide of benzo[*a*]pyrene is far less sensitive to change in pH than that from the *anti*-isomer. Thus, for the *syn*-isomer, over the pH range of 3–8, tetrol **C** (Scheme XVI), a product of *cis*-addition to C-10, is produced in roughly 85% yield, while tetrol **D** (Scheme XVI) is produced in approximately 10% yield. Less than 5% of the ketone **E** is detected. In contrast, hydrolysis of the *anti*-isomer **F** gives tetrols **H** and **I** in a ratio of approximately 8:2 under acid-catalyzed hydrolysis conditions but in roughly equal amounts at pH 7 or 8 where a spontaneous hydrolysis mechanism predominates. Ketone products are not observed in the hydrolysis of the *anti*-isomer (*533*).

The hydrolysis products of several other pairs of *syn*- and *anti*-bay-region dihydrodiol epoxides have been studied, and apparently three types of product distribution are obtained with *syn*-dihydrodiol epoxides. For these products, *cis*-addition (i.e., product **C** in Scheme XVI) may be predominant as found for the benzo[*a*]pyrene (pH 3–8) and acid-catalyzed benzo[*c*]phenanthrene derivative reactions (*464*). Second, roughly equal amounts of *cis*- and *trans*-addition (products **C** and **D**, respectively) may occur, as for the acid-catalyzed reactions of the phenanthrene and chrysene derivatives (*520*). Third, the ketone **E** may be the major product, as for the hydrolysis of the phenanthrene (*520*) and benzo[*c*]-phenanthrene (*464*) derivatives under neutral conditions.

For the *anti*-dihydrodiol epoxides, a ketone is never found (*520, 533*), and with the exception of the neutral hydrolysis of the benzo[*a*]pyrene derivative, where *cis*- and *trans*-addition (products **I** and **H**, respectively) occur in similar proportions, the *trans*-addition product has been found to be the major product. This includes the acid-catalyzed reaction of the benzo[*a*]pyrene, chrysene (*520*), phenanthrene (*520*), and benzo[*c*]phenanthrene (*464*) derivatives, as well as the neutral hydrolyses of the last two derivatives.

The hydrolysis of the tetrahydro epoxide analogs for some of these compounds has also been examined (*520*). These analogs can yield ketone under neutral conditions—a characteristic of the *syn*-dihydrodiol epoxides—but in the acid-catalyzed reaction, the chrysene and phenanthrene derivatives exhibit predominantly *trans*-addition that is more characteristic of the *anti*-dihydrodiol epoxides.

Kinetic analyses indicate that both specific and general acid-catalyzed hydrolysis mechanisms occur for the *syn*- and *anti*-dihydrodiol epoxide of benzo[*a*]pyrene (*531, 533–35*), and that, for hydrolysis in acid media, the rate-determining step involves carbon–epoxide oxygen bond cleavage from a pre-protonated epoxide ring to form a resonance-stabilized carbonium ion. However, both isomers also hydrolyze by a pH-independent mechanism (referred to as a spontaneous or water-catalyzed mechanism) under neutral- or alkaline-pH conditions (*533*). Furthermore, the relative rates for hydrolysis of the *syn*- and *anti*-isomers by the pH-independent mechanism differ from the relative rates under acid-catalyzed conditions. Thus, for hydrolyses below pH 5 (*531, 533*) where acid-catalyzed mechanisms predominate for both isomers, the *anti*-dihydrodiol epoxide of benzo[*a*]pyrene hydrolyzes 2–3 times more rapidly than the *syn*-isomer, but for hydrolyses by the spontaneous mechanism (e.g., at pH $>$ 7 for both isomers), the *syn*-isomer hydrolyzes nearly 30 times faster than the *anti*-isomer (*533*). Rates of hydrolysis for the *syn*-isomer are less sensitive to acid-catalyzed rate enhancement than are the rates for the *anti*-isomer. In concert with these findings, the *anti*-dihydrodiol epoxides of phenanthrene (*520*), chrysene (*520*), naphthalene (*524, 536*), and benzo[*c*]phenanthrene (*464*) hydrolyze more rapidly than the respective *syn*-isomers under acid-catalyzed conditions, but the corresponding *syn*-isomers react more rapidly than the *anti*-isomers in spontaneous hydrolyses.

Arguments concerning the differences in reactivity between the *syn*- and *anti*-dihydrodiol epoxides of benzo[*a*]pyrene have centered on the presence, in the *syn*-diastereomer, of the quasi-diaxial benzylic hydroxyl group at C-7. This group, as a result of its presence on the same face of the 7,8,9,10-ring as the epoxide oxygen, can donate a hydrogen bond to the epoxide oxygen (*537*). This hydrogen bond could offer electrophilic assistance to ring opening in the *syn*-isomer and enhance its reactivity relative to that of the *anti*-isomer, where such an intramolecular hydrogen bond cannot be formed. Other suggested effects are that this hydrogen bond lowers the basicity of the epoxide oxygen in the *syn*-isomer, and decreases its sensitivity to acid-catalyzed rate enhancement (*531*). However, rate differences have been found for the *syn*- and *anti*-diastereomers of *trans*-1,2-dimethoxy-3,4-epoxy-1,2,3,4-tetrahydronaphthalene (*524, 536*) in which the protons of the *trans*-hydroxyl groups have been replaced by methyl groups. Although the *trans*-methoxyl groups in these dihydrodiol epoxide analogs have been shown to adopt the quasi-diaxial and quasi-diequatorial conformation in the respective *syn*- and *anti*-isomers, an intramolecular hydrogen bond to the epoxide ring in the *syn*-dimethoxy analog is not possible. Nevertheless, the *syn*-dimethoxy isomer still hydrolyzes more rapidly than the *anti*-dimethoxy isomer by a spontaneous mechanism; this finding implies that basic conformational differences between the *syn*- and *anti*-isomers are likely to be more important in determining their relative rates of spontaneous hydrolysis than intramolecular hydrogen bonding (*524, 536*). As mentioned earlier, the *syn*-dihydrodiol epoxide of benzo[*c*]phenanthrene is exceptional in that the hydroxyl groups adopt the quasidiequatorial conformation (*464*). This conformation would make intramolecular hydrogen bonding between the benzylic hydroxyl group and the epoxide ring unfavorable even for the *syn*-isomer, but again, the rates of spontaneous hydrolysis for this isomer still exceed those of the *anti*-isomer (*464*).

There seems to be an agreement, then, that factors other than intramolecular hydrogen bonding in the *syn*-dihydrodiol epoxides are important in governing hydrolytic reactivity differences between the geometrical isomers. However, it is still likely that nucleophilic attack on the *syn*-isomers in nonaqueous media is facilitated by such a hydrogen bond (*370, 464, 524, 533*). For hydrolysis, aspects of conformation and possibly related effects on the basicity of the epoxide oxygens are currently regarded as important determinants of the reactivity differences between *syn*- and *anti*-dihydrodiol epoxides for both the acid-catalyzed and spontaneous mechanisms (*520, 524*). The rates for the acid-catalyzed hydrolysis of bay-region tetrahydro epoxides are much more rapid than the rates for either the *syn*- or *anti*-bay-region dihydrodiol epoxide analogs (*520, 524, 538*). Whalen et al. (*520*) have indicated that for the tetrahydro epoxides, both the rates of acid-catalyzed reaction and the ratio of *cis*- to *trans*-addition to the epoxide increase as the ability of the hydrocarbon residue to stabilize developing positive charge increases. However, for the dihydrodiol epoxides, relative rates of reaction are not paralleled by an analagous distribution of tetrols. An argument based on stereoelectronic factors and polar substituent effects has been invoked to rationalize the stereochemistry of hydrolysis and relative rate differences between tetrahydro epoxides and dihydrodiol epoxides (*520*). In view of the differences in carcinogenic activity for the kinds of compounds discussed and the difficulty of studying the reaction of such compounds in the cellular milieu, further developments in these challenging chemical investigations (*539*) will be followed with interest.

REACTIONS WITH NUCLEIC ACIDS. Despite extensive studies of hydrocarbon–nucleic acid interactions (discussed earlier), relatively few hydrocarbon–nucleoside interaction products have been reasonably well characterized. Early studies with the model compounds 7-bromomethylbenz[*a*]anthracene and 7-bromomethyl-12-methylbenz[*a*]anthracene (*323, 324*) identified the amino groups of nucleic acid bases as the most reactive sites toward these polycyclic aralkylating agents in aqueous solutions. The products of reaction with DNA for 7-bromomethylbenz[*a*]-anthracene were found to be N^2-(benz[*a*]anthracenyl-7-methyl)deoxyguanosine (**XII**A), N^6-(benz[*a*]anthracenyl-7-methyl)deoxyadenosine (**XIIB**), and N^4-(benz-[*a*]anthracenyl-7-methyl)deoxycytidine (**XIIC**). More recently, 6-chloromethyl-benzo[*a*]pyrene has been reported to modify the exocyclic amino groups of the nucleic acid bases (*540*), as have the simplest types of aralkylating agent, i.e., benzylating agents (*322, 541*). Also, an x-ray crystal structure of deoxyadenosine modified on its 6-amino group by 7-bromomethyl-12-methylbenz[*a*]anthracene (Structure **XII**B where R = CH_3) has been reported (*542*). Although an initial report suggested that the *K*-region epoxide of 7,12-dimethylbenz[*a*]anthracene reacted on the imidazole ring of guanine residues in polyguanylic acid (*543*), the amino group was later found to be the primary site of reaction (*544*).

The exocyclic amino groups of some nucleic acid bases are now known to be the principal sites of reaction for the bay-region dihydrodiol epoxide of benzo-[*a*]pyrene and are widely presumed to be the sites of reaction for dihydrodiol epoxide metabolites of other hydrocarbons. These reactions are more complex than those with the model compounds because the dihydrodiol epoxides are optically active compounds and the possibility of either *cis*- or *trans*-addition to the epoxide ring has to be considered in addition to identification of the sites of substitution on the nucleic acid bases. In 1976, Jeffrey et al. (*545*) demonstrated that reaction of benzo[*a*]pyrene bay-region racemic *anti*-dihydrodiol epoxide with polyguanylic acid produced a pair of diastereomeric products resulting from *trans*-addition of the exocyclic amino group (N^2) of guanosine residues to C-10 of the dihydrodiol epoxide. Similar studies by Koreeda et al. (*546*) of the reaction of the racemic *syn*-dihydrodiol epoxide with polyguanylic acid demonstrated production of two pairs of diastereomeric products resulting from both *cis*- and *trans*-addition of the exocyclic amino group of guanosine to C-10. Parallel studies of the in vitro binding of the racemic *anti*-dihydrodiol epoxide to DNA also indicated binding of the dihydrodiol epoxide to the exocyclic amino group of deoxyguanosine residues (*547*). Subsequently, the absolute configuration of the guanosine product (**XIII**A where R = OH) derived from *trans*-addition of $N^2$of guanosine to the (+)-*anti*-dihydrodiol epoxide of benzo[*a*]pyrene was assigned (*2, 548*), as was the

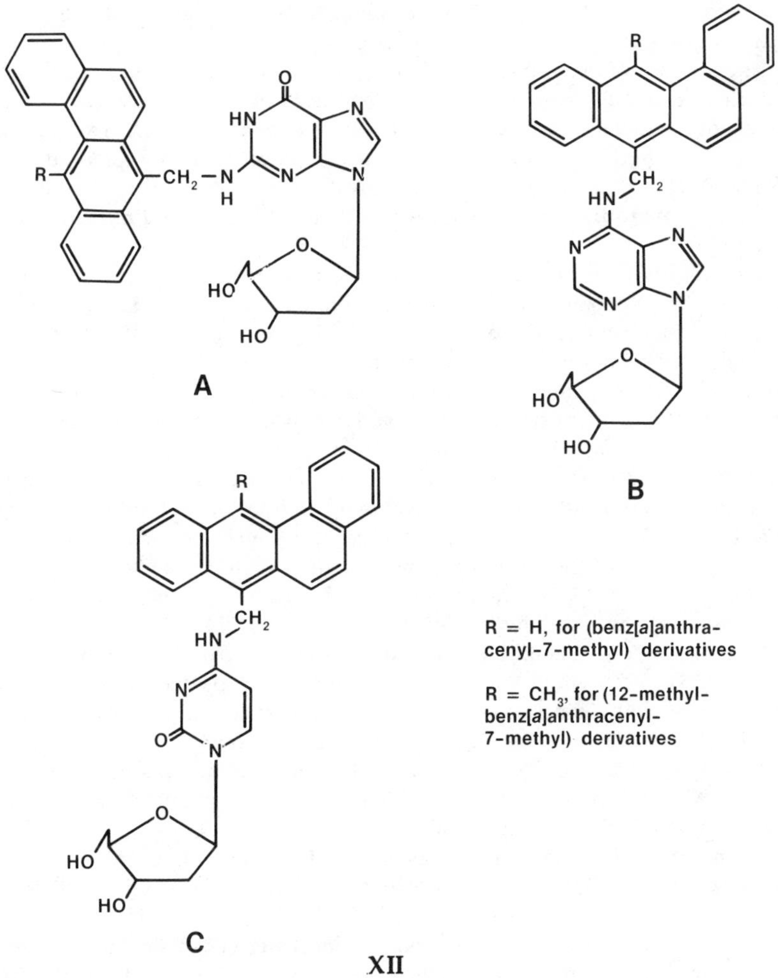

A

B

C

R = H, for (benz[*a*]anthracenyl-7-methyl) derivatives

R = CH_3, for (12-methylbenz[*a*]anthracenyl-7-methyl) derivatives

XII

configuration for the guanosine product (**XIII**B where R = OH) of *cis*-addition of N^2 to the same enantiomer (*548*). Furthermore, structures of guanosine adducts derived from both *trans*- and *cis*-addition to the (−)-*anti*-enantiomer (structures correspond to **XIII**A and **XIII**B, respectively, except the hydrocarbon residues bear a mirror image relationship to those illustrated) and *trans*- and *cis*-addition to both the (+)- and (−)-*syn*-enantiomers were also determined (*548*). The structure of the *trans*-addition product (**XIII**C) to the (+)-*syn*-enantiomer is illustrated.

Not all of these products of chemical reaction of benzo[*a*]pyrene bay-region dihydrodiol epoxides with guanine residues have been found in cells or tissues exposed to benzo[*a*]pyrene itself. The major product of benzo[*a*]pyrene–DNA binding (*228, 378–80, 384*) has been reported to be the result of *trans*-addition of the amino group of deoxyguanosine residues to C-10 of the (+)-*anti*-dihydrodiol epoxide in most systems (*see* Ref. 229 for exception).

For the case of benzo[*a*]pyrene binding to the RNA of mouse skin, the major products of reaction have been shown to be the result of *trans*- and *cis*-addition of the N^2 of guanosine residues to the (+)-*anti*-enantiomer, (**XIII**A and **XIII**B, respectively, where R = OH) as well as *trans*-addition to the (+)-*syn*-dihydrodiol epoxide (**XIII**C) (*228, 548*). These same products were formed in the binding of benzo[*a*]pyrene to the RNA of hamster embryo cells (*384*) and human bronchial tissue (*379*).

Benzo[*a*]pyrene modification of adenine residues in cellular RNA does not appear to be extensive (*379, 384*) although modified adenine residues were detected in hamster embryo cell DNA (*384*) and in in vitro reactions of benzo[*a*]pyrene dihydrodiol epoxide with ribo and deoxyribo homopolymers, as well as with DNA (*549–51*). In more recent chemical studies, the structure and stereochemistry of adenosine (R = OH) and deoxyadenosine (R = H) adducts with the (+)- and (−)-*anti*-7,8-dihydrodiol 9,10-epoxide of benzo[*a*]pyrene have been elucidated. These products have been shown to be a consequence of both *trans*- and *cis*-addition to C-10 of the dihydrodiol epoxide of benzo[*a*]pyrene by the N^6 exocyclic amino group of the adenine base; the structures of the *trans*-addition product (**XIII**D) and the *cis*-addition product (**XIII**E) to the (+)-*anti*-dihydrodiol epoxide are given (*552*). Interestingly, in in vitro reactions of the separate enantiomers of the *anti*-dihydrodiol epoxides with DNA, the major product of reaction of the (+)-enantiomer is with the amino group of deoxyguanosine residues (*551, 552*), while the exocyclic amino group of deoxyadenosine is the major site of DNA reaction with the (−)-enantiomer of the *anti*-dihydrodiol epoxide (*551, 552*). For the binding of benzo[*a*]pyrene with deoxyadenosine residues (R = H) in the DNA of mouse skin, only products resulting from *trans*-addition (**XIII**D) and *cis*-addition (**XIII**E) to the (+)-*anti*-dihydrodiol epoxide of benzo[*a*]pyrene have been detected so far (*553*).

As mentioned earlier, the involvement of the *syn*-dihydrodiol epoxide of benzo[*a*]pyrene in DNA binding has been clearly implicated in both in vitro reactions and in cellular systems (e.g., Refs. 229, 372, 373, 554). However, the structures and stereochemistry of DNA adducts derived from this geometrical isomer have not been as well defined as those for the adducts illustrated. Additionally, until more detailed spectroscopic characterizations are available, the structural assignments for products of the (−)-*anti*-dihydrodiol epoxide binding to DNA (*384*), of deoxycytidine-modified products (*384, 551*), or of minor products of dihydrodiol epoxide binding to sites other than the exocyclic amino groups of the DNA bases (*555, 556*) should probably be regarded as tentative at present. Difficulties in these structural characterizations stem from the limited availability of substantial quantities of well-characterized dihydrodiol epoxides, the low yields of nucleic products obtained and the consequent difficulty in obtaining extensive spectroscopic data, the complex chemistry that determines site selectivity in nucleic acid alkylation (*557–60*), and the complex reactivity and stereochemistry of the dihydrodiol epoxides discussed earlier.

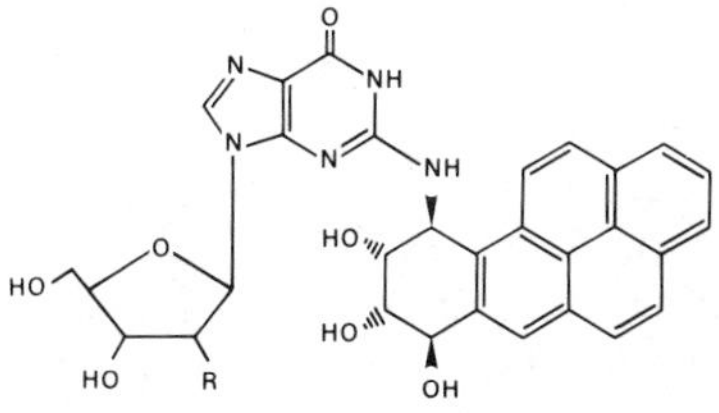

O NH N N N NH HO HO HO R HO OH

A. Product of *trans* addition of N^2 of guanosine (R = OH) and 2′-deoxyguanosine (R = H) to the (+) *anti* dihydrodiol epoxide of benzo[*a*]-pyrene.

O NH N N N NH HO HO OH HO HO OH

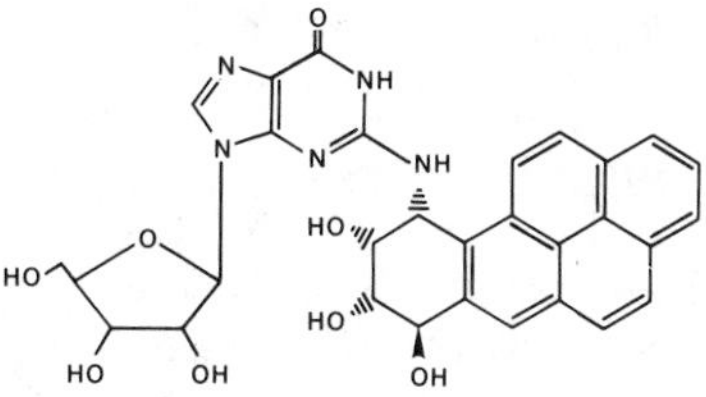

B. Product of *cis* addition of N^2 of guanosine to the (+) *anti* dihydrodiol epoxide of benzo[*a*]pyrene.

O NH N N N NH HO HO OH HO HO OH

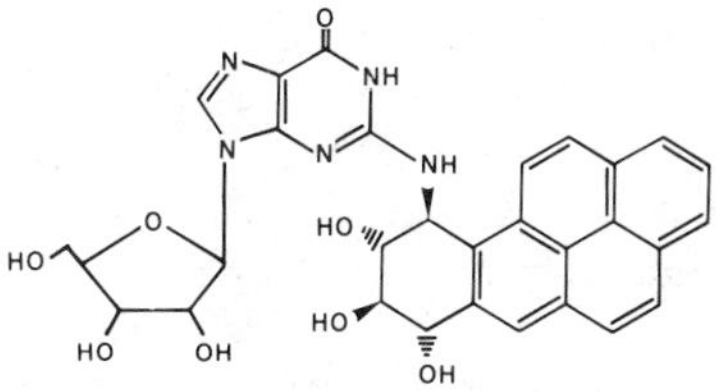

C. Product of *trans* addition of N^2 of guanosine to the (+) *syn* dihydrodiol epoxide of benzo[*a*]pyrene.

R OH OH O N N N N HN HO HO OH

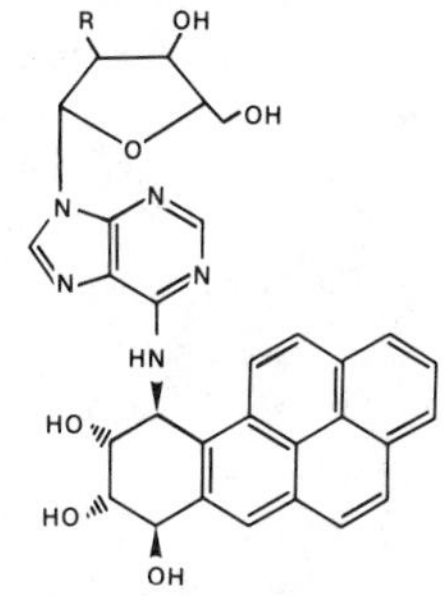

D. Product of *trans* addition of N^6 of adenosine (R = OH) and 2′-deoxyadenosine (R = H) to the (+) *anti* dihydrodiol epoxide of benzo[*a*]pyrene.

R OH OH O N N N N HN HO HO OH

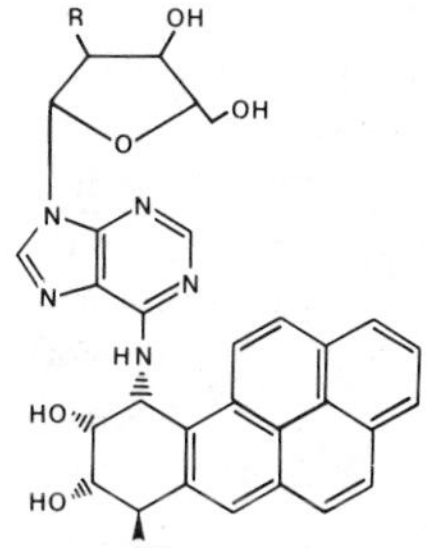

E. Product of *cis* addition of N^6 of adensoine (R = OH) and 2′-deoxyadenosine (R = H) to the (+) *anti* dihydrodiol epoxide of benzo[*a*]pyrene.

XIII

General Observations

During the last 7 or 8 years, research activity on the polycyclic aromatic hydrocarbons has been intense and, in order to limit the size of this chapter, a selection of material has been made. In making these choices, we have borne in mind that the subject matter is the polynuclear carcinogens themselves, not the process of carcinogenesis in general, and that the properties of this class of carcinogens that should be included are those that are most relevant to their carcinogenic properties. This latter judgment inescapably involves the authors' opinions or prejudices, which may not be shared by all our colleagues. Nevertheless, we have not reviewed all of the different cells, tissues, or microsomal preparations in which the metabolism of benzo[*a*]pyrene has been examined, nor have we reviewed the extensive studies of mutation, cytotoxicity, and DNA repair that have been undertaken with hydrocarbons or their derivatives. From our perspective, in the context of this volume, the key question for discussion is how the polynuclear carcinogens exert their carcinogenic or tumor-initiating effects. The developments in the field do not permit a discussion, as yet, of this whole process but rather focus attention on the metabolic activation of the carcinogen.

The recent burst of activity has been stimulated initially by the discovery by Sims et al. (*141*) of the dihydrodiol epoxide route of metabolism for polycyclic hydrocarbons. This finding created a need for the synthesis of dihydrodiols and dihydrodiol epoxides that has led to some fascinating chemistry and stereochemistry. Another major impact on the field was the bay-region dihydrodiol epoxide generalization by Jerina and Daly (*76*) that rationalized much of the structure–activity data that have been available for many years and gave direction to studies of hydrocarbons other than benzo[*a*]pyrene. With the benefit of hindsight, one wonders that this insight on structure–activity relationships was not recognized earlier and can only conclude that thinking about these relationships has been unconsciously restricted by the popular hypotheses of the day.

In thinking about the metabolic activation of hydrocarbon carcinogens, a conclusion that is difficult to avoid is that the most objective and useful criteria for examining activation, once routes of metabolism are known, are the data obtained in assays of the carcinogenic properties of various metabolites in relation to the carcinogenic properties of the parent hydrocarbons (Tables VI–IX). Through the efforts of several laboratories, and in particular through the productive collaboration between Jerina's and Conney's laboratories, extensive data are available. The carcinogenic properties of metabolites involved in the dihydrodiol epoxide pathway of metabolism strongly suggest an association between this pathway and the expression of carcinogenic activity. It is difficult, however, to look totally objectively at these data and conclude that it is proven that the ultimate carcinogen for most of the hydrocarbons listed in Tables VI–IX is the bay-region *anti*-dihydrodiol epoxide. This conclusion could only arise from a weighing of evidence for and against, which would necessarily be a subjective process.

These data were discussed earlier, but a more concise summary of the data obtained from the tumor initiation assays will permit discussion of a large group of hydrocarbons. Inclusive of benzo[*a*]pyrene, the activities of 12 hydrocarbons have been compared with the activities of the appropriate dihydrodiol precursor to the bay-region dihydrodiol epoxide in this system. For 10 of the hydrocarbons, the dihydrodiol exhibits activity equal to or higher than that of the parent hydrocarbon. The two exceptions are dibenz[*a,h*]anthracene, where the dihydrodiol exhibits only marginally lower activity than the parent hydrocarbon, and 3-methylcholanthrene, where the dihydrodiol exhibits only about 70% of the activity of the parent. However, in this latter case the activity of the dihydrodiol is increased by introducing a hydroxyl group in the 1-position (Table IX). Thus, for most of the cases examined, these dihydrodiols exhibit properties expected for proximate carcinogens. In seven cases, the activities of the hydrocarbons and bay-region dihydrodiol epoxides have been compared. In only two cases, benz[*a*]-anthracene and benzo[*c*]phenanthrene, the dihydrodiol epoxide is substantially more active than the parent hydrocarbon, and in these cases, it is also more active than its dihydrodiol precursor. In the remaining five cases, the dihydrodiol epoxide is substantially less active than the parent hydrocarbon and substantially less active than its dihydrodiol precursor. Thus, for most of these cases, the dihydrodiol epoxides do not exhibit the properties expected for ultimate carcinogens. This failure to meet expectation can be rationalized in a number of ways and, of course, in the newborn mouse system (Table VIII), the benzo[*a*]pyrene dihydrodiol epoxide does exhibit properties expected of an ultimate carcinogen. Nevertheless, it might be unwise to totally neglect the more direct interpretations of the findings discussed, i.e., although the dihydrodiols largely exhibit the properties of proximate carcinogens, the corresponding bay-region dihydrodiol epoxides largely do not exhibit the properties of ultimate carcinogens.

For example, one might conclude that more than one metabolite is required for initiation of carcinogenesis by hydrocarbons and although both of the required metabolites (one of these would presumably be the dihydrodiol epoxide) could be generated from the hydrocarbon or from the dihydrodiol, the dihydrodiol epoxide itself would not be a suitable precursor for the generation of the second metabolite in most cases. A second interpretation, which is analogous to some of our earlier work (*126*), might be that the ultimate carcinogen is really some reactive intermediate generated in the course of the metabolic conversion of the dihydrodiol to the dihydrodiol epoxide, such as a benzylic carbonium ion, akin to the intermediates discussed along with Schemes IV–VI. This possibility is not totally unrealistic for, given the complexity of the solvolytic reactivities of the dihydrodiol epoxides (discussed earlier), it is conceivable that those that do exhibit potent tumor-initiating activity could solvolyse primarily through the same intermediates that are generated metabolically; those dihydrodiol epoxides that are less potent initiators might solvolyze primarily through subtly different intermediates. Such a proposal would be consistent with the fact that the products of DNA binding in cellular systems are the same as those formed in in vitro reactions between DNA and bay-region dihydrodiol epoxides, but our model studies suggest that the distribution of products would be different (*557, 558*). However, the distribution of carcinogen adducts over the genome may well be a key factor in determining tumor initiation (*321, 322, 557*).

This discussion emphasizes the need for further detailed investigations of the chemistry of the dihydrodiol epoxides, because such efforts may well shed light on the mechanism of hydrocarbon carcinogenesis. Already, a fascinating story is developing with respect to the carcinogenic activities of the geometrical isomers of the bay-region dihydrodiol epoxides, apart from any relationship they might have to the carcinogenic activities of the parent hydrocarbons. Thus, for both bay-region *syn*- and *anti*-dihydrodiol epoxides, substantial carcinogenic activity seems to be associated with those dihydrodiol epoxides in which the hydroxyl groups prefer a quasi-diequatorial conformation and not with those in which the hydroxyl groups are quasi-diaxial. Moreover, even when the quasi-diequatorial conformation is preferred, as for the bay-region *anti*-dihydrodiol epoxide of benzo[*a*]pyrene, one enantiomer is a far more potent carcinogen than another. It is conceivable that the dihydrodiol function limits the carcinogenic potency of epoxides formed adjacent to a bay region; although, starting from the parent hydrocarbon, formation of the dihydrodiol serves the necessary purpose of saturating the neighboring double bond. Again, a quasi-diaxial conformation for these hydroxyl groups seems to be deleterious with respect to carcinogenic activity, and for benzo[*e*]pyrene and benz[*a*]anthracene, the dihydro analog of the dihydrodiol precursor of the bay-region dihydrodiol epoxide is a more potent tumor initiator than the dihydrodiol itself (Table IX).

The bay-region *syn*-dihydrodiol epoxide of benzo[*c*]phenanthrene is the only *syn*-dihydrodiol epoxide in which the hydroxyl groups prefer the quasi-diequatorial conformation and which exhibits carcinogenic potency comparable to that of the *anti*-diastereomer. Jerina has attributed this behavior to the steric presence of a benzo substituent in the bay region. A certain similarity exists between this steric situation and that of hydrocarbons with a methyl substituent in the bay region. For example, 7,12-dimethylbenz[*a*]anthracene, 5-methylchrysene, 15,16-dihydro-11-methylcyclopenta[*a*]phenanthrene-13-one and 11-methylbenzo[*a*]pyrene are all more potent carcinogens than the corresponding compound that lacks the bay-region methyl group. It will be of interest to see whether the bay-region dihydrodiol epoxides of these carcinogens exhibit any resemblance to those of benzo[*c*]phenanthrene.

In conclusion, the hydrocarbon field is in the midst of very exciting developments. The metabolic activation of the hydrocarbons is growing increasingly clear, and because of the availability of extensive series of related compounds, the possibility of defining some general rules for activation seems to be a realistic objective, which may be largely achieved already. After a comparatively stagnant period, the last decade has been turbulent and encouraging. Apart from the progress made toward understanding the metabolic activation of hydrocarbons—a major and welcome development in the authors' perception—has been the increase in the level of chemical characterization and sophistication. As researchers in this field, we have been fortunate to have experienced the recent exciting developments and look forward to the continuation of this high rate of progress in the future.

Acknowledgments

The authors express their thanks to Cheri Rhoderick and Carol Whipp for expert assistance in the preparation of this manuscript, to Wayne Levin for his advice on tumorigenicity data and for reviewing Tables VI, VII, and VIII, to Chris Michejda for discussions of chemistry, to Dijon Grunberger for copies of correspondence with Kurt Loening about nomenclature, and to Don Jerina, Bill Baird, Alan Jeffrey,

Ron Harvey, Phil Grover, Ercole Cavalieri, Bill Herndon, and other colleagues who graciously responded to our various inquiries. The authors' research is supported by contract NO1–CO–75380 with the National Cancer Institute, National Institutes of Health, Bethesda, Md.

Appendix A. Carcinogenic Activities of Unsubstituted Polycyclic Aromatic Hydrocarbons

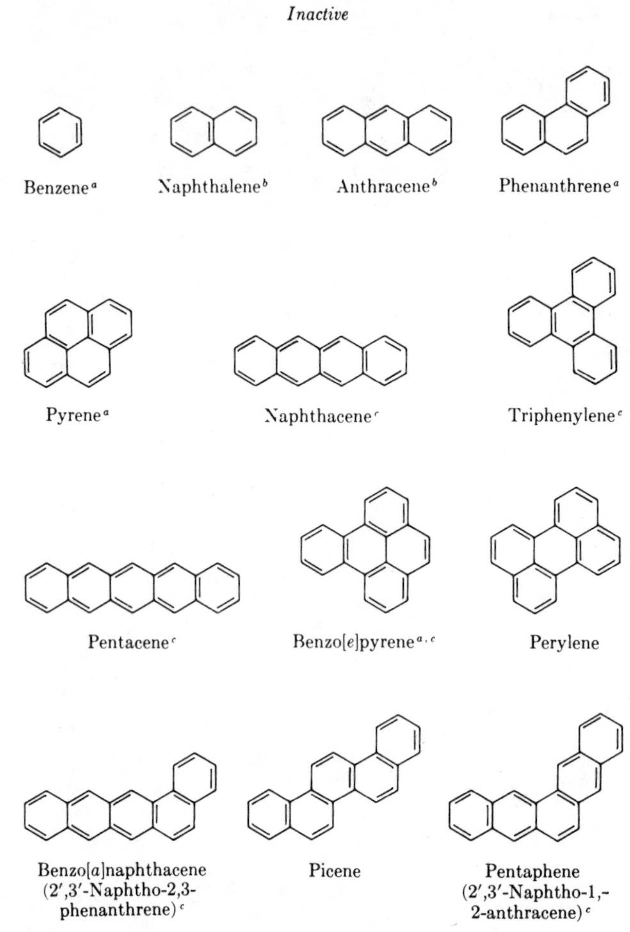

[a]Occasional skin papillomas reported.
[b]Tumors reported after very high doses.
[c]Subjected to limited testing only.
[d]Dibenzo[*de,qr*]naphthacene is referred to as naphtho[2,3:1,2]pyrene by Arcos and Argus (*24*) and is said to be inactive, although Hoffmann and Wynder (*39*) have demonstrated weak initiating activity.
[e]The activity exhibited by chrysene in early experiments (*40,41*) was subsequently attributed to impurities (*42*). Recently, however, Van Duuren et al. (*43*) found chrysene to be an effective initiator in the mouse skin system.
[f]Dibenz[*a,c*]anthracene, long regarded as inactive, recently exhibited some activity after topical application to mouse skin (*44, 45*) although it remains inactive if administered by subcutaneous injection to mice (*46*).

Disputed	*Moderate*	*High Activity*
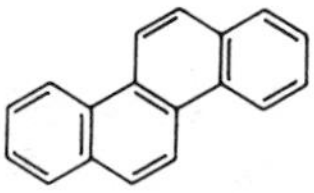 Chrysene[e]	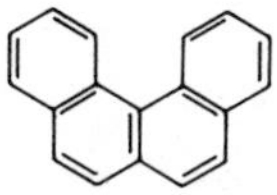 Benzo[*c*]phenanthrene (3, 4-Benzphenanthrene)	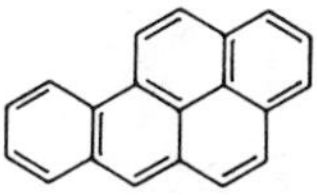 Benzo[*a*]pyrene
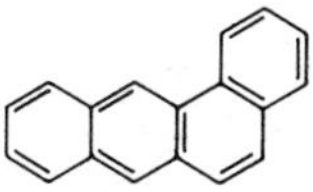 Benz[*a*]anthracene (1,2-Benzanthracene)	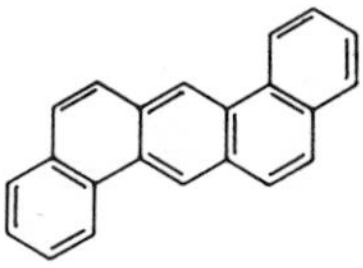 Dibenz[*a, h*]anthracene (1,2:5,6-Dibenzanthracene)[g]	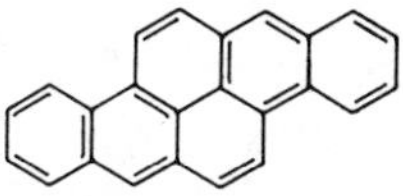 Dibenzo[*b, def*]chrysene (Dibenzo[*a, h*]pyrene)
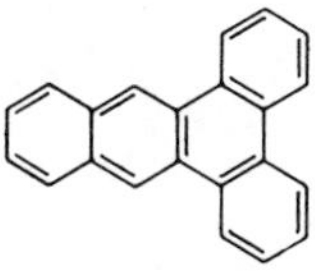 Dibenz[*a, c*]anthracene (1,2:3,4-Dibenzanthracene)[f]	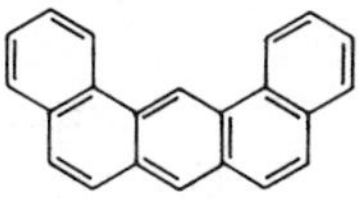 Dibenz[*a,j*]anthracene (1,2:7,8-Dibenzanthracene)[c,g]	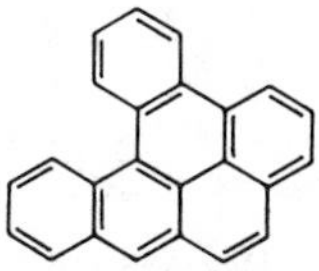 Dibenzo[*def,p*]chrysene (Dibenzo[*a,l*]pyrene)
	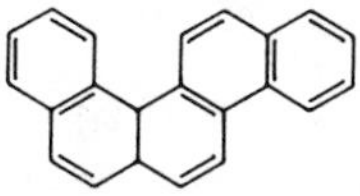 Benzo[*c*]chrysene (1,2:5,6-Dibenzphenanthrene)[c,h]	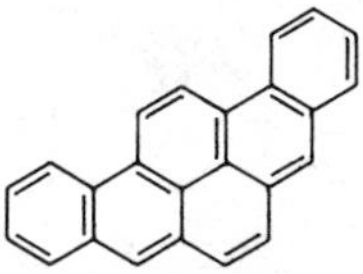 Benzo[*rst*]pentaphene (Dibenzo[*a,i*]pyrene)

[g]Dibenz[*a,j*]anthracene is less active than dibenz[*a,h*]anthracene (*44*).
[h]Benzo[*g*]chrysene is slightly more active than benzo[*c*]chrysene (*19*).
[i]*See* Lacassagne et al. (*37*).
[j]Produces leukemia and ovarian tumors but not sarcoma (*23*).

Continued on next page

Appendix A Continued

Inactive

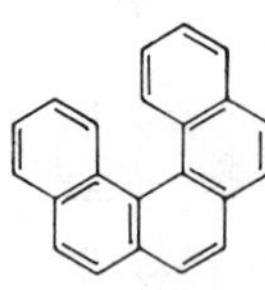

Dibenzo[*c,g*]phenanthrene (3,4:5,6-Dibenzphenanthrene)[c]

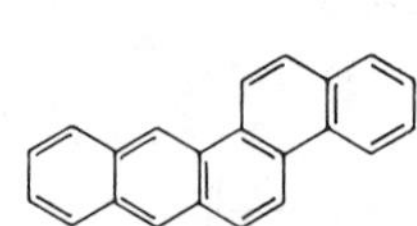

Benzo[*b*]chrysene(2′,3′-Naphtho-1,2-phenanthrene)[c]

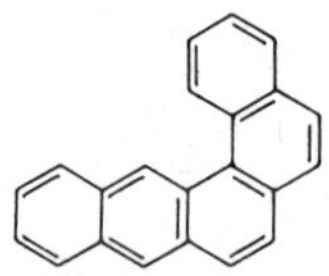

Dibenzo[*b,g*]phenanthrene(1,2-(1′,2′-Naphth)anthracene)[c]

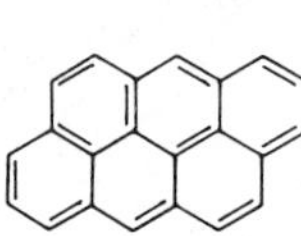

Dibenzo[*def,mno*]-chrysene (Anthanthrene)[a]

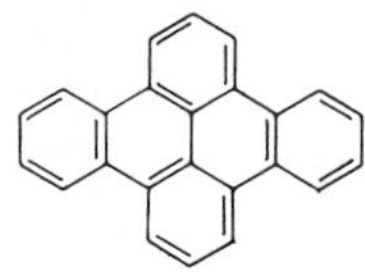

Dibenzo[*fg,op*]naphthacene (Dibenzo[*e,l*]pyrene)[c]

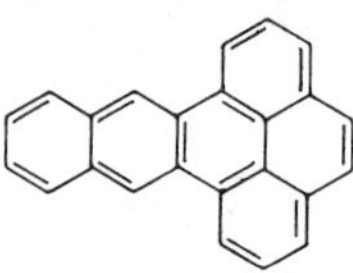

Dibenzo[*de,qr*]naphthacene(Naphtho-[2,3-*e*]pyrene)[c,d]

Dibenzo[*b,k*]chrysene

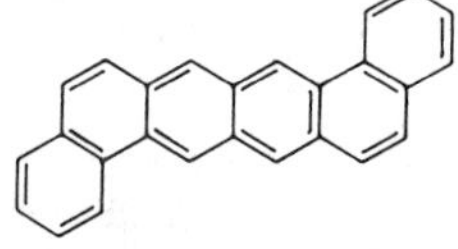

Dibenzo[*a,j*]naphthacene[c,i]

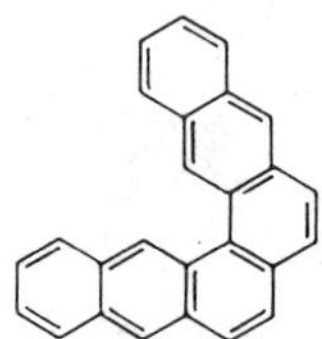

Anthra[1,2-*a*]anthracene

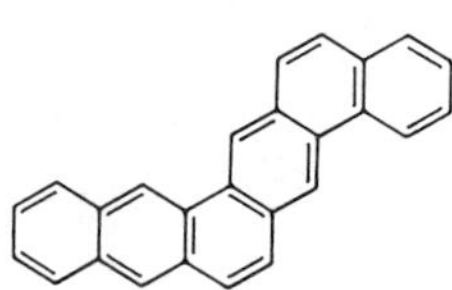

Benzo[c]penthaphene[c]

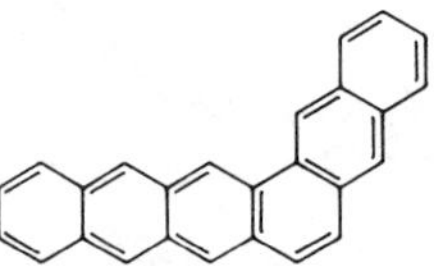

Benzo[*b*]pentaphene[c,i]

Naphtho[1,2-*b*]triphenylene

Disputed	*Moderate*	*High Activity*
	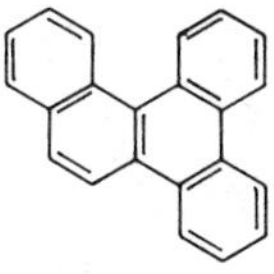 Benzo[*g*]chrysene(1,2:3,4-Dibenzphenanthrene)[h]	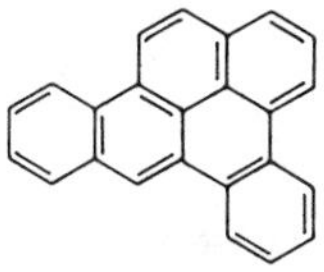 Naphtho[1,2,3,4-*def*]chrysene (Dibenzo[*a*,*e*]pyrene)
	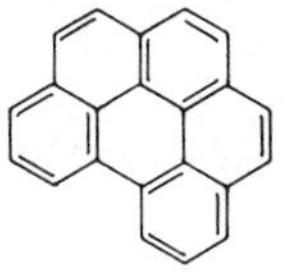 Benzo[*ghi*]perylene	
	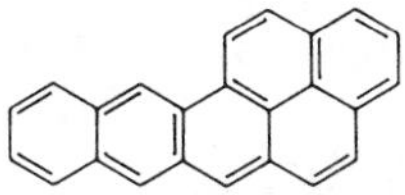 Naphtho[8,1,2-*cde*]naphthacene (Naphtho[2,3-*a*]pyrene)[c]	
	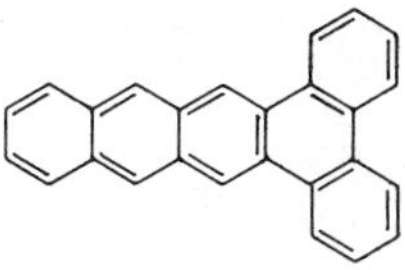 Dibenzo[*a*,*c*]naphthacene[i]	

Appendix B. Carcinogenic Activities of Monosubstituted Benz[*a*]anthracenes

Substituent Giving Rise to Compounds of Carcinogenic Activity:

Site of Substitution	*Inactive*
1	$-CH_3$[a,b,d]
2	$-CH_3$[a,c,d]
3	$-CH_3$[a,d]
4	$-CH_3$[a,d]; $-CH_2COOC_2H_5$[c]; $-OH$[a,b,c]; $-OCOCH_3$[b]; $-SO_2Cl$[c]; $-SO_3K$[c]; $-SO_3C_2H_5$[c]; $-OCH_3$[a,b,c]
5	$-CH_3$[d]; $-CH(CH_3)_2$[a]; $-OCH_2COOH$[b]; $-OCOC_6H_5$[b]; $-OCO(CH_2)_{16}CH_3$[b]; $-NCO$[b]; $-F$[a,b,c,i]
6	
7	$-CH_2CHCH_2$[b]; $-(CH_2)_2CH_3$[b]; $-CH(CH_3)_2$[a,b]; $-(CH_2)_3CH_3$[b]; $-(CH_2)_4CH_3$[b]; $-CH_2C_6H_5$[a]; $-CH_2COOH$[b,c]; $-CH_2COONa$[e]; $-CH_2CH(OCOC_6H_5)CH_2OCOC_6H_5$[b]; $-CH(OH)CH_3$[b]; $-CHO$[d]; $-CH_2Cl$[b]; $-CH_2OCH_3$[b]; $-CH_2OC_2H_5$[b]; $-COCH_3$[a,b]; $-COONa$; $-CH_2SH$[b]; $-CH_2SCH_2CH(NH_2)COOH$[b]; $-CH_2SCN$[b]; $-CH_2NCS$[b]; $-CH_2N(CH_3)_2$[b]; $-CH_2N(C_2H_5)_2$[b]; $-SCN$[b]; $-SCH_2CH(NH_2)COOH$[b]; $-NCO$[b]; $-NO_2$[b]; $-OH$[b]; $-Cl$[c]; $-Pb(C_6H_5)_3$[b]
8	$-(CH_2)_3CH_3$[c]; $-(CH_2)_4CH_3$[b]; $-(CH_2)_5CH_3$[b]; $-(CH_2)_6CH_3$[b]; $-CH_2COONa$[b]; $-COONa$[a,b,f]
9	$-CH_3$[d]; $-C_6H_5$[a]
10	$-CH_3$[a,d]; $-CH(CH_3)_2$[a]
11	$-CH_3$[b,c,d]; $-C_2H_5$[b]; $-CH(CH_3)_2$[b]; $-OH$[b]
12	

[a]Painting on mouse skin.
[b]Subcutaneous injection in mice.
[c]Subcutaneous injection in rats.
[d]Intramuscular injection in rats (*48*).
[e]Intravenous injection in mice.
[f]Intraperitoneal injection in mice.
[g]Tested for initiating activity in mouse skin (*49*).
[h]Subcutaneous injection in newborn mice (*50*).
[i]*See* Miller and Miller (*51*).

Substituent Giving Rise to Compounds of Carcinogenic Activity: Slight	Moderate	High
-CH_3[c]		
-CH_3[c]		
-CH_3[c]; -F[b,i]		-F[c,i]
-CH_3[a,c]; -OH[b]; -OCH_3[b]	-CH_3[b]	
-CH_3[a]		-CH_3[b,c,d]
-C_2H_5[d]; -CH_2CH_2OH[a,b]; -CH_2Br[g]; -CH_2CN[b]; -$CH_2OC_2H_5$[a]; -CH_2COONa[c]; -CN[a,b]; OCH_3[d]; -SH[b]; -Br[c]	-CH_3[a]; -CH_2OH[a]; -CHO[b]; -CH_2Br[h]; -CH_2OCOCH_3[a,b]; -CH_2COOH_3[b]; $COCl_3$[b,c]; -OCH_3[b]	-CH_3[b,c,d]; -C_2H_5[b]; -CH_2OH
-C_2H_5[a]; -$(CH_2)_2CH_3$[a]; -$CH(CH_3)_2$[a,b]; -$(CH_2)_3CH_3$[a]; -$(CH_2)_4CH_3$[a]; -$(CH_2)_5CH_3$[a]; -$(CH_2)_6CH_3$[a]; -C_6H_5[a]	-CH_3[a]; -OCH_3[b]	-CH_3[b,c,d]
-CH_3[a,c]	-$CH(CH_3)_2$[a]	
-CH_3[b,c]		
-CH_3[a]		
-CH_3[a]; -C_2H_5[d]	-CH_3[c,d]	-CH_3[b]

Appendix C. Carcinogenic Activities of Substituted Benz[*a*]anthracenes

Carcinogenic Activities of Dimethylbenz[a]*anthracenes*

Inactive	*Slight*
1,7[b]; 1,12[d]; 2, 9[a,b]; 2,10[a]; 3,9[a,d]; 3,10[a]; 4,7[d,m]; 4,12[d,m]; 5,12[b,d,m]; 8,11[b]	9,10[a,d]; 9,11[a]

Carcinogenic Activities of 7-Methylbenz[a]*anthracene Derivatives*

Inactive	*Slight*
1-CH_3[b]; 3-$CH(CH_3)_2$[b]; 4-CH_3[d,m]; 4-F[b,c,j]; 5-F[a,b,c]; 5-NCO[b]; 5-OH[b]; 9-$COOCH_3$[b]; 9-Cl[b]; 9-CN[b]; 9-COOH[b]; 10-$COOCH_3$[b]; 10-COOH[b]; 12-CH_2OH[h,u]; 12-SCN[b]; 2,3-di-CH_3[d,m]; 2,12-di-CH_3[d,m]; 3, 12-di-CH_3[d,m]; 4-OH, 12-CH_3[c,p]; 4-OCH_3, 12-CH_3[a,b,c,p]; 5-OCH_3,-12-CH_3[c,p]; 8-C_2H_5,12-CH_3[a,b]	3-F[a,g,k]; 4-F[g]; 5-F[g]; 9-F[b,c,k]; 10-Cl[b]; 12-$OCOCH_3$[b]; 5, 12-di-CH_3[d,m] 6, 12-di-CH_3[a,b]; 9, 10, 12-tri-CH_3[b]

Carcinogenic Activities of 7, 12-Disubstituted Benz[a]*anthracenes*

Inactive	*Slight*
7,12-di-C_2H_5[d,n]; 7,12-di-CN[d,m]; 7,12-di-OCH_3[b]; 7,12-di-CH_2OH[h]; 7,12-di-$(CH_2)_2CH_3$[b]; 7,12-di-C_6H_5[a]; 7,12-di-$OCOCH_3$[b]; 7-SCN,12-CH_3[b]; 7-$(CH_2)_2OH$,12-CH_3[d,l]; 7-$(CH_2)_3OH$,-12-CH_3[d,l]; 7-$(CH_2)_3CH_3$,12-CH_3[d,n]; 7-CH_2OCH_3,12-CH_3[d,n]; 7-CH_3,12-SCN[b]; 7-CH_3,12-CH_2OH[h,u]	7, 12-di-C_2H_5[a]; 7, 12-di-CH_2OH[b]; 7, 12-di-CH_2OCOCH_3[a,b]; 7-CH_2OH, 12-CH_3[d,l] 7-$CH(OH)CH_3$, 12-CH_3[d,l]; 7-CH_2OCH_3, 12-CH_3[c,p] 7-CH_2CHO, 12-CH_3[c,t]

Carcinogenic Activities of 7,12-Dimethylbenz[a]*anthracene Derivatives*

Inactive	*Slight*
2-CH_3[d,m]; 3-CH_3[d,m]; 4-OH[c,p]; 4-OCH_3[a,b,c,p]; 5-OCH_3[c,p]; 8-C_2H_5[a,b]	5-CH_3[d,m]; 6-CH_3[a,b]; 9,10-di-CH_3[b]; 5-F[v]

Carcinogenic Activities of Other Substituted Benz[a]*anthracenes*

Inactive	*Slight*
5,7-di-OCH_3[b]; 7,8-di-C_2H_5[d,o]; 7,9-di-C_2H_5[d,o]; 4-Cl,7-CH_2Br[b,g,r,s]; 5-OCH_3,7-$(CH_2)_2CH_3$[b,e]; 7-CH_2OH,5,12-di-CH_3[d,m]; 5-F,9-CH_3[v]	1-CH_3,7-CH_2Br[g,r]; 4-Br,7-CH_2Br[g,r]; 5-OCH_3,7-C_2H_5[b]; 7-CH_2OH,4,-12-di-CH_3[d,m]

[a] Painting on mouse skin.
[b] Subcutaneous injection in mice.
[c] Subcutaneous injection in rats.
[d] Intramuscular injection in rats.
[e] Intravenous injection in mice.
[f] Intraperitoneal injection in mice.
[g] Tested for initiating activity in mouse skin.
[h] Intragastric administration in rats giving mammary tumors.
[i] Intravenous injection in rats giving mammary tumors.
[j] Adequate testing was precluded by high toxicity.
[k] Miller and Miller (*51*).

Moderate	*High*
Carcinogenic Activities of Dimethylbenz*[a]*anthracenes	
6,7[b]; 6,12[b]; 7,8[b]; 7,11[b]	4,5[c]; 6,7[d]; 6,8[d]; 6,12[d]; 7,8[d]; 7,11[d,m]; 7,12[a,b,c,d,h]; 8,9[a]; 8,12[b,d]
Carcinogenic Activities of 7-Methylbenz*[a]*anthracene Derivatives	
3-F[b,c,k]; 5-OCH_3[b]; 6-F[b,k]; 6-CH_3[b]; 8-CH_3[b]; 8-OCH_3[b]; 8-$CONH_2$[b]; 9-F[a,g,k]; 10-F[a,b,c,g,k]; 10-CN[b]; 11-CH_3[b]; 12-C_2H_5[d,n]; 12-CH_2OH[b,t]; 8-CN, 12-CH_3[b]; 8-$(CH_2)_2CH_3$, 12-CH_3[a,b]; 9,12-di-CH_3[a,b]; 8,9,12-tri-CH_3[a,b]; 9,10,12-tri-CH_3[a]	6-F[a,c,k]; 6-CH_3[d]; 8-Cl[b]; 8-CN[b]; 8-CH_3[d]; 11-CH_3[d,m]; 12-CH_3[a,b,c,d,h]; 4,12-di-CH_3[d,m]; 6,8-di-CH_3[d]; 6,12-di-CH_3[d]; 8,12-di-CH_3[a,b,d,i]; 9,12,di-CH_3[d,m]; 10,12-di-CH_3[d,m]; 8-Br,12-CH_3[b]
Carcinogenic Activities of 7, 12-Disubstituted Benz*[a]*anthracenes	
7, 12-di-Cl[a]; 7,12-di-OCH_3[d,n]; 7-CN,12-CH_3[a,b]; 7-$CH_2OC_2H_5$, 12-CH_3[b]; 7-C_2H_5,12-CH_3[b]; 7-$(CH_2)_2CH_3$,12-CH_3[d,n]; 7-CH_2I, 12-CH_3[c,p]; 7-CH_2OH,12-CH_3[b,h,t,u]; 7-CH_2OCOCH_3,12-CH_3[b,t]; 7-CH_3,12-C_2H_5[d,n]; 7-CH_3, 12-CH_2OH[b,t]	7,12-di-CH_3[a,b,c,d,h]; 7-OC_2H_5,-12-CH_3[d]; 7-OCH_3,12-CH_3[d]; 7-CHO,12-CH_3[c,d,p]; 7-C_2H_5,12-CH_3[d,l]; 7-CH_2OH,12-CH_3[c,p]; 7-CH_2Br,12-CH_3[c,g,q,r]; 7-CH_2OCOCH_3, 12-CH_3[c,p]; 7-CH_2Cl, 12-CH_3[c,p]; 7-$CH_2OCOC_6H_5$, 12-CH_3[c,p]
Carcinogenic Activities of 7,12-Dimethylbenz*[a]*anthracene Derivatives	
8-CN[b]; 8-$(CH_2)_2CH_3$; 9-CH_3[a,b]; 8,9-di-CH_3[a,b]; 9,10-di-CH_3[a]	4-CH_3[d,m]; 6-CH_3[d]; 8-CH_3[a,b,d,i]; 8-Br[b]; 9-CH_3[d,m]; 10-CH_3[d,m]
Carcinogenic Activities of Other Substituted Benz*[a]*anthracenes	
8,12-di-C_2H_5[d,o]; 6-F, 7-CH_2Br[g,r]	6,8-di-C_2H_5[d,o]; 4,5,10-tri-CH_3[c]; 6,8,12-tri-CH_3[d]; 5-F,12-CH_3[v]

[l] Pataki and Huggins (*52*).
[m] Pataki et al. (*53*).
[n] Huggins et al. (*48*).
[o] Pataki and Balick (*54*).
[p] Flesher and Sydnor (*55*).
[q] Dipple and Slade (*56*).
[r] Dipple and Slade (*49*).
[s] Roe et al. (*50*).
[t] Boyland and Sims (*57*).
[u] Boyland et al. (*58*).
[v] Bergmann et al. (*59*).

Appendix D. Carcinogenic Activities of Tricyclic and Tetracyclic Aromatic Hydrocarbon Derivatives

Inactive

Anthracene Derivatives

1-C_6H_5[a]; 2-CH_3[a]; 2-C_6H_5[a]; 9-CH_3[a,b]; 9-C_2H_5[a]; 9-C_6H_5[a]; 9-(9′-anthryl)[a]; 1,2-di-CH_3[a,b]; 1,3-di-CH_3[a,b]; 1,4-di-CH_3[a,b]; 2,3-di-CH_3[a,b]; 9,10-di-CH_3[b]; 1,5-di-C(CH_2)CH_3[a]; 9,10-di-C_6H_5[a]; 9, 10-di-$CH_2C_6H_5$[a]; 9,10-di-(1′-naphthyl)[a]; 9-C_6H_5,10-$COOCH_3$[a]; 9-C_6H_5,10-COOH[a]; 9-C_6H_5,10-(1′-naphthyl)[a]; 2,9,10-tri-CH_3[b]; 3-CH_3,1,8,9-tri-OH[a]; 2,3,6,7-tetra-CH_3[a,b]

Phenanthrene Derivatives

1-CH_3,3-CH(CH_3)$_2$[b]; 1-CH_3,7-CH(CH_3)$_2$[a]; 1,9-di-CH_3[a,b]; 3,4-di-COOH[a]; 3,4-di-COONa[b]; 3,4-di-$COOCH_3$[b]; 1,2,3,4-tetra-CH_3[b]

Chrysene Derivatives

1-CH_3[a,b]; 1-OCH_3[b]; 1-OH[b]; 1-$OCOCH_3$[b]; 2-OCH_3[b]; 2-CH(CH_3)$_2$[a,b]; 3-OCH_3[b]; 4-OCH_3[b]; 4-OH[b]; 6-OCH_3[b]; 6-OH[b]; 2,3-di-CH_3[b]; 5,6-di-OCH_3[b]; 5,6-di-$OCOCH_3$[b]; 5,6-di-C_6H_5[a]

Benzo[c]phenanthrene Derivatives

3-CH_3[b]; 4-CH_3[b]; 5-CHO[a]; 5-(CH_2)$_2$$CH_3$[b]; 5-CH($CH_3$)$_2$[b]; 6-$CH_3$[b]; 6-CH($CH_3$)$_2$[a,b]; 2,3-di-$CH_3$[b]; 2-$CH_3$,6-COONa[b]; 5,8-di-$CH_3$[b]; 5,8-di-$C_2H_5$[b]

Inactive Derivatives of Pyrene

2-CH_3[a]; 3-O(CH_2)$_2$COOH[a]; 4-SO_3Na[a]; 3-OH,1,6,8-tri-SO_3Na[a]

[a]Painting on mouse skin.
[b]Subcutaneous injection in mice.

Slight	*Moderate*
Anthracene Derivatives	
9,10-di-CH_3[a]; 1,8,9-tri-OH[a]	
Phenanthrene Derivatives	
1-CH_3,3-$CH(CH_3)_2$[a]; 1,2,4-tri-CH_3[a]; 1,2,3,4-tetra-CH_3[a]	
Chrysene Derivatives	
3-OH[b]; 4-CH_3[b]; 6-CH_3[b]; 4,5-di-CH_3[b]; 5,6-di-CH_3[a,b]	5-CH_3[b]
Benzo[c]phenanthrene Derivatives	
2-CH_3[a,b]; 3-CH_3[a]; 4-CH_3[a]; 5-CHO[b]; 5-C_2H_5[a]; 5-$COCH_3$[a,b]	5-CH_3[a,b]; 5-$CH(CH_3)_2$[a]; 5-$(CH_2)_2CH_3$[a]; 6-CH_3[a]
Inactive Derivatives of	
Triphenylene	*Naphthacene*
1-CH_3[b]; 1,4-di-CH_3[b]	2-$CH(CH_3)_2$[a]; 5,6,11,12-tetra-C_6H_5[a]

Appendix E. Carcinogenic Activities of Pentacyclic and Hexacyclic Aromatic Hydrocarbon Derivatives

Inactive

Substituted Benzo[a]*pyrene Derivatives*

6-OH[a,b]; 6-NO_2; 6-CHC(CN)C_6H_4Br[b]; 7-OH[a,b]; 7-OCH_3[a,b]; 7-$OCOCH_3$[b]; 7-$OCOC_6H_4NH_2$[b]; 8-CH_3[a]; 11-OH[b]; 7,8-di-COOK[b]; 7,8-di-COONa[b,c]; 1,3,6-tri-Cl[a,b]

Substituted Dibenz[a,h]*anthracene Derivatives*

7-OH[a]; 7-$OCOCH_3$[a]; 7-NO_2[a]; 3,10-di-OH[b]; 3,11-di-OH[b]; 4,11-di-OH[m]; 5,12-di-OCH_3[a,b,l]; 5,12-di-$OCOCH_3$[a,b,l]; 7,14-di-OCH_3[b]

Derivatives of Other Compounds

Benzo[*g*]chrysene	9-CH_3[b]; 10-CH_3[b]
Picene	2,9-di-CH_3[b]
Benzo[*b*]chrysene	7,12-di-CH_3[b]
Perylene	3-CH_3[a,b]
Pentaphene	2,11-di-CH_3[a]
Dibenz[*a,c*]anthracene	9,14-di-CH_3[a,b]
Dibenz[*a,j*]anthracene	
Dibenzo[*b,def*]chrysene	7,14-di-CH_3[b,i]; 7,14-di-OSO_2Na[a,b]
Dibenzo[*def,p*]chrysene	10-C_6H_5
Benzo[*rst*]pentaphene	5,8-di-CH_3[b,i]
Benzo[*pqr*]picene	7-CH_3[b,h]
Naphtho[1,2,3,4-*def*]chrysene	
Anthanthrene	

[a]Painting on mouse skin.
[b]Subcutaneous injection in mice.
[c]Intraperitoneal injection in mice.
[d]Tested for initiating activity in mouse skin.
[e]Cook and Schoental (*60*).
[f]Lacassagne et al. (*61*).
[g]Bergmann et al. (*59*).
[h]Lacassagne et al. (*62*).
[i]Lacassagne et al. (*63*).

Slight	*Moderate*	*High*
	Substituted Benzo[a]*pyrene Derivatives*	
1-$COCH_3$[a]; 1-$C(CH_2)CH_3$; 3-OH[a,b]; 4-OCH_3[b]; 5-OH[b]; 5-Cl[a,b]; 6-OH[b,k]; 1, 6-di-OCH_3[b]; 3, 6-di-OCH_3[b]	5-CH_3[b]; 7-CH_3[b]; 1, 3, 6-tri-CH_3[b]	2-CH_3[b]; 3-CH_3[b,e]; 3-OCH_3[a,b]; 4-CH_3[b]; 6-CH_3[b]; 6-CHO[b]; 6-$CHCHC_6H_5$[b]; 11-CH_3[b]; 12-CH_3[b]; 1, 2-di-CH_3[b]; 1, 3-di-CH_3[b]; 1, 4-di-CH_3[b]; 1, 6-di-CH_3[b]; 2, 3-di-CH_3[b]; 3, 6-di-CH_3[b]; 3, 12-di-CH_3[b]; 4, 5-di-CH_3[b]
	Substituted Dibenz[a,h]*anthracene Derivatives*	
2-CH_3[a]; 3-CH_3[a]; 5-OCH_3[a,b,l]; 7-OCH_3[a]; 5, 6-di-OCH_3[a,b,l]; 7, 14-di-$(CH_2)_3CH_3$[a]	6-CH_3[a]; 7-OCH_3[a,l]; 7, 14-di-CH_3[a,b,l]	6-F[g]; 7-NCO[b]; 7-OCH_3[b,l]; 7-CH_3[b]
	Derivatives of Other Compounds	
10-CH_3[b]		
7-CHO, 14-CH_3[b,f]	7,14-di-CH_3[a,b]; 7-CH_3[b,i]; 7-CHO[b,f]	
10-CHO[b,j]		10-CH_3[b,j]
8-NO_2[b]; 5-CHO,8-CH_3[b,f]	5-CH_3[a,b,i]; 7-CH_3[d]	5-CHO[b,f]
	6-CH_3[b,j]	5-CH_3[b,j]
6-CH_3[b,d,i]; 6-CHO[b,f]; 6-CHO,12-CH_3[b,f]; 6,12-di-CH_3[b,i]		

[j] Lacassagne et al. (*38*).
[k] Nagata et al. (*64*).
[l] Heidelberger et al. (*65*).
[m] Badger (*20*).

Appendix F. Carcinogenic Activities of Some Hydrocarbon Derivatives Containing Five-Membered Rings

Inactive

Cholanthrene and Its Derivatives

1-oxo[b]; 11,12-dihydro[b]; 6-12b-dihydro[a]; 3-CH_3,8-OCH_3[b]; 3-CH_3,8-OH[b]; 3-CH_3,9-Cl[b]; 3-CH_3,9-OH[a,b]; 3-CH_3,9-OCH_3[a,b]; 3-CH_3,11-Cl[b]; 3-CH_3,11-CN[b]

*16,17-Dihydro-15*H*-cyclopenta*[a]*phenanthrene and Its Derivatives*

16,17-dihydro-15*H*-cyclopenta[*a*]phenanthrene[a,b,c]; 1-CH_3[a]; 2-CH_3[a]; 4-CH_3[a]; 6-CH_3[a,b]; 11-CH_3[b]; 12-CH_3[a,b]; 15-oxo[a,i]; 17-oxo[a,b,i]; 17-CH_3[a,b]; 2,12-di-CH_3[a,b]; 6,7-di-CH_3[a]; 4,12-di-CH_3[a]; 3-OCH_3, 17-CH_3[a,i]; 4,17-di-CH_3[a]; 6,17-di-CH_3[a,b]; 11-OCH_3,-17-CH_3[a,i]; 12,17-di-CH_3[a,i]; 2-CH_3,17-oxo[a,j]; 3-CH_3, 17-oxo[a,j]; 3-OCH_3,17-oxo[a,i]; 4-CH_3,17-oxo[a,j]; 6-CH_3,17-oxo[a,j]; 12-CH_3,-17-oxo[a,i]; 11,12-dihydro,11-CH_3,17-oxo[a,j]; 6,17,17-tri-CH_3[a,b]

Cyclopenta[a]*phenanthrene and Its Derivatives*

17*H*-cyclopenta[*a*]phenanthrene[a,i]; 17*H*,17-$C(CH_3)_2$[a,i]; 15*H*,3-OCH_3,17-CH_3[a,i]

[a]Painting on mouse skin.
[b]Subcutaneous injection in mice.
[c]Subcutaneous injection in rats.
[d]Intramuscular injection in rats.
[e]Intravenous injection in mice.
[f]Intraperitoneal injection in mice.
[g]Intragastric administration in rats giving mammary tumors.
[h]Oral administration to rats and mice.
[i]Coombs and Croft (*66*).
[j]Coombs et al. (*67*).

Slight	*Moderate*	*High*
Cholanthrene and Its Derivatives		
3-C(CH_3)[b]; 1-oxo,3-CH_3[a,b]	cholanthrene[a,c]; 3-CH(CH_3)$_2$[b]; 1,3-di-CH_3[b]; 1-OH,3-CH_3[b]	cholanthrene[b]; 3-CH_3[a,b,c,d,e,f,g,h]; 4-CH_3[b]; 5-CH_3[b]; 3-C_2H_5[b]; 2,3-di-CH_3[b]; 6,12b-dihydro[b]; 6,12b-dihydro, 3-CH_3[b]
*16,17-Dihydro-15*H*-cyclopenta*[a]*phenanthrene and Its Derivatives*		
7-CH_3[a]; 11-CH_3[a]; 17-CH_2[a,i]; 11,12-di-CH_3[a]; 11,17-di-CH_3[a,i]; 11,12,17-tri-CH_3[a,i]; 7-CH_3,17-oxo[a,j]; 11-C_2H_5,17-oxo[a,j]; 11-(CH_2)$_3$$CH_3$,17-oxo[a,j]; 11-OCO$CH_3$,17-oxo[a,i]; 11-$CH_3$,16-OH, 17-oxo[a,j]; 11-$CH_3$,15-oxo[a,j]	11-CH_3,17-OH[a,j]; 11-CH_3,-17-oxo[a,b,i]; 11-OCH_3,-17-oxo[a,i]; 6-OCH_3,-11-CH_3, 17-oxo[a,j]; 7-CH_3,-11-OCH_3,-17-oxo[a,j]; 11, 12-di-CH_3,-17-oxo[a,b,i]	
Cyclopenta[a]*phenanthrene and Its Derivatives*		
15*H*,17-CH_3[a,i]; 15*H*,12,17-di-CH_3[a,i]; 15*H*,11-OCH_3,17-CH_3[a,i]		15*H*,11,17-di-CH_3[a,i]; 15*H*,11,12,17-tri-CH_3[a,i]

Appendix G. Activities of Some Carcinogenic Heterocyclic Compounds

Slight

Dibenz[*a*,*h*]acridine

Dibenz[*c*,*h*]acridine

Dibenz[*a*,*j*]acridine

7*H*-Benzo[*a*]pyrido-[3,2-*g*]carbazole[a]

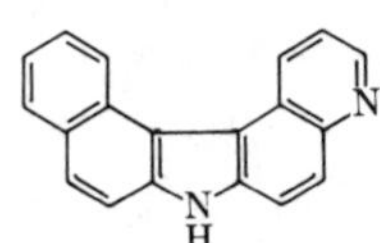

7*H*-Benzo[*c*]pyrido-[3,2-*g*]carbazole[a]

7*H*-Benzo[*g*]-γ-carboline[d]

11*H*-Benzo-[*a*]carbazole

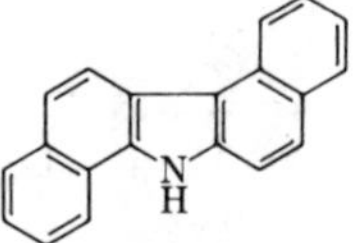

7*H*-Dibenzo-[*a*,*g*]carbazole

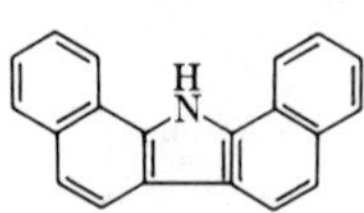

13*H*-Dibenzo-[*a*,*i*]carbazole

10-Azabenzo-[*a*]pyrene[c]

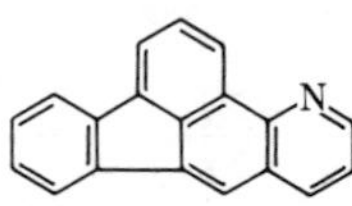

Fluoreno[9,9a,1-*gh*] quinoline[c]

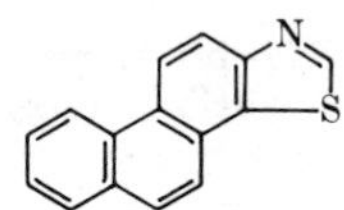

Phenanthro-[2,1-*d*]thiazole

Benzo[*h*]benzo[2,3]-thieno[3,2-*b*]quinoline

Benzo[*f*]benzo[2,3]-thieno[3,2-*b*]quinoline

Pyrido[2,3-*a*]thieno-[2,3-*i*]carbazole[d]

---

[a]Lacassagne et al. (*68*).
[b]Lacassagne et al. (*69*).
[c]Lacassagne et al. (*70*).
[d]Lacassagne et al. (*71*).
[e]Zajdela et al. (*72*).
[f]Sellakumar and Shubik (*73*).
[g]Lacassagne et al. (*74*).
[h]Lacassagne et al. (*75*).

Moderate	*High*
Benzo[*h*]naphtho-[1,2-*f*]quinoline[c]	7*H*-Benzo[*g*]pyrido-[3,2-*a*]carbazole[a]
7*H*-Benzo[*g*]pyrido-[2,3-*a*]carbazole[a]	7*H*-Dibenzo-[*c,g*]carbazole[f]
7*H*-Benzo[*c*]pyrido-[2,3-*g*]carbazole[b]	4,11-Diazadibenzo-[*b,def*]chrysene[a]
13*H*-Benzo[*a*]pyrido-[3,2-*i*]carbazole[b]	5-Oxo-5H-benzo[*e*]-isochromeno[4,3-*b*]indole[g]
1,12-Diazabenzo-[*rst*]pentaphene[e]	

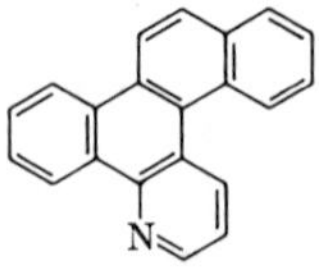

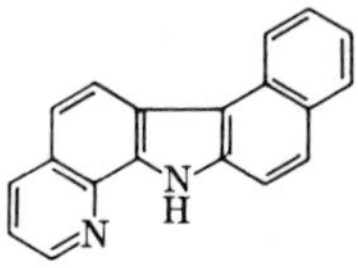

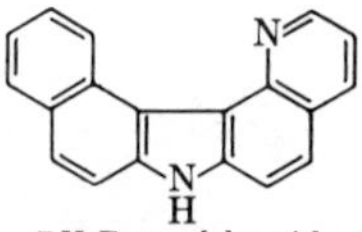

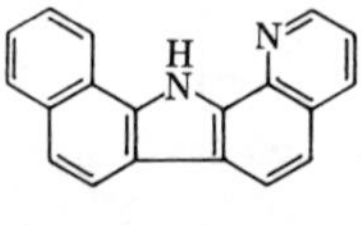

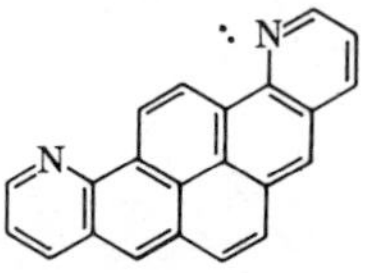

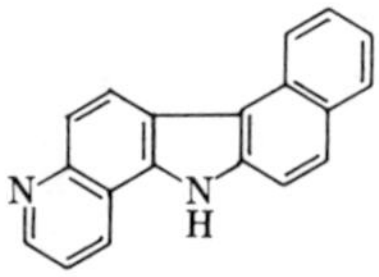

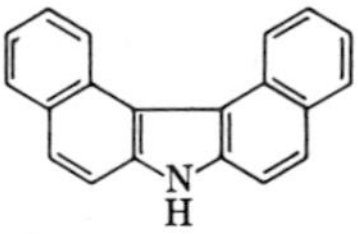

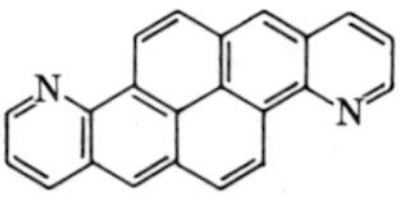

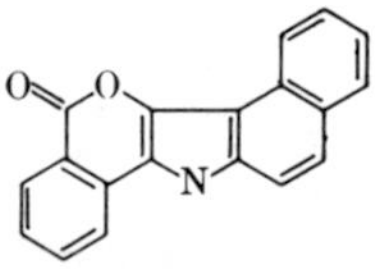

Continued on next page

Appendix G Continued

Slight		*Moderate*
5-Oxo-5*H*-benzo[*g*]-isochromeno[4,3-*b*]indole [h]	8-Oxo-8*H*-isochromeno-[3′,4′:4,5]pyrrolo[2,3-*f*]quinoline [g]	Tricycloquinazoline

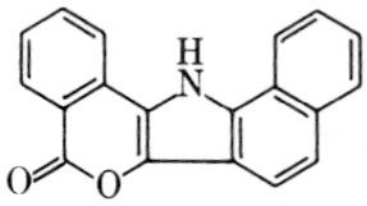

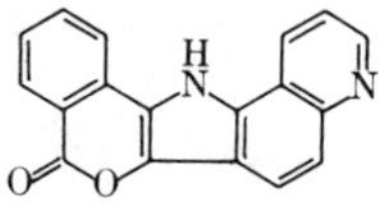

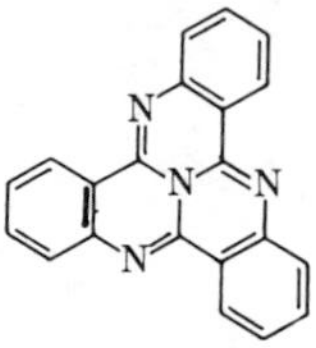

Appendix H. Carcinogenic Activities of Substituted Benzacridines

Inactive

Benz[a]*acridines*

9-CH_3[b]; 10-CH_3[a]; 10-C_6H_5[b]; 12-CH_3[a,b]; 12-CHO[b]; 8,9-di-CH_3[a,b]; 8-C_6H_5,-12-CH_3[b]; 9-Cl,12-C_2H_5[a]; 9-CF_3,12-CH_3[b]; 10-CH_3,12-$CH(CH_3)_2$[b]; 10-F,12-C_2H_5[b]; 10-F,12-$(CH_2)_2CH_3$[b]; 10-F,12-$(CH_2)_4CH_3$[b]; 10-F,-12-C_6H_5[b]; 2,9,12-tri-CH_3[b]; 8,9,12-tri-CH_3[a,b]; 8,11,12-tri-CH_3[a,b]; 9,11,12-tri-CH_3[a,b]; 2,9-di-CH_3,12-C_2H_5[b]; 2,12-di-CH_3,10-F[b]; 8,9-di-CH_3,12-$CH(CH_3)_2$[b]; 8,12-di-CH_3,9-Cl[b]; 9,12-di-CH_3,10-F[b]; 10,11-di-CH_3,12-$CH(CH_3)_2$[b]; 8-CH_3,9-Cl,12-C_2H_5[b]; 8-CH_3,9-Cl,12-$CH(CH_3)_2$[a,b]; 2,8,10,12-tetra-CH_3[b]; 3,8,10,12-tetra-CH_3[b]; 2,8,12-tri-CH_3,9-Cl[b]; 2,8,12-tri-CH_3,11-C_2H_5[b]; 2,3,8,10, 11-penta-CH_3[b]; 2,3,9,10,12-penta-CH_3[b]; 2,3,8,10,11,12-hexa-CH_3[b]

Benz[c]*acridines*

7-CHO[b]; 7-$(CH_2)_2CH_3$[a]; 8-CH_3[b]; 9-CH_3[a]; 9-C_6H_5[b]; 10-CH_3[b]; 5,7-di-CH_3[a,b] 10,11-di-CH_3[a,b]; 7-CH_3,9-C_2H_5[b]; 7-$CON(C_2H_5)_2$,9-CH_3[b]; 7-C_2H_5,-9-F[a,b]; 7-$(CH_2)_2CH_3$,9-F[b]; 7-$(CH_2)_4CH_3$,9-F[a,b]; 7-$CH_2C_6H_5$,9-F[b]; 7-CH_3,10-CF_3[b]; 7-C_2H_5,11-CH_3[a]; 5,7,11-tri-CH_3[b]; 7,8,11-tri-CH_3[b]; 7,9,10-tri-CH_3[b]; 7,11-di-CH_3,10-Cl[b]; 7-C_2H_5,10-Cl,11-CH_3[a]

Slight	*Moderate*	*High*
	Benz[a]*acridines*	
8,12-di-CH_3[b]; 9,12-di-CH_3[a]; 10-F,12-CH_3[a,b]; 3,8,12-tri-CH_3[b]; 8,12-di-CH_3,9-Cl[a]; 10-F,9,12-di-CH_3[a]	8,10,12-tri-CH_3[a]; 9,10,12-tri-CH_3[b]	
	Benz[c]*acridines*	
7-CN[b]; 7,11-di-CH_3[a,b]; 7-C_2H_5,9-CH_3[a]; 7-CH_3,9-C_6H_5[a]; 7-CH_3,11-F[b]; 5,7,11-tri-CH_3[a]; 7,8,11-tri-CH_3[a]; 7-C_2H_5,10-Cl,11-CH_3[b]; 7,8,9,11-tetra-CH_3[b]	7,9-di-CH_3[a,b]; 7,10-di-CH_3[a,b]; 7-CH_3,9-C_2H_5[a]; 7-CH_3,9-F[a,b]; 7-CHO,11-CH_3[b]; 7,9,10-tri-CH_3[a]; 7,9,11-tri-CH_3[a,b]	7-CH_3[a]; 7-CHO,9-CH_3[b]; 7,8,9,11-tetra-CH_3[a]

[a]Painting on mouse skin.

[b]Subcutaneous injection in mice.

Literature Cited

1. Kedzierski, B.; Thakker, D.R.; Armstrong, R.N.; Jerina, D.M. *Tetrahedron Lett.* **1981**, *22*, 405–8.
2. Nakanishi, K.; Kasai, H.; Cho, H.; Harvey, R.G.; Jeffrey, A.M.; Jennette, K.W.; Weinstein, I.B. *J. Am. Chem. Soc.* **1977**, *99*, 258–60.
3. Yagi, H.; Akagi, H.; Thakker, D.R.; Mah, H.D.; Koreeda, M.; Jerina, D.M. *J. Am. Chem. Soc.* **1977**, *99*, 2358–59.
4. Levin, W.; Buening, M.K.; Wood, A.; Chang, R.L.; Kedzierski, B.; Thakker, D.H.; Boyd, D.R.; Gadaginamath, G.S.; Armstrong, R.N.; Yagi, H.; Karle, J.M.; Slaga, T.J.; Jerina, D.M.; Conney, A.H. *J. Biol. Chem.* **1980**, *255*, 9067–74.
5. Pott, P. *Natl. Cancer Inst. Monogr.* **1963**, *10*, 7–13.
6. Yamagiwa, K.; Ichikawa, K. *Mitt. Med. Fak. Tokio* **1915**, *15*, 295–344.
7. Tsutsui, H. *Gann* **1918**, *12*, 17–21.
8. Bloch, B.; Dreifuss, W. *Schweiz. Med. Wochenschr.* **1921**, *51*, 1035–37.
9. Kennaway, E.L. *J. Pathol. Bacteriol.* **1924**, *27*, 233–38.
10. Kennaway, E.L. *Br. Med. J.* **1925**, *2*, 1–4.
11. Schroeter, G. *Ber. Dtsch. Chem. Ges.* **1924**, *57*, 1990–2003.
12. Kennaway, E.L. *Br. Med. J.* **1955**, *2*, 749–52.
13. Hieger, I. *Biochem. J.* **1930**, *24*, 505–11.
14. Kennaway, E.L.; Hieger, I. *Br. Med. J.* **1930**, *1*, 1044–46.
15. Clar, E. *Ber. Dtsch. Chem. Ges.* **1929**, *62*, 350–59.
16. Cook, J.W.; Hewett, C.L.; Hieger, I. *J. Chem. Soc.* **1933**, 395–405.
17. Prehn, R.T. *JNCI, J. Natl. Cancer Inst.* **1964**, *32*, 1–17.
18. Clayson, D.B. "Chemical Carcinogenesis"; Churchill: London, 1962.
19. Hueper, W.C.; Conway, W.D. "Chemical Carcinogenesis and Cancers"; Thomas: Springfield, IL, 1964.
20. Badger, G.M. *Br. J. Cancer* **1948**, *2*, 309–50.
21. Badger, G.M. *Adv. Cancer Res.* **1954**, *4*, 73–128.
22. Arcos, J.C.; Arcos, M. *Prog. Drug Res.* **1962**, *4*, 407–581.
23. Buu-Hoï, N.P. *Cancer Res.* **1964**, *24*, 1511–23.
24. Arcos, J.C.; Argus, M.F. *Adv. Cancer Res.* **1968**, *11*, 305–471.
25. Lacassagne, A.; Buu-Hoï, N.P.; Daudel, R.; Zajdela, F. *Adv. Cancer Res.* **1956**, *4*, 315–69.
26. Hartwell, J.L. "Survey of Compounds Which Have Been Tested for Carcinogenic Activity"; U.S. Public Health Service Publ. No. 149, Washington, D.C., 1951.
27. Shubik, P.; Hartwell, J.L. "Survey of Compounds Which Have Been Tested for Carcinogenic Activity," Supplement 1, U.S. Public Health Service Publ. No. 149, Washington, D.C., 1957.
28. *Ibid.* Supplement 2, U.S. Public Health Service, Publ. No. 149, Washington, D.C., 1969.
29. Thompson, J.I. et al. "Survey of Compounds Which Have Been Tested for Carcinogenic Activity," 1968–69 Volume, U.S. Public Health Service Publ. No. 149, Washington, D.C., 1968–69.
30. *Ibid.* 1970–71 Volume, U.S. Public Health Service Publ. No. 149, Washington, D.C., 1970–71.
31. Iball, J. *Am. J. Cancer* **1939**, *35*, 188–90.
32. Fieser, L.F. *Am. J. Cancer* **1938**, *34*, 37–124.
33. Berenblum, I. *Cancer Res.* **1945**, *5*, 561–64.
34. Scribner, J.D. *JNCI, J. Natl. Cancer Inst.* **1973**, *50*, 1717–19.
35. Lacassagne, A.; Buu-Hoï, N.P.; Zajdela, F.; Lavit-Lamy, D. *C.R. Hebd. Seances Acad. Sci.* **1961**, *252*, 826–28.

36. Van Duuren, B.L.; Sivak, A.; Langseth, L.; Goldschmidt, B.M.; Segal, A. *Natl. Cancer Inst. Monogr.* **1968**, *28*, 173–80.
37. Lacassagne, A.; Buu-Hoï, N.P.; Zajdela, F. *C.R. Hebd. Seances Acad. Sci.* **1960**, *250*, 3547–48.
38. Lacassagne, A.; Buu-Hoï, N.P.; Zajdela, F. *C.R. Hebd. Seances Acad. Sci.* **1964**, *259*, 3899–902.
39. Hoffmann, D.; Wynder, E.L. *Z. Krebsforsch.* **1966**, *68*, 137–49.
40. Barry, G.; Cook, J.W.; Haslewood, G.A.D.; Hewett, C.L.; Hieger, I.; Kennaway, E.L. *Proc. Roy. Soc. B* **1935**, *117*, 318–51.
41. Bottomley, A.C.; Twort, C.C. *Am. J. Cancer* **1934**, *20*, 781–88.
42. Bachmann, W.E.; Cook, J.W.; Dansi, A.; De Worms, C.G.M.; Haslewood, G.A.D.; Hewett, C.L.; Robinson, A.M. *Proc. R. Soc. London, Ser. B* **1937**, *123*, 343–68.
43. Van Duuren, B.L.; Sivak, A.; Segal, A.; Orris, L.; Langseth, L. *JNCI, J. Natl. Cancer Inst.* **1966**, *37*, 519–26.
44. Lijinsky, W.; Garcia, H.; Saffiotti, U. *JNCI, J. Natl. Cancer Inst.* **1970**, *44*, 641–49.
45. Van Duuren, B.L.; Sivak, A.; Goldschmidt, B.M.; Katz, C.; Melchionne, S. *JNCI, J. Natl. Cancer Inst.* **1970**, *44*, 1167–73.
46. Lacassagne, A.; Buu-Hoï, N.P.; Zajdela, F. *Eur. J. Cancer* **1968**, *4*, 123–27.
47. LaVoie, E.J.; Amin, S.; Hecht, S.S.; Furuya, K.; Hoffmann, D. *Carcinogenesis* **1982**, *3*, 49–52.
48. Huggins, C.B.; Pataki, J.; Harvey, R.G. *Proc. Natl. Acad. Sci. U.S.A.* **1967**, *58*, 2253–60.
49. Dipple, A.; Slade, T.A. *Eur. J. Cancer* **1971**, *7*, 473–76.
50. Roe, F.J.C.; Dipple, A.; Mitchley, B.C.V. *Br. J. Cancer* **1972**, *26*, 461–65.
51. Miller, J.A.; Miller, E.C. *Cancer Res.* **1963**, *23*, 229–39.
52. Pataki, J.; Huggins, C.B. *Biochem. Pharmacol.* **1967**, *16*, 607–12.
53. Pataki, J.; Duguid, C.; Rabideau, P.W.; Huisman, H.; Harvey, R.G. *J. Med. Chem.* **1971**, *14*, 940–45.
54. Pataki, J.; Balick, R. *J. Med. Chem.* **1972**, *15*, 905–9.
55. Flesher, J.W.; Sydnor, K.L. *Cancer Res.* **1971**, *31*, 1951–54.
56. Dipple, A.; Slade, T.A. *Eur. J. Cancer* **1970**, *6*, 417–23.
57. Boyland, E.; Sims, P. *Int. J. Cancer* **1967**, *2*, 500–504.
58. Boyland, E.; Sims, P.; Huggins, C. *Nature (London)* **1965**, *207*, 816–17.
59. Bergmann, E.D.; Blum, J.; Haddow, A. *Nature (London)* **1963**, *200*, 480.
60. Cook, J.W.; Schoental, R. *Br. J. Cancer* **1952**, *6*, 400–406.
61. Lacassagne, A.; Buu-Hoï, N.P.; Zajdela, F.; Lavit-Lamy, D. *C.R. Hebd. Seances Acad. Sci.* **1961**, *252*, 1711–13.
62. Lacassagne, A.; Buu-Hoï, N.P.; Zajdela, F.; Saint, Ruf, G. *C.R. Hebd. Seances Acad. Sci* **1968**, *266*, 301–4.
63. Lacassagne, A.; Buu-Hoï, N.P.; Zajdela, F. *C.R. Hebd. Seances Acad. Sci.* **1958**, *246*, 94–97.
64. Nagata, C.; Tagashira, Y.; Inomata, M.; Kodama, M. *Gann* **1971**, *62*, 419–21.
65. Heidelberger, C.; Baumann, M.E.; Griesbach, L.; Ghobar, A.; Vaughan, T.M. *Cancer Res.* **1962**, *22*, 78–83.
66. Coombs, M.M.; Croft, C.J. *Prog. Exp. Tumor Res.* **1969**, *11*, 69–85.
67. Coombs, M.M.; Bhatt, T.S.; Croft, C.J. *Cancer Res.* **1973**, *33*, 832–37.
68. Lacassagne, A.; Buu-Hoï, N.P.; Zajdela, F.; Périn, F.; Jacquignon, P. *Nature (London)* **1961**, *191*, 1005–6.
69. Lacassagne, A.; Buu-Hoï, N.P.; Zajdela, F.; Jacquignon, P.; Périn, F. *C. R. Hebd. Seances Acad. Sci.* **1963**, *257*, 818–22.
70. Lacassagne, A.; Buu-Hoï, N.P.; Zajdela, F.; Mabille, P. *C.R. Hebd. Seances Acad. Sci.* **1964**, *258*, 3387–89.
71. Lacassagne, A.; Buu-Hoï, N.P.; Zajdela, F.; Perrin-Roussel, O.; Jacquignon, P.; Périn, F.;

Hoeffinger, J.P. *C.R. Hebd. Seances Acad. Sci.* **1970**, *271*, 1474–79.
72. Zajdela, F.; Buu-Hoï, N.P.; Jacquignon, P.; Dufour, M. *Br. J. Cancer* **1972**, *26*, 262–64.
73. Sellakumar, A.; Shubik, P. *JNCI, J. Natl. Cancer Inst.* **1972**, *48*, 1641–46.
74. Lacassagne, A.; Buu-Hoï, N.P.; Zajdela, F.; Jacquignon, P.; Mangane, M. *Science (Washington, D.C.)* **1967**, *158*, 387–88.
75. Lacassagne, A.; Buu-Hoï, N.P.; Zajdela, F.; Stora, C.; Mangane, M.; Jacquignon, P. *C.R. Hebd. Seances Acad. Sci.* **1971**, *272*, 3102–4.
76. Jerina, D.M.; Daly, J.W. "Drug Metabolism"; Parke, D.V.; Smith, R.L., Eds.; Taylor and Francis: London, 1976; pp. 13–32.
77. Haddow, A.; Kon, G.A.R. *Br. Med. Bull.* **1947**, *4*, 314–26.
78. Williams, D.J.; Rabin, B.R. *Nature (London)* **1971**, *232*, 102–5.
79. Litwack, G.; Ketterer, B.; Arias, I.M. *Nature (London)* **1971**, *234*, 466–67.
80. Hewett, C.L. *J. Chem. Soc.* **1940**, 293–303.
81. Waravdekar, S.S.; Ranadive, K.J. *JNCI, J. Natl. Cancer Inst.* **1957**, *18*, 555–68.
82. Wynder, E.L. *Br. Med. J.* **1959**, *1*, 317–22.
83. Wynder, E.L.; Hoffmann, D. *Cancer* **1959**, *12*, 1194–99.
84. Clar, E. in "Polycyclic Hydrocarbons"; Academic: London, 1964; Vols. 1 & 2.
85. Coulson, C.A. in "Valence"; University: Oxford, 1952.
86. Pullman, A.; Pullman, B. *Adv. Cancer Res.* **1955**, *3*, 117–69.
87. Coulson, C.A. *Adv. Cancer Res.* **1953**, *1*, 1–56.
88a. Pullman, A. *C.R. Hebd. Seances Acad. Sci.* **1945**, *221*, 140–42.
88b. *C.R. Seances Soc. Biol. Ses Fil.* **1945**, *139*, 1056–58.
89. Pullman, A. *Ann. Chim. (Paris)* **1947**, *2*, 5–71.
90. Pullman, A. *C.R. Hebd. Seances Acad. Sci.* **1953**, *236*, 2318–20.
91. Schmidt, O. *Z. Phys. Chem.* **1938**, *39*, 59–82 (Pt. I).
92. *Ibid.* **1939**, *42*, 83–110; *44*, 185–93; *44*, 194–202.
93. Schmidt, O. *Naturwissenschaften* **1941**, *29*, 146–50.
94. Svartholm, N.V. *Arkiv. Kemi. Mineral. Geol.* **1941**, *A15*, No. 13, 1–13.
95. Buu-Hoï, N.P.; Daudel, P.; Daudel, R.; Lacassagne, A.; Lecocq, J.; Martin, M.; Rudali, G. *C.R. Hebd. Seances Acad. Sci.* **1947**, *225*, 238–40.
96. Greenwood, H.H. *Br. J. Cancer* **1951**, *5*, 441–57.
97. Pagés-Flon, M.; Buu-Hoï, N.P.; Daudel, R.; *C.R. Hebd. Seances Acad. Sci.* **1953**, *236*, 2182–84.
98. Coulson, C.A.; Daudel, P.; Daudel, R. *Rev. Sci.* **1947**, *85*, 29–32.
99. Berthier, G.; Coulson, C.A.; Greenwood, H.H.; Pullman, A. *C.R. Hebd. Seances Acad. Sci.* **1948**, *226*, 1906–8.
100. Baldock, G.; Berthier, G.; Pullman, A. *C.R. Hebd. Seances Acad. Sci.* **1949**, *228*, 931–33.
101. Pullman, B.; Pullman, A. *Nature (London)* **1963**, *199*, 467–71.
102. Pullman, B.; Pullman, A.; Umans, R.; Maigret, B. *Jerusalem Symp. Quantum Chem. Biochem.* **1969**, *1*, 325–38.
103. Matsen, F.A. *J. Chem. Phys.* **1956**, *24*, 602–6.
104. Hedges, R.M.; Matsen, F.A. *J. Chem. Phys.* **1958**, *28*, 950–53.
105. Lovelock, J.E.; Zlatkis, A.; Becker, R.S. *Nature (London)* **1962**, *193*, 540–41.
106. Kooyman, E.C.; Farenhorst, E. *Nature (London)* **1952**, *169*, 153–54.
107. Kooyman, E.C.; Heringa, J.W. *Nature (London)* **1952**, *170*, 661–62.
108. Pullman, A. *Bull. Soc. Chim. Fr.* **1954**, *21*, 595–603.
109. Koutecky, J.; Zahradnik, R. *Cancer Res.* **1961**, *21*, 457–62.
110. Flurry, R.L. *J. Med. Chem.* **1964**, *7*, 668–70.
111. Mainster, M.A.; Memory, J.D. *Biochim. Biophys. Acta* **1967**, *148*, 605–8.
112. Scribner, J.D. *Cancer Res.* **1969**, *29*, 2120–26.
113. Sung, S.S. *C.R. Hebd. Seances Acad. Sci.* **1971**, *273*, 1247–50.
114. *Ibid.* **1972**, *274*, 1597–600.

115. Herndon, W.C. *Trans. N.Y. Acad. Sci.* **1974**, *36*, 200–217.
116. Herndon, W.C. *Int. J. Quantum Chem.* Quantum Biology Symposium No. 1 **1974**, 123–34.
117a. Mason, R. *Br. J. Cancer* **1958**, *12*, 469–79.
117b. *Nature (London)* **1958**, *181*, 820–22.
118. Chalvet, O.; Mason, R. *Nature (London)* **1961**, *192*, 1070–72.
119. Szent-Györgyi, A.; Isenberg, I.; Baird, S.L. *Proc. Natl. Acad. Sci. U.S.A.* **1960,** *46*, 1444–49.
120. Allison, A.C.; Nash, T. *Nature (London)* **1963**, *197*, 758–63.
121. Epstein, S.S.; Bulon, I.; Koplan, J.; Small, M.; Mantel, N. *Nature (London)* **1964**, *204*, 750–54.
122. Laskowski, D.E. *Cancer Res.* **1967**, *27*, 903–11.
123. Pullman, A.; Berthier, G.; Pullman, B. *Acta Unio Int. Cancrum* **1951**, *7*, 140–48.
124. Jones, R.N. *J. Am. Chem. Soc.* **1940**, *62*, 148–52.
125. Kofahl, R.E.; Lucas, H.J. *J. Am. Chem. Soc.* **1954**, *76*, 3931–35.
126. Dipple, A.; Lawley, P.D.; Brookes, P. *Eur. J. Cancer* **1968**, *4*, 493–506.
127. Badger, G.M. *J. Chem. Soc.* **1950**, 1809–14.
128. Mottram, J.C.; Doniach, I. *Lancet* **1938**, *234*, 1156–59.
129. Santamaria, L. *Acta Unio Int. Cancrum* **1963**, *19*, 591–98.
130. Epstein, S.S.; Small, M.; Falk, H.L.; Mangel, N. *Cancer Res.* **1964**, *24*, 855–62.
131. Brock, N.; Druckrey, H.; Hamperl, H. *Arch. Exp. Pathol. Pharmakol.* **1938**, *189*, 709–31.
132. Weil-Malherbe, H. *Biochem. J.* **1946**, *40*, 351–63.
133. Liquori, A.M.; deLerma, B.; Ascoli, F.; Botré, A.; Trasciatti, M. *J. Mol. Biol.* **1962**, *5*, 521–26.
134. Boyland, E.; Green, B. *Br. J. Cancer* **1962**, *16*, 507–17.
135. Lerman, L. *J. Mol. Biol.* **1961**, *3*, 18–30.
136. Nagata, C.; Kodama, M.; Tagashira, Y.; Imamura, A. *Biopolymers* **1966**, *4*, 409–27.
137. Craig, M.; Isenberg, I. *Biopolymers* **1970**, *9*, 689–96.
138. Popp, F.A. *Arch. Geschwulstforsch.* **1977**, *47*, 97–105.
139. Veljković, V.; Lalović, D.I. *Experientia* **1977**, *33*, 1228–29.
140. Miller, E.C.; Miller, J.A. *Pharmacol. Rev.* **1966**, *18*, 805–38.
141. Sims, P.; Grover, P.L.; Swaisland, A.; Pal, K.; Hewer, A. *Nature (London)* **1974**, *252*, 326–28.
142. Harvey, R.G. *Acc. Chem. Res.* **1981**, *14*, 218–26.
143. Dewar, M.J.S. "The Molecular Orbital Theory of Organic Chemistry"; McGraw-Hill: New York, 1969.
144. Jerina, D.M.; Lehr, R.E.; Yagi, H.; Hernandex, O.; Dansette, P.M.; Wislocki, P.G.; Wood, A.W.; Chang, R.L.; Levin, W.; Conney, A.H. in "In Vitro Metabolic Activation in Mutagenesis Testing: Proceedings of the Symposium on the Role of Metabolic Activation in Producing Mutagenic and Carcinogenic Environmental Chemicals"; deSerres, F.J.; Fouts, J.R.; Bend, J.R.; Philpot, R.M., Eds.; Elsevier: Amsterdam, 1976; pp. 159–77.
145. Jerina, D.M.; Lehr, R.; Schaefer-Ridder, M.; Yagi, H.; Karle, J.M.; Thakker, D.R.; Wood, A.W.; Lu, A.Y.H.; Ryan, D.; West, S.; Levin, W.; Conney, A.H. in "Origins of Human Cancer: Cold Spring Harbor Conferences on Cell Proliferation"; Hiatt, H.H.; Watson, J.D.; Winsten, J.A., Eds.; Cold Spring Harbor: New York, 1977.
146. Lehr, R.E.; Yagi, H.; Thakker, D.R.; Levin, W.; Wood, A.W.; Conney, A.H.; Jerina, D.M. in "Polynuclear Aromatic Hydrocarbons"; Jones, P.W. ; Freudenthal, R.I., Eds.; Raven: New York, 1978.
147. Fu, P.P.; Harvey, R.G.; Beland, F.A. *Tetrahedron* **1978**, *34*, 857–66.
148. Smith, I.A.; Berger, G.D.; Seybold, P.G.; Servé, M.P. *Cancer Res.* **1978**, *38*, 2968–77.
149. Osborne, M.R. *Cancer Res.* **1979**, *39*, 4760–61.

150. Herndon, W.C. *Tetrahedron Lett.* **1981**, *22*, 983–86.
151. Loew, G.H.; Sudhindra, B.S.; Ferrell, J.E. *Chem.-Biol. Interact.* **1979**, *26*, 75–89.
152. Mason, H.S. *Adv. Enzymol. Relat. Subj. Biochem.* **1957**, *19*, 79–233.
153. Lu, A.Y.H.; West, S.B. *Pharmacol. Rev.* **1980**, *31*, 277–95.
154. Ryan, D.E.; Thomas, P.E.; Korzeniowski, D.; Levin, W. *J. Biol. Chem.* **1979**, *254*, 1365–80.
155. Alvares, A.P.; Schilling, G.; Levin, W.; Kuntzman, R. *Biochem. Biophys. Res. Commun.* **1967**, *29*, 521–24.
156. Sladek, N.E.; Mannering, G.T. *Biochem. Biophys. Res. Commun.* **1966**, *24*, 668–74.
157. Lu, A.Y.H. *Drug Metab. Rev.* **1979**, *10*, 187–208.
158. Estabrook, R.W.; Werringloer, J.; Capdevila, J.; Prough, R.A. "Polycyclic Hydrocarbons and Cancer"; Gelboin, H.V.; Ts'o, P.O.P., Eds.; Academic: New York, 1978; Vol. 1, pp. 285–319.
159. Griffin, B.W.; Peterson, J.A.; Estabrook, R.W. "The Porphyrins"; Dolphin, D., Ed.; Academic: New York, 1979; pp. 333–75.
160. White, R.E.; Coon, M.J. *Annu. Rev. Biochem.* **1980**, *49*, 315–56.
161. Nebert, D.W. *Mol. Cell. Biochem.* **1979**, *27*, 27–46.
162. Khandwala, A.S.; Kasper, C.B. *Biochem. Biophys. Res. Commun.* **1973**, *54*, 1241–46.
163. Gelboin, H.V. *Physiol. Rev.* **1980**, *60*, 1107–66.
164. Bresnick, E. *Drug Metab. Rev.* **1979**, *10*, 209–23.
165. Negishi, M.; Swan, D.C.; Enquist, L.W.; Nebert, D.W. *Proc. Natl. Acad. Sci. U.S.A.* **1981**, *78*, 800–804.
166. Bresnick, E.; Levy, J.; Hines, R.N.; Levin, W.; Thomas, P.E. *Arch. Biochem. Biophys.* **1981**, *212*, 501–7.
167. Oesch, F. *Prog. Drug Metab.* **1979**, *3*, 253–301.
168. Lu, A.Y.H.; Miwa, G.T. *Annu. Rev. Pharmacol. Toxicol.* **1980**, *20*, 513–31.
169. Guengerich, F.P.; Wang, P.; Mitchell, M.B.; Mason, P.S. *J. Biol. Chem.* **1979**, *254*, 12248–54.
170. Guengerich, F.P.; Wang, P.; Mason, P.S.; Mitchell, M.B. *J. Biol. Chem.* **1979**, *254*, 12255–59.
171. Guenthner, T.M.; Hammock, B.D.; Vogel, U.; Oesch, F. *J. Biol. Chem.* **1981**, *256*, 3163–66.
172. Gonzalez, F.J.; Kasper, C.B. *J. Biol. Chem.* **1981**, *256*, 4697–700.
173. Miller, J.A.; Miller, E.C. *JNCI, J. Natl. Cancer Inst.* **1971**, *47*, V-XIV.
174. Boyland, E. *Biochem. Soc. Symp.* **1950**, *5*, 40–54.
175. Williams, R.T. "Detoxication Mechanisms"; Wiley: New York, 1959.
176. Boyland, E.; Sims, P. *Biochem. J.* **1958**, *68*, 440–47.
177. *Ibid.* **1962**, *84*, 571–82.
178. Jeffrey, A.M.; Yeh, J.J.C.; Jerina, D.M.; DeMarinis, R.M.; Foster, C.H.; Piccolo, D.E.; Berchtold, G.A. *J. Am. Chem. Soc.* **1974**, *96*, 6929–37.
179. Jeffrey, A.M.; Jerina, D.M. *J. Am. Chem. Soc.* **1975**, *97*, 4427–28.
180. Newman, M.S.; Blum, S. *J. Am. Chem. Soc.* **1964**, *86*, 5598–600.
181. Boyland, E.; Sims, P. *Biochem. J.* **1965**, *97*, 7–16.
182. Sims, P. *Biochem. J.* **1966**, *98*, 215–28.
183. Jerina, D.M.; Daly, J.W.; Witkop, B.; Zaltzman-Nirenberg, P.; Udenfriend, S. *J. Am. Chem Soc.* **1968**, *90*, 6525–27.
184. Holtzman, J.; Gillette, J.R.; Milne, G.W.A. *J. Am. Chem. Soc.* **1967**, *89*, 6341–44.
185. Vogel, E.; Klärner, F.G. *Angew. Chem., Int. Ed. Engl.* **1968**, *7*, 374–75.
186. Jerina, D.M.; Daly, J.W.; Witkop, B.; Zaltzman-Nirenberg, P.; Udenfriend, S. *Biochemistry* **1970**, *9*, 147–56.
187. Hanzlik, R.P.; Edelman, M.; Michaely, W.J.; Scott, G. *J. Am. Chem. Soc.* **1976**, 98–1952–1955.

188. Guroff, G.; Daly, J.W.; Jerina, D.M.; Renson, J.; Witkop, B.; Udenfriend, S. *Science* **1967**, *157*, 1524–30.
189. Jerina, D.M.; Daly, J.W.; Witkop, B. *J. Am. Chem. Soc.* **1968**, *90*, 6523–25.
190. Boyd, D.R.; Daly, J.W.; Jerina, D.M. *Biochemistry* **1972**, *11*, 1961–66.
191. Kasperek, G.J.; Bruice, T.C.; Yagi, H.; Jerina, D.M., *J. Chem. Soc., Chem. Commun.* **1972**, 784–85.
192. Sims, P. *Biochem. J.* **1959**, *73*, 389–95.
193. Corner, E.D.S., Young L. *Biochem. J.* **1955**, *61*, 132–41.
194. Boyland, E.; Ramsay, G.S.; Sims, P. *Biochem. J.* **1961**, *78*, 376–84.
195. Sims, P. *Biochem. J.* **1964**, *92*, 621–31.
196. *Ibid.* **1962**, *84*, 558–63.
197. Boyland, E.; Sims, P. *Biochem. J.* **1962**, *84*, 564–70.
198. *Ibid.* **1964**, *90*, 391–98.
199. *Ibid.* *91*, 493–506.
200. *Ibid.* **1960**, *77*, 175–81.
201. Raha, C.R. *Bull. Soc. Chim. Biol.* **1970**, *52*, 105–7.
202. Pullman, A.; Pullman, B. *Jerusalem Symp. Quantum Chem. Biochem.* **1969**, *1*, 9–24.
203. Newman, M.S.; Olson, D.R. *J. Am. Chem. Soc.* **1974**, *96*, 6207–8.
204. Harvey, R.G.; Goh, S.H.; Cortez, C. *J. Am. Chem. Soc.* **1975**, *97*, 3468–79.
205. Dipple, A.; Levy, L.S.; Iype, P.T. *Cancer Res.* **1975**, *35*, 652–57.
206. Jerina, D.M.; Witkop, B.; McIntosh, C.L.; Chapman, O.L. *J. Am. Chem. Soc.* **1974**, *96*, 5578–80.
207. Pandov, H.; Sims, P. *Biochem. Pharmacol.* **1970**, *19*, 299–303.
208. Booth, J.; Keysell, G.R.; Sims, P. *Biochem. Pharmacol.* **1973**, *22*, 1781–91.
209. Booth, J.; Sims, P. *Biochem. Pharmacol.* **1974**, *23*, 2547–55.
210. Pearson, R.G.; Songstad, J. *J. Am. Chem. Soc.* **1967**, *89*, 1827–36.
211. Boyland, E.; Sims, P. *Biochem. J.* **1965**, *95*, 780–87.
212. *Ibid.* **1967**, *104*, 394–403.
213. McMahon, R.E.; Sullivan, H.R.; Craig, J.C.; Pereira, W.E. *Arch. Biochem. Biophys.* **1969**, *132*, 575–77.
214. Grandjean, C.; Cavalieri, E. *Biochem. Biophys. Res. Commun.* **1974**, *61*, 912–19.
215. Pataki, J.; Huggins, C.B. *Cancer Res.* **1969**, *29*, 506–9.
216. Sims, P. *Int. J. Cancer* **1967**, *2*, 505–8.
217. Boyland, E.; Levi, A.A. *Biochem. J.* **1935**, *29*, 2679–83.
218. Boyland, E.; Levi, A.A. *Biochem. J.* **1936**, *30*, 728–31.
219. Armstrong, R.N.; Levin, W.; Ryan, D.E.; Thomas, P.E.; Mah, H.D.; Jerina, D.M. *Biochem. Biophys. Res. Commun.* **1981**, *100*, 1077–84.
220. Hernandez, O.; Walker, M.; Cox, R.H.; Foureman, G.L.; Smith, B.R.; Bend, J.R. *Biochem. Biophys. Res. Commun.* **1980**, *96*, 1494–502.
221. Armstrong, R.N.; Kedzierski, B.; Levin, W.; Jerina, D.M. *J. Biol. Chem.* **1981**, *256*, 4726–33.
222. Thakker, D.R.; Yagi, H.; Levin, W.; Lu, A.Y.H.; Conney, A.H.; Jerina, D.M. *J. Biol. Chem.* **1977**, *252*, 6328–34.
223. Yang, S.K.; Roller, P.P.; Gelboin, H.V. *Biochemistry* **1977**, *16*, 3680–87.
224. Bellucci, G.; Berti, G.; Ingresso, G.; Mastrorilli, E. *J. Org. Chem.* **1979**, *45*, 299–303.
225. Yang, S.K.; McCourt, D.W.; Leutz, J.C.; Gelboin, H.v. *Science* **1977**, *196*, 1199–201.
226. Yang, S.K.; McCourt, D.W.; Roller, P.P.; Gelboin, H.V. *Proc. Natl. Acad. Sci. U.S.A.* **1976**, *73*, 2594–98.
227. Thakker, D.R.; Yagi, H.; Akagi, H.; Koreeda, M.; Lu, A.Y.H.; Levin, W.; Wood, A.W.; Conney, A.H.; Jerina, D.M. *Chem.-Biol. Interact.* **1977**, *16*, 281–300.
228. Koreeda, M.; Moore, P.D.; Wislocki, P.G.; Levin, W.; Conney, A.H.; Yagi, H.; Jerina, D.M. *Science* **1978**, *199*, 778–81.

229. Baird, W.M.; Diamond, L. *Biochem. Biophys. Res. Commun.* **1977**, *77*, 162–67.
230. Deutsch, J.; Vatsis, K.P.; Coon, M.J.; Leutz, J.C.; Gelboin, H.V. *Mol. Pharmacol.* **1979**, *16*, 1011–18.
231. Jerina, D.M.; Michaud, D.P.; Feldman, R.J.; Armstrong, R.N.; Vyas, K.P.; Thakker, D.R.; Yagi, H.; Thomas, P.E.; Ryan, D.E.; Levin, W. "Microsomes, Drug Oxidation and Drug Toxicity"; Sato, R.; Kato, R., Eds.; Japan Scientific Society Press: Tokyo, 1982; 195–201.
232. Miller, E.C. *Cancer Res.* **1951**, *11*, 100–8.
233. Wiest, W.G.; Heidelberger, C. *Cancer Res.* **1953**, *13*, 250–54.
234. Heidelberger, C.; Moldenhauer, M.G. *Cancer Res.* **1956**, *16*, 442–49.
235. Abell, C.W.; Heidelberger, C. *Cancer Res.* **1962**, *22*, 931–46.
236. Heidelberger, C.; Davenport, C.R. *Acta Unio Int. Cancrum* **1961**, *17*, 55–63.
237. Heidelberger, C. *J. Cell. Comp. Physiol.* **1964**, *64*, 129–48.
238. Brookes, P.; Lawley, P.D. *Nature (London)* **1964**, *202*, 781–84.
239. Miller, J.A.; Miller, E.C. *Adv. Cancer Res.* **1953**, *1*, 339–96.
240. Boveri, T.H. In "Zur Frage der Entstehung Maligner Tumoren"; Fischer: Jena, German Democratic Republ., 1914.
241. Grover, P.L.; Sims, P. *Biochem. J.* **1968**, *110*, 159–60.
242. Gelboin, H.V. *Cancer Res.* **1969**, *29*, 1272–76.
243. Haddow, A.J. *Pathol. Bacteriol.* **1938**, *47*, 581–91.
244. Vasiliev, J.M.; Gelfand, I.M. "Neoplastic and Normal Cells in Culture"; Cambridge University: Cambridge, 1981; pp. 38–40.
245. Diamond, L.; Defendi, V.; Brookes, P. *Cancer Res.* **1967**, *27*, 890–97.
246. Andrianov, L.N.; Belitsky, G.A.; Ivanova, O.J.; Khesina, A.Y.; Khitrovo, S.S.; Shabad, L.M.; Vasiliev, J.M. *Br. J. Cancer* **1967**, *21*, 566–75.
247. Gelboin, H.V.; Huberman, E.; Sachs, L. *Proc. Natl. Acad. Sci. U.S.A.* **1969**, *64*, 1188–94.
248. Iype, P.T.; Tomaszewski, J.E.; Dipple, A. *Cancer Res.* **1979**, *39*, 4925–29.
249. Wiebel, F.J. "Modifiers of Chemical Carcinogenesis", Slaga, T.J., Ed.; Raven: New York, 1980; pp. 57–84.
250. DiGiovanni, J.; Slaga, T.J.; Berry, D.L.; Juchau, M.R. "Modifiers of Chemical Carcinogenesis"; Slaga, T.J., Ed.; Raven: New York, 1980; pp. 145–68.
251. Wattenberg, L.W. "Modifiers of Chemical Carcinogenesis"; Slaga, T.J., Ed.; Raven: New York, 1980; pp. 85–98.
252. DiGiovanni, J.; Slaga, T.J. "Polycyclic Hydrocarbons and Cancer"; Gelboin, H.V.; Ts'o, P.O.P., Eds.; Academic; New York, 1981, vol. 3, pp. 259–92.
253. Wattenberg, L.W.; Leong, J.L. *Proc. Soc. Exp. Biol. Med.* **1968**, *128*, 940–43.
254. Diamond, L.; McFall, R.; Miller, J.; Gelboin, H.V. *Cancer Res.* **1972**, *32*, 731–36.
255. Slaga, T.J.; Thompson, S.; Berry, D.L.; DiGiovanni, J.; Juchau, M.R.; Viaje, A. *Chem.-Biol. Interact.* **1977**, *17*, 297–312.
256. Wattenberg, L.W.; Leong, J.L. *Cancer Res.* **1970**, *30*, 1922–25.
257. Gelboin, H.V.; Wiebel, F.; Diamond, L. *Science* **1970**, *170*, 169–71.
258. Kinoshita, N.; Gelboin, H.V. *Proc. Natl. Acad. Sci. U.S.A.* **1972**, *69*, 824–28.
259. Kinoshita, N.; Gelboin, H.V. *Cancer Res.* **1972**, *32*, 1329–39.
260. DiGiovanni, J.; Slaga, T.J.; Viaje, A.; Berry, D.L.; Harvey, R.G.; Juchau, M.R. *JNCI, J. Natl. Cancer Inst.* **1978**, *61*, 135–40.
261. Huggins, C.; Grand, L.; Fukunishi, R. *Proc. Natl. Acad. Sci. U.S.A.* **1964**, *51*, 737–42.
262. Hill, W.T.; Stanger, D.W.; Pizzo, A.; Riegel, B.; Shubik, P.; Waitman, W.B. *Cancer Res.* **1951**, *11*, 892–97.
263. Wheatley, D.N. *Br. J. Cancer* **1968**, *22*, 787–97.
264. Slaga, T.J.; Jecker, L.; Bracken, W.M.; Weeks, C.E. *Cancer Lett.* **1979**, *7*, 51–59.
265. Slaga, T.J.; Viaje, A.; Buty, S.G.; Bracken, W.M. *Res. Commun. Chem. Pathol. Pharmacol.* **1978**, *19*, 477–83.

266. Silinskas, K.C.; Okey, A.B. *JNCI, J. Natl. Cancer Inst.* **1975**, *55*, 653–57.
267. Berry, D.L.; Slaga, T.J.; DiGiovanni, J.; Juchau, M.R. *Ann. N.Y. Acad. Sci.* **1979**, *320*, 405–14.
268. Cohen, G.M.; Bracken, W.M.; Iyer, R.P.; Berry, D.L.; Selkirk, J.K.; Slaga, T.J. *Cancer Res.* **1979**, *39*, 4027–33.
269. DiGiovanni, J.; Bery, D.L.; Gleason, G.L.; Kishore, G.S.; Slaga, T.J. *Cancer Res.* **1980**, *40*, 1580–87.
270. Falk, H.L.; Kotin, P.; Thompson, S. *Arch. Environ. Health* **1964**, *9*, 169–79.
271. Wattenberg, L.W. *JNCI, J. Natl. Cancer Inst.* **1972**, *48*, 1425–30.
272. Slaga, T.J.; Bracken, W.M. *Cancer Res.* **1977**, *37*, 1631–35.
273. Wattenberg, L.W. *JNCI, J. Natl. Cancer Inst.* **1973**, *50*, 1541–44.
274. Shamberger, R.J. *JNCI, J. Natl. Cancer Inst.* **1970**, *44*, 931–36.
275. Ip, C. *Cancer Res.* **1981**, *41*, 4386–90.
276. Miyaji, T.; Moskowski, L.I.; Senoo, T.; Ogata, M.; Odo, T.; Kawai, K.; Sayama, Y.; Ishida, H.; Matsuo, H. *Gann* **1953**, *44*, 281–83.
277. Miller, E.C.; Miller, J.A.; Brown, R.R.; MacDonald, J.D. *Cancer Res.* **1958**, *18*, 469–77.
278. Miller, E.C.; Miller, J.A.; Hartmann, H.A. *Cancer Res.* **1961**, *21*, 815–24.
279. Miller, J.A.; Cramer, J.W.; Miller, E.C. *Cancer Res.* **1960**, *20*, 950–62.
280. Conney, A.H.; Miller, E.C.; Miller, J.A. *J. Biol Chem.* **1957**, *228*, 753–66.
281. Wattenberg, L.W.; Leong, J.L. *J. Histochem. Cytochem.* **1962**, *10*, 412–20.
282. Gelboin, H.V.; Blackburn, N.R. *Cancer Res.* **1964**, *24*, 356–60.
283. Wattenberg, L.W.; Page, M.A.; Leong, J.L. *Cancer Res.* **1968**, *28*, 934–37.
284. Nebert, D.W.; Gelboin, H.V. *J. Biol. Chem.* **1968**, *243*, 6250–61.
285. Bowden, G.T.; Slaga, T.J.; Shapas, B.G.; Boutwell, R.K. *Cancer Res.* **1974**, *34*, 2634–42.
286. Kouri, R.E. "Polynuclear Aromatic Hydrocarbons: Chemistry, Metabolism and Carcinogenesis"; Freudenthal, R.I.; Jones, P.W., Eds.; Raven: New York, 1976; pp. 139–51.
287. Diamond, L.; Gelboin, H.V. *Science* **1969**, *166*, 1023–25.
288. Wiebel, F.J.; Leutz, J.C.; Diamond, L.; Gelboin, H.V. *Arch. Biochem. Biophys.* **1971**, *144*, 78–86.
289. Huang, M.-T.; Johnson, E.F.; Muller-Eberhard, U.; Koop, D.R.; Coon, M.J.; Conney, A.H. *J. Biol. Chem.* **1981**, *256*, 10897–901.
290. Sullivan, P.D.; Calle, L.M.; Shafer, K.; Nettleman, M. "Polynuclear Aromatic Hydrocarbons"; Jones, P.W.; Freudenthal, R.I. Ed.; Raven: New York, 1978; pp. 1–8.
291. Slaga, T.J.; DiGiovanni, J., in Vol. II of this book, Chap. 00, pp. 000–00.
292. Speier, J.L.; Wattenberg, L.W. *JNCI, J. Natl. Cancer Inst.* **1975**, *55*, 469–72.
293. Lam, L.K.T.; Wattenberg, L.W. *JNCI, J. Natl. Cancer Inst.* **1977**, *58*, 413–17.
294. Benson, A.M.; Cha, Y.-N.; Bueding, E.; Heine, H.S.; Talalay, P. *Cancer Res.* **1979**, *39*, 2971–77.
295. Cha, Y.-N.; Bueding, E. *Biochem. Pharmacol.* **1979**, *28*, 1917–21.
296. Anderson, M.W.; Boroujerdi, M.; Wilson, A.G.E. *Cancer Res.* **1981**, *41*, 4309–15.
297. Ts'o, P.O.P.; Lu, P. *Proc. Natl. Acad. Sci. U.S.A.* **1964**, *51*, 272–80.
298. Rice, J.M. *J. Am. Chem. Soc.* **1964**, *86*, 1444–46.
299. Rapaport, S.A.; Ts'o, P.O.P. *Proc. Natl. Acad. Sci. U.S.A.* **1966**, *55*, 381–87.
300. Morreal, E.C.; Dao, T.L.; Eskins, K.; King, C.L.; Dienstag, J. *Biochim. Biophys. Acta* **1968**, *169*, 224–29.
301. Umans, R.S.; Lesko, S.A.; Ts'o, P.O.P. *Nature (London)* **1969**, *221*, 763–64.
302. Lesko, S.A.; Ts'o, P.O.P.; Umans, R.S. *Biochemistry* **1969**, *8*, 2291–98.
303. Udenfriend, S.; Clark, C.T.; Axelrod, J.; Brodie, B.B. *J. Biol. Chem.* **1954**, *208*, 731–39.
304. Hoffmann, H.D.; Lesko, S.A.; Ts'o, P.O.P *Biochemistry* **1970**, *9*, 2594–604.
305. Antonello, C.; Carlassare, F.; Musajo, L. *Gazz. Chim. Ital.* **1968**, *98*, 30–41.
306. Cavalieri, E.; Calvin, M. *Photochem. Photobiol.* **1971**, *14*, 641–53.

307. Blackburn, G.M.; Fenwick, R.G.; Thompson, M..H. *Tetrahedron Lett.* **1972**, *7*, 589–92.
308. Hoffmann, H.D.; Müller, W. *Jerusalem Symp. Quantum Chem. Biochem.* **1969**, *1*, 183–87.
309. Wilk, M.; Bez, W.; Rochlitz, J. *Tetrahedron* **1966**, *22*, 2599–608.
310. Rochlitz, J. *Tetrahedron* **1967**, *23*, 3043–48.
311. Wilk, M.; Girke, W. *Jerusalem Symp. Quantum Chem. Biochem.* **1969**, *1*, 91–105.
312. Jeftic, L.; Adams, R.N. *J. Am. Chem. Soc.* **1970**, *92*, 1332–37.
313. Fried, J.; Schumm, D.E. *J. Am. Chem. Soc.* **1967**, *89*, 5508–09.
314. Cavalieri, E. "Abstracts of Papers," 166th Natl. Meeting, ACS, 1973, Biol. 193.
315. Rogan, E.G.; Katomski, P.A.; Roth, R.W.; Cavalieri, E.L. *J. Biol. Chem.* **1979**, *254*, 7055–59.
316. Cavalieri, E.L.; Sinha, D.; Rogan, E.G. "Polynuclear Aromatic Hydrocarbons: Chemistry and Biological Effects"; Bjorseth, A.; Dennis, A.J., Eds.; Battelle: Columbus, OH, 1980; pp. 215–31.
317. Miller, E.C.; Miller, J.A. *Proc. Soc. Exp. Biol. Med.* **1967**, *124*, 915–19.
318. Flesher, J.W.; Sydnor, K.L. *Int. J. Cancer* **1970**, *5*, 253–59.
319. Lieberman, M.W.; Dipple, A. *Cancer Res.* **1972**, *32*, 1855–60.
320. Venitt, S.; Tarmy, E.M. *Biochim. Biophys. Acta* **1972**, *287*, 38–51.
321. Rayman, M.P.; Dipple, A. *Biochemistry* **1973**, *12*, 1538–42.
322. Dipple, A.; Moschel, R.C.; Hudgins, W.R. *Drug Metab. Rev.* **1982**, *13*, 249–68.
323. Dipple, A.; Brookes, P.; Mackintosh, D.S.; Rayman, M.P. *Biochemistry* **1971**, *10*, 4323–30.
324. Rayman, M.P.; Dipple, A. *Biochemistry* **1973**, *12*, 1202–7.
325. Lawley, P.D. *Prog. Nucleic Acid Res. Mol. Biol.* **1966**, *5*, 89–131.
326. Baird, W.M.; Dipple, A.; Grover, P.L.; Sims, P.; Brookes, P. *Cancer Res.* **1973**, *33*, 2386–92.
327. Nagata, C.; Kodama, M.; Tagashira, Y. *Gann* **1967**, *58*, 493–504.
328. Nagata, C.; Inomata, M.; Kodama, M.; Tagashira, Y. *Gann* **1968**, *59*, 289–98.
329. Inomata, M.; Nagata, C. *Gann* **1972**, *63*, 119–30.
330. Lorentzen, R.; Caspary, W.; Ts'o, P.O.P. "Abstracts of Papers," 162nd Natl. Meeting, ACS, 1971, Biol. 26.
331. Nagata, C.; Kodama, M.; Ioki, Y. "Polycyclic Hydrocarbons and Cancer Vol. 1," Gelboin, H.V.; Ts'o, P.O.P., Eds.; Academic: New York, 1978; pp. 247–60.
332. Van Duuren, B.L.; Langseth, L.; Orris, L.; Baden, M.; Kuschner, M. *JNCI, J. Natl. Cancer Inst.* **1967**, *39*, 1217–28.
333. Keysell, G.R.; Booth, J.; Sims, P.; Grover, P.L.; Hewer, A. *Biochem. J.* **1972**, *129*, 41p–42p.
334. Selkirk, J.K.; Huberman, E.; Heidelberger, C. *Biochm. Biophys. Res. Commun.* **1971**, *43*, 1010–16.
335. Grover, P.L.; Hewer, A.; Sims, P. *FEBS Lett.* **1971**, *18*, 76–80.
336. Grover, P.L.; Hewer, A.; Sims, P. *Biochem. Pharmacol.* **1972**, *21*, 2713–26.
337. Grover, P.L.; Sims, P. *Biochem. Pharmacol.* **1970**, *19*, 2251–59.
338. Grover, P.L.; Forrester, J.A.; Sims, P. *Biochem. Pharmacol.* **1971**, *20*, 1297–302.
339. Kuroki, T.; Huberman, E.; Marquardt, H.; Selkirk, J.K.; Heidelberger, C.; Grover, P.L.; Sims, P. *Chem.-Biol. Interact.* **1971/72**, *4*, 389–97.
340. Grover, P.L.; Sims, P.; Huberman, E.; Marquardt, H.; Kuroki, T.; Heidelberger, C. *Proc. Natl. Acad. Sci. U.S.A.* **1971**, *68*, 1098–101.
341. Marquardt, H.; Kuroki, T.; Huberman, E.; Selkirk, J.K.; Heidelberger, C.; Grover, P.L.; Sims, P. *Cancer Res.* **1972**, *32*, 716–20.
342. Huberman, E.; Kuroki, T.; Marquardt, H.; Selkirk, J.T.; Heidelberger, C.; Grover, P.L.; Sims, P. *Cancer Res.* **1972**, *32*, 1391–96.
343. Huberman, E.; Aspiras, L.; Heidelberger, C.; Grover, P.L.; Sims, P. *Proc. Natl. Acad. Sci. U.S.A.* **1971**, *68*, 3195–99.

344. Cookson, M.J.; Sims, P.; Grover, P.L.; *Nature(London) New Biol.* **1971**, *234*, 186–87.
345. Ames, B.N.; Sims, P.; Grover, P.L. *Science(Washington, D.C.)* **1972**, *176*, 47–49.
346. Fahmy, O.G.; Fahmy, M.J. *Cancer Res.* **1973**, *33*, 2354–61.
347. Flesher, J.W.; Harvey, R.G.; Sydnor, K.L. *Int. J. Cancer* **1976**, *18*, 251–353.
348. Flaks, A.; Sims, P. *Br. J. Cancer* **1975**, *32*, 604–9.
349. Grover, P.L.; Sims, P.; Mitchley, B.C.V.; Roe, F.J.C. *Br. J. Cancer* **1975**, *31*, 182–88.
350. Levin, W.; Wood, A.W.; Yagi, H.; Dansette, P.M.; Jerina, D.M.; Conney, A.H. *Proc. Natl. Acad. Sci., U.S.A.* **1976**, *73*, 243–47.
351. Huberman, E.; Sachs, L. *Proc. Natl. Acad. Sci., U.S.A.* **1976**, *73*, 188–92.
352. Wislocki, P.G.; Wood, A.W.; Chang, R.L.; Levin, W.; Yagi, H.; Hernandez, O.; Dansette, P.M.; Jerina, D.M.; Conney, A.H. *Cancer Res.* **1976**, *36*, 3350–57.
353. Maher, V.M.; McCormick, J.J. "Biology of Radiation Carcinogenesis"; Yuhas, J.M.; Tennant, R.W.; Regan, J.B., Eds.; Raven: New York, 1976; p. 129.
354. McCann, J.; Choi, E.; Yamasaki, E.; Ames, B.N. *Proc. Natl. Acad. Sci, U.S.A.* **1975**, *72*, 5135–39.
355. Malaveille, C.; Bartsch, H.; Grover, P.L.; Sims, P. *Biochem. Biophys. Res. Commun.* **1975**, *66*, 693–700.
356. Wislocki, P.G.; Wood, A.W.; Chang, R.L.; Levin, W.; Yagi, H.; Hernandez, O.; Jerina, D.M.; Conney, A.H. *Biochem. Biophys. Res. Commun.* **1976**, *68*, 1006–12.
357. Baird, W.M.; Harvey, R.G.; Brookes, P. *Cancer Res.* **1975**, *35*, 54–57.
358. Thompson, M.H.; Osborne, M.R.; King, H.W.S.; Brookes, P. *Chem.-Biol. Interact.* **1976**, *14*, 13–19.
359. Bigger, C.A.H.; Tomaszewski, J.E.; Dipple, A. *Biochem. Biophys. Res. Commun.* **1978**, *80*, 229–35.
360. King, H.W.S.; Osborne, M.R.; Brookes, P. *Int. J. Cancer* **1977**, *20*, 564–71.
361. Brookes, P.; Heidelberger, C. *Cancer Res.* **1969**, *29*, 157–65.
362. Duncan, M.; Brookes, P.; Dipple, A. *Int. J. Cancer* **1969**, *4*, 813–19.
363. Baird, W.M.; Brookes, P. *Cancer Res.* **1973**, *33*, 2378–85.
364. Borgen, A.; Darvey, H.; Castagnoli, N.; Crocker, T.T.; Rasmussen, R.E.; Wang, I.Y. *J. Med. Chem.* **1973**, *16*, 502–6.
365. Booth, J.; Sims, P. *FEBS Lett.* **1974**, *47*, 30–33.
366. Daudel, P.; Duquesne, M.; Vigny, P.; Grover, P.L.; Sims, P. *FEBS Lett.* **1975**, *57*, 250–53.
367. Ivanovic, V.; Geacintov, N.E.; Weinstein, I.B. *Biochem. Biophys. Res. Commun.* **1976**, *70*, 1172–78.
368. Grover, P.L.; Hewer, A.; Pal, K.; Sims, P. *Int. J. Cancer* **1976**, *18*, 1–6.
369. McCaustland, D.J.; Engel, J.F. *Tetrahedron Lett.* **1975**, *30*, 2549–52.
370. Yagi, H.; Hernandez, O.; Jerina, D.M. *J. Am. Chem. Soc.* **1975**, *97*, 6881–83.
371. Beland, F.A.; Harvey, R.G. *J. Chem. Soc. Chem. Commun.* **1976**, 84–85.
372. King, H.W. S.; Osborne, M.R.; Beland, F.A.; Harvey, R.G.; Brookes, P. *Proc. Natl. Acad. Sci., U.S.A.* **1976**, *73*, 2679–81.
373. Remsen, J.; Jerina, D.; Yagi, H.; Cerutti, P. *Biochem. Biophys. Res. Commun.* **1977**, *74*, 934–40.
374. Baer-Dubowska, W.; Alexandrov, K. *Cancer Lett.* **1981**, *13*, 47–52.
375. Eastman, A.; Sweetenham, J.; Bresnick, E. *Chem.-Biol. Interact.* **1978**, *23*, 345–53.
376. Wilson, A.G.E.; Kung, H.-C.; Boroujerd, M.; Anderson, M.W. *Cancer Res.* **1981**, *41*, 3453–60.
377. Weinstein, I.B.; Jeffrey, A.M.; Jennette, K.W.; Blobstein, S.H.; Harvey, R.G.; Harris, C.C.; Autrup, H.; Kasai, H.; Nakanishi, K. *Science (Washington, D.C.)* **1976**, *193*, 592–95.
378. Autrup, H.; Wefald, F.C.; Jeffrey, A.M.; Tate, H.; Schwartz, R.D.; Trump, B.F.; Harris, C.C. *Int. J. Cancer* **1980**, *25*, 293–300.

379. Jeffrey, A.M.; Weinstein, I.B.; Jennette, K.W.; Grzeskowiak, K.; Nakanishi, K.; Harvey, R.G.; Autrup, H.; Harris, C. *Nature* **1977**, *269*, 348–50.
380. Harris, C.C.; Autrup, H.; Stoner, G.D.; Trump, B.F.; Hillman, E.; Schafer, P.W.; Jeffrey, A.M. *Cancer Res.* **1979**, *39*, 4401–6.
381. Autrup, H.; Harris, C.C.; Trump, B.F.; Jeffrey, A.M. *Cancer Res.* **1978**, *38*, 3689–96.
382. Shinohara, K.; Cerutti, P.A. *Cancer Lett.* **1977**, *3*, 303–9.
383. Brown, H. S.; Jeffrey, A.M.; Weinstein, I.B. *Cancer Res.* **1979**, *39*, 1673–77.
384. Ivanovic, V.; Geacintov, N.E.; Yamasaki, H.; Weinstein, I.B. *Biochemistry* **1978**, *17*, 1597–603.
385. Ashurst, S.W.; Cohen, G.M. *Chem.-Biol. Interact.* **1980**, *29*, 117–27.
386. Lo, K.; Kakunaga, T. *Biochem. Biophys. Res. Commun.* **1981**, *99*, 820–29.
387. Baird, W.M.; Diamond, L. *Int. J. Cancer* **1978**, *22*, 189–95.
388. Swaisland, A.J.; Hewer, A.; Pal, K.; Keysell, G.R.; Booth, J.; Grover, P.L.; Sims, P. *FEBS Lett.* **1974**, *47*, 34–38.
389. Vigny, P.; Kindts, M.; Duquesne, M.; Cooper, C.S.; Grover, P.L.; Sims, P. *Carcinogenesis* **1980**, *1*, 33–36.
390. Cooper, C.S.; Ribeiro, O.; Farmer, P.B.; Hewer, A.; Walsh, C.; Pal, K.; Grover, P.L.; Sims, P. *Chem.-Biol. Interact.* **1980**, *32*, 209–31.
391. Cooper, C.S.; Ribeiro, O.; Hewer, A.; Walsh, C.; Pal, K.; Grover, P.L.; Sims, P. *Carcinogenesis* **1980**, *1*, 233–43.
392. Vigny, P.; Duquesne, M.; Coulomb, H.; Tierney, B.; Grover, P.L.; Sims, P. *FEBS Lett.* **1977**, *82*, 278–82.
393. King, H.W.S.; Osborne, M.R.; Brookes, P. *Chem.-Biol. Interact.* **1978**, *20*, 367–71.
394. Eastman, A.; Bresnick, E. *Cancer Res.* **1979**, *39*, 2400–5.
395. Phillips, D.H.; Grover, P.L.; Sims, P. *Int. J. Cancer* **1978**, *22*, 487–94.
396. Cooper, C.S.; Vigny, P.; Kindts, M.; Grover, P.L.; Sims, P. *Carcinogenesis* **1980**, *1*, 855–60.
397. Vigny, P.; Duquesne, M.; Coulomb, H.; Lacombe, C.; Tierney, B.; Grover, P.L.; Sims, P. *FEBS Lett.* **1977**, *75*, 9–12.
398. Moschel, R.C.; Hudgins, W.R.; Dipple, A. *Chem.-Biol. Interact.* **1979**, *27*, 69–79.
399. Tierney, B.; Hewer, A.; Walsh, C.; Grover, P.L.; Sims, P. *Chem.-Biol. Interact.* **1977**, *18*, 179–93.
400. Baird, W.M.; Dipple, A. *Int. J. Cancer* **1977**, *20*, 427–31.
401. Moschel, R.C.; Baird, W.M.; Dipple, A. *Biochem. Biophys. Res. Commun.* **1977**, *76*, 1092–98.
402. Ivanovic, V.; Geacintov, N.E.; Jeffrey, A.M.; Fu, P.P.; Harvey, R.G.; Weinstein, I.B. *Cancer Lett.* **1978**, *4*, 131–40.
403. Dipple, A.; Nebzydoski, J.A. *Chem. Biol. Interact.* **1978**, *20*, 17–26.
404. Chou, M.W.; Yang, S.K. *Proc. Natl. Acad. Sci. U.S.A.* **1978**, *75*, 5466–70.
405. Cooper, C.S.; Ribeiro, O.; Hewer, A.; Walsh, C.; Grover, P.L.; Sims, P. *Chem.-Biol. Interact.* **1980**, *29*, 357–67.
406. Vigny, P.; Kindts, M.; Cooper, C.S.; Grover, P.L.; Sims, P. *Carcinogenesis* **1981**, *2*, 115–19.
407. Dipple, A.; Tomaszewski, J.E.; Moschel, R.C.; Bigger, C.A.H.; Nebzydoski, J.A.; Egan, M. *Cancer Res.* **1979**, *39*, 1154–58.
408. MacNicoll, A.D.; Burden, P.M.; Ribeiro, O.; Hewer, A.; Grover, P.L.; Sims, P. *Chem.-Biol. Interact.* **1979**, *26*, 121–32.
409. Coombs, M.M.; Bhatt, T.S.; Young, S. *Br. J. Cancer* **1980**, *40*, 914–21.
410. Abbott, P.J.; Coombs, M.M. *Carcinogenesis* **1981**, *2*, 629–36.
411. Wiebers, J.L.; Abbott, P.J.; Coombs, M.M.; Livingston, D.C. *Carcinogenesis* **1981**, *2*, 637–43.

412. Phillips, D.H.; Grover, P.L.; Sims, P. *Int. J. Cancer* **1979**, *23*, 201–8.
413. Hewer, A.; Cooper, C.S.; Ribeiro, O.; Pal, K.; Grover, P.L.; Sims, P. *Carcinogenesis* **1981**, *2*, 1345–52.
414. Pelkonen, O.; Boobis, A.R.; Nebert, D.W. "Polynuclear Aromatic Hydrocarbons"; Jones, P.W.; Freudenthal, R.I., Ed.; Raven: New York, 1978; pp. 383–400.
415. Perin-Roussel, O.; Ekert, B.; Zajdela, F.; Jacquignon, P. *Cancer Res.* **1978**, *38*, 3499–504.
416. Perin-Roussel, O.; Croisy-Delcey, M.; Mispelter, J.; Saguem, S.; Chalvet, O.; Ekert, B.; Fouquet, J.; Jacquignon, P.; Lhoste, J.M.; Muel, B.; Zajdela, F.E. *Cancer Res.* **1980**, *40*, 1742–49.
417. MacLeod, M.C.; Cohen, G.M.; Selkirk, J.K. *Cancer Res.* **1979**, *39*, 3463–70.
418. King, H.W.S.; Thompson, M.H.; Brookes, P. *Cancer Res.* **1975**, *35*, 1263–69.
419. Bigger, C.A.H.; Moschel, R.C.; Dipple, A. "Chemical Analysis and Biological Fate: Polynuclear Aromatic Hydrocarbons"; Cooke, M.; Dennis, A.J., Ed.; Battelle: Columbus, OH, 1981; pp. 209–19.
420. Bigger, C.A.H.; Tomaszewski, J.E.; Dipple, A. *Carcinogenesis* **1980**, *1*, 15–20.
421. Bigger, C.A.H.; Tomaszewski, J.E.; Andrews, A.W.; Dipple, A. *Cancer Res.* **1980**, *40*, 655–61.
422. Bigger, C.A.H.; Tomaszewski, J.E.; Dipple, A.; Lake, R.S. *Science* **1980**, *209*, 503–5.
423. Pelkonen, O.; Boobis, A.R.; Levitt, R.C.; Kouri, R.E.; Nebert, D.W. *Pharmacology* **1979**, *18*, 281–93.
424. Baer-Dubowska, W.B.; Frayssinet, C.; Alexandrov, K. *Cancer Lett.* **1981**, *14*, 125–29.
425. Vigny, P.; Ginot, Y.M.; Kindts, M.; Cooper, C.S.; Grover, P.L.; Sims, P. *Carcinogenesis* **1980**, *1*, 945–50.
426. Levin, W.; Wood, A.W.; Wislocki, P.G.; Chang, R.L.; Kapitulnik, J.; Mah, H.D.; Yagi, H.; Jerina, D.M.; Conney, A.H. "Polycyclic Hydrocarbons and Cancer"; Gelboin, H.V.; Ts'o, P.O.P., Eds.; Academic: New York, 1978; Vol. 1, pp. 189–202.
427. Levin, W.; Wood, A.W.; Yagi, H.; Dansette, P.M.; Jerina, D.M.; Conney, A.H. *Proc. Natl. Acad. Sci. U.S.A.* **1976**, *73*, 243–47.
428. Levin, W.; Wood, A.W.; Yagi, H.; Jerina, D.M.; Conney, A.H. *Proc. Natl. Acad. Sci. U.S.A.* **1976**, *73*, 3867–71.
429. Wislocki, P.G.; Chang, R.L.; Wood, A.W.; Levin, W.; Yagi, H.; Hernandez, O.; Mah, H.D.; Dansette, P.M.; Jerina, D.M.; Conney, A.H. *Cancer Res.* **1977**, *37*, 2608–11.
430. Thakker, D.R.; Yagi, H.; Lehr, R.E.; Levin, W.; Buenning, M.; Lu, A.Y.H.; Chang, R.L.; Wood, A.W.; Conney, A.H.; Jerina, D.M. *Mol. Pharmacol.* **1978**, *14*, 502–13.
431. Levin, W.; Wood, A.W.; Wislocki, P.G.; Kapitulnik, J.; Yagi, H.; Jerina, D.M.; Conney, A.H. *Cancer Res.* **1977**, *37*, 3356–61.
432. Levin, W., unpublished data.
433. Kapitulnik, J.; Levin, W.; Yagi, H.; Jerina, D.M.; Conney, A.H. *Cancer Res.* **1976**, *36*, 3625–28.
434. Chang, R.L.; Wislocki, P.G.; Kapitulnik, J.; Wood, A.W.; Levin, W.; Yagi, H.; Mah, H.D.; Jerina, D.M.; Conney, A.H. *Cancer Res.* **1976**, *36*, 3625–38.
435. Slaga, T.J.; Viaje, A.; Berry, D.L.; Bracken, W.; Buty, S.G.; Scribner, J.D. *Cancer Lett.* **1976**, *2*, 115–22.
436. Chouroulinkov, I.; Gentil, A.; Grover, P.L.; Sims, P. *Br. J. Cancer* **1976**, *34*, 523–32.
437. Slaga, T.J.; Bracken, W.M.; Viaje, A.; Levin, W.; Yagi, H.; Jerina, D.M.; Conney, A.H. *Cancer Res.* **1977**, *37*, 4130–33.
438. Slaga, T.J.; Viaje, A.; Bracken, W.M.; Berry, D.L.; Fischer, S.M.; Miller, D.R.; Leclerc, S.M. *Cancer Lett.* **1977**, *3*, 23–30.
439. Levin, W.; Wood, A.W.; Chang, R.L.; Slaga, T.J.; Yagi, H.; Jerina, D.M.; Conney, A.H. *Cancer Res.* **1977**, *37*, 2721–25.

440. Slaga, T.J.; Bracken, W.J.; Gleason, G.; Levin, W.; Yagi, H.; Jerina, D.M.; Conney, A.H. *Cancer Res.* **1979**, *39*, 67–71.
441. Slaga, T.J.; Bracken, W.M.; Dresner, S.; Levin, W.; Yagi, H.; Jerina, D.M.; Conney, A.H. *Cancer Res.* **1978**, *38*, 678–81.
442. Wislocki, P.G.; Kapitulnik, J.; Levin, W.; Conney, A.H.; Yagi, H.; Jerina, D.M. *Cancer Lett.* **1978**, *5*, 191–97.
443. Kapitulnik, J.; Wislocki, P.G.; Levin, W.; Yagi, H.; Jerina, D.M.; Conney, A.H. *Cancer Res.* **1978**, *38*, 354–58.
444. Kapitulnik, J.; Wislocki, P.G.; Levin, W.; Yagi, H.; Thakker, D.R.; Akagi, H.; Koreeda, M.; Jerina, D.M.; Conney, A.H. *Cancer Res.* **1978**, *38*, 2661–65.
445. Buening, M.K.; Wislocki, P.G.; Levin, W.; Yagi, H.; Thakker, D.R.; Akagi, H.; Koreeda, M.; Jerina, D.M.; Conney, A.H. *Proc. Natl. Acad. Sci., U.S.A.* **1978**, *75*, 5358–61.
446. Kapitulnik, J.; Levin, W.; Conney, A.H.; Yagi, H.; Jerina, D.M. *Nature (London)* **1977**, *266*, 378–80.
447. Brookes, P. *Cancer Lett.* **1979**, *6*, 285–89.
448. Wood, A.W.; Chang, R.L.; Levin, W.; Ryan, D.E.; Thomas, P.E.; Mah, H.D.; Karle, J.M.; Yagi, H.; Jerina, D.M.; Conney, A.H. *Cancer Res.* **1979**, *39*, 4069–77.
449. Buening, M.K.; Levin, W.; Wood, A.W.; Chang, R.L.; Lehr, R.E.; Taylor, C.W.; Yagi, H.; Jerina, D.M.; Conney, A.H. *Cancer Res.* **1980**, *40*, 203–6.
450. Slaga, T.J.; Gleason, G.L.; Mills, G.; Elwald, L.; Fu, P.P.; Lee, H.M.; Harvey, R.G. *Cancer Res.* **1980**, *40*, 1981–84.
451. Levin, W.; Wood, A.W.; Chang, R.L.; Yagi, H.; Mah, H.D.; Jerina, D.M.; Conney, A.H. *Cancer Res.* **1978**, 1831–34.
452. Wood, A.W.; Levin, W.; Chang, R.L.; Lehr, R.E.; Schaefer-Ridder, M.; Karle, J.M.; Jerina, D.M.; Conney, A.H. *Proc. Natl. Acad. Sci., U.S.A.* **1977**, *74*, 3176–79.
453. Slaga, T.J.; Huberman, E.; Selkirk, J.K.; Harvey, R.G.; Bracken, W.M. *Cancer Res.* **1978**, *38*, 1699–704.
454. Levin, W.; Thakker, D.R.; Wood, A.W.; Chang, R.L.; Lehr, R.E.; Jerina, D.M.; Conney, A.H. *Cancer Res.* **1978**, *38*, 1705–10.
455. Buening, M.L.; Levin, W.; Wood, A.W.; Chang, R.L.; Yagi, H.; Karle, J.M.; Jerina, D.M.; Conney, A.H. *Cancer Res.* **1979**, *39*, 1310–14.
456. Levin, W.; Wood, A.W.; Chang, R.L.; Ittah, Y.; Croisy-Delcey, M.; Yagi, H.; Jerina, D.M.; Conney, A.H. *Cancer Res.* **1980**, *40*, 3910–14.
457. Chouroulinkov, I.; Gentil, A.; Tierney, B.; Grover, P.L.; Sims, P. *Int. J. Cancer* **1979**, *24*, 455–60.
458. Levin, W.; Buening, M.K.; Wood, A.W.; Chang, R.L.; Thakker, D.R.; Jerina, D.M.; Conney, A.H. *Cancer Res.* **1979**, *39*, 3549–53.
459. Chouroulinkov, I.; Gentil, A.; Tierney, B.; Grover, P.L.; Sims, P. *Br. J. Cancer* **1979**, *39*, 376–82.
460. Hecht, S.S.; Rivenson, A.; Hoffman, D. *Cancer Res.* **1980**, *40*, 1396–99.
461. Wislocki, P.G.; Fiorentini, K.M.; Fu, P.P.; Chou, M.W.; Yang, S.K.; Lu, A.Y.H. *Carcinogenesis* **1981**, *2*, 507–9.
462. Wislocki, P.G.; Gadek, K.M.; Chou, M.W.; Yang, S.K.; Lu, A.Y.H. *Cancer Res.* **1980**, *40*, 3661–64.
463. Slaga, T.J.; Gleason, G.L.; DiGiovanni, J.; Sukumaran, K.B.; Harvey, R.G. *Cancer Res.* **1979**, *39*, 1934–36.
464. Sayer, J.M.; Yagi, H.; Croisy-Delcey, M.; Jerina, D.M. *J. Am. Chem. Soc.* **1981**, *103*, 4970–72.
465. McCaustland, D.J.; Fischer, D.L.; Kolwyck, K.C.; Duncan, W.P.; Wiley, J.C.; Menon, C.S.; Engel, J.F.; Selkirk, J.K.; Roller, P.P "Polynuclear Aromatic Hydrocarbons:

Chemistry, Metabolism, and Carcinogenesis"; Freudenthal, R.I.; Jones, P.W., Eds.; Raven: New York, 1976; Vol. 1, pp. 349–411.
466. Jerina, D.M.; Yagi, H.; Hernandez, O.; Dansette, P.M.; Wood, A.W.; Levin, W.; Chang, R.L.; Wislocki, P.G.; Conney, A.H. "Carcinogenesis, Polynuclear Aromatic Hydrocarbons: Chemistry, Metabolism and Carcinogenesis"; Freudenthal, R.I.; Jones, P.W., Eds.; Raven: New York, 1976; Vol. 1, pp. 91–113.
467. Harvey, R.G.; Fu, P.P. "Polycyclic Hydrocarbons and Cancer"; Gelboin, H.V.; Ts'o, P.O.P., Eds.; Academic: New York, 1978, Vol. 1, pp. 133–65.
468. Sims, P.; Grover, P.L. "Polycyclic Hydrocarbons and Cancer"; Gelboin, H.V.; Ts'o, P.O.P., Eds.; Academic: New York, 1981; Vol. 3, pp. 117–81.
469. Goh, S.H.; Harvey, R.G. *J. Am. Chem. Soc.* **1973**, *95*, 242–43.
470. Harvey, R.G.; Goh, S.H.; Cortez, C. *J. Am. Chem. Soc.* **1975**, *97*, 3468–79.
471. Dansette, P.; Jerina, D.M. *J. Am. Chem. Soc.* **1974**, *96*, 1224–25.
472. Ishikawa, K.; Charles, H.C.; Griffin, G.W. *Tetrahedron Lett.* **1977**, 427–30.
473. Krishnan, S.; Kuhn, D.G.; Hamilton, G.A. *J. Am. Chem. Soc.* **1977**, *99*, 8121–23.
474. Cook, J.W.; Schoental, R. *J. Chem. Soc.* **1948**, 170–73.
475. Kitahara, Y.; Okuda, H.; Shudo, K.; Okamoto, T.; Nagao, M.; Seino, Y.; Sugimura, T. *Chem. Pharm. Bull.* **1978**, *26*, 1950–53.
476. Boux, L.J.; Cheung, H.T.A.; Holder, G.M.; Moldovan, L. *Tetrahedron Lett.* **1980**, *21*, 2923–26.
477. Berliner, E. *Org. React. (N.Y.)* **1949**, *5*, 229–89.
478. Johnson, W.S. *Org. React. (N.Y.)* **1944**, *2*, 114–77.
479. Fu, P.P.; Harvey, R.G. *Chem. Rev.* **1978**, *78*, 317–61.
480. Fu, P.P.; Harvey, R.G. *Tetrahedron Lett.* **1977**, 415–18.
481. Harvey, R.G. *Synthesis* **1970**, 161–72.
482. Waterfall, J.F.; Sims, P. *Biochem. J.* **1972**, *128*, 265–77.
483. Sims, P. *Biochem. J.* **1972**, *130*, 27–35.
484. Sims, P. *Biochem. J.* **1971**, *125*, 159–68.
485. Yagi, H.; Jerina, D.M. *J. Am. Chem. Soc.* **1973**, *95*, 243–44.
486. Yagi, H.; Jerina, D.M. *J. Am. Chem. Soc.* **1975**, *97*, 3185–92.
487. Jerina, D.M.; Yagi, H.; Daly, J.W. *Heterocycles* **1973**, *1*, 267–326.
488. Wilson, C.V. *Org. React. (N.Y.)* **1957**, *9*, 332–88.
489. Lehr, R.E.; Schaefer-Ridder, M.; Jerina, D.M. *J. Org. Chem.* **1977**, *42*, 736–44.
490. Fu, P.P.; Harvey, R.G. *Tetrahedron Lett.* **1977**, 2059–62.
491. Harvey, R.G.; Sukumaran, K.B. *Tetrahedron Lett.* **1977**, 2387–90.
492. Karle, J.M.; Mah, H.D.; Jerina, D.M.; Yagi, H. *Tetrahedron Lett.* **1977**, 4021–24.
493. Fu, P.P.; Harvey, R.G. *J. Chem. Soc. Chem. Commun.* **1978**, 585–86.
494. Lee, H.M.; Harvey, R.G. *J. Org. Chem.* **1980**, *45*, 588–92.
495. Gibson, D.T.; Mahadevan, V.; Jerina, D.M.; Yagi, H.; Yeh, H.J.C. *Science (Washington, D.C.)* **1975**, *189*, 295–97.
496. Lehr, R.E.; Taylor, C.W.; Kumar, S.; Mah, H.D.; Jerina, D.M. *J. Org. Chem.* **1978**, *43*, 3462–66.
497. Harvey, R.G.; Lee, H.M.; Shyamasundar, N. *J. Org. Chem.* **1979**, *44*, 78–83.
498. Lehr, R.E.; Kumar, S.; Cohenour, P.T.; Jerina, D.M. *Tetrahedron Lett.* **1979**, 3819–22.
499. Croisy-Delcey, M.; Ittah, Y.; Jerina, D.M. *Tetrahedron Lett.* **1979**, 2849–52.
500. Lee, H.M.; Harvey, R.G. *J. Org. Chem.* **1979**, *44*, 4948–53.
501. Harvey, R.G.; Fu, P.P.; Cortez, C.; Pataki, J. *Tetrahedron Lett.* **1977**, 3533–36.
502. Harvey, R.G.; Fu, P.P. *J. Org. Chem.* **1980**, *45*, 169–71.
503. Kitahara, Y.; Shudo, K.; Okamoto, T. *Chem. Pharm. Bull.* **1980**, *28*, 1958–61.
504. Fu, P.P.; Lai, C.C.; Yang, S.K. *J. Org. Chem.* **1981**, *46*, 220–22.

505. Amin, S.; Bedenko, V.; LaVoie, E.; Hecht, S.S.; Hoffmann, D. *J. Org. Chem.* **1981**, *46*, 2573–78.
506. Booth, J.; Boyland, E.; Turner, E.E. *J. Chem. Soc.* **1950**, 1188–90.
507. Jerina, D.M.; Selander, H.; Yagi, H.; Wells, M.C.; Davey, J.F.; Mahedevan, V.; Gibson, D.T. *J. Am. Chem. Soc.* **1976**, *98*, 5988–96.
508. Sukumaran, K.B.; Harvey, R.G. *J. Org. Chem.* **1980**, *45*, 4407–13.
509. Kundu, N.G. *J. Chem. Soc., Perkin/1 Trans.* **1980**, 1920–23.
510. Sukumaran, K.B.; Harvey, R.G. *J. Am. Chem. Soc.* **1979**, *101*, 1353–54.
511. Tierney, AB.; Abercrombie, B.; Walsh, C.; Hewer, A.; Grover, P.L.; Sims, P. *Chem.-Biol. Interact.* **1978**, *21*, 289–98.
512. Tierney, B.; Hewer, A.; MacNicoll, A.D.; Gervasi, P.G.; Rattle, H.; Walsh, C.; Grover, P.L.; Sims, P. *Chem.-Biol. Interact.* **1978**, *23*, 243–57.
513. Tierney, B.; Hewer, A.; Rattle, H.; Grover, P.L.; Sims, P. *Chem.-Biol. Interact.* **1978**, *23*, 121–35.
514. MacNicoll, A.D.; Burden, P.M.; Ribeiro, O.; Hewer, A.; Grover, P.L.; Sims, P. *Chem.-Biol. Interact.* **1979**, *26*, 121–32.
515. MacNicoll, A.D.; Burden, P.M.; Rattle, H.; Grover, P.L.; Sims, P. *Chem.-Biol. Interact.* **1979**, *27*, 365–79.
516. Yagi, H.; Thakker, D.R.; Lehr, R.E.; Jerina, D.M. *J. Org. Chem.* **1979**, *44*, 3439–42.
517. Zacharias, D.E.; Glusker, J.P.; Fu, P.P.; Harvey, R.G. *J. Am. Chem. Soc.* **1979**, *101*, 4043–51.
518. Chamberlain, P.; Roberts, M.L.; Whitham, G.H. *J. Chem. Soc. B.* **1970**, 1374–81.
519. Yagi, H.; Thakker, D.R.; Hernandez, O.; Koreeda, M.; Jerina, D.M. *J. Am. Chem. Soc.* **1977**, *99*, 1604–11.
520. Whalen, D.L.; Ross, A.M.; Yagi, H.; Karle, J.M.; Jerina, D.M. *J. Am. Chem. Soc.* **1978**, *100*, 5218–221.
521. Lehr, R.E.; Schaefer-Ridder, M.; Jerina, D.M. *Tetrahedron Lett.* **1977**, 539–42.
522. Fu, P.P.; Harvey, R.G. *J. Org. Chem.* **1979**, *44*, 3778–84.
523. Lee, H.; Harvey, R.G. *Tetrahedron Lett.* **1981**, *22*, 1657–60.
524. Becker, A.R.; Janusz, J.M.; Bruice, T.C. *J. Am. Chem. Soc.* **1979**, *101*, 5679–87.
525. Bruice, P.Y.; Bruice, T.C.; Selander, H.G.; Yagi, H.; Jerina, D.M. *J. Am. Chem. Soc.* **1974**, *96*, 6814–15.
526. Bruice, P.Y.; Bruice, T.C.; Yagi, H.; Jerina, D.M. *J. Am. Chem. Soc.* **1976**, *98*, 2973–81.
527. Keller, J.W.; Heidelberger, C. *J. Am. Chem. Soc.* **1976**, *98*, 2328–36.
528. Bruice, P.Y.; Bruice, T.C.; Dansette, P.M.; Selander, H.G.; Yagi, H.; Jerina, D.M. *J. Am. Chem. Soc.* **1976**, *98*, 2965–73.
529. Bruice, T.C.; Bruice, P.Y. *Acc. Chem. Res.* **1976**, *9*, 378–84.
530. Whalen, D.L.; Ross, A.M.; Dansette, P.M.; Jerina, D.M. *J. Am. Chem. Soc.* **1977**, *99*, 5672–76.
531. Keller, J.W.; Heidelberger, C.; Beland, F.A.; Harvey, R.G. *J. Am. Chem. Soc.* **1976**, *98*, 8276–77.
532. Yang, S.K.; McCourt, D.W.; Gelboin, H.V.; Miller, J.R.; Roller, P.P. *J. Am. Chem. Soc.* **1977**, *99*, 5124–30.
533. Whalen, D.L.; Montemarano, J.A.; Thakker, D.R.; Yagi, H.; Jerina, D.M. *J. Am. Chem. Soc.* **1977**, *99*, 5522–24.
534. Yang, S.K.; McCourt, D.W.; Gelboin, H.V. *J. Am. Chem. Soc.* **1977**, *99*, 5130–34.
535. Whalen, D.L.; Ross, A.M.; Montemarano, J.A.; Thakker, D.R.; Yagi, H.; Jerina, D.M. *J. Am. Chem. Soc.* **1979**, *101*, 5086–88.
536. Janusz, J.M.; Becker, A.R.; Bruice, T.C. *J. Am. Chem. Soc.* **1978**, *100*, 8269–71.
537. Hulbert, P.B. *Nature (London)* **1975**, *256*, 146–48.
538. Rogers, D.Z.; Bruice, T.C. *J. Am. Chem. Soc.* **1979**, *101*, 4713–19.

539. Becker, A.R.; Janusz, J.M.; Rogers, D.Z.; Bruice, T.C. *J. Am. Chem. Soc.* **1978**, *100*, 3244–46.
540. Royer, R.E.; Lyle, T.A.; Moy, G.G.; Daub, G.H.; Vander Jagt, D.L.V. *J. Org. Chem.* **1979**, *44*, 3202–7.
541. Shapiro, R.; Shiuey, S.J. *J. Org. Chem.* **1976**, *41*, 1597–600.
542. Carrell, H.L.; Glusker, J.P.; Moschel, R.C.; Hudgins, W.R.; Dipple, A. *Cancer Res.* **1981**, *41*, 2230–34.
543. Blobstein, S.H.; Weinstein, I.B.; Grunberger, D.; Weisgras, J.; Harvey, R.G. *Biochemistry* **1975**, *14*, 3451–58.
544. Jeffrey, A.M.; Blobstein, S.H.; Weinstein, I.B.; Beland, F.A.; Harvey, R.G.; Kasai, H.; Nakanishi, K. *Proc. Natl. Acad. Sci., U.S.A.* **1976**, *73*, 2311–15.
545. Jeffrey, A.M.; Jennette, K.W.; Blobstein, S.H.; Weinstein, I.B.; Beland, F.A.; Harvey, R.G.; Kasai, H.; Miura, I.; Nakanishi, K. *J. Am. Chem. Soc.* **1976**, *98*, 5714–15.
546. Koreeda, M.; Moore, P.D.; Yagi, H.; Yeh, H.J.C.; Jerina, D.M. *J. Am. Chem. Soc.* **1976**, *98*, 6720–22.
547. Osborne, M.R.; Beland, F.A.; Harvey, R.G.; Brookes, P. *Int. J. Cancer* **1976**, *18*, 362–68.
548. Moore, P.D.; Koreeda, M.; Wislocki, P.G.; Levin, W.; Conney, A.H.; Yagi, H.; Jerina, D.M. In "Drug Metabolism Concepts"; Jerina, D.M., Ed.; ACS Symposium Series No. 44; ACS: Washington, D.C., 1977; pp. 127–54.
549. Jennette, K.W.; Jeffrey, A.M.; Blobstein, S.H.; Beland, F.A.; Harvey, R.G.; Weinstein, I.B. *Biochemistry* **1977**, *16*, 932–38.
550. Meehan, T.; Straub, K.; Calvin, M. *Nature (London)*, **1977**, *269*, 725–27.
551. Meehan, T.; Straub, K. *Nature (London)* **1979**, *277*, 410–12.
552. Jeffrey, A.M.; Grzeskowiak, K.; Weinstein, I.B.; Nakanishi, K.; Roller, P.; Harvey, R.G. *Science* **1979**, *206*, 1309–11.
553. Ashurst, S.W.; Cohen, G.M. *Int. J. Cancer* **1981**, *27*, 357–64.
554. Shinohara, K.; Cerutti, P.A. *Proc. Natl. Acad. Sci., U.S.A* **1977**, *74*, 979–83.
555. Osborne, M.R.; Harvey, R.G.; Brookes, P. *Chem.-Biol. Interact.* **1978**, *20*, 123–30.
556. Osborne, M.R.; Jacobs, S.; Harvey, R.G.; Brookes, P. *Carcinogenesis* **1981**, *2*, 553–58.
557. Moschel, R.C.; Hudgins, W.R.; Dipple, A. *J. Org. Chem.* **1979**, *44*, 3324–28.
558. Moschel, R.C.; Hudgins, W.R.; Dipple, A. *J. Org. Chem.* **1980**, *45*, 533–35.
559. Moschel, R.C.; Hudgins, W.R.; Dipple, A. *Tetrahedron Lett.* **1981**, *22*, 2427–30.
560. Moschel, R.C., Hudgins, W.R., Dipple, A. *J. Am. Chem. Soc.* **1981**, *103*, 5489–94.

3

Soots, Tars, and Oils as Causes of Occupational Cancer

M. D. KIPLING[1]

Employment Medical Advisory Service, Department of Employment, Birmingham, England

M. A. COOKE

University of Aston in Birmingham, Department of Occupational Health and Safety, Birmingham, B4 7ET England
Firmenich and Co., Southall, Middlesex UB2 5NN England

Early History

THE INCREASED INCIDENCE OF SKIN CANCER in workers exposed to soot, tar, and oil and the induction of similar cancers in animals have resulted in worldwide research to isolate the active carcinogenic constituents. Population studies have been particularly fruitful in Britain where notification of occupational skin cancers to the Factory Inspectorate has been obligatory for over 50 years.

Cancer of the skin occurring in chimney sweeps caused by soot was first described in 1775 by Pott (*1*). Since then tar (*2*), pitch (*3*), and mineral oil (*4*) have been shown to be carcinogenic to the skin. Evidence also suggests that internal organs may be affected by these materials (*5–7*).

Domestic soots are products of imperfect combustion of carbonaceous materials such as wood, coal, and oil. They consist of finely divided carbon particles bound to hydrocarbons and tars. The presence of carcinogens in soots was first shown experimentally in mice (*8*). Later benzo[*a*]pyrene (formerly 3,4-benzpyrene) was identified as a carcinogenic constituent (*9*). Wood soot in a smoked-sausage factory was also shown to be carcinogenic (*10*). Industrial soots (carbon blacks in industry) are produced by the incomplete combustion of natural gas or oil residues and were also shown to contain benzo[*a*]pyrene (*11*).

[1] Deceased.

0065-7719/84/0182-0165$06.00/1

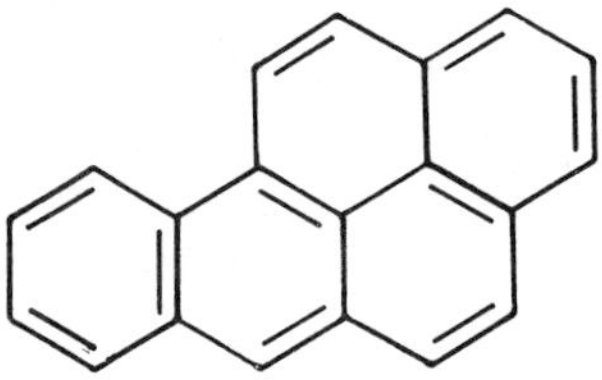

I

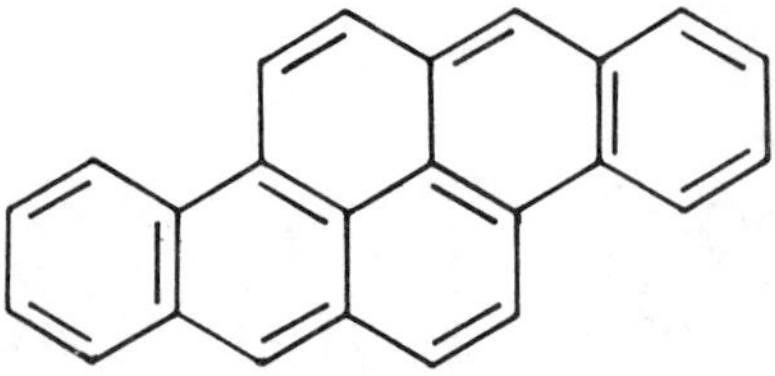

II

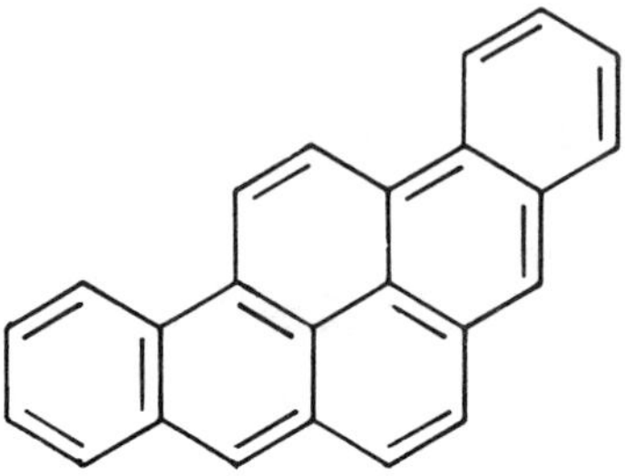

III

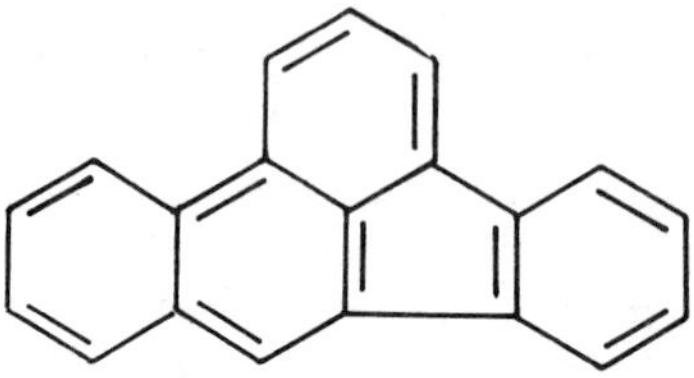

IV

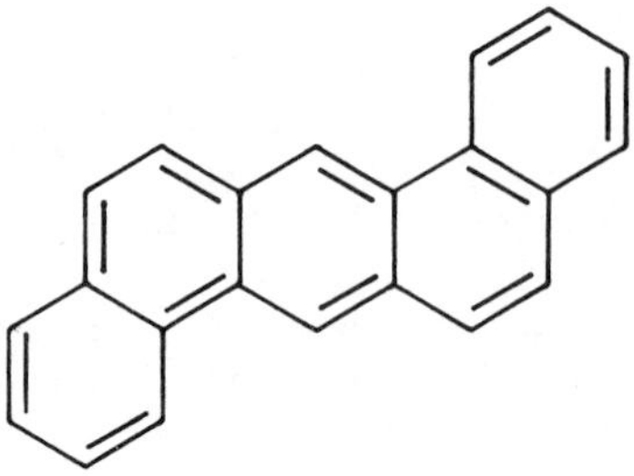

V

Coal tar and pitch are the residual products of coal distillation. Contact with these residues has also led to an increased incidence of skin cancer (*12*) and, in gas workers, lung cancer (*13, 14*).

Tar was first shown to be a carcinogen experimentally in 1915 by Yamagiwa and Ichikawa (*15*) who repeatedly painted the tar on rabbits' ears. Later, similar results were produced in mice (*16, 17*). Coal tar pitch (*18*), anthracene oil (*19*), and creosote derivatives of coal tar (*20*) were also shown to be carcinogenic, and skin cancers were produced from blast-furnace tar (*21*). Carcinogenic tars were manufactured synthetically from various sources such as isoprene, acetylene, skin, yeasts, and cholesterol. The carcinogenicity of tars increased coincidentally with the temperature involved in their distillation (*19*), and the carcinogenic potency of tars prepared at temperatures of 500, 600, and 750 °C materially increased with temperature (*22*).

A review in 1978 surveyed the literature on asphalt and coal-tar pitch, including their toxicity and carcinogenicity, and presented conclusions and recommendations (*23*).

In 1932, the observation that carcinogenic tars fluoresced with a spectrum similar to that of benz[*a*]anthracene led to the identification of benzo[*a*]pyrene (**I**) as a carcinogenic agent (*24*). Later, dibenzo[*a,h*]pyrene (**II**), dibenzo[*a,i*]pyrene (**III**), benzo[*b*]fluoranthene (**IV**), and dibenz[*a,h*]anthracene (**V**) also were shown to be carcinogenic constituents (*25*).

Shale Oil

Shale oil is derived from shale formed at the bottom of shallow lakes out of inorganic material and the debris of plants and aquatic organisms. The final composition of shale oil varies in different parts of the world. The oil crisis has renewed interest in oil-bearing shales, which are now likely to be increasingly worked on a large scale in the future.

The first case of carcinoma attributed to shale oil was described in 1876 (*4*). The oil's carcinogenicity was shown experimentally (*26*), and the presence of benzo[*a*]pyrene and other polycyclic hydrocarbons was demonstrated later (*27*). These substances could not be identified in the parent rock shale suggesting that the heat used in production was important in the formation of carcinogens. Shale oil distilled below 250 °C contained carcinogenic compounds other than benzo[*a*]-pyrene (*28*).

Petroleum Oils

Petroleum oils are formed by the decomposition of animal and vegetable matter affected by heat and pressure in the earth's crust. Petroleum oils vary in final composition in different parts of the world and consist of hydrocarbons (paraffinic and naphthenic) with compounds of sulfur, oxygen, and nitrogen. Sulfur is in the highest concentration (up to 6%) and nitrogen the lowest (about 0.1%). Benzo[*a*]-pyrene was isolated in a specimen of cracked oil (*29*) and its presence was demonstrated in crude oil (*30*).

In 1968, the Medical Research Council in the United Kingdom published its report, "The Carcinogenic Action of Mineral Oils," based on work done in several British universities (*31*). Crude oils from fields in Kuwait, Oklahoma, and Lagunillas were steam-distilled under reduced pressure to isolate specific carcinogens while minimizing decomposition. The most biologically active fractions (boiling range of 300–400 °C) were distilled further. Aliquots of the fractions (350–390 °C) obtained on a Stedman distilling apparatus were treated with maleic anhydride and picric acid, and were chromatographed on alumina (*32*). Other fractions (390–410 °C) were extracted in a small vacuum column. The carcinogenic activity appeared to lie in materials boiling above 350 °C (presence in lower-boiling fractions was possibly the result of azeotropism), and activity was still present in fractions boiling at 420 °C. The active compounds were extracted with acetone–water and appeared with the polycyclic aromatic fraction during absorption chromatography. Over 40 chemical compounds were isolated from mineral-oil fractions, many for the first time, by repeated chromatography, complexing with picric acid and trinitrobenzene, and fractional crystallization. Further studies of the nature of the active compounds did not identify any single highly potent carcinogen. Several of the compounds separated were structurally similar to very potent carcinogens, and the total activity of the oil could be caused by the combined effect of several individually weak carcinogens.

Compounds isolated included a wide range of aromatic hydrocarbons, such as dimethylnaphthalenes, trimethylnaphthalenes, tetramethylnaphthalenes, and phenanthrenes, chrysene and its methyl derivatives, perylene, triphenylene, and tetramethylfluorene. Heterocyclic compounds included dimethyldibenzothiophene, tetramethyldibenzothiophene, thiabenzofluorene, tetramethylcarbazole, and pentamethylcarbazole. Representative compounds that have been isolated from mineral-oil fractions are 2,3,6-trimethylnaphthalene (**VI**), 1,3,5,7-tetramethylanthracene (**VII**), 1,2,8-trimethylphenanthrene (**VIII**), 4-methylpyrene (**IX**), 4-methylbenzo[*a*]fluorene (**X**), 1,7-dimethylchrysene (**XI**), 1,2,7,8-tetramethyldibenzothiophene (**XII**), and 1,3,6,8-tetramethylcarbazole (**XIII**).

Three-ring hydrocarbons are generally not carcinogenic and the dimethylanthracenes isolated were all inactive except for 9,10-dimethylanthracene. Benz[*a*]-anthracene, although only weakly active, is the parent compound of several known carcinogens. For example, 10-methylbenz[*a*]anthracene, also isolated and positively identified, is weakly active on rabbit skin, but apparently not on mouse skin. Another member of this family, the weak carcinogen 9,10-dimethylbenz[*a*]anthracene, was possibly isolated but not positively identified. The isomeric 7,12-dimethylbenz[*a*]anthracene (formerly 9,10-dimethylbenz-1,2-anthracene) was never identified in the oil fractions but was used in this work as a standard strong carcinogen. The activity of chrysene, which was also identified, is variously reported in the literature; it may be slightly active. Several dimethyl derivatives of chrysene were identified in the oil, but these did not include the derivatives known to be active. Of the heterocyclic compounds separated from the oil, only 1,3,6,7-tetramethyldibenzothiophene is weakly active.

Certain straight-chain aliphatic compounds such as dodecane have been shown to enhance the carcinogenic activity of polycyclic aromatic compounds for mouse skin (*33*). Some sulfur compounds (*34*) and phenols (*35*) may act similarly.

Because it appeared that solvent or other comparable refining processes reduced the amounts of polycyclic aromatic hydrocarbons in oil, a 1971 review concluded that such refining processes would reduce or eliminate the risk of skin cancer (*30*). The reliability of tests for the total polycyclic aromatic content of oil or of those compounds that might cause skin cancer was therefore investigated. The results of new laborious techniques that isolate benzo[*a*]pyrene from crude oil were compared with the simpler measurement of UV absorbance (derived from FDA 121, 2589(c) of the United States Code of Federal Regulations, Title 21), measurement of total aromatic carbon by IR spectroscopy (*36*) or mass spectrometry (*37*). The measurement of UV absorbance was the most satisfactory and the IR determination of aromatic carbon content the least, but no method was accurate enough to be of value.

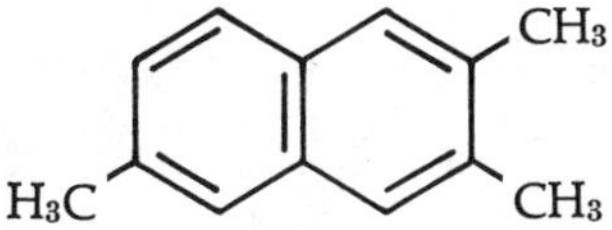

VI 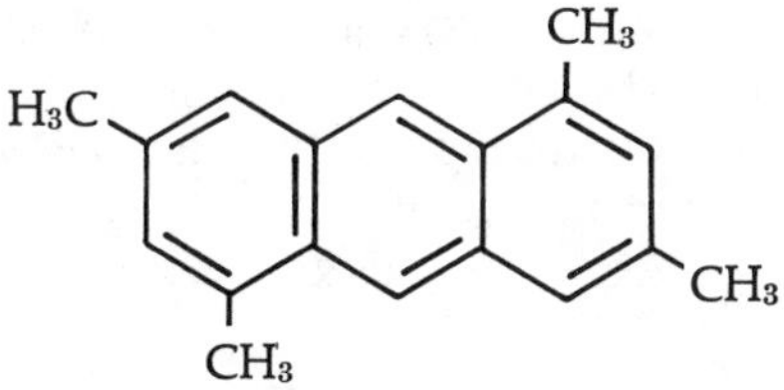 VII

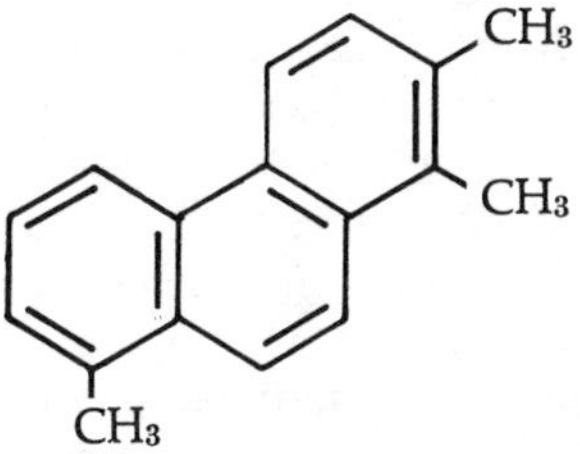

VIII 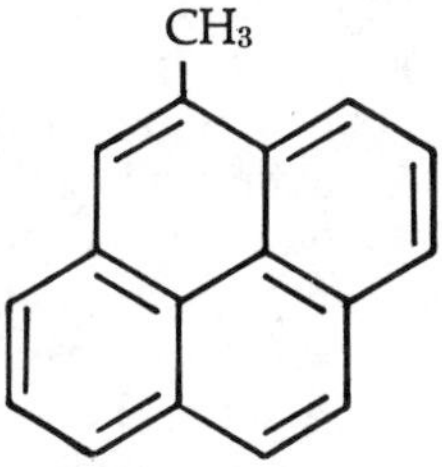 IX

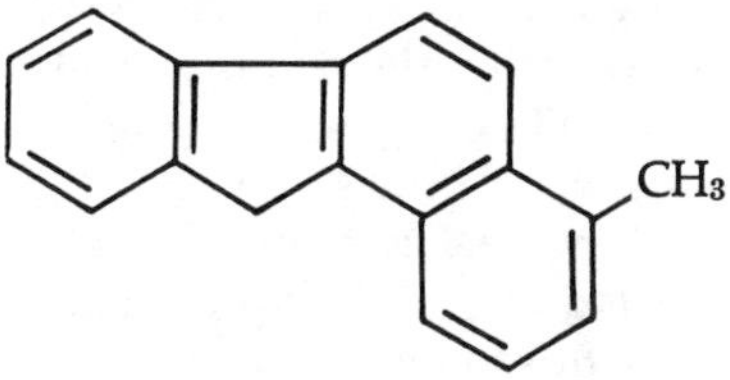

X 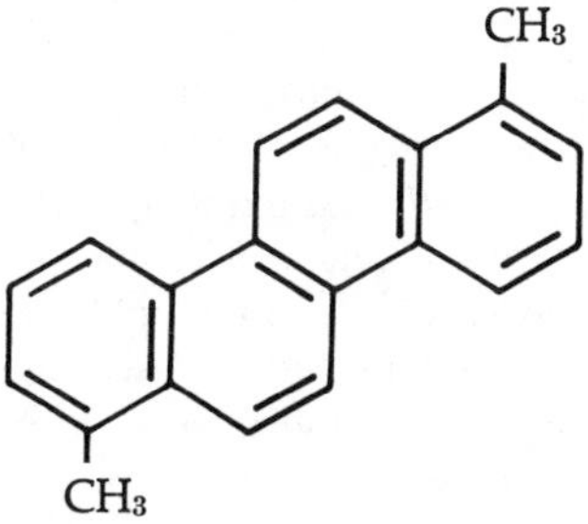 XI

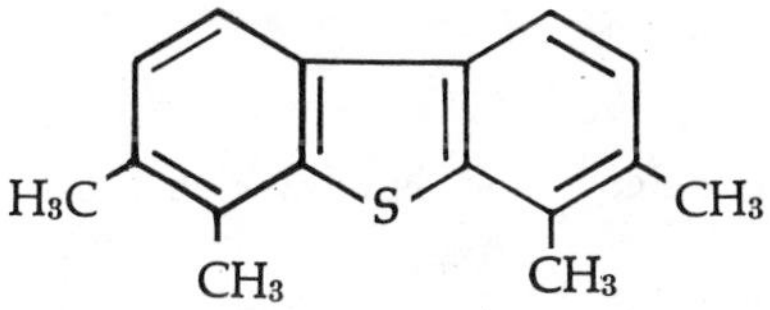

XII 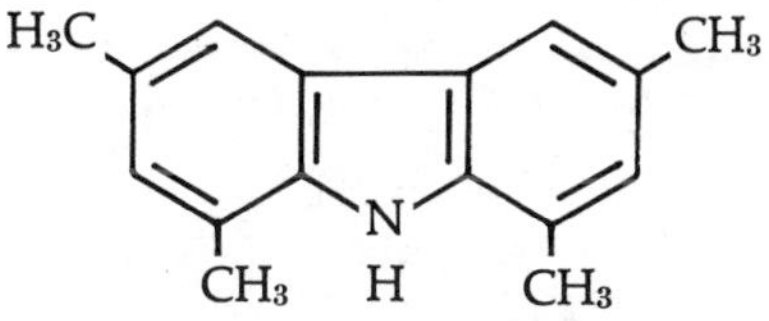 XIII

Soots

Today, exposure to domestic chimney soot is not significant, and chimney sweeps' cancer is rare. However, exposure to carbon black occurs among its manufacturers and users, notably rubber and paint makers. No increased incidence of cancer has been attributed to exposure to carbon black in this occupation, probably because polycyclic hydrocarbons are adsorbed onto the carbon black particles (*11*). It is not established that the polycyclics in rubber from carbon black and oil used as an extender are released by the action of heat and solvents in molding to produce a carcinogenic risk. An increased incidence of keratosis and leukoplakia of the oral mucous membrane has, however, been observed in workers exposed to soot (*38*).

Pitch and Tar

Exposure to pitch and tar occurs in the coal, gas, and coke industries; in steel-making plants; and in the manufacture of patent fuels. The development of pitch and tar warts is not uncommon in these industries. Sporadic cases of skin cancer occur among workers engaged in embedding optical lenses; jointing drain pipes; creosoting railroad sleepers; and manufacturing accumulator cases, carbon electrodes, brushes, pitch fiber pipes, and roofing material. Pipe benders and dippers and manufacturers of felt, crucibles, and clay pigeons from clay and pitch have also been affected. Attention has been drawn to the occurrence of growths on the lips of fishermen who hold the twine for net making in their teeth (*39*). Gas workers exposed to products of coal carbonization showed increased incidence of lung (and probably also bladder) cancer. Mortalities caused by lung cancer were 3.06 per 1000 for retort workers compared with 1.81 per 1000 in the comparable age and sex groups of the general population, and for bladder cancer, 0.31 per 1000 as compared with 0.14 per 1000. Work as topman on the retorts was a particular hazard (*40*). Among steelworkers in the United States, the mortality from respiratory cancer increased twofold in coke-oven workers (*13*).

An increase of UV light sensitization with increasing length of exposure to tar has been reported. This enhancement may indicate that carcinomatously transformed or pretransformed epidermal cells acquire an increased light sensitivity at the same time, and with continuing exposure to light, even without tar, the risk of developing skin epitheliomas rises (*41*). A personal susceptibility to pitch has also been suggested (*42*). The finding that topical application of coal tar solution induces aryl hydrocarbon hydroxylase in human skin could relate to the carcinogenic response of skin to this agent (*43*).

Lubricating and Cutting Oils

The first description of cancer of the scrotum in a Scottish shale-oil worker was in 1876 (*4*). Later, a user of shale oil in cotton mule spinning died from the disease (*44*). During 22 years, 19 cases of skin cancer, of which three were scrotal, occurred in paraffin process workers, and 46 cases, of which 28 were scrotal, occurred among the other workers such as retortmen and stillmen (*44*).

The cotton mule-spinning industry in Great Britain originally used shale oil to lubricate the spindles. Mules were machines on which a carriage moved back and forth requiring the operator to lean over so that his groin was contaminated by the spray from the spindles and from direct contact with oil on the carriage. From 1920 to 1943, there were 1303 recorded cases of skin cancer in the British textile industry, of which 824 were scrotal. There were 615 fatal cases of scrotal cancer recorded between 1911 and 1938 (*45*); 59% of mineral oil-induced cancer was found to be located on the scrotum (*46*).

Cancer from oil in the metal-working industry, particularly among workers in automatic machine shops, was first found to be an appreciable risk in a survey carried out in Birmingham, England (*47, 48*). Between 1950 and 1967, 187 cases of scrotal cancer occurred in this region, the majority of which could be attributed to oil (*49*). In 1966, for example, 16 of 19 recorded cases of scrotal cancer in Birmingham were caused by oil (*50*).

Toolsetters or setter operators in an automatic shop using neat (i.e., not emulsified) cutting oil run the greatest risk of skin cancer because their work constantly requires them to lean over the machine with subsequent oil contamination of the groin. In Birmingham, England, bar automatic machine workers showed a high incidence of cancer from oil. Other metal-working occupational sources of scrotal cancer include metal rolling, tube drawing, metal hardening, and general machine operating. Although the major risk is from exposure to neat oils, occasionally soluble emulsions have been incriminated. The industries with automatic shops and the nut and bolt manufacturers are affected most. Also, cases have arisen from exposure by changing transformer oil in electrical substations, painting or spraying of mold oil for brick and tile making or concrete molding, drop forging, rubber mixing, wire drawing, rope making in the jute industry, and from grease in metal working (*51*). No cases were found from handling oil in garages or from diesel oil (*52*).

In females, an increased incidence of cancer of the vulva was found in cotton operators in the United Kingdom and in silver polishers using cloths impregnated with mineral oil (*53*).

In the United States, studies of scrotal cancer victims showed that 9 out of 14 (*54*), 13 out of 27 (*55*), and 22 out of 28 (12 cotton workers and 10 machinists) (*56*) had been exposed to oil. Other cases occurred in a works pressing process (*57*). Out of five scrotal cancer cases reported in Australia, three were exposed to oil (two turners and one railway employee oiling axles), one was a gasworks stoker, and one had no occupational exposure (*58*). In Sweden, eight cases of scrotal cancer occurred among 250 automatic lathe operators in one Swedish engineering industry within 24 years (*59*).

In the valley of the river Arve in the Savoy Alps of France, at least 60 cases of scrotal cancer and many cases of skin cancer among the bar automatic machine workers (*décolleteurs*) were reported in 1970 as having occurred since 1955. The high incidence in the relatively small population of the valley occurred mainly among the self-employed workers or workers in small premises (*60*). Contact with neat cutting oils probably caused the epidemic, but other undetected factors might be involved because similar contact in many other centers did not cause a comparably high incidence (*61*).

An excess incidence of cancers other than skin (e.g., larynx, lung, and stomach) was attributed to oil mist in mule spinning (*46*). Recent evidence indicates that victims of scrotal cancer in engineering show a significant increase in cancers of the respiratory tract or upper digestive tract (*62*).

Exposure to mineral oil mists causes linear striations in the lungs in chest radiographs (*63*). The extent of more serious lesions is difficult to evaluate, but other bronchopulmonary diseases, including lipid pneumonia and carcinoma, are possibilities. The precise nature of the mist and the working conditions may materially affect the incidence of such disease. Although no respiratory cancer hazard was found for a group of workers in metal machining processes, there was an increase of cancers of the stomach and large intestine compared with the general U.S. population (*64*). If oil mist is carcinogenic, it seems to affect a susceptible subsection of the exposed population but the basis is unclear (*65*).

Preventive measures have reduced the incidence and severity of skin cancers in industry (*66*). In Britain, the Mule Spinning Regulations of 1952 ensured that after 1953 only oil drastically refined with sulfuric acid was used in cotton spinning and that mule spinners were examined medically every 6 months. These measures and the marked decline of mule spinning resulted in a sustained decline in the incidence of scrotal cancer in Britain (*67*). Voluntary medical examinations were provided in the shale oil and gas industries and, along with shower baths, are required by law in patent-fuel plants.

In the metal-working industry, routine medical examinations were arranged in a few plants where experience indicated a special risk. Warning leaflets (SHW 259A) with colored illustrations of the early stages of lesions caused by oil on the hands and scrotum are distributed to all people exposed to oil. This information has enhanced early detection and treatment in many cases of scrotal cancer. The use of solvent-refined oils is also strongly recommended. The award of damages in 1968 to the widow of a man who had scrotal cancer led to widespread publicity that has aided in educating workers and management. A high standard of cleanliness and the use of guards on the machinery are advised, but a survey of the hygienic conditions in machine shops showed the condition is not necessarily connected with poor hygiene among the workers (*51, 68*).

A 1970 comprehensive review of the carcinogenic potential of petroleum hydrocarbons documented the various approaches that can be used to reduce the hazard to workers (*69*). The incidence of skin disorders with exposure to cutting fluids has been reviewed (*70*).

The great disparity of the number of reported cancer cases caused by pitch, tar, and oil in the United Kingdom and other countries is not easily explained. Only in the French Alps has the incidence of scrotal cancer been comparable with that in England (*60*). The high incidence of skin cancer in British workers has been attributed to lack of hygiene, but a factor of real importance may be that legal notification since 1923, compensation by the State since 1910, and registration of tumors at the Regional Cancer Registries since 1936 have provided a greater knowledge of its occurrence than elsewhere. This theory is supported by the apparent great excess of bladder tumors in rubber workers and cancers from asbestos exposure in Great Britain as compared with other countries—an excess that cannot be attributed readily to other causes.

Prognosis and Prevention

The treatment of choice for scrotal cancer is wide and deep excision with removal of glands where there is incidence of metastasis (if necessary repeating 3–4 weeks after the initial operation) but leaving normal glands (*58*). The prognosis in tar- and oil-induced skin cancer is more serious for scrotal cancers than for those on other areas such as the hand, arm, and face, where the results of treatment are good. The serious prognosis for scrotal cancer, and the major nature of the operative therapy required, emphasize the importance of adequate hygiene control measures in the usage of the various recognized causative agents.

Literature Cited

1. Pott, P. "Chirurgical Works"; London, 1775; Vol. 5, p. 63.
2. Volkmann, R. *Beitr. Chirurg.* Leipzig **1875**, 370.
3. Manouviriez, A. *Ann. Hyg. Publique* **1876**, *45*, 459.
4. Bell, J. *Edinburgh Med. J.* **1876**, *22*, 135.
5. Butlin, H. T. *Br. Med. J.* **1892**, *1*, 1341.
6. Southam, A. *Rep. Int. Conf. Cancer* **1928**, 280.
7. Kennaway, E. L.; Kennaway, N. M. *Br. J. Cancer* **1947**, *1*, 260.
8. Passey, R. D. *Br. Med. J.* **1922**, *2*, 112.
9. Goulden, F.; Tipler, M. M. *Br. J. Cancer* **1949**, *3*, 157.
10. Sulman, E.; Sulman, F. *Cancer Res.* **1946**, *6*, 366.
11. Falk, H. L.; Steiner, P. E. *Cancer Res.* **1952**, *12*, 30.
12. Heller, J. *J. Ind. Hyg.* **1930**, *12*, 169.
13. Lloyd, J. W. *J. Occup. Med.* **1971**, *13*, 53.
14. Doll, R. *Br. J. Ind. Med.* **1952**, *9*, 180.
15. Yamagiwa, K.; Ichikawa, K. *J. Jpn. Path. Ges.* **1915**, *5*, 142.
16. Tsutsui, H. *Gann* **1918**, *12*, 17.
17. Murray, J. A. *Br. Med. J.* **1921**, *2*, 795.
18. Passey, R. D.; Woodhouse, J. L. *J. Pathol. Bacteriol.* **1925**, *28*, 145.
19. Kennaway, E. L. *Br. Med. J.* **1925**, *2*, 1.
20. Lenson, N. *N. Engl. J. Med.* **1956**, *254*, 520.
21. Bonser, G. M. *Lancet* **1932**, *1*, 775.
22. Twort, C. C.; Fulton, J. D. *J. Pathol. Bacteriol.* **1930**, *33*, 119.
23. Trosset, R. P.; Warshawsky, D.; Menefee, C. L.; Bingham, E. In "Investigation of Selected Potential Environmental Contaminants—Asphalt and Coal Tar Pitch"; U.S. Environmental Protection Agency, Contract No. 68-01-4188, 1978.
24. Cook, J. W.; Hewett, C.; Hieger, I. *Nature (London)* **1932**, *130*, 926.
25. Badger, G. M. In "The Chemical Basis of Carcinogenic Activity"; Thomas: Springfield, IL, 1962; p. 9.
26. Leitch, A. *Br. Med. J.* **1922**, *2*, 1104.
27. Berenblum, I.; Schoental, R. *Br. J. Exp. Pathol.* **1943**, *24*, 232.
28. Bogovski, P. *Vopr. Onkol.* **1959**, *5*, 486.
29. Tye, R.; Graf, M. J.; Horton, A. W. *Anal. Chem.* **1955**, *27*, 248.
30. Catchpole, W. M.; MacMillan, E.; Powell, H. *Ann. Occup. Hyg.* **1971**, *14*, 171.
31. Medical Research Council (Gr. Br.) *Spec. Rep. Ser.* **1968**, *306*.
32. King, P. J. *Ind. Lubric. Tribol.* **Aug. 1969**, 231.
33. Horton, A. W.; Denman, D. T.; Trosset, R. P. *Cancer Res.* **1957**, *17*, 758.
34. Horton, A. W.; Bingham, E. L.; Burton, M. J. G.; Tye, R. *Cancer Res.* **1965**, *25*, 1759.
35. Boutwell, R. K.; Bosch, D. K. *Cancer Res.* **1959**, *19*, 413.
36. Brandes, G. *Brennst–Chem.* **1956**, *37*, 263.
37. Gallegus, E. T. *Anal. Chem.* **1967**, *39*, 1833.
38. Smoliar, M.; Granin, A. V. *Stomatologiya (Moscow)* **1971**, *50*, 16.
39. Haddow, A. J. *Annu. Rep., Regional Cancer Committee*, Univ. of Glasgow, 8th, **1968**, *33*.
40. Doll, R.; Fisher, R. E. W.; Gammon, E. J.; Gunn, W.; Hughes, G. O.; Tyrer, F. H.; Wilson, W. *Br. J. Ind. Med.* **1965**, *22*, 1.
41. Gotz, H. *Aust. J. Dermatol.* **1976**, *17*, 57.
42. Hodgson, G. A.; Whiteley, H. J. *Br. J. Ind. Med.* **1970**, *27*, 160.
43. Bickers, D. R.; Kappas, A. *J. Clin. Invest.* **1978**, *62*, 1061.

44. Henry, S. A. In "Cancer of the Scrotum in Relation of Occupation"; Oxford Univ.: Oxford, England, 1946; p. 16.
45. Ibid., p. 43.
46. Henry, S. A. *Br. Med. Bull.* **1947**, *4*, 392.
47. Cruickshank, C. N. D.; Squire, J. R. *Br. J. Ind. Med.* **1950**, *7*, 1.
48. Cruickshank, C. N. D.; Gourevitch, A. *Br. J. Ind. Med.* **1952**, *9*, 74.
49. Waterhouse, J. A. H. *Ann. Occup. Hyg.* **1971**, *14*, 161.
50. Kipling, M. D. *Trans. Soc. Occup. Med.* **1969**, *19*, 39.
51. Kipling, M. D. *Ann. R. Coll. Surg. Engl.* **1974**, *55*, 74.
52. Kipling, M. D. *Ann. Rep., Her Majesty's Chief Inspector Factories* **1967**, **1968**, 113.
53. Cooke, M. A.; Kipling, M. D. *Arch. Mal. Prof. Med. Trav. Secur. Soc.* **1973**, *34*, 244.
54. Graves, R.; Flo, S. *J. Urol.* **1940**, *43*, 309.
55. Dean, A. L. *J. Urol.* **1948**, *61*, 511.
56. Kickham, C. J.; Dufresne, M. *J. Urol.* **1967**, *98*, 108.
57. Hendricks, N. V. *Arch. Ind. Hyg. Occup. Med.* **1959**, *19*, 524.
58. Milne, J. E. *Med. J. Aust.* **1970**, *2*, 13.
59. Avellan, L.; Breine, U.; Jacobsson, B.; Johanson, B. *Scand. J. Plast. Reconstr. Surg.* **1967**, *1*, 135.
60. Thony, C.; Thony, J. "Le Cancer du Décolleteur"; Centre de Médecine du Travail de Cluses, 1970.
61. Kipling, M. D. *Trans. Soc. Occup. Med.* **1971**, *21*, 73.
62. Holmes, J. G.; Kipling, M. D.; Waterhouse, J. A. H. *Lancet* **1970**, *11*, 214.
63. Jones, J. G. *Ann. Occup. Hyg.* **1961**, *3*, 264.
64. Decoufle, P. *JNCI, J. Natl. Cancer Inst.* **1978**, *61*, 1025.
65. Waldron, H. A. *Br. J. Cancer* **1975**, *32*, 256.
66. Kipling, M. D. *Ann. R. Coll. Surg. Engl.* **1974**, *55*, 79.
67. Waterhouse, J. A. H. *Ann. Occup. Hyg.* **1971**, *14*, 164.
68. Parkes, H. G. *Ind. Med. Surg.* **1970**, *39*, 78.
69. Bingham, E.; Trosset, R. P.; Warshawsky, D. "Carcinogenic Potential of Petroleum Hydrocarbons—A Critical Review"; Univ. of Cincinnati, Coll. of Med., Dept. of Environmental Health, OH, 1970.
70. Gellin, G. A. *Ind. Med. Surg.* **1970**, *39*, 65.

4

Carcinogenic Aromatic Amines and Related Compounds

R. C. GARNER and C. N. MARTIN

University of York, Cancer Research Unit, York, Y01 5DD, England

D. B. CLAYSON

Health and Welfare, Health Protection Branch, Tunney's Pasture, Ottawa, Ontario, KIA OL2, Canada

A CORRELATION BETWEEN AROMATIC AMINE EXPOSURE and human cancer was reported first by Rehn (*1*) in 1895. He observed that three men, who were employed making magenta (rosaniline, fuchsine) (**1**) from commercial aniline at the same factory in Basel, all had bladder cancer. A fourth bladder cancer patient was engaged in the same process at another factory. Bladder cancer is sufficiently rare to make a cluster of a few cases noteworthy. Rehn called this condition "aniline cancer," but we now know that this name is inappropriate. This occupational disease was reported subsequently in all countries with an established chemical industry. Experienced medical officers concluded that aniline (**2**), benzidine (4,4′-diaminobiphenyl) (**3**), 2-naphthylamine (**4**), and 1-naphthylamine (**5**) were the probable causative agents (*2*).

An epidemiological survey of bladder cancer in parts of the British chemical industry has greatly clarified this position. Case and his colleagues (*3*) listed all men who had worked in the industry making or using the suspect chemicals between 1921 and 1950. Those workers who had been employed for less than 6 months were excluded. The working histories of more than 4000 remaining names were assembled, and the men were divided into groups on the basis of the chemicals they worked with: aniline, benzidine, 2-naphthylamine, 1-naphthylamine, or a mixture of two or more of these chemicals. The incidence of the disease in each group was determined from death certificates, hospital records, reports of coroners' inquests, and by inquiry from the patient or his relatives. Death certificates are an unreliable way to determine the incidence of bladder cancer, because many cases have a long prognosis and patients may die of intercurrent disease while their tumor is in remission. In such cases bladder cancer is not shown

0065-7719/84/0182-0175$21.30/1

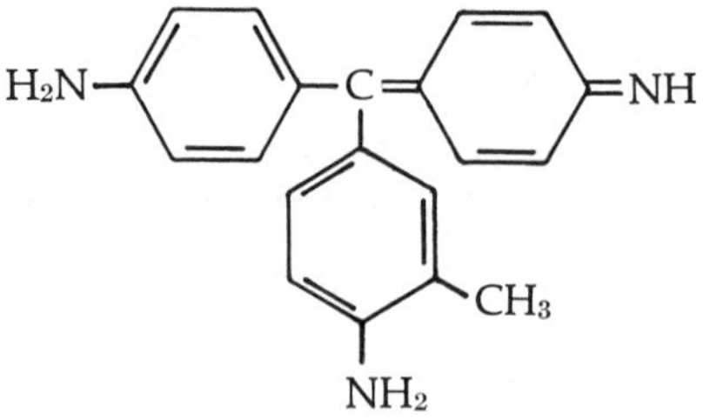

on the death certificate. As a control for this working population, Case and his colleagues used the entire male working population of England and Wales. The reason for this choice is referred to below; as a result, statistical comparisons could be made only between the number of death certificates for each group. Fortunately the position was sufficiently clearcut so that this limitation did not confuse the situation. This study first demonstrated that aniline induced excess bladder tumors only when used to manufacture auramine (**6**) and magenta (*4*).

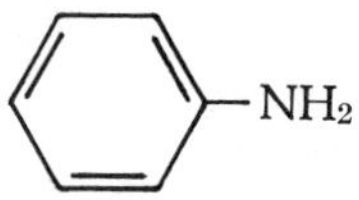

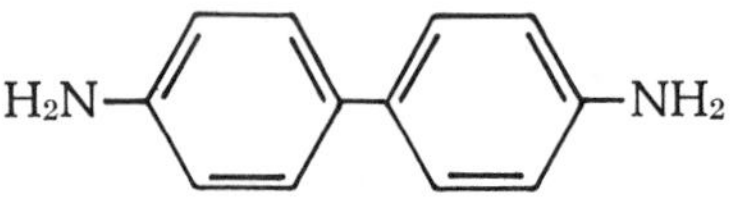

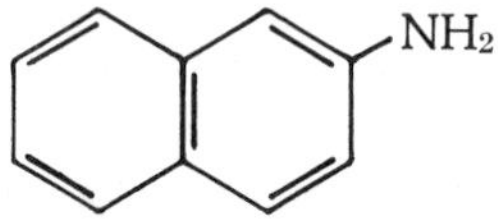

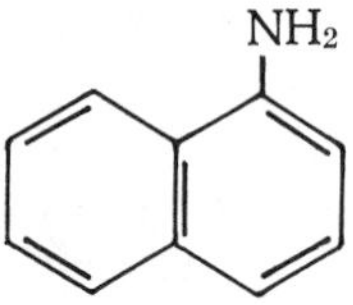

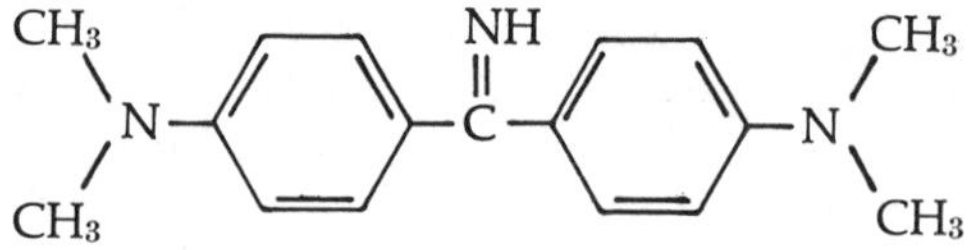

Subsequent work showed that a bladder cancer hazard was demonstrable in the manufacture of these two chemicals, but not with aniline in other circumstances. Therefore, the groups of men who had worked with the other suspect chemicals could be enlarged by adding those who had worked with aniline and only one other suspect chemical to the group exposed to the suspect chemical alone. 2-Naphthylamine was the most hazardous material, followed by benzidine and 1-naphthylamine. Even a 6-month exposure to 2-naphthylamine demonstrably increased the risk of bladder cancer, while 5 years or more appeared necessary for

1-naphthylamine. The average latent period from first entry into the industry to diagnosis was 17–18 years for 2-naphthylamine and benzidine and 22 years for 1-naphthylamine (*3*). Commercial 1-naphthylamine, in the time covered by the survey, normally contained 4–10% 2-naphthylamine. Apparently, the induction of bladder cancer by commercial 1-naphthylamine was probably due to the contaminating 2-naphthylamine; studies on pure 1-naphthylamine in dogs (*5*) have failed to demonstrate the carcinogenicity of this compound (*See* NAPHTHYLAMINES *on page 224*).

Case's first intention was to use the incidence of bladder cancer in men in an English county borough as a control population for the men in the chemical industry. He found that a section of this control population had an unexpectedly high incidence of the disease, and this was traced to men who had worked in a large rubber factory (*6*). The causative agent was identified as a rubber-compounding ingredient that contained 1- and 2-naphthylamines (Nonox S). Further research indicated that the manufacture of electric cables that were coated with rubber containing the same noxious compounding ingredient also led to bladder cancer (*7*). Later studies of workers employed in the rubber and cable-making industries suggest that excess bladder cancer incidence was not solely due to the use of naphthylamines, because an excess of bladder cancer incidence was noted for workers who had never been exposed to naphthylamines or who had joined the industry after their withdrawal (*8*).

Suspicion of human bladder cancer induced by aromatic amines was reported for rat catchers working with 1-naphthylthiourea (**7**); for medical personnel, chiefly nurses, who might have used benzidine to test for occult blood (*9*); for laboratory workers; and for tire remolders, who might have been exposed to aromatic amine fumes when the tires are heated. Furthermore, some patients receiving 2-naphthylamine mustard (**8**) for the blood condition polycythaemia vera succumbed to bladder cancer 2.5–11 years later (*10*). Confirmation of the industrial hazard in the manufacture of the naphthylamines and benzidine came from other countries (e.g., Japan, France, the United States, Russia, and Germany).

One further chemical, 4-biphenylamine (BPA; 4-aminobiphenyl) (**9**), has been shown to be a bladder carcinogen in humans (*11*). It was used in the United States between 1935 and 1954 when Melick and his colleagues reported that of the 171 men they knew had been exposed to the chemical, 19 developed bladder tumors. Since 1960, this series has been followed by exfoliative cytology (the examination of cells in freshly collected urine to see if their appearance after staining indicates that they may have come from a tumor). Of a population of 315 known to have been exposed, 53 have bladder tumors (*12, 13*).

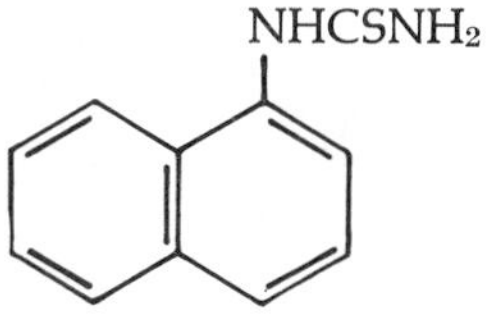

$NHCSNH_2$

7

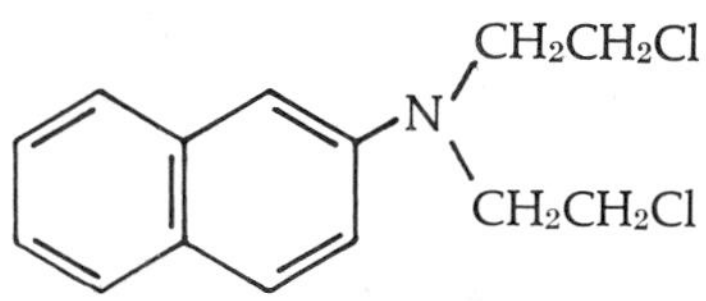

$N(CH_2CH_2Cl)_2$

8

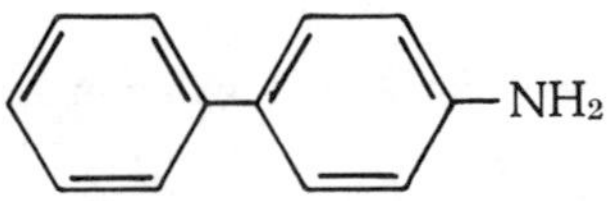

NH_2

9

The investigation of tumor induction in animals by the aromatic amines helped to confirm the epidemiological conclusions and provide experimental models for further study. Hueper et al. (*14*) provided the first successful model for human bladder cancer by injecting and then feeding large quantities of commercial 2-naphthylamine to dogs. After 2 years, bladder tumors were identified either at autopsy or cytoscopy in a substantial proportion of the animals. Partially purified and rigorously purified 2-naphthylamine were as effective bladder carcinogens as the commercial chemical (*15, 16*), thus the pure amine is likely to be the carcinogen rather than an impurity in it.

Further animal experiments proved the existence of many more carcinogenic aromatic amines since Hueper's classic experiment, and these studies are the basis of this chapter. Unlike the polycyclic aromatic hydrocarbons, aromatic amines do not induce tumors at the site of their administration but usually at a distant site such as the liver, intestine, or urinary bladder. Similarly, the response to aromatic amines is specific. 2-Naphthylamine, for example, is a potent bladder carcinogen in humans and dogs but is virtually noncarcinogenic in rabbits. These differences lead to the concept that the aromatic amines need metabolic activation to induce tumors, and this requirement has been demonstrated in detail by Miller and coworkers (*17*). On present evidence, *N*-hydroxylation is a prerequisite for carcinogenicity for this group of compounds; this reaction may be followed by esterification of the hydroxyl group in some but probably not all cases. The final intermediate is unstable and breaks down to an electrophile that interacts with the tissues (Scheme I). It might be expected that with this knowledge we could predict the stability and carcinogenicity of the activated metabolites of aromatic amines in animals, but this has yet to be achieved. Because metabolic activation explains the interrelationships among the chemicals discussed here, the mechanism of their activation is considered (1) by identification of certain structural features of aromatic amines important for carcinogenicity; and (2) by description of the known activation steps for some laboratory animal carcinogens. The details of the carcinogenicity of the various molecular species and the effects of different modifying factors follow.

Mechanism of Action of Some Aromatic Amines

In this section certain structural features of aromatic amines important for carcinogenicity are shown, and some of the known activation steps for some laboratory animal carcinogens are described.

Formation of *N*-Hydroxy Derivatives. Oxidation of primary and secondary aromatic amines is a long-recognized and well-documented reaction that takes place easily because of electron availability (*18*). Biological oxidation of foreign

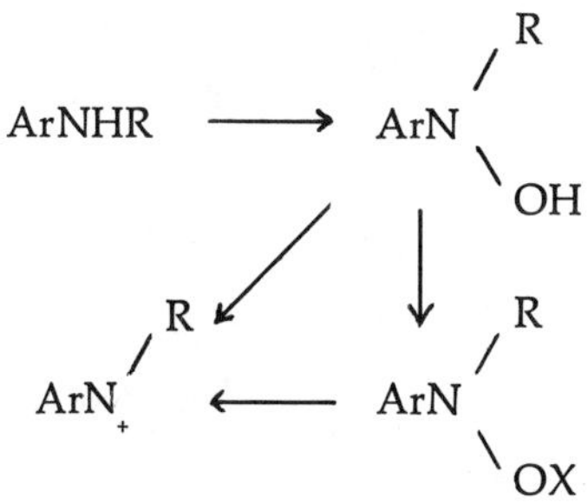

$$\mathrm{ArNHR} \longrightarrow \mathrm{ArN}(\mathrm{R})\mathrm{OH} \longrightarrow \mathrm{ArN}(\mathrm{R})\mathrm{OX} \longrightarrow \mathrm{ArN}^{+}\mathrm{R}$$

Scheme I. Metabolic activation of aromatic amines in which Ar = aryl group; R = H, aryl, or alkyl group; and X = ester group.

compounds has similarly been known for a number of years. Biological *N*-hydroxylation, however, has only been recognized relatively recently. In 1948, Brodie and Axelrod (*19*) suggested that phenylhydroxylamine might be formed during the metabolism of acetanilide (**10**) and assigned the methemoglobin production by acetanilide to this metabolite. Biological *N*-hydroxylation was then later demonstrated, again during studies on the mechanism of methemoglobin formation, by aromatic amines (*20*). Following these early observations, Uehleke (*21*) studied the metabolism of a series of *para*-substituted aniline derivatives and found that they were *N*-hydroxylated faster than aniline itself and that the resulting *N*-hydroxy derivative induced methemoglobinemia in proportion to the amount of *N*-hydroxylation. *N*-Hydroxylation is now known to be the first step in the conversion of aromatic amines to their ultimate carcinogenic form, that is, to a metabolite that is directly responsible for tumor formation (*22*). From the evidence available to date, apparently all carcinogenic aromatic amines must be converted to *N*-hydroxy compounds, although all *N*-hydroxy compounds are not necessarily carcinogenic. Hence *N*-phenylhydroxylamine (**11**), *N*-ethyl-*N*-phenylhydroxylamine (**12**), and *N*-hydroxy-*N*-1-fluorenylacetamide (**13**) (*23*) were all noncarcinogenic when tested. There are two major routes to *N*-hydroxy derivatives: (1) oxidation of a primary or secondary amino group, or (2) reduction of a nitro, nitroso, or *N*-oxide group.

OXIDATION. Oxidation of either a primary or a secondary aromatic amine is the major route to *N*-hydroxy compounds in animals. The oxidation can occur within a

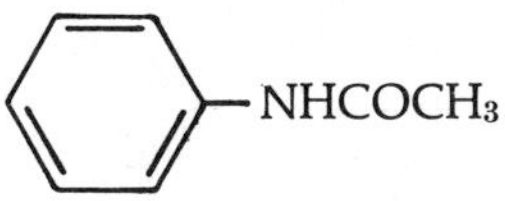

$C_6H_5NHCOCH_3$ **10**

$C_6H_5N(H)OH$ **11**

$C_6H_5N(C_2H_5)OH$ **12**

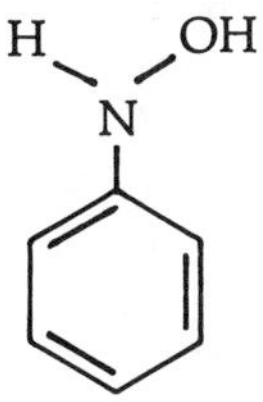

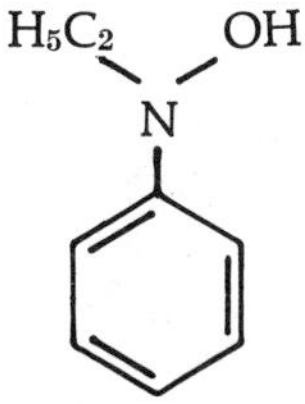

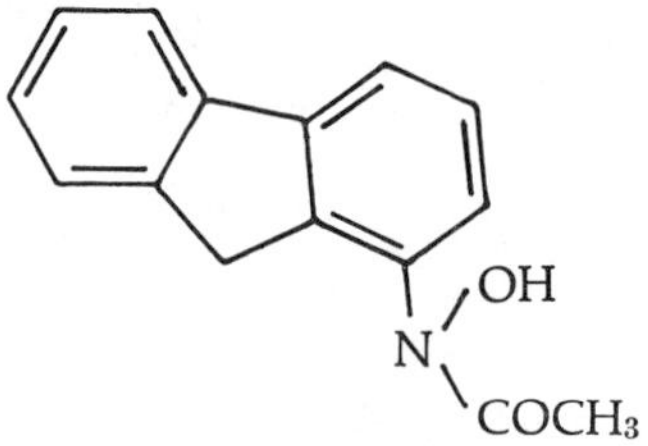

OH N COCH3

13

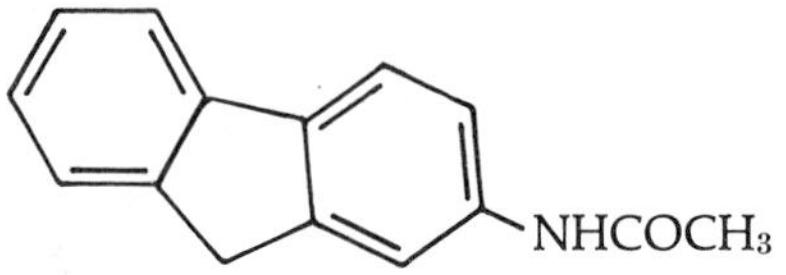

NHCOCH3

14

OH N COCH3

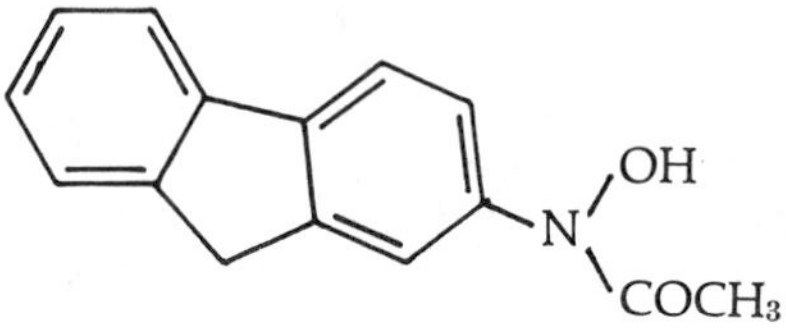

15

number of organs in the body, but it takes place primarily in the liver. The enzymes responsible for oxidation in the liver are in a network of intracellular membranes known as the endoplasmic reticulum. These membranes have a number of functions but are important chiefly as sites of protein synthesis. They can be obtained by centrifugation of liver postmitochondrial supernate at $100{,}000g \times 60$ min that precipitates them as a pellet at the bottom of the centrifuge tube. The pellet consists of endoplasmic reticulum membrane fragments together with bound ribosomes known as microsomes. Microsomes are artifacts of the preparation procedure but are capable of carrying out many enzymic conversions if supplemented with the necessary cofactors. The endoplasmic reticulum membranes contain an electron transport system collectively known as the mixed-function oxidases (monooxygenases) that can metabolize a variety of drugs, carcinogens, steroids, and so forth. By using the microsomal fraction, these conversions can be carried out in vitro as shown by Kiese and Uehleke (*20*). The microsomal fraction has to supplemented with NADPH or an NADPH-generating system, and atmospheric oxygen is required for the oxidation of foreign compounds.

Historically, the study of metabolism of 2-fluorenylacetamide (2-FAA) (**14**) led to the definitive demonstration of in vivo *N*-hydroxylation to aromatic amines (*24*). *N*-Hydroxy-2-FAA (fluorenyl-2-acethydroxamic acid) (**15**) was detected in the urine of rats treated with 2-FAA. The metabolite was present almost entirely as its glucuronic acid conjugate. *N*-Hydroxy-2-FAA was tested for carcinogenicity (*25*) and was more potent in the rat than the parent compound. In the guinea pig, *N*-hydroxy-2-FAA induced tumors at the site of injection, whereas 2-FAA did not (*26*). The guinea pig is also refractory to the liver carcinogenicity of 2-FAA, and it was suggested that this result might be due to an inability of the species to effect *N*-hydroxylation. The low amounts of this metabolite found in the urine of treated animals appeared to result, however, from a poor ability of guinea pigs to

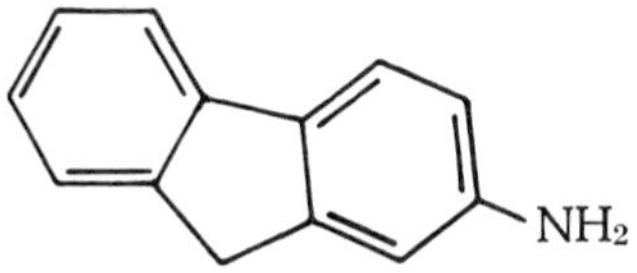

16

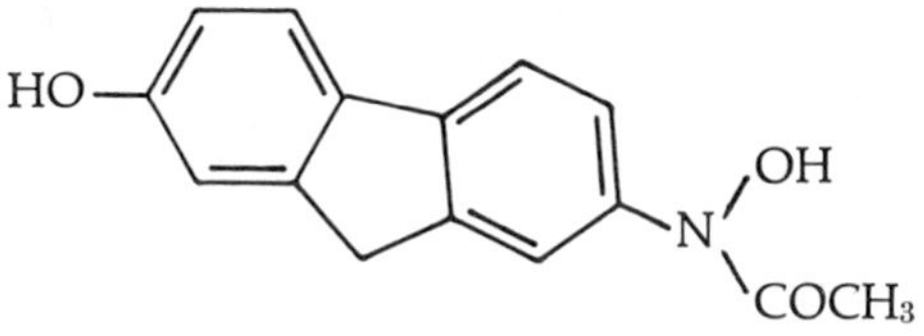

17

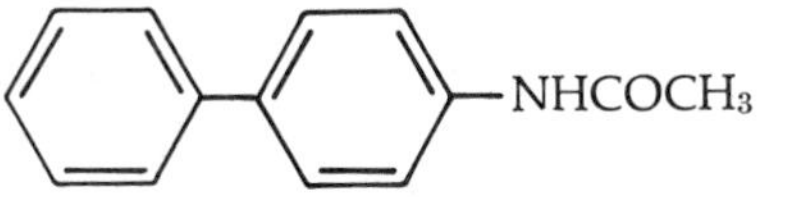

18

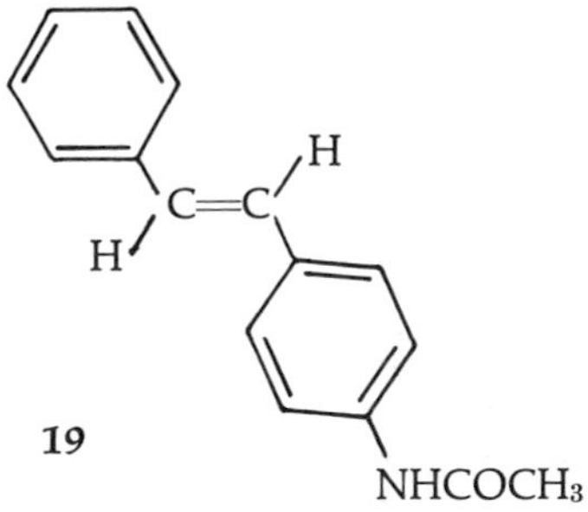

19

N-hydroxylate 2-FAA in vivo coupled with a high capacity for N-deacetylation (*27*). The 2-fluorenamine (2-FA) (**16**) resulting from this reaction is N-hydroxylated proficiently (*28*). Takeishi et al. (*29*) have since demonstrated that guinea pig liver homogenates efficiently N-hydroxylate 2-FAA, but the intact liver has a high level of detoxifying enzymes.

A variety of factors can affect the rate and extent to which aromatic amines are N-hydroxylated. Repeated exposure to an aromatic amine carcinogen, for instance, can sometimes increase the rate of metabolism. Thus, if rats are exposed repeatedly to 2-FAA, a gradual increase in the amount of N-hydroxy-2-FAA excreted in the urine is seen until a ninefold increase is reached at 18 weeks (*30*). This rate increase may be an important consideration when the metabolism of compounds in animals is investigated, because repeated exposure can possibly alter the relative amounts of toxic and nontoxic metabolites formed. Substrate specificity can also affect the extent of N-hydroxylation of aromatic amines. Some amines cannot be enzymically N-hydroxylated and hence are noncarcinogenic. However, if the N-hydroxy derivative is prepared chemically, tumors can be induced; this distinction is true of N-hydroxy-7-OH-2-FAA (**17**) (*23*). N-Hydroxylation can also be increased by suitable ring substitution. 7-OH-2-FAA is one of the main detoxification products of 2-FAA; if, however, the 7-position is fluorinated, which blocks hydroxylation at that position, then N-hydroxylation and carcinogenic activity are increased.

Such treatments that affect the rate and extent of N-hydroxylation also provide valuable evidence as to the importance of this oxidation in the carcinogenic process. Further evidence is provided by the increased carcinogenicity of N-hydroxylated metabolites over their parent amines, e.g., 4-biphenylacetamide (BPAA) (**18**) (*31*), 4-stilbenylacetamide (SAA) (**19**) (*32*), and 2-phenanthrenylacetamide (PAA) (**20**) (*32*). Treatment of animals with 3-methylcholanthrene

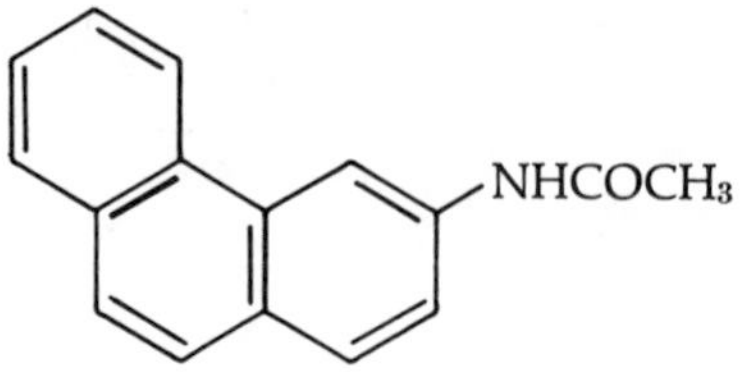

NHCOCH$_3$

20

decreases the carcinogenicity of 2-FAA; however, the compound has no effect on the carcinogenicity of *N*-hydroxy-2-FAA (*33*). Enzyme induction by the hydrocarbon reduces the production of the *N*-hydroxy compound, and this finding once again shows the importance of this oxidation for the carcinogenicity of aromatic amines.

Reduction. *N*-Hydroxy derivatives can also be formed by reductases, some of which can reduce nitro, nitroso, or *N*-oxide groups to *N*-hydroxy derivatives. Perhaps the best characterized of these reductases are those that act on 2-FAA congeners. 2-Nitrosofluorene (**21**), a metabolic product of 2-FAA and *N*-hydroxy-2-FAA, can be converted to *N*-hydroxy-2-FA (**22**). Hamster and rabbit liver soluble enzymes had considerably more activity in carrying out this reduction than those from the rat (*34*).

4-Nitroquinoline 1-oxide (NQO) (**23**) is a potent carcinogen in the rat and mouse. Repeated subcutaneous injection of 4-hydroxyaminoquinoline 1-oxide (HAQO) (**24**) results in more local sarcomas than injection of the parent compound (*35*). A single injection of HAQO induced tumors, while the nitro derivative did not (*36*); both observations suggest that HAQO is a proximate carcinogenic species of NQO. NQO is a potent mutagen for *Salmonella typhimurium* but is unable to mutate phage (*37*). On the other hand, HAQO is mutagenic for both. A reductase was identified in *Salmonella* that reduces NQO to its *N*-hydroxy derivative. A similar enzyme was identified in rat liver soluble fraction. NQO is also active in the unscheduled DNA synthesis assay in HeLa cells in the absence of a rat liver metabolizing preparation; this finding suggests that these cells possess a nitro-reducing capability (*38*). One of the enzymes identified appears to be a diaphorase and not the nitroreductase responsible for *p*-nitrobenzoic acid reduction (*39*).

Japanese workers have carried out numerous structure–activity studies on NQO and its derivatives. Apparently the nitro group must be in the 4-position for carcinogenicity.

Reduction of a nitro group also appears to be important for the carcinogenicity of some nitrofuran compounds. Urinary bladder tumors were found after feeding *N*-[4-(5–nitro-2-furyl)-2-thiazolyl]formamide (**25**) to rats and mice (*40*). The same compound induced both bladder and renal pelvic tumors in the dog (*41*). Many other 5-nitrofuran compounds have been tested for carcinogenicity; certain structural features are important for activity. Several enzymes are capable of reducing nitrofurans to their corresponding *N*-hydroxy derivative. One of these

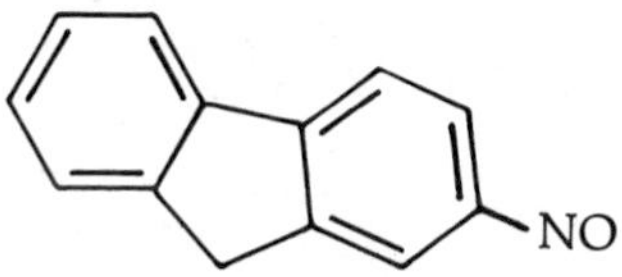

21 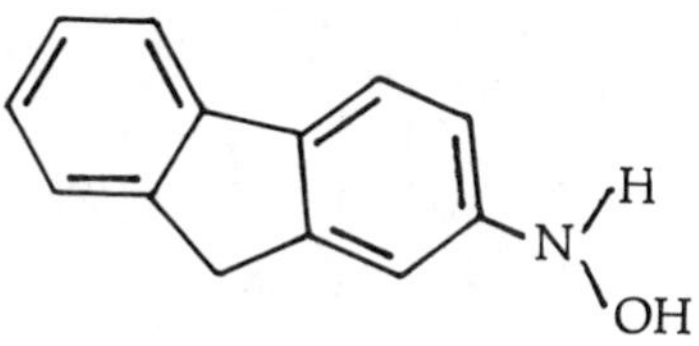 **22**

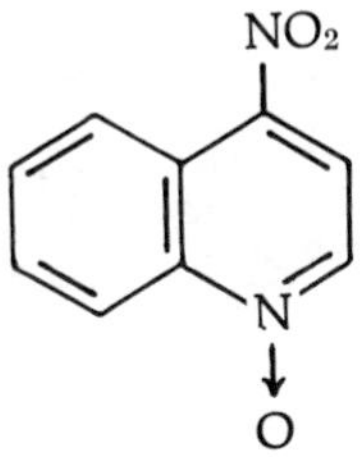

23 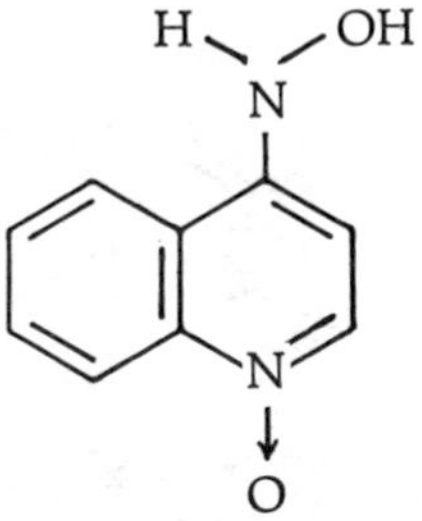 **24**

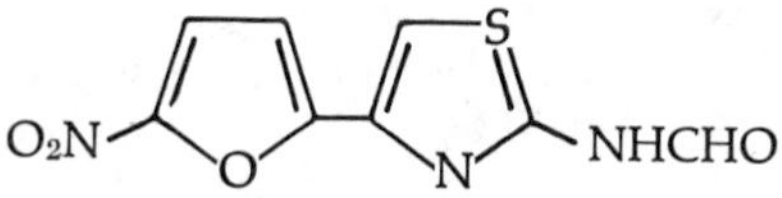

25 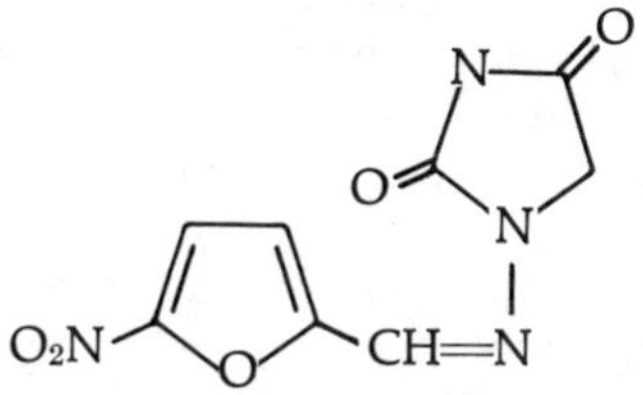 **26**

enzymes occurs in the liver soluble fraction and requires NADPH (*42*). Two other enzymes capable of reducing nitrofurazone (**26**) and furazolidone (**27**) were found in the liver microsomal fraction. One of these appeared to be xanthine oxidase, because it was inhibited by allopurinol, and the other was NADPH–cytochrome *c* reductase (*43*).

ESTERIFICATION. If *N*-hydroxy derivatives were the ultimate form of the carcinogen, then they should react in vitro with cellular macromolecules to give derivatives similar to those found in vivo after administration of the parent compound, but there are only a few reports in the literature of *N*-hydroxy derivatives binding to macromolecules in vitro (*44, 45*). Under acidic conditions, however, reaction can occur in certain cases (*46, 47*), and this finding had led in part to the proposal that the acidity of urine may play a role in the bladder carcinogenicity of certain aromatic amines. In general, *N*-hydroxy derivatives are not usually the ultimate

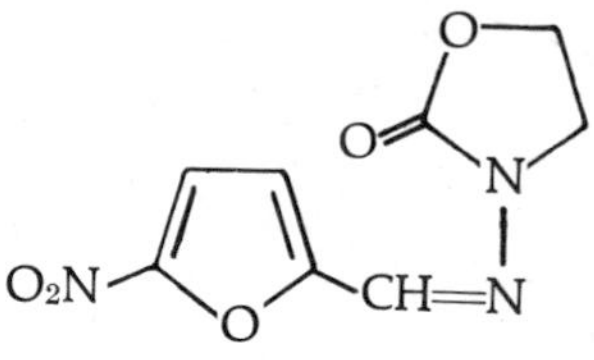

27 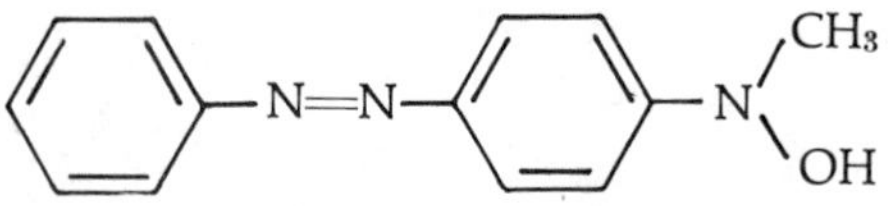 **28**

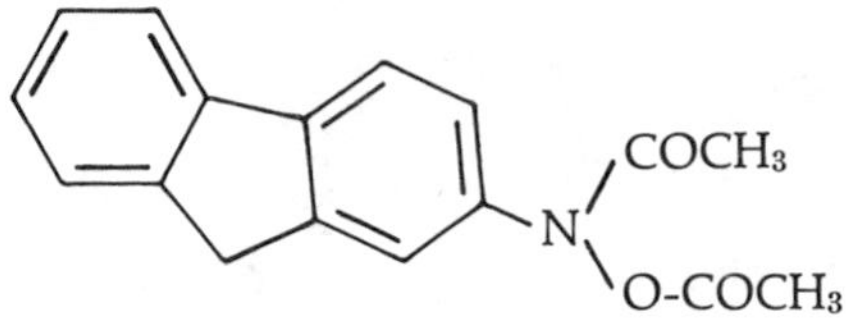

29 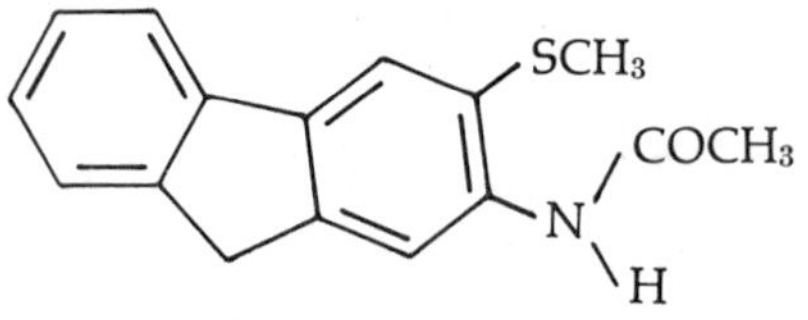 **30**

carcinogenic forms of aromatic amines under physiological conditions but are proximate forms that must be further metabolized.

A clue to these further metabolites was provided when Miller and coworkers (*48*) were attempting to synthesize *N*-hydroxymethylaminoazobenzene (*N*-hydroxy-MAB) (**28**). They found that the synthesis [since achieved by Kadlubar et al. (*49*)] failed due to instability of the product, and therefore they synthesized the benzoyloxy ester. The idea was that the ester would break down in the tissues to yield *N*-hydroxy-MAB. When the ester was tested for carcinogenicity, it was found to be extremely potent, particularly at the site of injection. Incubation of the benzoyloxy ester with macromolecules in vitro gave covalently bound derivatives that were similar to those found following MAB administration in vivo (*50*). This experiment gave the first indication that esters might be the ultimate form of carcinogenic aromatic amines. Since these early observations, a variety of esters of various carcinogens have been extracted or identified by enzyme–substrate experiments. The major groups are discussed briefly below.

ACETATE ESTERS. Following the realization that esters of *N*-hydroxy compounds might be the ultimate forms of these carcinogens, the *N*-acetoxy ester of 2-FAA (**29**) was synthesized. This compound was an extremely potent carcinogen subcutaneously; tumors were induced at the injection site. It was equipotent with the polycyclic hydrocarbons, the most potent compounds known at that time. Also, *N*-acetoxy-2-FAA reacted in vitro with cellular macromolecules to give covalently bound derivatives identical with those found after administration of 2-FAA to animals. For example, *N*-acetoxy-2-FAA reacts with methionine to yield 3-methylmercapto-2-FAA in vitro (**30**) (*51*). 3-Methylmercapto-2-FAA is also found on alkaline hydrolysis of liver protein after 2-FAA administration in vivo. *N*-Acetoxy-2-FAA also reacts with guanosine monophosphate to give 8-guanyl-2-FAA in vitro. A similar conjugate was isolated from a hydrolysate of DNA after 2-FAA administration (*50*).

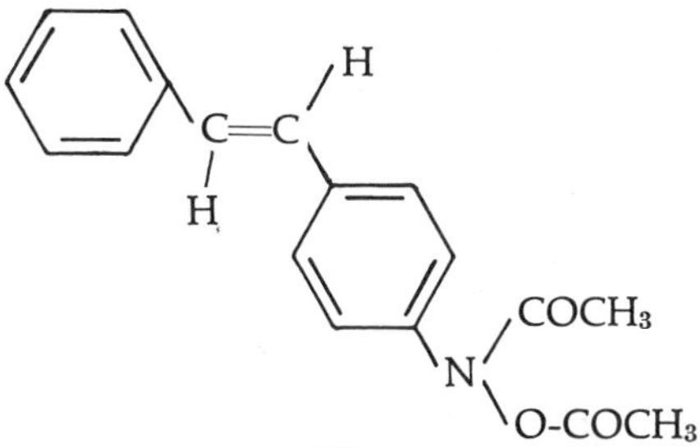

31

In a study of the mechanism of nucleophilic attack in a series of acetohydroxamic acids, *N*-acetoxy-FAA and *N*-acetoxy-SAA (**31**) underwent unimolecular dissociation to form acetate ions and carbonium ions, whereas the corresponding biphenyl and phenanthrene compounds underwent bimolecular dissociation (*51*).

Esterification by acetate is a common conjugation mechanism in the metabolism of amines, sulfonamides, and some aromatic amino acids. It can take place nonenzymically as in the reaction of *N*-hydroxy-2-FAA with acetyl CoA (*52*). However, the pH optimum for this reaction is about 10.0, so that at physiological pH, only a small amount of ester can be formed.

Only two mechanisms of enzymic acetylation of *N*-hydroxy compounds have been described. *N*-Hydroxy-2-FAA is converted to a free nitroxide radical by a one-electron oxidation process. Both potassium ferricyanide and moist silver oxide catalyze the reaction to produce the radical form (*see* Scheme II). The two nitroxide ions formed dismutate to yield one molecule of 2-nitrosofluorene and one molecule of *N*-acetoxy-2-FAA (*53*). Both molecules have carcinogenic activity. The reaction can be catalyzed by various peroxidases: both human myeloperoxidases and lactoperoxidases are active (*54*). The importance of peroxidase activity for organ specificity of carcinogens is discussed later. Other acethydroxamic acids can also undergo one-electron oxidation.

Bartsch et al. reported another activation enzyme that is found in liver cell sap and esterifies hydroxamic acids (*55*). It can transfer an acetyl group from a molecule of *N*-hydroxy-2-FAA to a molecule of *N*-hydroxy-2-FA. The acetyl donor need not be *N*-hydroxy-2-FAA. Other carcinogenic acethydroxamic acids such as *N*-hydroxy-4-acetoxy-BPAA can be used (*56*). Such systems have been found in tissues other than liver; King et al. isolated an *N,O*-acyltransferase from the mammary tissue of rats (*57*).

Acetylation does not always lead to increased carcinogenicity. Diacetylhydroxyaminoquinoline (**32**) is much more reactive with nucleophiles in vitro than NQO but is less carcinogenic than NQO (*58*). Possibly the molecule is so reactive that it is unable to reach the critical target within the cell to initiate tumors; instead, it reacts with noncritical nucleophiles.

SULFATE ESTERS. Although various synthetic esters of *N*-hydroxy-2-FAA were found to be extremely reactive, these did not appear to be the ones actually generated within the cell. Miller et al. (*59*) and King and Phillips (*60*) independently

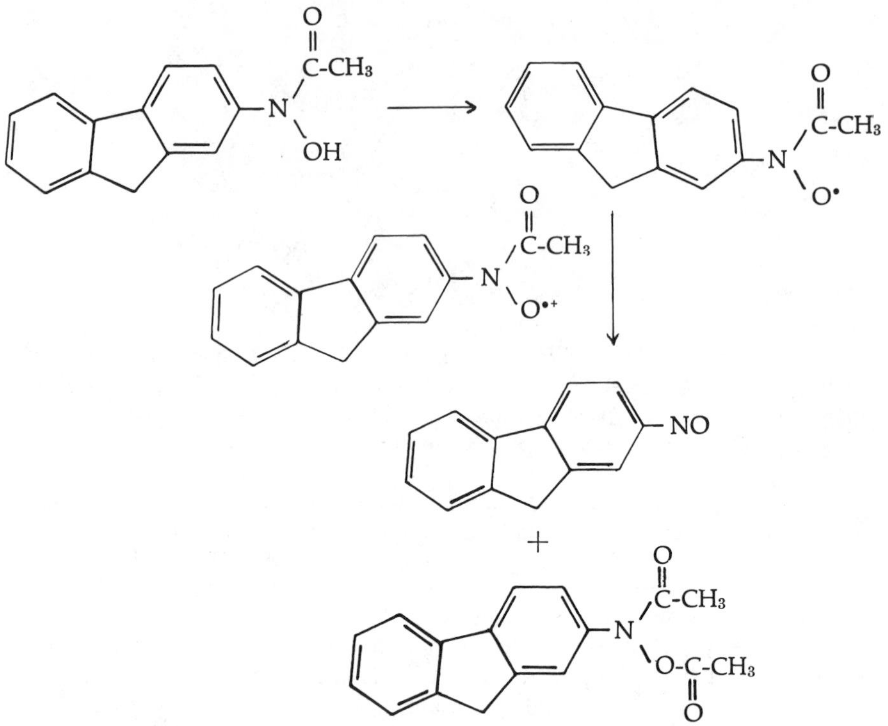

Scheme II. Formation of N-2-*acetoxy-FAA by one-electron oxidation process.*

demonstrated that *N*-hydroxy-2-FAA could be esterified with 3′-phosphoadenosine 5′-phosphosulfate by an enzyme in the soluble fraction of the liver cell. The enzyme activity of this sulfotransferase differed between the sexes and between species. Male rats had a higher activity than females, and activity was directly related to the species' sensitivity to the carcinogenic action of 2-FAA (*61*). The guinea pig, for example, resists the carcinogenic activity of 2-FAA and has low sulfotransferase activity. The guinea pig therefore not only poorly *N*-hydroxylates

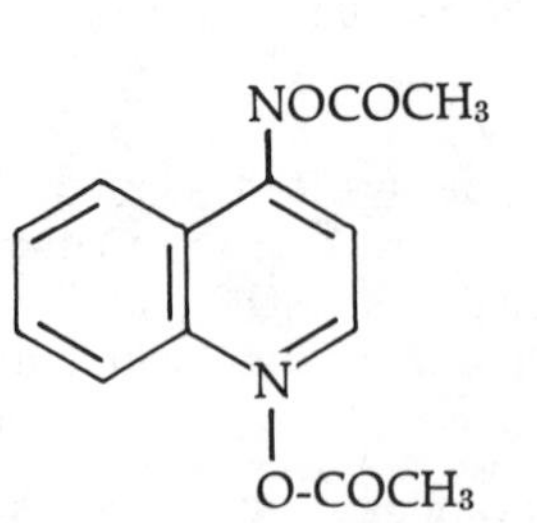

32

2-FAA (due to efficient detoxification) but is also unable to esterify any *N*-hydroxy compound formed. These two low enzyme activities probably account for this species' resistance to liver tumor induction by 2-FAA.

The synthetic *N*-sulfate of 2-FAA is extremely reactive and has a half-life of about 1 min in water. When this compound was tested for carcinogenicity either subcutaneously in rats or on the skin of mice or rats, very few tumors were obtained; the ester most likely breaks down on reaction with extracellular materials before it can reach critical cellular targets. Confirmatory evidence for the involvement of the *N*-sulfate in carcinogenesis was the discovery that depletion of the intracellular sulfate level with acetanilide reduces the carcinogenicity of 2-FAA (*62*). Also, the toxicity and reactivity of *N*-hydroxy-2-FAA are increased by simultaneous administration of sulfate ion (*63*).

CARBAMATE ESTERS. *N*-Carbamate esters of *N*-hydroxy compounds are formed nonenzymically by reaction with a suitable donor. Carbamyl phosphate formed carbamate esters with *N*-hydroxy-2-FAA; the pH optimum of the reaction was 4.5 (*64*), and negligible reaction occurred at physiological pH. At pH 7.0, acetylation by acetyl CoA produces more esterification of *N*-hydroxy-2-FAA than carbamylation by carbamyl phosphate, in contrast to *N*-hydroxy-4-SAA or *N*-hydroxy-2-PAA, with which one obtains more carbamate ester.

PHOSPHATE ESTERS. Activation of *N*-hydroxy-2-FAA has been found with orthophosphate (*65*). Activation of HAQO was thought to occur by phosphate esterification in vivo (*66*). Transfer of a phosphate group from ATP to the hydroxamic acid is catalyzed in vitro by a soluble enzyme of the liver. The resulting phosphate ester reacts with nucleophiles to form adducts identical to those obtained in vivo after administration of the parent compound.

GLUCURONIDES. The importance of glucuronidation as an activation mechanism for aromatic amines is under debate. Glucuronidation of the *N*-hydroxy group is one of the major routes for excretion of *N*-hydroxy-2-FAA. The *N*-glucuronide of *N*-hydroxy-2-FAA, *N*-glu-2-FAA, will react in vitro with nucleophiles although the reaction rate is much slower than with either *N*-acetoxy-2-FAA or *N*-2-FAA-*N*-sulfate (*44*). This glucuronide also has a much lower carcinogenic potency than *N*-hydroxy-2-FAA (*67*) and no mutagenic activity (*68*). The *N*-glucuronide of 2-FA might be formed by deacetylation of *N*-glu-2-FAA or by esterification of *N*-hydroxy-2-FA. This glucuronide is considerably more reactive with nucleophiles than *N*-glu-2-FAA in vitro (*69*). It is also a potent mutagen for bacteria-transforming DNA (*70*). However, it is less carcinogenic than *N*-glu-2-FAA. This finding can be explained in the same way as the weak carcinogenicity of *N*-2-FAA-*N*-sulfate. The *N*-glucuronides of *N*-hydroxy-2-naphthylamine, *N*-hydroxy-1-naphthylamine, and *N*-hydroxy-4-BPA at pH 5 were capable of conversion to reactive derivatives that could bind covalently to nucleic acids (*71*).

Metabolic Activation of Some Important Aromatic Amines. ANILINES. As already discussed, activation of most aromatic amines as a general rule is initiated via *N*-hydroxylation and this includes single-ring compounds. Acetaminophen (**33**) is known to arylate macromolecules, and in large doses it causes liver necrosis in humans; activation is through the *N*-hydroxide (*72*). Phenacetin (4-ethoxyace-

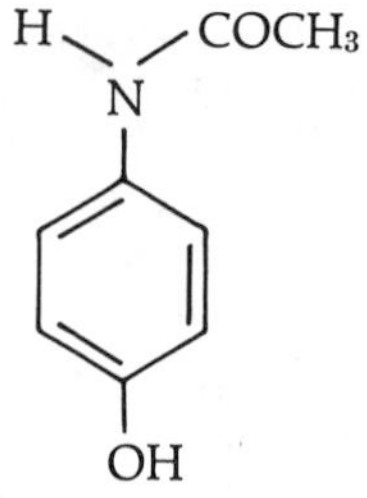

H COCH3 N OH

33

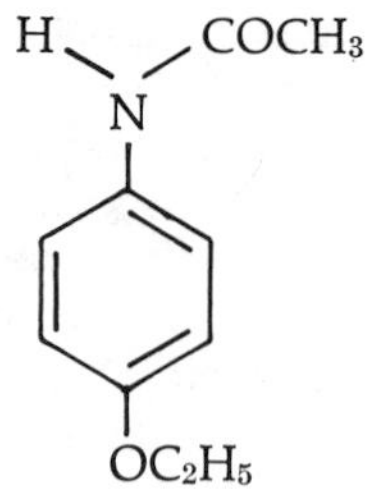

H COCH3 N OC2H5

34

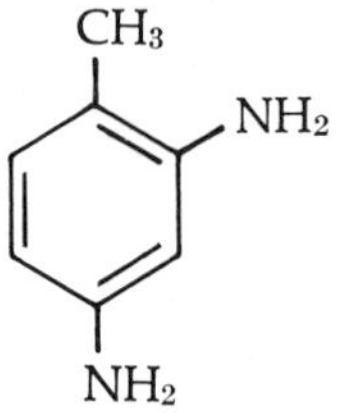

CH3 NH2 NH2

35

OCH3 NH2 NH2

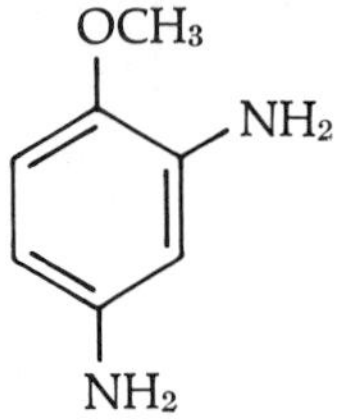

36

tanilide) (**34**) is similarly activated (*73, 74*), possibly to some extent via *N*-hydroxylation of acetaminophen (*75*) produced by *O*-deethylation. The second stage in the activation process appears to be deacetylation of *N*-hydroxyphenacetin (*76*).

The mouse is refractory to the rat carcinogen 2,4-diaminotoluene (**35**). *N*-Hydroxylation is suggested to be at a low level in the mouse because of a high degree of *N*-acetylation of the *p*-amino group (*77*).

The following compounds are also biologically active via *N*-hydroxylated metabolites: *N,N*-dimethylaniline (*78*), *p*-chloroaniline and *p*-chloro-*N*-methylaniline (*79*), *p*-chloroacetanilide (*80, 81*), and *N*-ethyl-*N*-methylaniline (*82*). *N*-Hydroxylation is also suggested as the initial reaction in the activation of 2,4-diaminoanisole (**36**) to a mutagen and carcinogen (*83*).

EXTENDED ANILINES. *4-Biphenylamine (BPA).* This compound was shown to be *N*-hydroxylated by rabbit and dog liver microsomes (*84*). *N*-Hydroxy metabolites have also been identified in the urine of animals treated with the parent amine (*85, 86*). The hydroxylamine metabolite rather than the hydroxamic acid seems to be implicated in the activation process in bladder carcinogenesis (*87*). Acceptance of the hydroxylamine metabolite as being involved in this process was initially impeded by the fact that it is insoluble and unstable in aqueous media. This obstacle was removed, however, by the discovery of a glucuronide conjugate of *N*-hydroxy-4-BPA in the urine of dogs fed the parent amine (*87*). The conjugate was sensitive to acid pH but was stable at physiological pH; therefore, its transport from liver to bladder is possible. This glucuronide was isolated from urine (*88*), synthesized (*89*), and characterized as the *N*-glucuronide of *N*-hydroxy-4-BPA.

4-Biphenylacetamide (BPAA). This compound can be deacetylated by dog liver (*90*) to release 4-BPA that can be further metabolized as described in the previous section. BPAA may also be activated by direct *N*-hydroxylation (*31*). The *N*-hydroxide can then act as an acetyl donor for liver *N,O*-acyltransferases in rats (*56, 91*). When *N*-hydroxy-BPA, produced by deacetylation and subsequent *N*-hydroxylation, acts as an acyl receptor, the highly reactive species *N*-acetoxy-BPA may be formed (*56*). Also, *N*-hydroxy-BPAA may be reduced back to the parent amine by gut bacteria in the rat and aid detoxification in vivo (*92*).

Benzidine. Benzidine has received relatively little attention in recent years, and, consequently, less is known about the metabolic activation of this compound. Martin and Ekers (*93*) suggested that benzidine was activated by *N*-hydroxylation and that the synthesis of this unstable intermediate could be circumvented by synthesis of the more stable *N*-benzoyloxy ester. *N*-Benzoyloxybenzidine itself proved too unstable for characterization, but the presumed compound was shown to react with DNA. On hydrolysis of the DNA, the adduct was shown to cochromatograph with the adduct generated in rat liver DNA by intraperitoneal injection of [^{3}H]benzidine. Experiments using rat liver metabolizing systems in vitro (*94, 95*) have demonstrated production of *N*-hydroxy-*N,N'*-diacetylbenzidine, which is chemically more stable than the postulated *N*-hydroxybenzidine and can be synthesized and isolated. The in vitro work also showed that *N*-hydroxy-*N,N'*-diacetylbenzidine could act as substrate for both *N,O*-acyltransferase and sulfotransferase to produce reactive esters. Recent pH-dependent solvent partitioning experiments (*96*) have shown that the adduct generated by *N*-benzoyloxybenzidine is different from that generated by benzidine in vivo. Also, intraperitoneal injection of either benzidine or *N*-acetylbenzidine into rats was shown to result in production of a single DNA adduct, viz., *N*-(deoxyguanosine-8-yl)-*N'*-acetylbenzidine. The injection of *N,N'*-diacetylbenzidine resulted in barely detectable levels of binding. The adduct produced could have arisen via a variety of routes. *N*-OH-*N'*-acetylbenzidine was shown to give the same adduct when reacted with DNA at pH 5. This hydroxylamine could be further activated in vivo by sulfotransferase enzymes or by intermolecular N→O acyl transfer. Alternatively, *N*-OH-*N,N'*-diacetylbenzidine may be produced by acetylation of this molecule and itself further activated by intramolecular *N*→*O* acyl transfer. Sulfotransferase activation of this metabolite is ruled out as the product of reaction with DNA would be diacetylated.

4-Stilbenylacetamide (SAA). *N*-Hydroxylation of SAA results in production of a more potent carcinogen than the parent amide with a wider range of tumors produced (*32, 97–99*). Stilbenamine is similarly hydroxylated (*100*). Epoxidation of the stilbene double bond leads to deactivation, and the product is nonmutagenic in bacteria (*101*). Synthetic esters of *N*-hydroxy-SAA react with nucleophiles as do esters of *N*-hydroxy-2-FAA, though less extensively (*50, 51*). Such studies suggest that the activation of SAA and SA is likely to follow similar routes to that of BPAA and PAA, or FAA and FA, respectively.

FUSED-RING AMINES. *2-Fluorenylacetamide (2-FAA).* Following *N*-hydroxylation, this compound can be activated in a variety of ways. In the presence of 3′-phosphoadenosyl 5′-phosphosulfate and sulfotransferase enzymes, the highly reactive *N*-sulfate is formed (*17, 61, 102*). Peroxidase enzymes can produce a nitroxide free radical (*53, 103*) that dismutates with a second radical molecule to form *N*-acetoxy-2-FA and nitrosofluorene that can then be further metabolized. *N,O*-Acyltransferase enzymes can transpose the acetyl group from the *N*-hydroxy-2-FAA donor to a deacetylated *N*-hydroxy-2-FA acceptor to produce *N*-acetoxy-2-FA. Esters can also be formed with the O atom of the *N*-hydroxy group leading, for example, to *O*-glucuronide formation in vivo in the presence of glucuronyltransferase enzymes (*104*). The most active of the metabolites produced in vivo is probably *N*-sulfate (*for reviews of the metabolism of FAA see* Ref. 17 *and* 105).

2-Naphthylamine (2-*NA*). As in the case of 4-BPA, *N*-hydroxylation of 2-naphthylamine leads to a reactive product that is transported to the bladder as the *N*-glucuronide (*106, 107*), which is itself unstable at low pH values (*71*). 1-Naphthylamine appears to be noncarcinogenic, most likely because ring hydroxylation occurs at the expense of *N*-hydroxylation. If, however, *N*-hydroxy-1-naphthylamine is synthesized, it acts as a substrate for glucuronyltransferase enzymes in rat microsomes that are fortified with uridine 5′-diphosphoglucuronic acid, as does *N*-hydroxy-2-naphthylamine (*71*). *N*-Glucuronides of aromatic amines are thought to act as proximate bladder carcinogens through the release of *N*-hydroxy compounds at the acidic pH of urine in humans and dogs (*46*). However, whether the *N*-hydroxide reacts directly with bladder tissue or requires further metabolism is not known.

AMINOAZO DYES. N-*Methylaminoazobenzene (MAB).* As mentioned previously, the early inability to synthesize the *N*-hydroxy derivative of MAB led to difficulties in pursuing metabolic studies on the activation of this compound. This problem was partially circumvented by the synthesis of the benzoic acid ester *N*-benzoyloxy-MAB (**37**) in vitro. Reaction products of this compound with nucleic acids were identical to those obtained in vivo following administration of MAB (*108*). Following the later synthesis of *N*-hydroxy-MAB (*49*), microsomal *N*-oxidation of MAB was shown to occur. It was further demonstrated that this compound was a substrate for microsomal sulfotransferase yielding a reactive species, the presumed MAB-*N*-sulfate (*109*), and that it gave identical reaction products with nucleic acid to those obtained on administration of MAB to animals. Evidence has been presented that implicates the enzymic production of a nitroxide free radical from *N*-hydroxy-MAB in the activation of MAB (*110*).

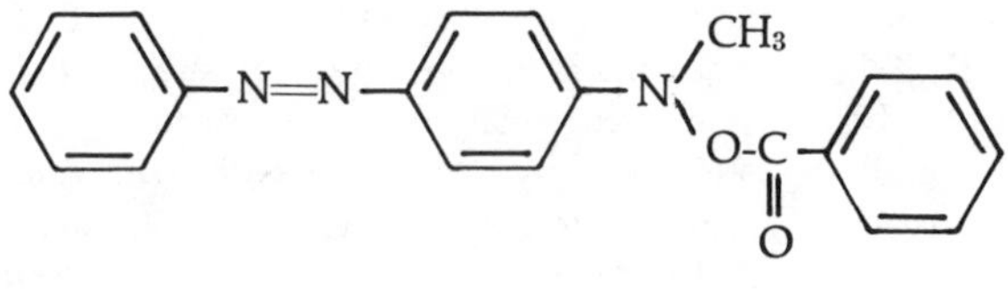

CH_3 N=N N O-C O

37

Benzidine-Derived Azo Dyes. Dyes derived from benzidine have been shown to be potent carcinogens in rats (*111*). Free benzidine and its *N*-acetylated metabolites have been detected in the urine of monkeys (*112*), rats, and humans (*113*) treated with or, in the last case, industrially exposed to, this type of compound. The azo reduction leading to release of the amine can be carried out by both gut bacteria (*114*) and mammalian liver azo reductases (*115*). Recent work has indicated, however, that the part played by liver azo reductases may be significant though quantitatively small (*116, 117*). Three dyes, direct black 38, direct blue 6, and direct brown 95, were all shown to be reduced to benzidine by rat liver in vivo. Trypan blue, Chicago sky blue, and congo red were not reduced. All six dyes are reduced to a far greater extent in the gut. The direct dyes, however, are potent animal liver carcinogens (*111*); thus the small contribution by the liver in releasing the free amine may be more significant than that of the gut microflora in carcinogenesis of the liver.

HETEROCYCLIC AMINES. *4-Nitroquinoline 1-Oxide (4-NQO).* 4-NQO is activated to 4-HAQO by nitroreductase enzymes present in both the cytosolic and microsomal fractions of rat liver (*39*). 4-HAQO does not however react with nucleophiles in vitro and thus is not the ultimate carcinogen. Phosphotransferase enzymes were initially implicated in the further activation of 4-HAQO (*66*). The enzyme responsible now appears to be seryl tRNA synthetase (*118*). Activation occurs via aminoacylation of the *N*-hydroxy compound yielding a directly acting metabolite. Other aminoacyl tRNA synthetases including prolyl tRNA may also play a role in activation to an ultimate carcinogen via aminoacylation of 4-HAQO.

Nitrofurans. Nitrofurans are reduced by xanthine oxidase (*42, 119, 120*), aldehyde oxidase (*121*), and liver microsomes (*120, 122*), probably through cytochrome c reductase. Reduction of the nitro group is essential for biological activity, and *N*-hydroxylamine production is presumed to be responsible (*123*).

Detoxification Mechanisms. All the activation mechanisms described use enzymes normally involved in the detoxification of foreign compounds. The enzymes carrying out these reactions sometimes generate reactive metabolites but usually produce less toxic derivatives. For example, hydroxylation generally produces a less toxic compound as in the conversion of aniline to *p*-aminophenol, whereas *N*-hydroxylation gives a much more toxic compound. Detoxification enzymes convert a foreign compound to a more polar molecule and thus facilitate its excretion in the urine and feces. Sulfate esterification of *N*-hydroxy-2-FAA yields the highly reactive *N*-sulfate. Sulfate esterification of phenols to give ethereal sulfates leads to a less toxic and more rapidly excreted product. Because ring hydroxylation is the predominant metabolic route for aromatic amines, a balance will result between activation and deactivation reactions. This balance can be altered, for example, by pretreatment with 3-methylcholanthrene, which increases the rate of ring hydroxylation of 2-FAA without a proportional increase in *N*-hydroxylation; thus the carcinogenicity of 2-FAA in the rat is reduced by prior 3-methylcholanthrene administration.

ORTHO-HYDROXYLATION. The major detoxification pathway for aromatic amines is ring hydroxylation, particularly at the position *ortho* to the amino group. This step was

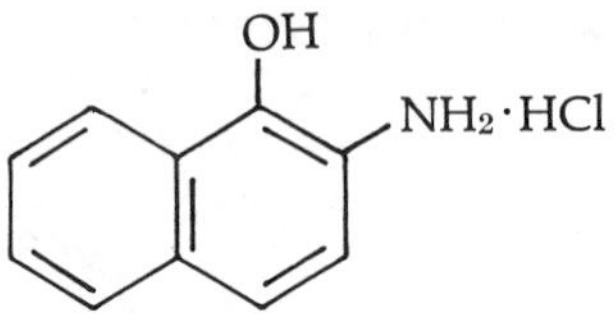

38 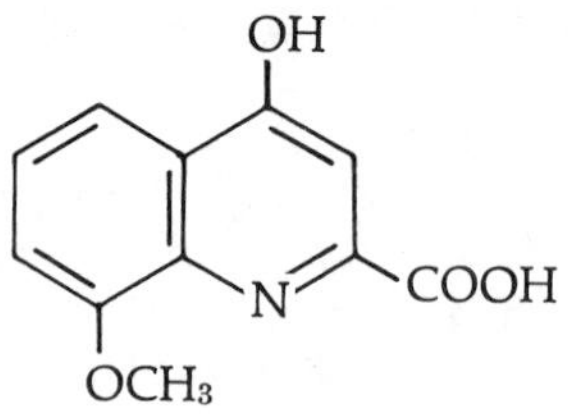 **39**

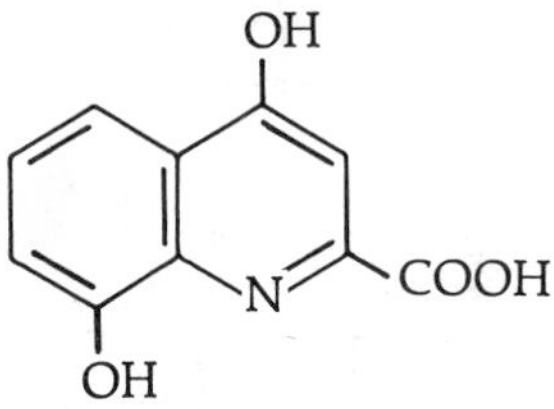

40 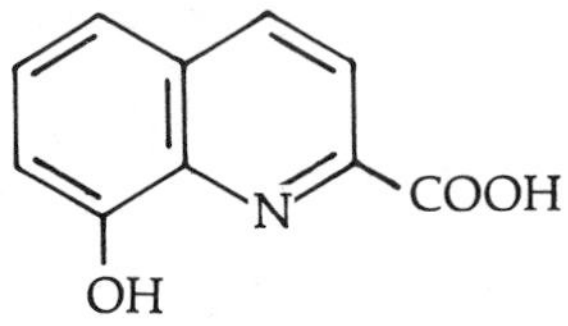 **41**

once thought to be the prime activation mechanism for several aromatic amines (*124*). This interpretation was based on the observation that a number of *ortho*-hydroxy aromatic amines induced bladder tumors in 40–50 weeks when implanted in a paraffin or cholesterol pellet in the bladder lumen. For example, 2-amino-1-naphthol hydrochloride (**38**) induced tumors in this test but 2-naphthylamine did not. The validity of such tests was questioned because the paraffin or cholesterol pellet itself produces profound changes in the bladder epithelium with variable tumor induction (*125–28*).

In a series of tests in mice, the cholesterol pellet induced an 8% bladder tumor incidence, while 8-methylxanthurenic acid (**39**), xanthurenic acid (**40**), 8-hydroxyquinaldic acid (**41**), 3-hydroxy-L-kynurenine (**42**), and 3-hydroxyanthranilic acid (**43**) (all metabolites of tryptophan) gave a significantly higher incidence. When 8-methylxanthurenic acid, which gave a 30% bladder tumor incidence when implanted in a cholesterol pellet, was injected into animals with a cholesterol

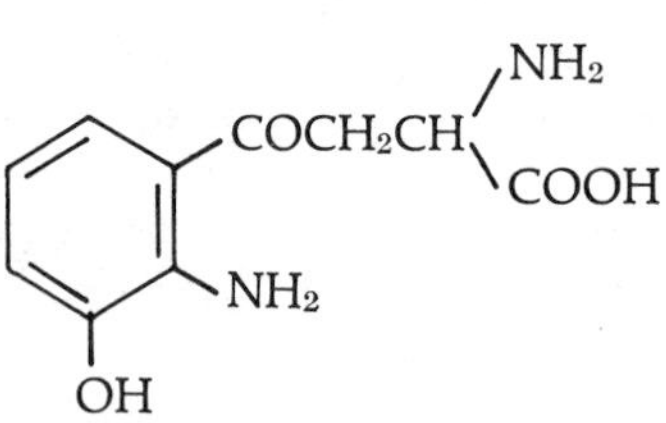

42 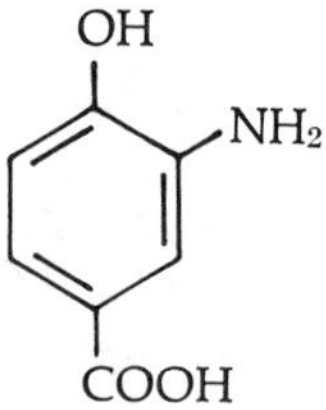 **43**

bladder implant, a similar bladder tumor incidence was obtained (*129*). Jill (*130*) showed that implanted pellets without added chemicals led to a 50% yield of bladder carcinoma in 2 years.

Among other changes, a pellet induces a hyperplastic and an inflammatory response (*125*) and significantly increases the mitotic rate in the bladder epithelium (*126*). Apparently, the presence of the pellet leads to a carcinogenic response by the epithelium. This response may be because of a cocarcinogenic action of the pellet or because the bladder is sensitized to the action of low levels of extraneous carcinogens present in the urine.

Bladder cancer patients who have not been occupationally exposed to carcinogens may have an abnormal tryptophan metabolism with emphasis on the niacin pathway. The tumors were thought to be induced by tryptophan or one of its metabolites, because these compounds were active in the bladder implantation test. DL-Tryptophan induced marked hyperplasia of the bladder transitional epithelium (*131*), and this condition might be associated with a promoting action (*See* TRYPTOPHAN AND INDOLE on page 255).

ortho-Hydroxylation can occur by transfer of the hydroxyl group from the hydroxylamine. Incubation of *N*-hydroxy-2-FAA with rat liver microsomes leads to a transfer of the hydroxyl group to the 3-position. A similar reaction is found with the *N*-hydroxy derivative of BPAA (*132*).

DEACETYLATION AND DEHYDROXYLATION. Administration of ring-labeled 2-FAA to animals causes a higher binding of radioactivity to liver macromolecules than 2-FAA labeled in the acetyl side chain. This difference is the result of deacetylation of 2-FAA to give 2-FA-bound residues. Some enzymes identified can deacetylate both 2-FAA and *N*-hydroxy-2-FAA.

One such enzyme in rats is localized in the liver cell soluble fraction and can be inhibited by fluoride ions (*133*). Two deacetylating enzymes have been identified in guinea pig microsomes. One of these enzymes deacetylates *N*-hydroxy-2-FAA 265 times faster than 2-FAA, while the other enzyme has a similar activity for both substrates (*134*). A dehydroxylating enzyme has also been found in the cell soluble fraction of rat liver. It was comparatively labile and lost activity after a 60-min incubation at 37 °C (*132*). Deacetylation could be considered under certain circumstances to be an activation step, particularly in organs where transacetylation could occur.

Reactions of Aromatic Amines with Macromolecules. 2-FLUORENYLACETAMIDE. Reaction of 2-FAA with macromolecules was first demonstrated by Williard and Irving (*135*) and Marroquin and Farber (*136*) using [9-^{14}C]2-FAA or [9-^{14}C]2-fluorenylacetylhydroxamic acid. The nature of the binding was established by Lotlikar et al. (*137*), who reacted *N*-acetoxy-2-FAA with glycylmethionine and methionine and deduced that a methionium intermediate was formed and, in the former instance, split and rearranged to 3-methylmercapto-2-FAA (**30**) and homoserine lactone in equimolar amounts. Similar experiments by Kriek et al. (*138*) with *N*-acetoxy-2-FAA and guanosine revealed *N*-2-(8-guanyl)-FAA (**44**) as the major bound form, after the mild acid hydrolysis to remove the ribose group.

Esters of *N*-hydroxy-2-FAA have been used to synthesize marker compounds to characterize the nucleic acid adducts formed in vivo after administration of

2-FAA or its hydroxamic acid. Using [9-^{14}C]*N*-hydroxy-2-[2′-^{3}*H*]acetylaminofluorene, Irving et al. (*139*) demonstrated that 70% of the covalently bound adducts with DNA in rat liver did not carry the acetyl group. The deacetylated adduct appears not to arise from deacetylation of the acetyl adduct, because no deacetylase activity could be detected in rat liver nuclei. Approximately 80% of the 2-FAA residues in rat liver DNA have been identified as *N*-2-(8-deoxyguanosyl)-FAA (**44**) (*140–42*). The remaining fraction of the FAA residues in rat liver DNA have been identified by Westra et al. (*143*) as 3-(*N*-deoxyguanosyl)-2-FAA (**45**). The deacetylated derivative of 2-FAA is unstable but has been characterized as *N*-2-(8-deoxyguanosyl)-FA (**46**) (*144*). This adduct breaks down under alkaline conditions to form two pyrimidine derivatives through breakage of the 7,8-guanine bond.

Studies on the removal of the various 2-FAA adducts from rat liver DNA have demonstrated that the *C*-adduct has a half-life of 7 d while the *N*-adduct is persistent. Decomposition of the *C*-fluorenylamine adduct may occur in vivo leading to the possible formation of apurinic sites. In vitro the ring-opening reaction is catalyzed by an alkaline pH, by Mg^{2+} and Mn^{2+} ions, and by alkaline phosphatase from *Escherichia coli* (*144*).

Formation of the *C*-guanine-FA adduct in DNA could occur either through direct reaction of *N*-hydroxy-2-FA with DNA, which is unlikely under physiological conditions (*44*), or through some reactive ester of *N*-hydroxy-2-FA such as the *O*-glucuronide (*27*) or acetoxy ester (*56*).

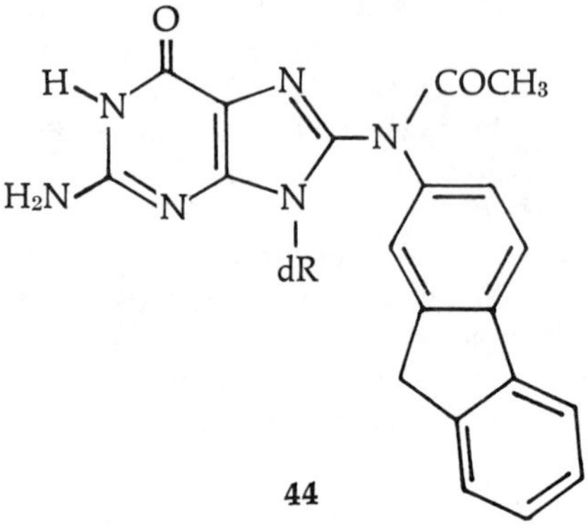

44

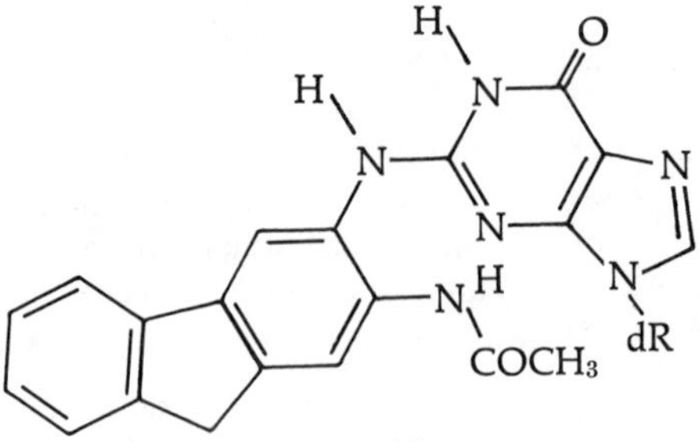

45

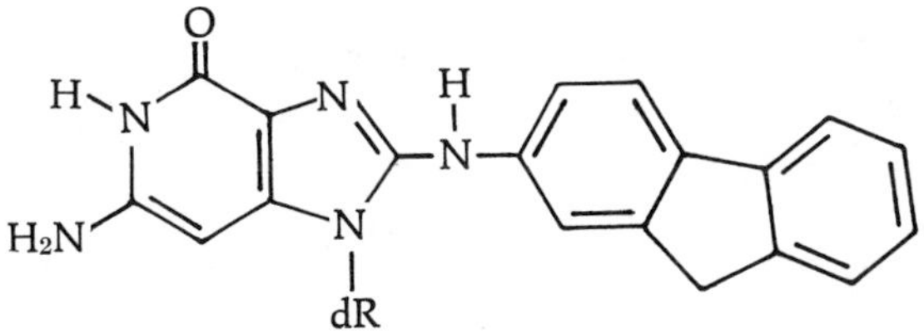

46

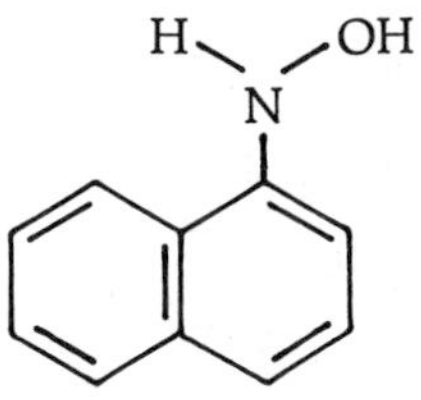

47

1-NAPHTHYLAMINE (1-NA). Reaction of *N*-hydroxy-1-naphthylamine (**47**) with DNA in vitro under slightly acidic conditions yields three adducts that have been characterized by Kadlubar et al. (*46*). The reaction proceeds via a nitrenium ion with overall second-order kinetics; the rate is dependent on both the hydroxylamine and the DNA concentration. Binding occurred in the following order: DNA > polyguanylic acid > denatured DNA and ribosomal DNA > polyadenylic acid. The major adduct formed in DNA was characterized as *N*-(*O*-deoxyguanosinyl)-1-naphthylamine (**48**) and a minor adduct as 2-(*O*-deoxyguanosinyl)-1-naphthylamine (**49**), together with a decomposition product. No evidence has yet been published showing these adducts to be formed on administration of 1-naphthylamine or its oxidation products to animals.

2-NAPHTHYLAMINE. *N*-Hydroxy-2-naphthylamine reacts with a variety of macromolecules under mildly acidic conditions (*47*). The extent of reaction is in the order polyguanylic acid > DNA > protein > RNA > polyadenylic acid > polyuridylic acid. At pH 7, reaction only occurred with protein. Enzymic hydrolysis of DNA that had reacted with *N*-hydroxy-2-NA revealed three nucleoside adducts. These adducts have been identified as 1-(*N*-deoxyguanosinyl)-2-NA (**50**), 2(*N*-deoxyguanosinyl)-2-NA (**51**), and a purine ring-opened derivative of *N*-(8-deoxyguanosinyl)-2-NA, tentatively identified as 1,5-(2,6-diamino-4-oxo)pyrimid-

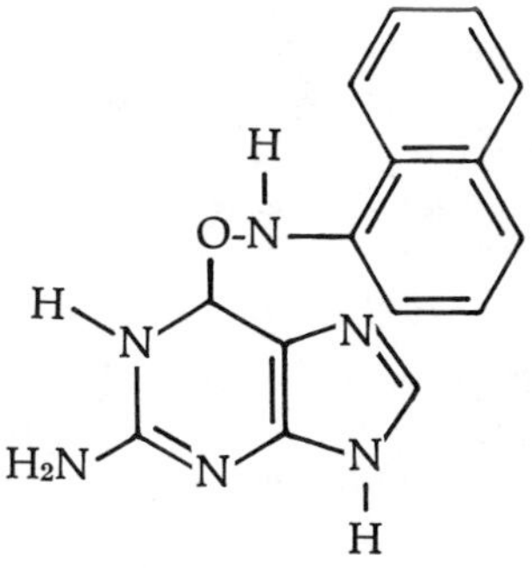

48

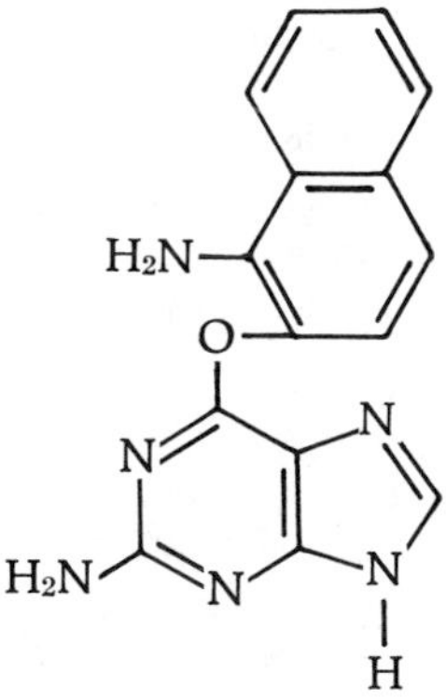

49

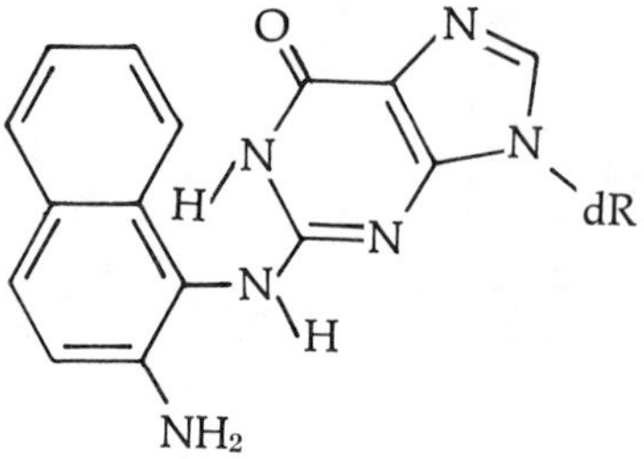

50

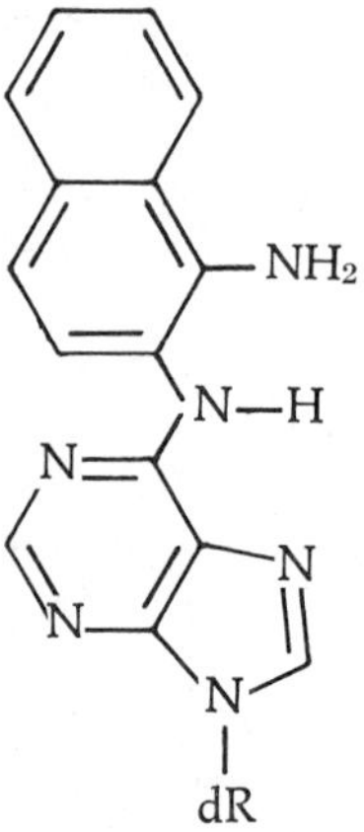

51

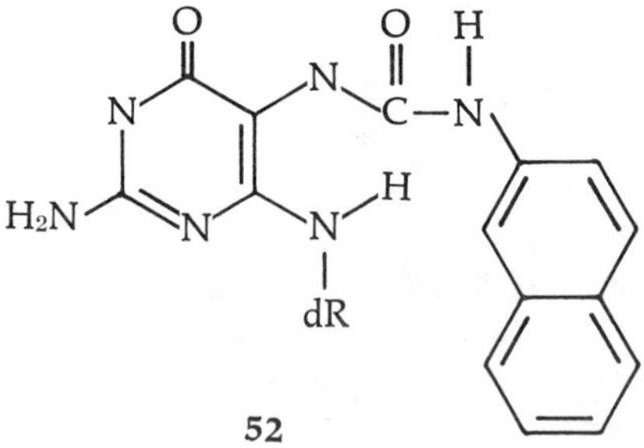

52

inyl-*N*-deoxyriboside-3-(2-naphthylurea) (**52**). Similar adducts to those obtained in vitro have not as yet been identified in vivo after 2-NA administration.

2-PHENANTHRYLACETAMIDE (PAA). *N*-Acetoxy-2-PAA reacts more slowly than its fluorene analog with methionine and guanosine (*145*); therefore, *N*-acetoxy-2-PAA reacts with adenosine and guanosine with equal affinity. The guanosine reaction occurs at the *C*-position to yield *N*-(8-deoxyguanosinyl)-2-PAA (**53**), while with adenosine the major adduct is 1-(*N*-deoxyadenosinyl)-2-PAA (**54**). These adducts are also formed when *N*-acetoxy-2-PAA reacts with DNA. Similar adducts have not been found in rat liver DNA after administration of 2-PAA (*146*).

N,N-DIMETHYL-4-PHENYLAZOANILINE (4-DIMETHYLAMINOAZOBENZENE; DAB). Reaction of *N*-benzoyloxy-*N*-methyl-4-phenylazoaniline, a synthetic ester of DAB, with deoxyguanosine yields a number of products, including *N*-methyl-*N*-(8-deoxyguanosinyl)-4-phenylazoaniline (**55**) (*108*). A similar adduct is found in liver DNA when DAB is fed to rats (*147*). A further major guanine adduct is found in vivo, however, in which the guanine is substituted at the extra-amino nitrogen, i.e., *N*-methyl-3-(*N*-

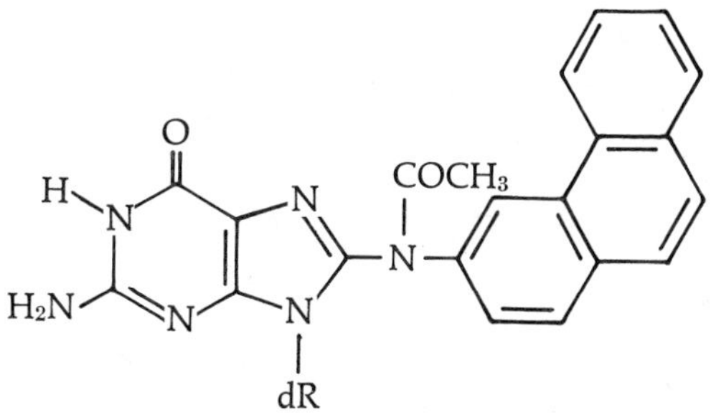

53

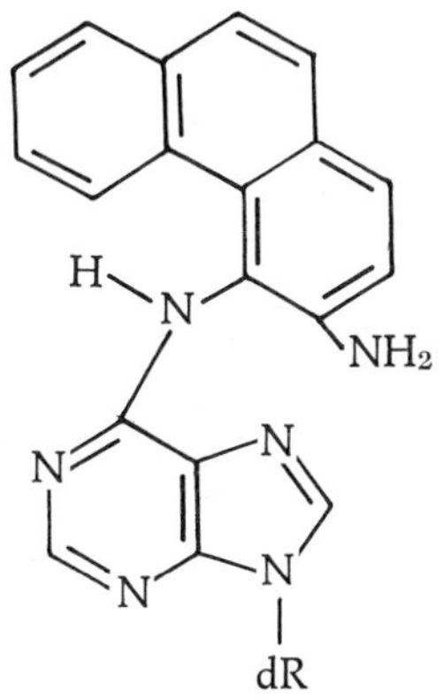

54

deoxyguanosinyl)-4-phenylazoaniline (**56**) (*148*). The *N*-benzoyloxy ester also reacts in vitro with deoxyadenosine but the structure of the adduct has not been elucidated (*149*).

4-BIPHENYLACETAMIDE. Both the sulfate esters of *N*-hydroxy-4-BPAA and its 4′-fluoro derivative react with DNA in vitro to give *C*- or *N*-deoxyguanosine adducts (**57**) and (**58**) (*105, 150*). Levels of binding for these two esters are considerably lower than those seen with the equivalent FAA ester. Administration of *N*-hydroxy-4-BPAA to rats gives the same esters, but binding levels to DNA are some 20 times lower than those seen with *N*-hydroxy-2-FAA.

4-STILBENYLACETAMIDE (SAA). *N*-Acetoxy-4-SAA yields a large number of derivatives in reactions with guanosine, adenosine, or cytidine in aqueous solution (*151*). Some of these derivatives have been characterized. Reaction with cytidine yields a deaminated product in which the stilbene residue is attached at a bridgehead carbon (**59**). Reaction with guanosine also gives a bridgehead reacted adduct at the *N*-position of guanine (**60**). Two adenosine derivatives are found; one adduct is unusual in the formation of a new five-membered ring (**61**), and the other adduct is formed through attack of the extra amino group by a carbonium ion at a bridgehead carbon (**62**). The cytidine and one of the adenine adducts formed in vitro are also found in vivo after administration of 4-SAA (*152*). The types of adduct formed with this carcinogen are not typical of those seen for other aromatic amines and resemble those more usually seen with alkylating agents.

BENZIDINE. *N*-OH-*N*′-acetylbenzidine (**63**) has been synthesized as a model to generate the presumptive ultimate carcinogenic nitremium ion. Reaction with DNA in vitro followed by enzymic hydrolysis to the nucleoside level has resulted in the generation of a single adduct. This adduct has been identified by mass and NMR spectroscopy as *N*-(deoxyguanosin-8-yl)-*N*′-acetylbenzidine. The same adduct was shown to be produced in rat liver DNA following intraperitoneal administration of benzidine to male Sprague–Dawley rats (*96*).

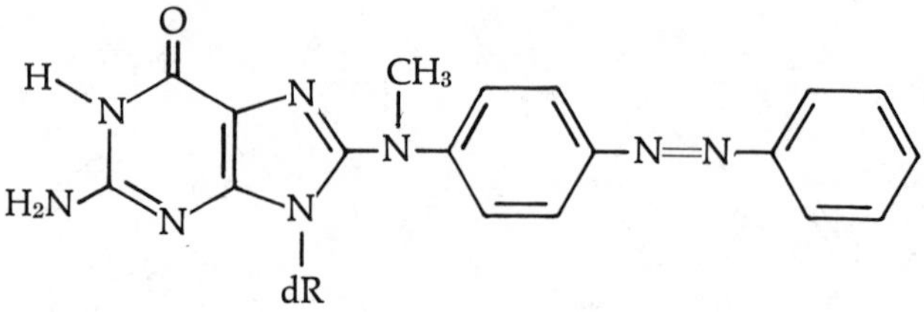

H N O N CH3 N N=N H2N N N dR

55

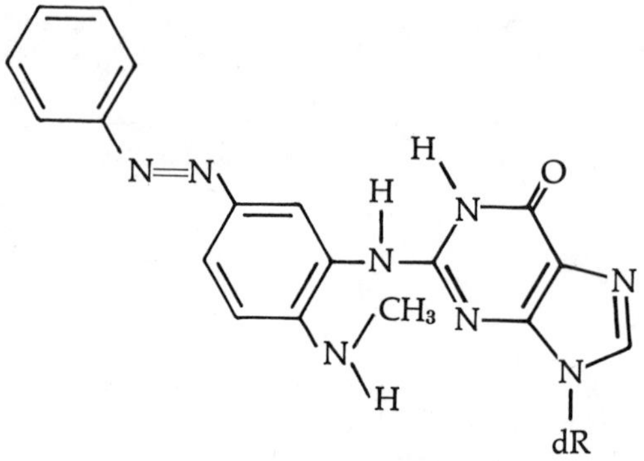

N=N H H O N N CH3 N N N H dR

56

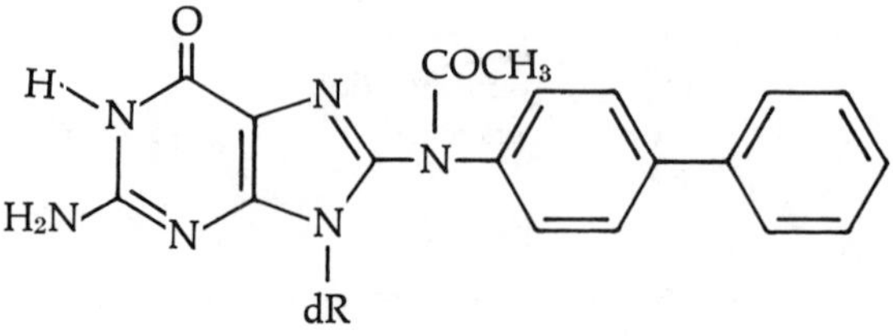

O COCH3 H N N N H2N N N dR

57

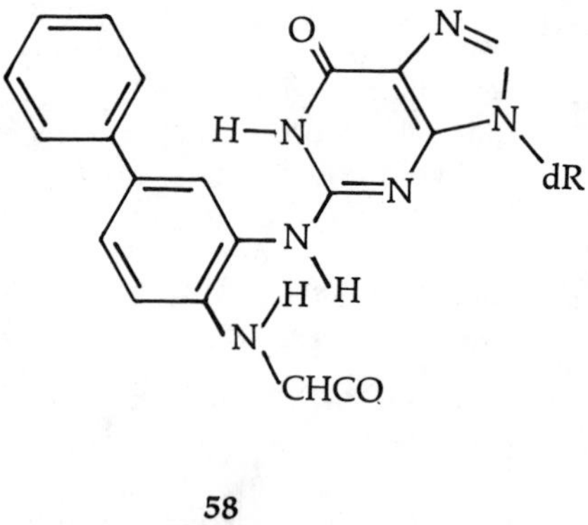

O N= H—N N dR N N H H N CHCO

58

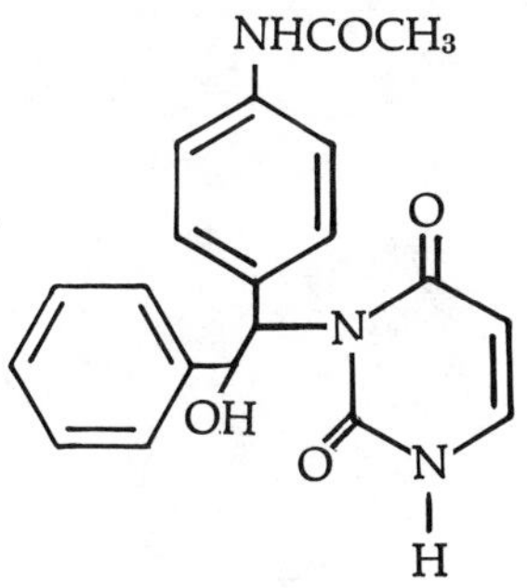

NHCOCH3 OH O N O N H

59

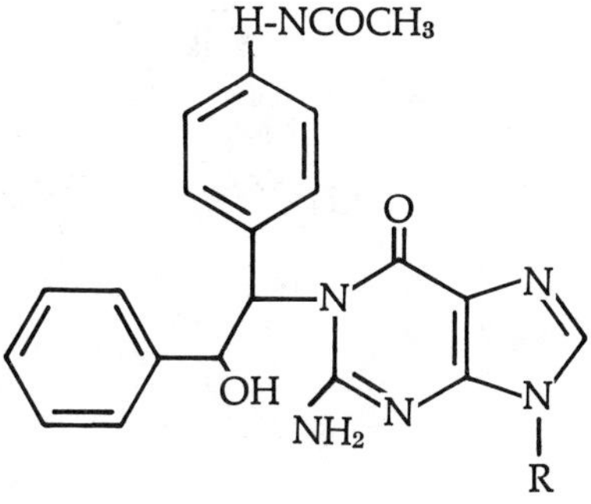

H-NCOCH3 O N N OH NH2 N N R

60

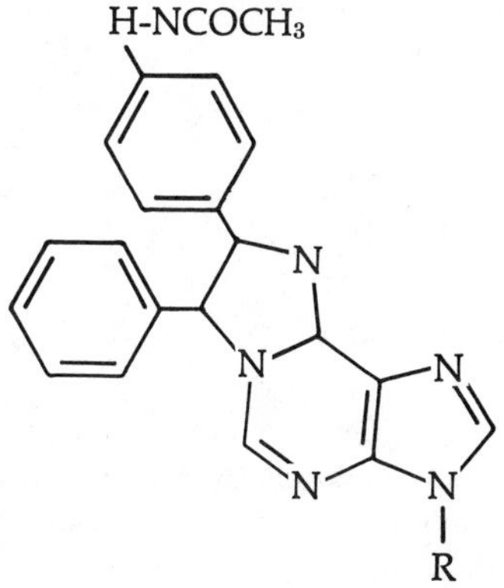

H-NCOCH3 N N N N N R

61

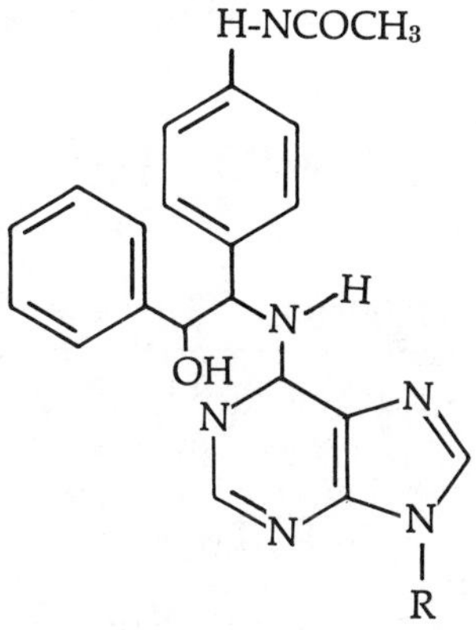

H-NCOCH3 N H OH N N N N R

62

H2N OH H N O C O

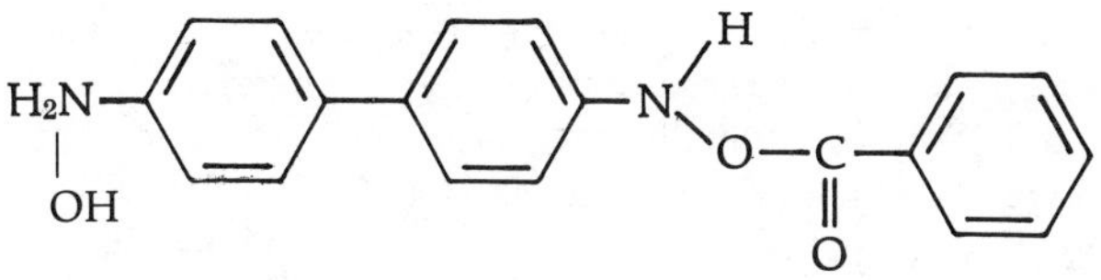

63

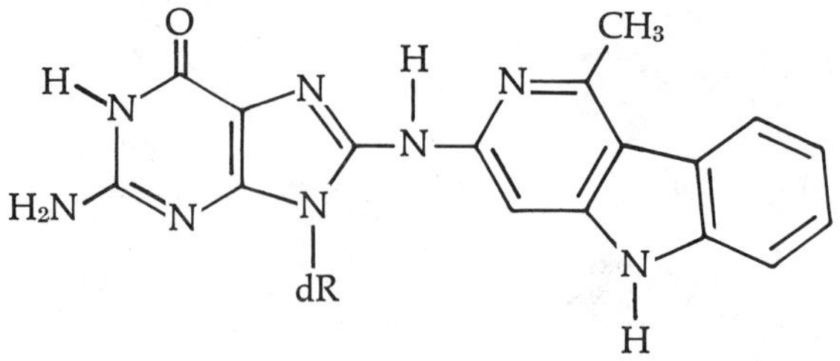

64

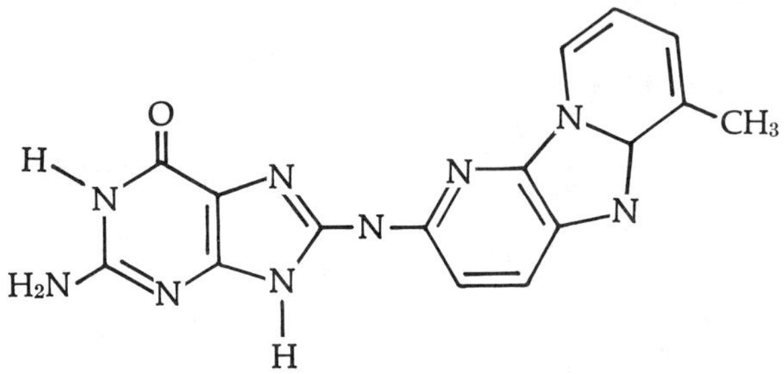

65

Heterocyclic Amines. Although a large number of heterocyclic amines are known and some have produced tumors on feeding to animals, only a few have been investigated as to their DNA reaction products. 3-Amino-1-methyl-5*H*-pyrido[4,3-*b*]indole (Trp-P-2), a pyrolysis product of tryptophan, binds to DNA in vitro after microsomal metabolism to give as one of the adducts guanine substituted at the *C*-position (*153*). This product has been characterized and assigned the structure 3-(*C*-guanyl)amino-1-methyl-5*H*-pyrido[4,3-*b*]indole (**64**). Another pyrolysis product, 2-amino-6-methylpyrido[1,2-*a*:3′,3′-*d*]imidazole (Glu-P-1), this time from glutamine, also binds to DNA in a rat liver microsomal mediated reaction to give a guanine adduct substituted at the C-8 position, namely 2-(C^8-guanyl)amino-6-methyldipyrido[1,2-*a*:3′,2′-*d*]imidazole (**65**) (*154*).

The nitrofurans represent another class of heterocyclic amines with proven carcinogenicity. Although a large number of these compounds have been tested for carcinogenicity by Bryan and colleagues, little attention has been directed toward analyzing the products of reaction with nucleic acids. 1-(2-Hydroxyethyl)-2-methyl-5-nitroimidazole (**66**) has been shown to be activated by reducing agents such as sodium dithionite. The compounds generated are unstable and react specifically with either guanine or cytosine in DNA (*155*).

4-Nitroquinoline 1-oxide (NQO) does not react covalently with DNA in vitro, but it does associate with DNA and various polynucleotides. The magnitude of binding decreased in the following order: native DNA > polyA > apyrimidinic acid > denatured DNA > apurinic acid. This finding indicates that NQO associates with purine rather than pyrimidine bases (*156*). Analysis of DNA after reaction

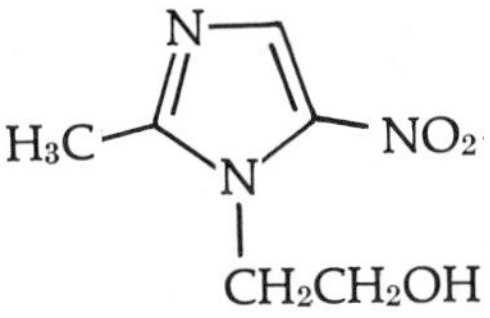

66

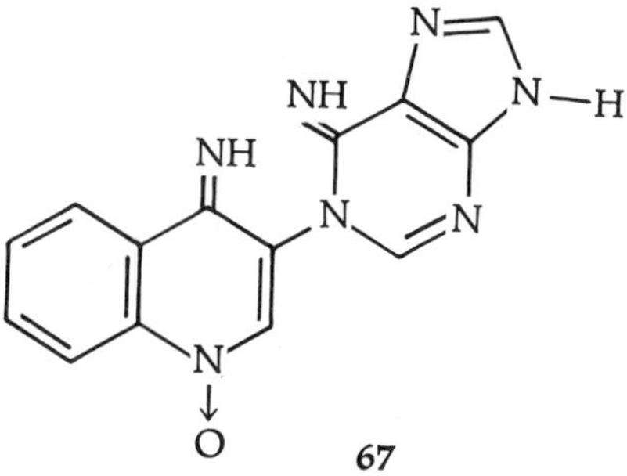

67

with 4-HAQO, a postulated active metabolite of NQO, revealed the presence of three adducts, two of which were with guanine and one with adenine. The adenine adduct, which is the major one, is 4-nitroquinoline-3-(1-adenyl)-2-oxide (**67**) (*157*).

Structure–Activity Relationships

The carcinogenic potential of the many aromatic amines that have been tested for their ability to induce cancer is discussed in this section. The basic information is recorded in the various volumes published by the U.S. Public Health Service, the scientific literature, the technical reports of the American National Cancer Institute bioassay program, and the International Agency for Research on Cancer monographs.

The different molecular types discussed in this section all have one thing in common: in each case they are metabolically activated to aryl hydroxylamines or related compounds. In compiling data on these compounds that have been shown to be carcinogenic, we have eliminated results in which insufficient numbers of animals were used and those in which the authors, for one reason or another, failed to maintain the animals for enough time to develop tumors. Furthermore, certain techniques and types of tumors—such as local sarcomas formed in response to the subcutaneous injection of some test substances and bladder tumors after bladder implantation—present difficulties in interpretation. What remains is not claimed to be comprehensive, but demonstrates the major groups of active compounds so far identified.

Anilines. Early experiments that purported to show that aniline was carcinogenic were disputed by Bonser (*158*), who drew attention to the inadequacy of the histopathological description of the lesions. Further investigation of this substance was discouraged by the demonstration, which used epidemiological methods, that aniline was not a bladder carcinogen in workers exposed during its manufacture, purification, or use (*4*). This finding does not discount aniline-induced cancer at other sites. Recent animal studies have shown that aniline is indeed a carcinogen; it induces tumors of the spleen in rats but not in mice (Table I).

The consumption of excessive quantities of analgesics containing phenacetin (**34**), antipyrine (**68**), and caffeine (**69**), particularly in Sweden, may be an example of a single-ring aromatic amine inducing cancer in humans. Analgesic abuse

Table I

Carcinogenicity of Aniline and Its Derivatives

			Sites of Tumor Induction[a]							
Compound	*Species*	*Adequacy*[b]	*Local*	*Bladder*	*Kidney*	*Liver*	*Intestine*	*Ear Duct*	*Breast*	*Other*
Analine	rat	NCI	–	–	–	–	–	–	–	spleen (?)
	mouse	NCI	–	–	–	–	–	–	–	–
o-Toluidine	rat	NCI,S	–	+	–	–	–	–	+[c]	spleen(?)
	mouse	NCI,S	–	–	–	+	–	–	–	vascular,(SC)
m-Toluidine	rat	S	–	–	–	–	–	–	–	–
	mouse	S	–	–	–	+	–	–	–	–
p-Toluidine	rat	S	–	–	–	–	–	–	–	–
	mouse	S	–	–	–	+	–	–	–	–
2,4-Xylidine	rat	S	–	–	–	–	–	–	–	–
	mouse	S	–	–	–	–	–	–	–	lung(?)
2,5-Xylidine	rat	S	–	–	–	–	–	–	–	–
	mouse	S	–	–	–	?	–	–	–	vascular(?)
2,4,5-Trimethylaniline	rat	S	–	–	–	–	–	–	–	–
	mouse	S	–	–	–	+	–	–	–	–
2,4,6-Trimethylaniline	rat	NCI,S	–	–	–	+	–	–	–	lung
	mouse	SCI,S	–	–	–	+	–	–	–	vascular
p-Chloroaniline	rat	NCI	–	–	–	–	–	–	–	spleen
	mouse	NCI	–	–	–	–	–	–	–	vascular
3-Chloro-*p*-toluidine	rat	NCI,A	–	–	–	–	–	–	–	–
	mouse	NCI,A	–	–	–	–	–	–	–	–

4-Chloro-*o*-toluidine	rat	NCI,A	−	−	−	−	−	−	−	−
	mouse	NCI,A	−	−	−	−	−	−	−	vascular
5-Chloro-*o*-toluidine	rat	NCI	−	−	−	−	−	−	−	−
	mouse	NCI	−	−	−	−	−	−	−	vascular
2,4,6-Trichloroaniline	rat	S	−	−	−	−	−	−	−	−
	mouse	S	−	−	−	−	−	−	−	vascular
2,3,5,6-Tetrachloro-4-nitroanisole	rat	NCI	−	−	−	−	−	−	−	−
	mouse	NCI	−	−	−	−	−	−	−	−
2-Nitrochlorobenzene	rat	S	−	−	−	−	−	−	−	−
	mouse	S	−	−	−	−	−	−	−	vascular
o-Anisidine	rat	NCI	−	−	−	−	−	−	−	skin; lung
	mouse	NCI	−	−	−	−	−	−	−	−
m-Cresidine	rat	NCI	−	+	−	−	−	−	−	−
	mouse	NCI	−	−	−	−	−	−	−	−
p-Ethoxyacetanilide	rat	S	−	−	−	−	−	+	+(?)	−
N-Hydroxy-*p*-ethoxyacetanilide	rat	S	−	−	−	+	−	−	−	−
p-Cresidine	rat	NCI	−	+	−	−	−	−	−	olfactory
	mouse	NCI	−	+	−	+	−	−	−	−
2,4-Dimethoxyaniline	rat	NCI	−	−	−	−	−	−	−	−
	mouse	NCI	−	−	−	−	−	−	−	−
4-Nitroanthranilic acid	rat	NCI	−	−		−	−	−	−	−
	mouse	NCI	−	−	−	−	−	−	−	−

NOTE: All compounds were administered orally.
[a]+, tumors reported; −, tumors not reported; and ?, evidence equivocal.
[b]A, tested in more than one institute; S, evidence less convincing; and NCI, tested as part of the bioassay program.
[c]Benign tumors only.

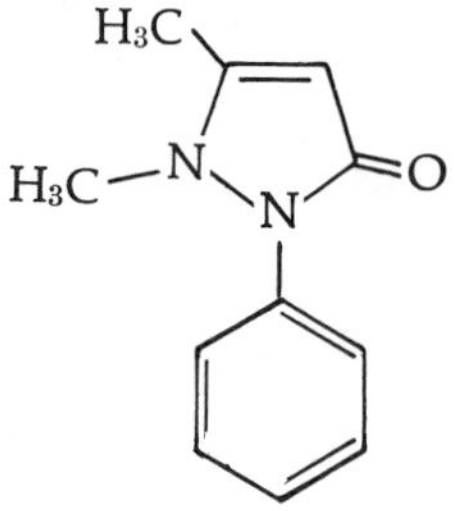

68

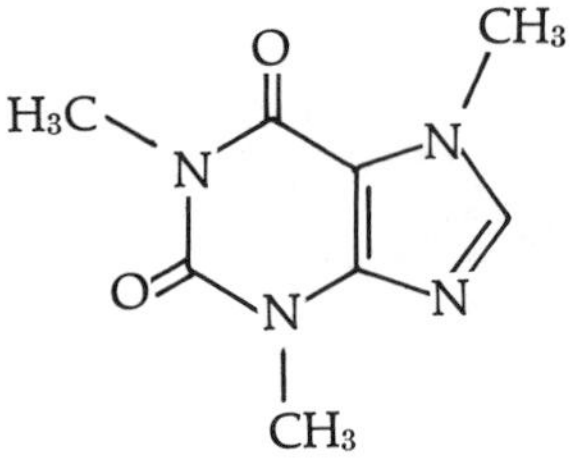

69

became part of folk medicine in some districts of Sweden after World War I. Some individuals are known to have ingested amounts in excess of 1 kg over several years. These quantities may result in renal papillary necrosis. Bengsston et al. (*159*) noted that renal pelvic cancer was also associated with excessive consumption of the drug. Of 242 patients with renal papillary necrosis, 142 were abusers. All cases of renal pelvic cancer occurred in the latter group, thus establishing a correlation between analgesic abuse and this form of cancer; there were also a few instances of bladder cancer. Bengsston and colleagues also showed that renal pelvic cancer in abusers occurred at an earlier age than similar tumors in instances where the etiology was unknown. There are two difficulties in assessing this evidence. First, little information is available about similar conditions in countries other than Sweden, although cases of urinary tract carcinoma associated with excessive consumption of analgesics have been reported from Australia (*160*) and the United States (*161*). Second, no evidence suggests which components in the analgesic lead to the tumors. Bengsston et al. (*159*) indicted phenacetin, and this speculation is supported by the known predilection of the carcinogenic aromatic amines for the urinary tract in humans.

Further support for indicting phenacetin as a human carcinogen has come from Australia, where in a series of 88 cases of kidney carcinoma, 42% were considered to be chronic analgesic users. Other compounding factors such as smoking or long-standing urinary tract infection could not be discounted (*162*).

The potent mutagenicity of various single-ring aromatic amines (*163, 164*) indicates that this group of chemicals may as a class be animal carcinogens. However, no satisfactory evidence to date has shown that any of them are human carcinogens. Nevertheless, the animal studies suggest that care should be taken in handling and using single-ring aromatic amines.

Both aniline hydrochloride (**70**) and *p*-chloroaniline (**71**) induced splenic tumors in rats (Table I). In earlier experiments that used small numbers of animals, phenylhydroxylamine (**11**) was noncarcinogenic, as were two of its analogs (*22*). These experiments were inadequate because of the short survival time of the animals. *N*-Hydroxyphenacetin (**72**), on the other hand, induced liver tumors (*165*) rather than splenic tumors in rats. Phenylhydroxylamines can oxidize hemoglobin to methemoglobin, and because the spleen is intimately involved in red blood cell metabolism, it is perhaps not surprising that tumors of the spleen arise through aniline exposure.

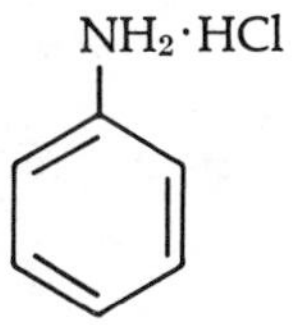

$NH_2 \cdot HCl$ NH_2 CH_3CO OH N Cl OC_2H_5

70 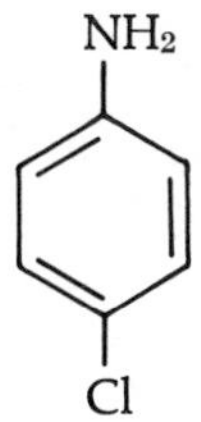 **71** 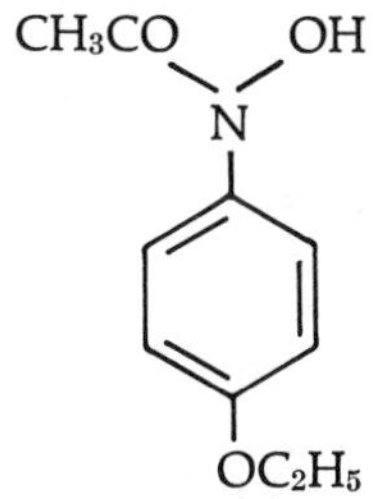 **72**

Phenacetin is carcinogenic to the ear duct and probably the mammary gland in rats (*166*). It is converted in vivo to *N*-hydroxyphenacetin, which induces liver tumors. Why the parent compound induces tumors in one organ and its derivative, the postulated carcinogenic species, induces tumors in another organ is not known.

A wide range of single-ring aromatic amines has been tested for carcinogenic potential in the National Cancer Institute bioassay program, and the results obtained are listed in Tables I and II (*167*). No common structural features are immediately obvious for this group of compounds, although the reactive species are likely to be hydroxylamines. Factors that would effect carcinogenicity for this group would include lipid solubility, blocked positions to ring hydroxylation, electron withdrawing or donating nature of ring substituents, etc.

Extended Anilines. 4-BIPHENYLAMINES (BPAs). The carcinogenicity of 4-BPA in humans has already been mentioned. This chemical provides a useful example of a substance that produces varied responses in different experimental species, and this characteristic indicates that the substance needs metabolic activation to exert its action. Thus Walpole and his colleagues (*168*) showed that BPA was a powerful bladder carcinogen in dogs. In rats, BPA induced mainly intestinal and mammary tumors later in life (*169*). The results in dogs were confirmed by Deichmann et al. (*170*), who also demonstrated that as little as 1 mg/kg body weight/d of BPA induced bladder carcinomas and papillomas within 33 months in all six dogs tested (*171*), but that a single dose was ineffective (*172*). 2-Naphthylamine, which is also a powerful bladder carcinogen in dogs (*see* page 211), was not effective under the former conditions. The same workers also showed that 4-nitrobiphenyl was carcinogenic to the dog bladder (*173*). BPA is only weakly carcinogenic in mice; it induced a low incidence of bladder tumors in two strains of mice and liver tumors in one strain (*174, 175*). In rabbits, however, BPA induced bladder tumors in 2 to 5 years (*176*).

Results of experiments that tested the derivatives of BPA (Table III) illustrate some of the apparent generalizations that apply to other types of aromatic amines. For example, the position of the amino group relative to the biphenyl appears to be important. Miller et al. (*177*) demonstrated that both BPA and 4-BPAA have moderate carcinogenicity in the rat, but in the same experiment, 3- and 2-BPAA appeared to be only weakly carcinogenic in the rat, the only species tested. This result reflects the general observation that aromatic amines that have a conjugated

Table II

Carcinogenicity of Phenylenediamines and Related Substances

Compound	Species	Adequacy[b]	Sites of Tumor Induction[a]							
			Local	Bladder	Kidney	Liver	Intestine	Ear Duct	Breast	Other
o-Phenylenediamine	rat	S	–	–	–	?	–	–	–	–
	mouse	S	–	–	–	+	–	–	–	–
m-Phenylenediamine	rat	S	–	–	–	–	–	–	–	–
	mouse	S	–	–	–	–	–	–	–	–
p-Phenylenediamine	rat	NCI	–	–	–	–	–	–	–	–
	mouse	NCI	–	–	–	–	–	–	–	–
Tetrafluoro-*m*-phenylenediamine	rat	S	–	–	–	–	–	–	–	–
	mouse	S	–	–	–	+	–	–	–	–
2,4-Toluenediamine	rat	NCI,S	–	–	–	+	–	–	+	subcutaneous
	mouse	NCI,S	–	–	–	–	–	–	–	vascular lymph(?)
2,5-Toluenediamine	rat	NCI,S	–	–	–	–	–	–	–	–
	mouse	NCI	–	–	–	–	–	–	–	–
2,6-Toluenediamine	rat	NCI	–	–	–	–	–	–	–	–
	mouse	NCI	–	–	–	–	–	–	–	–
2,4-Diaminoanisole	rat	NCI	–	–	–	–	–	–	–	skin; thyroid
	mouse	NCI	–	–	–	–	–	–	–	thyroid
5-Nitro-*o*-toluidine	rat	NCI	–	–	–	–	–	–	–	–
	mouse	NCI	–	–	–	–	–	–	–	vascular
5-Nitro-*o*-anisidine	rat	NCI	–	–	–	–	–	+	–	various glands
	mouse	NCI	–	–	–	–	–	–	–	–
2,4-Dinitrotoluene	rat	NCI	–	–	–	–	–	–	+[c]	–
	mouse	NCI	–	–	–	–	–	–	–	–

4-Nitro-*o*-phenylenediamine	rat	NCI	–	–	–	–	–	–	–	–
	mouse	NCI	–	–	–	–	–	–	–	–
2-Nitro-*p*-phenylenediamine	rat	NCI	–	–	–	–	–	–	–	–
	mouse	NCI	–	–	–	–	–	–	–	–
4-Chloro-*o*-phenylenediamine	rat	NCI	–	–	–	–	–	–	–	forestomach
	mouse	NCI	–	–	–	–	–	–	–	–
4-Chloro-*m*-phenylenediamine	rat	NCI	–	–	–	–	–	–	–	adrenal
	mouse	NCI	–	–	–	+	–	–	–	–
2-Chloro-*p*-phenylenediamine	rat	NCI	–	–	–	–	–	–	–	–
	mouse	NCI	–	–	–	–	–	–	–	–
1-Chloro-2,4-dinitrobenzene	rat	S	–	–	–	–	–	–	–	–
	mouse	S	–	–	–	–	–	–	–	–
3-Nitro-*p*-acetophenetidine	rat	NCI	–	–	–	–	–	–	–	–
	mouse	NCI	–	–	–	+	–	–	–	–
N-Phenyl-*p*-phenylenediamine	rat	NCI	–	–	–	–	–	–	–	–
	mouse	NCI	–	–	–	–	–	–	–	–
4-Amino-2-nitrophenol	rat	NCI	–	+	–	–	–	–	–	–
	mouse	NCI	–	–	–	–	–	–	–	–

NOTE: All compounds were administered orally.
[a]+, tumor reported; –, tumor not reported; and ?, evidence equivocal.
[b]A, tested in more than one institute; S, evidence less than convincing; and NCI, tested as part of the bioassay program.
[c]Benign tumors only.

Table III

Carcinogenicity of 4-Biphenylamine and Its Derivatives

Compound	Species	Route[b]	Adequacy[c]	Site of Tumor Induction[a]							
				Local	*Bladder*	*Kidney*	*Liver*	*Intestine*	*Ear Duct*	*Breast*	*Other*
4-Biphenylamine	mouse	o	S	−	?	−	+	−	−	−	−
	rat	o	A	−	−	−	?	?	−	+	−
	hamster	o		−	−	−	−	−	−	−	−
	rabbit	o	S	−	+	−	−	−	−	−	−
	dog	o	A	−	+	−	−	−	−	−	−
4-Biphenylhydroxylamine	mouse (newborn)	s.c.	S	−	−	−	+	−	−	−	−
N-Acetoxy-4-biphenyl-acetamide	rat	s.c.	S	+	−	−	−	−	−	−	−
4-Biphenylacetamide	rat	o	A	−	−	−	−	+	+	+	−
4-Biphenyldimethylamine	rat	o	S	−	−	−	−	+	+	+	−
4-Nitrobiphenyl	dog	o	A	−	+	−	−	−	−	−	−
4-Biphenylacethydroxamic acid	rat	o	A	+	−	−	−	−	+	+	−
2-Fluoro-4-biphenylamine	rat	o	S	−	−	−	−	−	−	+	−
2-Chloro-4-biphenylamine	rat	s.c.	S	−	−	−	−	−	−	−	−
3′-Fluoro-4-biphenylamine	rat	o	S	−	−	−	−	−	−	+	−

4′-Fluoro-4-biphenylamine	mouse	o	S	−	−	−	+	−	−	−	−
	rat	s.c.	A	−	−	+	+	+	−	−	pancreas
2-Methyl-4-biphenylamine	rat	o	S	−	−	−	−	+	+	−	−
3-Methyl-4-biphenylamine	rat	o	S	−	−	−	−	−	−	−	−
2′-Methyl-4-biphenylamine	rat	o	S	−	−	−	−	−	−	−	−
4′-Methyl-4-biphenylacetamide	rat	o	S	−	−	−	−	−	−	−	−
2′,3-Dimethyl-4-biphenylamine	rat	s.c./o	A	−	+	−	−	+	+	+	salivary gland
3,3′-Dimethyl-4-biphenylamine	rat	s.c.	S	−	−	−	−	+	−	−	salivary gland
2′,3,5′-Trimethyl-4-biphenylamine	rat	s.c.	S	−	−	−	+	+	−	−	−
2′,3,4′,6′-Tetramethyl-4-biphenylamine	rat	s.c.	S	−	−	−	+	+	−	−	−
3-Methoxy-4-biphenylamine	rat	s.c.	S	−	+	−	−	−	−	−	−
4-Chloro-4′-aminobiphenyl ether	mouse	o	S	−	+	−	−	−	−	−	vascular
	rat	o	S	−	−	−	+	−	−	−	−
4-Chloro-4′-nitrobiphenyl ether	mouse	o	S	−	−	−	−	−	−	−	−
	rat	o	S	−	−	−	−	−	−	−	pancreas

[a] +, tumors reported; −, tumors not reported; and ?, evidence equivocal.
[b] o, oral; and s.c., subcutaneous injection.
[c] A, tested in more than one institute; and S, evidence less than convincing.

para-substituent in the same ring tend to be more carcinogenic than amines that do not have a *para*-substituent (*178*).

Substitution of a methyl group that is *ortho* to an aromatic group often enhances the carcinogenicity of an aromatic amine. The potency of 3,2′-dimethyl-BPA in the rat intestine illustrates this generalization; intestinal tumors were formed with a latency of less than 300 d in 75% of male Wistar rats after the chemical was injected subcutaneously to a total dose of 2.8–4.0 g/kg body weight (*169*). Tumors of other tissues, such as the ear duct, were also present. 1,2-Dimethylhydrazine hydrochloride, cycasin, and methylazoxymethanol acetate were also shown to induce lower intestinal tract tumors (*13*). A surgically prepared, isolated segment of colon was not susceptible to 3,2′-dimethyl-BPA-induced tumorigenesis. The result indicated that the presence of feces was necessary for tumor formation, but whether the fecal metabolite content, the mechanical properties of the feces, or the absence of gut bacteria were responsible could not be determined (*179*).

When 3,2′-dimethyl-BPA was given by subcutaneous injection to Wistar rats for limited periods, the intestinal cancer yield was almost abolished, and only a small number of bladder papillomas occurred instead. In Slonaker rats, more bladder tumors were found (*180*).

The importance to the carcinogenic action of the methyl group at the position *ortho* to the amino group is confirmed by studies of other compounds. 3-Methyl-4-BPA; 3,3′-dimethyl-4-BPA; 3,2′,5′trimethyl-4-BPA; and 3,2′,4′,6′-tetramethyl-4-BPA are carcinogenic to intestinal tract and other tissues (*169, 181, 182*), whereas 2- and 2′-methyl-BPA and their acetylated derivatives failed to induce tumors in similar experiments (*169, 177, 181*).

The effect of *ortho*-substitution other than methyl in BPA is varied. 3-Methyl-BPA is a bladder carcinogen in rats, but 3-chloro-BPA and 3-hydroxy-BPA apparently have no effect (*177, 181, 182*).

The bond between a carbon atom in an aromatic ring and fluorine is usually very strong, and fluorine substitution has been used to block metabolic hydroxylation. Ring-C-hydroxylation is believed to be a detoxification mechanism, and the finding that fluorine substitution in the ring positions where detoxifying hydroxylation occurs leads to more potent carcinogens seems to support this theory. For example, 4′-fluoro-4-BPA (**73**) with blocked 4′-hydroxylation is a more potent carcinogen than BPA. It produced tumors in most of the rats tested. These tumors included hepatomas, cholangiomas, and renal tumors, which developed within 6 months, as well as injection-site sarcomas, intestinal tract adenocarcinomas, and pancreatic and testicular tumors. Some of the pancreatic and testicular tumors were possibly unrelated to the chemical, because no untreated animals were kept as a control (*183, 184*).

N Hydroxylation of BPA as an activating step is further supported by the finding that *N*-hydroxy-BPAA induces more mammary tumors in female weanling rats than does BPAA. BPA, in contrast to some other aromatic amines, is a relatively potent toxin, and the finding that it induces methemoglobinemia in dogs is a further indication of conversion to an *N*-hydroxy derivative.

In contrast to 2-FAA, coadministration of 3-methylcholanthrene with BPAA does not greatly influence the yield of tumors induced by the amide carcinogen.

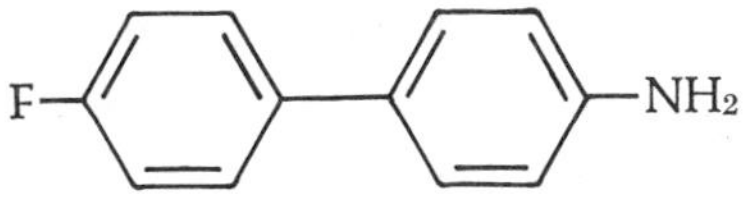

F—C6H4—C6H4—NH_2

73

N-Acetoxy-BPAA is a potent, locally acting carcinogen. BPA is a bladder carcinogen in dogs, but because this species does not acetylate aromatic amines, *N*-hydroxy-BPAA is probably not a link in the pathway leading to metabolic activation in this species. Radomski and colleagues (*185*) showed by chromatographic analysis of both classes of compound that arylhydroxylamines are easily oxidized to nitroso compounds under biological conditions. In dogs, the fraction of the dose of BPA, 2-naphthylamine, and 1-naphthylamine that was converted to hydroxylamines and nitroso compounds combined was, in this limited series, proportional to the carcinogenicity of the parent amines to the dog bladder (i.e., BPA > 2-naphthylamine > 1-naphthylamine). The active metabolite of BPA in dogs is likely to be the glucuronide of *N*-hydroxy-BPA (*87,88*), which has been obtained in solution from dog urine but decomposes on concentration. BPA serves as a model for amino derivatives of several important ring systems such as 2-FAA, 3-aminobenzofuran, and 3-aminodibenzothiophene and its oxides; FAA induces bladder tumors in mice and liver tumors in rats; 3-aminodibenzothiophene causes tumors of the pancreas in rats.

BENZIDINE (4,4′-DIAMINOBIPHENYL). Benzidine is not only carcinogenic to people who make, purify, or use it in the chemical industry (*3, 186*) but also is carcinogenic in certain animal species. The pattern, however, differs from that found with 4-BPA. Bladder tumors were found in the dog (*187*) but only in a proportion of animals after a latent period of 7 to 9 years and at a time in a dog's life when spontaneously occurring tumors are common. In rats, subcutaneously injected benzidine induced liver tumors, ear duct carcinomas, and a few adenocarcinomas of the intestine (*181*), while only hepatomas were induced in mice (*187*). In rabbits, the toxicity of benzidine prevented the administration of the dose given to other species, and comparable results could not be obtained (*176*).

Several derivatives of benzidine, such as *o*-tolidine, 3,3′-dichlorobenzidine (**74**), and *o*-dianisidine (3,3′-dimethoxybenzidine) (**75**), are important as dye intermediates and rubber- and plastic-compounding ingredients. They are often produced in batches in benzidine plants and may contribute to the environmental carcinogenic load associated with benzidine in humans. Each derivative was investigated experimentally in some depth, especially by Pliss (*188–91*) who used rats as his test species (Table IV) and induced tumors with each compound. The industrial precursor of benzidine, hydrazobenzene, is carcinogenic to rats and mice and induces a spectrum of tumors similar to those induced by benzidine. Presumably the hydrazobenzene can rearrange under the acid conditions of the stomach to benzidine.

4,4′-METHYLENEDIANILINE (DAPM) AND ANALOGS. 4,4′-Methylenedianiline (**76**) and 4,4′-methylenebis(2-chloroaniline) (DACPM, MOCA) (**77**) are used exten-

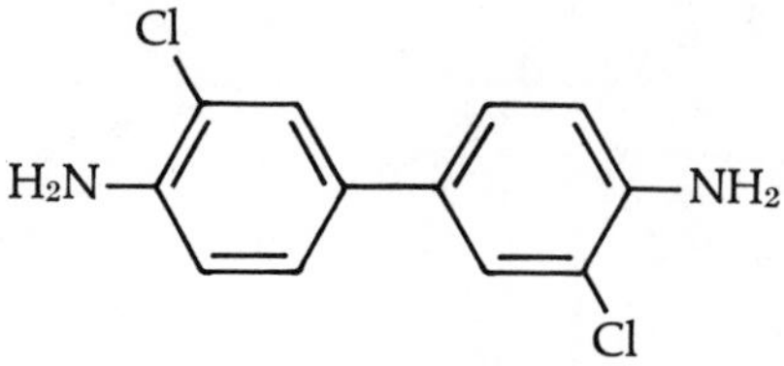

74 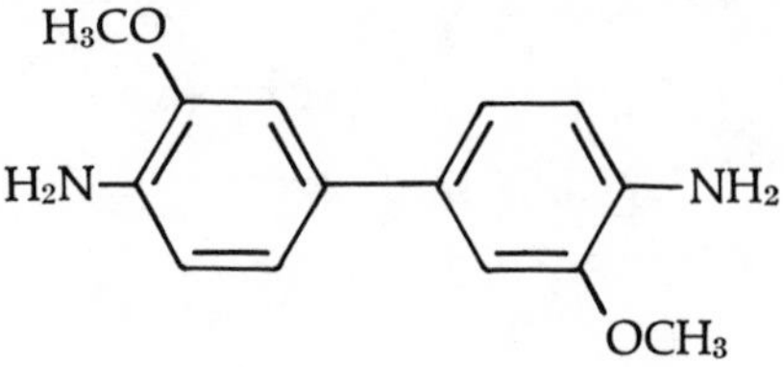 **75**

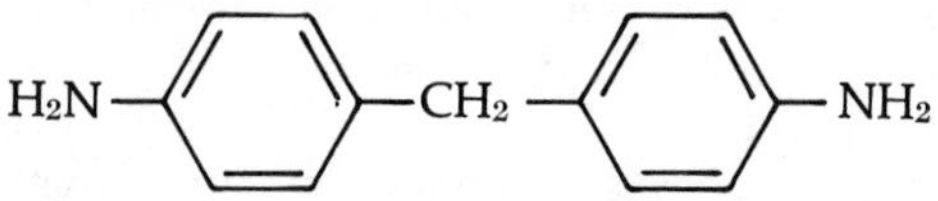

76

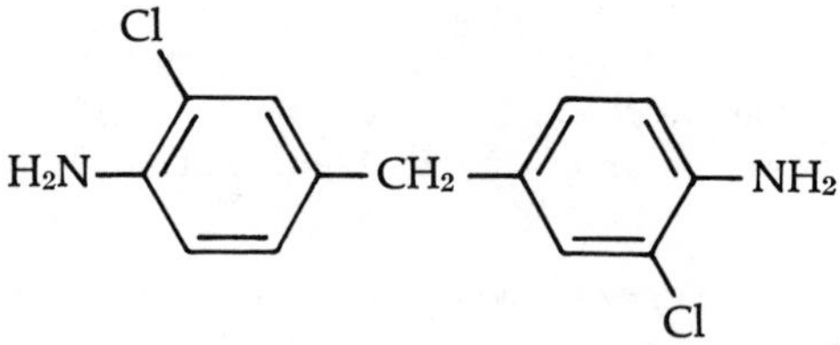

77

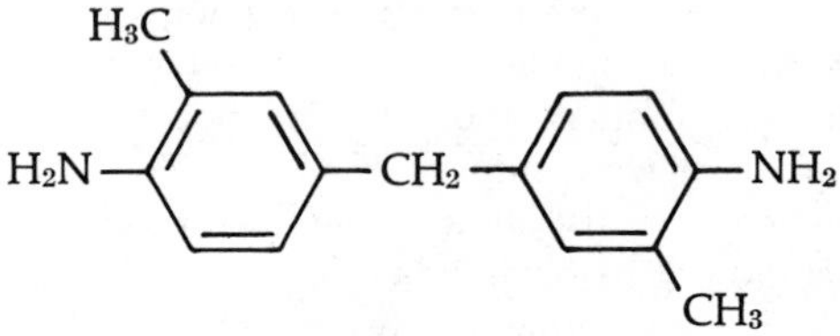

78

sively in the plastics industry, especially after conversion to the diisocyanate in the manufacture of polyurethane foams and resins. 4,4′-Methylenebis(2-methylaniline) (DAMPM) (**78**) (*192*) was used experimentally for this purpose but is not manufatured on as large a scale. These chemicals are also used to make dyes such as *p*-rosaniline.

DACPM and DAMPM are carcinogenic when high levels are administered (Table V). DAPM is hepatotoxic and therefore cannot be fed at high levels. The chance DAPM contamination of flour which was made into bread led to 84 cases of jaundice and hepatocellular necrosis in the population of an Essex town (*193*). Munn (*194*) reported that DAMPM was far more carcinogenic than DAPM in rats,

Table IV

Carcinogenicity of Benzidine and Its Derivatives

Compound	Species	Route[b]	Adequacy[c]	Site of Tumor Induction[a]							
				Local	Bladder	Kidney	Liver	Intestine	Ear Duct	Breast	Other
Benzidine	dog	o	A	−	+(?)	−	−	−	−	−	−
	hamster	o	S	−	−	−	+	−	−	−	−
	rat	s.c.	A	−	−	−	+	+	+	−	−
Diacetylbenzidine	rat	o	S	−	−	−				?	
o,o'-Tolidine	rat	s.c.	A	+	−	−	−	−	+	+	lymphoma; skin
o,o'-Dianisidine	hamster	o	S	−	?	−	−	−	−	−	forestomach
	rat	o	S	−	−	−	−	−	?	−	−
3,3'-Dichlorobenzidine	rat	o/s.c.	A	−	+	−	−	+	+	+	lymphoma; skin
	hamster	o	S	−	+	−	+	−	−	−	bone
	dog	o	S	−	+	+	−	−	−	−	−
3,3'-Diaminobenzidine	rat	o	S	−	−	+	−	−	−	−	−
	mouse	o	S	−	−	−	−	−	−	−	lung
3,3'-Dihydroxybenzidine	rat	o/s.c./top.	S	−	−	−	−	−	−	−	−
3,3'-Benzidinedicarboxylic acid	rat	s.c.	S	−	−	−	?	−	−	?	?
2-Methyldiacetylbenzidine	rat	o	S	−	−	−	−	+	+	+	−
4,4'-Thiodianiline	rat	o	NCI	−	−	−	+	+	−	−	ear canal
	mouse	o	NCI	−	−	−	+	−	−	−	thyroid glands
Hydrazobenzene	rat	o	NCI	−	−	−	+	−	+	−	
	mouse	o	NCI	−	−	−	+	−	−	−	vascular

[a] +, tumors reported; −, tumors not reported; and ?, evidence equivocal.
[b] o, oral; s.c., subcutaneous injection; and top., topical application.
[c] A, tested in more than one institute; and S, evidence less than convincing.

Table V

Carcinogenicity of Methylenedianiline and Related Compounds

				Site of Tumor Induction[a]							
Compound	*Species*	*Route*[b]	*Adequacy*[c]	*Local*	*Bladder*	*Kidney*	*Liver*	*Intestine*	*Ear Duct*	*Breast*	*Other*
4,4′-Methylenedianiline	rat	o/s.c.	A	–	–	–	?	–	–	–	–
	dog	o	S	–	–	–	–	–	–	–	–
4,4′-Methylenebis(2-methylaniline)	rat	o	A	–	–	–	+	–	–	+	lung; skin
4,4′-Methylenebis(2-chloroaniline)	rat	o.s.c.	A	–	–	–	+	–	–	–	lung
	mouse	o	S	–	–	–	+	–	–	–	hemangio-
	dog	o	S	–	+	–	–	–	–	–	sarcoma
4,4′-Methylenebis-(2-carbomethoxyaniline)	rat	o	S	–	–	+	+	–	–	–	–
4-Aminodiphenylamine	mouse	s.c.	S	–	–	–	–	–	–	–	–
Auramine	rat	o/s.c.	S	+	–	–	+	?	–	–	–
	mouse	o	S	–	–	–	+	–	–	–	–

[a] +, tumors reported; –, tumors not reported; and ?, evidence equivocal.
[b] o, oral; and s.c., subcutaneous injection.
[c] A, tested in more than one institute: and S, evidence less than convincing.

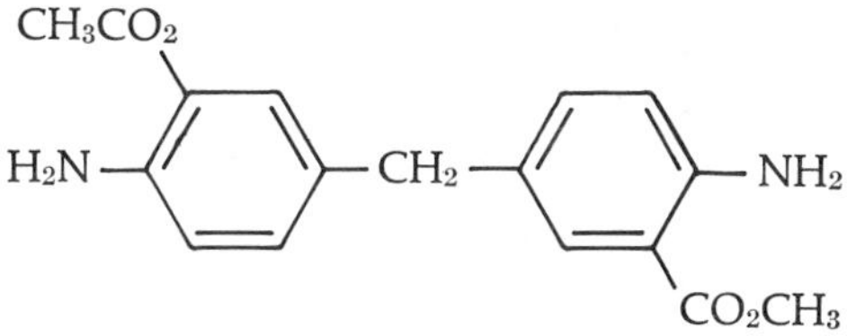

CH_3CO_2

H_2N — — CH_2 — — NH_2

CO_2CH_3

79

but because the experiment was uncontrolled, the carcinogenicity of DAPM could not be assessed. Steinhoff and Grundmann (*195*) approximately doubled the background incidence of benign and malignant tumors by the subcutaneous administration of DAPM to a total dose of 1.4 g/kg body weight over 1000 d, but whether DAPM is truly carcinogenic is not known.

Evidence for the carcinogenicity of DACPM and DAMPM comes from experiments using oral and subcutaneous administration. DACPM led to vascular and liver tumors in mice and liver and lung tumors in rats. The amount of DACPM used was high: 1000 ppm in one feeding experiment and a total dose of 25–27 g/kg of body weight in another (*196, 197*). DAMPM led to tumors of the lung, liver, mammary gland, and skin after administration by gavage to rats at a total dose of 10.2 g/kg of body weight. A third feeding experiment at 200 ppm in the diet was reported in these references, but the results were difficult to assess. A related compound, 4,4′-methylenebis(2-carbomethoxyaniline) (**79**) induced tumors of the kidney and liver when fed to rats (*197*). An epidemiological evaluation of the effect of DACPM was negative (*198*). However, because the population risk consisted of only 31 workers with defined exposure of 6 months to 16 years and 178 other DACPM workers of unstated duration of exposure who were examined cytologically, any conclusion from this study is tentative. The presence of a small unsanitary chemical plant in Adrian, Michigan, has led to widespread pollution of the locality with DACPM. Analysis demonstrated levels of 590 ppm of DACPM in surface soil samples taken from near the factory, up to 55 ppm in garden samples, and up to 18 ppm in house dust from vacuum cleaners (*199*). Values in waste water ranged from 1500 ppm in the settling lagoon sludge to 10 ppm in the Raison River (*200*). The level of human exposure is unknown (*201*), but a prospective epidemiological study in this heavily exposed population should be undertaken.

Another methylenebisaniline derivative, auramine, induces bladder cancer in humans (*3,4*). Williams and Bonser (*202*) showed that this substance was hepatocarcinogenic to rats and mice. Attempts to induce tumors in dogs (*203*) or rabbits (*176*) were unsuccessful.

Two further compounds in this series were examined by feeding rats 1.62 nmol/kg in the diet (*204*). 3-Benzylacetanilide (**80**) was without activity, whereas 4-phenylthioacetanilide (**81**) gave single tumors of the breast and intestine in nine male and nine female rats by 10 months.

STILBENAMINES. The carcinogenic activities of derivatives of 4-stilbenamine (SA) (4-aminostilbene) (**82**) and 4-stilbenylacetamide (SAA) (**19**) are listed in Table VI.

Table VI

Carcinogenic Activity of Stilbenamines and Related Compounds

Compound	*Species*	*Route*[a]	*Adequacy*[c]	*Site of Tumor Induction*[a]							
				Local	*Bladder*	*Kidney*	*Liver*	*Intestine*	*Ear Duct*	*Breast*	*Other*
4-*N*-Stilbenamine	rat	s.c./o	A	?	−	−	−	−	+	+	−
4-*N*-Stilbenylacetamide	rat	s.c./o	A	−	−	−	−	−	+	+	−
	mouse	top.	S	+	−	−	−	−	−	−	−
N-(4-Styrylphenyl)hydroxylamine	rat	s.c.	S	+	−	−	−	?	?	−	−
N-Hydroxy-4,*N*-stilbenylacetamide	rat	s.c./o/ top.	A	+	−	−	−	?	+	+	−
N-Acetoxy-4,*N*-stilbenylacetamide	rat	s.c.	S	+	−	−	−	−	+	−	−
4-Stilbenyl-*N*,*N*-dimethylamine	rat	o	A	−	−	−	−	−	+	−	−
4-Stilbenyl-*N*,*N*-diethylamine	rat	s.c.	S	−	−	−	−	−	+	−	−
2-Methyl-4-stilbenamine	rat	s.c.	S*	+	−	−	−	−	−	−	−
3-Methyl-4-stilbenamine	rat	s.c.	S*	+	−	−	−	−	−	−	−
N,*N*,2′-Trimethyl-4-stilbenamine	rat	o	S	S							
N,*N*,3′-Trimethyl-4-stilbenamine	rat	o	S	−	−	−	−	−	+	−	−
N,*N*,4′-Trimethyl-4-stilbenamine	rat	o	S	−	−	−	−	−	?	−	−
	mouse	o	S	−	−	−	+	−	−	−	−
4-(2,5-Dimethoxy)stilbenamine	rat	s.c./o	A	−	−	−	+	−	+	−	−
2′-Fluoro-4-stilbenyl-*N*,*N*-dimethylamine	rat	o	S	−	-	−	+	−	+	+	−

4′-Fluoro-4-stilbenamine	rat	s.c.	S*	−	−	−	+	+	+	−	−
4′-Fluoro-4-stilbenyl-*N,N*-dimethylamine	rat	o	S	−	−	−	−	−	+	−	−
2′-Chloro-4-stilbenyl-*N,N*-dimethylamine	rat	o	S	−	−	−	−	−	+	?	sarcomas (?)
3′-Chloro-4-stilbenyl-*N,N*-dimethylamine	rat	o	S	−	−	−	?	−	+	?	
4′-Chloro-4-stilbenyl-*N,N*-dimethylamine	rat	o	S	−	−	−	−	−	+	−	−
4′-Nitro-4-stilbenyl-*N,N*-dimethylamine	rat	o	S	−	−	−	−	−	?	−	−
4,4′-Diaminostilbene	rat	s.c.	S*	?	−	−	+	−	−	−	−
3,3′-Dichloro-4,4′-diaminostilbene	rat	s.c.	S*	+	−	−	−	−	−	−	−
2,2′-Dichloro-4,4′-diaminostilbene	rat	s.c.	S*	?	−	−	+	?	−	−	−
2-Cyano-4-stilbenamine	rat	s.c.	S	−	−	−	+	−	−	−	lung
2-(4,*N,N*-Dimethylaminostyryl)-quinoline	rat	o	S	−	−	−	−	−	+	−	stomach(?)
	mouse	i.v.	S	−	−	−	+	−	−	−	leukemia(+); ovary(?)

[a] +, tumors reported; −, tumors not reported; and ?, evidence equivocal.
[b] o, oral; top, topical; s.c., subcutaneous injection; and i.v., intravenous injection.
[c] A, tested in more than one institute; S, evidence less than convincing; and S*, preliminary communication or abstract.

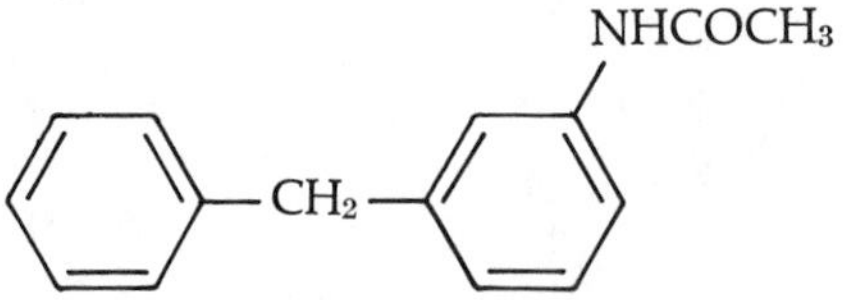

80

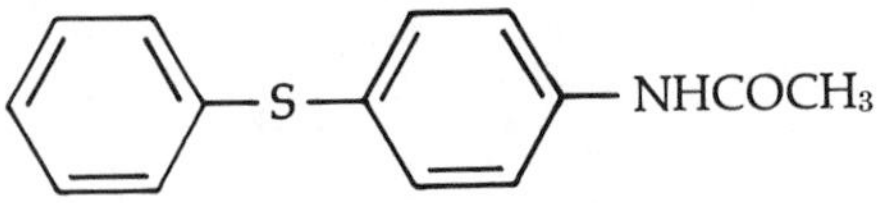

81

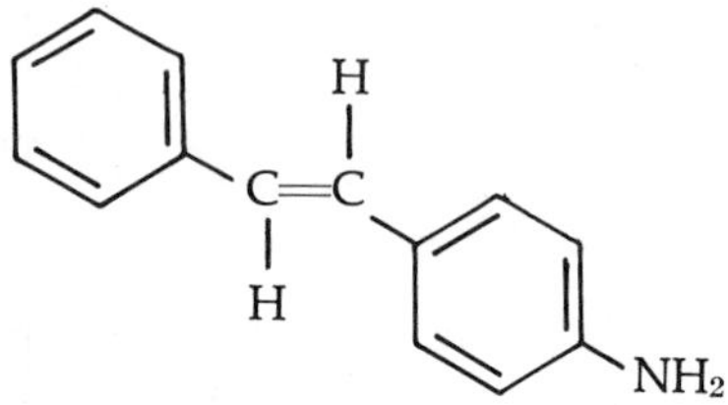

82

Attention was first drawn to this group by Haddow and his colleagues (*205*), who examined them as possible antineoplastic agents. The main feature of the stilbenamines is their ability to induce acoustic duct carcinomas in rats; Druckrey (*206*) employed this characteristic in the study of dose–response relationships in carcinogenesis. The acoustic duct carcinoma is particularly useful for the purpose, because it becomes clinically apparent early in its development. In Druckrey's experiment the smallest dose, 0.5 mg/kg body weight/d of 4-stilbenyldimethylamine, led to 39 carcinomas in 50 rats in 560 d.

Comparatively little work has been done on the critical structure for SA carcinogenesis. The ethylenic bond (–CH=CH–) appears to be useful insofar as its replacement by anil (–CH=N–) removes carcinogenicity. 4-Dibenzylamine is a very weak carcinogen (*51*).

N-Hydroxy-SAA induces sarcomas on subcutaneous injection in only a few treated rats and is a more effective mammary gland carcinogen than SAA on feeding to weanling female rats. It should be considered a proximate carcinogen. *N*-Acetoxy-SAA was prepared and induced sarcomas and acoustic duct tumors on subcutaneous injection (*51*). Some evidence suggests that epoxidation of the ethylenic bond of stilbene occurs, and this reaction possibly contributes to the carcinogenicity of the stilbenamines (*207, 208*).

Fused-Ring Amines. 2-Fluorenylacetamide (2-FAA; 2-acetylamino- or 2-acetamidofluorene; 2-AAF). 2-FAA was proposed as an insecticide to replace the highly toxic lead, arsenic, and fluorine sprays that were used before 1940. Tumors of the liver, bladder, renal pelvis, acoustic duct, and in single instances, of the colon, lung, and pancreas arose in male and female Slonaker rats given 0.03–0.125% 2-FAA in their diet for 95–333 d (*209*). World War II delayed the fuller publication of these results until 1947 (*210–13*). These publications described tumors that were induced by

2-FAA in mice. Tumors of liver, bladder, and kidney were produced in C57, C3H, and Bagg albino mice. In rats, the importance of the amino group in the action of 2-FA and 2-FAA was demonstrated; 2-chlorofluorene, fluorene, fluorenone, and xanthone did not induce tumors.

Different species respond to chronic administration of 2-FAA in different ways (Table VII). Both guinea pigs and monkeys fail to develop tumors after treatment; with monkeys, the correct dosage and length of experiment possibly has not yet been achieved. Guinea pigs may be deficient in the enzyme necessary for the first step of aromatic amine activation. The sites of tumors induced by 2-FAA in other species are variable. For example, bladder and liver tumors have been induced in dogs, mice, and rats; liver tumors (but not bladder tumors) in chickens, fish, cats, and hamsters; and bladder tumors (but not liver tumors) in rabbits.

Also, variations in the response to 2-FAA in different colonies of inbred animals within a species have been observed. Bielschowsky (*214, 215*) found that 2-FAA induced intestinal cancer in Piebald rats, whereas the Wistar strain was less susceptible to this tumor. This finding is in contrast with the bladder tumors described in the Slonaker rat (*209*). In mice, Armstrong and Bonser (*216*) examined the effect of 2-FAA in five inbred strains (Table VIII). The variations were reported in comparatively small numbers of mice; nevertheless, the differences were convincing. Large-scale experiments using BALB/c and C57 mice confirmed these results; the incidence of bladder papillomas was both sex and strain dependent (*217, 218*). Similar studies on a compound related to 2-FAA, 2-fluorenyldiacetamide, revealed strain differences in susceptibility in male rats that were fed 0.025% in a semisynthetic diet. Sprague–Dawley and NIH black rats were the most susceptible and Osborne Mendel male rats were the least (*219*).

Chemical structure and carcinogenic activity relationships in the 2-FAA series, the metabolism of these compounds in rats, and so forth were reviewed by Weisburger and Weisburger in 1958 (*220*). In rats, an equilibrium is set up between the enzymic deacetylation of 2-FAA and the reacetylation of 2-FA; therefore, any fluorene derivative that may be converted enzymically to FA or FAA is carcinogenic, as illustrated by *N*-2-fluorenylmethylamine and 2-nitrofluorene (Table VII). *N*-Fluorenylphthalamic acid led to the induction of smaller yields of transplantable hepatomas that superficially appear to be similar to normal liver. Enzyme measurements, however, have demonstrated important differences between normal liver tissue and each of these so-called "Morris" hepatomas (*221, 222*). Compounds with other substituents on the nitrogen, for example, *N*-fluorenyl-2-benzenesulfonamide or *N*-fluorenyl-2-*p*-toluenesulfonamide, failed to induce tumors, because they were not hydrolyzed in vivo.

The effects of ring substituents on the carcinogenicity of 2-FAA (Table VII) were similar to those with 4-BPA. A study on a series of seven carcinogenic fluoro derivatives of 2-FAA indirectly demonstrates that *C*-hydroxylation of 2-FAA does not lead to tumor formation (*223*).

Studies on the metabolism of FAA established the most prominent metabolites of 2-FAA were *C*-hydroxylated derivatives conjugated with glucuronide or sulfate. These metabolites are not involved with carcinogenesis but instead are the detoxification products of 2-FAA. The isolation and characterization of these metabolites and the study of their conjugation with sulfate and glucuronic acid

Table VII

Carcinogenic Activity of 2-Fluorenamine and Related Compounds

Compound	Species	Route[b]	Adequacy[c]	Site of Tumor Induction[a]							
				Local	Bladder	Kidney	Liver	Intestine	Ear Duct	Breast	Other
2-Fluorenamine (2-FA)	mouse	v	A	–	?	–	+	–	–	–	–
	rat	v	A	–	–	–	+	+	+	+	lung
2-Fluorenylacetamide (2-FAA)	mouse	v	A	–	+	–	+	–	–	+	–
	rat	v	A	–	+	+	+	+	+	+	various
	hamster	v	A	–	–	–	+	–	–	–	–
	guinea pig			–	–	–	–	–	–	–	–
	rabbit	o	A	–	+	–	–	–	–	–	ureter
	cat	o	S	–	–	–	+	–	–	–	lung
	dog	o	S	–	+	–	+	–	–	–	–
	monkey[d]			–	–	–	–	–	–	–	–
	fish		S	–	–	–	+	–	–	–	–
	chicken		S	–	–	+	+	–	–	–	fallopian tube; ovary
9-Hydroxy-2-FAA	rat	o	S	–	–	–	+	–	–	?	–
9-Oxo-2-FAA	rat	o	S	–	–	–	+	?	?	+	–
2-Fluorenyldimethylamine	rat	o	A	–	–	–	+	+	+	+	–
2-Fluorenyldiethylamine	rat	o	S	–	–	–	–	+	–	–	lung
2-Fluorenylmonomethylamine	rat	o	A	–	–	–	+	–	+	+	lung
N-Acetoxy-FAA	rat	s.c.	S	+	–	–	–	–	?	–	–
N-Benzoyloxy-FAA	rat	s.c.	S	+	–	–	–	–	?	–	–
2-Fluorenyldiacetamide	rat	o	A	–	?	–	+	–	+	+	orbital and Harderian gland tumors
2-Nitrofluorene	rat	o	S	–	–	–	–	?	–	–	?
N-Hydroxy-2-FAA (fluorenyl-2-acethydroxamic acid)	mouse	v	A	+	+	–	+	–	–	+	–

	rat	v	A	+	–	–	+	+	+	+	–
	hamster	v	A	+	–	–	+	?	–	–	–
	rabbit	v	A	+	+	–	–	?	–	–	–
	guinea pig	v	A	+	–	–	–	+	–	–	–
2-Fluorenylhydroxylamine	rat	s.c.	S	+	–	–	–	–	+	+	–
2-Nitrosofluorene	rat	s.c.	S	+	–	–	–	–	+	–	–
N-Fluorenyl-2-benzamide	rat	i.p.	S	–	–	–	–	–	–	–	–
N-Fluorenyl-2-benzohydroxamic acid	rat	i.p.	S	+	–	–	–	+ (small)	–	+	–
N-2-Fluorenylformamide	rat	o	S	–	–	–	–	–	+	+	–
N-Fluorenyl-2-phthalimic acid	rat	o	S	–	–	–	+	–	–	–	–
N-Fluorenyl-2-benzenesulfonamide	rat	i.p.	S	–	–	–	–	–	–	–	–
N-Hydroxy-*N*-fluorenylbenzene-sulfonamide	rat	i.p.	S	+	–	–	–	–	–	+	lung(?)
N-2-Fluorenyl(2′-carboxybenz)amide	rat	o	A	–	–	–	+	–	–	–	–
N-2-Fluorenylsuccinamic acid	rat	o	S	–	–	–	+	–	–	–	–
N-2-Fluorenyl-*p*-toluenesulfonamide	rat	o	S	–	–	–	–	–	–	–	–
N-(2-Fluorenyl)-2,2,2-trifluoroacetamide	rat	o	S	–	–	–	+	–	+	+	–
N-3-Glycylaminofluorene	rat	o	S	–	–	–	+	–	–	–	–
1-Fluoro-2-FAA	rat	o	S	–	–	–	–	–	+	+	–
3-Fluoro-2-FAA	rat	o	S	–	–	–	+	–	+	+	–
4-Fluoro-2-FAA	rat	o	S	–	–	–	–	–	+	+	–
5-Fluoro-2-FAA	rat	o	S	–	–	–	–	–	+	+	–
6-Fluoro-2-FAA	rat	o	S	–	–	–	+	+	+	+	–
7-Fluoro-2-FAA	rat	o	A	–	–	–	+	–	+	+	–
8-Fluoro-2-FAA	rat	o	S	–	–	–	+	?	+	+	–
7-Fluoro-2-*N*-(fluorenyl)acethydroxamic acid	rat	o	S	+	–	–	+	+	+	+	–
7-Chloro-2-FAA	rat	o	A	–	–	–	?	–	–	–	–
3-Iodo-2-FAA	rat	o	S	–	–	–	–	–	+	–	–
7-Iodo-2-FAA	rat	o	S	–	–	–	–	–	–	–	–
1-Methoxy-2-FA	rat	o	A	–	–	–	+	+	?	–	–
3-Methoxy-2-FA	rat	o	A	–	–	–	–	–	–	–	–
1-Methoxy-2-FAA	rat	o	A	–	–	–	–	?	–	?	–
3-Methoxy-2-FAA	rat	o	A	–	–	–	–	–	–	–	–
7-Methoxy-2-FAA	rat	o	A	–	–	–	+	–	+	+	–

Continued on next page

Table VII Continued

				Site of Tumor Induction[a]							
Compound	*Species*	*Route*[b]	*Adequacy*[c]	*Local*	*Bladder*	*Kidney*	*Liver*	*Intestine*	*Ear Duct*	*Breast*	*Other*
2,5-Dinitrofluorene	rat	o	S	–	–	–	–	–	–	?	–
2,7-Dinitrofluorene	rat	o	S	–	–	–	–	–	–	+	–
2,7-Fluorenyldiamine	rat	o	S	–	–	–	–	–	–	+	–
2,5-Fluorenylenebisacetamide	rat	o	S	–	–	–	–	–	–	+	–
2,7-Fluorenylbisacetamide	mouse	o	S	–	–	–	+	–	–	–	–
	rat	o	A	–	–	–	+	+	+	+	various[e]
1-Fluorenylacetamide	rat	i.p.	A	–	–	–	–	–	–	+	–
1-Fluorenylacethydroxamic acid	rat	i.p.	S	–	–	–	–	–	–	+	–
3-Fluorenylacetamide	rat	i.p.	S	–	–	–	–	–	–	+	–
3-Fluorenylacethydroxamic acid	rat	i.p.		–	–	–	–	–	–	+	–

[a] +, tumors reported; –, tumors not reported; and ?, evidence equivocal.
[b] o, oral; s.c., subcutaneous injection; i.p., intraperitoneal injection; and v, various routes.
[c] A, tested in more than one institute; and S, evidence less than convincing.
[d] In experiments with monkeys, there is doubt whether the chronic toxicity tests were terminated before tumors could have appeared.
[e] Includes jejunum, lung, glandular, and stomach tumors.

Table VIII

Carcinogenicity of 2-Fluorenylacetamide in Mice: Effect of Mouse Strain

	Mouse Strain				
	CBA	*IF*	*R111*	*White Label*	*Strong A*
Number of mice surviving 20 weeks (male and female)	18	20	21	24	25
Percent of hepatomas [a]	73	44	16	10	5
Percent of bladder tumors[a]	78	70	48	22	22

[a]Percent yields based on number of mice examined histologically.

have been summarized (*24*):

1. *N*-Hydroxy-2-FAA leads to a greater yield of tumors than an equimolar level of 2-FAA, especially in the mammary gland of weanling rats (*25, 26*).
2. *N*-Hydroxy-2-FAA induces local tumors (e.g., in the forestomach on feeding or in the subcutaneous tissues especially on injection, as the cupric chelate (*224*).
3. *N*-Hydroxy-2-FAA induces tumors in guinea pigs, whereas 2-FAA is without effect in this species.
4. The effect of feeding a variety of substances with 2-FAA on the tumor yield is explicable by the levels of *N*-hydroxy-2-FAA produced from 2-FAA under these conditions (*see* **Modification of Aromatic Amine Carcinogenesis**, p. 258).
5. The failure of *N*-hydroxy-FAA to react nonenzymically with DNA, RNA, and protein in vitro clearly indicates that this compound is a proximate rather than ultimate carcinogen (*17*).
6. The synthesis and demonstration of the carcinogenicity of the highly reactive *N*-acetoxyarylacetamides and *N*-benzoyloxyarylacetamides suggest that the ultimate carcinogen might be an ester of *N*-hydroxy-2-FAA (*51*).
7. There is evidence that in the liver the sulfate ester of *N*-hydroxy-FAA is not a powerful carcinogen (*59, 61*), possibly because it reacts with nonspecific targets.

The observation that continuous feeding of 2-FAA increases the urinary levels of *N*-hydroxy-2-FAA but markedly reduces sulfotransferase activity indicates that the sulfate ester is less likely to be the ultimate carcinogen in the bladder (*225*). In other tissues even less is known about the ultimate carcinogen, because sulfotransferase is not present (*226*). The phosphate (*17*) and the acetate (*54–56*) of 2-FAA, *N*-nitroso-2-fluorene, 2-fluorenylhydroxylamine, the *O*-glucuronide of fluorenylhydroxylamine or *N*-hydroxy-2-FAA (*227*), and free radicals (*228*) were all suggested as possible carcinogens. The ultimate carcinogen may have to be determined in each tissue that responds to 2-FAA.

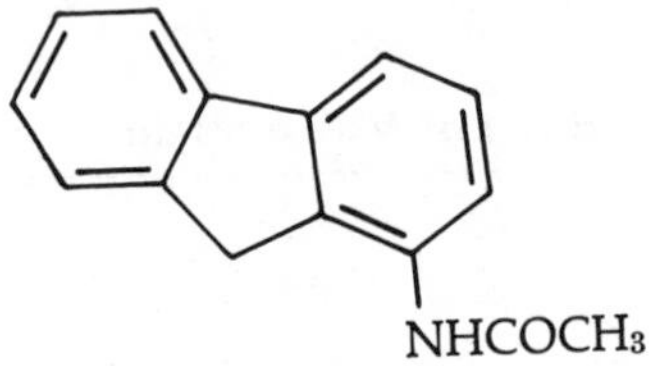

$NHCOCH_3$

83

$NHCOCH_3$

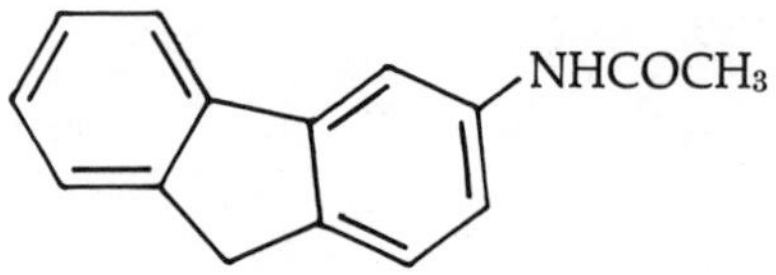

84

Certain substituents on the amino groups of FA are inimical to its enzymic hydroxylation. Thus, *N*-2-fluorenylbenzamide (*23*) is inactive, whereas *N*-2-fluorenylbenzhydroxamic acid induces tumors locally in the small intestine and breast tissue on intraperitoneal injection (Table VII). Similarly, *N*-hydroxy-*N*-2-fluorenylbenzenesulfonamide induces tumors at the injection site in the breast and in the lung, whereas the *N*-2-fluorenylbenzenesulfonamide is not active (*23*, *229*). In subsequent studies, *N*-hydroxy-*N*-2-fluorenylbenzenesulfonamide was shown to convert to *N*-2-fluorenylhydroxylamine in vivo (*230*).

The positional isomers of 2-FAA, namely 1-FAA (**83**) and 3-FAA (**84**) are carcinogenic, especially to the mammary glands of female Holtzman rats (*229*).

Yost and Gutmann (*231*) compared the carcinogenicity of 2-, 3-, and 4-fluorenylacethydroxamic acids and showed that the 2-isomer and 3-isomer had approximately equal carcinogenicities and that both were much more carcinogenic than the 4-isomer; the 1-isomer has an intermediate level of carcinogenicity (*229*). By examination of the reactivity of the *N*-acetoxyfluorenylacetamides with methionine, tRNA, guanosine, and adenosine, they concluded that the carcinogenicity of the positional isomers could not be rationalized on the basis of the reactivity of the corresponding *N*-acetoxyarenamides. Because most tumors in the carcinogenicity tests were in the mammary gland of female rats and because sulfotransferase is not present in females (*226*), the *O*-sulfate of 2-FAA is not likely to be involved in mammary carcinogenesis in the rat; an acyl transferase may be the activating enzyme in this tissue (*56*).

NAPHTHYLAMINES. In the 1930s, the growing realization that 2-naphthylamine (2-NA) (**4**) was a bladder carcinogen in occupationally exposed workmen led to intensive attempts to reproduce the human disease in laboratory animals. Hueper et al. (*14*) effectively demonstrated the susceptibility of the dog to this chemical in 1938. In their only report—an interim statement that appeared about 26 months after the experiment began—they reported that 13 out of 16 dogs developed bladder tumors after subcutaneous injection and later after oral administration of 2-NA. Tumors were detected in two dogs at autopsy; the others were found by cytoscopy. This experiment involved the relatively impure commercial chemical, but in later tests (*16*), rigorously purified 2-NA gave similar results. More recent results showed that the tumor response depended on the dose of 2-NA (*232*).

The way in which different species respond to 2-NA is shown in Table IX. The hamster (when subjected to high levels), the dog, the rat, and the monkey all develop bladder tumors similar to those found in humans. The mouse develops

Table IX

Carcinogenicity of Aromatic Amines and Their Derivatives with Fused Aromatic Rings

Compound	Species	Route[b]	Adequacy[c]	Site of Tumor Induction[a]							
				Local	Bladder	Kidney	Liver	Intestine	Ear Duct	Breast	Other
1-Naphthylamine	mouse	o	S[d]	–	–	–	?	–	–	–	–
	hamster	o	S	–	–	–	–	–	–	–	–
	dog	o	A	–	–	–	–	–	–	–	–
2-Naphthylamine	mouse	o	A	–	–	–	+	–	–	–	–
	rat	o	A	–	–	–	–	–	–	–	–
	hamster	o	S	–	+	–	–	–	–	–	–
	rabbit	o	S	–	–	–	–	–	–	–	–
	cat	o	S	–	–	–	–	–	–	–	–
	dog	o/s.c.	A	–	+	–	–	–	–	–	–
	monkey	o	S	–	+	–	–	–	–	–	–
1-Naphthylacetamide	mouse	o	S	–	–	–	–	–	–	–	–
1-Naphthylhydroxylamine	mouse	top.	S	+	–	–	–	–	–	–	–
	rat	o	S	+	–	–	–	–	–	–	–
1-Naphthylacethydroxamic acid	rat	i.p./s.c.	S	–	–	–	–	–	–	–	–
1-Nitronaphthalene	mouse	o	NCI	–	–	–	–	–	–	–	–
	rat	o	NCI	–	–	–	–	–	–	–	–
1-Nitrosonaphthalene	mouse	s.c.	S	–	–	–	+	–	–	–	lung
	rat	top.	S	–	–	–	–	–	–	–	skin
1,5-Diaminonaphthalene	mouse	o	NCI	–	–	–	+	–	–	–	thyroid; lung
	rat	o	NCI	–	–	–	–	–	–	–	uterus
2-Naphthylhydroxylamine	mouse	top.	S	+	–	–	–	–	–	–	–
	rat	i.p.	A	+	–	–	–	–	–	–	–
2-Nitrosonaphthalene	mouse			–	–	–	+	–	–	–	–
	rat	i.p.	S	–	–	–	–	–	–	–	–
N-Phenyl-2-naphthylamine	hamster	o	S	–	–	–	–	–	–	–	–
1-Fluoro-2-naphthylamine	mouse	s.c.	S	–	–	–	–	–	–	–	–
1-Methoxy-2-naphthylamine	mouse	s.c.	S	–	–	–	–	+	–	–	–
3-Methyl-2-naphthylamine	rat	o/s.c.		+	–	?	–	+	–	+	skin
3-Nitro-2-naphthylamine	rat	o	S	–	–	–	–	–	?	–	skin

Continued on next page

Table IX Continued

Compound	Species	Route[b]	Adequacy[c]	Site of Tumor Induction[a] Local	Bladder	Kidney	Liver	Intestine	Ear Duct	Breast	Other
N,N-Bis(2-chloroethyl)-2-naphthylamine	mouse	i.p.	S	–	–	–	–	–	–	–	lung
1-Anthramine	rat	top.	S	–	–	–	–	–	–	–	–
2-Anthramine	mouse	s.c.	S	–	–	–	+	–	–	–	–
	rat	top./s.c.	A	+ (top.)	–	–	–	–	–	+	–
	hamster	top.	A	+	–	–	–	–	–	–	–
9-Anthramine	rat	s.c.	S	–	–	–	–	–	–	–	–
2-Anthranylacetamide	rat	s.c.	S	–	–	–	–	–	–	–	–
1-Phenanthrylamine	mouse	o	S	–	–	–	–	–	–	–	–
	rat	o	S	–	–	–	–	–	–	+[e]	–
2-Phenanthrylamine	mouse	o	S	–	–	–	–	–	–	–	–
	rat	o	S	–	–	–	–	–	–	+[e]	–
3-Phenanthrylamine	mouse	o	S	–	–	–	–	–	–	–	–
	rat	o	S	–	–	–	–	–	–	+[e]	–
9-Phenanthrylamine	mouse	o	S	–	–	–	–	–	–	–	–
	rat	o	S	–	–	–	–	–	–	+[e]	–
1-Phenanthrylacetamide	mouse	i.m.[f]	S	–	–	–	–	–	–	–	–
	rat	o[g]	S	–	–	–	–	–	–	–	–
9,10-Dihydro-2-phenanthramine	rat	o	A	–	–	–	–	+	+	+	–
2-Phenanthrylacetamide	mouse	i.m.	S	–	–	–	–	–	–	–	–
	rat	o	A	–	–	–	–	+	+	+	leukemia
2-Phenanthrylacethydroxamic acid	rat	s.c.	S	+	–	–	–	–	–	+	–
9-Phenanthrylacetamide	mouse	i.m.[g]	S	–	–	–	–	–	–	–	leukemia(?)
	rat	o[f]	A	–	–	–	–	–	–	–	–
N-Acetoxy-4-phenanthrylacetamide	rat	s.c.	S	+	–	–	–	–	–	–	–

[a]+, tumors reported; –, tumors not reported; and ?, evidence equivocal.
[b]o, oral; s.c., subcutaneous injection; i.p., intraperitoneal injection; top., topical; and i.m., intramuscular injection.
[c]A, tested in more than one institute; S, evidence less than convincing; and S*, preliminary communication or abstract.
[d]Earlier results not included because 1-isomer was often contaminated with 2-naphthylamine.
[e]Three doses.
[f]One dose only.
[g]Two doses only.

liver tumors, whereas other species fail to respond. The failure of 2-NA to induce a significant incidence of tumors in rabbits was demonstrated in several independent experiments.

Commercial 1-naphthylamine (1-NA) (**5**) in the United Kingdom, at least at one time, contained 4–10% of 2-NA. In about 1950, using the analytical methods of Butt and Strafford (*233*), Clayson found 3.5% of 2-NA in a purified sample of 1-NA. Because of this contamination, the earlier attempts to induce tumors with 1-NA, which sometimes gave positive results, are not emphasized. For example, Gehrmann et al. (*234*) fed 300–350 mg of 1-NA to five dogs five times weekly without inducing bladder tumors; Bonser et al. (*235*) reported a bladder papilloma in one of two surviving dogs fed 500 mg of 1-NA three times weekly for life. Rigorously purified 1-NA (a 2-NA content of 0.04% or less) administered to beagles for approximately 9 years induced neither pathological lesions nor cancer of the bladder (*5*). Analysis of the urine revealed the presence of small amounts of *N*-oxidation products. In the young adult mouse, Clayson and Ashton (*236*) gave mice 1-NA (free from 2-NA) in their drinking water at a level of 0.1% for 70 weeks and obtained a barely significant incidence of hepatomas only in females. Newborn mice gave similarly inconclusive results (*237*). The Syrian golden hamster was not affected by 1-NA at levels of 0.1 or 1.0% in the diet (*238, 239*). This evidence strongly suggests that 1-NA is not a carcinogen for the dog or humans, despite its mutagenicity in bacteria.

In a series of studies relating metabolism of 1- and 2-NA to tumor susceptibility or resistance, Boyland and his colleagues (*240*), as well as Troll and Nelson (*241*), demonstrated the presence of 2-naphthylhydroxylamine in the urine of dogs fed 2-NA. The former group showed that this compound induces local sarcomas on intraperitoneal injection. Nevertheless, despite the fact that nearly all dogs develop bladder cancer when fed 2-NA, not all dogs excrete 2-NA in their urine as 2-naphthylhydroxylamine (*242*). This discrepancy was explained by identifying 2-nitrosonaphthalene as a metabolite formed by the reduction of the hydroxylamine in tissues. The nitroso and hydroxylamino derivatives of 1-NA and 2-NA were tested for carcinogenicity in dogs by intravesicular distillation, i.e., the transfer of a dimethyl sulfoxide solution of the test solution by catheter into the bladder lumen. These substances were also tested by intraperitoneal injection in rats or by subcutaneous injection in newborn mice within the first 24 h and on the third and fifth day after birth. In dogs, no tumors were formed after instillation of 2-NA, but 2-naphthylhydroxylamine induced three cases of bladder carcinomas in four dogs (*237*). In mice, an excessive incidence of hepatomas and pulmonary adenomas was found after administering 1- and 2-naphthylhydroxylamine and, in male mice only, after 1- and 2-nitrosonaphthalene. Rats were susceptible only to 1-naphthylhydroxylamine and 1-nitrosonaphthalene.

An interesting derivative of 2-NA (Table IX), 2-naphthylamine mustard (2-bis(2′-chloroethyl)aminonaphthalene) (**8**), was marketed under the name chlornaphazin. It was originally intended for patients with leukemia and Hodgkin's disease, both of which had a poor prognosis at that time. Unfortunately this drug found favor in Scandinavia for treating polycythemia vera, a disease involving overproduction of red blood cells for which there is a more favorable prognosis. In a series of 61 patients, of whom 27 survived, 13 had bladder cancer and 5 more had abnormal cells in their urine, which suggests a developing bladder tumor (i.e., abnormal urinary cytology). Polycythemia alone does not predispose to bladder cancer, nor does the ^{32}P administered to most of these patients concomitantly with the chlornaphazin. The dose required to induce abnormal urinary cytology or tumors ranged from 2 to 350 g; the mean latent period of the tumors was 5.5 years (range 2.5–11)—a much shorter period than that associated with industrial bladder cancer. This alkylating drug induces lung adenomas in mice (*243*). It probably derives its carcinogenic action by being converted to derivatives of 2-naphthylamine. Boyland and Manson (*244*) showed that in the rat it was converted to 2-amino-1-naphthyl hydrogen sulfate and 2-acetamidonaphthalene hydrogen sulfate. The chlornaphazin used for treatment is likely to have contained up to 10% 2-NA as an impurity of the synthetic procedure. No attempt was made to remove the contaminating 2-NA. Possibly the impurity was responsible for the bladder cancer induction, because *N*-dechloroethylation of both chloroethyl groups is not a known metabolic reaction.*

ANTHRAMINES. 1-Anthramine (**85**) and 9-anthramine (**86**) have not induced tumors in limited tests in rats (Table IX). 2-Anthramine (**87**), however, is unusual because it is one of the few aromatic amines that leads to skin tumors when painted on the skin of rats or hamsters (*245, 246*). These tumors resemble the range of tumors found in human skin and were used for pathological studies (*247*). No evidence has been reported on the metabolic activation of 2-anthramine in skin.

PHENANTHRAMINES. Most of the phenanthrene derivatives recorded in Table IX were investigated only in the Huggins system in which one, two, or three large doses of a carcinogen are given by intubation to 50-day-old female Sprague–Dawley rats, and the incidence of breast tumor is used as an index of carcinogenicity (*248*).

2-Phenanthrylacetamide (2-PAA) (**88**), which is carcinogenic (*41*), has been studied in more detail to provide a firmer base for the general theory of aromatic amine activation (*31*). Small quantities of *N*-hydroxy-2-PAA were found in the urine of 2-PAA-treated rats and the synthetic compound induced mammary adenocarcinomas in female Holtzmann rats.

OTHER ARYLAMINES. Higher arylamines, e.g., 7-benz[*a*]anthramine, have been recorded in the carcinogenesis literature. These compounds are not discussed in this chapter because there is no adequate work on their carcinogenicity or mechanisms of action.

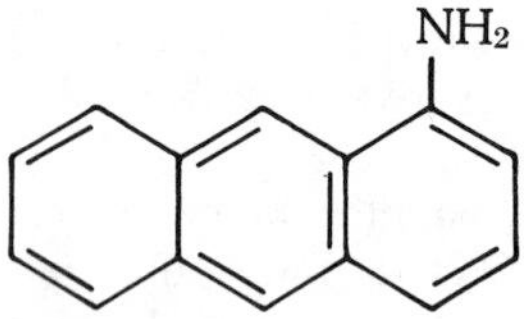

NH_2 NH_2

85 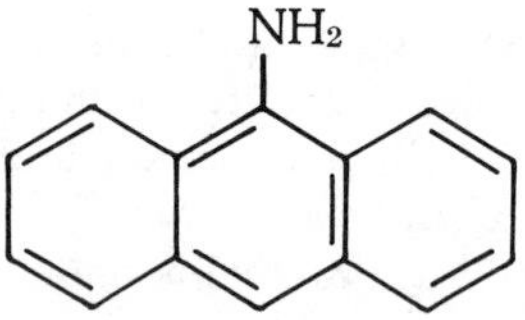 **86**

*T.A. Connors, personal communication.

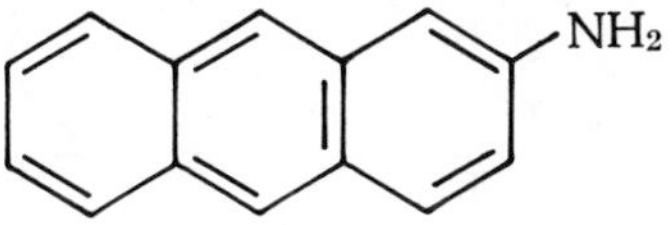

87

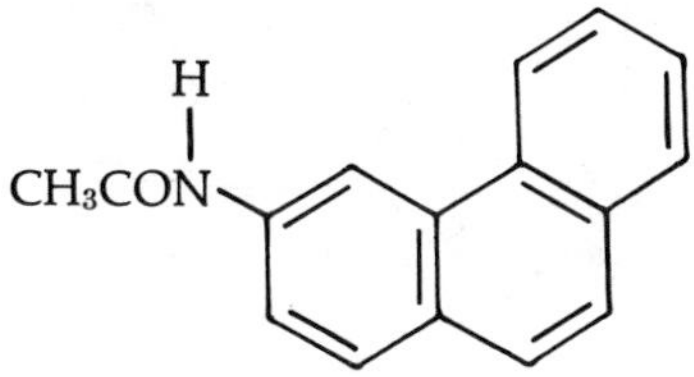

88

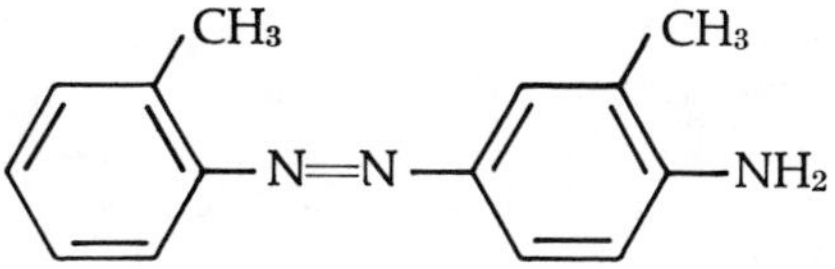

89

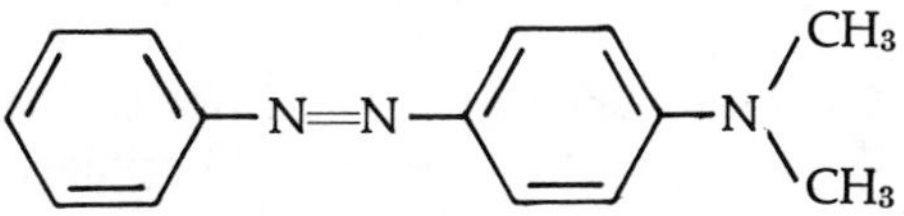

90

Aminoazo Compounds and Related Azo Dyes. This group of carcinogens is so large that it is more convenient to consider it under three headings: (1) those dyes that have an unsubstituted amino group, such as 4-(*o*-tolylazo)-*o*-toluidine (**89**); (2) dyes in which the amino group is methylated, as with *N,N*-dimethyl-4-phenylazoaniline (**90**); and (3) various azo dyes that have been tested for carcinogenicity because they are required for use in food, medicine, or other applications. These azo dyes may not necessarily be aromatic amines, but in each example, amines may be produced as a result of in vivo reduction.

DERIVATIVES OF 4-PHENYLAZOANILINE. 4-Phenylazoaniline (4-aminoazobenzene) (AB) (**91**) was tested for carcinogenicity in several species. Generally the data suggest that AB and 4-phenylazoacetanilide (AAB) are not carcinogenic. However, only in a few experiments was the maximum tolerated dose of chemical given for the major part of the life span of a substantial number of animals. Kirby and Peacock (*249*) reported liver tumors in rats. They fed the highest tolerated dose of AB (0.2–0.3%) in the diet to 16 male rats on a low-protein diet and induced two metastasizing liver cell carcinomas and five hepatomas. No liver tumors were reported in eight male and eight female control rats. Also, injection of AB into the kidney of frogs (*Rana pipiens*) leads to kidney tumors (*250*). Because the latent

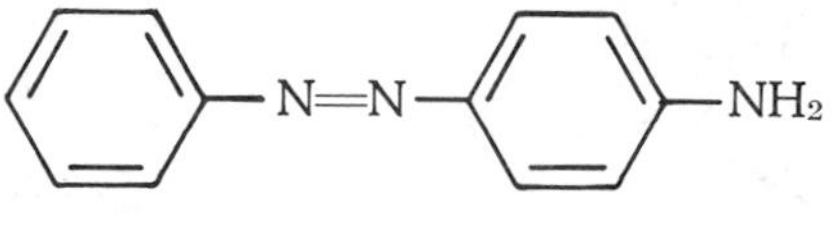

C_6H_5—N=N—C_6H_4—NH_2

91

period of these tumors was as short as 3 weeks, they were probably induced by the Lucke virus, which is known to produce tumors in this species.

The oncogenicity of AB derivatives was compared by feeding them at a level that was equivalent, on a molar basis, to 0.05% *N*-methyl-AB for 54 weeks (*251*). This schedule adequately demonstrates whether or not these compounds are potently carcinogenic but does not exclude the possibility that they are weakly carcinogenic. No tumors were induced by *N*-hydroxy-4-phenylazoacetanilide (*N*-hydroxy-ABB), its cupric chelate. *N*-hydroxy-AB, AB, AAB, or *N*-acetoxy-AAB. AAB, *N*-hydroxy-AAB, 3-hydroxy-AAB, and 4′-hydroxy-AAB were all shown to be present (often in relatively small amounts) in the urine of rats fed AAB, *N*-hydroxy-AAB, AB, *N*-methyl-AB (MAB), *N,N*-dimethyl-AB (DAB), or *N*-hydroxy-AB. These metabolic data confirm previous observations on these compounds (*252*).

On the other hand, the carcinogenicity of 4-(*o*-tolylazo)-*o*-toluidine (*o*-aminoazotoluene) is well documented (Table X). Historically, this was the first carcinogenic azo compound to be discovered. Yoshida reported that it induced hepatomas in rats in 1932 (*253*). It is more carcinogenic in mice than in rats, and has induced hepatomas, pulmonary adenomas, and hemangioendotheliomas in several tissues and, from only one report, bladder tumors. It is also carcinogenic in hamsters, dogs, and possibly in rabbits (Table X). The azo compound appears to be *N*-hydroxylated in vivo, because 4,4′-bis(*o*-tolylazo)-2,2′-dimethylazobenzene (**92**) has been isolated from the liver of mice treated with 4-(*o*-tolylazo)-*o*-toluidine (*254*). This metabolic activation is confirmed indirectly by the demonstration that 4-(*o*-tolylazo)-*o*-toluidine interacts in vivo with DNA, RNA, and protein (*255–57*).

Five positional isomers of 4-(*o*-tolylazo)-*o*-toluidine were tested for carcinogenicity in groups of 17–27 rats and 11–15 mice (*258*). Only 2-(*o*-tolylazo)-*p*-toluidine (**93**) was carcinogenic to the liver of both species while 4-(*p*-tolylazo)-*m*-toluidine (**94**) gave hepatomas in mice.

N-Methyl- and *N,N*-dimethyl-4-(phenylazo)-*o*-anisidine are unusual among the derivatives of *N,N*-dimethyl-4-(phenylazo)aniline insofar as they induce extrahepatic tumors, i.e., ear duct, intestinal, and skin carcinomas. 2-Methoxy-AB behaves similarly (*259*). Fare et al. (*260*) first used these compounds to elucidate the possible protective effect of dietary copper acetate on hepatocarcinogenesis. This treatment apparently protected the liver from tumors but not the skin or ear duct.

N,N-Dimethyl-4-(phenylazo)-*o*-anisidine induced keratinitis and a variety of skin tumors by direct painting on rat skin (*261*). Ear duct carcinomas were the only other tumor to be induced. Finally, Fare (*262*) demonstrated that painting AB,

Table X

Carcinogenicity of Derivatives of 4-Phenylazoaniline

Compound	Species	Route[b]	Adequacy[c]	Site of Tumor Induction[a]: Local	Bladder	Kidney	Liver	Intestine	Ear Duct	Breast	Other
4-(Phenylazo)aniline	rat	top./o	A	+ (top.)	–	–	–[d]	–	–	–	–
	frog	intrarenal	S	–	–	+	–	–	–	–	–
4-(Phenylazo)acetanilide	rat	o	A	–	–	–	–	–	–	–	–
4-(Phenylazo)diacetanilide	rat	o	S	–	–	–	–	–	–	–	–
4-(Phenylazo)-*N*-phenylhydroxylamine	rat	s.c.	S	–	–	–	–	–	–	–	–
4-(Phenylazo)*N*-phenylacethydroxamic acid	rat	o/i.p.	S	–	–	–	–	–	–	–	–
4-(Phenylazo)-*o*-anisidine	rat	o/top.	A	+ (top.)	–	–	+	?	+	–	skin(o)
4-[(*p*-Methoxyphenyl)azo]-*o*-anisidine	rat	o	S	–	–	–	+	+	?	–	–
4-(*m*-Tolylazo)aniline	rat	o	S	–	–	–	–	–	–	–	–
4-(*m*-Tolylazo)acetanilide	rat	o	S	–	–	–	–	–	–	–	–
4-(*o*-Tolylazo)-*o*-toluidine	mouse		A	–	+	–	+[e]	–	–	–	lung, hemangio-endothlioma
	rat		A	–	–	–	+	–	–	–	–
	rabbit		A	–	?	–	–	–	–	–	–
	hamster		S	–	+	–	+	–	–	+	–
	dog		S	–	+	–	?	–	–	–	gall bladder
2-(*o*-Tolylazo)-*p*-toluidine	mouse	o	S	–	–	–	–	–	–	–	–
	rat	o	A	–	–	–	–	–	–	–	–
4-(*o*-Tolylazo)-*m*-toluidine	rat	o	S	–	–	–	–	–	–	–	–
2-(*p*-Tolylazo)-*p*-toluidine	mouse	o	S	–	–	–	+	–	–	–	–
	rat	o	S	–	–	–	+	–	–	–	–
4-(*m*-Tolylazo)-*m*-toluidine	mouse	o		–	–	–	–	–	–	–	–
	rat	o		–	–	–	–	–	–	–	–

Continued on next page

Table X Continued

Compound	Species	Route[b]	Adequacy[c]	Site of Tumor Induction[a]							
				Local	Bladder	Kidney	Liver	Intestine	Ear Duct	Breast	Other
4-(*p*-Tolylazo)-*m*-toluidine	mouse	o		–	–	–	+	–	–	–	–
	rat	o		–	–	–	–	–	–	–	–
4-(*p*-Tolylazo)-*o*-toluidine	mouse	o		–	–	–	–	–	–	–	–
	rat	o		–	–	–	–	–	–	–	–
4-(*o*-Tolylazoxy)-*o*-toluidine	rat	o	S	–	–	–	–	–	–	–	–
1-[4-(*o*-Tolylazo)-*o*-tolylazo]-2-naphthol (Scarlet Red)				abnormal proliferative lesions only							
4′-Fluoro-*p*-phenylaniline	rat	o	S	–	–	–	–	–	–	–	–
1-(Phenylazo)-2-naphthylamine	rat	o/s.c.	A	–	–	–	–	–	–	–	–
1-(*o*-tolylazo)-2-naphthylamine	mouse	o	S	–	–	–	–	–	–	–	–
	rat	o/s.c.	A	–	–	–	–	–	–	–	–
	dog	o	S	–	–	–	–	–	–	–	–

NOTE: *N,N*-Dimethyl derivatives are not included.
[a] +, tumors reported; –, tumors not reported; and ?, evidence equivocal.
[b] o,oral; top., topical; s.c., subcutaneous injection; and i.p., intraperitoneal injection.
[c] A, tested in more than one institute; and S, evidence less than convincing.
[d] One author claims to have induced hepatomas (*see* text).
[e] Possibly on rice diet (*124*).

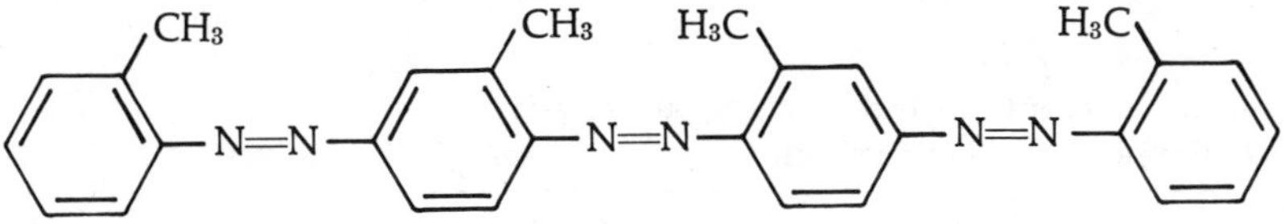

92

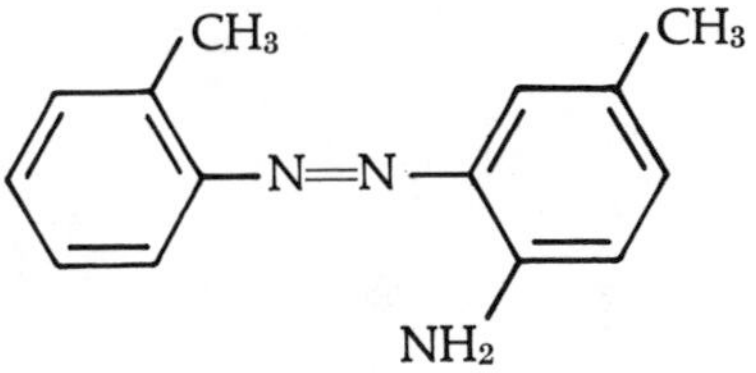

93

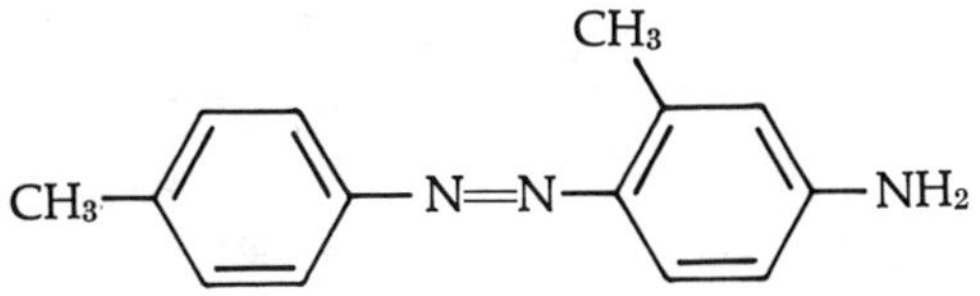

94

N-methyl-AB, *N,N*-dimethyl-AB, and the 3-methoxy derivatives of these compounds on the skin of male rats gave a range of skin tumors; a similar experiment in mice was not successful.

These results could be important in a number of ways. The fact that AB is definitely carcinogenic on painting but is, at the most, weakly carcinogenic on feeding seemingly contradicts the idea that some of the compound travels to the liver to be metabolically activated and the idea that the active metabolite is then "liberated" in the skin. On the other hand, the ability of *N,N*-dimethyl-4-(phenylazo)-*o*-anisidine to induce skin tumors, whether fed or painted, seemingly supports these ideas. Possibly rat skin contains *N*-hydroxylating enzymes and therefore activates these compounds. Alternatively, there may be another pathway for the activation of these azo dyes. These observations demonstrate the need for skin-painting studies in addition to feeding studies for aromatic amines, and the need for more detailed examination of the transport mechanisms and the enzyme distribution that activate these carcinogens.

The tumors induced by these azo compounds and by 2-anthramine (*see* previous section ANTHRAMINES) closely resemble those observed in human skin. They included keratocanthoma, squamous carcinoma, basal carcinoma, anaplastic carcinoma, and several miscellaneous tumors.

DERIVATIVES OF *N,N*-DIMETHYL-4-PHENYLAZOANILINE. *N,N*-Dimethyl-4-phenylazoaniline, often known as 4-dimethylaminoazobenzene (DAB) or butter yellow, was used to give a yellow color to hair creams in Scandinavia (*263*), as well as in many other technical applications. DAB and related compounds induce liver tumors in rats when the compounds are fed continuously in the diet. DAB itself was tested in several species and led to invasive bladder tumors in two dogs fed 20 mg/kg body weight/d for 3–4 years (*264*). A quarter of this dose was ineffective. The chemical induced liver tumors in mice with a latent period of more than 1 year, but negative

Table XI

Effect of Substituents on the Carcinogenic Activity of *N,N*-Dimethyl-*p*-phenylazoaniline

	Position										
Substituent	*2*	*3*	*2′*	*3′*	*4′*	*2,3′*	*2,4′*	*2,6*	*3,4′*	*3,5′*	*2′,4′,6′*
$-CH_3$	−	+	+	+	+	−	−		+	−	
$-C_2H_5$			−	+	+				+		
$-CF_3$			−	−	−						
−F	+	+	+	+	+			−		+	+
−Cl			+	+	+				+		
−Br				−							
−OH	−	−	−	−	−						
$-OCH_3$	±	+[a]	+	+	+						
$-OC_2H_5$				±							
$-NO_2$			+	+	−						
$-NH_2$					−						
$-SO_3H$					−						
$-CO_2H$			±[b]	±							

[a]Ear duct, skin, and intestinal tumors, but no hepatomas.
[b]Bladder papillomas and hepatomas possibly induced (*see* text).

results were obtained with squirrels, chickens, guinea pigs, hamsters, chipmunks, and cotton rats. Some of these negative results may have resulted more from the inadequate, early carcinogenicity protocols than from the resistance of the species. The work on derivatives of DAB, described in Table XI and the accompanying list, is almost entirely confined to changes in the rat liver in tests that are usually relatively short. In other words, compounds reported as noncarcinogenic in these tests may prove to be carcinogenic if fed for a longer period or at higher levels.

The azo group in DAB is essential to the carcinogenic action of the chemical. Kensler et al. (*265*) postulated that the split products, in which the azo group is reduced to two amino groups, might be carcinogenic. Nevertheless, feeding rats with mixtures of the hydrochlorides of aniline, *N,N*-dimethyl-4-phenylenediamine, or *N*-methyl-4-phenylenediamine (**95**) or with mixtures of *m*-toluidine (**96**) and *N,N*-dimethyl-4-phenylenediamine failed to induce tumors (*266–69*). Furthermore, riboflavin in the diet inhibits DAB carcinogenesis in rat liver. Riboflavin is a component of a flavine adenine dinucleotide that acts as an essential cofactor for the enzyme azo reductase (*270*). The azo group could be lost also by reduction to a hydrazine and by conversion in an acid medium to benzidines or semidines, and these products could be carcinogenic (*see* previous section BENZIDINE). This hypothesis however was shown to be unlikely by the synthesis of four of the five possible derivatives (**97–101**), and the consequent demonstration that they were not carcinogenic to rats (*271*). Because 2′,4′,6′-trifluoro-DAB is a more potent carcinogen than DAB itself and because the C–F bond is unlikely to be broken in

Liver Carcinogenicity of *N,N*-Dimethyl-*p*-phenylazoanilines in Rats

Positive	*Negative*
N,N-Dimethyl-4-(4′-benzimidazolylazo)aniline	2-Dimethylamino-5-(phenylazo)pyridine
N,N-Dimethyl-4-(6′-benzthiazolylazo)aniline	*N,N*-Dimethyl-4-(5′-benzimidazolylazo)aniline
N,N-Dimethyl-4-(7′-benzthiazolylazo)aniline	*N,N*-Dimethyl-4-(2′-dibenzofuranylazo)aniline
N,N-Dimethyl-4-[4′-(2′,6′-dimethylpyridyl-1′-oxide)azo]aniline	*N,N*-Dimethyl-4-(1′-dibenzothienylazo)aniline
N,N-Dimethyl-4-(6′-1*H*-indazylazo)aniline	*N,N*-Dimethyl-4-(2′-dibenzothienylazo)aniline
N,N-Dimethyl-4-(4′-isoquinolinylazo)aniline	*N,N*-Dimethyl-4-(3′-dibenzothienylazo)aniline
N,N-Dimethyl-4-(5′-isoquinolinylazo)aniline	*N,N*-Dimethyl-4-(3-dibenzothienylazo)aniline
N,N-Dimethyl-4-(7′-isoquinolinylazo)aniline	*N,N*-Dimethyl-4-(4′-benzthiazylazo)aniline
N,N-Dimethyl-4-(5′-isoquinolyl-2′-oxide)azoaniline	*N,N*-Dimethyl-4-(5′-benzthiazylazo)aniline
N,N-Dimethyl-4-[4′-(2′,5′-lutidyl)azo]aniline	*N,N*-Dimethyl-4-(2-fluorenylazo)aniline
N,N-Dimethyl-4-[4′-(2′,6′-lutidyl-1′-oxide)azo]aniline	*N,N*-Dimethyl-4-(3′-1*H*-indazylazo)aniline
N,N-Dimethyl-4-[4′-3′,5′-lutidyl-1′-oxide)azo]aniline	*N,N*-Dimethyl-4-(4′-1*H*-indazylazo)aniline
N,N-Dimethyl-4-[4′-(2′-methylpyridyl)azo]aniline	*N,N*-Dimethyl-4-(5′-1*H*-indazylazo)aniline
N,N-Dimethyl-4-[2′-methylpyridyl-1′-oxide)azo]aniline	*N,N*-Dimethyl-4-(7′-1*H*-indazylazo)aniline
N,N-Dimethyl-4-[4′-(3′-methylpyridyl-1′-oxide)azo]aniline	*N,N*-Dimethyl-4-[2′-(4′-methylpyridyl)azo]aniline
N,N-Dimethyl-4-[4′-(3′-methylpyridyl-1′-oxide)azo]aniline	*N,N*-Dimethyl-4-[2′-(6′-methylpyridyl)azo]aniline
N,N-Dimethyl-4-[4′-(2′-methylpyridyl-1′-oxide)azo]aniline	*N,N*-Dimethyl-4-(7′-quinolylazo)aniline
N,N-Dimethyl-4-[4′-(2′-methylpyridyl-1′-oxide)azo]-*o*-toluidine	*N,N*-Dimethyl-4-(8′-quinolylazo)aniline
N,N-Dimethyl-4-[5′-(3′-methylquinolyl)azo]aniline	*N,N*-Dimethyl-4-[(2′-quinolyl-1′-oxide)azo]aniline
N,N-Dimethyl-4-[5′-(6′-methylquinolyl)azo]aniline	*N,N*-Dimethyl-4-[(3′-quinolyl-1′-oxide)azo]aniline
N,N-Dimethyl-4-[5′-(7′-methylquinolyl)azo]aniline	*N,N*-Dimethyl-4-[(7′-quinolyl-1′-oxide)azo]aniline
N,N-Dimethyl-4-[5′-(8′-methylquinolyl)azo]aniline	*N,N*-Dimethyl-4-[(8′-quinolyl-1′-oxide)azo]aniline
N,N-Dimethyl-4-(2′-naphthylazo)aniline	*N,N*-Dimethyl-4-[2′-(4′-methylpyridyl-1′-oxide)azo]aniline
N,N-Dimethyl-4-[(3′-picolyl-1′-oxide)azo]-*o*-toluidine	*N,N*-Dimethyl-4-[2′-(6′-methylpyridyl-1′-oxide)azo]aniline
N,N-Dimethyl-4-[(3′-picolyl-1′-oxide)azo]-*m*-toluidine	
N-N-Dimethyl-4-[(4′-pyridyl-1′-oxide)azo]-2,3-xylidine	
N,N-Dimethyl-4-[(4′-pyridyl-1′-oxide)azo]-2,5-xylidine	
N,N-Dimethyl-4-[(4′-pyridyl-1′-oxide)azo]-3,5-xylidine	
N,N-Dimethyl-4-(3′-pyridylazo)aniline	
N,N-Dimethyl-4-[(4′-pyridyl-1′-oxide)azo]aniline	
N,N-Dimethyl-4-(5′-quinaldylazo)aniline	

Continued on next page

Liver Carcinogenicity of *N,N*-Dimethyl-*p*-phenylazoanilines in Rats Continued

Positive
N,N-Dimethyl-4-(3′-quinolylazo)aniline
N,N-Dimethyl-4-(4′-quinolylazo)aniline
N,N-Dimethyl-4-(5′-quinolylazo)aniline
N,N-Dimethyl-4-(6′-quinolylazo)aniline
N,N-Dimethyl-4-[(4′-quinolyl-1′-oxide)azo]aniline
N,N-Dimethyl-4-[(5′-quinolyl-1′-oxide)azo]aniline
N,N-Dimethyl-4-[(6′-quinolyl-1′-oxide)azo]aniline
N,N-Dimethyl-4-(5′-quinolylazo)-*m*-toluidine
N,N-Dimethyl-4-(2′-quinoxalylazo)aniline
N,N-Dimethyl-4-(5′-quinoxalylazo)aniline
N,N-Dimethyl-4-(6′-quinoxalylazo)aniline

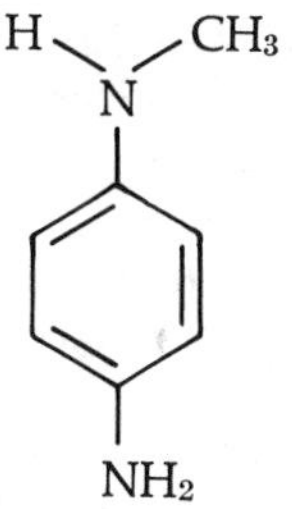

95 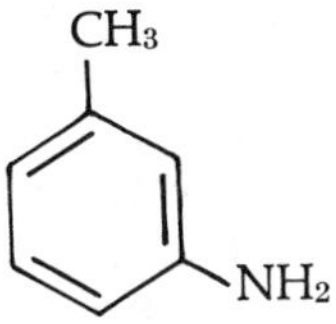 **96** 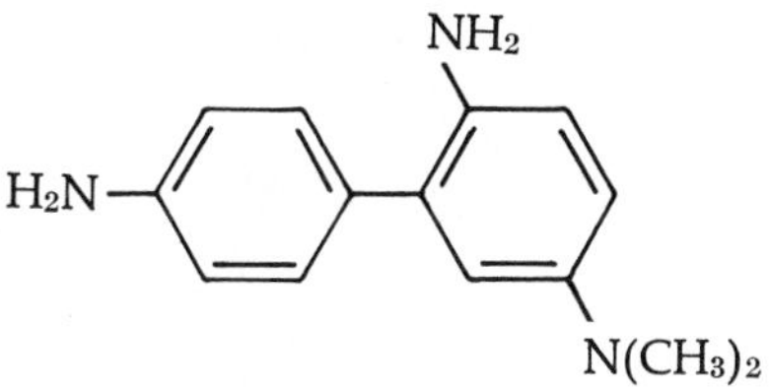 **97**

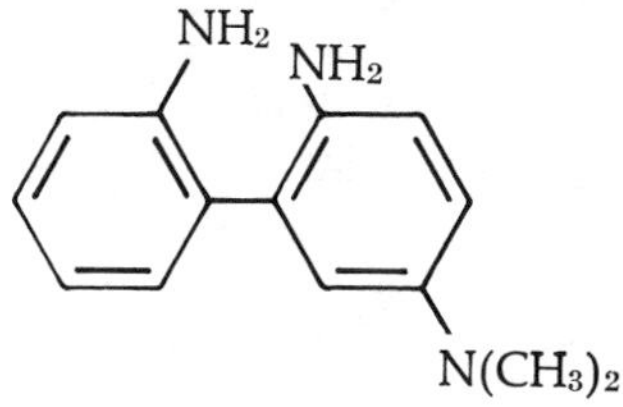

98 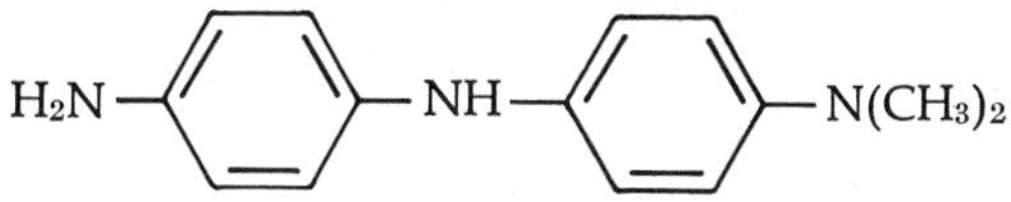 **99**

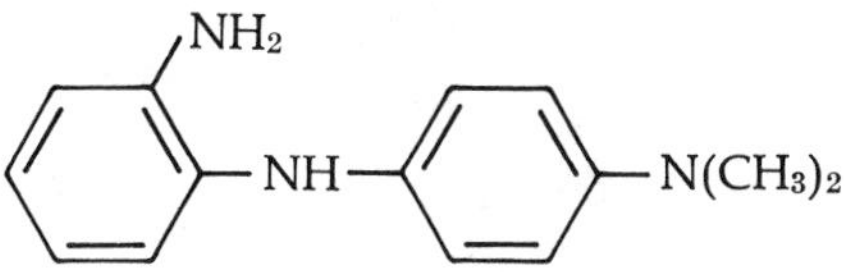

100 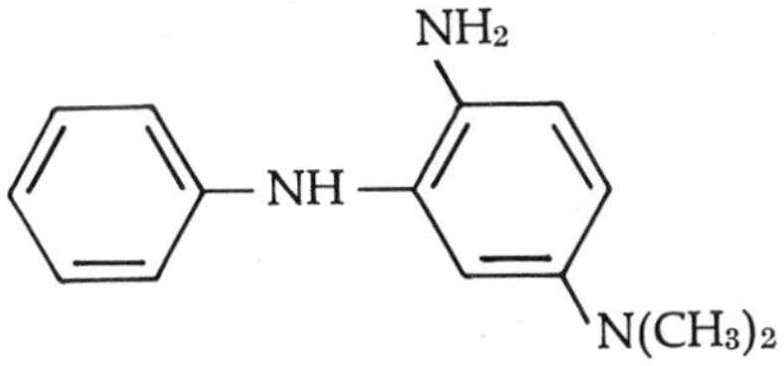 **101**

the mild conditions of a benzidine transformation, it is unlikely that **97–100** participate in the carcinogenicity of DAB.

N-Methylaminoazobenzenes are, in most cases, equipotent to the corresponding DAB derivatives, whereas AB itself is apparently noncarcinogenic on feeding. Thus, at least one methyl group seems to be essential for carcinogenicity to rat liver. This hypothesis is confirmed by considering the carcinogenic activity of a series of *N,N*-dialkyl-AB derivatives and a further series of *N*-alkyl-*N*-methyl derivatives. Although DAB is carcinogenic, none of the following derivatives gives tumors on feeding to rats: *N,N*-diethyl-AB, *N,N*-di-*n*-propyl-AB, *N,N*-di-*n*-butyl-AB,

N,N-di-*n*-amyl-AB, and 4-(phenylazo)formalinide. On the other hand, *N*-ethyl-*N*-methyl-AB and *N*-methyl-4-(phenylazo)formanilide are both potent carcinogens. This rule of thumb may not apply to all derivatives of DAB, because 4-([4-(diethylamino)phenyl]azo)pyridine 1-oxide (**102**), for example, is carcinogenic to rat liver. However, examples of this nature need not be regarded as contraindicating the significance of the *N*-methyl group, because the exceptions may induce cancer by mechanisms different from those that can be described for other DAB derivatives. Further confirmation of a difference in carcinogenicity between *N*-methyl and *N*-ethyl analogs is provided by the much lower activity of *N*-hydroxy-EAB compared with *N*-hydroxy-MAB (*272*). The former compound is less reactive than the latter and less amenable to sulfation.

DAB derivatives that were tested for carcinogenicity are given in Tables XI and XII. A similar but smaller table could be drawn up for derivatives of *N*-monomethyl-4-phenylazoaniline (MAB), but the carcinogenicity of each MAB derivative would not differ appreciably from that of the DAB derivative.

The number of DAB derivatives, which were tested by feeding to rats, is large and probably reflects their ease of synthesis and testing rather than their importance to our environment or to the development of theories of carcinogenesis. To help quantify this data, Miller and Miller (*271*) introduced the concept of an index of relative activity of carcinogenic azo dyes, and it is defined as

$$\text{relative activity} = \frac{6 \times M_{DAB} \times \%_{tc}}{M_{tc} \times \%_{DAB}}$$

where M_{DAB} is the months of feeding with DAB, $\%_{tc}$ is the percent of tumors with the test chemical, M_{tc} is the months of feeding with the test chemical, and $\%_{DAB}$ is the percent of tumors with DAB. While DAB itself has a relative activity of 6, other derivatives vary from 0 to 200 or more. If not too much emphasis is placed on the absolute figures, this index can be used to grade carcinogens according to activity.

The carcinogenic derivatives of DAB usually induce hepatomas in rats, the only species to be tested. Feeding 3-methoxy-DAB leads to skin, ear duct, and intestinal tumors, whereas 2′-carboxy-DAB (*273*) (methyl red) was reported to yield bladder papillomas and hepatomas. This result, however, must be regarded with caution, because a subsequent study (*274*) failed to confirm the finding, while a third experiment led to only a single hepatoma (*275*). The DAB derivatives in which the prime ring is replaced by a heterocyclic ring system maybe hepatocarcarcinogenic. For example, 6-([*p*-(dimethylamino)phenyl]azo) quinoxaline (**103**) at 0.3% in the diet led to 10 histologically confirmed hepatomas in 10 rats in 2 months, whereas the 2-isomer (**104**) was inactive at 8 months after feeding at the same level in the diet (*276*). Nevertheless, heterocyclic derivatives are not necessarily more potently carcinogenic, because *N,N*-dimethyl-4-(2,3-xylylazo)aniline (**105**) fed in the diet at a level of 0.06% gave 10 histologically confirmed hepatomas in 10 rats by the end of 1 month (*277*). The structural features necessary for this group of chemicals to be carcinogenic has been fully elucidated. In vitro cell transformation data indicate that 4-(*N*-pyrrolidinyl)azobenzene (PyAB) (**106**) is a more potent carcinogen that DAB (*278*), but carcinogenicity data in the rat show

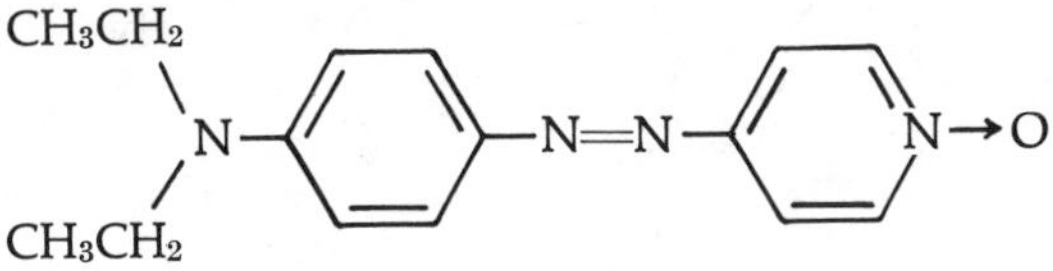

102

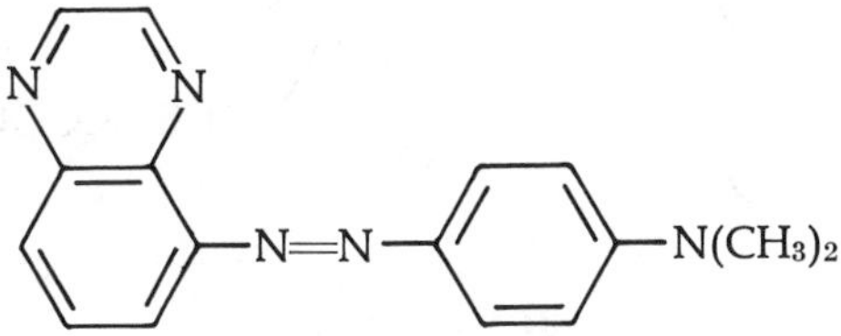

103

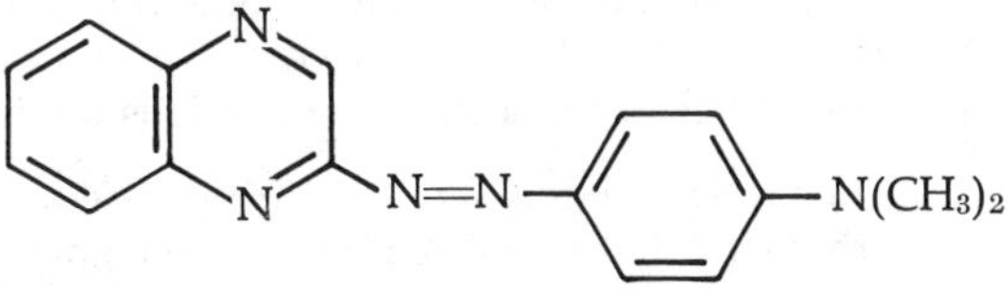

104

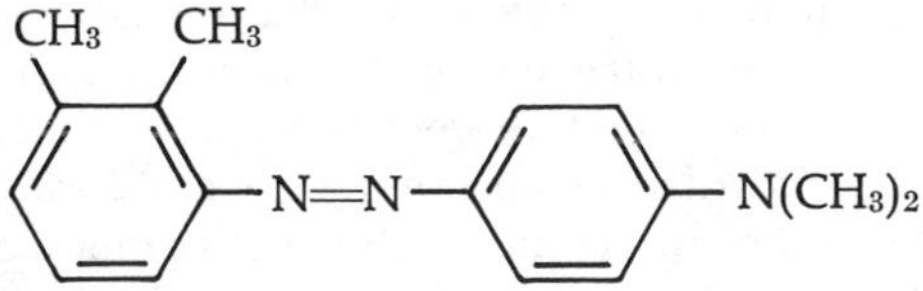

105

that it is less active as a hepatocarcinogen. Tumors developed with DAB administration by 10 months, while none were seen by PyAB (*279*).

The details of the mechanisms by which azo dyes might induce cancer have been worked out consequent to the synthesis of *N*-hydroxy-MAB (*49*). The synthesis of this proximate carcinogen using the Cope elimination enabled Miller et al. to test its carcinogenicity. Feeding *N*-hydroxy-MAB for a 5-week period to rats resulted in the appearance of hepatic tumors some 18–22 months later in approximately 25% of the animals. Rats given phenobarbitone in their drinking water subsequent to *N*-hydroxy-MAB administration had twice as many tumors compared with those given *N*-hydroxy-MAB alone. *N*-Hydroxy-MAB, but not MAB, also induced multiple papillomas of the forestomach in approximately 50% of the animals. *N*-Hydroxy-EAB and EAB proved to be less potent than their respective methyl analogs, a result that confirmed previous findings (*272*).

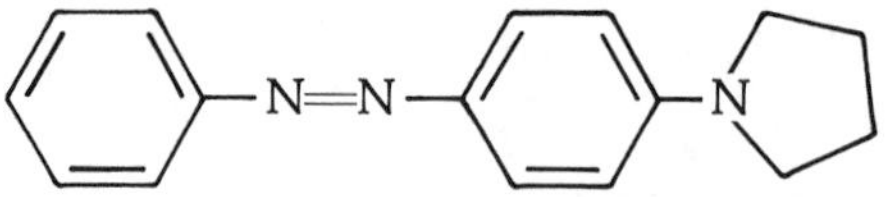

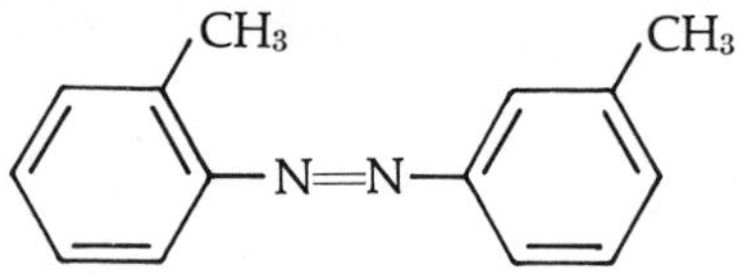

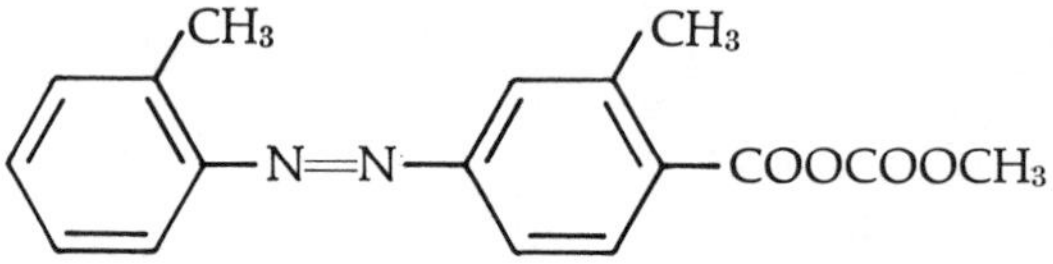

o-TOLYLAZO-*m*-TOLUENE. *o*-Tolylazo-*m*-toluene (**107**) and 4-(*o*-tolylazo)-2-methylbenzoic acid methylcarbonate (**108**) induced bladder papillomas when fed to rats at a level of 0.1–0.3% in their food (*280, 281*). Strombeck (*282*) at first failed to confirm the result with *o*-tolylazo-*m*-toluene. However, when he used a polished-rice diet, as favored by earlier Japanese workers, he obtained bladder papillomas that were often accompanied by bladder stones. Because neither of these earlier experiments was properly controlled, Strombeck and Ekman (*283–85*) administered the azo dye, *o*-toluidine, *p*-aminophenol, *o*-aminobenzoic acid, aniline, and 2-FAA separately to groups of rats on semisynthetic diets and obtained a number of bladder papillomas. Similar tumors were obtained without any added chemical. Urinary calculi were recorded at necropsy in about 50% of the animals with bladder tumors. The difficulties in interpreting the significance of bladder tumors in the presence of bladder stones have been summarized (*128*).

PHENYLAZONAPHTHOL DYES. Derivatives of phenylazonaphthol are important as dyes in food and in other products. Several derivatives have led to bladder tumors after bladder implantation in mice (*286, 287*), but the significance of these observations is difficult to assess.

Substances intended for use as food dyes, which include derivatives of 1-phenylazo-2-naphthol, should be assayed for carcinogenic activity by oral administration and preferably by inclusion in the diet. This type of assay is important for reasons other than mimicking the route of human exposure. First, the gut flora reductively degrade the azo group (*288*). For tartrazine and other water-soluble azo dyes, bacterial reduction is more important to the overall reduction of the dye than hepatic azo reductase (*289–91*). The reaction was studied in vitro, and the relevant enzyme was isolated (*290, 292*). Second, parenteral administration, especially by subcutaneous injection, leads to problems with nonchemically induced sarcomas (*293–95*). This complication is particularly well illustrated by Patent Blue V, a triphenylmethane dye that gave no tumors on feeding at the maximum tolerated level. The sodium salt of Patent Blue V gave sarcomas on injection, whereas the calcium salt did not (*296*). Golberg et al. showed that sarcomas at the injection site did not depend on the chemical structure of the test substance but instead on the physical properties of the solution; surfactant solutions, for example, led to sarcomas (*295, 297*). For these reasons, oral administration of derivatives of 1-phenylazo-2-naphthol will be emphasized.

There have been few attempts to assess the carcinogenicity of the "oil-soluble" derivatives of 1-phenylazo-2-naphthol (**109**) by conventional methods. Injection of 1-phenylazo-2-naphthol into the subcutaneous tissue of stock mice led to 7 hepatomas in 24 animals that survived for 15 months; the males were more sensitive than the females. Unfortunately, no proper controls were kept. Only 5 hepatomas occurred in 449 similar mice that were used in other experiments (*297*). Bonser was unable to confirm this observation in CBA mice although two bladder papillomas were induced in rabbits. 1-*o*-Tolylazo-2-naphthol (**110**) induced tumors of the ileo–caecal junction in mice fed or injected with this compound (*187*). Thirteen untreated mice of this stock, which is no longer available, developed one papilloma of the ileocaecal region. Citrus Red No. 2, i.e., 1-(2,5-dimethoxyphenylazo)-2-naphthol (**111**), led to bladder epithelial hyperplasia and a low incidence of bladder papillomas and carcinomas on feeding to rats and mice (*298*). The carcinogenicity associated with each of these components must be regarded as equivocal. Sharratt (*299*) confirmed the carcinogenicity of Citrus Red No. 2 in female mice, but not male mice.

Grice et al. (*300*) fed 0.3, 1.0, and 5.0% Ponceau 3R—Food Red No. 66, the disodium salt of 3-hydroxy-4-[(2,4,5-trimethylphenyl)azo]-2,7-naphthalenedisulfonic acid (**112**)—to groups of 30 rats for 65 weeks. Although there was a dose-related incidence of trabecular cell carcinomas of the liver (0, 7, and 24%), the result was not statistically significant. In another experiment, 5.0, 2.0, 1.0, and 0.5% of the dye was fed to large groups of weanling Osborn Mendel rats of both sexes, and it was demonstrated unequivocally that the substance was a liver carcinogen in rats (*301*). Unfinished experiments on mice that are being fed levels of 2.0, 1.0,

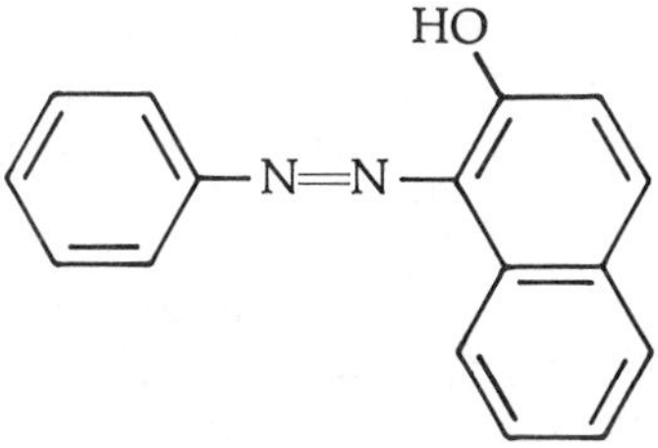

HO, N=N

109

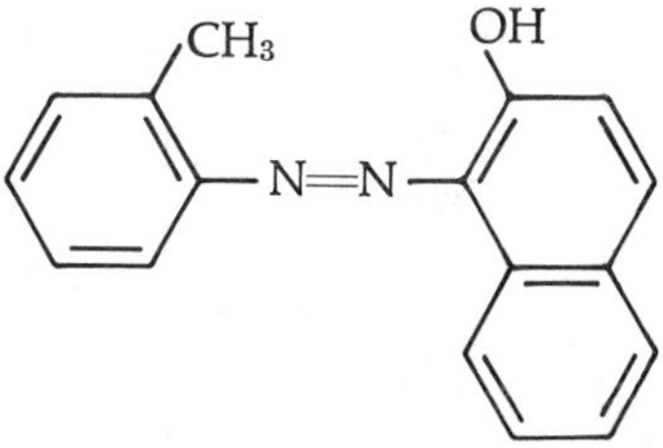

CH_3, OH, N=N

110

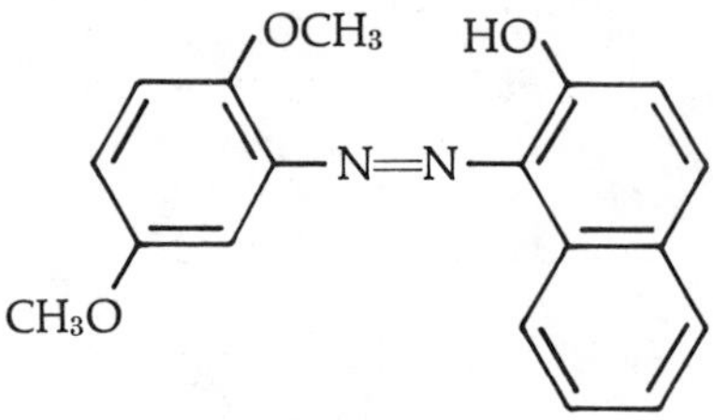

111

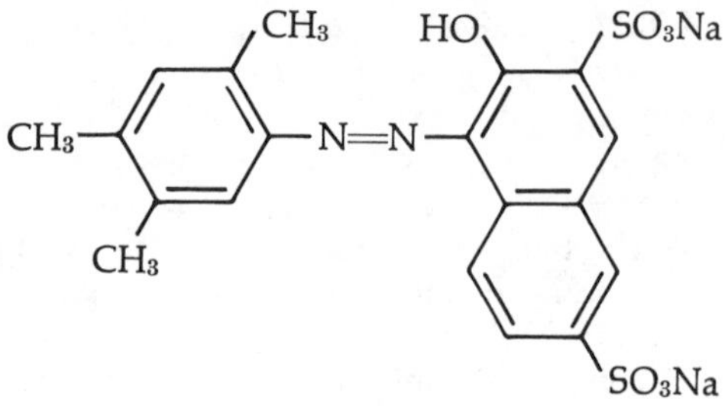

112

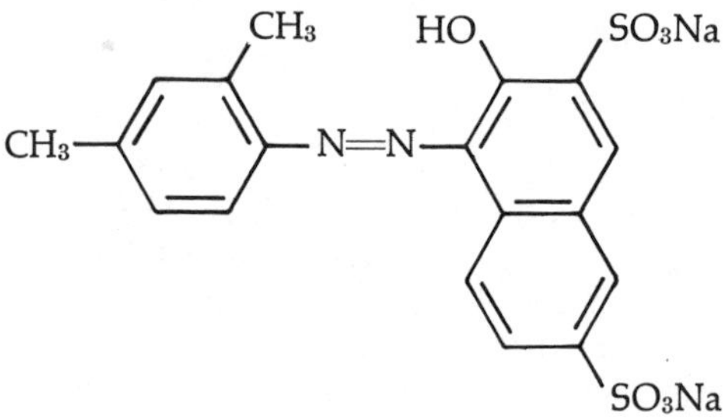

113

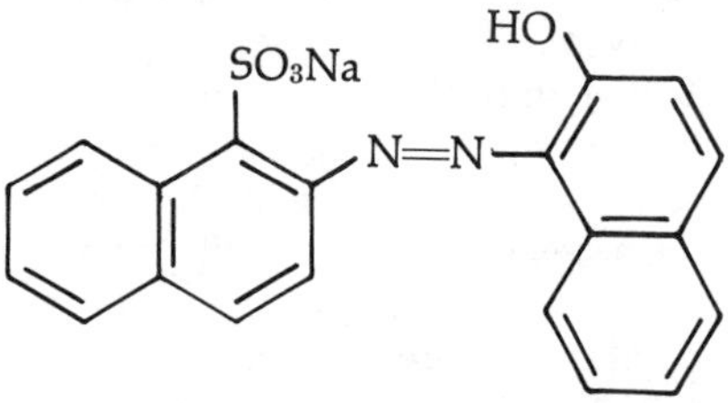

114

and 0.5% of the dye also suggest that Ponceau 3R is hepatocarcinogenic. Mannell (*302*) provided further corroborative information and, by examining the trimethylaniline after reduction of the azo group, demonstrated the gross lack of specificity in structure of the food dye.

When a similar substance named Ponceau MX—the disodium salt of 3-hydroxy-4-(2,4-xylylazo)-2,7-naphthalenedisulfonic acid (**113**)—was fed to rats at levels of 0.27, 1, and 3%, it led to a dose-related incidence of liver changes (*303*). The original workers diagnosed these lesions as tumors, but this conclusion was disputed (*304*). A further large experiment led to the induction of similar lesions also with a disputed diagnosis (*305, 306*). Similar lesions were found in mice (*307*). Prudence suggests that this substance is unsuitable for addition to food.

Other similar compounds did not induce tumors in large-scale feeding experiments: D and C Red No. 10—the monosodium salt of 1-(1-naphthalenesulfonic acid)azo-2-naphthol (**114**)—was negative in rats (*300*); Ponceau SX—the disodium salt of 4-hydroxy-3-[(5-sulfo-2,4-xylyl)azo]-1-naphthalenesulfonic acid (**115**)—was negative in rats and mice (*308*); Chocolate Brown FB—the coupling product of diazotized naphthionic acid and a mixture of 2′,3′,4′,6,7-pentahydroxyflavone and pentahydroxybenzophenone—were also negative in rats and mice (*309*); and Black PH—the tetrasodium salt of 2-(7-sulfo-4-*p*-phenylsulfonylazo-1-naphthylazo)-1-naphthol-3,5-disulfonic acid (**116**)—was negative in rats (*310*). Other compounds were reported to be inactive in less extensive tests.

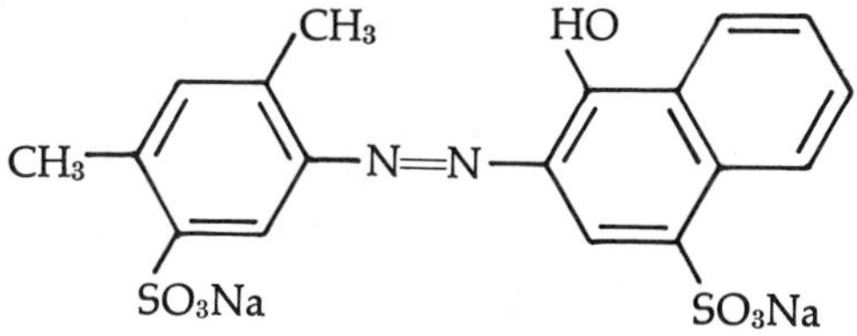

115

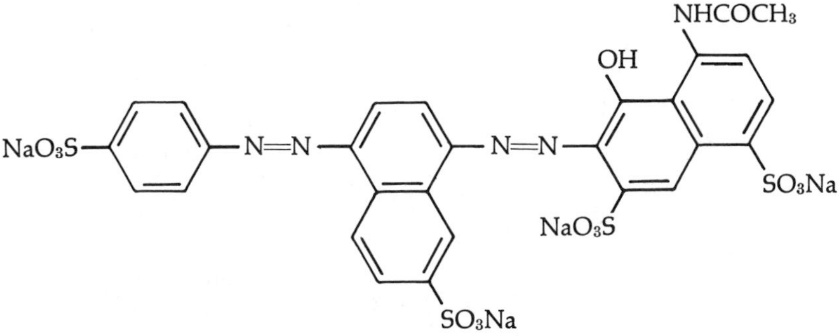

116

TRYPAN BLUE. When Trypan Blue—the tetrasodium salt of 3,3′-[(3,3′-dimethyl-4,4′-biphenylylene) bis (azo)] bis (5-amino-4-hydroxy-2,7-naphthalenedisulfonic acid) (**117**)—is injected into pregnant rats it induces abnormalities in the fetuses that closely resemble those seen in human pregnancies, and it is used as a model teratogen for experimental studies. When Trypan Blue is repeatedly injected into normal rats, it is absorbed by serum albumin and taken up by the reticuloendothelial system. Malignant tumors of this tissue appeared after only 100 d (*311, 312*).

The structural features necessary for the carcinogenecity of Trypan Blue were examined. Although Evans Blue (the tetrasodium salt of 6,6′-[(3,3′-dimethyl-4,4′-biphenylylene)bis(azo)]bis(4-amino-5-hydroxy-1,3-naphthalenedisulfonic acid (**118**) is active, Vital Red (the tetrasodium salt of 1,1′-(3,3′-dimethyl-4,4′-biphenylylene)bis(azo)bis(2-amino-3,6-naphthalenedisulfonic acid)) (**119**) and benzopurpurin 4B (the disodium salt of 2,2′-(3,3′-dimethyl-4,4′-biphenylylene)bis(azo)bis(1-amino-4-naphthalenesulfonic acid)) (**120**) are without carcinogenic activity (*313*). Semi-Trypan Blue (2-(*o*-tolyl)azo-4-hydroxy-8-amino-3,6-naphthalenedisulfonic acid) (**121**) is also without activity (*314*).

Limited metabolism studies on the phenylazonaphthols gave little indication of their metabolic activation (*315*). The simple suggestion that reduction of the azo group leads to liberation of a carcinogenic aromatic amine could explain the results obtained with the oil-soluble derivatives Ponceau 3R and Ponceau MX, from which

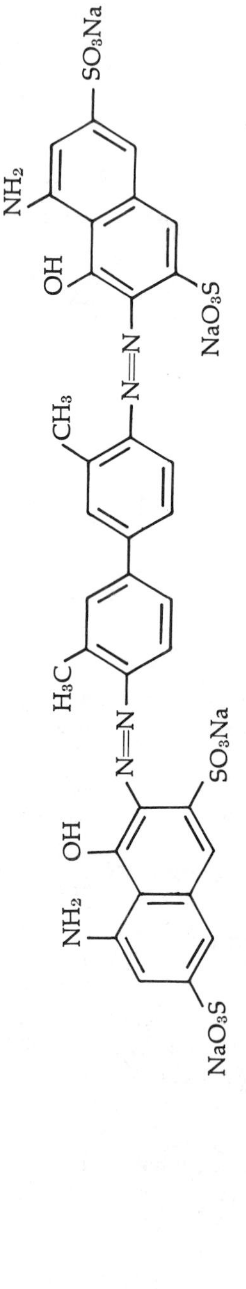

117

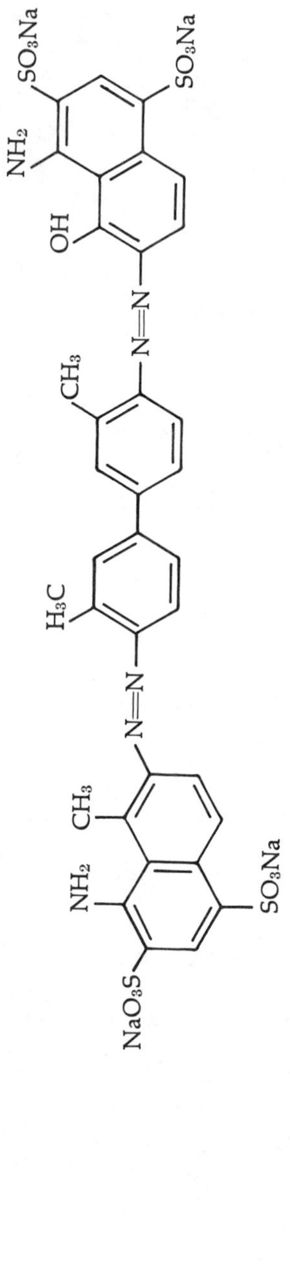

118

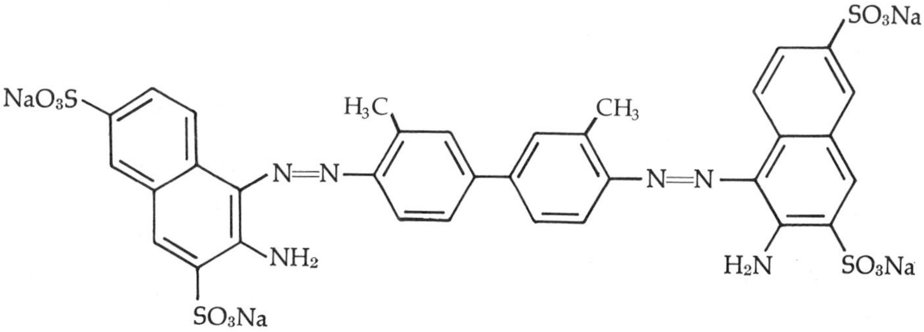

NaO_3S SO_3Na H_3C CH_3 $N{=}N$ NH_2 H_2N SO_3Na SO_3Na

119

NH_2 H_3C CH_3 NH_2 $N{=}N$ SO_3Na SO_3Na

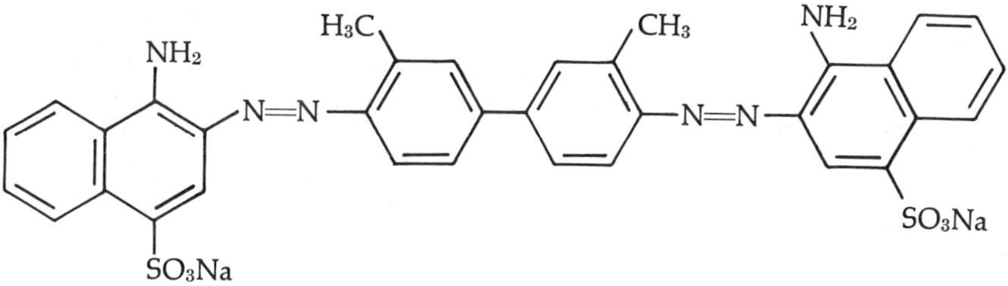

120

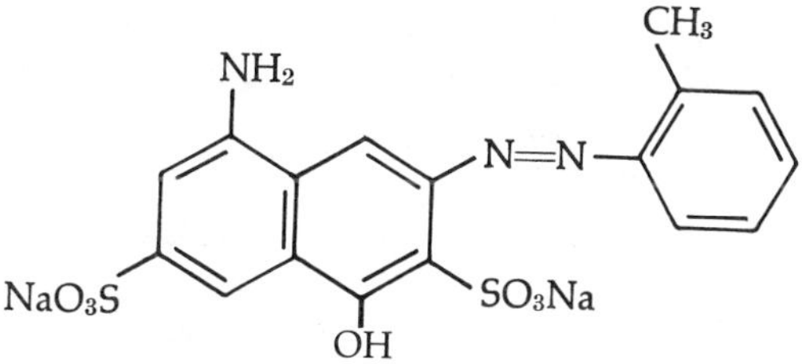

CH_3 NH_2 $N{=}N$ NaO_3S SO_3Na OH

121

122

123

124

analogs of the well-known but weak carcinogen *o*-toluidine are liberated (*see* previous section BENZIDINE). Nevertheless, the fact that Trypan Blue induces histiocytic or Kupfer cell tumors of the liver, whereas the aromatic amine derived from it, *o*-toluidine, does not (Table I) seemingly contradicts the hypothesis that *o*-toluidine is responsible for the carcinogenicity of Ponceau 3R and Ponceau MX.

OTHER AZO DYES. Three dyes, Direct Blue 6 (**122**), Direct Black 38 (**123**), and Direct Brown 95 (**124**), have been tested as part of the Carcinogenesis Testing Program of the National Cancer Institute, because they are derived from benzidine. In a 13-week subchronic toxicity test usually performed prior to a life-time study, neoplastic lesions, including hepatocellular carcinoma, were found for all three dyes in rats, whereas none were found in mice given diets containing the same concentrations of these dyes (*111*). Feeding of benzidine to parallel groups of animals did not induce any tumors in this time period. Clearly these benzidine-based dyes are powerful carcinogens in rats. Whether other benzidine- or congener-related dyes are of equal potency remains to be established.

Other commercially important dyes have been tested for carcinogenicity under more or less rigorous conditions. Substances such as 1-phenylazo-2-naphthylamine (**125**) and 1-*o*-tolylazo-2-naphthylamine (F, D, and C Yellow No. 4) (**126**) failed to induce tumors in several tests. This absence of tumors could be grossly misleading as an index of safety to humans unless great care is taken to ensure that each batch is free from 2-naphthylamine residue.

A number of azo compounds such as amaranth (*316*) and tartrazine (*317*) are used as food dyes; the former compound is claimed to be a carcinogen, but the experimental evidence is unconvincing.

Heterocyclic Compounds. 4-NITROQUINOLINE 1-OXIDE (NQO) (**23**) AND ITS DERIVATIVES. NQO has a low degree of electrophilic reactivity. The nitro group can be replaced in vitro by alkoxyl, aryloxyl, mercapto, and hydroxyl groups, halogens, and amino acids.

Although initially NQO was thought to react directly with DNA, RNA, and protein in vivo to induce carcinogenic transformation, the reaction product, 4-hydroxylaminoquinoline 1-oxide (HAQO), was determined to be the more likely proximate carcinogen.

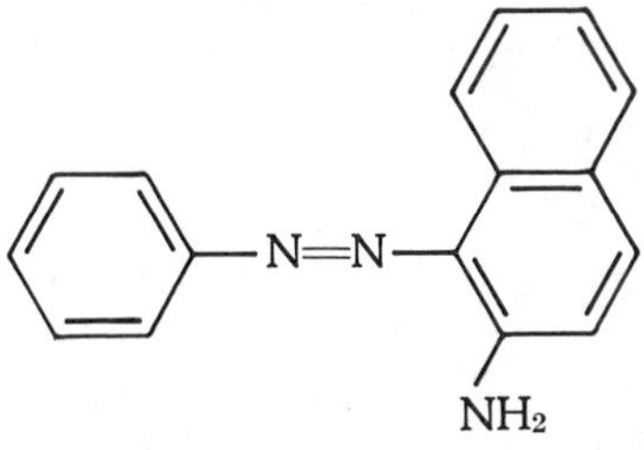

N=N NH_2

125

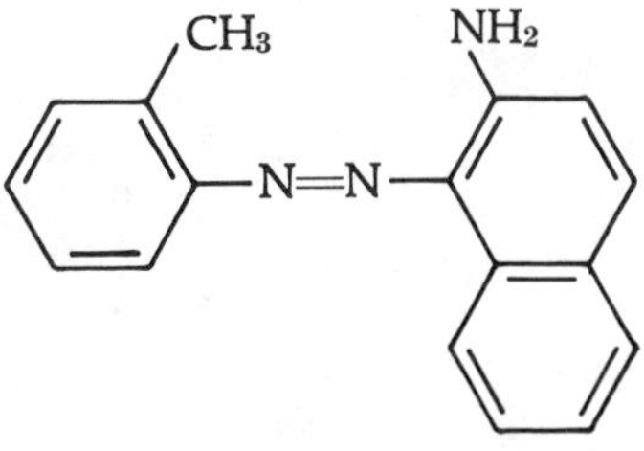

CH_3 NH_2 N=N

126

Table XII

Substituted 4-Nitroquinoline 1-Oxide and 4-Hydroxylaminoquinoline 1-Oxide Derivatives Tested for Carcinogenic Activity in Mice

	Position							
Substituent	*2*	*3*	*5*	*6*	*7*	*8*	*6,7-Di*	*6,8-Di*
4-Nitro								
Fluoro		+				+	+	
Chloro		+	+	+			+	−
Bromo		+	+	+	+			
Methoxy	+	−	+	+				
Methyl	+	−	+	+	+	+	+	
Ethyl	−							
Nitro			−	+	−	−		
Carboxylic acid				+				
Cyclohexyl				−				
n-Hexyl				+				
n-Butyl				−				
4-Hydroxylamino								
Chloro			+	+	+		+	
Methoxy		−						
Methyl	+	+	+	+	+	+		
Nitro				+	+			
Carboxylic acid				+				
Cyclohexyl				−				
n-Butyl				+				
tert-Butyl				−				

The carcinogenicity of NQO, HAQO, and their analogs is set out in Tables XII and XIII. Both NQO and HAQO act locally on skin painting, subcutaneous injection, gastric intubation, or esophageal infusion thus demonstrating that many tissues probably possess the enzymes required to activate these compounds. NQO is also carcinogenic in a range of animal species, including the mouse, rat, lovebird, guinea pig, and hamster.

Table XIII indicates the molecular specificity necessary for the carcinogenic activity of NQO. Loss of the nitro group, the 1-oxide, or the second benzene ring (as in 4-nitropyridine 1-oxide) leads to inactive compounds. Addition of a further benzene ring, as in 9-nitroacridine 1-oxide, likewise gives an inactive compound. Similarly, the positional isomers 3- and 5-nitroquinoline 1-oxide are not carcinogenic. 4-Aminoquinoline 1-oxide has not induced tumors. On the other hand, many substituted derivatives of NQO are potent carcinogens (Table XII).

The overall evidence suggests that the metabolic activation of NQO to HAQO is important. The failure of 3-methyl-NQO and 3-methoxy-NQO to give tumors in

Table XIII

Carcinogenic Activity of 4-Nitroquinoline 1-Oxide Analogs

Compound	*Species*	*Route*[b]	*Adequacy*[c]	*Site of Tumor Induction*[a]							
				Local	*Bladder*	*Kidney*	*Liver*	*Intestine*	*Ear Duct*	*Breast*	*Other*
4-Nitroquinoline 1-oxide (NQO)	rabbit	s.c.	A								
	guinea pig	top.	S	+	–	–	–	–	–	–	lung
	hamster	top.	S	+	–	–	–	–	–	–	–
	rat	v	A	+	–	–	–	–	–	–	lung
	mouse	v	A	+	–	–	–	–	–	–	lung adenomas; leukemia
4-Aminoquinoline 1-oxide	rat	s.c.	A	–	–	–	–	–	–	–	–
	mouse	s.c.	S	–	–	–	–	–	–	–	–
Quinoline 1-oxide	mouse	s.c.	S	–	–	–	–	–	–	–	–
4-Hydroxylaminoquinoline 1-oxide	rat	o	A	+	–	–	–	–	–	+	lung; glandular stomach
	mouse	s.c./o	A	+	–	–	–	–	–	–	glandular stomach; lung
3-Hydroxylaminoquinoline 1-oxide	rat	s.c.	S	–	–	–	–	–	–	–	–
	mouse	s.c.	S	–	–	–	–	–	–	–	–
5-Hydroxylaminoquinoline 1-oxide	rat	s.c.	S	–	–	–	–	–	–	–	–
	mouse	s.c.	S	–	–	–	–	–	–	–	–
4-Nitropyridine 1-oxide	rat	s.c.	S	–	–	–	–	–	–	–	–
	mouse	s.c.	S	–	–	–	–	–	–	–	–
4-Hydroxylaminopyridine 1-oxide	rat	s.c.	S	–	–	–	–	–	–	–	–
	mouse	s.c.	S	–	–	–	–	–	–	–	–
9-Nitroacridine 9-oxide	mouse	s.c.	S	–	–	–	–	–	–	–	–

[a] +, tumors reported; and –, tumors not reported.
[b] o, oral; s.c., subcutaneous injection; top., topical; and v, various routes.
[c] A, tested in more than one institute; and S, evidence less than convincing.

animals may be because these NQO derivatives are difficult to convert to HAQO derivatives enzymically, whereas NT-diaphorase can readily reduce 2-methyl-NQO, 6,7-dichloro-NQO, or 8-methyl-NQO in the presence of reduced pyridine nucleotide; 3-methyl-NQO, 3-methoxy-NQO, 3-chloro-NQO, and 3-bromo-NQO are only slightly reduced. Of the latter compounds, 3-methyl-NQO, 3-chloro-NQO, and 3-methoxy-NQO are not carcinogenic, whereas the 3 bromo derivative may be hydrolyzed before reduction in vivo (*318*).

Enomoto et al. showed that the *N,O*-diacetyl-4-hydroxylaminoquinoline 1-oxide (*58, 319*) reacts covalently with DNA, RNA, and polynucleotides to a greater extent than HAQO. It also reacts with methionine. This substance would therefore appear to be a candidate for the ultimate carcinogenic form of NQO if it or *O*-acetyl-HAQO was found in vivo. However, carcinogenicity studies using this compound showed it to be less active than NQO, possibly because of its ready action with noncritical nucleophiles (*319*).

PURINE OXIDES. The demonstration that the subcutaneous injection of unspecified "oxides" of xanthine and purine induces local sarcomas in rats has led to another example where *N*-hydroxylation is a determining factor in carcinogenesis. 3-Hydroxyxanthine and 3-hydroxyguanine were effective carcinogens, but 3-hydroxyadenine was not. The carcinogenicity of various derivatives is given in Table XIV (*320*).

The discovery that 8-methylmercaptoxanthine and 8-methylmercaptoguanine were present as metabolites of the carcinogenic 3-acetoxypurines (*320*) along with the information gathered from a study of the chemistry of these compounds (*321*) led to the proposed mechanisms for metabolic activation illustrated in Scheme III. The 8- or 9-methyl derivatives of the 3-hydroxypurines are not carcinogenically active, because the methyl interferes with the activation of the 8-position. Formation of a sulfate ester is unlikely to be the final activating step for these oxides. Incubation in vitro of a cell extract containing sulfotransferase and [^{35}S] 3′-phosphoadenosylsulfate was performed with each 3-hydroxypurine derivative that has been tested for carcinogenicity. The liberated sulfate that was measured as free $^{35}SO_4$ produced by the sulfation of the 3-hydroxy groups and their rapid reaction with nucleophiles did not correspond with the carcinogenicity of the purine used (*322*). Acetoxy derivatives of these purines, on the other hand, inactivate and mutate *B. subtilis* transforming DNA (*323, 324*).

There has been much speculation on the possibility of endogenous carcinogenesis, i.e., the production of carcinogens within the body that may be responsible for cancer of "natural" or unknown origin. To the best of our knowledge no evidence exists for the production of 3-hydroxypurines in vivo.

AMINO AND NITRO DERIVATIVES OF FIVE-MEMBERED HETEROCYCLIC RING COMPOUNDS. Furan (**127**), pyrrole (**128**), thiophene (**129**), and several other heterocyclic five-membered ring systems are aromatic because they have two unsaturated bonds and a hetero atom that contributes a lone pair of electrons to make up an aromatic sextet. Their nitro and amino derivatives therefore are included in this chapter.

Compounds of this nature play an important role in human and veterinary medicine. The observation that some of these derivatives are carcinogenic is an obstacle for the development of efficient drugs.

Table XIV

Carcinogenicity of Hydroxypurine Derivatives by Subcutaneous Injection in Rats

Compound	*Activity*[a]
3-Hydroxyxanthine	+++
3-Acetoxyxanthine	++
3-Hydroxy-1-methylxanthine	+++
3-Hydroxy-7-methylxanthine	0
3-Hydroxy-8-methylxanthine	0
3-Hydroxy-9-methylxanthine	0
3-Hydroxy-8-azaxanthine	0
3-Hydroxy-7,9-dimethylxanthine	0
3-Hydroxyguanine	++
3-Hydroxy-1-methylguanine	++
3-Hydroxy-7-methylguanine	0
3-Hydroxy-8-methylguanine	0
3-Hydroxy-9-methylguanine	0
1-Hydroxyxanthine	0
7-Hydroxyxanthine	++
9-Hydroxyxanthine	0
Hypoxanthine 3-oxide	++
Adenine 1-oxide	+
Purine 3-oxide	++

[a] +++, highly carcinogenic; ++, carcinogenic; +, moderately carcinogenic; and 0, not carcinogenic.

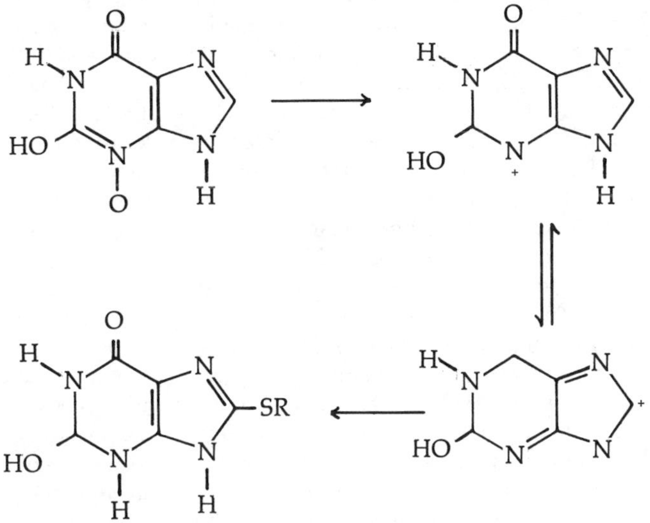

Scheme III. Proposed mechanisms for the metabolic activation of 8-methylmercaptoxanthine and 8-methylmercaptoguanine.

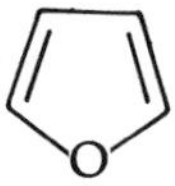

O N S

127 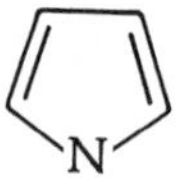 128 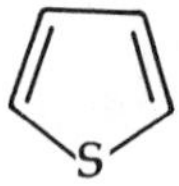 129

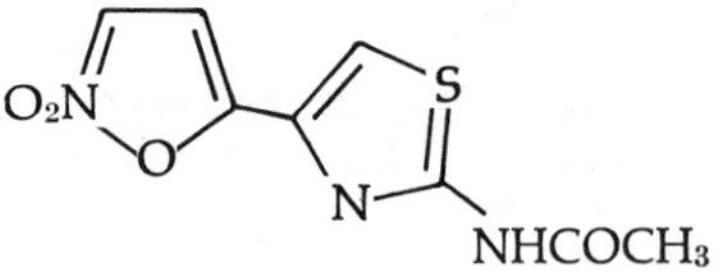

O_2N O S N $NHCOCH_3$

130

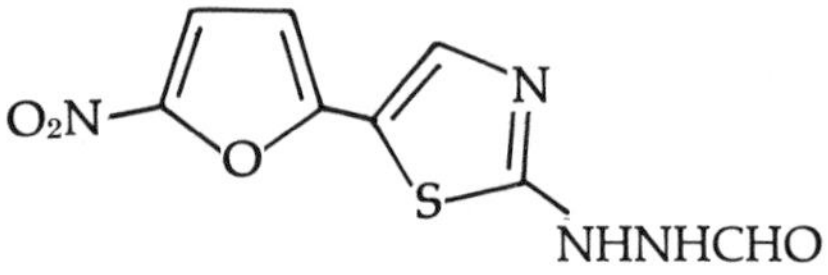

O_2N O N S NHNHCHO

131

O_2N O CH=N N S

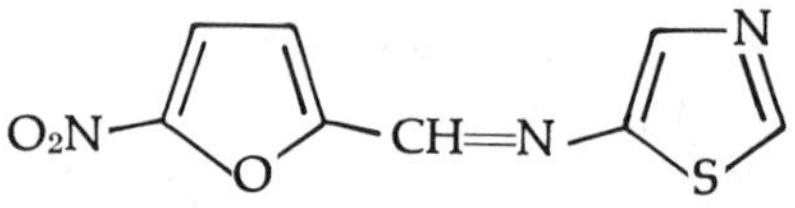

132

The first observations on 2-nitro-5-furyl derivatives were carried out by Price et al. (*325*) and Stein et al. (*326*). The demonstration that *N*-[4-(5-nitro-2-furyl)-2-thiazolyl]formamide (**25**) is an exceedingly potent bladder carcinogen in mice, dogs, and hamsters established interest in this group of compounds (*40, 41, 327, 328*). This particular compound is one of the most potent bladder carcinogens known in the rat (*329*).

A related compound, *N*-[4-(5-nitro-2-furyl)-2-thiazolyl]acetamide (**130**) was used pharmaceutically in some countries against human infectious disease. It was tested in female rats and, unlike the formamide, led to mammary gland adenocarcinoma, renal pelvic tumors, lung adenocarcinoma, and salivary gland adenocarcinoma. In dogs and hamsters, the formamide and acetamide induced similar tumor types, while in mice the acetamide led to leukemia and tumors of the forestomach (*41, 330–32*). The other compound of this series which has been tested with equal thoroughness is formic acid 2-[4-(5-nitro-2-furyl)-2-thiazolyl] hydrazide (**131**). It is one of a series of drugs whose routine testing for carcinogenicity led to the discovery of this group of compounds. In rats, the hydrazide led to tumors of the renal pelvis, tubular epithelium, and renal stroma (*333*). In mice, stomach, lung, and mammary tumors occurred, while urinary tract tumors predominated in hamsters (*330, 333*).

The other 5-nitro-2-furyl compounds were tested in rats and occasionally in mice (Table XV). They show the structural features necessary for carcinogenic activity. In general, compounds containing two directly joined heterocyclic rings are among the most active. This proximity of two rings with aromatic character makes these compounds similar to aromatic amines of the biphenylamine and benzidine series—a hypothesis that is confirmed by the demonstration that 2-hydrazino-4-(4-aminophenyl)thiazole and 2-hydrazino-4-(4-nitrophenyl)thiazole are active in rats (*334*). A second carcinogenic structure helps to demonstrate the variety of systems that may be involved (**132**). In the heterocyclic series, linkage by the –CH=N– bond produces carcinogenic derivatives, in contrast to the obser-

Table XV

Carcinogenicity of 2-Nitrofuryl Compounds and Related Substances by Oral Administration

			Site of Tumor Induction[a]							
Compound	*Species*	*Adequacy*[b]	*Local*	*Bladder*	*Kidney*	*Liver*	*Intestine*	*Ear Duct*	*Breast*	*Other*
2-Amino-5-(5-nitro-2-furyl)thiazole	rat	A	–	–	–	–	–	–	+	salivary gland; various other tissues
	mouse	S	–	?	?	–	–	–	–	stomach
Formic acid, 2-[4-(5-nitro-2-furyl)-2-thiazolyl]hydrazide	rat	S	–	–	+	?	–	–	+	lung(?); skin(?); stomach
	hamster	S	–	+	–	–	–	–	–	stomach(?)
	mouse	S	–	–	–	–	–	–	+	lung(?)
2-Hydrazino-4-(5-nitro-2-furyl)thiazole	rat	S	–	–	?	–	–	–	+	stomach(?)
	mouse	S	–	–	–	–	–	–	+	stomach(?)
2-Hydrazino-4-(4-nitrophenyl)thiazole	rat	S	–	–	–	–	–	–	+	skin(?); salivary gland(?)
	mouse	S	–	–	–	–	–	–	–	stomach(?)
N-[4-(5-Nitro-2-furyl)-2-thiazolyl]formamide	dog[c]	A	–	+	–	–	–	–	+	gall bladder
	rat	A	–	+	+	–	–	–	+	–
	hamster	S	–	+	–	–	–	–	–	stomach
	mouse	S	–	+	–	–	–	–	–	lung(?)
5-Acetamido-3-(5-nitro-2-furyl)-6*H*-1,2,4-oxadiazine	rat	S	–	–	–	+	–	–	–	lung, mesentery (hemangioendotheliosarcomas)
5-Nitro-2-furaldehyde semicarbazone	rat	S	–	–	–	–	–	–	?	–
N-[4-(5-Nitro-2-furyl)-2-thiazolyl]acetamide	rat	S	–	–	+	–	–	–	+	lung; salivary gland
	hamster	S	–	+	–	–	–	–	–	–
	mouse	S	–	–	–	–	–	–	–	leukemia
1-(5-Nitro-2-furylidene)aminohydantoin	rat		–	–	–	–	–	–	–	–

Continued on next page

Table XV. Continued

Compound	Species	Adequacy[b]	Site of Tumor Induction[a]: Local	Bladder	Kidney	Liver	Intestine	Ear Duct	Breast	Other
4-Methyl-1-[5-nitrofurylido)-amino]-2-imidazolidinone	rat	S	–	–	–	–	–	–	+	–
1-5-Morpholinomethyl-3-[(5-nitro-2-furylidene) amino]-2-oxazolidine	rat	S	–	–	–	–	–	–	+	lymphoma
1-(2-Hydroxyethyl)-3-[5-nitrofurylidene)amino]-2-imidazoline	rat	S	–	–	–	–	–	–	+	–
5-Nitro-2-furamidoxime	rat	S	–	–	–	–	–	–	–	–
4,6-Diamino-2-(5-nitro-2-furyl)-*s*-triazine	rat	S	–	–	–	–	–	–	+	–
N,N'-[6-(5-Nitro-2-furyl)-*s*-triazine-2, 4-diyl]bisacetamide	rat	S	–	–	–	–	–	–	+	–
Hexamethylmelamine	rat	S	–	–	?	–	–	–	?	–
2-Hydrazino-4-phenylthiazole	rat	S	–	–	–	–	–	–	–	–
D-(–)–*threo*-1-(*p*-Nitrophenyl)-2-dichloroacetamido-1,3-propanediol	rat	S	–	–	–	–	–	–	–	–
1-(2,Hydroxyethyl)-2-methyl-5-nitroimidazole	rat	S	–	–	–	–	–	–	+	–
1,2-Dimethyl-5-nitroimidazole	rat	S	–	–	–	–	–	–	+	–
2-Amino-5-phenyl-2-oxazolin-4-one + $Mg(OH)_2$	rat	S	–	–	–	–	–	–	?	–
3-Aminotriazole	rat	A	–	–	–	+	–	–	–	thyroid
	mouse	A	–	–	–	+	–	–	–	thyroid
1-(2-Hydroxy)ethyl-2-methyl-5-nitroimidazole	mouse	S	–	–	–	–	–	–	–	lymphoma; lung
2-Quino-5-(5-nitro-2-furyl)thiazole	rat	S	–	+	+	–	–	–	–	stomach; mammary gland
1-(5-Nitro-2-thiazolyl)-2-imidazolidinone	rat	S	–	–	+	–	–	–	–	stomach
2,4-Diamino-6-phenyl-5-triazine	rat	S	–	–	–	–	–	–	–	–
	mouse	S	–	–	–	–	–	–	–	–
2,4-Dichloro-6-[(*o*-chloranilo)5-triazine]	rat	NCI	–	–	–	–	–	–	–	testis; glands
	mouse	NCI	–	–	–	+	–	–	–	glands
3-Amino-9-ethylcarbazole	mouse	NCI	–	–	–	+	–	–	–	–

[a]+, tumors reported; –, tumors not reported; and ?, evidence equivocal. [b]A, tested in more than one institute; S, evidence less than convincing; and NCI, tested as part of the bioassay program. [c]Both subcutaneous injection and oral administration used.

vations in the carbocyclic series with stilbenamine analogs, where the –CH=N– group between the two carbocyclic aromatic rings does not lead to carcinogenic compounds.

Single-ring 2-nitro-5-furyl and other nitroheterocyclic compounds present some interesting problems. 5-Nitro-2-furanidoxine and 5-nitro-2-furanoethanediol diacetate are inactive, while 5-nitro-2-furaldehyde semicarbazone has induced only fibromas of the rat mammary gland. Mammary fibromas are considered benign by many pathologists, but Bryan et al. (*334*) believe them to be malignant, because they were transplantable into untreated rats—one of the classical properties associated with malignancy. However, with the increasing use of pure line and other relatively inbred animals, the significance of this property has been undermined. The standing of the mammary fibroma in carcinogenicity tests is important, because the possible carcinogenicity of some valuable substances depends on it: 5-nitro-2-furaldehyde semicarbazone, which is an important antiseptic for the urinary tract known as Furadantin; nitrofurantoin; and 1,2-dimethyl-5-nitroimidazole, which is a veterinary medicine (*335*). 1-(2-Hydroxymethyl)-3-methyl-5-nitroimidazole, known as Flagyl or metronizadole, was used in the treatment of infectious vaginitis and leprosy. This compound was tested in mice and induced an excess of lymphomas and lung tumors (*336, 337*). In rats, this drug significantly increased the incidence of mammary tumors and hepatomas in females, and at the highest dose, it increased Leydig cell tumors of the testes and pituitary adenomas in males (*338*). In our view, the carcinogenicity of the five-membered single-ring aromatic heterocyclics has many similarities to that of the derivatives of single-ring carbocyclic aromatic amines; high doses of both are required to demonstrate carcinogenicity. There is a diversity of chemical structures leading to carcinogenicity, including the imidazole and triazole structures. 3-Aminotriazole is a goitrogen, but unlike the other goitrogens, it apparently induces tumors of the rat liver. We therefore prefer to relate the carcinogenicity of this class of compounds to an amino or nitro group attached to a suitable heterocycle than merely to the possession of a 2-nitrofuryl group.

TRYPTOPHAN AND INDOLE. The essential amino acid, tryptophan, and two related compounds, indole and indoleacetic acid, enhance the incidence of bladder cancer in certain closely defined situations. Dunning et al. (*338, 339*) showed that rats fed 2-FAA in the diet with 1.4 or 4.9% DL-tryptophan (**133**), 0.8 or 1.6% indole (**134**), or 1.0% indoleacetic acid (**135**) developed bladder tumors, whereas those fed 2-FAA alone did not. This experiment has been repeated, although attempts to substitute other aromatic amines such as benzidine or 2-naphthylamine for 2-FAA (*340*) or to use DL-tryptophan and 3-aminobenzofuran in female IF × C57 mice did not lead to bladder tumors. In hamsters, indole or DL-tryptophan and 2-FAA gave slightly more bladder tumors than did 2-FAA by itself (*341, 342*). Feeding 2-FAA with a vitamin B deficient diet also enhanced bladder tumor induction (*343*).

A possible explanation of these results is that the additive protects the liver against tumorigenesis. In a study in which the two strains of rat did not develop bladder cancer after feeding with 2-FAA and excess DL-tryptophan, the most noteworthy result was a reduced incidence of liver tumors (*344*). This finding was confirmed and extended to show that rats fed 2-FAA alone developed aggressive trabecular cell carcinomas of the liver after a few months, but when there was a

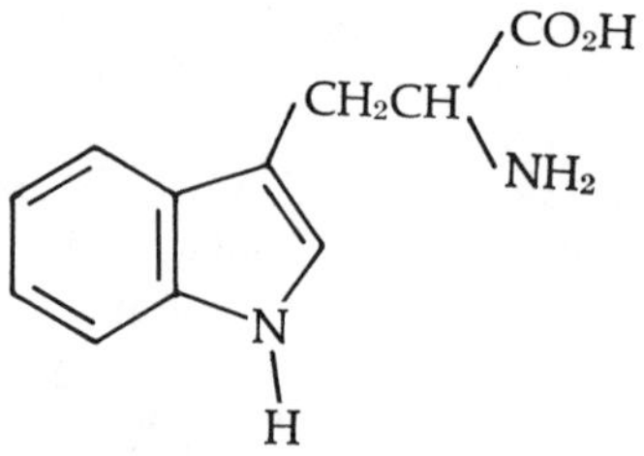

133 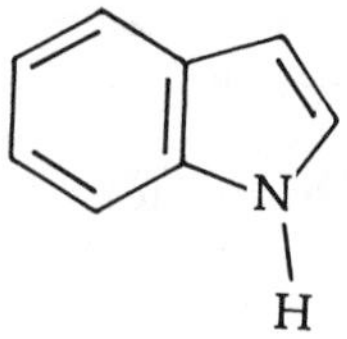 **134** 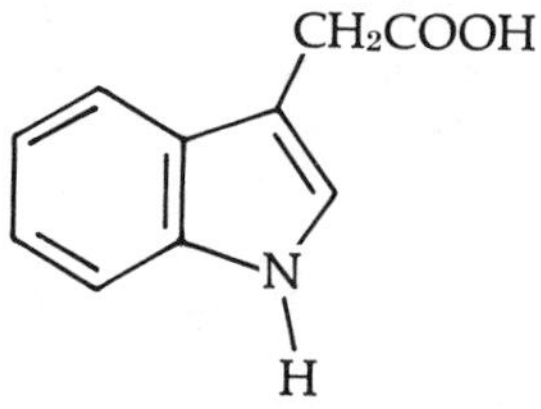 **135**

dietary supplement, these early tumors did not develop; instead, relatively benign cystic tumors of the liver appeared at a later date. The latent period of the bladder tumors was such that they were induced later than the trabecular cell tumors. The experiments in hamsters (*342*) suggested that DL-tryptophan or indole protected against cholangiofibrosis and cholangiosarcoma. DL-Tryptophan was without effect on the induction of bladder tumors by *N*-nitrosodibutylamine in rats, but it inhibited liver tumor induction by the nitrosamine (*345*).

Boyland et al. (*345*) noted that those metabolites of tryptophan that lie on the niacin pathway were *o*-aminophenol derivatives and *o*-aminophenols and they were postulated to be active metabolites of the aromatic amines at the time; they tested some of the metabolites for carcinogenicity by bladder implantation. 3-Hydroxykynurenine (**42**), 3-hydroxyanthranilic acid (**43**) (in a cholesterol but not a paraffin wax pellet), and 2-amino-3-hydroxyacetophenone (**136**) were carcinogenic. The fact that these *o*-aminophenols were carcinogenic when suspended in cholesterol but not in paraffin wax was further established in other experiments (*346, 347*). Many reservations have been expressed about the meaning of tumors produced by bladder implantation. The pellet is believed to participate in tumor formation. This role was demonstrated by Bryan and Springberg (*129*), who showed that bladder-implanted xanthurenic acid-8-methyl ether gave bladder tumors in mice, whereas the same chemical was ineffective when injected, unless there was a cholesterol pellet in the bladder lumen. This compound led to an increased incidence of lymphoreticular tumors in rats that were injected three times weekly with 1 mg for about 600 d (*348*). To the best of our knowledge, no suspect tryptophan metabolite has been shown to induce tumors as a result of testing by a conventional feeding or injection experiment; therefore, the significance of these bladder implantation results is in question.

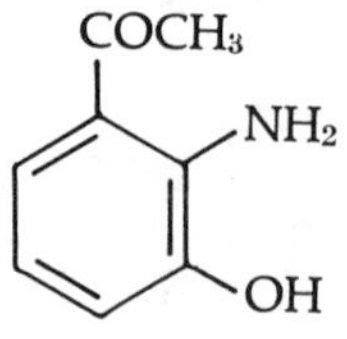

136

Price et al. (*349*) reasoned that because aromatic amines were the only known causative agents of human bladder cancer, the spontaneous disease might be induced by endogenous aromatic amines. The only naturally occurring aromatic amines in human urine were metabolites of tryptophan. They therefore developed methods for the quantitation of the metabolites. Patients with bladder cancer excreted significantly more kynurenic acid, acetylkynurenine, kynurenine, and 3-hydroxykynurenine after ingesting a loading dose of L-tryptophan than did control subjects with no known disease. Half of the patients with nonindustrial bladder cancer excreted an excess of these metabolites after a loading dose of L-tryptophan, but 10 industrial bladder cancer patients did not (*350*). Conflicting results were obtained in other centers (*351–54*), possibly because of the technical difficulty of the analysis. An attempt by the original authors to repeat their observations using patients from the area surrounding Boston, Massachusetts, instead of from Wisconsin gave unconvincing results (*355*). To explain these differences, it was suggested that tryptophan had a relatively weak influence on the development of bladder cancer that was easily overlaid by other factors such as traces of bladder carcinogens in urban environments. Cohen et al. (*356*) showed that DL-tryptophan acted as a tumor-promoting agent in rat bladders previously exposed to a limited dose of a bladder carcinogen.

Abnormal tryptophan metabolism is not specific to bladder cancer patients. It was reported in patients with nonmalignant genitourinary tract disease (*354*), other forms of cancer (*357*), neurological conditions (*358*), scleroderma (*359*), rheumatoid arthritis (*360*), and pregnancy (*361*). Thus, although abnormal tryptophan metabolism may be found in some patients with bladder cancer, the significance of this observation to the natural history of the disease is obscure.

Some progress toward determining the effect of tryptophan and its metabolites has been published. Radomski et al. (*126*) fed dogs seven times the normal dietary concentration of DL-tryptophan for 7 years and demonstrated that there was hyperplasia of the bladder epithelium, but no tumors occurred between 3 months and 7 years. Similarly, Miyakawa and Yoshida (*362*) found transitional cell hyperplasia and increased proliferation that was demonstrated autoradiographically after the injection of tritiated thymidine in rats given a tryptophan supplement. In our view, these two papers constitute the only direct evidence for the interaction of the resting bladder epithelium with tryptophan or its metabolites. Indirect evidence of bladder cancer induction by tryptophan or its metabolites was adduced in experiments on the effect of dietary modification on spontaneous tumor incidence (*363*). The incidence of most spontaneous tumors was reduced in rats fed a high-protein diet (51.0% casein) compared with that in rats receiving 22.0 and 10.0% casein, despite increased longevity in the high-protein group. Benign bladder papillomatosis and tumors of the lymphoid tissue, however, were more frequent in the high-protein groups. Because this protein is the main source of the essential amino acid tryptophan, it is possible but not ascertained that tryptophan is involved in the formation of these tumors. The solution to the problem may lie in the synthesis of the *N*-hydroxy derivatives of tryptophan and its metabolites and their specific identification in the urine of patients and animals receiving high doses of L-tryptophan. Tryptophan may play another role in aromatic amine carcinogenesis as a promoting agent. Experiments demonstrating the possible role of tryptophan in promotion are described later in this chapter.

OTHER HETEROCYCLIC AROMATIC AMINES. The remaining compounds are analogs of two- or, generally, three-ringed carbocyclic aromatic amines with one or more oxygen, nitrogen, or sulfur atoms replacing –CH– in the ring system. Most of the compounds recorded in Table XVI are analogs of FA or FAA (*175, 203, 364*). Little work has been carried out to determine the mode of action of these compounds; however, these compounds further indicate the range of aromatic-ring systems which, when substituted with an amino group, are carcinogenic in animals. As mentioned in the section on DNA adducts of aromatic amines, pyrolysis products of both tryptophan and glutamine have been shown to bind to DNA (*see* previous section HETEROCYCLIC AMINES).

These products, which can also be formed from cooked foods, are mutagenic to *Salmonella typhimurium* and have been shown to be carcinogenic. 3-Amino-1,4-dimethyl-5*H*-pyrido[4,3-*b*]indole (Trp-P-1) and 3-amino-1-methyl-5*H*-pyrido[4,3-*b*]indole (Trp-P-2), pyrolysis products of tryptophan, induce hepatocellular carcinomas in mice fed 200 ppm in the diet (*365*). Trp-P-1 is present in cigarette-smoke condensate at a level of 80 ng/cigarette, while its acetyl derivative is present at around 7 ng/cigarette. The levels in grilled beef approach 650 ng of Trp-P-1/g of beef and 64 ng of the acetyl ester/g of beef—the highest level of these compounds so far reported (*366*). Considering the amounts of food consumed and cigarettes smoked, human exposure to these agents might be substantial.

Modification of Aromatic Amine Carcinogenesis. The complete and quantitative analysis of the way in which aromatic amine carcinogenesis may be modified requires an understanding of the pharmacokinetics of the action of each agent, i.e., the concentrations of an aromatic amine and its metabolites in each of the body compartments (blood, urine, bile, etc.) and the activity of each of the metabolizing enzymes (*367*). The laborious nature of such investigations was illustrated in the stilbenamine series (*368*). The information considered here is more fragmentary.

During metabolism, the extent to which all the metabolizing enzymes act on a foreign compound is determined by the available concentrations of the compound and its metabolites, the activity of the enzymes, and their affinity for each substrate. If a specific detoxifying enzyme is affected by a modifying agent, the concentration of carcinogen and its time of availability to the tissues may be different from that obtained in the absence of the modifying agent. For example, the riboflavin concentration in the diet was shown to be inversely related to the carcinogenicity of DAB to rat liver. The concentration of riboflavin determined the concentration of a flavin–adenine cofactor which in turn determined the activity of the enzyme azo reductase. This enzyme detoxified DAB: the lower the enzyme activity, the more DAB available for conversion to the proximate carcinogen (*270*). Nevertheless, 2′- and 3′-methyl-DAB were unaffected by higher levels of dietary riboflavin because of the reduced ability of the liver to store riboflavin during the feeding of these compounds (*270*). Other vitamins, which do not contribute to cofactors essential for these metabolizing enzymes, have no effect.

One form of modification is enzyme induction, in which the modifying agent increases the synthesis of some microsomal metabolizing enzymes. Enzyme-inducing agents consist of a spectrum of different chemical structures such as polycyclic aromatic hydrocarbons and quinones, barbiturates, steroids, certain

Table XVI

Carcinogenicity of Other Heterocyclic Aromatic Amines and Their Analogs

				Site of Tumor Induction[a]							
Compound	*Species*	*Route*[b]	*Adequacy*[c]	*Local*	*Bladder*	*Kidney*	*Liver*	*Intestine*	*Ear Duct*	*Breast*	*Other*
2-Carbazolylacetamide	rat	o	S	−	−	−	−	−	−	?	−
3-Carbazolylacetamide	rat	o	S	−	−	−	−	−	−	−	−
3-Dibenzofuranylacetamide	rat	o	S	−	−	−	−	−	+	+	−
3-Dibenzofuranylamine	mouse	o	S	−	+	−	+	−	−	−	−
2-Dibenzothiophenylacetamide	rat	o	S	−	−	−	−	+	+	+	−
3-Dibenzothiophenylacetamide	rat	o	S	−	−	−	−	+	+	+	−
2-Methoxy-3-benzofuranylamine	rat	o	S	−	+	+	−	−	+	+	−
S-Oxydibenzothiophenyl-2-acetamide	rat	o	S	−	−	−	−	−	+	?	−
6-[(1-Methyl-4-nitroimidazol-5-yl) thio]purine, Azathioprine	mouse	i.m.	S	−	+[d]	+[d]	−	−	−	−	+[d]
	rat	o	S	−	−	−	−	−	+	−	thymoma
3,6-Bis(dimethylamino)acridine HCl, Acridine orange	mouse	top./s.c.	S	−	−	−	?	−	−	−	−
	rat	o	S	−	−	−	+	−	−	−	−
2-Amino-9,10-anthracenedione	rat	o	NCI	−	−	−	+	−	−	−	−
	mouse	o	NCI	−	−	−	+	−	−	−	−
1-Amino-2-methyl-9,10-anthracenedione	rat	0	NCI	−	−	−	+	−	−	−	−
	mouse	o	NCI	−	−	−	−	−	−	−	−
2-Methyl-1-nitro-9,10-anthracenedione	rat	o	NCI	−	−	−	+	−	−	−	−
	mouse	o	NCI	−	−	−	−	−	−	−	hemangio-sarcoma

[a] +, tumors reported; −, tumors not reported; and ?, evidence equivocal.
[b] o, oral; s.c., subcutaneous injection; i.m., intermuscular injection and top., topical.
[c] A, tested in more than one institute; S, evidence less less convincing.
[d] In NB × NZW strain.

chlorocarbons, and so on (*369*). Enzyme induction and carcinogenicity can be, but are not necessarily, properties of the same molecule.

3-Methylcholanthrene is an enzyme-inducing agent as well as a carcinogen. Feeding 3-methylcholanthrene and the potent hepatocarcinogen 3′-methyl-DAB in the diet to rats inhibited the appearance of liver tumors until after 25 weeks, whereas 3′-methyl-DAB alone gave a 98% tumor yield in 15–29 weeks (*370, 371*). The route of administration of the hydrocarbon was immaterial, as inhibition followed intravaginal, oral, subcutaneous, or intraperitoneal administration, but the greatest inhibition occurred when both compounds were given in the diet. This observation was repeated many times with different derivatives of DAB; inhibition was produced if 3-methylcholanthrene feeding was started no later than 6 weeks after the beginning of the azo dye feeding (*372*). 3-Methylcholanthrene may be successfully replaced by benzo[*a*]pyrene, dibenz[*a,h*]anthracene, benz[*a*]-anthracene, dibenz[*a,h*]anthracene-7,14-quinone, and dibenz[*a,h*]anthracene-5,6-quinone (*373–75*). The level of protein binding was also inhibited by the enzyme-inducing agent, indicating that the amount of metabolically activated carcinogen was reduced (*373*). The levels of azo reductase and *N*-demethylase measured in vitro were increased several-fold as a result of treatment by the enzyme-inducing agents (*374*).

2-FAA-induced hepatocarcinogenesis in rats was also inhibited by the use of dietary 3-methylcholanthrene as an enzyme-inducing agent (*370*). In an extension of these findings, the feeding of 3-methylcholanthrene with 2-FAA to rats was shown to result in a reduced urinary excretion of *N*-hydroxy-2-FAA (*33*). To circumvent the problem of the exact nature of the active ester of 2-FAA, Irving et al. (*376*) studied the in vivo binding to rat liver nucleic acids of [9-^{14}C]2-FAA and *N*-hydroxy-[9-^{14}C]2-FAA. If 3-methylcholanthrene were fed to rats before 2-FAA to induce the metabolizing enzymes, the binding level was lower in the hydrocarbon-plus-2-FAA-treated rat livers than in those using 2-FAA alone. The hydrocarbon did not affect the level of binding when the hydroxamic acid was used. This observation clearly indicates that the hydrocarbon-mediated enzyme induction was concerned with the hydroxylation step of 2-FAA activation. If higher levels of the hydrocarbon were injected prior to a single dose of 2-FAA or *N*-hydroxy-FAA, both amine and hydroxylamine binding levels were reduced. This finding demonstrated that enzyme induction inhibited both *N*-hydroxylation and esterification under these conditions. The position is further complicated by changes in the excretion of hydroxamic acid derivatives during continuous feeding of 2-FAA. Rats excreted about 20% of a single dose of 2-FAA in the bile as the glucuronide of *N*-hydroxy-2-FAA and 1% of this metabolite in the urine. Moreover, when the glucuronide was administered, it was excreted unchanged in the rat bile, but was excreted in a variously metabolized form in the rat urine (*377*). Irving (*376*) suggested that the increased urinary excretion in the rat of *N*-hydroxylated 2-FAA with the time of feeding was the result of impaired biliary excretion of the *N*-glucuronide. This finding was consistent with the observed impairment of biliary secretion in 2-FAA-fed rats (*378*) and with electron microscopic demonstration of changes at the borders of the bile ducts (*379*). This finding also explained why feeding 3-methylcholanthrene with 4-BPAA failed to affect the tumor incidence in rats (*31*). The absence of liver injury when BPA was fed meant that no change occurred in the excretion pattern of *N*-hydroxy-4-BPAA. The concept that liver injury may affect the proportion of *N*-hydroxy-2-FAA derivatives that are produced from 2-FAA and excreted in the urine is further supported by studies concerning the feeding of the hepatotoxins 2-FAA, 3′-methyl-DAB, thioacetamide, thermally oxidized oils, as well as those excreted from surgical or chemical (carbon tetrachloride-induced) partial hepatectomy (*380–82*).

Despite the inhibition of 2-FAA tumorigenesis brought about by inducing hydrocarbons in vivo, hydrocarbon induction of rat liver raises the levels of the microsomal *N*-hydroxylating enzymes measured in vitro several-fold (*383*). The balance of the effective activities of all the metabolizing enzymes is the relevant factor in vivo.

Phenobarbital as an inducing agent increased the excretion of *N*-hydroxy-2-FAA glucuronide by rats (*384, 385*). It modified the carcinogenicity of 2-FAA in two ways (*386*): (1) when it was fed simultaneously with 2-FAA, it reduced the incidence of hepatomas because, as suggested by Weisburger and Weisburger (*387*), it induced a high level of *N*-glucuronyltransferase so that the glucuronide was readily cleared in the bile; and (2) when phenobarbital was given after feeding 2-FAA for 11–26 d, the incidence of hepatomas significantly increased. The phenobarbital-increased proliferation rate returned to normal values in hepatocytes and littoral cells in less than 70 d. Similar effects to those seen with phenobarbital are found with butylated hydroxytoluene, an antioxidant, and DDT, a pesticide. Both these chemicals are liver enzyme-inducing agents that behave in a similar manner to phenobarbital. The mechanism of the enhancing effect has been studied extensively by Peraino et al. (*388–91*). They liken the process of enhancing 2-FAA carcinogenicity to the mouse skin promotion system of polycyclic hydrocarbons and croton oil. The promoting effects of phenobarbital can be seen for as long as 120 d after cessation of 2-FAA feeding. From their studies, Peraino et al. conclude that phenobarbital has no initiating activity and that promotion by phenobarbital involves primarily an increase in the probability that hepatocytes that are initiated by 2-FAA will express their malignant phenotype (*391*). A similar enhancement to that seen with 2-FAA is also found with DAB; therefore, phenobarbital may be a general promoting agent for hepatocarcinogens (*392*).

A similar promoting action may also occur in the bladder. Administration of DL-tryptophan to dogs that have been given a previous dose of either 4-BPA or 2-NA appears to lead to an enhanced tumor incidence. DL-Tryptophan alone does not give tumors (*393*). Radomski et al. suggest that DL-tryptophan or its metabolites irritate the bladder and cause the production of tumors of this area. In this manner, tryptophan could be acting as a tumor promoter for other environmental aromatic amines and thereby could promote cancer in nonoccupationally exposed populations. As mentioned previously, Cohen et al. (*356*) have demonstrated that DL-tryptophan acted as a promoting agent for rat bladder tumors that were initiated with a carcinogen.

Enzyme-inducing studies that use 3-methylcholanthrene have been conducted in species other than the rat. The proportion of the dose excreted as *N*-hydroxy-2-FAA derivatives was increased by feeding 3-methylcholanthrene to rabbits or hamsters (*394*). In contrast to the rat, the rabbit excretes all but a trace of the *N*-glucuronide of *N*-hydroxy-2-FAA that is produced from 2-FAA in the urine

(*395*). In the hamster, the incidence of tumors induced by 2-FAA was increased by 3-methylcholanthrene. Mice maintained a similar level of *N*-hydroxy-2-FAA derivatives with or without hydrocarbon induction (*387*).

Feeding a 40-*M* excess of acetanilide with 2-FAA to rats inhibited the appearance of hepatomas that would have been expected with 2-FAA alone (*396*). The hepatotoxic effects of 2-FAA were also inhibited, and this finding suggested that acetanilide might be interfering with the metabolism and possibly the *N*-hydroxylation of 2-FAA. The experiment was confirmed, and *m*-acetotoluidine and *m*-aminobenzoic acid, but not the *o*- and *p*-isomers of these chemicals, were shown to mimic acetanilide. *N*-Hydroxy-2-FAA carcinogenicity, however, was also inhibited by acetanilide; therefore, the *N*-hydroxylation step was not necessarily affected. As predicted (*17*), the *p*-hydroxy acetanilide formed from acetanilide competed with *N*-hydroxy-2-FAA for sulfate ions. Feeding excess sulfate overrode the inhibition induced by acetanilide on *N*-hydroxy-2-FAA, but not on 2-FAA, and led to liver tumors (*61*). Because the liver tumors induced by 2-FAA with added sulfate were not as advanced and the toxic effects were not as pronounced as with 2-FAA alone, further experiments with higher levels of sulfate were conducted. All surviving animals had large multiple hepatomas (*62*). 8-Hydroxyquinoline also inhibited 2-FAA hepatocarcinogenesis and may act by the same mechanism as acetanilide (*397*).

Thus, many compounds are likely to affect some aspect of the metabolism of the aromatic amines and thereby alter their toxic or carcinogenic response. Matsushima and Weisburger (*398*), in addition to the substances already discussed, examined the effect of prefeeding chloroamphenicol, indole, L-tryptophan, L-methionine, L-tyrosine, guanosine, and inosine for 4 weeks on *N*-hydroxy-FAA-induced alterations to body and liver weight, binding to DNA and other fractions, and tumorigenicity. Chloramphenicol and indole decreased *N*-hydroxy-FAA binding to liver nuclear DNA and were inhibitors of hepatocarcinogenesis. Chloramphenicol increased the proportion of *N*-2-fluorenyldiacetamide excreted as the *N*-hydroxy glucuronide (which is readily excreted in the bile) and probably decreased the amount available for esterification to the ultimate carcinogen (*399*). Blunck (*400*) showed that prefeeding chloramphenicol for 7–20 d also inhibited 3′-methyl-DAB hepatocarcinogenesis. She then demonstrated that the protein binding of 3′-methyl-DAB was not significantly changed by chloroamphenicol (*401, 402*). Nevertheless, the livers were grossly enlarged between 4 and 20 d, and the RNA–DNA ratio was elevated in chloramphenicol-fed animals. Azo reductase, normally suppressed by 3′-methyl-DAB, was returned to more normal levels. Unfortunately, DNA-to-dye binding was not measured in these experiments.

Hormonal changes brought about by endocrine ablation and/or injection of appropriate hormones affect the metabolism of aromatic amines and thereby affect their carcinogenicity. For example, the male rat liver is more susceptible than the female rat liver to carcinogenesis by 2-FAA and *N*-hydroxy-2-FAA. The esterification step is of overriding importance, because male rat liver has much higher levels of sulfotransferase than female rat liver (*61*). Castration alone, or followed by the injection of testosterone propionate, had little effect on the sulfotransferase activity in the liver of either sex. On the other hand, injection of 17β-estradiol into castrated animals of either sex resulted in at least a 50% depression in sulfotransferase activity 14 weeks after the operation (*61, 403, 404*).

Adrenalecotomy inhibited hepatocarcinogenesis in 2-FAA-treated rats as first demonstrated by Symeonidis et al. (*405*). It inhibited the *N*-hydroxylation of 2-FAA but had little effect on sulfotransferase activity (*403*). Replacement therapy with cortisone and deoxycorticosterone restored *N*-hydroxylation to near normal levels (*403*). Hypophysectomy inhibited both *N*-hydroxylation and sulfotransferase levels. Adrenocorticotrophic hormone restored *N*-hydroxylation and carcinogenicity (*61, 406, 407*). Surgical thyroidectomy had an inhibiting effect on sulfotransferase activity but not on *N*-hydroxylation and inhibited 2-FAA carcinogenesis (*408*). Similar studies have been reported for other carcinogens, especially the aminoazo dyes (*409–14*).

These studies relating to the effects of hormones or steroids on carcinogenicity have been directed toward alterations in aromatic amine metabolism. However, these endogenous substances need not exert their action only at the initiating phase of carcinogenesis, but also at the tumor progression stage by altering the tumor latency period.

Certain lessons must be drawn from this brief discussion of exogenous and endogenous modifiers of carcinogenesis. First, the two-stage activation of 2-FAA and related compounds leads to a variety of effects—changes in *N*-hydroxylation or sulfotransferase or both. If some of the postulated second activation steps other than sulfate esterification are effective, as appears to be the case with certain extrahepatic tumors, further types of modification may be found. Second, in vitro studies are of only limited use in this area. The amount of the compound which is metabolically activated depends on the relative activities of the activating and detoxifying enzymes and the concentrations of their substrates. In vivo, these concentrations vary with time. Third, exogenous and endogenous factors may have variable effects. Fourth, although some of the modifying agents might be able to reduce the carcinogenicity of an agent to humans over a short period, there is as yet nothing acceptable to inhibit carcinogenesis on a long-term basis. The information given in this section may imply that the effectiveness of a potential inhibitor of carcinogenesis would have to be evaluated directly in humans.

Finally, an experiment in which 2-FAA was fed and croton oil was painted concurrently on to the skin should be mentioned. The finding that skin papillomas were induced shows not only that 2-FAA is a carcinogen at many sites, but also that it "initiates" tumor cells in the skin and possibly elsewhere (*415*).

Conclusions

There is strong evidence that *N*-hydroxylation is the primary stage in conversion of aromatic amines to their ultimate carcinogenic forms. Such *N*-hydroxy derivatives can be formed either through oxidation of an amino group or reduction of a nitro or nitroso group. With certain compounds, there is also sound evidence that a further activation step is necessary. Whether this second stage occurs is to some extent dependent on the reactivity of the initial *N*-hydroxy derivative.

Ar-N(OX)(R)

137

Ar = aromatic structure

R = H, alkyl or aryl

X = H or esterifying group

Ar(R)N^+

138

Aromatic amine carcinogenesis is the result of bioactivation to the ultimate carcinogenic form (**137**) and then dissociation of the reactive spec es to give a nitrenium ion (**138**).

Predicting the effect of aromatic structures, alkyl or aryl groups, or different esters on the activation and dissociation stages is still impossible. Nevertheless, some generalizations can be made from the extensive literature:

1. Potent carcinogenicity is associated with aromatic groups consisting of two or more conjugated or fused aromatic rings. Single aromatic or nonconjugated ring systems may be carcinogenic in some cases, but apparently much higher doses are often required.
2. Substituents on the amino nitrogen can modify the carcinogenicity of an aromatic amine by interfering with *N*-hydroxylation. The effect of R on carcinogenicity becomes progressively less activating in the order OX > OH(NO) > H, $COCH_3$, CH_3, NO_2 > COA > A > COPh > SOPh, where X = esterifying group, A = alkyl other than methyl, Ph = aromatic ring, and NO_2 = nitroarene. More evidence is required before it can be determined whether heterocyclic aromatic amines will resemble the carboxylic compounds in this respect.
3. The influence of substituents on the aromatic ring on biological activation is not predictable. The effects of these are (a) to block ring positions to hydroxylation; (b) to affect lipid solubility and therefore the occurrence of *N*-oxidation; (c) to influence possible delocalization of charge; and (d) to affect reactivity of the nitrenium ion.

The aromatic amines are one of the few classes of chemical carcinogens for which there is convincing evidence that some members induce cancer in humans; therefore, there are convincing reasons why animal tests with these compounds must be taken as having a particular relevance to humans, who are able to *N*-hydroxylate. Nevertheless, the single-ring aromatic amines that need to be fed in large quantities to induce tumors pose more difficult questions. To the best of our knowledge, *o*-toluidine has never been convincingly demonstrated to induce bladder or other tumors in humans despite its use as a basic industrial chemical for many decades. Our present qualitative approach to carcinogenesis prevents us from answering questions of this nature without extensive and expensive epidemiological investigations, probably made more than a generation after the original large-scale use of the substance under consideration.

To protect workers from exposure to carcinogens, the suspect compound can now be screened quickly and cheaply using short-term tests for carcinogenicity. We have not mentioned these tests in this chapter because the literature on them is already voluminous. Suffice it to say that structure–activity studies can be carried out quickly using these tests, but they will not provide a measure of carcinogenic potency.

Furthermore, a multitude of new aromatic amine or heterocyclic amino compounds will most likely be discovered in the foreseeable future, such as those found in cooked foods (*416, 417*), in carbon black (*418*), or in urban environments (*419*). All of these new compounds will have to be studied if we are seriously concerned about reducing the incidence of human cancer.

What questions should be asked quantitatively to understand the differences between the carcinogenic responses of humans and animals? The first series of questions should surely concern the relative exposure by all routes of the test species and the human species. The second series of questions concerns genetic factors that are now slowly being dissected into single phenomena. The questions of enzymic activation and detoxification of aromatic amine carcinogens and the effects of induction and other modifying effects on them were discussed at length in this chapter. Other factors, such as the ability to repair genetic and tissue damage or the competence of the immune system to remove precancerous cells, are intrinsic to the biology of the host and are important if carcinogenesis is to be put on a quantitative footing, especially in relation to apparently weak carcinogenic stimuli.

Acknowledgment and Apologia

We thank Mrs. Ray Nixon and Mrs. Yvonne Cook for typing the manuscript.

In compressing the vast amount of information in the aromatic amine field, we have had to select ruthlessly despite the space allotted to us by the editor. We wholeheartedly apologize to those authors who feel that we have ignored or paid too little attention to their work.

Abbreviations

AAB	phenylazoacetanilide
AB	phenylazoaniline, aminoazobenzene
BPA	biphenylamine
BPAA	biphenylacetamide
DAB	dimethylaminoazobenzene, *N,N*-dimethyl-4-phenylazoaniline
DACPM	methylenebis(2-chloroaniline)
DAMPM	methylenebis(2-methylaniline)
DAPM	methylenedianiline
FAA	fluorenylacetamide
HAQO	hydroxyaminoquinoline 1-oxide
MAB	methylaminoazobenzene
MOCA	*See* DACPM
NA	naphthalamine
NADPH	reduced form of nicotinamide adenine dinucleotide phosphate
NQO	nitroquinoline 1-oxide
PAA	phenanthrenylacetamide
PyAB	4-*N*-pyrrolidinylazobenzene
SA	stilbenamine

SAA stilbenylacetamide
Trp-P-1 3-amino-1,4-dimethyl-5*H*-pyrido[4,3-*b*]indole
Trp-P-2 3-amino-1-methyl-5*H*-pyrido[4,3-*b*]indole

Literature Cited

1. Rehn, L. *Arch. Klin. Chir.* **1895**, *50*, 588.
2. Hueper, W. C. "Occupational Tumors and Allied Diseases"; Thomas: Springfield, IL, 1942.
3. Case, R. A. M.; Hosker, M. E.; McDonald, D.B.; Pearson, J.T. *Br. J. Ind. Med.* **1954**, *11*, 75.
4. Case, R. A. M.; Pearson, J. T. *Br. J. Ind. Med.* **1954**, *11*, 213.
5. Radomski, J. L.; Deichmann, W.B.; Altman, N. H.; Radomski, T. *Cancer Res.* **1980**, *40*, 3537.
6. Case, R. A. M.; Hosker, M. E. *Br. J. Prev. Soc. Med.* **1954**, *8*, 39.
7. Davies, J. *Lancet* **1965**, *ii*, 143.
8. Fox, A. J.; Collier, P. F. *Br. J. Ind. Med.* **1976**, 249.
9. Anthony, H. M.; Thomas, G. M. *JNCI, J. Natl. Cancer Inst.* **1971**, *45*, 879.
10. Thiede, T.; Christensen, B. C. *Acta Med. Scand.* **1969**, *185*, 133.
11. Melick, W. F.; Escue, H. M.; Naryka, J. J.; Mezera, R. A.; Wheeler, E. P. *J. Urol.* **1955**, *74*, 760.
12. Melick, W. F.; Naryka, J. J.; Kelly, R. E. *J. Urol.* **1971**, *106*, 220.
13. IARC Monograph, **1972**, *1*, 74.
14. Hueper, W. C.; Wiley, F. H.; Wolfe, H. D. *J. Ind. Hyg.* **1938**, *20*, 46.
15. Bonser, G. M. *J. Pathol. Bacteriol.* **1943**, *55*, 1.
16. Bonser, G. M.; Clayson, D. B.; Jull, J. W.; Pyrah, L. N. *Br. J. Cancer* **1956**, *10*, 533.
17. Miller, J. A. *Cancer Res.* **1970**, *30*, 559.
18. Smith, P. A. S. "The Chemistry of Open Chain Nitrogen Compounds"; Benjamin: New York, 1965; Vol. 1; Chap. 3, p. 85.
19. Brodie, B. B.; Axelrod, J. *J. Pharmacol. Exp. Ther.* **1948**, *94*, 29.
20. Kiese, M.; Uehleke, H. *Naunyn-Schmiedebergs Arch. Exp. Pathol. Pharmakol.* **1961**, *242*, 117.
21. Uehleke, H. *Proc. Int. Pharmacol. Meet., 1st* **1962**, *6*, 31.
22. Miller, E. C.; Lotlikar, P. D.; Pitot, H. C.; Fletcher, T. L.; Miller, J. A. *Cancer Res.* **1966**, *26*, 2239.
23. Gutmann, H. R.; Galitski, S. B.; Foley, W. A. *Cancer Res.* **1967**, *27*, 1443.
24. Cramer, J. W.; Miller, J. A.; Miller, E. C. *J. Biol. Chem.* **1960**, *235*, 885.
25. Miller, E. C.; Miller, J. A.; Hartman, H. A. *Cancer Res.* **1961**, *21*, 815.
26. Miller, E. C.; Miller, J. A.; Enomoto, M. *Cancer Res.* **1964**, *24*, 2018.
27. Irving, C. C. *Cancer Res.* **1966**, *26*, 1390.
28. Kiese, M.; Reuner, G.; Wiedermann, I. *Naunyn-Schmiedebergs Arch. Exp. Pathol. Pharmakol.* **1965**, *251*, 88.
29. Takeishi, K.; Okuno-Kaneda, S.; Seno, T. *Mutat. Res.* **1979**, *62*, 425.
30. Miller, J. A.; Cramer, J. W.; Miller, E. C. *Cancer Res.* **1960**, *20*, 950.
31. Miller, J. A.; Wyatt, C. S.; Miller, E. C.; Hartmann, H. A. *Cancer Res.* **1961**, *21*, 1465.
32. Andersen, R. A.; Enomoto, M.; Miller, E. C.; Miller, J. A. *Cancer Res.* **1964**, *24*, 128.
33. Lotlikar, P. D.; Enomoto, M.; Miller, J. A.; Miller, E.C. *Proc. Soc. Exp. Biol. Med.* **1967**, *125*, 341.
34. Lotlikar, P. D.; Miller, E. C.; Miller, J. A.; Margreth, A. *Cancer Res.* **1965**, *25*, 1743.

35. Shirasu, Y. *Gann* **1963**, *54*, 487.
36. Endo, H.; Kume, F. *Gann* **1965**, *56*, 261.
37. Yamamoto, N.; Fukada, S.; Takebe, H. *Cancer Res.* **1970**, *30*, 2532.
38. Martin, C. N.; McDermid, A. C.; Garner, R. C. *Cancer Res.* **1978**, *38*, 2621.
39. Kato, R.; Takuhashi, A.; Ochima, T. *Biochem. Pharmacol.* **1970**, *19*, 45.
40. Erturk, E.; Price, J. M.; Morris, J. E.; Cohen, S. M.; Leith, R. S.; von Esch, A. M.; Crovetti, A. J. *Cancer Res.* **1967**, *27*, 1998.
41. Erturk, E.; Atassi, S. A.; Yoshida, O.; Cohen, S. M.; Price, J. M.; Bryan, G. T. *JNCI J. Natl. Cancer Inst.* **1970**, *45*, 535.
42. Akao, M.; Kuroda, K.; Mujaki, K. *Biochem. Pharmacol.* **1971**, *20*, 3091.
43. Feller, D. R.; Morita, M.; Gillette, J. R. *Proc. Soc. Exp. Biol. Med.* **1971**, *137*, 433.
44. Marroquin, F.; Coyote, N. *Chem.- Biol. Interact.* **1970**, *2*, 151.
45. Irving, C. C.; Veazey, R. A.; Hill, J. T. *Biochim. Biophys. Acta* **1969**, *179*, 189.
46. Kadlubar, F. F.; Miller, J. A.; Miller, E. C. *Cancer Res.* **1978**, *38*, 3628.
47. Kadlubar, F. F.; Unruh, L. E.; Beland, F. A.; Straub, K. M.; Evans, F. E. *Carcinogenesis* **1980**, *1*, 139.
48. Poirier, L. A.; Miller, J. A.; Miller, E. C.; Sato, K. *Cancer Res.* **1967**, *27*, 1600.
49. Kadlubar, F. F.; Miller, J. A.; Miller, E. C. *Cancer Res.* **1976**, *36*, 1196.
50. Miller, J. A.; Miller, E. C. *Prog. Exp. Tumor Res.* **1969**, *11*, 273.
51. Scribner, J. D.; Miller, J. A.; Miller, E. C. *Cancer Res.* **1970**, *30*, 1570.
52. Lotlikar, P. D.; Luha, L. *Mol. Pharmacol.* **1971**, *7*, 381.
53. Bartsch, H.; Traut, M.; Hecker, E. *Biochim. Biophys. Acta* **1972**, *237*, 556.
54. Bartsch, H.; Miller, J. A.; Miller, E. C. *Biochim. Biophys. Acta* **1972**, *273*, 40.
55. Bartsch, H.; Dworkin, M.; Miller, J. A.; Miller, E. C. *Biochim. Biophys. Acta* **1972**, *286*, 272.
56. Bartsch, H.; Dworkin, M.; Miller, E. C.; Miller, J. A. *Biochim. Biophys. Acta* **1973**, *304*, 42.
57. King, C. M.; Traub, N. R.; Lortz, M.; Thissen, M. R. *Cancer Res.* **1979**, *39*, 3369.
58. Enomoto, M.; Miller, E. C.; Miller, J. A. *Proc. Soc. Exp. Biol. Med.* **1971**, *136*, 1206.
59. DeBaun, J. R.; Rowley, J. Y.; Miller, E. C.; Miller, J. A. *Proc. Soc. Exp. Biol. Med.* **1968**, *129*, 268.
60. King, C. M.; Phillips, B. *Science (Washington, D. C.)* **1968**, *159*, 1351.
61. DeBaun, J. R.; Miller, E. C.; Miller, J. A. *Cancer Res.* **1970**, *30*, 577.
62. Weisburger, J. H.; Yamamoto, R. S.; Williams, G. M.; Grantham, P. H.; Matsushima, T.; Weisburger, E. K. *Cancer Res.* **1972**, *32*, 491.
63. DeBaun, J. R.; Smith, J. Y. R.; Miller, E. C.; Miller, J. A. *Science (Washington, D. C.)* **1970**, *167*, 184.
64. Lotlikar, P. D.; Luha, L. *Biochem. J.* **1971**, *124*, 69.
65. Lotlikar, P. D.; Wasserman, M. B. *Biochem. J.* **1970**, *120*, 661.
66. Tada, M.; Tada, M. *Biochem. Biophys. Res. Commun.* **1972**, *46*, 1025.
67. Irving, C. C.; Wiseman, R. *Cancer Res.* **1971**, *31*, 1645.
68. Maher, V. M.; Miller, E. C.; Miller, J. A.; Szybalski, W. *Mol. Pharmacol.* **1968**, *4*, 411.
69. Irving, C. C.; Russell, L. T. *Biochemistry* **1970**, *9*, 2471.
70. Maher, V. M.; Reuter, M. *Proc. Am. Assoc. Cancer Res.* **1971**, *12*, 72.
71. Kadlubar, F. F.; Miller, J. A.; Miller, E. C. *Cancer Res.* **1977**, *37*, 805.
72. Mitchell, J. R.; Jollow, D. J.; Potter, W. Z.; Davis, D. C.; Gillette, J. R.; Brodie, B. B. *J. Pharmacol. Exp. Ther.* **1973**, *187*, 185.
73. Hinson, J. A.; Mitchell, J. R. *Drug Metab. Dispos.* **1976**, *4*, 430.
74. Carro-Ciampi, G. *Toxicology* **1978**, *10*, 311.
75. Gemborys, M. W.; Gribble, G. W.; Mudge, G. H. *J. Med. Chem.* **1978**, *21*, 649.
76. Wirth, P. J.; Dybing, E.; von Bahr, C.; Thorgeirsson, S. S. *Mol. Pharmacol.* **1980**, *18*, 117.

77. Glinsuken, T.; Benjamin, T.; Grantham, P. H.; Weisburger, E. K.; Roller, P. P. *Xenobiotica* **1975**, *5*, 475.
78. Hlavica, P.; Kehl, M. *Biochem. J.* **1977**, *164*, 487.
79. An, H. P.; Fouts, J. R.; Devereaux, T. R. *Xenobiotica* **1979**, *9*, 441.
80. Hinson, J. A.; Mitchell, J. R.; Jollow, D. J. *Mol. Pharmacol.* **1975**, *11*, 462.
81. Watabe, T.; Sawahata, T. *Biochem. Pharmacol.* **1976**, *25*, 599.
82. Gorrod, J. W.; Temple, D. J.; Beckett, A. H. *Xenobiotica* **1975**, *5*, 453.
83. Dybing, E.; Aune, T.; Nelson, S. D. *Biochem. Pharmacol.* **1979**, *28*, 43.
84. Brill, E.; Radomski, J. L. *Xenobiotica* **1971**, *1*, 35.
85. Boyland, E.; Manson, E. *Biochem. J.* **1966**, *99*, 189.
86. Brill, E.; Radomski, J. L. *Life Sci.* **1967**, *6*, 2293.
87. Radomski, J. L.; Rey, A. A.; Brill, E. *Cancer Res.* **1973**, *33*, 1284.
88. Radomski, J. L.; Hearn, W. L.; Radomski, T.; Moreno, H.; Scott, W. E. *Cancer Res.* **1977**, *37*, 1757.
89. Moreno, H. R.; Radomski, J. L. *Cancer Lett.* **1978**, *4*, 85.
90. Lower, G. M.; Bryan, G. T. *J. Toxicol. Environ. Health* **1976**, *1*, 421.
91. Olive, C. W.; King, C. M. *Chem.- Biol. Interact.* **1975**, *11*, 599.
92. Wheeler, J. A.; Soderberg, F. B.; Goldman, P. *Cancer Res.* **1975**, *35*, 2962.
93. Martin, C. N.; Ekers, S. F. *Carcinogenesis* **1980**, *1*, 101.
94. Morton, K. C.; King, C. M.; Baetke, K. P. *Cancer Res.* **1979**, *39*, 3107.
95. Morton, K. C.; Beland, F. A.; Evans, F. E.; Fullerton, N. F.; Kadlubar, F. F. *Cancer Res.* **1980**, *40*, 751.
96. Martin, C. N.; Beland, F. A.; Roth, R. W.; Kadlubar, F. F. *Cancer Res.* **1982**, *42*, 2678–86.
97. Baldwin, R. W.; Smith, W. R. D.; Surtees, S. J. *Nature (London)* **1963**, *199*, 613.
98. Baldwin, R. W.; Cunningham, G. J.; Smith, W. R. D.; Surtees, S. J. *Br. J. Cancer* **1968**, *22*, 133.
99. Baldwin, R. W.; Smith, W. R. D. *Br. J. Cancer* **1965**, *19*, 433.
100. Scribner, J. D.; Naimy, N. K. *Proc. Am. Assoc. Cancer Res.* **1977**, *18*, 521.
101. Glatt, H. R.; Metzler, M.; Neumann, H. G.; Oesch, F. *Biochem. Biophys. Res. Commun.* **1976**, *73*, 1025.
102. Weisburger, J. H.; Yamamoto, R. S.; Grantham, P. H.; Weisburger, E. K. *Proc. Am. Assoc. Cancer Res.* **1970**, *11*, 82.
103. Floyd, B. A.; Soong, L. M.; Walker, R. N.; Stuart, M. *Cancer Res.* **1976**, *36*, 2761.
104. Hill, J. T.; Irving, C. C. *Biochemistry* **1967**, *6*, 3816.
105. Kriek, E.; Westra, J. G. In "Chemical Carcinogens and DNA"; Grover, P. L., Ed.; CRC: Boca Raton, FL, **1979**; Vol. II, p. 1.
106. Radomski, J. L.; Brill, E. *Science (Washington, D. C.)* **1970**, *167*, 992.
107. Radomski, J. L.; Conzelman, G. M.; Rey, A. A.; Brill, E. *JNCI, J. Natl. Cancer Inst.* **1973**, *50*, 989.
108. Lin, J. K.; Schmall, B.; Sharpe, I. D.; Muira, I.; Miller, J. A.; Miller, E. C. *Cancer Res.* **1975**, *35*, 832.
109. Kadlubar, F. F.; Miler, J. A.; Miller, E. C. *Cancer Res.* **1976**, *36*, 2350.
110. Kimura, T.; Kodama, M.; Nagata, C. *Biochem. Pharmacol.* **1979**, *28*, 557.
111. Robens, J. F.; Dill, G. S.; Ward, J. M.; Joiner, J. R.; Griesemer, R. A.; Douglas, J. F. *Toxicol. Appl. Pharmacol.* **1980**, *54*, 431.
112. Rinde, E.; Troll, W. *JNCI, J. Natl. Cancer Inst.* **1975**, *55*, 181.
113. Lowry, L. K.; Tolos, W. P.; Boeniger, M. F.; Nony, C. R.; Bowman, M. C. *Toxicol. Lett.* **1980**, *7*, 29.
114. Walker, R. *Food Cosmet. Toxicol.* **1970**, *8*, 659.
115. Martin, C. N.; Kennelly, J. C. *Carcinogenesis* **1981**, *2*, 308–12.
116. Morita, M.; Feller, D. R.; Gillette, J. R. *Biochem. Pharmacol.* **1971**, *20*, 217.

117. Wang, C. Y.; Behrens, B. C.; Ichikawa, M.; Bryan, G. T. *Biochem. Pharmacol.* **1974**, *23*, 3395.
118. Tada, M.; Tada, M. *Nature (London)* **1975**, *255*, 510.
119. Wolpert, M. K.; Althaus, J. R.; Johns, D. G. *J. Pharmacol. Exp. Ther.* **1973**, *185*, 202.
120. McCalla, D. R.; Reuners, A.; Kaiser, C. *Biochem. Pharmacol.* **1971**, *20*, 3532.
121. Tatsumi, K.; Kitamura, S.; Yashimiura, H. *Arch. Biochem. Biophys.* **1976**, *175*, 131.
122. Wang, C. Y.; Chiu, C. W.; Bryan, G. T. *Drug Metab. Dispos.* **1975**, *3*, 89.
123. Wang, C. Y.; Chiu, C. W.; Kaiman, B.; Bryan, G. T. *Biochem. Pharmacol.* **1975**, *24*, 29.
124. Clayson, D. B. "Chemical Carcinogenesis"; J. & A. Churchill: London, 1962.
125. Bonser, G. M.; Jull, J. W. *J. Pathol. Bacteriol.* **1956**, *72*, 489.
126. Clayson, D. B.; Pringle, J. A. S. *Br. J. Cancer* **1961**, *20*, 564.
127. Clayson, D. B.; Cooper, E. H. *Adv. Cancer Res.* **1970**, *13*, 271.
128. Clayson, D. B. *JNCI, J. Natl. Cancer Inst.* **1974**, *52*, 1685.
129. Bryan, G. T.; Springberg, P. D. *Cancer Res.* **1966**, *26*, 105.
130. Jill, J. W. *Cancer Lett.* **1981**, *6*, 21–25.
131. Radomski, J. L.; Glass, E. M.; Deichmann, W. B. *Cancer Res.* **1971**, *31*, 1690.
132. Gutmann, H. R.; Erickson, R. R. *J. Biol. Chem.* **1972**, *247*, 660.
133. Grantham, P. H.; Weisburger, E. K.; Weisburger, J. H. *Biochim. Biophys. Acta* **1965**, *107*, 414.
134. Jarvinen, M.; Santti, R. S. S.; Hopsu-Havu, V. K. *Biochem. Pharmacol.* **1971**, *20*, 2971.
135. Williard, R. F.; Irving, C. C. *Fed. Proc. Fed. Am. Soc. Exp. Biol.* **1964**, *23*, 167.
136. Marroquin, F.; Farber, E. *Cancer Res.* **1965**, *25*, 1262.
137. Lotlikar, P. D.; Scribner, J. D.; Miller, J. A.; Miller, E. C. *Life Sci.* **1966**, *5*, 1263.
138. Kriek, E.; Miller, J. A.; Juhl, U.; Miller, E. C. *Biochemistry* **1967**, *6*, 177.
139. Irving, C. C.; Veazey, R. A.; Russell, L. T. *Chem.- Biol. Interact.* **1969**, *1*, 19.
140. Kriek, E. *Chem.- Biol. Interact.* **1969**, *1*, 3.
141. Kriek, E. *Cancer Res.* **1972**, *32*, 2042.
142. Irving, C. C.; Veazey, R. R. *Cancer Res.* **1969**, *29*, 1799.
143. Westra, J. G.; Kriek, E.; Hittenhausen, H. *Chem.- Biol. Interact.* **1976**, *15*, 149.
144. Kriek, E.; Westra, J. G. *Carcinogenesis* **1980**, *1*, 459.
145. Scribner, J. D.; Naimy, N. K. *Cancer Res.* **1975**, *35*, 1416.
146. Scribner, J. D.; Koponen, G. *Chem.- Biol. Interact.* **1979**, *28*, 201.
147. Lin, J. K.; Miller, J. A.; Miller, E. C. *Cancer Res.* **1975**, *35*, 844.
148. Beland, F. A.; Tullis, D. L.; Kadlubar, F. F.; Straub, K. M.; Evans, F. E. *Chem.- Biol. Interact.*, in press.
149. Tarpley, W. G.; Miller, J. A.; Miller, E. C. *Cancer Res.* **1980**, *40*, 2493.
150. Kriek, E.; Hengeveld, G. M. *Chem.- Biol. Interact.* **1978**, *21*, 179.
151. Scribner, N. K.; Scribner, J. D.; Smith, D. L.; Schram, K. H.; McCloskey, J. A. *Chem.- Biol. Interact.* **1979**, *26*, 27.
152. Gaugler, B. J. M.; Neumann, H. G.; Scribner, N. K.; Scribner, J. D. *Chem.- Biol. Interact.* **1979**, *27*, 335.
153. Hashimoto, Y.; Shudo, K.; Okamoto, T. *Chem. Pharm. Bull.* **1979**, *27*, 1058.
154. Hashimoto, Y.; Shudo, K.; Okamoto, T. *Chem. Pharm. Bull.* **1979**, *27*, 2532.
155. LaRusso, N. F.; Tomasz, M.; Muller, M.; Lipman, R. *Mol. Pharmacol.* **1977**, *13*, 872.
156. Nagata, C.; Kodama, M.; Tagashira, Y.; Imamura, A. *Biopolymers* **1966**, *4*, 409.
157. Kawazoe, Y.; Aroki, M.; Huong, G. F.; Okomoto, T.; Tada, M.; Tada, M. *Chem. Pharm. Bull.* **1975**, *23*, 3041.
158. Bonser, G. M. *Br. Med. Bull.* **1947**, *4*, 379.
159. Bengsston, U.; Angervall, L.; Ekman, H.; Lehmonn, L. *Scand. J. Urol. Nephrol.* **1968**, 2, 145.
160. Begley, M.; Chadwick, J. M.; Jepson, R. P. *Med. J. Aust.* **1970**, *11*, 1133.
161. Mannion, R. A.; Susmano, D. *J. Urol.* **1971**, *106*, 692.

162. Mahony, J. F.; Storey, B. G.; Ibanez, R. C.; Stewart, J. H. *Aust. N. Z. J. Med.* **1977**, *7*, 463.
163. Ames, B. N.; Kammen, H. O.; Yamasaki, E. *Proc. Nat. Acad. Sci. U.S.A.* **1975**, *72*, 2423.
164. Garner, R. C.; Nutman, C. A. *Mutat. Res.* **1977**, *44*, 9.
165. Calder, J. C.; Goss, D. E.; Williams, J. J.; Funder, C. C.; Green, C. R.; Ham, K. N.; Tange, J. R. *Pathology* **1976**, *8*, 1.
166. Johannson, S.; Angervall, L. *Acta Pathol. Microbiol. Scand.* **1976**, *84*, 375.
167. Weisburger, E. K.; Russfield, A. B.; Homburger, F.; Weisburger, J. H.; Boyer, E.; von Dongen, C. G.; Chu, K. C. *J. Environ. Pathol. Toxicol.* **1978**, *2*, 325.
168. Walpole, A. L.; Williams, M. H. C.; Roberts, D. C. *Br. J. Ind. Med.* **1954**, *11*, 105.
169. Walpole, A. L.; Williams, M. H. C.; Roberts, D. C. *Br. J. Ind. Med.* **1952**, *9*, 255.
170. Deichmann, W. B.; Radomski, J. L.; Anderson, W. A. D.; Coplan, M. M.; Woods, F. M. *Ind. Med. Surg.* **1958**, *27*, 25.
171. Deichmann, W. b.; Radomski, J. L.; Anderson, W. A. O.; Coplan, M. M.; Glass, E.; Woods, F. M. *Ind. Med. Surg.* **1965**, *34*, 640.
172. Deichmann, W. B.; McDonald, W. E. *Food Cosmet. Toxicol.* **1968**, *6*, 143.
173. Deichmann, W. B.; McDonald, W. M.; Coplan, M. M.; Woods, F. M.; Anderson, W. A. D. *Ind. Med. Surg.* **1958**, *27*, 634.
174. Clayson, D. B.; Lawson, T. A.; Santana, S.; Bonser, G. M. *Br. J. Cancer* **1965**, *19*, 297.
175. Clayson, D. B.; Lawson, T. A.; Pringle, J. A. S. *Br. J. Cancer* **1967**, *21*, 755.
176. Bonser, G. M. In "The Morphological Precursors of Cancer"; Severi, L., Ed.; Perugia, 1962; p. 435.
177. Miller, E. C.; Sandin, R. B.; Miller, J. A.; Rutsch, H. P. *Cancer Res.* **1956**, *16*, 525.
178. Clayson, D. B. *Br. J. Cancer* **1953**, *7*, 460.
179. Cleveland, J. C.; Cole, J. W. *Surg. Forum* **1966**, *17*, 314.
180. Walpole, A. L.; Williams, M. H. C.; Roberts, D. C. *Br. J. Cancer* **1955**, *9*, 170.
181. Walpole, A. L.; Williams, M. H. C. *Br. Med. Bull.* **1958**, *14*, 141.
182. King, E. S. J.; Varasdi, G. *Aust. N. Z. J. Surg.* **1959**, *29*, 38.
183. Hendry, J. A.; Matthews, J. J.; Walpole, A. L.; Williams, M. H. C. *Nature (London)* **1955**, *175*, 1131.
184. Matthews, J. J.; Walpole, A. L. *Br. J. Cancer* **1956**, *10*, 539.
185. Radomski, J. L.; Brill, E. *Arch. Toxicol.* **1971**, *28*, 159.
186. Goldwater, L. J.; Rosso, A. J.; Kleinfold, M. *Arch. Environ. Health* **1965**, *11*, 814.
187. Bonser, G. M.; Clayson, D. B.; Jull, J. W. *Br. J. Cancer* **1956**, *10*, 653.
188. Pliss, G. B. *Acta Unio Int. Cancrum* **1963**, *19*, 499.
189. Pliss, G. B. *Gig. Tr. Prof. Zabol.* **1965**, *9*, 18.
190. Pliss, G. B. *Vopr. Onkol.* **1959**, *5*, 524191.
191. Pliss, G. B.; Zabezhinsky, M. A. *JNCI, J. Natl. Cancer Inst.* **1970**, *45*, 283.
192. "The Evaluation of Carcinogenic Risk of Chemicals to Man, IARC Monographs, 1974, Vol. 4, p. 78.
193. Kopelman, H.; Robertson, M. H.; Sanders, P. G.; Ash, I. *Br. Med. J.* **1966**, *1*, 514.
194. Munn, A. "Bladder Cancer—A Symposium"; Deichmann; Lampe, Eds.; Aesculapius: Birmingham, 1967; p. 187.
195. Steinhoff, D.; Grundmann, E. *Naturwissenschaften* **1971**, *58*, 578.
196. Russenfield, A. B.; Homburger, F.; Boger, E.; Weisburger, E. K.; Weisburger, J. H. *Toxicol. Appl. Pharmacol.* **1975**, *31*, 4.
197. Stula, E. F.; Sherman, H.; Zapp, J. A.; Clayton, J. W. *Toxicol. Appl. Pharmacol.* **1975**, *31*, 159.
198. Linch, A. L.; O'Connor, G. B.; Barner, J. R.; Killian, A. S.; Neeld, W. E. *Am. Ind. Hyg. Assoc. J.* **1971**, *32*, 802.
199. Michigan Department of Natural Resources, "Summary of Investigations 1–9," 1979, Air Quality Division, Lansing, MI.

200. Walkington, T. Michigan Department of Natural Resources, Meeting with the City (Adrian) April, 1979. Adrian–Anderson Development Co. File, May 4, 1979.
201. U.S. National Research Council National Academy of Sciences, "Aromatic Amines: An Assessment of the Biological and Environmental Effects," 1981," National Academy: Washington, D. C., in press.
202. Williams, M. H. C.; Bonser, G. M. *Br. J. Cancer* **1962**, *16*, 87.
203. Walpole, A. L. *Acta Unio Int. Cancrum* **1963**, *19*, 483.
204. Miller, J. A.; Sandin, R. B.; Miller, E. C.; Rusch, H. P. *Cancer Res.* **1955**, *15*, 188.
205. Haddow, A.; Harris, R. J. C.; Kon, G. A. R.; Roe, E. M. F. *Philos. Trans. R. Soc. London* **1941**, *A241*, 167.
206. Druckrey, H. "Carcinogenesis: Mechanism of Action", Ciba Foundation Symposium, Wolstenholme; O'Connor, Eds.; Churchill: London, 1959; p. 110.
207. Watabe, T.; Akamatsu, K. *Biochem. Pharmacol.* **1974**, *23*, 1845.
208. Metzler, M.; Neumann, H. C. *Xenobiotica* **1977**, *7*, 117.
209. Wilson, R. H.; De Eds, F.; Cox, A. J. *Cancer Res.* **1941**, *1*, 595.
210. Wilson, R. H.; De Eds, F.; Cox, A. J. *Cancer Res.* **1947**, *7*, 444.
211. Wilson, R. H.; De Eds, F.; Cox, A. J. *Cancer Res.* **1947**, *7*, 450.
212. Wilson, R. H.; De Eds, F.; Cox, A. J. *Cancer Res.* **1947**, *7*, 453.
213. Cox, A. J.; Wilson, R. H.; De Eds, F. *Cancer Res.* **1947**, *7*, 647.
214. Bielschowsky, F. *Br. J. Exp. Pathol.* **1944**, *25*, 1.
215. Bielschowsky, F. *Br. J. Exp. Pathol.* **1946**, *27*, 135.
216. Armstrong, E. C.; Bonser, G. M. *J. Pathol. Bacteriol.* **1947**, *59*, 19.
217. Littlefield, N. A.; Cento, C.; Davis, A. K.; Medlock, K. *Proc. Soc. Toxicol.* **1974**, *63*.
218. Frith, C. H.; Jaques, W. E. *Proc. Soc. Toxicol.* **1974**, *63*.
219. Reuber, M. D. *JNCI, J. Natl. Cancer Inst.* **1976**, *57*, 111.
220. Weisburger, E. K.; Weisburger, J. H. *Adv. Cancer Res.* **1958**, *5*, 331.
221. Morris, H. P. *Adv. Cancer Res.* **1965**, *9*, 227.
222. Weber, G. "Liver Cancer: Proceedings"; World Health: Albany, 1969.
223. Clayson, D. B. *Br. J. Cancer* **1953**, *7*, 460.
224. Miller, J. A.; Enomoto, M.; Miller, E. C. *Cancer Res.* **1962**, *22*, 1381.
225. Irving, C. C.; Veazey, R. A. *Cancer Res.* **1971**, *31*, 19.
226. Irving, C. C.; Janss, D. H.; Russell, L. T. *Cancer Res.* **1971**, *31*, 387.
227. Irving, C. C. *Xenobiotica* **1971**, *1*, 387.
228. Scribner, J. D.; Naimy, N. K. *Cancer Res.* **1973**, *33*, 1159.
229. Gutmann, H. R.; Leaf, D. S.; Yost, Y.; Rydell, R. E.; Yost, Y. *Cancer Res.* **1970**, *30*, 1485.
230. Malejka-Giganti, D.; Gutmann, H. R.; Rydell, R. E.; Yost, Y. *Cancer Res.* **1971**, *31*, 778.
231. Yost, Y.; Gutmann, H. R. *Proc. Am. Assoc. Cancer Res.* **1974**, *15*, 21.
232. Conzelman, G. M.; Moulton, J. E. *JNCI, J. Natl. Cancer Inst.* **1972**, *49*, 193.
233. Butt, L. T.; Stafford, N. *J. Appl. Chem.* **1956**, *6*, 525.
234. Gehrmann, G. H.; Foulger, J. H.; Fleming, A. J. *Proc. Int. Congr. Ind. Med., 9th* **1948**, 472.
235. Bonser, G. M.; Clayson, D. B.; Jull, J. W. *Br. Med. Bull.* **1958**, *14*, 146.
236. Clayson, D. B.; Ashton, M. J. *Acta Unio Int. Cancrum* **1963**, *19*, 539.
237. Radomski, J. L.; Brill, E.; Deichmann, W. B.; Glass, E. M. *Cancer Res.* **1971**, *31*, 1461.
238. Saffiotti, U.; Cefis, F.; Montesano, R.; Sellakumar, A. R. "Bladder Cancer—A Symposium"; Deichmann & Lampe, Eds.; Aesculapius: Birmingham, 1967, p. 129.
239. Sellakumar, A. R.; Montesano, R.; Saffiotti, U. *Proc. Am. Assoc. Cancer Res.* **1969**, *10*, 78.
240. Boyland, E.; Dukes, C. E.; Grover, P. L. *Br. J. Cancer* **1963**, *17*, 79.
241. Troll, W.; Nelson, N. *Fed. Proc. Fed. Am. Soc. Exp. Biol.* **1961**, *20*, 41.
242. Brill, E.; Radomski, J. L. "Bladder Cancer—A Symposium"; Deichmann & Lampe, Eds.; Aesculapius: Birmingham, 1967; p. 90.

243. Shimkin, M. B.; Weisburger, J. H.; Weisburger, E. K.; Gubareff, N.; Santzell, V. *JNCI, J. Natl. Cancer Inst.* **1966**, *36*, 915.
244. Boyland, E.; Manson, D. A. R. *Annu. Rep.—Cancer Res. Campaign* **1963**, *41*, 69.
245. Bielschowsky, F. *Br. J. Exp. Pathol.* **1946**, *27*, 54.
246. Schubik, P.; Pietra, G.; Della Porta, G. *Cancer Res.* **1960**, *20*, 100.
247. Lennox, B. *Br. J. Cancer* **1955**, *9*, 631.
248. Dannenbuerg, H.; Huggins, C. *Z. Krebsforsch.* **1969**, *72*, 321.
249. Kirby, A. H. M.; Peacock, P. R. *J. Pathol. Bacteriol.* **1947**, *59*, 1.
250. Strauss, E.; Mateyko, G. M. *Cancer Res.* **1964**, *24*, 1969.
251. Sato, K.; Poirier, L. A.; Miller, J. A.; Miller, E. C. *Cancer Res.* **1966**, *26*, 1678.
252. Ishidate, M.; Tanura, Z.; Nakajima, T.; Sanejima, K. *Chem. Pharm. Bull.* **1962**, *10*, 75.
253. Yoshida, T. *Proc. Jpn. Acad.* **1932**, *8*, 464.
254. Matsumoto, M.; Terayama, H. *Gann* **1965**, *56*, 339.
255. Lawson, T. A. *Biochem. J.* **1968**, *109*, 917.
256. Lawson, T. A. *Chem.- Biol. Interact.* **1970**, *2*, 9.
257. Lawson, T. A.; Dzhioev, F. K. *Chem.- Biol. Interact.* **1970**, *2*, 165.
258. Crabtree, H. G. *Br. J. Cancer* **1949**, *3*, 387.
259. Miller, J. A.; Miller, E. C. *Cancer Res.* **1961**, *21*, 1068.
260. Fare, G.; Howell, J. S. *Cancer Res.* **1964**, *24*, 1279.
261. Fare, G.; Orr, J. W. *Cancer Res.* **1965**, *25*, 1784.
262. Fare, G. *Cancer Res.* **1966**, *26*, 2406.
263. Williams, M. H. C. *Acta Unio Int. Cancrum* **1962**, *18*, 676.
264. Nelson, A. A.; Woodward, G. *JNCI, J. Natl. Cancer Inst.* **1953**, *13*, 1497.
265. Kensler, C. J.; Dexter, S. O.; Rhoads, C. P. *Cancer Res.* **1942**, *2*, 1.
266. Miller, J. A.; Miller, E. C. *J. Exp. Med.* **1948**, *87*, 139.
267. Kinosita, R. *Yale J. Biol. Med.* **1940**, *12*, 287.
268. Sugiura, K.; Halter, C. R.; Kensler, C. J.; Rhoads, C. P. *Cancer Res.* **1945**, *5*, 235.
269. White, F. T.; White, J. *JNCI, J. Natl. Cancer Inst.* **1946**, *7*, 99.
270. Mueller, G. C.; Miller, J. A. *J. Biol. Chem.* **1950**, *185*, 145.
271. Miller, J. A.; Miller, E. C. *Adv. Cancer Res.* **1953**, *1*, 339.
272. Miller, E. C.; Kadlubar, F. F.; Miller, J. A.; Pitot, H. C.; Drinkwater, N. R. *Cancer Res.* **1979**, *39*, 3411.
273. Kinosita, R. *Gann* **1936**, *30*, 423.
274. Kinosita, R. *Trans. Jpn. Pathol. Soc.* **1937**, *27*, 665.
275. Crabtree, H. G. *Br. J. Cancer* **1955**, *9*, 310.
276. Brown, E. V.; Fisher, W. M. *J. Med. Chem.* **1969**, *12*, 1113.
277. Brown, E. V. *J. Med. Chem.* **1968**, *11*, 1234.
278. Ashby, J.; Styles, J. A.; Paton, D. *Carcinogenesis* **1980**, *1*, 1.
279. Scribner, J. D.; Miller, J. A.; Miller, E. C. *Carcinogenesis* **1980**, *1*, 419.
280. Otsuka, I.; Nagao, N. *Gann* **1939**, *30*, 561.
281. Nagao, N.; Hashimoto, T. *Gann* **1939**, *33*, 196.
282. Strombeck, J. P. *J. Pathol. Bacteriol.* **1946**, *58*, 275.
283. Strombeck, J. P.; Ekman, B. *Acta Pathol. Microbiol. Scand.* **1949**, *26*, 480.
284. Ekman, B.; Strombeck, J. P. *Acta Pathol. Microbiol. Scand.* **1949**, *26*, 447.
285. Ekman, B.; Strombeck, J. P. *Acta Pathol. Microbiol. Scand.* **1949**, *26*, 472.
286. Clayson, D. B.; Jull, J. W.; Bonser, G. M. *Br. J. Cancer* **1958**, *12*, 222.
287. Bonser, G. M.; Boyland, E.; Busby, E. R.; Clayson, D. B.; Grover, P. L.; Jull, J. W. *Br. J. Cancer* **1963**, *17*, 127.
288. Childs, I. J.; Nakajima, C.; Clayson, D. B. *Biochem. Pharmacol.* **1967**, *16*, 1555.
289. Jones, R.; Ryan, A. J.; Wright, S. E. *Food Cosmet. Toxicol.* **1966**, *4*, 213.
290. Roxon, J. J.; Ryan, A. J.; Wright, S. E. *Food Cosmet. Toxicol.* **1966**, *4*, 419.

291. Daniel, J. W. *Food Cosmet. Toxicol.* **1967**, *5*, 533.
292. Roxon, J. J.; Ryan, A. J.; Wright, S. E. *Food Cosmet. Toxicol.* **1967**, *5*, 645.
293. Grasso, P.; Goldberg, L. *Food Cosmet. Toxicol.* **1966**, *4*, 297.
294. Grasso, P.; Goldbergh, L. *Food Cosmet. Toxicol.* **1966**, *4*, 269.
295. Gangolli, S. D.; Grasso, P.; Goldberg, L. *Food Cosmet. Toxicol.* **1967**, *5*, 601.
296. Truhaut, R. *Aliment. Vie* **1962**, *50*, 77.
297. Grasso, P.; Gangolli, S. D.; Gaunt, I. F. *Food Cosmet. Toxicol.* **1971**, *9*, 1.
298. Dacre, J. C. *Proc. Univ. Otago Med. Sch.* **1965**, *43*, 31.
299. Sharratt, M.; Frazer, A. C.; Paranjoti, I. S. *Food Cosmet. Toxicol.* **1966**, *4*, 493.
300. Grice, H. C.; Mannell, W. A.; Allmark, M. G. *Toxicol. Appl. Pharmacol.* **1961**, *3*, 509.
301. Hansen, W. H.; Davis, K. J.; Fitzhugh, O. G.; Nelson, A. A. *Toxicol. Appl. Pharmacol.* **1963**, *5*, 105.
302. Mannell, W. A. *Food Cosmet. Toxicol.* **1964**, *2*, 169.
303. Ikeda, Y.; Horiuchi, S.; Furuya, T.; Omori, Y. *Food Cosmet. Toxicol.* **1966**, *4*, 485.
305. Grasso, P.; Landsdown, A. B. G.; Kiss, I. S.; Gaunt, I. F.; Gangolli, S.D. *Food Cosmet. Toxicol.* **1969**, *7*, 425.
306. Bonser, G. M.; Roe, F. J. C. *Food Cosmet. Toxicol.* **1979**, *8*, 477.
307. Ikeda, Y.; Horiuchi, S.; Kobuyashi, K.; Furaja, T.; Kohgo, K. *Food Cosmet. Toxicol.* **1968**, *6*, 591.
308. Davis, K. J.; Nelson, A. A.; Zwickey, R. E.; Hanson, W. H.; Fitzhugh, O. G. *Toxicol. Appl. Pharmacol.* **1966**, *8*, 306.
309. Gaunt, I. F.; Brantom, P. G.; Grasso, P.; Creasey, M.; Gangolli, S. D. *Food Cosmet. Toxicol.* **1972**, *10*, 3.
310. Gaunt, I. F.; Corpanini, F. M. B.; Grasso, P.; Kiss, I. S.; Gangolli, S. O. *Food Cosmet. Toxicol.* **1922**, *10*, 17.
311. Gillman, J.; Gillman, T.; Gilbert, C. *S. Afr. J. Med. Sci.* **1949**, *14*, 21.
312. Gillman, J.; Gillman, T. *Cancer* **1952**, *5*, 792.
313. Brown, D. V.; Norlind, L. M. *Arch. Pathol.* **1961**, *72*, 251.
314. Marshall, A. H. E. *Acta Pathol. Microbiol. Scand.* **1953**, *33*, 1.
315. Fujita, K.; Iwase, S.; Matusubara, T.; Ishigura, I.; Matsui, H.; Mizuno, T.; Arai, T.; Takayanagi, T.; Sugiyama, Y.; Shirafugi, K. *Gann* **1956**, *47*, 181.
316. Childs, I. J.; Clayson, D. B. *Biochem. Pharmacol.* **1966**, *15*, 1247.
317. Rubenchik, B. L. *Vopr. Pitan.* **1962**, *21*, 72.
318. Kawazoe, Y.; Tachibana, M.; Aoki, K.; Nakahara, W. *Biochem. Pharmacol.* **1967**, *16*, 631.
319. Enomoto, M.; Sato, K.; Miller, E. C.; Miller, J. A. *Life Sci.* **1968**, *7*, 1025.
320. Brown, G. B.; Sugiura, K.; Cresswell, R. M. *Cancer Res.* **1965**, *25*, 986.
321. Brown, G. B.; Teller, M. N.; Smullgan, I.; Birdsall, N. J. M.; Lee, T. C.; Parham, J. C.; Stohrer, G. *Cancer* **1973**, *33*, 1113.
322. Birdsall, N. J. M.; Parham, J. C.; Wolke, U.; Brown, G. B. *Tetrahedron* **1972**, *28*, 3.
323. McDonald, J. J.; Stohrer, G.; Brown, G. B. *Cancer Res.* **1973**, *33*, 3319.
324. McCuen, R. W.; Stohrer, G.; Sirotno, F. M. *Cancer Res.* **1974**, *34*, 378.
325. Price, J. M.; Morris, J. E.; Lalich, J. J. *Fed. Proc. Fed. Am. Soc. Exp. Biol.* **1966**, *25*, 419.
326. Stein, R. J.; Yost, D.; Petroliunas, F.; von Esch, A. *Fed. Proc., Fed. Am. Soc. Exp. Biol.* **1966**, *25*, 291.
327. Erturk, E.; Cohen, S. M.; Bryan, G. T. *Cancer Res.* **1970**, *30*, 1309.
328. Croft, W. A.; Bryan, G. T. *JNCI, J. Natl. Cancer Inst.* **1973**, *51*, 941.
329. Erturk, E.; Cohen, S. M.; Price, J. M.; Bryan, G. T. *Cancer Res.* **1969**, *29*, 2219.
330. Cohen, S. M.; Erturk, E.; Bryan, G. T. *Cancer Res.* **1970**, *30*, 2320.
331. Erturk, E.; Cohen, S. M.; Bryan, G. T. *Cancer Res.* **1970**, *30*, 936.
332. Erturk, E.; Cohen, S. M.; Bryan, G. T. *Cancer Res.* **1970**, *30*, 2098.

333. Cohen, S. M.; Erturk, E.; Bryan, G. T. *Cancer Res.* **1970**, *30*, 906.
334. Cohen, S. M.; Erturk, E.; von Esch, A. M.; Crovetti, A. J.; Bryan, G. T. *JNCI, J. Natl. Cancer Inst.* **1973**, *51*, 403.
335. Morris, J. E.; Price, J. M.; Lalich, J. J.; Stein, R. J. *Cancer Res.* **1973**, *29*, 2145.
336. Rustia, M.; Shubik, P. *JNCI, J. Natl. Cancer Inst.* **1972**, *48*, 721.
337. Cohen, S. M. "Carcinogenesis, Nitrofurans 4"; Bryan, G. T., Ed.; Raven: New York, 1978; pp. 171–231.
338. Dunning, W. F.; Curtis, M. R.; Mann, M. E. *Cancer Res.* **1950**, *10*, 454.
339. Dunning, W. F.; Curtis, M. R. *Proc. Soc. Exp. Biol. Med.* **1958**, *99*, 91.
340. Boyland, E.; Harris, J.; Horning, E. S. *Br. J. Cancer* **1954**, *8*, 647.
341. Oyasu, R.; Sumie, H.; Burg, H. E. *JNCI, J. Natl. Cancer Inst.* **1970**, *45*, 853.
342. Oyasu, R.; Kitajima, T.; Hopp, M. L.; Sumie, H. *Cancer Res.* **1972**, *32*, 2027.
343. Morris, H. P.; Sidranky, H.; Wagner, B. P. *Proc. Am. Assoc. Cancer Res.* **1960**, *3*, 136.
344. Dunning, W. F.; Curtis, M. R. *Cancer Res.* **1954**, *14*, 299.
345. Allen, M. J.; Boyland, E.; Dukes, C. E.; Horning, E. S.; Watson, J. G. *Br. J. Cancer* **1957**, *11*, 212.
346. Bryan, G. T.; Brown, R. R.; Price, J. M. *Cancer Res.* **1964**, *24*, 582.
347. Bryan, G. T.; Brown, R. R.; Price, J. M. *Cancer Res.* **1964**, *24*, 596.
348. Bryan, G. T. *Cancer Res.* **1968**, *28*, 183.
349. Price, J. M. *Proc. Can. Cancer Res. Conf.* **1966**, *6*, 224.
350. Price, J. M.; Brown, R. R. *Acta Unio Int. Cancrum* **1962**, *18*, 684.
351. Abul-Fadl, M. A. M.; Khalafallah, A. S. *Br. J. Cancer* **1961**, *15*, 479.
352. Trout, G. E.; Gillman, J.; Prates, M. D. *Acta Unio Int. Cancrum* **1962**, *18*, 575.
353. Quagliariello, E.; Tancredi, F.; Fedele, L.; Saccone, C. *Br. J. Cancer* **1961**, *15*, 367.
354. Benassi, C. A.; Serissinotto, B.; Allegri, G. *Clin. Chim. Acta* **1963**, *8*, 822.
355. Brown, R. R.; Price, J. M.; Friedell, G. H.; Bierney, S. W. *JNCI, J. Natl. Cancer Inst.* **1969**, *43*, 295.
356. Cohen, S. M.; Aria, M.; Jacobs, J. B.; Freidell, G. H. *Cancer Res.* **1979**, *39*, 1207.
357. Leppanen, V. V. E.; Oka, M. *Ann. Med. Exp. Biol. Fenn.* **1963**, *41*, 123.
358. Price, J. M.; Brown, R. R.; Peters, H. A. *Neurology* **1959**, *9*, 456.
359. Price, J. M.; Brown, R. R.; Rukavina, J. G.; Mendelson, C.; Johnson, S. A. M. *J. Invest. Dermatol.* **1957**, *29*, 289.
360. Flinn, J. H.; Price, J. M.; Yess, N.; Brown, R. R. *Arthritis Rheum.* **1964**, *7*, 201.
361. Brown, R. R.; Thornton, M. J.; Price, J. M. *J. Clin. Invest.* **1961**, *40*, 617.
362. Miyakawa, M.; Yoshida, O. *Gann* **1973**, *64*, 411.
363 Ross, M. H.; Bras, G. *J. Nutr.* **1973**, *64*, 411.
364. Radomski, J. L.; Brill, E.; Glass, E. M.; *JNCI, J. Natl. Cancer Inst.* **1967**, *39*, 1069.
365. Matsukara, N.; Kawachi, T.; Morino, K.; Ohgaki, H.; Sugimura, T.; Takayama, S. *Science (Washington, D. C.)* **1981**, *213*, 346.
366. Matsumoto, T.; Yoshida, D.; Tomita, H. *Cancer Lett.* **1981**, *12*, 105.
367. Weusburger, J. H.; Grantham, P. H.; Weisburger, E. K. *Jerusalem Symp. Quantum Chem. Biochem.* **1969**, *1*, 262.
368. Groth, U.; Neumann, H. G. *Chem.- Biol. Interact.* **1971**, *4*, 409.
369. Conney, A. H. *Pharmacol. Rev.* **1967**, *19*, 317.
370. Richardson, H. L.; Stier, A. R.; Barsos-Nachtnebel, E. *Cancer Res.* **1952**, *12*, 356.
371. Miyaji, T.; Moszkowski, L. I.; Senoo, T.; Ogata, M.; Oda, T.; Kawai, K.; Sayama, Y.; Ishida, H.; Matsuo, H. *Gann* **1953**, *44*, 281.
372. Meecham, R. J.; McCafferty, D. E.; Jones, R. S. *Cancer Res.* **1953**, *13*, 802.
373. Miller, E. C.; Miller, J. A.; Brown, R. R.; MacDonald, J. C. *Cancer Res.* **1958**, *18*, 469.
374. Conney, A. H.; Miller, E. C.; Miller, J. A. *Cancer Res.* **1956**, *16*, 450.
375. Arcos, J. C.; Conney, A. H.; Buu-Hoi, N. G. *J. Biol. Chem.* **1961**, *236*, 1291.

376. Irving, C. C.; Peeler, T. C.; Veazey, R. A.; Wiseman, R. *Cancer Res.* **1971**, *31*, 1468.
377. Irving, C. C.; Wiseman, R.; Hill, J. T. *Cancer Res.* **1967**, *27*, 2309.
378. Morris, H. P.; Wagner, B. P.; Lombard, L. S. *JNCI, J. Natl. Cancer Inst.* **1958**, *20*, 1.
379. Mikata, A.; Luse, S. A. *Am. J. Pathol.* **1964**, *44*, 455.
380. Sugai, M.; Witting, L. A.; Tsuchiyama, H.; Kummerow, F. A. *Cancer Res.* **1962**, *22*, 510.
381. Weisburger, J. H.; Weisburger, E. K. *Acta Unio Int. Cancrum* **1963**, *19*, 513.
382. Magreth, A.; Lotlikar, P. D.; Miller, E. C.; Miller, J. A. *Cancer Res.* **1964**, *24*, 920.
383. Lotlikar, P. D.; Wasserman, M. B.; Luka, L. *Proc. Soc. Exp. Biol. Med.* **1973**, *144*, 445.
384. Wyatt, P. L.; Cramer, J. W. *Cancer Res.* **1970**, *11*, 83.
385. Matsushima, T.; Grantham, P. H.; Weisburger, E. K.; Weisburger, J. H. *Biochem. Pharmacol.* **1972**, *21*, 2043.
386. Peraino, C.; Fry, R. J. M.; Staffeldt, E. *Cancer Res.* **1971**, *31*, 1506.
387. Weisburger, J. H.; Weisburger, E. K. *Pharmacol. Rev.* **1973**, *25*, 1.
388. Peraino, C.; Fry, R. J. M.; Staffeldt, E. *Cancer Res.* **1977**, *37*, 3623.
389. Peraino, C.; Fry, R. J. M.; Staffeld, E.; Christopher, J. P. *Cancer Res.* **1975**, *35*, 2884.
390. Peraino, C.; Fry, R. J. M.; Staffeldt, E.; Kisieleski, W. E. *Cancer Res.* **1973**, *23*, 2701.
391. Peraino, C.; Staffeldt, E.; Haugen, D. A.; Lombard, L. S.; Stevens, F. J.; Fry, M. R. J. *Cancer Res.* **1980**, *40*, 3268.
392. Kitagawa, T.; Sugano, H. *Gann* **1977**, *68*, 255.
393. Radomski, J. L.; Radomski, T.; MacDonald, W. E. *JNCI, J. Natl. Cancer Inst.* **1977**, *58*, 1831.
394. Ulland, B. M.; Weisburger, J. H.; Yamamoto, R. S.; Weisburger, E. K. *Toxicol. Appl. Pharmacol.* **1972**, *22*, 281.
395. Enomoto, M.; Miyake, M.; Sato, K. *Gann* **1968**, *59*, 177.
396. Yamamoto, R. S.; Glass, R. M.; Frankel, H. H.; Weisburger, E. K.; Weisburger, J. H. *Toxicol. Appl. Pharmacol.* **1968**, *13*, 108.
397. Yamamoto, R. S.; Williams, G. M.; Frankel, H. H.; Weisburger, J. H. *Toxicol. Appl. Pharmacol.* **1971**, *19*, 687.
398. Matsushima, T.; Weisburger, J. H. *Chem.- Biol. Interact.* **1969–70**, *1*, 211.
399. Weisburger, J. H.; Shirasu, Y.; Grantham, P. H.; Weisburger, E. K. *J. Biol. Chem.* **1967**, *242*, 372.
400. Blunck, J. M. *Pathology* **1971**, *3*, 99.
401. Blunck, J. M. *Chem.- Biol. Interact.* **1970**, *2*, 217.
402. Blunck, J. M.; Leeds, B. J.; Masden, N. P. *Chem.- Biol. Interact.* **1971–72**, *4*, 219.
403. Lotlikar, P. D.; Enomoto, M.; Miller, E. C.; Miller, J. A. *Cancer Res.* **1964**, *24*, 1835.
404. Weisburger, E. K.; Grantham, P. H.; Weisburger, J. H. *Biochemistry* **1964**, *3*, 808.
405. Symeonidis, A.; Mulay, A. S.; Burgoyne, F. H. *JNCI, J. Natl. Cancer Inst.* **1954**, *14*, 805.
406. O'Neal, M. A.; Hoffman, H. E.; Dodge, B. G.; Griffin, A. C. *JNCI, J. Natl. Cancer Inst.* **1958**, *21*, 1161.
407. Reuber, M. D. *Fed. Proc. Fed. Am. Soc. Exp. Biol.* **1964**, *23*, 336.
408. Bielschowsky, F.; Hall, W. H. *Br. J. Cancer* **1953**, *7*, 358.
409. Griffin, A. C.; Richardson, H. L.; Robertson, C. H.; O'Neal, M. A.; Spain, J. D. *JNCI, J. Natl. Cancer Inst.* **1955**, *15*, 1623.
410. Ward, D. N.; Spain, J. D. *Cancer Res.* **1957**, *17*, 623.
411. Fujita, K.; Iwase, S.; Ito, T.; Arai, T.; Takayanagi, T.; Sugiyama, Y.; Matsuyama, M.; Takagi, C.; Ohmae, T.; Mine, T. *Gann* **1957**, *48*, 277.
412. Spain, J. D.; Clayton, C. C. *Cancer Res.* **1958**, *18*, 155.
413. Takashi, M.; Iwase, S. *Nature (London)* **1958**, *181*, 1211.
414. Mulay, A. S.; O'Gara, R. W. *Proc. Soc. Exp. Biol. Med.* **1959**, *100*, 320.
415. Ritchie, A. C.; Saffiotti, U. *Cancer Res.* **1955**, *15*, 84.

416. Yamazoe, Y.; Ishii, K.; Kamataki, T.; Kato, R.; Sugimura, T. *Chem.- Biol. Interact.* **1980**, *30*, 125.
417. Takeda, K.; Shudo, K.; Okamoto, T.; Nagao, M.; Wakabayashi, K.; Sugimura, T. *Carcinogenesis* **1980**, *1*, 889.
418. Rosenkranz, H. S.; McCoy, E.; Sanders, D. R.; Butler, M.; Kiriazides, D. K.; Mermelstein, R. *Science (Washington, D. C.)* **1980**, *209*, 1039.
419. Pitts, J. N.; Cauwenberghe, K. A.; Grosjean, D.; Schmid, J. P.; Fitz, D.; Belser, W. L.; Knudson, G. B.; Hynds, P. M. *Science (Washington, D. C.)* **1978**, *202*, 515.

5

Epidemiology of Aromatic Amine Cancers

H. G. PARKES

British Rubber Manufacturers' Association Ltd., Health Research Unit, Scala House, Holloway Circus, Birmingham B1 1EQ England

A. E. J. EVANS

Imperial Chemical Industries PLC, Organics Division, P. O. Box 42, Hexagon Tower, Blackley, Manchester M9 3DA England

THE ROLE OF THE EPIDEMIOLOGIST is to study the interaction of humans and their environment. The epidemiologist is concerned with the statistical analysis of the incidence of different diseases, but only insofar as that incidence can be related to an expected frequency. If it can be established that a selected population has experienced a significantly excessive incidence of a particular disease, the conclusion can be drawn that some environmental factor is or has been in operation to create the excess. The detection and identification of such environmental causes of disease are the main aims of all epidemiological studies.

The chemical induction of cancer has been the subject of intensive study since 1932 when Cook et al. (*1*) first reported the experimental production of cancer in mice by dibenz[*a,h*]anthracene, but the involvement of chemical substances in the etiology of certain types of cancer was established by the epidemiologist many years earlier. By the end of the last century, the carcinogenic properties of soot, tar, pitch, and shale oil were already appreciated. In 1895, the first report linking bladder cancer with a group of chemical workers soon led to the incrimination of certain aromatic amines.

Since the discovery of aniline in 1826, the commercial potential of the aromatic amino and nitro compounds has been progressively explored by chemists. The theoretical number of such compounds—if one includes primary, secondary, and tertiary derivatives—is almost infinite. Today they represent a large and still expanding group of commercially important compounds extensively used in a wide variety of industrial processes.

The toxicity of the aromatic amines, which is closely linked with the toxicity of the related nitro compounds, has been recognized since the early industrial use of

0065-7719/84/0182-0277$07.25/1

aniline when the clinical picture of "anilism" was first seen. Cystitis, hematuria, methemoglobinemia, and dermatitis were the principal manifestations of this toxicity, but such symptoms and signs were in most cases speedily resolved by improved manufacturing practices.

Although industrial exposure to aromatic amines has been linked with occupational bladder cancer since the end of the last century, the present understanding of the problem dates from the epidemiological studies of Case et al. (2). In vitro and in vivo testing has now shown conclusively that many aromatic amines have the potential to cause cancer; therefore, vigilance must be maintained to ensure that the currently accepted "nonindustrial" tumors are not due to unrecognized industrial exposure. This observation is, of course, relevant to cancers generally and not merely those of the genitourinary system.

Current toxicological screens may enable industry to filter out some of the potential human carcinogens, but complete success is an ideal that will remain unrealized irrespective of the extent and complexity of the screening protocol. Nevertheless, the availability and the successful application of epidemiological techniques in the identification of occupational cancer hazards may contribute significantly in the future to our ability to monitor and thus diminish the risk of human exposure to potential carcinogens.

When attention became focused on the potential carcinogenicity of aromatic amines, aniline was the first to come under suspicion. The tumors that were found were bladder tumors and were thought to result from the hemorrhagic cystitis associated with aniline exposure. They were therefore described originally as aniline tumors, and the misnomer persisted in medical textbooks until recent times. In fact, the experimental evidence that finally incriminated other aromatic amines and cleared aniline of suspicion was not reported until 1938 when Hueper et al. (3) successfully induced bladder tumors in female dogs after prolonged oral administration of commercial 2-naphthylamine. The earlier attempts to demonstrate the carcinogenic activity of 2-naphthylamine had failed because the compound had been tested in the wrong animal species and because of insufficient understanding of the lengthy latent period of tumor induction. The experimental carcinogenicity of 2-naphthylamine in dogs was confirmed by the experiments of Bonser in 1943 (4).

With the accumulation of experimental evidence to indicate the potent carcinogenicity of 2-naphthylamine, investigators made an intensive survey of related chemical compounds. From 1950 onward, growing numbers of aromatic amines were carefully studied, and although very few proved to have the carcinogenic potency of 2-naphthylamine, several were nevertheless revealed as carcinogens. Furthermore, although the experiments with dogs had established the bladder as the principal target organ, tests with other species provided evidence of cancer induction in many different sites. As a result of this work, for which much of the credit must go to Bonser et al., currently accepted theories were formulated regarding the mode of action of the aromatic amines in the carcinogenic process (5). These theories are discussed in detail in Chapter 4.

The practical importance of these studies will be more readily apparent when they are considered in the context of the industrial use of aromatic amines. Although their commercial origins are deeply rooted in the manufacture of dyestuffs, many of these amines have since been found to have important applications in other industries. They have been used on a large scale in the rubber and cablemaking industries, in textile dyeing and printing, and in the manufacture of pigments, paints, and plastics. The most important members of the series from the standpoint of industrial epidemiology are 1-naphthylamine, 2-naphthylamine, benzidine, 4-biphenylamine, 4,4′-methylenebis(2-chloroaniline), 3,3′-dichlorobenzidine, and diphenylamine. Among these are the aromatic amines that have proved responsible for all of the known incidence of occupational bladder cancer.

Aromatic Amines of Industrial Importance

1-Naphthylamine (α-Naphthylamine) (I). 1-Naphthylamine was extensively used in industry in the manufacture of azo dyes and in the chemical construction of antioxidants for the rubber industry. It is not easily produced in pure form but usually contains a small proportion of 2-naphthylamine. Within the United States, 1-naphthylamine manufacture after 1953 supposedly did not produce more than 0.5% of 2-naphthylamine impurity, but certain grades of European origin probably contained up to 10% until 1-naphthylamine manufacture was finally abandoned.

Doubts regarding the carcinogenicity of pure 1-naphthylamine have been expressed. Scott (*6*) recorded a total of 56 cases of bladder cancer that he attributed to exposure to commercial 1-naphthylamine. In a study by Bonser et al., experimentally "pure" 1-naphthylamine induced a single bladder papilloma in two dogs after lifetime exposure (9 years) (*7*). More recent work by Radomski (*8*) and Purchase (*9*) strongly supports the conclusion that pure 1-naphthylamine is not a carcinogen and that any carcinogenic potential attributed to this chemical has been due to contamination by the 2-isomer. The fact that these two compounds should, despite their structural similarity, have such dissimilar potency is fascinating and illustrates the potential pitfalls inherent in structure–function analogy. A possible explanation of this difference in biological activity is the hypothesis that the 2-isomer is able to bind with urothelial DNA and persist in the urothelium. The work of Kadlubar et al. (*10*) supports this theory.

1-Naphthylthiourea (ANTU) (II). This rodenticide is made by reacting 1-naphthylamine and thiocyanate salts and the development of this compound has been described by Richter (*11*). Subsequent to laboratory development, extensive field trials confirmed the efficacy of the compound.

Evidence indicates that ANTU was used in the United Kingdom from 1946, and comment was made as early as 1954 by Case in his unpublished Joseph Henry

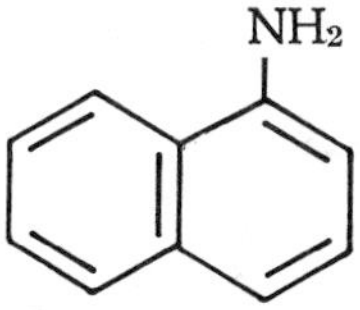

NH_2

I

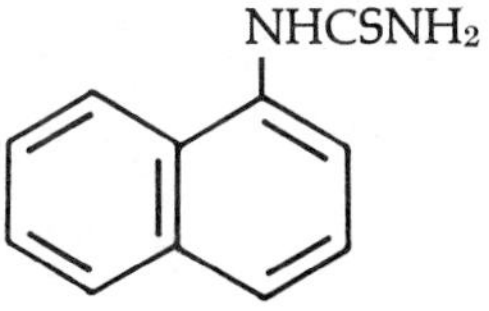

$NHCSNH_2$

II

Lecture to the Royal College of Surgeons of the possibility of a carcinogenic hazard arising from this compound. The carcinogenic potential was deduced from the presence of unreacted amine in ANTU. Analysis of various samples subsequently showed that up to 2% of unreacted naphthylamine could be present, with as much as one-fifth being the 2-isomer. During succeeding years, sporadic cases of bladder cancer in rodent-control operators indicated that the compound could possibly be a human carcinogen. This risk was sufficient for the U.K. Ministry of Agriculture, Food, and Fisheries to ban the use of this compound early in 1967.

A detailed study has been done by Davies, Thomas, and Manson (*12*) who show that the evidence does implicate ANTU as a bladder carcinogen. They comment on the low level of exposure and the small amount of naphthylamine impurity and suggest the possibility that ANTU itself is being metabolized to a potential carcinogen. They have proposed that this hypothesis should be examined in animal studies.

2-Naphthylamine (β-Naphthylamine) (III). The commercial uses of 2-naphthylamine have been similar to those of 1-naphthylamine, but its most significant use was in dyestuffs manufacture and the large-scale manufacture of antioxidants for the rubber industry. As already stated, the carcinogenicity of this compound is not disputed, and it is recognized as one of the most potent of the industrial bladder carcinogens.

2-Naphthylamine was the first aromatic amine to be established as an experimental carcinogen by Hueper in 1938 (*3*), and the epidemiological evidence that is discussed later is conclusive. Because of its commercial value and importance, attempts were made to devise safe procedures for its manufacture and use, but as these proved ineffectual, the industrial use of the compound diminished, and its manufacture was gradually abandoned. 2-Naphthylamine manufacture ceased in Britain in 1949, but regrettably continued on a limited scale for many years thereafter in other parts of the world. The last U.S. plant to manufacture 2-naphthylamine was not closed until 1970, and some production continued in Japan until 1972. Since that date the available evidence is that commercial manufacture has completely ceased.

Benzidine (4,4′-Diaminobiphenyl) (IV). Benzidine, which has been manufactured on an industrial scale for nearly 100 years, was mainly used in the dyestuffs industry as the starting point for the making of azo dyes. Unlike the naphthylamines, its use in the rubber industry was very limited, although it was also a hardener and a constituent of some adhesives and plastics. It had valuable properties that were used in the textile printing industry; it was used in the production of security paper; and it was, for many years, the essential chromogen

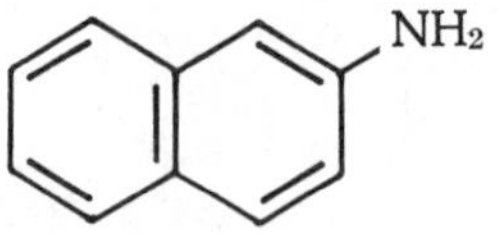

NH_2

III

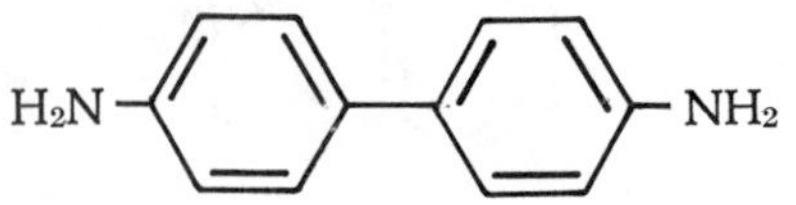

H_2N — — NH_2

IV

in the standard hospital laboratory test for occult blood (Chapter 6). Although epidemiological evidence implicating benzidine was already accumulating (*13*), it was not until 1950 when Spitz et al. (*14*) published their report on the induction of bladder tumors in dogs that its carcinogenicity was experimentally confirmed. Unlike 2-naphthylamine, its industrial use was not thereafter abandoned. Production ceased in Britain in October 1962, but substantial manufacture continues, predominantly in Eastern Europe and the Far East.

The role of benzidine in the causation of bladder cancer has again come under scrutiny as a result of positive animal-feeding studies with the benzidine-based dyes Direct Black 38, Direct Blue 6, and Direct Brown 95. These dyes contained less than 4 ppm of residual benzidine. Subsequent analysis of the rodent urines showed quite clearly that metabolic breakdown was occurring with formation of the free amine (*15*).

As a result of the findings in these experimental studies—now of questionable significance due to the possible misdiagnosis of liver carcinoma (*16*)—a comprehensive survey of work situations was undertaken in the United States in those areas where benzidine-based dyes were handled. This study indicated that benzidine or its metabolites could be detected in the workers' urine, but only in those situations where there was poor industrial hygiene (*17*). A recent British survey demonstrated the absence of any such benzidine metabolites in urine in good working conditions (*18*).

To date only one instance has been reported in which human bladder cancer has been attributed to exposure to benzidine-based dyes (*19*). However, in this study of silk dyers and painters, benzidine-based dyes were not the only dyestuffs to which the workers were exposed.

Until recent findings can be properly evaluated, it would seem prudent to accept that these dyes may be a potential cancer hazard and to insist on good standards of industrial hygiene, on all occasions, during the handling of these compounds.

4-Biphenylamine (4-Aminobiphenyl; 4-Aminodiphenyl; Xenylamine; 4-ADP) (V). The history of the industrial use of 4-ADP differs in some important respects from that of the naphthylamines and of benzidine. Unlike these compounds, which had their major application in the dyestuffs industry at the turn of the century, 4-ADP manufacture was not started until 1935 when it was used in the rubber industry as an antioxidant. It was then produced only in the United States, and production continued for 19 years before evidence of its carcinogenic potential was revealed in the reports of Melick et al. (*20*) who found 19 cases of bladder tumor in a population of 171 men. The fact that no fewer than 11% of those exposed developed tumors within such a short space of time was evidence enough of the highly carcinogenic nature of the compound. In a more recent study, Melick (*21*) has reported 53 cases in a population of 315 men. In Britain, a similar tragedy was averted by the foresight of Walpole et al. (*22*) who published in 1952 the first experimental proof of its carcinogenicity. In 1954, they confirmed their work with dog experiments and warned that the compound could be expected to cause bladder tumors in exposed workers. For this reason, manufacture of 4-ADP in Britain was never started, although limited amounts of the imported material were used for a time in the British rubber industry. Existing epidemiological evidence seems to indicate now that the carcinogenic potency of 4-ADP is at least equal to, and is possibly even greater than, that of 2-naphthylamine.

4,4′-Methylenedianiline (4,4′-Diaminodiphenylmethane; MDA; DADPM) (VI). MDA, which is usually made by the reaction of formaldehyde with aniline, has been manufactured and used on a commercial scale for more than half a century. The compound has a variety of applications, such as a laboratory analytical agent in tungsten determination, a corrosive inhibitor, and an intermediate in nylon yarn production. Today it is chiefly used as an intermediate in the manufacture of diphenylmethane diisocyanate and as a curing agent for polyurethane elastomers and epoxy resins. For some applications MDA is accepted as a useful substitute for 4,4′-methylenebis(2-chloroaniline) (MBOCA), which is suspected as being a possible human carcinogen.

Until recently the data did not indicate that MDA was an animal carcinogen (*23–27*). However, review of the data shows that many of the experimental protocols are unsatisfactory and unacceptable when compared with current standards; therefore, the findings must be interpreted with reservation. Results of the National Toxicology Program (NTP) bioassay vindicate this cautious approach because the study shows that MDA is an experimental carcinogen in both mice and rats; it produced tumors affecting several different organs including urinary bladder transitional cell papillomas in female rats (*28*).

Interestingly, MDA in rats administered either with a proven carcinogen or in the "post-initiation" stage has reduced the incidence of malignant tumors. The mechanism of action is not known but it could either be a nonspecific toxic effect (i.e., inhibition of food consumption with reduced growth) or a result of the inhibition of DNA synthesis (*29*).

The major human interest in the compound is related to the so-called Epping Jaundice outbreak in 1966 (*30*). This outbreak occurred in England following the accidental contamination of a sack of flour with MDA. Bread baked from this flour in an Epping bakery was subsequently identified as a source of the outbreak, which affected 84 people. Fortunately no deaths were reported, but some of the victims experienced a severe hepatotoxic effect.

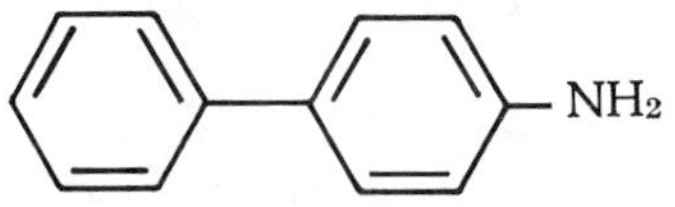

NH_2

V

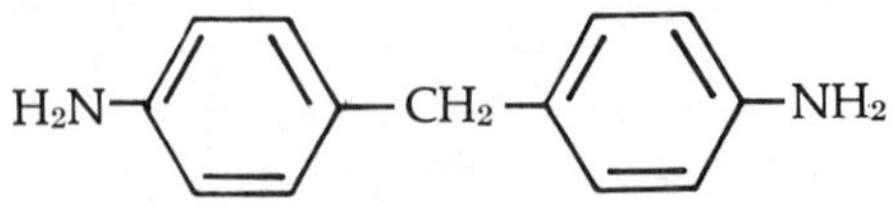

H_2N — CH_2 — NH_2

VI

The hepatotoxicity of this compound has been amply confirmed by both human and animal studies (*31*).

Limited epidemiological evidence suggests that under good conditions of commercial manufacture and use, MDA does not represent a carcinogenic hazard to humans (*32, 33*).

3,3′-Dichlorobenzidine (DCB) (VII). DCB has been produced commercially for over 40 years and has been substantially used as an intermediate in the dyestuffs industry. It has also been used as a curing agent for polyurethane elastomers.

Using various routes of administration, the compound has been shown to be an animal carcinogen in a variety of species. It induces tumors of the skin, Zymbal glands, mammary gland, and intestines in the rat (*34*). Work by Stula et al. (*35*) has shown DCB to be both a bladder and liver carcinogen in the dog.

In view of its accepted animal carcinogenicity and structural similarity to benzidine, DCB has been implicated as a potential human bladder carcinogen. However, epidemiological studies by Gerarde (*36*), Gadian (*37*), and McIntyre (*38*) show that exposure in plant manufacture has not caused bladder cancer. Although the data could not be regarded as conclusive, these studies have practical import.

These apparently conflicting results can be reconciled by understanding that the level of exposure in manufacturing practice is low enough to prevent the carcinogenic effect of the compound.

In the United Kingdom, DCB is a controlled substance under the U.K. Carcinogenic Substances Regulations 1967—Statutory Instrument No. 879 (*18*). Like MBOCA, it is subject in the United States to a permanent standard of the Department of Labor.

4,4′-Methylenebis(2-chloroaniline) (MBOCA, DACPM) (VIII). This compound has been important industrially for approximately 20 years, and its most significant industrial application is as a curing agent for polyurethane elastomers. It is an

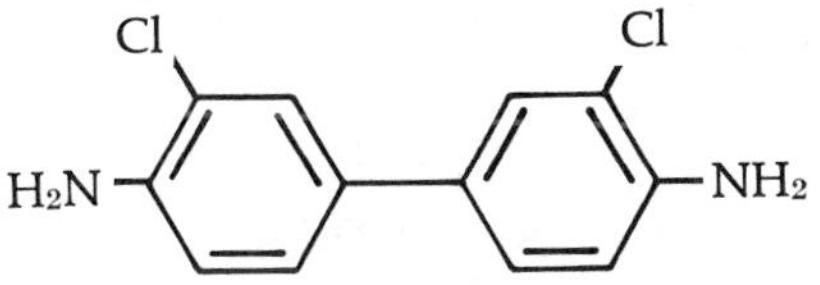

Cl Cl

H_2N NH_2

VII

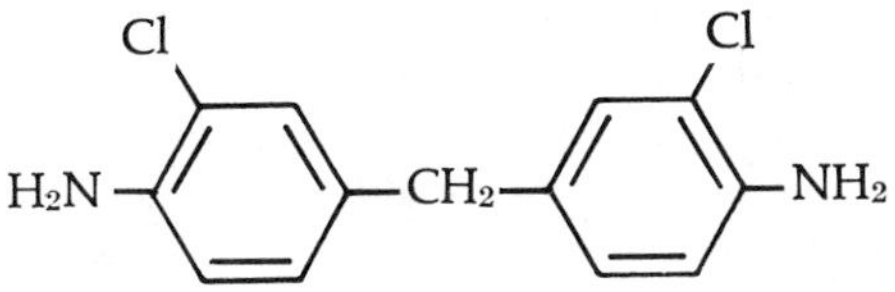

Cl Cl

H_2N CH_2 NH_2

VIII

extremely versatile and efficient compound in this role, and there has been heavy demand to stimulate production. It is synthesized by reacting formaldehyde with *o*-chloroaniline.

Routine testing of MBOCA for carcinogenicity showed that the compound is carcinogenic on both oral and subcutaneous administration in rats. It induced a variety of malignant tumors including lung and liver carcinomas (*39, 40*). The compound has also produced liver tumors in the mouse (*41*). However, experimental studies in the dog have caused the major concern; all five of the animals completing the study developed carcinomas of the urinary endothelium and four had the bladder as the target organ (*42*).

At present, insufficient epidemiological evidence is available to make any reliable assessment of the human carcinogenicity of this compound; but because of strong suspicions aroused by the experimental evidence, many British manufacturers, on the recommendation of the British Rubber Manufacturers Association, have refrained from its use. Furthermore, within the past 10 years, at least one major manufacturer has ceased production. Since October 1983, MBOCA has been on the list of suspect aromatic amines in the U.K. Schedule of Prescribed Industrial Diseases. The compound is listed as a suspect human carcinogen in the Threshold Limit Values publication, 1983–84, of the American Conference of Governmental Industrial Hygienists (ACGIH) and in the Health and Safety Executive (HSE) Guidance Note EH 15/80. In both publications an 8-h time weighted average (TWA) for airborne contamination is 0.02 ppm (0.22 mg/m^3). Skin absorption is also a very important route of entry for this compound, as is emphasized in each publication.

The potential of the compound to affect the urinary system is confirmed by observation on a case of acute exposure that resulted from contamination with hot liquid. Examination of the urine indicated damage to the renal tubules, but the observed abnormality returned to normal within 3 weeks (*43*).

Diphenylamine (*N*-Phenylbenzeneamine) (IX). The inclusion of diphenylamine in a short list of industrially important aromatic amines would not be justified solely on the grounds of its possible carcinogenicity. Indeed, no substantive evidence exists, either experimental or epidemiological, on which it can at present be indicted. However, two features connected with this compound give grounds for some concern: first, commercial diphenylamine usually contains a small amount of 4-biphenylamine as an impurity, and second, the industrial use of diphenylamine is still expanding. Although its original use in the early years of this century was largely confined to the dyestuffs industry, diphenylamine has been extensively used for the past 20 years in the manufacture of rubber industry antioxidants. This last application may once again be greatly expanded. Many rubber manufacturers, confronted with the medical and legal problems connected with the use of antioxidants containing trace quantities of 2-naphthylamine have now abandoned these antioxidants in favor of others that are not subject to this criticism. Some of the alternatives are the condensation products of acetone and diphenylamine. If the trend continues, then the manufacture and use of diphenylamine is certain to be increased dramatically. In 1962 Scott (*6*) pointed to the need to maintain a careful watch on what could prove to be a dangerous manufacture. Thus far such fears do not appear to have been realized.

***N*-Phenyl-2-naphthylamine (PBNA) (X).** This compound has many and varied uses, e.g., as a component of rocket fuel and as a stabilizer in electrical insulating silicone enamels, but its major use, dating from its industrial introduction in the late 1920s, has been as an antioxidant in rubber processing and also in certain lubricating oils.

However this use as a rubber antioxidant, although still appreciable, has been declining since the mid 1960s and its role as a stabilizer in staining products of synthetic rubbers has been largely replaced by the phenolic antioxidants.

The compound, as manufactured, contains a varying quantity of 2-naphthylamine as an impurity, although present use is generally confined to PBNA with less than 1 ppm of this impurity. In view of this and its structural similarity to 2-naphthylamine, the compound has been suspected of having carcinogenic potential. Experimental studies in mice both by oral administration and by single subcutaneous injection suggest that the compound may be carcinogenic, but no firm conclusions could be drawn due to the inadequate protocols used (*44*). A 4.5-year feeding study on three dogs reported by Gehrmann (*45*) did not show any tumor formation, but the small number of animals and the limited observation period make the study inconclusive.

Studies in human volunteers (*46*) have shown that this compound is metabolized by *N*-dephenylation to 2-naphthylamine, and experiments in the dog by Batten and Hathway (*47*) have also demonstrated this metabolic pathway. In the dog study, the strictly limited formation of 2-naphthylamine by *N*-dephenylation is discussed, and the authors conclude that the level of 2-naphthylamine is unlikely to present a carcinogenic risk. In addition, the presumed ultimate carcinogen, namely 2-naphthylhydroxylamine, was not detected in the urine, which suggests that this important further metabolic step does not occur.

A recent study using the Syrian golden hamster did not show the compound to be carcinogenic and supports the conclusion drawn from the metabolic studies (*48*).

Probably the most important and relevant finding is that epidemiological studies (*49–52*) have not shown an increased incidence of bladder tumors among operatives involved either in the manufacture or in commercial use of *N*-phenyl-2-naphthylamine in the rubber industry over many years.

***o*-Toluidine (XI).** Commercial manufacture of *o*-toluidine dates back 100 years in the United Kingdom. This compound is also produced in the United States, Western Europe, and Japan. *o*-Toluidine and its hydrochloride are used mainly as

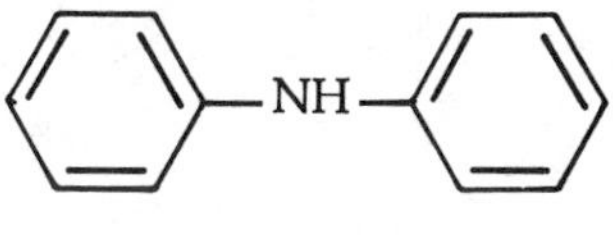

NH

IX

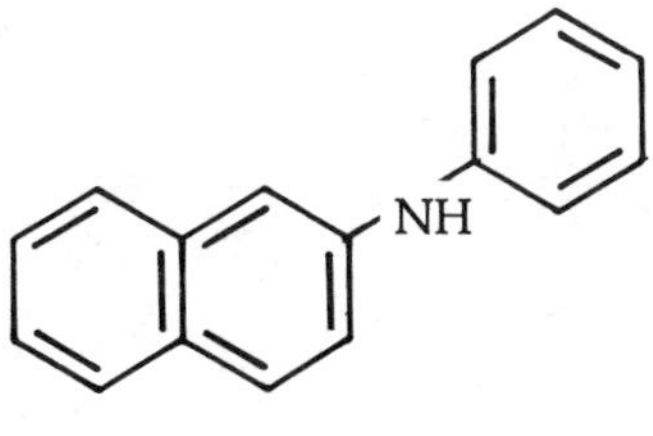

NH

X

intermediates in the manufacture of dyestuffs, but they are also used in the manufacture of pigments and rubber chemicals (*53*).

o-Toluidine is absorbed via the skin and respiratory tract. Acute poisoning is known to cause irritation of the kidneys and bladder with the development of hematuria.

Administration to animals by various routes of exposure has produced a variety of tumors; bladder tumors were noted in the rat, guinea pig, and rabbit (*53*). The compound had also been assessed experimentally in the rat and mouse by the U.S. National Cancer Institute where tumors affecting many organs were found in both species (*54*). Included in these findings was a significant increase in bladder tumors in the female rat. From the many animal studies, this compound is clearly indicted as an animal carcinogen.

Despite the accepted animal carcinogenicity, nothing in published epidemiological studies seriously challenges the inference of the Case study that this compound is not a carcinogenic hazard to humans. This assessment is supported by the critical evaluation of the biological and epidemiological evidence published by the International Agency for Research on Cancer (IARC) (*53*).

***m*-Toluidine (XII).** The available animal experimental results indicate that this compound is not an animal carcinogen.

***p*-Toluidine (XIII).** The animal studies on this compound are equivocal, and although *p*-toluidine cannot be classed as noncarcinogenic, the evidence indicates that its action, at worst, is only weakly carcinogenic.

The difference in carcinogenic potential of the three toluidine isomers is somewhat unexpected and may well be explained by the fact that the most active compound, namely *o*-toluidine, is not as readily metabolized as the *m*- and *p*-isomers. This hypothesis is discussed by Cheever et al. (*55*).

Epidemiology of Bladder Cancer

What has been said so far demonstrates that the epidemiology of the aromatic amine cancers is, for all practical purposes, synonymous with the epidemiology of industrial bladder cancer. Before this relation is considered further, brief reference to the epidemiology of bladder cancer in a general way without special reference to the question of its industrial etiology is helpful.

Figures published in the United States in 1981 and drawn from 11 regional cancer registries illustrate the major geographical difference in bladder cancer

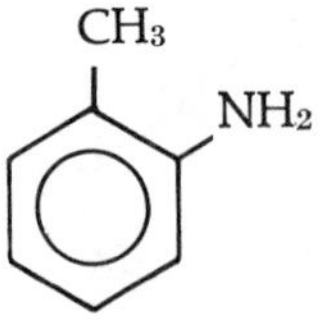

CH_3 NH_2

XI

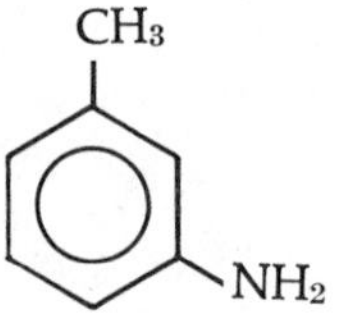

CH_3 NH_2

XII

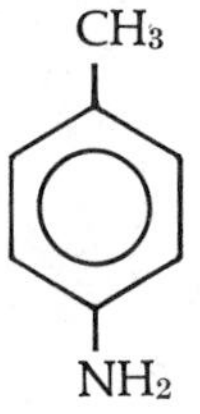

CH_3 NH_2

XIII

incidence. Average annual age-adjusted incidence rates per 100,000 population (males) are shown to vary from a low of 7.5 in Puerto Rico to a high of 17.1 in Connecticut (*56*).

In England and Wales, bladder cancer ranks as the seventh commonest cause of cancer death for the male population (*see* Table I) and has an average annual age-adjusted incidence rate of 13.3 for 100,000 population.

More interesting, however, is the observation that bladder cancer mortality rates have been steadily rising. This increase can be seen in Table II, which sets out the crude death rates per million population for England and Wales from 1950 to 1978.

A number of theories have been advanced to explain this increasing incidence, but the etiology is complex. At present, substantial evidence confirms a positive correlation with cigarette smoking, especially in males, and a dose–response relationship is demonstrable in both sexes. A reduction of risk associated with the use of filter cigarettes compared to nonfilter cigarettes has been reported. An increased incidence of bladder cancer has also been observed in pipe smokers (*59*). Additionally, an increased incidence of the disease has been correlated with the consumption of coffee and of artificial sweeteners. A further study has identified an association of the disease with abnormal tryptophan metabolism. Evidently, a number of factors could be influencing the overall increase in bladder cancer rates, but the major interest is still concentrated in the more readily definable area of industrial exposure to carcinogenic aromatic amines. However, industrial exposure and smoking are unlikely to account for most bladder cancers, and other possible factors such as diet, drugs, genetic predisposition, and immune status should continue to be explored. The importance of adopting this wider approach has again been emphasized by the findings of Doll and Peto (*60*).

Table I

Bladder Cancer Ranked with Other Sites in Males in England and Wales in 1979

ICD No.	*Cancer Site*	*Crude Death Rates/ Million People*
162	Lung and bronchus	1120
151	Stomach	274
185	Prostate	202
153	Colon	180
154	Rectum	143
157	Pancreas	129
188	Bladder	122
150	Esophagus	85
204–208	Leukemia	74
189	Other genitourinary organs	60
191	Brain	54

SOURCE: Ref. 57.

Table II

Bladder Cancer: Crude Death Rates/Million People in England and Wales from 1950 to 1978

Sex	*1950*	*1954*	*1958*	*1962*	*1966*	*1970*	*1974*	*1978*
Males	79	87	92	103	107	113	119	123
Females	34	37	37	39	41	45	50	52

SOURCE: Ref. 58.

Industrial Bladder Cancer

This form of cancer has a specific and identifiable industrial etiology. The etiology is important for those investigators who wish to determine what proportion of all bladder tumors can rightly be attributed to occupational exposure, and to achieve this end, one should consider how those tumors that are of industrial origin may be correctly identified. Thus far no evidence suggests that any significant pathological, biochemical, or immunological differences exist between tumors of industrial origin and tumors described as idiopathic. The presenting features are likewise identical and one must, therefore, take into account evidence that is nonspecific and circumstantial. The most important piece of evidence—namely that of occupational exposure to aromatic amines—is still too frequently missed, usually as a result of inadequate records but sometimes because of a failure to realize that exposure may occur in occupations other than those found in the chemical and rubber industries. For example, it was reported in the medical press that three cases of bladder tumor had been identified in anglers. The inference was drawn that, because anglers were known to use chrysoidine bait dye, the observed association could be causal (*61*). However, without careful consideration of the detailed occupational history of each affected individual, such an inference cannot be substantiated.

The necessity of obtaining a proper occupational history cannot be overemphasized and involves checking the patients' claims. A patient's recollection of events some 20–30 years ago is frequently vague, and it is easy to confuse chemical names, which may sound similar but have quite different potential toxic effects. In making the assessment of cause and effect, the help of medical personnel with special expertise in this area is advisable.

Another important factor that may provide a clue to an occupational etiology is the age of the patient. Although cancer of the bladder is among the 10 most frequent forms of malignant disease, the impact is chiefly on those between 65 and 74 years old (Table III). Because it is rare below the age of 45, bladder cancer in a man aged 50 or younger should arouse instant suspicion of an occupational etiology and provoke a detailed inquiry into his work history. Because of the lack of any absolute distinguishing features, widely differing estimates of the frequency of occupational tumors are given. Although many would concede that the environmental and social factors are important in the etiology of bladder cancers, it is widely held that tumors attributable directly to aromatic amine exposure constitute no more than 5% of the total.

Table III

Malignant Bladder Neoplasms (ICD 188) in England and Wales in 1979

	Number of Deaths			*Rate per Million*	
Age	*Male*	*Female*	*Age*	*Male*	*Female*
All ages	2917	1285	All ages	122	51
1–4	—	—	1–4	—	—
5–9	1	1	5–14	0[a]	0[a]
10–34	—	—	15–34	—	—
35–39	8	4	35–44	7	4[a]
40–44	13	6	45–54	40	20
45–49	27	20	55–64	176	57
50–54	85	35	65–74	576	160
55–59	204	64	75–84	1228	295
60–64	260	101	85+	2024	536
65–69	531	179			
70–74	618	236			
75–79	553	234			
80–84	376	205			
85–89	168	140			
90–94	66	51			
95+	7	9			

[a]Rates calculated from fewer than 20 deaths: a warning to the user that their reliability as a measure may be affected by the small number of events.
SOURCE: Ref. 57.

Epidemiology of Industrial Bladder Cancer

That the aromatic amines are deeply involved in the epidemiology of industrial bladder cancer is today a matter of historical record. It took, however, more than 50 years before the full implications of this involvement were properly understood and before Scott and Williams published in 1953 the first effective Code of Practice designed to protect workers against hazardous exposure to carcinogenic amines (*62*).

The starting point of this lengthy epidemiological investigation can be accurately placed in 1895, when a Congress of the German Surgical Society received a report from a Frankfurt surgeon, Rehn (*63*), on the effects of exposure of a group of chemical workers to certain aromatic amines. Rehn noted chiefly the frequency of cyanosis and hematuria but drew attention also to the unexpected finding of four cases of bladder tumor. All the men involved had been working in the manufacture of fuchsin (rosaniline) for periods of up to 20 years. At the time, Rehn suggested that all these observed effects probably resulted from aniline exposure, but his conclusion was contested by some of his contemporaries who asserted that aniline would not cause bladder tumors. In 1898, Leichtenstern (*64*) suggested for the first time that exposure to "naphthylamines" could cause bladder tumors. During the next few years, evidence to support this conclusion was gradually accumulated, and in 1906 Rehn (*65*) reported 38 cases of bladder tumor and suggested the possible involvement of naphthylamine and benzidine. By this time interest in the industrial etiology of bladder tumors was aroused in other European countries, and in 1912 Leuenberger (*66*) reported an extended series of cases among aniline dye workers in Basel, Switzerland. By a comparison of his findings with data obtained from the general population, he showed that the male dye worker experienced 33 times the risk of other industrial employees. At this point the chain of investigation was unfortunately broken by the First World War. Although the existing evidence and state of knowledge were extensively reviewed in an International Labor Organization (ILO) report in 1921 (*67*), interest had waned to a point that allowed the establishment of the developing dyestuffs industries of Britain, France, Italy and the United States, without any real appreciation or understanding of the hazards being introduced.

The first reference to industrial bladder cancer in Britain was made by Wignall in 1929 (*68*) when he referred to the discovery of 14 cases of tumor among 1-naphthylamine and benzidine workers. However, the reports of Goldblatt in 1947 (*69*) and 1949 (*70*) first drew attention to the gravity of the problem. These reports reviewed in detail the evidence that had accumulated during the years of the Second World War and established beyond doubt the existence of a major health hazard in the British industry. His findings provided the compelling reasons for the appointment in 1948 of Case as a research fellow charged with conducting a full epidemiological investigation of the dyestuffs industry.

In the meantime, cases of industrial bladder cancer appeared elsewhere in the world. Gehrmann in 1934 (*71*) reported 27 cases in the United States, and in 1949 Gehrmann et al. (*72*) attributed those tumors to 2-naphthylamine exposure. Concurrently, in 1949, di Maio (*73*) and Barsotti and Vigliani (*74*) reported cases from Italy, and Billiard-Duchesne (*75*) reported cases from France.

Thus, a great mass of evidence, both experimental and epidemiological, had accumulated by the late 1940s to support the conclusion that exposure to certain aromatic amines, notably 2-naphthylamine, benzidine, and 1-naphthylamine, would inevitably constitute a serious bladder cancer hazard. The responsibility fell to the lot of one man to provide the ultimate proof and to reveal the risk of involving as yet unsuspected groups of industrial workers. This proof was achieved by one of the most careful and comprehensive epidemiological studies ever carried out that even today stands as a model.

The Work of R. A. M. Case

The classic studies of Case and his colleagues followed his appointment as a Research Fellow at the Chester Beatty Research Institute in London to carry out an investigation of the incidence and causes of industrial bladder cancer for the Association of British Chemical Manufacturers. Case's first task was to construct, from factory records, a nominal roll of all those men who had been employed in the dyestuffs industry and who had been in contact with one or more of the suspect carcinogens for longer than 6 months. It was possible to trace 4622 names of men meeting these criteria. Steps were then taken to identify, within this population, all those who had either died as a result of or who had been treated for bladder tumors. In the "at risk" population, 341 such cases were found. Case then conducted a careful search of all local hospital records and examined mortality data provided by the Registrar General to establish the number of males in the area population dying between 1921 and 1949 who were known to have had bladder tumors. He then analyzed these data by "comparative composite cohort analysis." Case describes this as

> a technique whereby the actual occurrence of an event in a population defined by individual name and working environment, with the age and date of entry into the environment, is observed, and the result compared with what would be expected from a general population, or population not exposed to a specific risk of the event, observed for the same length of time. Thus the unit of the analysis is the cohort which is defined by two or more characteristics, each defining a sub-cohort, e.g., age, environment, and date of entry into environment. These sub-cohorts are later combined by summation of the expected frequency of the event introducing the composite elements.

Case points out that the particular advantage of this type of analysis when applied to environmental problems is that much more data can be used than in alternative techniques because withdrawal from the environment does not affect the method of estimation. The only difficulty with successful application of this technique is that the willing and unstinted cooperation of the industry or manufacturers concerned in the investigation must be secured, because free access to personnel records is an indispensable prerequisite.

Case's work greatly advanced existing knowledge of occupational bladder tumors. In addition to establishing the precise incidence of the disease, he showed that the risk of contracting bladder tumors was 30 times as great for the exposed chemical worker as for the general population, and he also ranked the suspected chemicals in order of carcinogenic potency. He showed the relative potencies for 2-naphthylamine, benzidine, and 1-naphthylamine were in the ratios of 5, 1.7, and 1, respectively, and mixed exposures gave a result of 2.7. He could not find any evidence to incriminate aniline as a carcinogen. 2-Naphthylamine, therefore, stood at last revealed—at least in the British dyestuffs industry—as the principal carcinogenic amine. Williams (*76*) later substantiated this conclusion with the dramatic finding that the bladder tumor incidence among a small group of 18 men working for longer than 5 years on the distillation of benzidine and 2-naphthylamine had risen to 94%.

The application of Case's comprehensive analytical technique to the problems of the British dyestuffs industry allowed him to extend his original frame of reference and thereby greatly increase the value of his contribution. In particular, he devised a statistical method for the estimation of the expected number of cases of bladder tumor in both an exposed (*2*) and a nonexposed (*77*) population. He showed that the availability of such information could be invaluable in detecting hitherto unsuspected hazards.

Much of the complexity of the epidemiological techniques such as those described by Case derives from the necessity to extend the time scale of the investigation retrospectively over many years as a result of the lengthy induction period of occupational tumors. Researchers involved in the investigation of industrial bladder cancer have provided evidence about the length of this latent period. The *latent period* is defined as the interval of time that elapses between the date of first exposure to or contact with the known or suspect carcinogen and the date of the first established onset of disease. In this context, Case reporting his observations on the British Dyestuffs Chemical industry in 1954 (*2*) found the average latent period for mixed exposures to be 18 years with a standard deviation of 7 years. He further pointed out that although the latent period most frequently observed lay between 15 and 20 years, tumors had been shown to occur within 5 years and after 45 years from first exposure to risk, so that the overall range of induction times is very wide. Furthermore, any new case of bladder cancer diagnosed later than 1980 but occurring among men whose occupational exposure to aromatic amines dates from 1950 or earlier must, by definition, have a latent period of induction in excess of 30 years. Consequently, as each new case is added to the total, there is a resultant lengthening of the average latency of the series. At the present time (1982), the average latency of occupational bladder cancer affecting the population of United Kingdom rubber and chemical workers exposed prior to 1950 has risen to more than 25 years.

One further element in Case's study requires particular mention because it represents what was possibly his most important discovery. Until 1949, the hazard of industrial bladder cancer resulting from exposure to the aromatic amines was generally believed to be confined within the chemical industry to the dyestuff manufacturers. Case was the first to show that the hazard extended beyond the confines of chemical manufacture and that it also involved other major manufacturing operations. Had it not been for the element of chance combined with the astute perception of the epidemiologist, this important discovery could well have been delayed many more years.

During the early days of his investigation in the chemical industry, Case sought to establish a suitable control population against which to match his study population. For this purpose he explored at first the possibility of establishing such a population within a large concentration in a different geographical location. When he came to examine the incidence of bladder cancer within this control population, he was astonished to discover an incidence in excess of national expectation that itself seemed to merit further inquiry. He therefore proceeded to note the last recorded occupation of the bladder cancer cases in this area and immediately observed that a disproportionate number of them appeared to have occurred in men listed as rubber workers.

Following this line of investigation, he soon discovered that many of these men had been employed in a large tire factory situated in the area. From this point it was a relatively short step to the realization that the suspect carcinogen 2-

naphthylamine was an important chemical component of a rubber antioxidant then in use and that the existence of a major industrial health hazard was now likely to be uncovered in a considerable number of rubber factories spread throughout the country. The full extent of this discovery was not really appreciated until 1957, and by that time Case's inquiry had already extended to other areas of manufacture in which the use of benzidine and 2-naphthylamine had been demonstrated. Laboratory workers, rodent exterminators, textile printers, makers of security paper, cobblers, and gas retort house workers had all attracted early suspicion, and more recent epidemiological studies such as those of Anthony and Thomas (*78*) and Cole et al. (*79)* now indicate the possible extension of the hazard to include such diverse occupations as weavers, tailors' cutters, hairdressers, cooks, and kitchen workers. Nevertheless, the major share of the hazard still remains with the dyestuffs workers and with the rubber and cable manufacturers.

If the findings of the Case enquiry were important and dramatic, the consequences were more so. Certainly the most important consequence of all was the decision taken by the British chemical manufacturers in 1949 to abandon the further production of 2-naphthylamine promptly. This action was followed, on the advice of the chemical manufacturers, by the decision of the rubber manufacturers to discontinue use of the suspect rubber antioxidants containing 2-naphthylamine immediately and to return or destroy all existing stocks. As has already been noted, the production of benzidine continued until some years later, because such production was thought to be entirely free from risk by the careful implementation of the Code of Practice described by Scott and Williams (*60*). In 1962 this assumption was finally thrown into question by the occurrence of a case of bladder cancer in a benzidine worker and only then was the decision taken to cease benzidine production in Britain. Other and more remote consequences, which will be discussed in greater detail later, included the provision of financial support by the manufacturers for the victims of industrial bladder cancer and the acceptance and recognition that the disease was of industrial origin. In 1953, bladder cancer became officially prescribed in Britain as "Industrial Disease No. 39" under the National Insurance (Industrial Injuries) Act (*80*). Many years later, under the British Carcinogenic Substances Regulations 1967 (*81*), the manufacture and use of the principal carcinogenic amines were specifically prohibited in the United Kingdom subject only to certain exemptions.

These more recent developments have focused attention upon the grave hazards of industrial exposure to the carcinogenic amines, the manufacture and use of which have been generally abandoned during the past decade. The need, however, for continuing epidemiological study of the industrial workers at risk has become increasingly apparent to establish that no unidentified carcinogens have remained in use. Only during the past few years with the growing availability of more sophisticated analytical techniques has it been recognized that a number of industrial chemicals in widespread use do in fact contain as impurities trace quantities of carcinogenic amines such as 2-naphthylamine; therefore, a matter of urgent concern is to verify that the impurity level in such cases has not been sufficient to allow of any extension of the bladder cancer hazard.

Screening

Although appropriate steps are now being implemented to achieve proper epidemiological control of industrial bladder cancer, all possible measures should also be taken to protect those known to have been at risk and to compensate those now suffering from bladder cancer as a result of industrial exposure. Unhappily, protection in this context is limited to the provision of adequate medical supervision and routine diagnostic screening procedures, because past exposure is clearly irreversible. Nevertheless, cytodiagnostic screening programs offer at least the opportunity for early treatment in a high proportion of cases and may thereby exert a favorable effect on prognosis. Comprehensive cytological screening facilities of this nature have been generally available to all "at risk" workers in the British chemical and rubber industries for over 25 years; cytodiagnostic facilities were provided first for chemical workers in 1951 and subsequently for rubber workers in 1957. To date, these services have detected more than 300 new cases of bladder cancer in a population of approximately 25,000 employees, the great majority of whom had been exposed at some time to contact with carcinogenic aromatic amines.

In recent years evidence has been accumulating to suggest that the incidence of new cases of bladder cancer of industrial origin is now declining. However, this trend has not resulted in any observable reduction in cancer morbidity because of the sharply age-related increase now affecting the screened population. This finding is in line with the expected morbidity rates for a substantial proportion of all forms of malignant disease in an aging population.

Immunological techniques have been investigated recently as a potential screening method. Chemical workers with a known history of exposure to urinary carcinogens have been identified, and the toxicity of their lymphocytes to a culture of bladder cancer cells has been measured. Results show that the lymphocytes from these exposed workers had an increased ability to kill these cancer cells (*82, 83*). Subsequent study of this group, measuring antibody (*84*) and tissue polypeptide antigen (*85*), also gave abnormal findings. These preliminary studies have given interesting results, but considerably more work is required before these methods could justifiably be adopted for routine screening in the industrial setting.

For the future the possibility of identifying, prior to any exposure to aromatic amines, those who may be at increased risk is currently being examined (*86*).

Compensation

A victim of industrial bladder cancer cannot be adequately compensated for the infliction of an injury that will in many cases cost him his life. Nevertheless, his entitlement at least to some relief from financial hardship must be recognized even though the scale and mode of obtaining such compensation will vary considerably according to custom and practice in different parts of the world. When the condition of occupational bladder cancer was prescribed in Britain as an industrial disease in 1953, the relevant social security legislation allowed those affected to claim state benefits in respect of industrial injury. Also, private schemes have been set up by a number of British chemical and rubber manufacturers that provide for additional ex gratia payments to be made, and the broad intention of such schemes is to protect the affected worker against loss of earnings. However, the victim cannot expect to recover any substantial sum from either of these sources, and he may therefore seek to bring a common law action for damages against his employer in the courts. The possibility of a successful outcome to such litigation remained in doubt until recent times, when an important test case involving both a manufacturer and a user of carcinogenic aromatic amine compounds was successfully fought by the plaintiffs in the British High Court; the judgment of that court was subsequently upheld on appeal. The circumstances of this case are of wider than usual interest in that the judgment defines, and appears to establish, some important and legal principles concerned with a manufacturer's liability.

Legal Liability

The High Court Action in the British Courts (*87*) was brought by two Dunlop workers suffering from industrial bladder cancer who claimed that they had contracted their disease through exposure to carcinogenic aromatic amines that were manufactured by Imperial Chemical Industries Ltd. (ICI) and sold to Dunlop. They alleged negligence against ICI on the grounds that the carcinogenic properties of the antioxidant Nonox S were recognized prior to 1949, when the compound was ultimately withdrawn, and against Dunlop on the grounds that the company had failed to provide, at a sufficiently early date, cytodiagnostic screening facilities in accordance with recommendations generally accepted by the industry in 1957. The High Court judge awarded each plaintiff £1000 against Dunlop and a total of £21,000 for the two plaintiffs against ICI. On appeal, ICI submitted that at no time prior to 1949 could they have known that the free amines in their compound Nonox S would give rise to cases of bladder cancer among workers in Dunlop factories. Their Lordships concluded, however, that contemporaneous documentation showed that ICI had known from 1942 on that very small amounts of the free amines could constitute a grave hazard to health, and appropriate steps had then been taken by ICI to protect their own workers. They held that ICI should then have given thought to the risks to Dunlop workers and should either have withdrawn the product or given due warning to Dunlop of the danger that existed. They held also that ICI owed a duty to Dunlop employees in respect of Nonox S, the extent of that duty being to take all reasonable steps to satisfy themselves that Nonox S would be a safe product to use in the expected conditions.

"Safe" in this context, as defined by the Court of Appeal, means that

> there was no substantial risk of any substantial injury to health on the part of persons who were likely to use it or to be brought into contact with its use, the method of use being such as was intended or contemplated or was at least reasonably to be expected as a normal and proper use.

This judgment appears to extend very significantly the previously held view of common law liability and introduces the concept of a strict liability for the safety of a product. Apparently, the British courts are now prepared to hold not only that a manufacturer must fully satisfy himself that a product will not constitute a hazard to his own employees in the production process, but also that a product can be safely used by the purchaser. The implication of this responsibility is that the manufacturer must have knowledge of and give adequate consideration to those processes in which his product may subsequently be used. In setting out the duty of a manufacturer in respect to products that might constitute a health hazard, the appeal court stated that "if a manufacturer discovers that his product is unsafe or if he has reason to believe that it might be unsafe, his duty may be to cease forthwith to manufacture or supply the product in its unsafe form." In this context, a satisfactory definition of what is to be regarded as an unsafe product becomes all-important. The trial judge Mr. Justice O'Connor in the High Court judgment said:

> The duty of a manufacturer of chemical products can be simply stated. It is to take reasonable care that the product is safe in use. . . . If a manufacturer chooses to use a chemical which he knows to be a dangerous carcinogen in the manufacture of a product and knows or ought to know that the product contains a proportion of the carcinogen, and if he chooses to market the product without giving warning of the presence of the carcinogenic material, then I hold that the law imposes a very high duty indeed upon him to satisfy himself that the product will not prove dangerous when used for the purpose for which it is supplied. The discharge of the duty requires that he should inform himself of the circumstances in which the product will be used, the quantities in which it will be used and the possibilities of exposure to which men may be subjected. If in the state of knowledge at the time he cannot say positively that the proportion of carcinogen present in the product will be harmless, then I hold that he cannot market it without giving adequate warning of the presence of the carcinogenic material.

Little comfort is found in these words for either the manufacturer or the user of chemical compounds that may contain trace quantities of suspect carcinogens. Although the existence of an exposure threshold below which contact with chemical carcinogens may be regarded as safe can be reasonably postulated, in practice the threshold itself can rarely be determined. In the particular case of the aromatic amines, such quantification has not even been attempted. Furthermore, although it is indicated that complete withdrawal or abandonment of a potentially carcinogenic product may not necessarily be required and that an adequate warning of its dangerous properties may suffice, the judge had no doubt about the course that should have been adopted in this case. In a later passage from the judgment he states, "the alternative of giving an appropriate warning of its possible carcinogenicity is really an academic consideration because it is common ground that any such warning would have made it unsaleable."

We are left therefore with the conclusion that the recognized presence of any quantity of a suspect carcinogen in a manufacturer's product may force its withdrawal from the market. No doubt exceptions to this generalization will be encountered, e.g., asbestos products, but the threatened application of strict legal liability will certainly influence future manufacturing and marketing policies.

Legislation

The influence that government action by legislation may have on the manufacture and use of carcinogenic or suspect carcinogenic materials must be considered. Experience suggests that effective action in this field is likely to be impeded as much by the complexity of the problem as by ignorance of its full extent. Some precedent for legislative intervention exists. This precedent allied with increasing expression of popular concern led in 1967 in Britain to the passage of the Carcinogenic Substances Regulations (*88*) and in January 1974 in the United States to the publication by the Occupational Safety and Health Administration (OSHA) of the Department of Labor of new Occupational Health and Safety Standards relating to the manufacture and use of certain carcinogens (*89*).

The effect of the British regulations together with the Prohibition of Importation order (*82*), which came into operation on the same date, has been to prohibit the importation, manufacture, or use of the major carcinogens in the aromatic amine series (e.g., 2-naphthylamine, benzidine, and 4-biphenylamine) and to impose strict controls on other compounds in the same series such as 1-naphthylamine, *o*-toluidine, dianisidine, 3,3′-dichlorobenzidine, auramine, and magenta. Some provision for exemption from the regulations exists in special circumstances, and the regulations as stated do not apply in any case where the compound is present as a by-product of a chemical reaction in any other substance in a total concentration not exceeding 1%. This last proviso has caused some confusion about the correct interpretation of the regulations. It was also a matter of some concern to the High Court, where it was suggested that the use of the antioxidant Nonox S would still be lawful because the 2-naphthylamine impurity would only be present in that compound as a by-product of a chemical reaction and would in any case be within the permitted 1%. This submission was not accepted by the judge who held that the 2-naphthylamine impurity was present not as a by-product but as an unreacted material which was part of the original constituents. He declined also to infer that the regulations implied that % 2-naphthylamine was harmless. On the contrary he stated that "if any conclusion is to be drawn from the regulation it is the exact opposite."

In spite of such difficulties in construction and interpretation, the Carcinogenic Substances Regulations have probably made an important contribution to the final elimination from the industrial scene in Britain of bladder cancer attributable to aromatic amine exposure.

In the United States, the more recently promulgated permanent OSHA standards relate to 14 listed compounds that are either already accepted as being or are currently under suspicion of being important industrial carcinogens. The standard contains control measures and designated work practices designed to protect employees from industrial exposure to these compounds. Considerable variation is present in the degree of carcinogenic potential that is currently attributed to these listed carcinogens. At one end of the scale are the potent and established carcinogens such as 2-naphthylamine and 4-biphenylamine, whereas at the other end are such compounds as 4,4′-methylenebis(2-chloroaniline) and ethyleneimine. The case for including all these compounds together in the same listing rests on acceptance of the view that the same degree of protection should be given to workers exposed to substances found only to be carcinogenic in experimental animals and that a safe level of exposure for any of the 14 listed compounds cannot be established in the present state of knowledge. This view of the situation would appear to correspond with that expressed in the British High Court. In one important respect, however, the U.S. standard goes further than the British regulation insofar as it requires employers to provide for the indoctrination and training of their employees in the nature of carcinogenic hazards that may exist in the establishment. Information relating to the training and education that may be required is specified in the standards listed for each chemical compound.

Legislation that is intended to protect workers who may be in a risk situation as a result of potential exposure at work to carcinogenic chemicals is not confined only to the United States and the United Kingdom. Similar steps are being or have already been taken in many other countries. For example, draft legislation is currently in preparation within the European Economic Community for more stringent regulatory control of known or suspected occupational hazards.

Finally, it is hoped that some profit may be gained from our past experience of dealing with a major chemical cancer hazard. We have learned much about the mechanisms of chemical carcinogenesis and the techniques of epidemiological investigation. This knowledge, properly applied, should enable us to anticipate, or at least detect in its early stages, any similar threat that may emerge in the future (*90*). It cannot be too often emphasized that the role of the occupational physician is primarily one of prophylaxis.

Literature Cited

1. Cook, J. W.; Hieger, I.; Kennaway, E. L.; Mayneord, W. V. *Proc. R. Soc. London, Ser. B* **1932**, *111*, 455.
2. Case, R. A. M.; Hosker, M. E.; McDonald, D. B.; Pearson, J. T. *Br. J. Ind. Med.* **1954**, *11*, 75.
3. Hueper, W. C.; Wiley, F. H.; Wolfe, H. D. *J. Ind. Hyg.* **1938**, *20*, 46.
4. Bonser, G. M. *J. Pathol. Bacteriol.* **1943**, *55*, 1.
5. Bonser, G. M.; Clayson, D. B.; Jull, J. W.; Pyrah, L. N. *Br. J. Cancer* **1952**, *6*, 412.
6. Scott, T. S. "Carcinogenic and Chronic Toxic Hazards of Aromatic Amines"; Elsevier: Amsterdam, 1962.
7. Bonser, G. M.; Clayson, D. B.; Jull, J. W. *Br. Med. Bull.* **1958**, *14*, 147.
8. Radomski, J. L.; Deichmann, W. B.; Allman, N. H.; Radomski, T. *Cancer Res* **1980**, *40*, 3537.
9. Purchase, I. F. H.; Kalinowski, A. E.; Ishmael, J.; Wilson, J.; Gore, C. W.; Chart, I. S. *Br. J. Cancer* **1981**, *44*, 892.
10. Kadlubar, F. F.; Anson, J. F.; Dooley, K. L.; Beland, F. A. *Carcinogenesis* **1981**, *2* 467–70.
11. Richter, C. P. *JAMA, J. Am. Med. Assoc.* **1945**, *129*, 927–31.
12. Davies, J. M.; Thomas, H. F.; Manson, D. *Br. Med. J.* **1982**, *285*, 927–31.
13. Hueper, W. C. In "Occupational Tumors and Allied Diseases"; Thomas: Springfield, IL, 1942.
14. Spitz, S.; Maguigan, W. H.; Dobriner, K. *Cancer* **1950**, *3*, 789.
15. "Carcinogenesis Technical Report," National Cancer Institute, 78–1358, 1978.

16. "Status of the Current Testing of Dyes," National Toxic Program BAB Dye Initiative, **1982**, June.
17. Bueniger, Mark "Technical Report: The Carcinogenicity and Metabolism of Azo Dyes, Especially those derived from Benzidine," DHHS (NIOSH), 80–119, 1980, July.
18. Meal, P. F.; Cocker, J.; Wilson, H. K.; Gilmour, J. M. *Br. J. Ind. Med.* **1981**, *38*, 191.
19. Yoshida, O.; Myakoga, M. "Etiology of Bladder Cancer: Metabolic Aspects, Analytical and Experimental Epidemiology of Cancer"; Baltimore Univ.: Baltimore, 1973; pp. 31–39.
20. Melick, W. F.; Escue, H. M.; Naryka, J. J.; Mezera, R. A.; Wheeler, E. P. *J. Urol.* **1955**, *74*, 760.
21. Melick, W. F.; Naryka, J. J.; Kelly, R. E. *J. Urol.* **1971**, *106*, 220.
22. Walpole, A. L.; Williams, M. H. C.; Roberts, D. C. *Br. J. Ind. Med.* **1952**, *9*, 255.
23. Schoental, R. *Nature (London)* **1968**, *219*, 1162–3; *Isr. J. Med. Sci.* **1968**, *4*, 1146–58.
24. Munn, A. In "Bladder Cancer"; Deichman, W.; Lampe, K. F., Eds.; Birmingham, Alabama: Aesculapius, 1967; p. 187.
25. Deichmann, W. B.; MacDonald, W. E.; Copan, F.; Woods, F.; Blum, E. *Toxicol.* **1978**, *11*, 185–8.
26. Griswold, D., Jr.; Casey, A. E.; Weisburger, E. K.; Weisburger, J. H. *Cancer Res.* **1968**, *28*, 924–33.
27. Steinhoff, D.; Grundmann, E. *Naturwissenschaften* **1970**, *57*, 247–8.
28. "NTP Draft Technical Report," 1981, NTP-81-143, 82, 2504.
29. Fukushima, S.; Hirose, M.; Hagiwara, A.; Hasegawa, R; Ito, N. *Carcinogenesis* **1981**, *2*, 1033–37.
30. Kopelman, H.; Robertson, M. H.; Saunders, P. G.; Ash, I. *Br. Med. J. 1966, 1*, 514.
31. Kopelman, H.; Scheuer, P. J.; Williams, R. *Q. J. Med.* **1966**, *35*, 553.
32. ACGIH Documentation of TLV's update, 1977.
33. ICI Organics Division, unpublished data.
34. Stula, E. F.; Sherman, H.; Zapp, J. A. *Toxicol. Appl. Pharmacol.* **1971**, *19*, 380.
35. Stula, E. F.; Barnes, J. R.; Sherman, H.; Reinhardt, C. F.; Zapp, J. A., Jr. *J. Environ. Pathol. Toxicol.* **1978**, *1*, 475.
36. Gerarde, H. W.; Gerarde, D. F. *J. Occup. Med.* **1974**, *16*, 332.
37. Gadian, T. *Chem. Ind. (London)* **1975**, *4*, 821.
38. McIntyre, I. *J. Occup, Med.* **1975**, *17*, 23.
39. Stula, E. F.; Sherman, H.; Zapp, J. A. In "Experimental Neoplasia in ChR-CD Rats with the Oral Administration of 3,3'-Dichlorobenzidine, 4,4'-Methylene-bis (2-chloroaniline), and 4,4'-Methylenebis (2-methylaniline)," Soc. Toxicol. 10th Annu. Meet., Washington, D.C., 1971; p. 39.
40. Steinhoff, D.; Grundmann, E. *Naturwissenschaften* **1971**, *58*, 578.
41. Russfield, A. B.; Homburger, F.; Boger, E.; Van Dongen, C. G.; Weisburger, E. K.; Weisburger, J. H. *Toxicol. Appl. Pharmacol.* **1975**, *31*, 47.
42. Stula, E. F.; Barner, J. R.; Sherman, H.; Reimhardt, C. F.; Zapp, J. A., Jr. *J. Environ. Pathol. Toxicol.* **1977**, *1*, 31.
43. Hosein, H. R.; Van Roosonalen, P. B. *Am. Ind. Hyg. Assoc. J.* **1978**, *39*, 496–502.
44. "Evaluation of the Carcinogenic Risk of Chemicals to Man"; IARC Monograph, 1978, Vol. 16, 325.
45. Gehrmann, G. H.; Foulger, J. H.; Fleming, A. J. Proceedings of the 9th International Congress of Industrial Medicine, 1948, p. 472.
46. Kummer, R.; Tordoi, W. F. *Tijdschr. Geneeskd.* **1975**, *53*, 415–9.
47. Batten, P. L.; Hathway, D. E. *Br. J. Cancer* **1977**, *35*, 342–6.
48. Green, U.; Holste, J.; Spikermann, A. R. J. *J. Cancer Res. Clin. Oncol.* **1979**, *95*, 51–55.

49. Veys, C. A., M.D. Thesis, Book 1, Univ. of Liverpool, 1973.
50. Fox, A. J.; Lindars, D. C.; Owe, R. *Br. J. Ind. Med.* **1974**, *31*, 140–51.
51. Parkes, H. G.; Veys, C. A.; Waterhouse, J. A. H.; Peters, A. *Br. J. Ind. Med.* **1982**, *39*, 209–20.
52. "Evaluation of the Carcinogenic Risk of Chemicals to Man"; IARC Monograph, 1982, Vol. 28.
53. IARC Monograph, "Evaluation of the Carcinogenic Risk of Chemicals to Man"; 1978, Vol. 16, 349.
54. "Bioassay of o-Toluidine Hydrochloride," National Cancer Institute, 1979, (NIH) 79–1709.
55. Cheever, K. L.; Richards, D. G.; Plotnick, H. B. *Toxicol. Appl. Pharmacol.* **1980**, *56*, 361.
56. Young, J. L.; Percy, C. L.; Asire, A. J. "Surveillance Epidemiology and End Results: Incidence and Mortality Data 73–77" National Cancer Institute Monograph 57, 1981, 81–2330.
57. Mortality Statistics, 1979: Cause, Series DH2, No. 6, Table 3, pp. 84–85, HMSO, 1980.
58. Registrar General's Statistical Review for England and Wales, Part 1 for 1960 and 1970, Table 8, HMSO *and* Mortality Statistics: Cause for Years 1974 and 1978, Series DH2, Nos. 1 and 5, HMSO.
59a. Howe, G. R.; Burch, J. D.; Miller, A. B.; Cook, G. M.; Esteve, J.; Morrison, B. et al. *JNCI, J. Natl. Cancer Inst.* **1980**, *64*, 701.
59b. Price, J.M.; Bladder Cancer Canadian Cancer Conference. **1966**, 6, 244.
60. Doll, Richard; Peto, Richard In "The Causes of Cancer: Quantitative Estimates of Avoidable Risks of Cancer in the United States Today; Oxford Univ.: Oxford, 1981.
61. Searle, C. E.; Teale, J. *Lancet* **1982**, *I*, 564.
62. Scott, T. S.; Williams, M. H. C. *Br. J. Ind. Med*, **1957**, *14*, 150.
63. Rehn, L. *Arch. Klin. Chir.* **1895**, *50*, 588.
64. Leichtenstern, O. *Dtsch. Med. Wochenschr.* **1898**, *24*, 709.
65. Rehn, L. *Verh. Dtsch. Ges. Chir.* **1906**, *35*, 313.
66. Leuenberger, S. C. *Bruns Beitr. Klin. Chir*, **1912**, *80*, 208.
67. Studies and Reports, Series F, International Labour Office, 1921, No. 1, p. 6.
68. Wignall, T. H. *Br. Med. J.* **1929**, *2*, 258.
69. Goldblatt, M. W. *Br. Med. Bull.* **1947**, *4*, 405.
70. Goldblatt, M. W. *Br. J. Ind. Med.* **1949**, *6*, 65.
71. Gehrmann, G. H. *J. Urol.* **1934**, *31*, 126.
72. Gehrmann, G. H.; Foulger, J. H.; Fleming, A. J. *Proc. Int. Congr. Ind. Med., 9th* **1948**, 472.
73. di Maio, G. *Proc. Int. Congr. Ind. Med., 9th* **1948**, 476.
74. Barsotti, M.; Vigliani, E. C. *Med. Lav.* **1949**, *40*, 129.
75. Billiard-Duchesne, J. F. *Proc. Int. Congr. Ind. Med., 9th* **1948**, 507.
76. Williams, M. H. C. In "Cancer", Raven, R. W., Ed.; Butterworths: London, 1958, Vol. 3, p. 377.
77. Case, R. A. M. *Br. J. Prev. Soc. Med.* **1953**, *7*, 14.
78. Anthony, H. M.; Thomas, G. M. *JNCI, J. Natl. Cancer Inst.* **1970**, *45*, 879.
79. Cole, P. T.; Hoover, R.; Friedell, G. H. *Cancer* **1972**, *29*, 1250.
80. National Insurance (Industrial Injuries) Act, Her Majesty's Stationery Office, London, 1946.
81. Carcinogenic Substances (Prohibition of Importation) Order, Statutory Instrument No. 1675, Her Majesty's Stationery Office, London, 1967.
82. Kumar, S.; Taylor, G.; Wilson, P., Hurst, W. *Br. Med. J.* **1980**, *280*, 512–13.

83. Kumar, S.; Taylor, G.; Huston, W.; Wilson, P.; Costello, C. B. *Br. J. Ind. Med.* **1981**, *38*, 167.
84. Kumar, S.; Wilson, P. B.; Costello, C. B. *Oncology* **1982**, *39*, 65.
85. Kumar, S.; Wilson, P.; Brenchley, P.; Taylor, G.; Bjorklund, B.; Eklund, G. *Int. J. Cancer* **1978**, *22*, 542.
86. Lower, G. M., Jr.; Nilsson, T.; Nelson, C. R.; Wolf, H.; Gamsky, T. E.; Bryon, G. T. *Environ. Health Persp.* **1979**, *29*, 71–79.
87. "Cassidy v Imperial Chemical Industries Ltd., Wright v Same. Before Lord Justice Sachs, Lord Justice Megaw, and Lord Justice Lawton," *The Times EHP*, London, Law Report, November 1, 1982.
88. Carcinogenic Substances Regulations, Statutory Instrument No. 879. Her Majesty's Stationery Office, London, 1967.
89. "Occupational Safety and Health Standards," U.S. Government Dept. of Labor, U.S. Federal Register, 1974, 39, 20.
90. Parkes, H. G. *Practitioner* **1975**, *214*, 80.

Chemical Carcinogens as Laboratory Hazards

C. E. SEARLE

University of Birmingham, Department of Cancer Studies, The Medical School, Birmingham B15 2TJ, England

THE CONTINUALLY INCREASING ATTENTION paid in recent years to environmental aspects of chemical carcinogens has tended to focus on chemical risks encountered on a large scale in industry, as environmental pollutants, or as dietary additives and contaminants. Carcinogenic hazards may also be encountered, however, in smaller-scale laboratory work, where workers are also becoming subject to controls to reduce such risks.

The potent carcinogens of the polycyclic aromatic hydrocarbon type were the first chemical carcinogens identified just over 50 years ago. Their usage in purified form has for all practical purposes been confined to cancer research laboratories, where they have been widely used with considerably less regard to safety than is now considered essential. Not very long ago, large numbers of mice were repeatedly skin-painted with benzo[*a*]pyrene or related substances at concentrations as high as 0.5% in an oil or solvent, and the result was heavy contamination of cages, bedding, walls, and personnel. Perhaps such practices have not yet entirely died out.

Outside cancer research, little thought was given to hazards from carcinogenic chemicals in laboratories until soon after World War II. Then Case's extensive epidemiological studies of the causes of bladder cancer in British factory workers clearly incriminated several aromatic amines, particularly 2-naphthylamine and benzidine, as human carcinogens. This work and its far-reaching implications were described by Case in his Michael Williams Lecture (*1*). Unlike the carcinogenic aromatic hydrocarbons, the carcinogenic aromatic amines were common chemicals, widely used for many laboratory purposes as well as in chemical manufacture. The industrial findings thus showed that laboratory workers in various fields could also be subjected to some degree of carcinogenic hazard. Moreover, many more chemicals used in laboratories have since been recognized as carcinogens, including a wide range of alkylating agents, *N*-nitroso compounds, and some solvents.

0065-7719/84/0182-0303$06.25/1

Because laboratory work involves use of chemicals on a generally small scale when compared with the manufacturing industry, it seems reasonable that any carcinogenic hazards are correspondingly less. This assumption cannot be taken for granted, however, and one can envisage the possibility of workers being in fact at greater risk in a poorly run laboratory than in a factory maintaining a high standard of industrial hygiene.

At present there is relatively little epidemiological evidence on which to base conclusions about actual carcinogenic hazards in the laboratory. Clinical impression led Case to the view that some urinary tract tumors in laboratory workers had resulted from their handling carcinogenic aromatic amines (*2*). Williams suggested that nurses might be at risk through their use of benzidine in testing for occult blood in urine and feces (*3*). This suggestion received some support from the study of occupations of 1030 patients with papilloma and carcinoma of the bladder in the Leeds area of England during 1959–67 carried out by Anthony and Thomas (*4*). This study indicated an increased risk of bladder cancer in some medical workers, particularly in nurses and laboratory technicians, although the number of cases was small.

Laboratory uses of carcinogens have, of course, not been confined to clinical chemistry, and moreover the range of known carcinogens of various chemical classes is continually expanding. Therefore suspicions that some chemists might develop cancer as a result of their work are warranted, and several epidemiological studies have now been carried out to investigate this possibility. It has been largely impossible, however, for such studies to take any account of the actual work experience of the chemists, or of other important relevant factors such as their smoking and dietary habits.

Epidemiological Studies of Chemists

United States. The first serious attempt to study the mortality of chemists was made by Li et al. (*5*), who reported on the causes of death of 3637 members of the American Chemical Society (ACS) who died between 1948 and 1967. Most members were males who were studied in two groups. The 2152 dying between the ages of 20 and 64 were compared with a control group of 9957 U.S. professional men who died between the same ages during 1950 only. The 1370 members who died over the age of 64 were compared with U.S. males who died over 64 during 1959. Only 112 female ACS members were in the study, and these women were compared with white females who died in 1959.

Both groups of male chemists showed a significantly increased mortality from cancer. The difference was most marked in the younger age range (Table I) where there were 444 observed cancer deaths compared with the expected number of 354. The individual cancers that showed significant increases were malignant tumors of the lymphoid system (lymphomas) and cancer of the pancreas, but not cancer of the bladder as would previously have been thought the most probable. The commonest cause of death, diseases of the circulatory system, occurred with almost identical frequency in the chemists and their controls, but deaths from respiratory diseases and cirrhosis of the liver were significantly reduced in chemists. For the female chemists, breast cancer mortality was doubled, a result

Table I

Causes of Death of Male Members of the American Chemical Society Between the Ages of 20 and 64 from 1948 to 1967

Cause	*Observed*	*Expected*[a]
All causes	2152	2152
All cancers	444	354[b]
Stomach	20	24
Intestine, rectum	68	59
Liver, biliary	13	12
Pancreas	36	22[c]
Respiratory system	74	64
Urinary system	24	21
Bladder, etc.	10	10
Lymphoma and leukemia	94	59[b]
Lymphosarcoma, etc.	61	34[b]
Leukemia	33	25
Others	109	84
Circulatory diseases	1112	1105
Respiratory diseases	30	50[c]
Diabetes	21	26
Cirrhosis of liver	17	41[b]
Accidents	155	165
Suicide	97	83
All other causes	276	328

[a]On basis of comparison with 9957 other professional males who died aged 20–64 in 1950.
[b]$P < 0.001$
[c]$P < 0.01$
SOURCE: Based on Ref. 5.

more likely derived from the relatively high proportion of unmarried women and higher socioeconomic class than from chemical exposure.

Despite the disparities in the time span studied of the chemists' and the control groups' deaths, and other unavoidable weaknesses of the study, Li et al. considered it unlikely that the increased mortalities from certain cancers seen in both age groups were by chance. New studies of the mortality of male and female ACS members are now in progress (personal communication from Dr. J. Walrath, National Cancer Institute).

A recent retrospective study has compared the causes of death of chemists employed by the Du Pont Company (U.S.) with those of salaried nonchemists in the same company and with the general U.S. population (*6*). Cancer incidence rates in those aged 20–64 were also compared with the same groups.

Of the 3686 men and 75 women employed as chemists or in similar work in 1959, 198 died during 1964–77. Based on the company's nonchemists, the expected deaths would have totalled 241. There were markedly fewer deaths than expected from arteriosclerotic disease and from lung cancer, and the total cancer deaths were 43 (expected 62.4).

In this study, no evidence was seen of an increased incidence of lymphoma in chemists, although the numbers were small. Leukemia and lymphoma deaths together totalled nine, and the expected numbers were 7.5 or 9.1 depending on the control population chosen.

Sweden. In 1976 Olin (*7*) published the first of a number of reports describing mortality studies of male Swedish chemists. Those studied were graduates of the Royal College of Technology in Stockholm, and though the numbers were very much smaller than in the ACS study, the follow-up was almost complete. During the years 1930–50, 857 men graduated, of whom 67 died before the end of 1974. The controls were the general male population of Sweden.

Although comparisons between the two very different studies are difficult to make and the number of persons studied was small, Olin also observed an increased liability of chemists to die from tumors of the lymphoid system: six from lymphoma and leukemia (1.7 expected) and three from Hodgkin's disease (0.3 expected).

In an extension of this work by Olin and Ahlbom (*8*), the mortality of chemists graduating from 1930 to 1959 who had died by the end of 1977 was again compared with that of the general male population of Sweden, but a smaller number of graduates in architecture was now also included in the study. The architects form a very valuable group for comparison, having had similar socioeconomic and educational backgrounds, but without comparable exposure to chemicals at work.

Both professional groups suffered fewer total deaths than expected by comparison with Swedish males, the difference being more marked in the architects: 83 chemists (103.8 expected) and 59 architects (87.8 expected). The chemists had, however, a few more cancer deaths than expected (32; expected, 24.2; $P < 0.05$) while architects had significantly fewer (11; expected, 20.5; $P < 0.01$). The numbers of deaths observed and expected among the chemists are listed in Table II.

In addition to the increase in lymphoma deaths noted in 1976, Olin and Ahlbom (*8*) now reported that deaths from brain tumors were also significantly increased in chemists (Table II) in comparison with the general population, although not in comparison with the architects. Again, small numbers were involved in forming this conclusion compared, for example, with the chemists' markedly lower rate for deaths from circulatory diseases. There is now some controversy in the United States over the possibility that brain tumors may sometimes result from industrial exposure to chemicals.

In their latest report (*9*) Olin and Ahlbom extended their comparison to Swedish graduate mining engineers/metallurgists, whose overall cancer death rate did not differ from that expected. They also suggested a possible association between the brain tumors (gliomas) in chemists and the former use of the rat neural carcinogen *N*-methyl-*N*-nitrosourea in organic chemistry courses.

Table II

Causes of Death of Swedish Chemists Who Graduated Between 1930 and 1959

Cause	*Observed*	*Expected*[a]
All causes	83	103.8[b]
All cancers	32	24.2
Digestive system	8	9.2
Pancreas	2	1.6
Respiratory system	3	4.0
Prostate	3	1.5
Urinary system	3	1.8
Brain	5	1.2[c]
Lymphoma and leukemia	7	3.2[b]
Hodgkin's disease	3	0.7[b]
Circulatory system	22	40.4[c]
Accidents and suicide	15	21.9
All other causes	14	17.3

NOTE: Data compiled through the end of 1977.

[a]On basis of comparison with general male population of Sweden.

[b]$P < 0.5$

[c]$P < 0.01$.

SOURCE: Based on Reference 8.

United Kingdom. The first steps toward a study of the mortality of chemists in the United Kingdom were taken in 1976. The study was confined to those who held the qualification of Fellow or Member of the Royal Institute of Chemistry, but could then only cover deaths from 1965 to 1975 because records of those who died before 1965 had been destroyed.

To date, only a brief report of some preliminary findings has been published (*10*). During an 11-year period, 1332 deaths occurred, of which 291 (21.8%) were from cancer. There were 19 deaths from lymphoma, an unduly high proportion (6.5%) of all cancer deaths. National experience indicates an expected number of 8.7 ($P < 0.05$). This result appeared to confirm the raised lymphoma risk observed in the earlier studies, and there were suspicions of an undue proportion of cancer deaths occurring under 50 years of age.

In 1980 the Institute amalgamated with the Chemical Society to form the Royal Society of Chemistry, with possibilities of greatly extending the range of epidemiological studies, both retrospective and prospective, and of correlating causes of diseases with chemical exposure. As part of a projected U.K. prospective study, British chemists completed detailed questionnaires on personal habits (such as smoking and alcohol, tea, and coffee consumption), illnesses, and chemicals to which they have had significant exposure. The answers showed exposures decreasing with time for chemicals such as benzidine, mustard gas, and DDT, and increasing for others including 1,4-dioxane, acrylonitrile, and hexamethylphosphoramide. A disturbing aspect of replies in the first report (*11*) was the high level of adverse health effects attributed by chemists themselves to the chemicals they had encountered at work.

Future studies should have comparable professional control groups without chemical exposure, as in the most recent Swedish report (*9*) and should also pay particular attention to age at death. Especially valuable, though more difficult than retrospective mortality studies, would be prospective studies of the actual incidence of cancers and other diseases. Because leukemias and lymphomas are now frequently treated more successfully than many other cancers, studies based only on mortality data may increasingly underestimate the proportions of these diseases actually occurring.

Studies of Some Other Chemically Exposed Populations

In some other populations, increased lymphoma incidence has been associated with chemical exposure, or such a relationship has at least been suspected. Because of their possible relevance to the studies of chemists, these will also be described briefly.

Hospital Practice. Large numbers of persons working in operating room environments have had heavy and prolonged exposure to a variety of volatile anesthetics. Many publications have linked such exposures with adverse effects on health, particularly in respect to increased incidence of miscarriages and congenital abnormalities in children born to women who have had occupational exposure to anesthetics during pregnancy.

Certain earlier studies suggested a possible increased incidence of cancers attributable to volatile anesthetics. Bruce et al. (*12*) reported that over a 20-year period, deaths among members of the American Society of Anesthesiologists had shown an abnormally high proportion of lymphoid tumors, but the numbers studied were small. According to Corbett et al. (*13*), the cancer incidence in Michigan nurse–anesthetists had increased more than threefold, while Cohen et al. (*14*) also reported an increased cancer incidence in female operating room personnel. In contrast, a prospective study of anesthetists (*15*), in which the causes of 211 deaths were compared with those occurring in insurance policy holders, found no excess of cancer deaths. A later joint study by the American Society of Anesthetists and the American Cancer Society (*16*) also found no evidence of a different death rate for anesthesiologists.

In the United Kingdom, a 20-year prospective study of the causes of mortality of doctors in respect to their smoking habits permitted comparisons between the causes of death of doctors in different occupations. Doll and Peto (*17*) found that anesthetists had a lower overall death rate than expected among physicians, but they had more deaths from cancer of the pancreas (5; expected, 1.7). Bearing in mind the results of Li et al. (*5*) for chemists, this result might not, as the authors considered, have been only due to chance.

If there is indeed any carcinogenic hazard for operating room personnel, it also raises the serious possibility of risks for transplacental carcinogenesis when women are exposed to anesthetics during pregnancy. Two studies (*18,19*) have reported on cases of cancer in children born to operating room personnel, but once again the numbers are too small to assess their significance.

Analysis of long-term effects of anesthetics on humans is complicated by the great changes that have occurred in the volatile anesthetics used over the years; only nitrous oxide has remained in continuous use. Of the now discontinued anesthetics, some evidence suggests very weak carcinogenicity of chloroform and possibly trichloroethylene in animals (*20*). Of fluorinated agents, some anesthetics with vinyl groups, but apparently not others, give positive results in the Ames test for mutagenicity in the presence of metabolizing enzymes (*21*), and are hence under some suspicion of being carcinogenic. Halothane and nitrous oxide were found to be mutagenic for *Drosophila* (*21*) and a teratogenic action of nitrous oxide in rats has been reported (*22*).

The real effects, if any, of anesthetic exposure on cancer incidence of personnel and their children remain to be elucidated, but the recognition of their other harmful effects is stimulating the provision of much higher standards of ventilation in operating rooms. Corbett (*23*) reviewed the possible carcinogenic hazards of anesthetics.

A study of the causes of death of 310 hospital pathologists and technicians in Britain by Harrington and Shannon (*24*) showed a small but significant increase in non-Hodgkin's lymphoma (8; expected 3.3; $P < 0.01$), but no increase in Hodgkin's disease, leukemia, or other cancers. Fewer cases of bladder cancer occurred than were expected.

Chemicals to which such personnel are regularly exposed include various stains, ethanol, xylene, and formaldehyde. There is no reason to suspect ethanol or xylene of a direct carcinogenic action, but formaldehyde has long been known to be mutagenic and was therefore under some suspicion of being carcinogenic. In 1980, uncompleted inhalation tests of formaldehyde were reported to have induced carcinomas in the nasal passages of a high proportion of rats exposed to 15 ppm in air, a level that also caused severe tissue damage (*25*). Few tumors occurred in rats at 6 ppm, or in mice at 15 ppm. These results were of great concern to the chemical industry and for companies installing urea–formaldehyde foam insulation, and a warning was issued by the National Institute of Occupational Safety and Health (NIOSH) recommending that formaldehyde be handled in the workplace as a potential occupational carcinogen (*26*). The rat findings have been confirmed in another study carried out for the Chemical Industry Institute of Toxicology (*27*), and the subject has been reviewed by the International Agency for Research on Cancer (IARC) (*28*). The question of whether the rat experiments indicate that formaldehyde is a real carcinogenic hazard in the industrial, laboratory, or domestic situation remains controversial, but may be clarified by fuller epidemiological studies of exposed industrial and laboratory workers.

Exposure to Solvent Pollution. A small population in Little Elk Valley, Maryland, was exposed to very heavy pollution from an organic solvent recovery plant during 1961–71. Atmospheric solvent levels and causes of sickness and death in the inhabitants were reported by Capurro (*29,30*). About 30 solvents were identified in the air surrounding the plant and some, including benzene, were determined in the blood of patients.

Capurro reported that, in the most heavily exposed community of 117 person, there had been seven cancer deaths (expected, 1.23) over a 6-year period (*29*). Of these, three (expected, 0.04) had been from reticulum cell sarcoma or lymphosarcoma. In the larger valley population of about 1000, there had been 10 cases of lymphoma diagnosed during an 11-year period (expected, 0.09). The case histories included three deaths that may have been from pancreatic cancer (*30*).

Reduced Immunity and Cancer. Patients treated with immunosuppressive drugs to prevent rejection of organ transplants suffer a greatly enhanced risk of developing lymphoma. For example, in a recent report of a collaborative United Kingdom–Australasian study (*31*) of 3825 renal transplant patients, there was a 60-fold increase in non-Hodgkin's lymphoma. The incidence of skin carcinomas and mesenchymal tumors was also elevated, but there was no evidence for an increase in the common cancers.

The increased risk of lymphoma is unfortunately now a well-recognized hazard of such treatments, but at present it has to be accepted because the operations are undertaken to relieve life-threatening conditions. A remarkable feature of the cases that have been recorded in such patients is that lymphoma appears within an extremely short time from the start of treatment, sometimes within the first year. This period is much shorter than the induction period generally seen in chemically induced cancers in humans. Although the agents used (azathioprine, cyclophosphamide, and chlorambucil) have shown carcinogenic activity, the effect seems more understandable in terms of a depressed immune system being unable to resist progression of a previously latent cancer, possibly of viral origin. According to earlier views of immune surveillance by the body's natural defenses, as elaborated by Burnet (*32*), immune suppression would have been expected to permit progression of the whole spectrum of human tumors, but this does not in fact occur.

A number of inherited immunodeficiency disorders are also associated with increased risks of various malignancies. Subjects with the rare inherited condition of ataxia telangiectasia are abnormally sensitive to x-rays. They also have a raised incidence of cancers, of which a major proportion are lymphomas.

Chromosome Studies Following Chemical Exposure. Exposure to ionizing radiation and chemical mutagens can be detected through damage to chromosomes of blood lymphocytes, though such studies are laborious and not very sensitive. The newer but poorly understood procedure of counting sister chromatid exchanges (SCEs) in lymphocyte chromosomes was applied to studies of some factory and laboratory personnel in Sweden by Funes-Cravioto et al. (*33*). Mean numbers of SCEs per cell ranged from 6.3 to 9.9 in various groups of chemically exposed workers, compared with 4.8 in controls. No clear correlation with actual chemicals was found. Possible harmful effects on 14 children of mothers who worked during pregnancy were indicated by their mean SCE levels of 9.4 per cell, compared with only 2.4 in seven control children, providing further evidence of the special need to minimize chemical exposures of pregnant women.

Lambert and Lindblat (*34*) reported a study of SCE levels and chromosome abnormalities in lymphocytes of laboratory workers and of smokers. Chemical exposure and smoking caused comparable increases in SCE levels, but the effects were not simply additive. The authors thought it reasonable to suspect working conditions, such as solvent exposure, as being a cause of increases in SCE levels.

Carcinogenic Reagents in Clinical Chemistry. Despite the wide range of carcinogens now known, none have been of more concern as general laboratory hazards than benzidine and some other aromatic amines. In clinical chemistry laboratories, a number of important tests formerly relied on the use of benzidine, *o*-tolidine, and *o*-dianisidine as chromagens, but various other methods have now been devised to replace potentially hazardous procedures, or have been adopted in the course of normal development. In one of a series of papers on laboratory safety, George (*35*) recommended that the use of liquid reagents containing these carcinogens was no longer justified, and raised the question of the legal position of the head of a department where potential carcinogens had not been eliminated if a laboratory worker develops a bladder tumor.

However, hospital laboratories have special problems, not faced by other laboratories, in that with constantly increasing workloads, they have to carry out various analyses on patient specimens that may carry tuberculosis, infective or serum hepatitis, or other serious sources of infection. Precautions essential to protect personnel against such infections are so important as to overshadow the possible long-term hazards from carcinogenic reagents, which received no mention in one account of precautions necessary in hospital biochemistry laboratories (*36*).

Fecal Occult Blood. The detection of gastrointestinal bleeding is of major importance to both clinician and patient. The order of sensitivity of the chromagens used to detect occult blood has been *o*-tolidine > benzidine > phenolphthalein > guaiac. As benzidine and *o*-tolidine are carcinogenic, the choice now lies between phenolphthalein, guaiac, or a method such as Deadman and Timms' modification of the blood glucose method using 2,6-dichlorophenolindophenol (*37*).

3,3′,5,5′-Tetramethylbenzidine, recommended as a sensitive alternative to benzidine for the detection of blood, gave no tumors when injected into rats in doses greater than those in which benzidine or *o*-tolidine gave a high yield of neoplasms (*38*), and was also inactive in the Ames bacterial mutagenicity test (*39*).

Steinberg (*40*) drew attention to the hazards to criminal justice personnel from the continuing use of benzidine for blood detection and fingerprinting. The carcinogen was said to be employed in preference to other reagents and without adequate safety precautions.

Glucose and Other Determinations. An extensive bibliography has grown up around blood glucose determinations (*41*). Newer procedures use 2,2′-diazobis(3-ethylbenzothiazolidine-6-sulfonic acid) as the chromagen or the hexokinase method, but unfortunately the carcinogenic *o*-tolidine has many advantages and gives values closely approximating "true glucose."

The method of Ratcliff and Hardwicke (*42*) for estimation of haptoglobins on Sephadex G100 columns gives simple, reproducible results. It correlates well with the comparison method and obviates the use of benzidine or *o*-tolidine as chromagen. Immunological methods for haptoglobin estimation are also available.

In the preparation of protein aggregates, bis-diazotized dapsone (4,4′-diaminodiphenyl sulfone) was used satisfactorily to crosslink γ-globulin in place of bis-diazotized benzidine (*43*). Subsequently dapsone, an important drug for treating leprosy and some other diseases, was found to be carcinogenic in the male rat only (*44*). Unlike the corresponding sulfide and sulfoxide, dapsone was not mutagenic in the Ames test.

Myeloperoxidase Determination. For determining leukocyte myeloperoxidase in blood or bone marrow, benzidine was replaced by 3,3′-diaminobenzidine and later, 2,7-fluorenediamine. This chemical is, however, also carcinogenic, though diaminobenzidine appears not to be, as discussed later. Laycock et al. (*45*) described a method using catechol with *p*-phenylenediamine, which has given negative results in various carcinogenicity tests, but which is unfortunately a potent sensitizing agent.

Antineoplastic Drugs. However successfully carcinogens are eliminated from hospital and other laboratories, certain potently carcinogenic drugs used in treating cancer patients will continue to be handled for the foreseeable future by pharmacists, doctors, and nurses. Following reports of mutagenic activity in the urine of nurses administering cytotoxic drugs (albeit at much lower levels than in the urine of treated patients), guidelines for handling such drugs have been recommended (*46,47*).

Other Analytical Uses of Carcinogenic Amines

The use of benzidine and related compounds in analysis has been widespread because of the ease of their oxidation to colored quinonoid products. Feigl and Anger (*48*) stated that benzidine was used in some 60 spot-test procedures. Following a warning by the Society for Analytical Chemistry against the use of benzidine, these authors reported the replacement of benzidine by copper ethylacetoacetate and tetra base, bis(4-dimethylaminophenyl)methane, as spot-tests for cyanide and cyanogen (*48*). Other methods for cyanide determination use pyridine in conjunction with *p*-phenylenediamine (*49*) or with 3-methyl-1-phenyl-5-pyrazolone (*50*).

Important analyses that depended on the use of benzidine and *o*-tolidine included the analysis of chlorine in water at water supply undertakings and swimming pools. The *N,N*-diethyl-*p*-phenylenediamine (DPD) methods of Palin (*51*) are now well established for chlorine determination, and also for the determination of chlorite, bromine, iodine, and ozone in water. Similarly, 1-naphthylamine has been replaced by Cleve's acid (8-aminonaphthalene-2-sulfonic acid) in the determination of nitrites in water (*52*). As with dapsone mentioned earlier, these alternatives are undoubtedly safer than the reagents they replace, even though they cannot confidently be stated to be entirely risk-free.

Nevertheless, *o*-tolidine reagent has remained available, and is supplied as a 0.1% solution ready for use. With suitable precautions, the hazards of using such solutions are probably extremely small, but it would seem responsible to use noncarcinogenic alternatives wherever satisfactory ones exist. It is perhaps strange that the relatively small-scale laboratory use of such materials has been of such concern while these amines have continued in large-scale industrial use as sources of valuable azo dyes. Apparently these dyes themselves may be hazardous through enzymic reduction in the body to yield the parent amines, and it has consequently been recommended that their production in the United States should now cease (*53*).

Possible Carcinogenicity of Some Other Reagents

Once attention has been drawn to possible risks from known carcinogenic chemicals, it is not surprising that anxieties should also arise about possibilities of hazards from many other chemicals encountered in the laboratory. Doubts have been raised, for example, over the safety of using magenta, diphenylamine, diaminobenzidine, ninhydrin, and formaldehyde in hospital, educational, and other laboratories.

The manufacture of magenta was found early on to carry a carcinogenic hazard to workmen, leading to its control by legislation (*54*), but the carcinogenicity was almost certainly due to amines used in its manufacture or present as contaminants. There is still no evidence that magenta itself is carcinogenic (*55*). The chief risk from diphenylamine appears to be from possible contamination with the highly carcinogenic 4-biphenylamine. Diaminobenzidine (3,3′,4,4′-tetraaminobiphenyl), widely used in histology laboratories, has been tested twice for carcinogenicity. One experiment was inadequate, and the second suggested that it is, at the most, a very weak carcinogen (*56*).

No carcinogenicity tests on ninhydrin have been carried out, but it has toxic and irritant properties and should be handled with caution, particularly avoiding inhalation if it is used as a chromatographic spray reagent. Ninhydrin has recently been subjected to short-term tests, but proved negative in the Ames test using *Salmonella typhimurium*, strain TA 100 (*57*). The evidence that high levels of formaldehyde are carcinogenic for the rat nasal epithelium has already been cited.

The range of chemicals to which laboratory workers may be exposed is extremely large, and of these very many are well-known to have considerable toxicity. The studies of anesthetists already discussed have shown how heavy exposure even to chemicals generally regarded as innocuous may nevertheless have harmful effects on health. Possibly, the increases in lymphomas reported in chemists could similarly be caused not by identifiable carcinogens, but could be an indirect consequence of adverse effects (on, for example, the immune system) of prolonged exposure to high levels of some of the many widely used volatile solvents. Threshold limit values of some solvents of low toxicity are currently very high, and breathing air containing such concentrations would thus lead to very substantial intakes. Even in light work, some 5 m^3 of air is inhaled during a working day, which could result in intakes of up to 6 g for diethyl ether and 12 g for acetone, or more during heavier work. Assuming that such intakes are entirely innocuous may not be justifiable. As Quickenden (*58*) concluded in a thoughtful article on toxic hazards of the laboratory: "The most important single reform which is greatly overdue in most laboratories is the provision of adequate ventilation systems and the proper provision of fume hoods which operate efficiently under practical working conditions."

Potency and Volatility of Chemical Carcinogens

The degree of hazard posed by chemical carcinogens in the laboratory, as elsewhere, varies greatly. Major factors include their potencies and ease of entrance into the body. Carcinogen potencies cover a range of approximately six orders of magnitude, from aflatoxin B_1, carcinogenic for the rat at a daily dose of 1 μg/kg body weight, at one extreme, to agents such as saccharin or trichloroethylene, giving barely detectable responses at over 1 g/kg (*59*).

Also of outstanding importance are factors, particularly volatility, that determine to what extent the substance may enter the body via the lungs or skin. The volatility of the carcinogenic aromatic amines, for example, played an important part in their dangers as bladder carcinogens in industry. Other industrial carcinogens have included the volatile liquids bis(2-chloroethyl) sulfide (mustard gas) and bis(chloromethyl) ether and the gas vinyl chloride. In contrast 1,2-oxathiolane 2,2-dioxide (1,3-propane sultone), a compound of industrial value that is an effective animal carcinogen, is a nondusty solid of low volatility, and would correspondingly be expected to be much less hazardous in use.

The volatile liquid carcinogen *N*-nitrosodimethylamine was investigated by Magee and Barnes after it had caused liver injury to two out of three men who had used it as a solvent in an industrial research laboratory. After confirming the hepatotoxicity of the nitrosamine in rats, they discovered its strong carcinogenicity (*60*), and thus initiated the tremendous amount of research on *N*-nitroso carcinogens which has since been carried out. Apart from its outstanding importance to various areas of cancer research and environmental safety, this compound clearly demonstrated the great hazards that widespread industrial or laboratory use of many nitroso compounds would involve. The volatility of *N*-nitrosodimethylamine under laboratory conditions was strikingly demonstrated by Hubermann et al. (*61*) during experiments on carcinogenesis in vitro. Up to 25% of the carcinogen added to culture medium in petri dishes in an incubator was lost, and its presence could be demonstrated in dishes to which it had not been added.

Laboratory Precautions with Carcinogens

There are two main aspects to the problem of eliminating chemical carcinogens in the laboratory setting. One aspect concerns intentional or unavoidable work with known or potential carcinogens in situations such as cancer research laboratories. Here it is essential to draw up and enforce rules to protect the operator and other persons from all foreseeable carcinogenic hazards in a manner that was barely considered until quite recently. Sometimes this requirement is now legal as well as moral.

The second aspect is to a large extent educational: to ensure that laboratory workers in general receive information on chemical carcinogens because of the possibility, or likelihood, that they may be handling carcinogens in completely different fields of work. This has, of course, long been the case with the aromatic amine reagents already referred to in relation to analytical laboratories.

Laboratory Use of Potent Carcinogens. After realizing that aromatic amines would continue to be used in laboratories for some time and that they might have caused some bladder cancer in laboratory workers (*2*), workers at the Chester Beatty Research Institute in London published a booklet drawing attention to the carcinogenicity of various aromatic amines and nitro compounds (*62*) and the risk of their absorption through the lungs or skin. The booklet also gave advice on safety measures such as avoiding all skin contact and using protective clothing, impervious bench surfaces, and copious cold water for removing contamination.

The Carcinogenic Substances Regulations came into effect in the United Kingdom in 1967 (*54*). These regulations imposed a complete ban on industrial manufacture or use of 2-naphthylamine, benzidine, 4-biphenylamine, and 4-nitrobiphenyl and controlled the use of related compounds such as 3,3′-dimethylbenzidine (*o*-tolidine), 3,3′-dimethoxybenzidine (*o*-dianisidine), and 3,3′-dichlorobenzidine.

Nonindustrial laboratories, such as those in hospitals, colleges, and schools, were then outside the scope of the regulations, but these institutions have more recently come under the Health and Safety at Work etc. Act 1974 (*63*). Under the act, obligations for minimizing hazards were imposed both on employers and employees. The Commission of the European Communities is expected to issue a directive on chemical carcinogens, also applying to all places of work. The member countries of the Community will then be required to enact their own legislation to bring the directive into effect.

Meanwhile organizations in various countries have drawn up recommendations on carcinogen handling. The U.S. National Cancer Institute issued interim safety standards in 1975 (*64*) for suspected chemical carcinogens and other toxic substances. These standards were described in an American Chemical Society publication by Barbeito (*65*); he summarized the key principles in protecting employees, including proper use of equipment, establishment of good personnel practices, and employment of safe laboratory procedures.

Recommendations were made regarding protective clothing; showers; bans on eating, drinking, and smoking in laboratories; and in some cases medical surveillance. Access to laboratories should be controlled; carcinogens should be labelled "DANGER—CHEMICAL CARCINOGENS"; and potentially hazardous chemicals should be handled only in adequately ventilated fume hoods, biological safety cabinets, or glove-box systems. Pipetting should be done using approved pipetting aids. Contamination should of course be avoided, but provision must be made for clean-up procedures in the event of an accident, as well as for safe disposal of carcinogenic waste.

The U.S. National Institutes of Health (NIH) guidelines on handling laboratory carcinogens were published by the Department of Health and Human Services (DHHS) in 1981 (*66*). A two-volume multiauthor compilation concerned with handling carcinogens and other chemicals with short- and long-term risks has also been published (*67*).

In the United Kingdom, a committee of the Medical Research Council (MRC) drew up guidelines on carcinogen handling (*68*), primarily for use in MRC laboratories. These guidelines were clearly stated to be intended for work involving substantial amounts of potent carcinogens, such as a number of specified polycyclic aromatic hydrocarbons, aromatic amines, alkylating agents, and *N*-nitroso compounds. Considerable discretion is allowed for laboratories to decide on the precautions appropriate for less hazardous work. The MRC recognizes that excessive restrictions on experimentation with compounds with relatively much smaller hazards could be counterproductive and might well impede identification of other carcinogens and causes of human disease. The guidelines give particular attention to the difficult problems of safety in animal-feeding experiments with carcinogens and in disposal of contaminated animal wastes.

The International Agency for Research on Cancer (IARC) (*69*) defined the problems of laboratory use of carcinogens, and briefly described suitable operational practices, emergency procedures, and methods for storing, handling, monitoring, and disposing of carcinogens. Inadequacies of present information on a number of matters were pinpointed, particularly with regard to safe methods of destroying and disposing of the very disparate range of carcinogens that may be encountered in laboratory work.

Because carcinogens are of many different types with very different chemical, physical, and biological properties, laying down detailed rules applicable to all of them is not practical, particularly with respect to methods of decontamination and waste disposal. For example, many alkylating agents can be relatively easily destroyed by interaction with water, thiosulfate, or other readily available reagents, and nitrosamines can be reduced to amines prior to disposal. The polycyclic aromatic hydrocarbons present more difficult problems owing to their persistence and chemical stability, making it generally necessary to destroy them by incineration. The use of concentrated sulfuric acid–dichromate mixture is sometimes recommended, but this process introduces additional hazards. Valuable information on carcinogen reactivity is contained in a book by Slein and Sansone (*70*); for aflatoxins and nitroso carcinogens, more detailed guidance is available from the IARC (*71,72*).

Polycyclic Aromatic Hydrocarbons. Because of the very widespread use of these carcinogens in cancer research, Darlow et al. (*73*) investigated the extent to which the carcinogens might become dispersed into the atmosphere during animal skin-painting experiments. These researchers simulated the application of a carcinogen solution with an acetone suspension of *Bacillus globigii* spores that could subsequently be detected on culture plates by the pigmentation of the resultant colonies. Very high air and surface counts were obtained for 6 h after a single application to the skin of 30 mice. Counts then fell sharply, but rose again many days later when the animals' hair was clipped, their bedding was changed, or the floor was swept. Factors other than carcinogenic potency important in relation to the actual degree of hazard in such work were also listed. These factors included the compound's solubility, volatility, and ease of absorption into the body; the vehicle used for its administration; and variables in caging the animals (e.g., changing their bedding, and the size, ventilation, and methods of cleaning the rooms where they were housed).

In further tests of contamination during skin-painting experiments, Sansone and Losikoff (*74*) treated mouse skin with anthracene in acetone in a laminar flow hood. Then samples were taken for determination of this noncarcinogenic hydrocarbon over a 17-d period from the hood, the room with the hood, the corridors, and the room where the mice were kept. Nearly all of the anthracene and all of the solvent were retained in the hood. Most of the contamination arose from the animals' maintenance and transport. This finding is in contrast with the wide dispersal found by Darlow et al. (73) using bacteria in the open laboratory. Sansone and Losikoff considered that the hoods would provide an adequate safeguard. However, in experiments involving repeated skin applications of carcinogens such as benzo[*a*]pyrene, the very considerable risk of widespread contamination probably would be reduced, but not prevented, by carrying out the actual applications in hoods.

Carcinogen Handling in General Chemical Laboratories. As indicated at the beginning of this chapter, recognizing that certain widely used compounds such as benzidine are potent human carcinogens also meant recognizing that workers in a very wide range of laboratories are likely to be exposed to carcinogenic hazards at work. The list of known carcinogens that may be encountered in the laboratory has now become so extensive that, in any laboratory handling chemicals, there should ideally be someone present with adequate information in this field.

Carcinogenicity is, of course, only one sort of toxic action that may be encountered in a chemical, but in many important instances it is a property of chemicals that had long been regarded as relatively harmless. Carcinogenic chemicals were thus used extensively and with little care for many years before their long-term dangers to health became apparent.

Other types of carcinogens, such as alkylating agents, have short-term irritant and toxic actions that should themselves enforce a greater degree of caution in usage. This concern is even greater for the methylating agents diazomethane and methyl fluorosulfonate ("magic methyl") for which serious toxicity considerations are paramount. Nevertheless, it is worth repeating the caution that diazomethane should be prepared from *N*-methyl-*N*-nitroso-4-toluenesulfonamide and not from the other possible but carcinogenic reagents *N*-methyl-*N*-nitrosourea, *N*-methyl-*N'*-nitro-*N*-nitrosoguanidine (MNNG), or the still more hazardous *N*-methyl-*N*-nitrosourethane.

The increased appreciation of the range of potential carcinogenic hazards now indicates that simple warnings to avoid specific hazards of important carcinogens have become inadequate. Practical information on the wide range of recognized carcinogens is needed; this information should enable laboratory workers not only to identify any carcinogens that they may be handling, but also to form some estimate of the actual degree of hazard and the precautions that are appropriate.

Unfortunately, though the literature on chemical carcinogenesis is so voluminous, the laboratory worker may have considerable difficulty in finding the sort of published guidance required. Many carcinogens are listed among other hazards in such valuable sources as the volumes by Sax (*75*) and Steere (*76*). Two safety handbooks for chemical laboratories give quickly accessible data on fire and explosion hazards and on toxicity and disposal of a smaller range of chemicals, but have relatively limited information on carcinogenicity (*77,78*). Chemical suppliers though are giving more indication of carcinogenicity in their catalogs, on labels, or in separate publications (*79*).

Most likely many organizations, nowadays much more aware of carcinogen safety problems, are having to study the literature and tackle the problems piecemeal as best as they can, sometimes with little appreciation of the complexities involved. I can only comment on investigations of the problems with which I have been involved at one of the universities in the United Kingdom. Some groups at least have been attempting to formulate rules for the use of carcinogens in their universities to ensure compliance with the requirements of the Health and Safety at Work Act (*63*)—a very difficult task for a safety representative, particularly in institutions where no unit carries out cancer research, as is usually the case. In at least one university, a long document was written that included warnings against hazards of esoteric heterocyclic carcinogens most unlikely ever to be encountered, but had no reference to the risks from much more widely used and therefore important carcinogenic chemicals.

At the University of Birmingham, the existence of a Department of Cancer Studies has facilitated the task of giving practical guidance to the variety of other laboratories on the campus, while clearly illustrating some of the problems involved. The safety subcommittee concerned with carcinogens and other toxic substances composed a document that included background information on the wide range of known carcinogens, their human hazards where recognized, and existing or projected legislation for their control (*80*). Carcinogens were discussed in major groups, and the most important ones were listed.

However, the relative hazards of carcinogens cover such a wide range that the subcommittee felt it essential to include a grading system to indicate the degree of hazard and the precautions appropriate in specific cases. A system of star-rating for each chemical was used, as follows:

no star	carcinogenicity weak or possible
*	carcinogenicity established, but little hazard with reasonable care
**	significant carcinogenic hazard
***	high carcinogenic hazard

In addition, an "H" was appended to those agents recognized as having caused human cancer. The subcommittee emphasized that carcinogens without this mark are not necessarily less hazardous, and also that current concern over long-term risks from chemical carcinogens must not detract from precautions against other manifold and immediate hazards of scientific laboratories, such as fire, explosion, electrical accidents, or direct toxicity of chemicals.

For carcinogens carrying a single star, no specific precautions were recommended. Rules were laid down for use of carcinogens with two stars. Carcinogens with three stars may only be used with the agreement of the Safety Unit and with strict adherence to written rules concerning handling and disposal.

The ratings, which attempted to allow for factors such as volatility as well as carcinogenic potency, were acknowledged as subjective in nature and liable to be considerably amended in the light of future knowledge or legislation. Nevertheless, this sort of system is of much greater practical value in a laboratory than simple listings of carcinogens, however comprehensive.

Carcinogens in Science Education

Aromatic Amines in Schools. Apparently, the first realization of carcinogenic hazards in school chemistry teaching was the discovery of a bottle of benzidine in the chemical store of an English Midlands school in 1966. By that time, benzidine was being labeled "carcinogenic", and the bottle had been left unopened. However, its suspected original purpose was as a chromatographic spray, surely one of the most hazardous uses for such a chemical in a laboratory.

The risks for school children handling carcinogens were then brought to the attention of educational authorities in the Midlands. In Birmingham, the Education Department carried out a survey of carcinogen stocks in schools under its jurisdiction. While most schools had none, some schools had sufficient stocks of benzidine and naphthylamines to make it clear that action was needed on a national scale (*81*). Information about carcinogen hazards was then sent to schools, teacher-training colleges, and further education establishments from the Department of Education and Science in London (*82*) or from its counterparts in Scotland and Northern Ireland. Teachers also received information directly through the journal of the Association for Science Education (*83*). An editorial in another educational journal pointed out the carcinogenicity of some aromatic amines and the high toxicity of nitrobenzene and aniline and concluded that "for the chemistry teacher, the safest precaution is, presumably, to ban experiments with aromatic amines. After all, are any of them really necessary to an understanding of chemistry?" (*84*).

A convincing demonstration of the need for greater awareness of chemical carcinogens was the publication in a teachers' journal of a suggested experiment for students in which benzidine was to be prepared and converted to a dye with an unspecified naphthalene derivative, and the product was then to be used for dyeing cotton. This experiment had been proposed by an industrial correspondent in 1967, the year in which use of benzidine in British factories became illegal.

In Kentucky, observation of benzidine in a chemical laboratory similarly led to a survey of aromatic amines and other carcinogens in 350 high schools and 41 institutions of higher education (*85*). As in the survey in Birmingham, England, benzidine and the naphthylamines were the carcinogens most frequently found. Chemistry professors unanimously agreed that chemical principles could be illustrated equally well with safer chemicals.

Also in 1976, a report appeared that 190 kg of carcinogens were being stored or used in 79 high schools, 64 community colleges, and 56 colleges and universities in California (*86*). The carcinogens surveyed were those subject to regulation under state and federal Occupational Safety and Health Acts, comprising nine aromatic amines or related compounds, *N*-nitrosodimethylamine, and five alkylating agents. No evidence was stated that students were being unduly exposed, but schools were advised to arrange for sale and lawful disposal of the carcinogens. Sansone and Lijinsky (*87*) deplored this situation and thought that the chemicals should be required to be disposed of by degradation, deactivation, or incineration. They pointed out the likelihood that very great quantities of the regulated and other carcinogens would still be present in schools throughout the country, and that such materials would still be used without precautions and in ignorance of their hazards.

Other Carcinogens in Education. Students may be exposed to hazards from various other carcinogens as well as aromatic amines, particularly simple nitrosamines produced in tests to distinguish aliphatic amines, asbestos, and benzene and other solvents. The risks of nitrosamines and benzene are such that their use in schools should certainly be avoided, and considerable care needs to be exercised also with respect to chloroform and tetrachloromethane. Nevertheless, a survey of 246 British schools in 1976 (*88*) showed that use of benzene, chloroform, and tetrachloromethane in schools was common, often at frequent intervals and in the open laboratory, producing atmospheric concentrations very much higher than those regarded as acceptable in industry even for short periods. Such solvents are also liable to be used in other parts of schools, such as workshops or art rooms, where their hazards are even less likely to be appreciated.

Undoubtedly, improving information and working conditions with chemicals in schools is essential. The Association for Science Education in the United Kingdom has recently reviewed possible hazards from school use of a range of organic and inorganic carcinogens, including asbestos (*89*). Because of the more frequent exposures for teachers, they are at greater risk than their pupils, though understandably attention has been focused on the students.

The conclusion that a range of potent carcinogens should not be used or kept in schools is inescapable, and thus considerable education on carcinogenic hazards is required. However, for those continuing to study science at more advanced levels, the situation is less well defined, and learning to handle potentially hazardous chemicals and processes safely is an essential part of a chemical training.

The range of known carcinogens is now so great that their complete elimination from the environment is clearly impracticable. Nevertheless in many situations, substitution of carcinogens by safer materials is possible. Where carcinogens of significant risk still have to be used, it must be with full knowledge and observance of the safety precautions now regarded as essential to protect both the operator and other people. The suggestion of Haddow (*90*) that an introduction to chemical carcinogenesis should form part of the education of chemists is more pertinent now than when it was made.

Acknowledgments

I wish to acknowledge the cooperation of W. H. S. George (deceased 1979) of the City Hospital, Derby, England, in writing the original version of this chapter.

Literature Cited

1. Case, R.A.M. *Proc. R. Soc. Med.* **1969**, *62*, 1061–66.
2. Case, R.A.M. *Ann. Rep. Br. Empire Cancer Campaign* **1966**, *44*, 56; **1967**, *45*, 90.
3. Williams, M.H.C. In "Cancer"; Raven, R., Ed.; Butterworths: London, 1957; Vol. 3, p. 337.
4. Anthony, H.M.; Thomas, G.M. *JNCI, J. Natl. Cancer Inst.* **1970**, *45*, 879–95.

5. Li, F.P.; Fraumeni, J.F., Jr.; Mantel, N.; Miller, R.W. *JNCI, J. Natl. Cancer Inst.* **1969**, *43*, 1159–64.
6. Hoar, S.K.; Pell, S. *J. Occup. Med.* **1981**, *23*, 495–501.
7. Olin, R. *Lancet* **1976**, *II*, 916.
8. Olin, G. R.; Ahlbom, A. *Environ. Res.* **1980**, *22*, 154–61.
9. Olin, R.; Ahlbom, A. *Ann. N.Y. Acad. Sci. U.S.A.* **1982**, *381*, 197–201.
10. Searle, C.E.; Waterhouse, J.A.H.: Henman, B.A.; Bartlett, D.; McCombie, S. *Br. J. Cancer* **1978**, *38*, 192–93.
11. Royal Society of Chemistry, First report "RSC Effects of Chemicals Assessment Programme" Royal Society of Chemistry, London, 1980.
12. Bruce, D.L.; Eide, K.A.; Linde, H.W.; Eckenhoff, J.E. *Anesthesiology* **1968**, *29*, 565–69.
13. Corbett, T.H.; Cornell, R.G.; Lieding, K.; Endres, J.L. *Anesthesiology* **1973**, *38*, 260–63.
14. Cohen, E.N.; Brown, B.W.; Bruce, D.L. et al. *Anesthesiology* **1974**, *41*, 321–40.
15. Bruce, D.L.; Eide, K.A.; Smith, N.J.; Seltzer, F.; Dykes, M.H.M. *Anesthesiology* **1974**, *41*, 71–74.
16. Law, E.A. *Anesthesiology* **1979**, *51*, 195–99.
17. Doll, R.; Peto, R. *Br. Med. J.* **1977**, *1*, 1433–36.
18. Corbett, T.H.; Cornell, R.G.; Endres, J.L.; Lieding, K. *Anesthesiology* **1974**, *41*, 341–44.
19. Tomlin, P.J. *Br. Med. J.* **1979**, *1*, 779–84.
20. "The Evaluation of the Carcinogenic Risk of Chemicals to Humans"; IARC Monograph, IARC: Lyon, 1979; Vol. 20, pp. 401–17; 545–72.
21. Baden, J.M.; Simmon, V.F. *Mutat. Res.* **1980**, *75*, 169–89.
22. Lane, G.A.; Nahrwold, M.A.; Tait, A.R. et al. *Science (Washington, D.C.)* **1980**, *210*, 899–901.
23. Corbett, T.H. in "Occupational Hazards to Operating Room and Recovery Room Personnel"; Cottrell, J.E., Ed.; Little, Brown: Boston, 1981; pp. 99–120.
24. Harrington, J.M.; Shannon, H.S. *Br. Med. J.* **1975**, *4*, 329–32.
25. Swenberg, J.A.; Kerns, W.D.; Mitchell, R.I.; Gralla, E.J.; Pavkov, K.L. *Cancer Res.* **1980**, *40*, 3398–402.
26. "Formaldehyde: Evidence of Carcinogenicity," National Institute for Occupational Safety and Health, Current Intelligence Bulletin *34*, 1981.
27. Albert, R.E.; Sellakumar, A.R.; Laskin, S.; Kuschner, M.; Nelson, N.; Snyder, C.A. *JNCI, J. Natl. Cancer Inst.* **1982**, *68*, 597–603.
28. "Some Industrial Chemicals and Dyestuffs"; IARC Monograph No. 29, IARC: Lyon, 1982; pp. 345–89.
29. Capurro, P.U.; Eldridge, J.E. *Lancet* **1978**, *i*, 942.
30. Capurro, P.U. *Clin. Toxicol.* **1979**, *14*, 285–94.
31. Kinlen, L.J.; Sheil, A.G.R.; Peto, J.; Doll, R. *Br. Med. J.* **1979**, *2*, 1461–66.
32. Burnet, F.M. *Br. Med. J.* **1965**, *1*, 338–42.
33. Funes-Cravioto, F.; Zapata-Gayon, C.; Kalmodin-Hedman, B. et al. *Lancet* **1977**, *ii*, 322–25.
34. Lambert, B.; Lindblad, A. *J. Toxicol. Environ. Health* **1980**, *6*, 1237–43.
35. George, W.H.S. *Ann. Clin. Biochem.* **1971**, *8*, 130–2.
36. Neill, D.W.; Doggart, J.R. in "Hazards in the Chemical Laboratory"; 2nd ed., Muir, D.G., Ed.; Chem. Soc.: London, 1977; pp. 437–45.
37. Deadman, N.M.; Timms, B.G. *Clin. Chim. Acta* **1969**, *26*, 369–70.
38. Holland, V.R.; Saunders, B.C.; Rose, F.L.; Walpole, A.L. *Tetrahedron* **1977**, *30*, 3299–302.
39. Garner, R.C.; Walpole, A.L.; Rose, F.L. *Cancer Lett. Shannon, Irel..* **1975**, *1*, 39–42.
40. Steinberg, H. NBH Spec. Publ. U.S. No. 480–21, 1977.
41. Chernoff, H.N. "Monographs on Proficiency Testing," National Communicable Diseases Center, DHEW, Atlanta, GA, 1970

42. Ratcliff, A.P.; Hardwicke, J. *J. Clin. Pathol.* **1964**, *17*, 676–9.
43. Stanworth, D.R.; Coombes, E. Unpublished data, 1972.
44. Griciute, L., Tomatis, L. *Int. J. Cancer* **1980**, *25*, 123–29.
45. Laycock, B.J.; Britton, J.A.; Lilleyman, J.S. *J. Clin. Pathol.* **1980**, *33*, 194–6.
46. Knowles, R.S.; Virden, J.E. *Br. Med. J.* **1980**, *281*, 589–91.
47. Zimmerman, P.F.; Larsen, R.K.; Barkley, E.W.; Gallelli, J.F. *Am. J. Hosp. Pharm.* **1981**, *38*, 1693–5.
48. Feigl, F.; Anger, V. *Analyst* **1966**, *91*, 282–4.
49. Bark, L.S.; Higson, H.G. *Talanta* **1964**, *11*, 621–31.
50. "Standard Methods for the Examination of Water and Wastewater," 11th ed.; Am. Pub. Health Assoc.: New York, 1965.
51. Palin, A.T. *J. Inst. Water Eng.* **1967**, *21*, 537–47.
52. Bunton, N.G.; Crosby, N.T.; Patterson, S.J. *Analyst* **1969**, *94*, 585–88.
53. "Special Hazard Review for Benzidine-Based Dyes," National Institute for Occupational Safety and Health, DHEW (NIOSH) Publ. No. 80–109, 1980.
54. "The Carcinogenic Substances Regulations 1967", S.I. No. 879, Her Majesty's Stationery Office, London, 1967.
55. Green, U.; Holste, J.; Spikermann, A.R. *J. Cancer Res. Clin. Oncol.* **1979**, *95*, 51–55.
56. Weisburger, E.K.; Russfield, A.B.; Homburger, F. et al. *J. Environ. Pathol. Toxicol.* **1978**, *2*, 325–56.
57. Bjeldanes, L.F.; Chew, H. *Mutat. Res.* **1979**, *67*, 367–71.
58. Quickenden, T.I. *Chem. Aust.* **1980**, *47*, 119–27.
59. Fox, J.L. *Chem. Eng. News* **1977**, *12 Dec.*, 34–46.
60. Magee, P.N.; Barnes, J.M. *Br. J. Cancer* **1956**, *10*, 114–22.
61. Hubermann, E.; Traut, M.; Sachs, L. *JNCI, J. Natl. Cancer Inst.* **1970**, *44*, 395–402.
62. "Precautions for Laboratory Workers Who Handle Carcinogenic Aromatic Amines"; Chester Beatty Research Institute, London, 1966; reprinted with notes, 1971.
63. The Health and Safety at Work etc. Act 1974. Her Majesty's Stationery Office, London, 1974.
64. "Safety Standards for Research Involving Chemical Carcinogens," DHEW Publ. No. (NIH) 76–900, Bethesda, MD, 1975.
65. Barbeito, M.S. in "Toxic Chemical and Explosives Facilities." ACS Symposium Series No. 96, ACS: Washington, D.C., 1979; pp. 191–214.
66. "NIH Guidelines for the Laboratory Use of Chemical Carcinogens," U.S. Department of Health and Human Services, NIH Publication No. 81–2385, 1981.
67. "Safe Handling of Chemical Carcinogens, Mutagens, Teratogens, and Highly Toxic Substances"; Walters, D.B., Ed.; Ann Arbor Science: Ann Arbor, MI, 1980.
68. "Guidelines for Work with Chemical Carcinogens in Medical Research Council Establishments," Medical Research Council, London, 1981.
69. "Handling Chemical Carcinogens in the Laboratory: Problems of Safety"; Montesano, R.; Bartsch, H.; Boyland, E. et al., Eds.; IARC Sci. Publ. No. 33, IARC: Lyon, 1979.
70. Slein, Milton W.; Sansone, Eric B. "Degradation of Chemical Carcinogens: An Annotated Bibliography"; Van Nostrand Reinhold: New York,1980.
71. "Laboratory Decontamination and Destruction of Aflatoxins B_1, B_2, G_1, G_2 in Laboratory Wastes"; Castegnaro, M.; Hunt, D.C.; Sansone, E.B. et al., Eds.; IARC Sci. Publ. No. 37; IARC: Lyon, 1980.
72. "Laboratory Decontamination and Destruction of Carcinogens in Laboratory Wastes: Some Nitrosamines"; Castegnaro, M.; Ellen, G.; Keeter, L. et al., Eds.; IARC Sci. Publ. No. 43; IARC: Lyon, 1982.
73. Darlow, H.M.; Simmons, D.J.C.; Roe, F.J.C. *Arch. Environ. Health* **1969**, *18*, 883–93.

74. Sansone, E.B.; Losikoff, A.M. *Food Cosmet. Toxicol.* **1979**, *17*, 349–52.
75. Sax, N.I. in "Dangerous Properties of Industrial Materials", 5th ed.; Van Nostrand-Reinhold: New York, 1979.
76. "Handbook of Laboratory Safety, CRC," 2nd ed.; Steere, Norman V., Ed.; CRC: Boca Raton, 1971.
77. Green, M.E.; Turk, A. in "Safety in Working with Chemicals"; Macmillan: New York, 1978.
78. "Hazards in the Chemical Laboratory", 3rd ed.; Bretherick, L., Ed.; Royal Soc. Chem.: London, 1981.
79. "Handling of Carcinogens and Hazardous Compounds," Technical Bulletin, Calbiochem–Behring Corp., La Jolla, CA.
80. Searle, C.E.; Teale, O.J. "Prevention of Occupational Cancer International Symposium: Proceedings of the International Symposium on the Prevention of Occupational Cancer, Helsinki, April 21–24, 1981"; Int. Labour Office: Geneva, 1982; No. 46, pp. 594–600.
81. Searle, C.E. *Ann. Rep. Br. Empire Cancer Campaign* **1968**, *46*, 247–48.
82. "Avoidance of Carcinogenic Aromatic Amines in Schools and Other Educational Establishments," Department of Education and Science, Administrative Memorandum No. 3/70, 1970.
83. Searle, C.E. *Sch. Sci. Rev.* **1969**, *51*, 282–88.
84. *Educ. Chem.* **1969**, *6*, 163.
85. Block, J.B. *J. Coll. Sci. Teach.* **1976**, *6*, 24–26.
86. *Occup. Safety Health Rep.* **1976**, *6*, 501.
87. Sansone, E.B.; Lijinsky, W. *Science (Washington, D.C.)* **1977**, *196*, 1271, 1358.
88. Dewhurst, F.; Cassells, W.M. *Br. J. Cancer* **1979**, *40*, 817.
89. Association for Science Education, *Educ. Sci.* **1979**, 17–20.
90. Haddow, A. *New Sci.* **1965**, *25*, 348–49.

7

Carcinogenesis by Alkylating Agents

P. D. LAWLEY

Pollards Wood Research Station, Chester Beatty Research Institute, Institute of Cancer Research, Royal Cancer Hospital, Nightingales Lane, Chalfont St. Giles, Bucks, HP8 4SP, United Kingdom

ALKYLATING AGENTS ARE CONSIDERED TO BE ARCHETYPAL CARCINOGENS. The primary carcinogen is the alkylating agent, not one of its metabolic products; alkylating agents react with significant receptors in vivo the same way as in vitro. In fact the majority of other chemical carcinogens are only active after being metabolized to alkylating or aralkylating agents; prominent examples are aflatoxins, dialkylnitrosamines, polycyclic aromatic hydrocarbons, and vinyl chloride. Thus, in the study of alkylating agents, the influence of specific chemical reactions in the carcinogenic process can be determined both qualitatively and quantitatively. In view of the well-established mutagenic properties of the alkylating agents, their effects on the genetic material, in particular the DNA template, have been investigated predominantly. The influence of DNA repair processes known to be important in modification of the initial alkylation effects of DNA can also be studied. Chemical analyses of alkylated DNA have also played an important part in such studies.

Chemical Reactivity as a Factor Determining Carcinogenic Potency

The first specific definition of a chemical reaction of a carcinogen with nucleic acids in vivo was the demonstration (*1*) that mustard gas (**1**), often considered to be the first well-defined chemical mutagen (*2*), alkylated the N-7 position of guanine in vitro and in nucleic acids of the mouse in vivo.

This example typifies the shift in generally accepted concepts of the carcinogenic process that occurred around 1960. Until this period the long-standing somatic mutation theory of cancer (reviewed in Ref. 3) had fallen somewhat into abeyance. Mustard gas, although recognized as a mutagen, was not originally suspect as a potent carcinogen on the basis of conventional animal tests, for example, induction of lung adenoma in strain A mice (*4, 5*). In fact, mustard gas was shown to have inhibitory action on carcinogenesis in the mouse skin system

0065-7719/84/0182-0325$27.10/1

$Cl\,CH_2\,CH_2\,S\,CH_2\,CH_2\,Cl$ $Cl\,CH_2\,CH_2\,S\,CH_2\,CH_2\,OH$

Mustard gas Hemi-sulfur mustard

1

(*6*), but in retrospect this finding reflects its potent cytotoxic action on dividing cells. However in 1968, evidence implicating mustard gas as a potent human carcinogen came from assessment of the incidence of respiratory tract cancer in Japanese workers who were involved in mustard gas manufacture for military purposes (*7*).

A once widely accepted view, contrary to the somatic mutation theory, was that carcinogens affected epigenetic processes and probably acted on essential protein receptors as hormones did. This view seemed to be consistent with the properties of an extensive and, at that time, archetypal class of carcinogens: the polycyclic aromatic hydrocarbons. Such concepts began to lose acceptance when Brookes and Lawley (*8*) compared the covalent reactions of a spectrum of such compounds with proteins and nucleic acids of mouse skin. They found a positive quantitative correlation between reaction with DNA and carcinogenic potency of the hydrocarbons, but no such correlation emerged for RNA or protein as receptors. Subsequently the nature of the reactions involved has been clarified by studies of hydrocarbon metabolism, notably by the findings of Sims et al. (*9*). They determined that the essential activations occur through diol epoxide aralkylating metabolites (for details *see* Chapters 1 and 8).

Loveless (*10*) indicated the importance of specific chemical reactions with DNA in the mechanism of carcinogenesis. After examining the comparative studies of alkylating agents as mutagens and as carcinogens, he deduced that alkylation of guanine in DNA at the extranuclear O-6 atom potentiated mutations by direct miscoding of O^6-alkylguanines with thymine, rather than the normal Watson–Crick pairing of guanine with cytosine. This concept is consistent with the somatic mutation hypothesis in the sense that a good positive quantitative correlation has been found (*11*) between the promutagenic O^6-alkylation of guanine in mouse thymus DNA and the yield of induced thymic lymphoma by alkylating agents of various reactivities. This correlation is illustrated in Figure 1.

The *y*-axis in this figure represents the number of carcinogenic hits based on a dose- and time-dependence study of tumor induction following a single intraperitoneal injection of alkylating agent; this was derived empirically showing the following equation:

$$-\ln\,(1-p_t) = (kD)^n(t-t_0) \tag{1}$$

where p_t is the probability of induction of thymoma at time t after injection; D is the dose administered; k is a constant for a given strain of mice and a given alkylating agent; and t_0 is a minimal latent period of about 70 d.

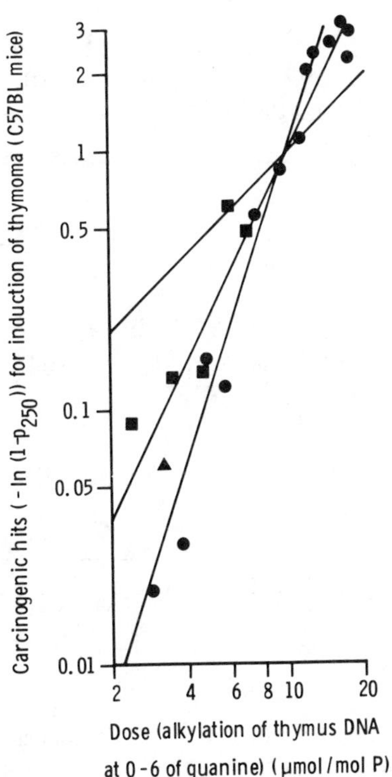

Figure 1. Correlation between induction of thymic lymphoma in C57BL/cbi mice and extent of alkylation of O-6 of guanine in thymus DNA in vivo. Key: ■, N-*ethyl*-N-*nitrosourea, one hit;* ▲, *ethyl methanesulfonate, two hits; and* ●, N-*methyl*-N-*nitrosourea, three hits.*

The *x*-axis represents an effective dose to target thymus DNA obtained from the determination of the extent of alkylation of DNA at O-6 of guanine at a short time (about 1 h) after injection of the dose *D*; over the range of doses used, the effective dose was proportional to the actual dose.

The exponent *n* represents the slope of the graph as both axes are logarithmic; from Poisson statistics, *n* represents the number of dose-dependent hits required to cause the tumor, in addition to one time-dependent hit. From analyses of alkylated DNA, O^6-alkylation was the only reaction shown to correlate for the four agents used (methyl methanesulfonate cannot be shown; it induced no tumors because of the relatively low proportion of O^6-methylguanine induced). The value of *n* appears to be 2–3.

This example emphasizes the importance of the reactivity of alkylating agents as a determinant of carcinogenic potency. The more electrophilic the reagent, the more it will react with weaker nucleophiles. Thus, as electrophilic reactivity increases, a wider spectrum of reactive sites will be affected. Comparative studies of alkylating mutagens by Ehrenberg et al. (*12*) showed a clear positive correlation between electrophilic reactivity and mutagenic potency. However, this positive

Table I

Yield of Thymic Lymphoma in C57BL Female Mice After Single Intraperitoneal Injection of Alkylating Carcinogens in Relation to Extent of Alkylation of DNA of Thymus

			Alkylation of Guanine in DNA of Thymus	
Agent	*Dose (mmol/kg)*	*Yield of Thymoma (%)*	*O-6 Alkylation (μmol/mol DNA-P)*	*Ratio of O-6/N-7 Alkylation*
Methyl methanesulfonate	1.0	0	0.2	0.003
Ethyl methanesulfonate	2.4	2	1	0.02
N-Methyl-*N*-nitrosourea	0.2	3	3	0.1
	0.8	83	18	
N-Ethyl-*N*-nitrosourea	2.1	38	8	0.6

NOTE: Mice were injected at 8–10 weeks of age, and the yields of tumors refer to groups of 50 or more mice at 250 d after injections. The minimal latent period for induction of thymomas was about 70 d; no tumors were found in 100 controls. Alkylation was measured by analyzing DNA isolated 1 h after injection of [^{14}C]alkyl-labeled carcinogen. For details *see* Ref. 11.

correlation holds only to a limited extent in vivo, because excessive reactivity permits extensive removal of reagent by solvolysis; in other words, the need for the reagent to penetrate to essential receptor DNA by diffusion through a medium containing weak nucleophiles, such as water, limits the extent of reaction with the genetic material.

This effect is also clear in carcinogenesis. As shown in Figure 1, the most potent carcinogen of the series of alkylating agents used is *N*-methyl-*N*-nitrosourea, whereas *N*-ethyl-*N*-nitrosourea is the most reactive (Tables I and II). The reason is that the extent of alkylation of DNA in vivo per unit dose of the ethyl homolog is only about one-fifth of that for the methylating agent. The limitations on achieving a sufficiently high extent of alkylation of DNA in vivo are therefore due to a combination of factors: the limited doses that can be used because of toxicity to the animal and either too low a reactivity (as with methyl or ethyl methanesulfonates) or too high a reactivity (as with *N*-ethyl-*N*-nitrosourea) with concomitantly high solvolysis.

Another example was found in a comparative study of alkyl bromides as inducers of injection-site sarcoma in the rat (*13*). The aralkyl bromides 7-bromomethylbenz[*a*]anthracene and 7-bromomethyl-12-methylbenz[*a*]anthracene, compounds with intermediate electrophilic activity, were the most effective carcinogens of the series; the more reactive triphenylmethyl (trityl) bromide and the less reactive ethyl and isopropyl bromides failed to yield tumors by single injection under the conditions in which the benzanthracenyl bromides were effective (Table III).

Table II
Representative Alkylating Agents Classified According to Their Values of the Substrate Constant (*s*) of Swain and Scott (*26*) and Their Suggested Reaction Mechanism

Alkylating Agent	k_0' (h^{-1})	$t_{1/2}$ (*h*)	s	*Mechanism*	*Remarks*
2-Oxopropyl methanesulfonate	0.3	2.3	1.9[a]	S_N2	For a discussion of the effect of β-carbonyl substituents, leading to relatively high *s* values, *see* Ref. 34
Iodoacetate			1.33[b]	S_N2	
Methyl iodide			1.15[b]	S_N2	Ethyl also reacts mainly by S_N2 mechanism; reactivity of RX increases in order $X = F \ll Cl < Br < I$ (*19*)
Methyl bromide	0.0059	116	1.00[c]	S_N2	
Glycidol	0.0068	102	0.96[c,d]	S_N2	Ring-opening reaction; $R \cdot \underset{\diagdown O \diagup}{CH \cdot CH_2} + Y^- \rightarrow$ $R \cdot CHOH \cdot CH_2Y$ by S_N2 mechanism (*35*)
Mustard gas	~33[e]	~0.02			Shows S_N1-type kinetics (*36*) but may react through S_N2 mechanism; for discussion of *S,N*-mustards, *see* the text.
Mustard gas cation			0.95[e]	?	
Trimethyl phosphate			0.8[d]	S_N2	Only one methyl group reacts under pseudo-physiological conditions (*19*)
β-Propiolactone	0.68[g]	1.0	0.77[c]	S_N2	Nucleophilic attack on β-*C*-atom.
Methyl methanesulfonate	0.072[h]	9.5	0.83[a]	S_N2	Dimethyl sulfate closely similar, one methyl group reacting under pseudo-physiological conditions (*19*)
n-Butyl methanesulfonate	0.05[h]	13.8	0.68[a]	S_N2	
Ethyl methanesulfonate	0.06[h]	11.5	0.67[a]	mainly S_N2	"S_N1/S_N2 borderline" mechanism (*37*)
Isopropyl methanesulfonate	3.1	0.22	0.29[a]	mainly S_N1	
N-Methyl-*N*-nitrosourea	2.74[i]	0.25	0.42[j]	partly S_N1 (?)	Reacts via $CH_3N_2^+ [\rightarrow CH_3^+ \text{ (?)}]$

Continued on next page

Table II Continued

Alkylating Agent	k'_0 *(h^{-1})*	$t_{1/2}$ *(h)*	s	*Mechanism*	*Remarks*
N-Ethyl-*N*-nitrosourea	2.36[i]	0.29	0.26[j]	partly S_N1 (?)	Reacts via $C_2H_5N_2^+[\rightarrow C_2H_5^+$ (?)]; the alkylnitrosourea decompositions are alkali-catalyzed; "exact mechanisms are in doubt" (*38*); reviewed (*39*); *see also* Scheme III and Refs. 40 and 41 for *N*-*n*-propyl-*N*-nitrosourea mechanisms.

NOTE: Also given are the first order rate constants for reaction with water at 37 °C (k'_o), and the half-life of hydrolysis ($t_{1/2}$). The value of $s = 1.00$ for methyl bromide is the reference standard, in the relationship log $(k_y/k_o) = s\S n_y$, where k_y denotes the second order rate constants for reaction of a nucleophile of nucleophilic constant n with the alkylating agent, and k_o is the corresponding constant for water; $k'_o = k_o\,[H_2O] = 55.5\,k_o$.
[a]Ref. 12. [b]Ref. 25. [c]Ref. 26. [d]Ref. 27. [e]Ref. 28. [f]Ref. 29. [g]Ref. 30. [h]Ref. 31 (interpolated values). Cited in Ref. 19. [i]Ref. 32. [j]Ref. 33.

Table III
Yield of Injection Site Sarcomas in Female CB Hooded Rats After Single Subcutaneous Injection of Alkyl or Aralkyl Bromides

Agent	*Dose (mmol/kg)*	*Yield of Injection Site Sarcoma (%)*
Isopropyl bromide	0.83–8.3	0
Ethyl bromide	1.25–12.5	0
Benzyl bromide	0.083–0.83	0
7-Bromomethylbenz[*a*]anthracene	0.025	5
	0.083	25
	0.25	35
7-Bromomethyl-12-methyl-benz[a]anthracene	0.0056	5
	0.0185	65
	0.056	75
Triphenylmethyl bromide	0.025–0.25	0

NOTE: Rats were injected at 6 weeks of age, and yields of tumors refer to groups of 20 rats per dose level at 90 weeks after injection. Minimal latent periods were about 20 weeks for the most potent carcinogen; controls showed no injection site sarcoma. The order of compounds is the same as the order of increasing reactivity as measured by rate of alkylation of a standard nucleophile 4-(*p*-nitrobenzyl)pyridine. For details *see* Ref. 13.

In another comparative study of alkyl halides, Poirier et al. (*14*) used multiple intraperitoneal injections into strain A mice (Table IV). Relatively high total doses of 10 halides, out of the 17 studied, gave significantly higher yields of lung tumors than those seen in control animals. Some correlation between carcinogenic potency and chemical reactivity was noted. For example, following the concepts developed by Ingold (*15*), one concludes that chain-branching in the structure of isomeric alkyl halides confers higher electrophilic reactivity (or ability to react through the S_N1 mechanism, *see* Table II), and reactivity increases from chlorides through bromides to iodides. For the series of halides of Table IV, a general trend is for branched-chain halides to be more carcinogenic than the unbranched-chain isomers (e.g., *tert*-butyl chloride and *sec*-butyl chloride were active, whereas *n*-butyl chloride was inactive). The more reactive *tert*-butyl iodide was also inactive. Again, compounds of intermediate reactivity appear to be the most potent carcinogens.

In general, the reactivity of the alkylating agents can be discussed according to several classical concepts. Ingold (*15*) introduced the concept of reaction mechanism through the unimolecular (S_N1) and bimolecular (S_N2) pathways in nucleophilic substitution reactions, and the preference for one mechanism over the other has been the subject of several reviews (*16–24*), some of which include particular reference to biological aspects (*18–24*).

These mechanisms may be regarded as limiting cases of a common mechanism in which alkylating agents are believed to react through ion pairs (*25*) (*see* Scheme I). Agents classified as reacting through the S_N1 mechanism will generally show lower sensitivity to the nucleophilicity of the attacking agents because of the

Table IV

Pulmonary Tumor Response of A/He Mice to Alkyl Halides

Agent	*Total Dose (mmol/kg)*	*Average No. of Lung Tumors/Mouse*
	Positive Response	
Methyl iodide	0.31	0.55
n-Propyl iodide	17.6	0.70
Isopropyl iodide	7.0	0.53
	35.3	0.58
sec-Butyl chloride	35.0	1.20
tert-Butyl chloride	32.4	0.73
	65	1.00
Isobutyl bromide	43.7	0.75
sec-Butyl bromide	21.8	1.00
	43.7	1.15
tert-Butyl bromide	21.8	0.73
	43.7	0.78
n-Butyl iodide	2.6	0.63
	6.6	0.60
	13.1	0.63
sec-Butyl iodide	32.6	0.63
	Statistically Not Significant	
Ethyl bromide	11–55	0.21–0.35
Ethyl iodide	7.7–38.4	0.20–0.15
n-Butyl chloride	12.9–65	0.15–0.31
n-Butyl bromide	0.24–1.2	0.12–0.16
tert-Butyl iodide	0.2–0.42	0.20–0.42
Benzyl chloride	4.7–15.8	0.26–0.50
1-Chloromethylnaphthalene	1.4–7	0.22–0.47

NOTE: Male and female mice (6–8 weeks old) were injected by the intraperitoneal route three times weekly for up to 8 weeks, and the experiments were terminated at 24 weeks after the first injection. For details *see* Ref. 14.

high reactivity of the postulated carbonium ion intermediates (*15*). These properties of the alkylating agent (considered as the substrate) and of the attacking nucleophiles can be expressed quantitatively by Swain and Scott's (*26*) parameters *s* and *n*, respectively. Values of nucleophilicity for some representative groups are given in Table V. An alternative measure of the nucleophilicity parameter was used for reactions of nucleic acids and derivatives with the *N,N*-diethyleneimmonium ion (**2**), which is derived from the nitrogen mustard (**3**) (*21*). This measure is the competition factor *F* and it is related to *n* by the following equations:

$$\log F_y = \log (k_y/k_o) - \log [H_2O] \tag{2}$$

(a) $$\text{R-X} \xrightarrow{k_1} \text{R}^+ + \text{X}^-;\ \text{R}^+ + \text{Y}^- \xrightarrow{k_2[\text{Y}]} \text{RY}$$
$$k_1 << k_2[\text{Y}];\ \text{unimolecular kinetics}$$

(b) $$\text{Y}^- + \text{R-X} \rightarrow [\text{Y}^{\delta-} \ldots \text{R}^{\delta+} \ldots \text{X}^{\delta-}] \rightarrow \text{Y-R} + \text{X}^-$$
$$\text{Rate} = k_2\ [\text{RX}]\ [\text{Y}^-];\ \text{bimolecular kinetics}$$

(c) $$\text{RX} \underset{k_{-1}}{\overset{k_1}{\rightleftharpoons}} \text{R}^+\text{X}^- \begin{cases} \xrightarrow{k_S} \text{ROH} \\ \xrightarrow{k_Y[\text{Y}]} \text{RY} \end{cases}$$

(d) $$k_{-1}/k_S \rightarrow 0;\ \text{resembles } S_N1$$
$$k_{-1}/k_S \rightarrow \infty;\ \text{resembles } S_N2$$

Scheme I. S_N1 (a) and S_N2 (b) mechanisms (15), *unified mechanism (c)* (63), *and limiting cases (d).*

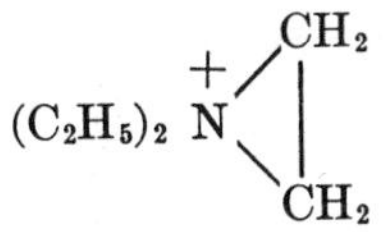

$(C_2H_5)_2\overset{+}{N}<(CH_2)_2$ (aziridinium ring)

2

$(C_2H_5)_2N \cdot CH_2CH_2Cl$

3

$$s\ n_y = \log\ (k_y/k_o) \quad (3)$$

$$\log F_y = s\ n_y - 1.74 \quad (4)$$

Pearson and Songstad (*42*) classified nucleophiles as "hard" and "soft" Lewis bases; these categories approximate Swain and Scott's division of low- and high-*n* reagents (*26*) (Table V). The electrophilic (acidic) components were classified in order of increasing hardness as $CH_3^+ < R_2CH^+ < R_3C^+, ROCH_2^+ < RCO^+$. Soft acids react rapidly with soft bases and hard acids with hard bases. In biological material, hydroxyl, phosphate, carboxylate, and aliphatic amino groups are "hard;" ring-nitrogen or aromatic amino groups are "borderline"; and thiol groups are "soft." Generally, the harder alkylating agents are those of lower *s* factor.

Alkylating agents of the mustard type present some special features in the classification of their reaction mechanisms, and these features are explained by the "neighboring group effect" (*16, 38, 43*). This effect is illustrated for the cases of mustard gas and nitrogen mustards in Scheme II.

The mechanism is generally considered to consist of two successive S_N2 reactions (*38, 43*). However, Ross (*19*) believed that mustard gas reacts by the S_N1

Table V

Nucleophilic Constants, Competition Factors, and Hard and Soft Character of Bases

Nucleophile (Y)	n_y	*Class*	*log* F_y
H_2O	0.00	hard	
CH_3COO^-	2.72	hard	
Cl^-	3.04	borderline	
Pyridine	3.6	borderline	
OH^-	4.2	hard	
Aniline	4.49	borderline	
I^-	5.04	soft	
HS^- (or cysteine)	5.1	soft	
$S_2O_3^{2-}$	6.36	soft	
$H_2PO_4^-$	2.8		
DNA (per P atom) (average of all sites)	2.5–3.0		
DNA (N-7 of guanine)	~3.5		
DNA (O-6 of guanine)	~1.2		
DNA (dTpdT, phosphodiester)	~1		
Adenine, N-1			3.34
Adenine, N-3			3.88
Adenine, N-9			3.21
Adenosine, N-1			2.93
5′-Adenylic acid, N-1			2.91
5′-Adenylic acid, phosphate			4.06
Poly (A), N-1			3.29
Poly (A), phosphodiester			4.10
Guanosine, N-7			3.54
Guanylic acid, N-7			3.45
Guanylic acid, phosphate			3.97
Deoxycytidine, N-3			~2.70
Thymidine, N-3			1.6
DNA, N-7 of guanine			5.18

NOTE: The nucleophilic constant n_y is defined by Swain and Scott (*26*) according to the equation $\log (k_y/k_o) = sn_y$ (*cf.* Table I), and the value n for H_2O is assigned as 0.00. The competition factor F_y is related to n_y by the relationship $\log F_y = sn_y - 1.74$. The values reported refer to alkylation by the *N,N*-diethylethyleneimmonium ion at pH 7, 37° (*21*). The values of n_y are from Swain and Scott (*26*) except for $H_2PO_4^-$ and DNA (per P atom) which are from Osterman–Golkar et al. (*12*). The classification of nucleophiles as hard or soft Lewis bases is from Pearson and Songstad (*42*). The values for N-7, O-6 of guanine in DNA, and for the phosphodiester group were derived from studies on methylation and ethylation of DNA (*53,54,56*) and comparisons with the average n_y value for DNA of Ref. 41.

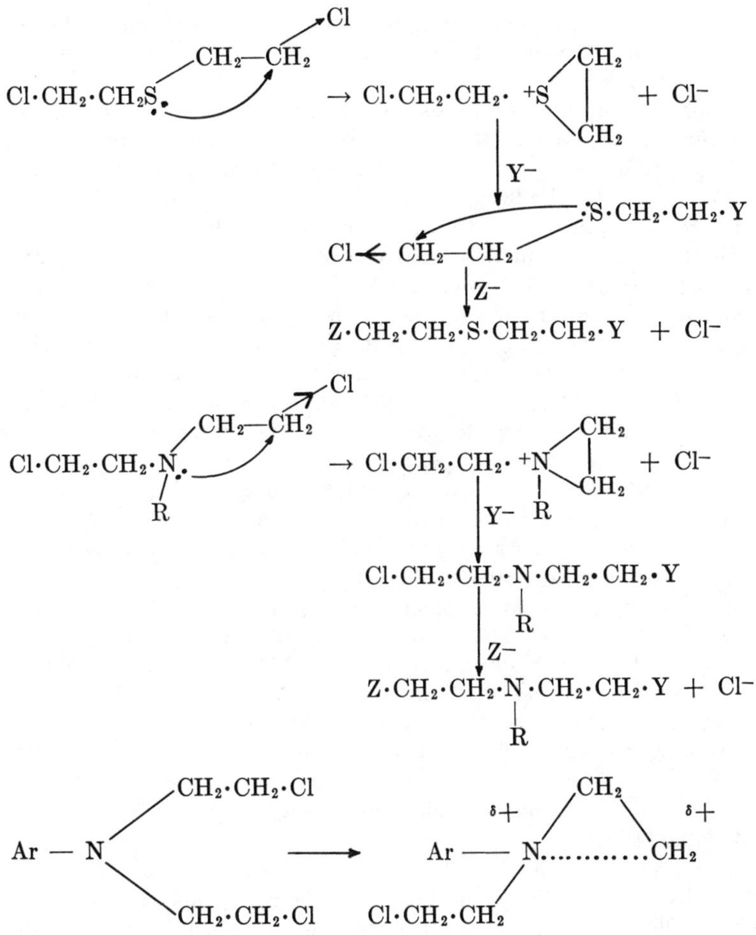

$$Cl{\cdot}CH_2{\cdot}CH_2S{:}\ (CH_2{-}CH_2{\rightarrow}Cl) \rightarrow Cl{\cdot}CH_2{\cdot}CH_2{\cdot}\ {}^{+}S\langle{CH_2 \atop CH_2}\rangle + Cl^-$$

$$\downarrow Y^-$$

$$Cl \leftarrow CH_2{-}CH_2 \ \ {:}S{\cdot}CH_2{\cdot}CH_2{\cdot}Y$$

$$\downarrow Z^-$$

$$Z{\cdot}CH_2{\cdot}CH_2{\cdot}S{\cdot}CH_2{\cdot}CH_2{\cdot}Y + Cl^-$$

$$Cl{\cdot}CH_2{\cdot}CH_2{\cdot}N(R){:}\ (CH_2{-}CH_2{\rightarrow}Cl) \rightarrow Cl{\cdot}CH_2{\cdot}CH_2{\cdot}\ {}^{+}N(R)\langle{CH_2 \atop CH_2}\rangle + Cl^-$$

$$\downarrow Y^-$$

$$Cl{\cdot}CH_2{\cdot}CH_2{\cdot}N(R){\cdot}CH_2{\cdot}CH_2{\cdot}Y$$

$$\downarrow Z^-$$

$$Z{\cdot}CH_2{\cdot}CH_2{\cdot}N(R){\cdot}CH_2{\cdot}CH_2{\cdot}Y + Cl^-$$

$$Ar{-}N(CH_2{\cdot}CH_2{\cdot}Cl)_2 \longrightarrow Ar{-}\overset{\delta+}{N}(CH_2{\cdot}CH_2{\cdot}Cl)\langle CH_2 \rangle \cdots \overset{\delta+}{C}H_2$$

Scheme II. The neighboring-group mechanism for sulfur and nitrogen mustards.

mechanism. This belief follows the opinion of Ogston (*36*), who showed that the reaction kinetics of this mustard gas were consistent with ionization as the rate-controlling step, as required by the S_N1 mechanism. Streitweiser (*16*) stated that the cyclic sulfonium intermediates have real carbonium ion character. The reaction rate of mustard gas in aqueous media at 37 °C is rapid with a $t_{1/2}$ of about 2 min. On the other hand, the mustard cation has a fairly high Swain–Scott *s* factor (0.95) and was included by Swain and Scott (26) in a group of S_N2 agents (*20*). However, agents that react through the S_N1 mechanism can show a considerable range of competition factors that increase as the stability of the derived carbonium ion increases. Thus triphenylmethyl (trityl) halides give the relatively stable trityl cation $(Ph)_3C^+$. This cation shows a very high discrimination between nuceophiles (*44*) and corresponds to an *s* value of about 0.61. *tert*-Butyl chloride, which again reacts through the S_N1 mechanism but yields a less stable cation, shows a much lower range of competition factors (*36*) and corresponds to an *s* value of about 0.4.

Aliphatic nitrogen mustards, which are typified by bis(2-chloroethyl)-methylamine, are generally thought to react mainly through the S_N2 mechanism, although Ludlum (*45*) obtained evidence that suggests an S_N1 reaction with polynucleotide phosphodiester groups. This path was confirmed by Shooter (*46*), but the S_N1 component was thought to be a relatively small contribution to the overall alkylations. Aromatic nitrogen mustards generally tend toward the S_N1 mechanism because of the lower basicity of the nitrogen atom (*19, 28*). Ross (*28*) showed that the effects of substituents in the aromatic moiety supported this concept; electron-releasing substituents *ortho* or *para* to the mustard group enhanced the hydrolysis rate, while electron-withdrawing groups had the opposite effect. Bardos et al. (*23*) developed a method for comparing the relative abilities of aromatic mustards to alkylate the reagent 4-(*p*-nitrobenzyl)pyridine (an S_N2 reaction) and to undergo solvolysis (an S_N1 reaction). Their comparison between reactivities and antitumor activities agreed with Ross' previous deduction (*28*) that reaction by the S_N1 mechanism correlated positively with biological activity.

This correlation may also apply to simple alkylating agents with respect to mutagenic action. Ehrenberg et al. (*12*) drew a parallel conclusion from their comparisons of mutagenic effectiveness of a series of alkyl methanesulfonates in barley. Also the results of studies with a range of alkylating mutagens—including *N*-methyl- and *N*-ethyl-*N*-nitrosoureas that react through alkyldiazonium ions—in *Escherichia coli* and *Arabidopsis thaliana* were consistent with this correlation. The more efficient mutagens had low values of the Swain–Scott constant *s*, whereas alkylating agents with higher *s* values were either nonmutagenic or inefficient mutagens. Linear dose–response relationships could be shown with the agents of lower *s*, but dose–response relationships for agents of $s > 0.55$ were described as exponential (*47, 48*).

Osterman-Golkar et al. (*12*) pointed out that reagents of high *s*—which are typified by the β-carbonyl-substituted alkylating agents such as 2-oxopropyl methanesulfonate or iodoacetamide—react more extensively in vivo with nucleophiles of high *n*, such as thiol groups, or with the more nucleophilic groups in DNA; therefore, they concluded that the groups in DNA of lower nucleophilicity were more specifically alkylated by the efficient mutagens. Alkylation of groups of higher *n* was indicated to be lethal.

Alkylation of DNA in Relation to Carcinogenic Potency of Alkylating Agents: Induction of Directly Miscoding Bases

As a result of the increasing recognition that cancer may originate from somatic mutations (*3, 49, 50*), emphasis has been placed on DNA as the significant in vivo target of chemical carcinogens. Therefore, special attention should be given to those aspects of reactivity of alkylating agents that influence their reaction with DNA.

As already noted, the ability of alkylating carcinogens to react with the less nucleophilic sites in DNA (notably the O-6 atom of guanine) is positively associated with carcinogenic potency in certain cases (*11*). Figure 2 shows the

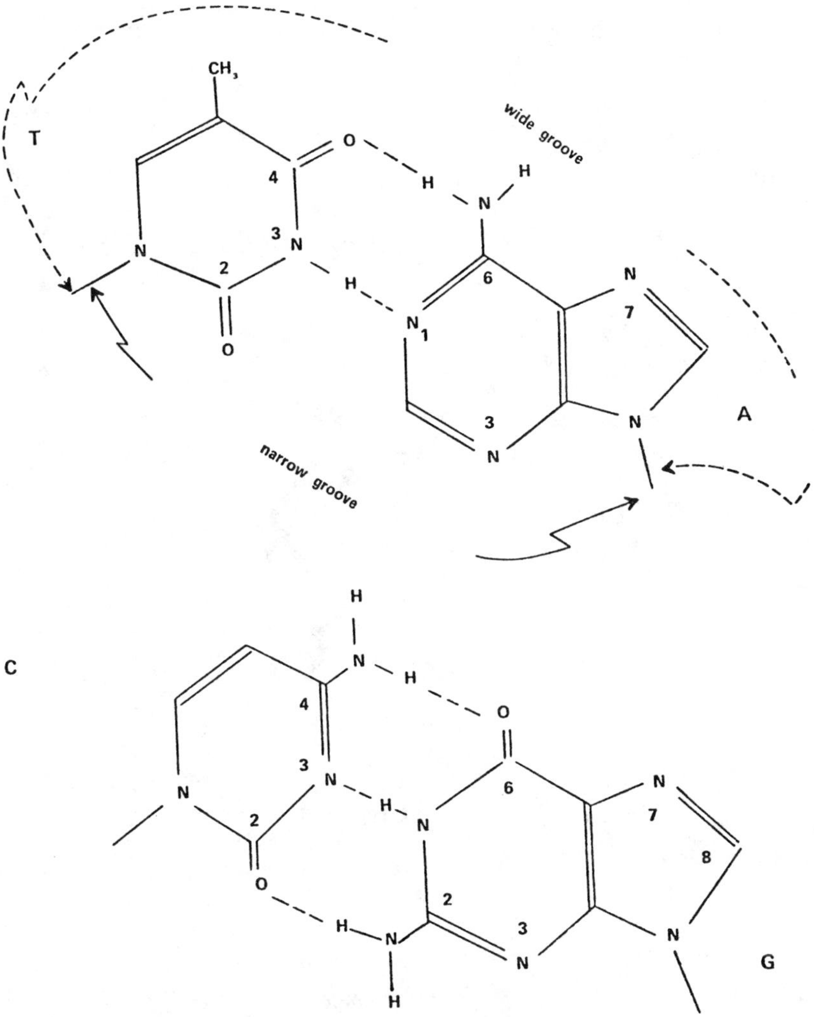

Figure 2. Sites of alkylation of base pairs in double-helical DNA according to the Watson–Crick model. Key to bases: A, adenine; C, cytosine; G, guanine; and T, thymine.

The sites of O-2 of pyrimidines and N-2 or N-3 of purines are situated in the narrow groove of the double helix. The sites of O-4 of thymines or N-4 of cytosine, at N-6 of adenine or O-4 of guanine, at N-7 of adenine or guanine, and at C-8 of guanine are situated in the wide groove of the helix, as are the C-5, C-6 double bonds of the pyrimidines that are involved in formation of pyrimidine dimers. The sites at N-3 of pyrimides and N-1 of purines are involved in hydrogen bonding.

$ClCH_2CH_2N(NO)CONHR \longrightarrow [ClCH_2CH_2N_2]^+ \longrightarrow$

(a)

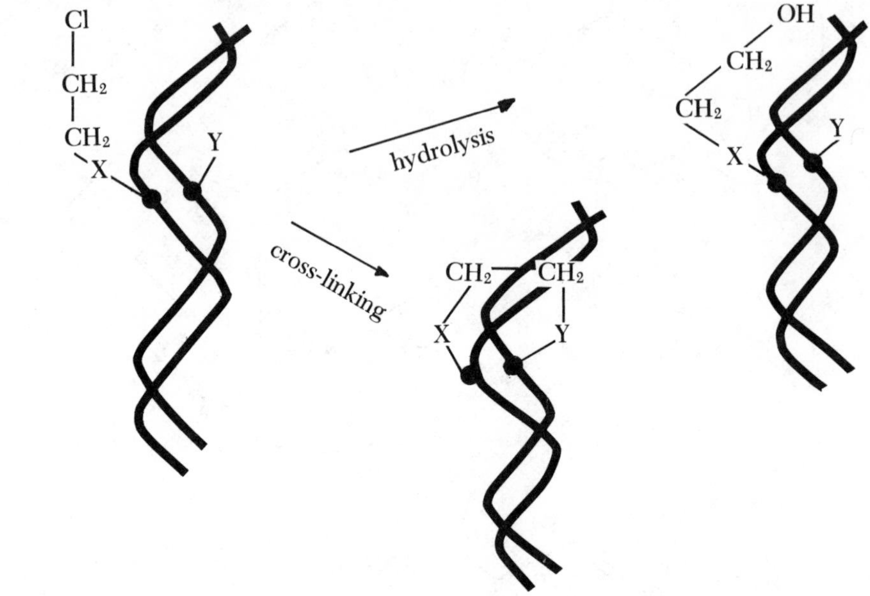

(b)

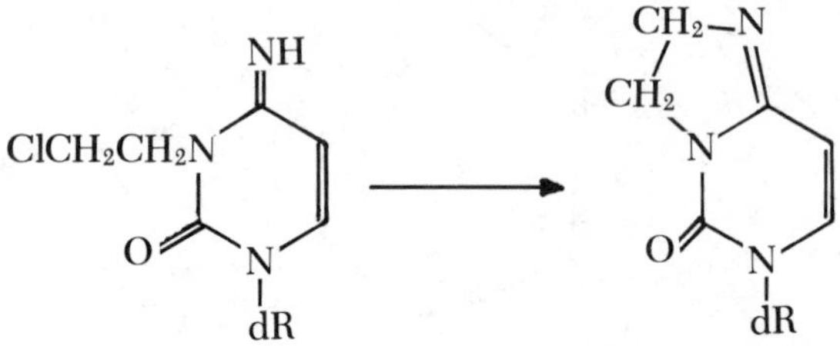

3,N^4-ethanodeoxycytidine

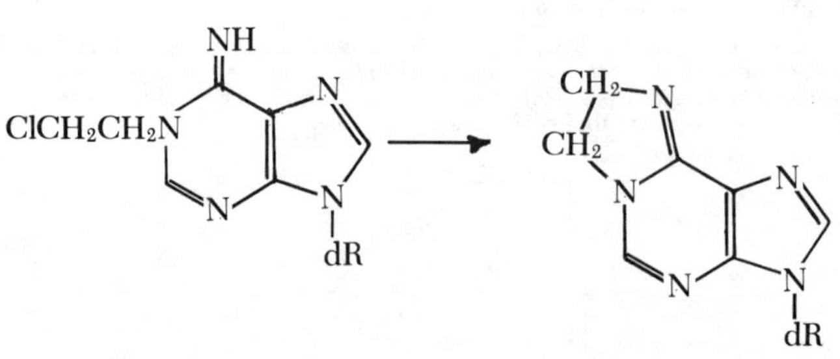

1,N^6-ethanodeoxyadenosine

various sites in the DNA double helix that have been shown to be reactive toward alkylating agents. The most nucleophilic site is the N-7 atom of guanine and the principal next most reactive is the N-3 atom of adenine. These positions are the main sites of alkylation by typical S_N2 agents such as methyl methanesulfonate or dimethyl sulfate.

As the electrophilic reactivity of alkylating agents increases or as the Swain–Scott *s* factor decreases, reaction at the less nucleophilic O-atom sites becomes more prominent.

Steric factors have also been invoked to account for some apparent anomalies in considerations of relative nucleophilicities of sites in DNA. For example, the basic groups of adenine at the N-1 position and cytosine at the N-3 position are more reactive towards protons in the respective isolated nucleotides than in the less basic N-7 atom of guanine; however, this last site is the most nucleophilic in DNA in reactions with typical S_N2 agents such as dimethyl sulfate. Evidently the involvement of the adenine and cytosine basic sites in Watson–Crick hydrogen bonding reduces their nucleophilic reactivity. However, in certain cases—such as with the cancer chemotherapeutic agent 1,3-bis(2-chlorethyl)-1-nitrosourea and related 1-(2-haloethyl)-1-nitrosoureas—the alkylation of cytosine in DNA appears to be an important reaction that induces a potentially miscoding base, 3-N^4-ethanocytosine, in addition to O^6-(2-hydroxyethyl)guanine. The alkylation also results in cross-links between the DNA strands that are important in the cytotoxic action (*see* Scheme III) (*51, 52*).

Conversely, the weakly basic and weakly nucleophilic phosphate groups in the phosphodiester linkages between the deoxyribonucleoside units on the outside of the DNA chain are relatively more reactive towards alkylating agents with larger alkyl moieties. Thus, their reactivity increases through the series of agents introducing methyl < ethyl < isopropyl groups, somewhat more than would be expected on grounds of decreasing *s* values through this series.

This order is illustrated in Figure 3, in which the relative reactivities toward a spectrum of methylating and ethylating agents of the N-7 atom of guanine in DNA are compared with the reactivities at the O-6 atom of guanine (sterically near to the N-7 atom) and the reactivities at a representative phosphodiester group, thymidylyl-3′,5′-thymidine. Attack at the latter site would yield the corresponding alkyl dithymidylyl phosphotriester.

The relative reactivities, in terms of the Swain–Scott equations, applied to two nucleophiles, *Y* and *Z*, that react with two alkylating agents, *A* and *B*, are as follows. If n_y and n_z denote the respective nucleophilicities, and s_A and s_B denote the respective Swain–Scott substrate constants of the reactants, then the relative extents of reaction at the two sites for the two reagents will be given by:

$$\log (k_y/k_z)_A - \log (k_y/k_z)_B = (s_A - s_B)(n_y - n_z) \tag{5}$$

◁ *Scheme III. Reactions of chloroethylnitrosoureas with DNA. The groups X identified are N-1 of adenine, N-3 of cytosine, and O-6, N-7 of guanine* (51, 52). *Interstrand cross-linkages (a) between X,Y = N−7 of guanine have been identified* (52).

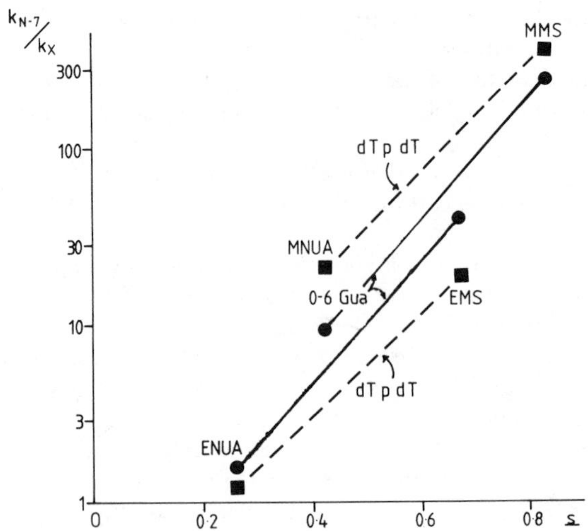

Figure 3. Relative reactivities of O-6 of guanine and of a typical phosphodiester site dTpdT in DNA toward alkylating agents according to the correlations of Swain and Scott (26).

The y-axis represents the difference between the nucleophilicities (Swain–Scott n*) of N-7 of guanine, the major nucleophilic center, and of the groups X = O-6 of guanine or dTpdT. The x-axis represents the substrate constant (or selectivity) of the alkylating agents (Swain–Scott factor* s*) as determined with a range of standard nucleophiles* (12). *The standard values are* n = 0 *for water and* s = 1 *for methyl bromide. According to the Swain–Scott equation log* $(k_y/k_0)_A = n_y s_A$ *where* k *is the second-order rate constant for reaction of a nucleophile* ($_y$) *of nucleophilicity* n_Y *with an alkylating agent* (A) *of substrate constant* s_A*, and* k_o *is the rate constant for reaction of* A *with solvent.*

Therefore a plot of the log of relative extents of reaction at sites *Y* and *Z*, log (k_y/k_z) vs. *s* for various alkylating agents, should be a straight line through the origin of slope equal to the difference in nucleophilicities of *Y* and *Z*.

As seen in Figure 3, this prediction is borne out to some extent by the data, and the apparent nucleophilicities of the sites in DNA toward the methylating and ethylating carcinogens have been estimated: N-7 atom of guanine, 3.5; O-6 atom of guanine, 1.2; and the typical phosphodiester group, dTpdT, 1 (*53, 54*). These apparent nucleophilicities are based on the value 2.5 for an average DNA nucleotide unit (*55*).

Evidently deviations from the simple Swain–Scott predictions occur; in particular the influence of decreasing Swain–Scott *s* factors is more marked for the ethylating than for the methylating agents, and is also more marked for the phosphodiester group than for the O-6 atom of guanine. The isopropylation of DNA has not been studied in such detail, but about 90% of the products from isopropyl methanesulfonate and DNA could not be accounted for as alkylated bases (*56*), and are therefore most probably phosphotriesters.

Two factors can be invoked to account for these comparative data. First, the reaction at O-atom sites is additionally favored by a component of S_N1 reactivity; second, this tendency can be reinforced by the steric factor, as results with branching of the alkyl chain, which, according to Ingold's concepts, enhances S_N1 reactivity.

The involvement of a component of S_N1 reactivity in DNA alkylations has apparently been contraindicated to some extent by studies with propylating carcinogens conducted by Park et al. (*41, 42*) (Scheme IV). They point out that reaction through the *n*-propylcarbonium ion [more strictly termed carbenium ion, according to Olah (*57*)] would permit partial isomerization to the isopropyl derivative, which could then be detected in the products. The products from hydrolysis of the propyldiazonium intermediate generated either by metabolic activation of *N*-nitrosodi(*n*-propyl)amine or by chemical activation in aqueous solution of *N*-*n*-propyl-*N*-nitrosourea did show a considerable proportion (17–39%) of isopropyl alcohol. However, an appreciable extent of isomerization was not detected in the product from DNA alkylated at N-7 of guanine. This finding accords with S_N2 alkylation by the alkyldiazonium ion or its precursors as the predominant mechanism. It would be interesting to determine whether such isomerization was more marked during reactions at O-atom sites in DNA, because these sites are expected to effect a higher S_N1 component of reaction than at the more nucleophilic N-7 site.

See also the "Note Added in Proof," page 467.

A comprehensive review of the relative reactivities of the methylated and ethylated sites in DNA has been given by Swenson (*58*) and is summarized in Table VI. Available data show that these relative reactivities also apply to alkylation in vivo shortly after administration of the alkylating agents, but an important proviso with regard to subsequently observed extents of alkylation is that the sites and therefore reactivity may be modified by DNA repair processes.

These considerations lead to a discussion of the biological consequences of the various DNA alkylations that appear to be of particular significance in determining carcinogenic potency. One of the most important consequences for carcinogenesis is the ability of alkylating carcinogens to act as directly miscoding mutagens. Figure 4 shows some significant modes of miscoding of alkylated bases. The available evidence suggests that miscoding of O^6-alkylguanines with thymine is the most important cause of such mutations, with the complementary miscoding of O^4-alkylthymines as the principal secondary source of mutation.

Other suggestions have encompassed almost all other alkylations (*62*) and subsequent hydrolytic removals of alkylated bases from DNA, such as depurination of 3- and 7-alkylpurines (*63, 64*). No doubt all these processes have their appropriate repair systems, so that the net effects of alkylation will be complex to interpret in terms of detailed processes.

An overall expression of the salient factors in mutagenesis induced by direct miscoding of altered bases can be expressed as follows:

$$\frac{M}{Z} = n_M \times \sum_i \left(f_i \times p_{M,i} \frac{(1 - r_{M,i})}{g_i} \right) \quad (6)$$

where M is the mutations induced per surviving cell, phage, and so on; Z is the extent of overall alkylation per nucleotide unit (P atom) of DNA; n_M is the number

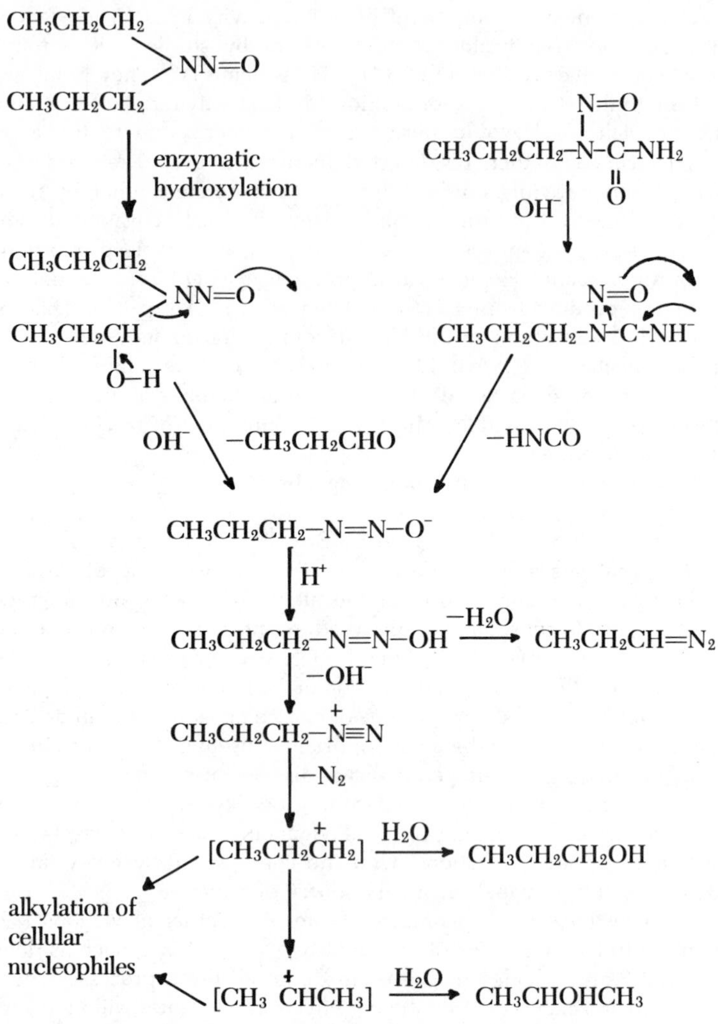

Scheme IV. Mechanism for the microsomal metabolism of N-*nitrosodi*-n-*propylamine and the base-catalyzed decomposition of* N-n-*propyl*-N-*nitrosourea.*

The mechamisms are analagous to those suggested for the simpler N-*nitrosodialkylamines and* N-*alkyl*-N-*nitrosoureas in general* (see also *Scheme V). If the* n-*propyldiazonium ion, $CH_3CH_2CH_2N_2^+$, reacts through the S_N2 mechanism, isomerization will not result. If the carbenium (often formerly termed carbonium) ion $CH_3CH_2CH_2^+$ is generated by the S_N1 mechanism, some isomerization to the isopropyl ion will occur. With water as the nucleophilic reactant, about 30% of the total propanols formed were isopropyl alcohol* (40)*; with RNA, of the total 7-propylguanine formed, only a "minor" proportion was 7-isopropylguanine; and with DNA it was considered that the S_N1 mechanism was "probably not involved"* (41). See also *the "Note Added in Proof"*

Table VI

Relative Reactivities of Sites in DNA Toward Methylating and Ethylating Carcinogens

Site in DNA	*Methyl Methanesulfonate*	*Ethyl Methanesulfonate*	N-*Methyl*-N-*nitrosourea*	N-*Ethyl*-N-*nitrosourea*
Adenine N-1	1.9	1.7	0.9	0.3
N-3	11.3	4.2	8.4	2.8
N-6[a]	n.d.	n.d.	n.d.	n.d.
N-7	1.8	1.9	2.0	0.4
Cytosine O-2[a]	n.d.	0.3	n.d.	2.9
N-3	0.7	0.4	0.5	0.2
Guanine N-1	n.d.	n.d.	n.d.	n.d.
N-2	0.6	n.d.	n.d.	n.d.
N-3	0.3	0.3	0.6	0.6
O-6[a]	0.2	2.1	6.0[b]	7.9
N-7	81.4	58.4	66.4[b]	11.0
Thymidine O-2[a]	n.d.	n.d.	0.1	7.8
N-3	0.08	n.d.	n.d.	n.d.
O-4[a]	n.d.	n.d.	0.7	1.0
Phosphodiester[c]	0.82	12.0	12.1	55.4

NOTE: For details of methods and other relevant references, *see* Ref. 58; values are expressed as percentage of total alkylation products.
n.d.: Not detected in this series of determinations.
[a]Extranuclear atom.
[b]The ratio for O^6-methylguanine/7-methylguanine reported in Ref. 58 is somewhat lower than the generally observed value of 0.11 (*see* Refs. 59 and 60).
[c]Based on a value assuming random alkylation of phosphodiester sites of 13.7 × alkylation of thymidylyl-3′,5′-thymidine phosphodiester site; for a detailed discussion, *see* Ref. 54.

of nucleotide sites at which mutation can be induced; f_i is the fraction of total alkylations at a site assumed to cause miscoding (e.g., O-6 of guanine); g_i is the proportion of total DNA bases of type "*i*", e.g., the molar proportion of guanine in mammalian DNA is 0.21; $P_{m\,i}$ is the probability that the assumed reaction "*i*" will cause miscoding; and $r_{M,i}$ is the proportion of assumed miscoding base removed from DNA by repair enzymes before alkylated DNA replicates.

As an example of the experimental possibilities for specification of these various factors, Lawley and Martin (*65*) used [^{14}C]ethyl methanesulfonate as the mutagen and obtained a quantitative correlation between extent of alkylation of a bacteriophage (T4rIIAP72) and induced reversion mutation to wild-type T4; Krieg (*66*) had previously shown that this mutation occurs by GC → AT transition at a single base-pair site. From experimental data, M, Z, f_i (in this case 0.026 for O^6-ethylguanine), and g_i (0.17) were obtained, and n_M, as stated, was taken as unity. The value of the product of the remaining factors, $p_{M,i}$ $(1 - r_{M,i})$, that emerged was 0.36 ± 0.11. Apportionment between the separate factors remained speculative. Because the host bacterium *Escherichia coli* had been found to remove O^6-alkylguanine from DNA by enzymic repair (*67, 68*), ethylated phage would probably effect the same removal, and $r_{M,i}$ would then be significantly positive. With regard to the probability of the miscoding, $p_{M,i}$, a value of less than unity was found for the analogous O^6-methylguanine by Abbott and Saffhill (*69*) in a study of

(a) THE NORMAL BASE PAIRS

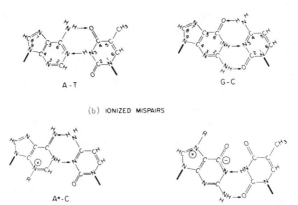

A - T

G - C

(b) IONIZED MISPAIRS

A*-C

G*-T

(c) MISPAIRS WITH ALKYLATED BASES

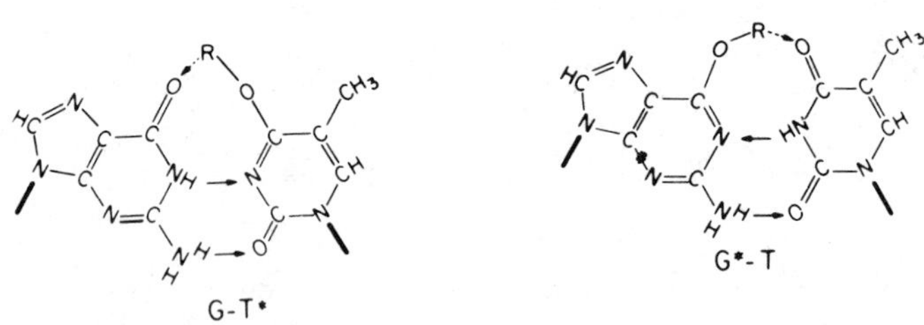

(d) EFFECT OF $\underline{N}^2$-ARALKYLATION OF GUANINE

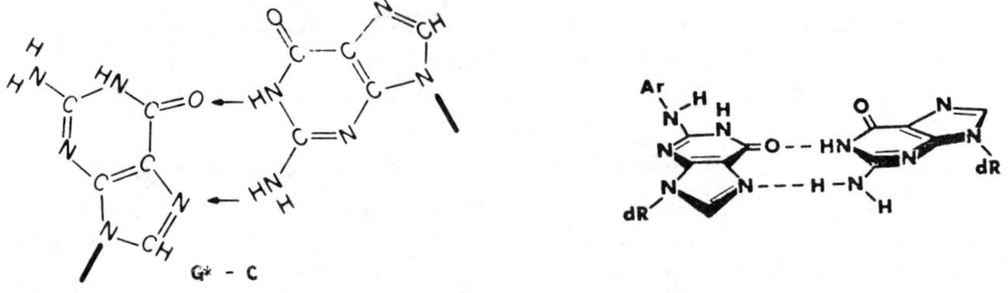

Figure 4. Normal Watson–Crick base pairs and suggested anomalous base pairs in which there is virtually no distortion of the overall dimensions. (Reproduced with permission from Refs. 62 and 132.)

Key for b: alkylated bases (R = alkyl) A, 3-alkyladenine* (66) *and G*, 7-alkylguanine* (135). *Key for c: G*, O^6-alkylguanine* (10) *and T*, O^4-alkylthymine* (131). *Key for d: G*, guanine rotated about the* N-*glycosidic linkage to the DNA chain* (132). See also *the "Note Added in Proof."*

N-methyl-*N*-nitrosourea-methylated poly(dG-dC) as a template for DNA polymerase I (DNA nucleotidyltransferase) of *E. coli,* and this probability value might also apply to the phage polymerase.

Newbold et al. (*70*) correlated alkylation of cellular DNA by dimethyl sulfate (DMS) or *N*-methyl-*N*-nitrosourea (MNU) in the V79-4 line of Chinese hamster cells with induced forward mutation to 8-azaguanine resistance. These data support the view that, at low doses and high survival, methylation of DNA at the O-6 atom of guanine is the principal cause of mutation, whereas methylation of adenine at the N-3 atom appears to be the principal cause of cytotoxic action.

In this case the relationships between induced mutation for each survivor and administered dose, *D* (m*M*), deviated significantly from linearity

$$M_A = a_A D_A + b_A D_A^{\ 2} + \ldots \qquad (6)$$

where subscript *A* denotes a mutagenic agent, and a_A and b_A are constants characteristic of that agent. Survival of colony-forming ability for the two compounds followed similar nonlinear functions of dose, and the ratio of equisurvival doses was about 6; DMS was the more effective cytotoxic agent.

On the other hand, MNU was the more effective mutagenic agent and, for the range of low dose and high survival, the ratio $a_{MNU}:a_{DMS}$ was about 4. In terms of Equation 6, these coefficients represent values of $(M/Z)_A \times (Z/D)_A$ as $Z \rightarrow 0$. To correlate mutation and alkylation, the extents of formation per unit dose of O^6-methylguanine, 7-methylguanine, and 3-methyladenine in cellular DNA were determined by chemical analysis, i.e., values were determined for $(f_{O\text{-}6} \times Z/D)_A$. Because both DMS and MNU methylated DNA at the same chemical sites but in different proportions, probably the values of the remaining parameters of Equation 6—target size, probability of miscoding, and repair of DNA—are the same for both agents.

Because removal of O^6-methylguanine from DNA of these cells by the rapid DNA repair mechanism (possibly demethylation) could not be detected (*71*), the factor $r_{M,\,O\text{-}6}$ can be put as zero, and Equation 6 then becomes

$$\left(\frac{M}{f_{O\text{-}6} \times z}\right)_{MNU} = \left(\frac{M}{f_{O\text{-}6} \times z}\right)_{DMS} = \frac{n_M \times p_{M,O\text{-}6}}{g} \qquad (8)$$

The observed values of these experimentally determined quantities were about 230 for MNU and about 300 for DMS, i.e., approximately equal within reasonable limits of experimental error. With the assumption that p_M would be about 4, because four cell divisions occurred during the measurements of mutation frequency, the apparent target size n_M could thus be estimated as about 13 guanine deoxyribonucleotide units in cellular DNA. This result is much smaller than the number of guanines (about 300) in the gene coding for a subunit of the enzyme that is inactivated by the mutations (*72*), but this discrepancy might be reasonably accounted for by assuming a lower probability of miscoding or by assuming that most miscoding would not cause sufficient modification of the gene product to eliminate enzymic activity.

A somewhat analogous conclusion that the methylation of target DNA at the O-6 atom of guanine is a major source of mutagenesis in mammalian cells was reached by Sega et al. (*73*) from results of a study of alkylation-induced dominant lethal mutations in germ cells of male mice. This type of mutation appears to be caused either by alkylation of protamine in the target sperm cells (essentially a cytotoxic action) that was the principal mode of action with the S_N2 agents methyl and ethyl methanesulfonates, or by alkylation of O-atoms in DNA that appeared to be the predominant significant action of MNU.

Comparative determinations of extent of methylation of DNA and protamine in sperm heads from 4 h to about 15 d after intraperitoneal injection of alkylating agents were made for chemical dosimetry. The correlations between the time courses of the alkylations and of the induced dominant lethal mutations showed that MNU was about 17 times as effective a mutagen per sperm head methylation as methyl methanesulfonate, but was much less able to methylate protamine. This approach suggests strongly that overall ability of carcinogens to induce dominant lethal mutations (including the essentially cytotoxic component) will not correlate quantitatively with carcinogenic potency, whereas ability to induce such mutations through alkylation of DNA, rather than of protein, might correlate better.

Alkylating agents in general can induce dominant lethal mutations in male mice (*73–83*) (*see* Table VII), and in view of the previous remarks, a quantitative positive correlation between these effects and carcinogenic potency of the agents seems unlikely.

Table VII

Induction of Dominant Lethal Mutations in Male Mammals by Alkylating Agents

	Type of Cell Affected			
Compound	*Spermatozoa (weeks 1–2)*	*Spermatids (weeks 3–5)*	*Spermatocytes (weeks 6–8)*	*References*
Methyl methanesulfonate	++	++	−	74,75
Ethyl methanesulfonate				
mouse	++	++	−	74
rat	++	++	−	76
n-Propyl methanesulfonate	++	++	−	77
Isopropyl methanesulfonate				
mouse	+	+	++	77
rat	+	+	++	76
Trimethyl phosphate	++	++		78
N-Methyl-*N*′-nitro-*N*-nitrosoguanidine	−	−	−	74
ICR-170 (**4**)	−	−	−	74
Butadiene dioxide	−	−	−	79
	++	+	+	80
Myleran (**5**)	++	−	++	80
TEM	++	++	+	81
	++	++	+	80
Tepa, thio Tepa (**6**)	+	+	−	79
Trenimon (**7**)	+	+	−	82
Cyclophosphamide (**8**)	+	+	−	83

NOTE: Except where indicated, the animal tested was the mouse. "Mutagenic" effects refer to measurements of preimplantation loss.

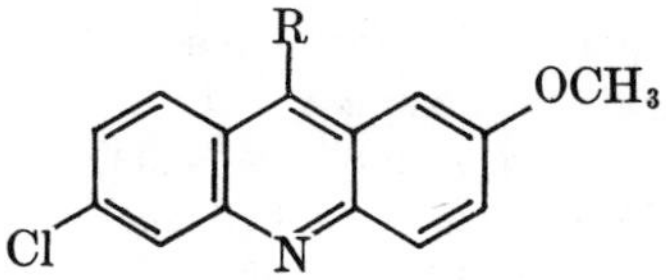

Acridine (quinacrine) mustards—
ICR-49, R = $—NH(CH_2)_3N(CH_2CH_2Cl)_2$;
ICR-50a, R = $—NH\ CH(CH_3)(CH_2)_3N(CH_2CH_2Cl)_2$;
ICR-170, R = $—NH\ (CH_2)_3N(C_2H_5)CH_2CH_2Cl$;
ICR-191, R = $—NH(CH_2)_3\ NH\ CH_2CH_2Cl$

4

$CH_3SO_2O(CH_2)_nOSO_2CH_3$ Methylene dimethanesulfonate, $n = 1$;
Myleran (Busulphan), $n = 4$

5

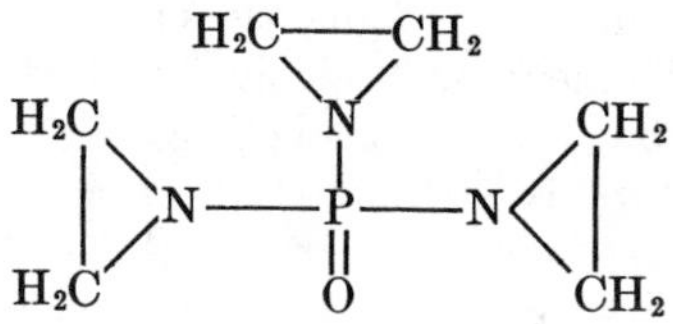

6

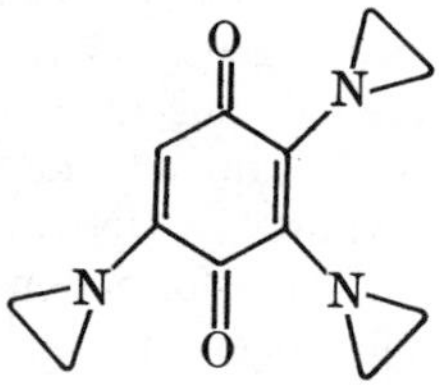

7

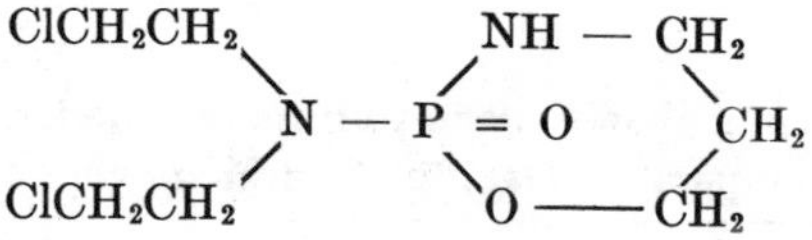

8

More recent interest in methods for study of mammalian mutagenesis has therefore been directed increasingly towards detection of more subtle changes in the genetic material, such as point mutations, which might result from miscoding at single base-pair sites. The correlations between chemistry of the alkylation of DNA and carcinogenic potency of alkylating agents have indicated that this miscoding is important. This area of research has been reviewed fairly extensively (*84, 85*), but so far insufficient quantitative data are available to warrant detailed discussion here of any chemical correlates. Russell et al. (*86*) consider *N*-ethyl-*N*-nitrosourea to be "by far the most potent mutagen yet discovered in the mouse." It is about five times as effective as X-radiation. A dose of 250 mg/kg of this chemical carcinogen to male mice induced temporary sterility, but mutant offspring could be obtained after this period from matings with females of a specific locus test strain, with 87 times the spontaneous mutation frequency. This finding may presage a correlation between alkylation-induced point mutations in mammals and O^6-alkylation of guanine in DNA.

The important cytogenetic technique of detection of sister chromatid exchange (SCE) (*87*, reviewed in Ref. 88) allows rapid screening of carcinogens in mammalian cells, including human cells (principally applied to lymphocytes). This phenomenon might be assumed a priori to be a reflection of cytotoxic damage and therefore, as with the induction of dominant lethals, unlikely to correlate with induced DNA miscoding. However mutagens that react more extensively at the O-6 atom of guanine did appear to be outstandingly effective inducers of SCE (*89*). A more detailed correlation with DNA alkylation has been started by Swenson et. al. (*90*). This rapid screening test may therefore prove to have some degree of quantitative correlation with carcinogenic potency. However, relatively weak carcinogens such as methyl methanesulfonate are to some extent effective inducers of SCE; thus, quantitative correlation with the amount of miscoding bases in DNA seems unlikely to be absolute, and 3-methyladenine (and possibly 3-methylthymine) in DNA were considered as other possible lesions causing SCE.

Transformation of mammalian cells in culture is often termed "in vitro carcinogenesis" because the transformed cells, assessed by criteria of changed morphological growth pattern or of ability to grow indefinitely on culture in semisolid media such as soft agar, can be shown to yield injection site tumors after appropriate culture in vitro. This screening test is widely advocated for environmental carcinogens. Representative results from a recent compilation (*91*) are shown in Table VIII. Again the wide spectrum of effective compounds failed to

Table VIII

Transformation of Mammalian Cells in Culture by Alkylating Agents and Related Compounds, with Comparative Data for Noncarcinogens

Compound	*Cryopreserved Hamster Embryo Cells (Pienta)*	*Baby Hamster Kidney BHK 21/Cl 13 Cells (Styles)*	*Enhancement of Adenovirus Transformation in Hamster Embryo Cells (Casto)*
Acetamide	+		
Benzyl chloride	+		
Bis(chloromethyl) ether		+	+
1,4-Butane sultone	+		
Cisplatin (*cis*-Dichlorodiammine platinum) (II) (**9**)			+
Chlorambucil		+	
Chloroform		−	−

Table VIII Continued

Compound	*Cryopreserved Hamster Embryo Cells (Pienta)*	*Baby Hamster Kidney BHK 21/Cl 13 Cells (Styles)*	*Enhancement of Adenovirus Transformation in Hamster Embryo Cells (Casto)*
Cyclophosphamide	+		
1,2-Dichloroethane		+	+
1,2,3,4-Diepoxybutane	+		
Dimethylcarbamoyl chloride (**10**)	+		
1,2-Epoxybutane	+		
DL-Ethionine (**11**)	+	+	
Ethyl carbamate (urethane)	–[a]		
Ethylene dibromide			+
Ethylenethiourea		+	
Ethyl methanesulfonate		+	+
Ethyl *p*-toluenesulfonate	+		
Glycidaldehyde	+		
Glycidol	+		
Hexamethylphosphoramide (**12**)		+	
Methyl iodide	+		
Methyl methanesulfonate			+
Mitomycin C (**13**)		+	
Naphthylamine mustard			+
Nitrogen mustard (HN2)		+	
1,3-Propane sultone	+	+	+
β-Propiolactone		+	
Propyleneimine	+		
Propylene oxide			+
Succinic anhydride	+		
Thioacetamide	+		
Uracil mustard	+		
Vinyl chloride		+	
	Noncarcinogenic Controls		
Caffeine		–	+
ε-Caprolactone	–		
Cyclohexylamine		–	+
DDT		–	
Dicyclohexylamine		–	
Dieldrin		–	
Diethylthiourea		–	
Dimethylformamide	–	–	
Dimethyl sulfoxide	–		
Ethanol	–		–
Ethylene glycol			–
Hexachlorocyclohexane		–	
Hydroxylamine hydrochloride	–		+
Maleimide			–
Methyl carbamate	–		
Phenobarbital		–	
Thiourea			–

NOTE: Blank denotes not investigated in this study. For details, *see* Ref. 91.
[a]Reported positive using metabolic activation with liver microsomes.

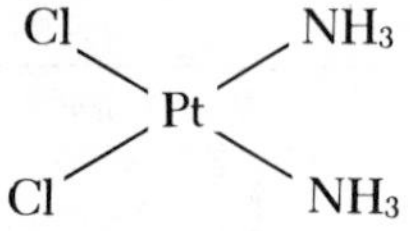

$Cl_2Pt(NH_3)_2$

9

$(CH_3)_2NCOCl$

10

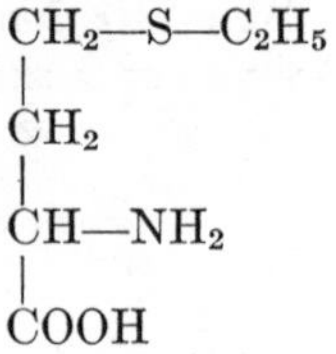

$CH_2—S—C_2H_5$
CH_2
$CH—NH_2$
$COOH$

11

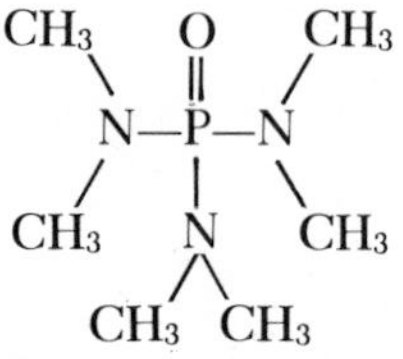

$[(CH_3)_2N]_3P{=}O$

12

H_2N, H_3C, O, O, CH_2OCONH_2, OCH_3, N, NH

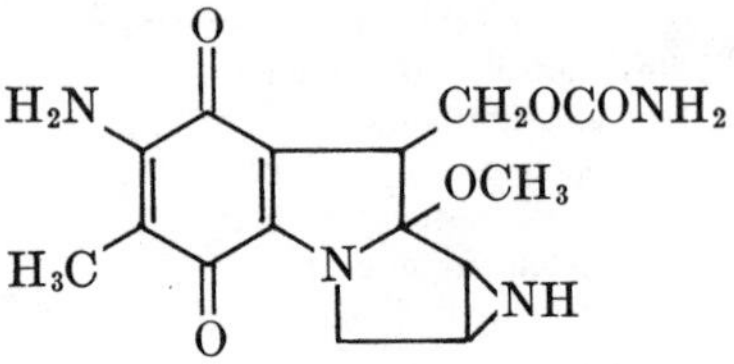

13

suggest any quantitative correlations with carcinogenic potency, although excellent concordance was found between simple ability of a compound to act as a mutagen and as a transforming agent.

Several apparently unresolved questions emerge on the relationship between these studies in vitro and carcinogenesis in vivo. Styles (*92*), in accord with the views expressed here concerning the relevance of chemical reactivity to carcinogenic potency, considered that transformation in vitro "appears to detect DNA-reactive compounds and is probably registering a mutational event," but apparently is "not capable of predicting carcinogenic potency."

Price and Mishra (*93*) used Fischer rat embryo cells infected with a murine leukemia (type-C) virus that is adapted to grow in rat cells and tested the ability of carcinogens and related compounds to cause their transformation. They considered that "complex biologic promotion by the very ubiquitous type-C virus most certainly exists in most if not all mammalian species, including man." Di Paolo and Casto (*94, 95*) developed a test system in which enhancement of adenovirus-induced transformation by chemical carcinogens is assayed. Their results indicate that cocarcinogenic action of chemicals and tumor virus (whether the genetic material is RNA, as with murine leukemia virus, or DNA, as with adenovirus) may be required for efficient in vitro transformation. However, according to Heidelberger (*96*), this synergism is not essential.

Transformation of cells of the 3T3 line derived from the Balb/c strain of mice has also been used extensively in tests of chemical carcinogenesis in vitro (*97*). An analogous cell line derived from NIH Swiss mice has been used to demonstrate that transformation can be effected by DNA extracted from other transformed cell lines (*98*), including some where a chemical carcinogen (3-methylcholanthrene) was used as the transforming agent.

These experiments can therefore be interpreted as showing that some modification of cellular DNA is involved in transformation in certain cases. For example, in one series of experiments, 5 out of 15 DNAs extracted from mouse or rat cell lines that were transformed by 3-methylcholanthrene induced transformed foci in NIH-3T3 cells (*98*). The effective part of the transfecting DNA was indicated to contain a single small fragment of less than 30×10^3 base pairs, i.e., about the size of a single gene.

The main progress in this field has been made by using viral transformation, but the essential *onc* genes responsible for transformation are homologous to genes of the host animal cells. A human *onc* gene homologous to the transforming gene of a simian sarcoma virus has been detected (*99*).

The relationship between transformation of cells in vitro and carcinogenesis in vivo remains unresolved (*100*). Apparently, multiple discrete stages occur in carcinogenesis in vivo; transformation of a cell line may represent one of these stages, possibly a single mutation. Also, transformation appears to be associated with an increased level of expression of *onc* genes in certain cases. The nature of the target genes for chemical mutagens in transformation and their relationship to the *onc* genes is still undefined.

See also the "Note Added in Proof," page 467.

Because the rapid screening tests for carcinogens are thought to be essentially indirect tests of the ability of chemicals to react with DNA in target cells, it remains possible that the essential action of mutagens in carcinogenesis is not in fact to act as conventional mutagens, but to produce some associated biological effect. In a screening test (*101*) using appropriate strains of *Drosophila melanogaster* to indicate the ability of chemicals to cause somatic eye-color "mutations" at relatively high frequencies (on the order of 10% or more), X-rays and ethyl methanesulfonate showed positive results.

Subsequently, Fahmy and Fahmy (*102*) studied a wider variety of carcinogens, and dose–response relationships were determined for certain aflatoxins, nitroso compounds, and polycyclic aromatic hydrocarbons. These experiments show "experimental evidence for the high efficiency of carcinogens in effecting alterations in the transcriptional activity of this system during the growth and differentiation of eye tissue" (*103*). They suggest that the induced changes are epigenetic and involve induced aberrant differentiation, perhaps mediated by changes in the orientation of transposable elements in the genome. This interpretation has been challenged by Auerbach (*104*), who considered that the results could be attributed to a mutation that causes deletion of the transposing element.

The question of quantitative correlations between carcinogenicity of alkylating agents and results of tests using activation of tumor virus from mammalian cells or bacteriophage from bacterial cells also remains unresolved. Teich et al. (*105*) compared the ability of various mutagens and inhibitors of DNA synthesis to induce murine leukemia virus from cultured AKR mouse embryo cell lines and found that methyl and ethyl methanesulfonates were ineffective. The more potent alkylating carcinogens such as *N*-methyl-*N*-nitrosourea were not tested.

In analogous bacterial tests, the induction of lysogeny in *E. coli* (λ) strains (*106*) has been used with a variety of alkylating agents (reviewed in Refs. 107 and 108). Loveless (*107, 109*) concluded that difunctional and polyfunctional alkylating agents were better inducers of *E. coli* K12 (λ) than monofunctional agents, and this finding accords with their greater cytotoxicity but not with mutagenicity or carcinogenicity. Prophage λ induction in *E. coli* K12 *enVA uvrB* was proposed as a highly sensitive test for potential carcinogens (*110*), but was considered to be inferior for this purpose when compared with the straightforward mutagenicity tests (*111*); a preferred test would be the Ames test that uses induced reversions of auxotrophic *Salmonella* strains (*112, 113*).

A very comprehensive comparative study of rapid-screening test systems (*114*) examined 10 pairs of chemically related "carcinogens" and "noncarcinogens" (appropriately defined); the prophage λ "inductest" correctly registered 12 out of 25 carcinogens and incorrectly registered 3 out of 17 noncarcinogens (*115*). The alkylating agents chosen for pairing were β-propiolactone (**14**) (carcinogen) versus γ-butyrolactone (**15**) (noncarcinogen); cyclophosphamide (**8**) and epichlorhydrin

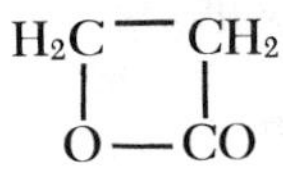

H_2C—CH_2 / O—CO (four-membered ring)

14

H_2C—CH_2 / CH_2, CO / O (five-membered ring)

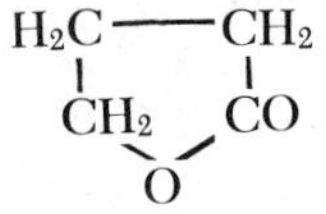

15

(**16**) were used as miscellaneous carcinogens, and the supposed acylating agent dimethylcarbamoyl chloride (**10**) (carcinogen) was paired with dimethylformamide (**17**) (noncarcinogen). β-Propiolactone gave "clear positive responses" in

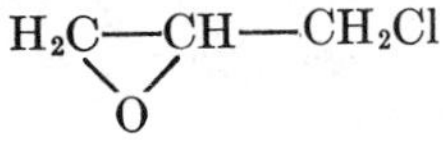

H_2C—CH—CH_2Cl (epoxide, O bridging H_2C and CH)

16

$HCON(CH_3)_2$

17

90% of the in vitro systems (*116*). γ-Butyrolactone—which is generally regarded as a nonreactive lactone, because it does not have the ring strain conferred by the β-lactone structure—was negative in 80% of the assays, although, somewhat surprisingly, it proved a positive transforming agent for BHK cells. Epichlorhydrin and dimethylcarbamoyl chloride behaved as directly acting mutagens in all tests, and cyclophosphamide required metabolic activation in the in vitro microbial test systems but gave positive results in the test that used eukaryotic cells and yeast. Dimethylformamide was negative in all tests as expected.

Several studies of the reactions of β-propiolactone with DNA in vitro and in vivo have been conducted. Initially, the principal reactive center was shown to be the N-7 atom of guanine, as expected for this reagent because of its relatively high Swain–Scott *s* factor of 0.77 (*117*).

In a comparative study of several alkylating agents, which included a spectrum of carcinogenic potencies, the relative abilities to alkylate DNA and protein of a target tissue, mouse skin, were assessed (*118, 119*). β-Propiolactone (a potent initiator of skin tumors) reacted much more extensively with DNA than did 3-iodopropionic acid (a weaker initiator) and much more extensively than 3-chloropropionic acid and iodacetamide (noninitiators). This relatively weak affinity for reaction with DNA but high affinity for reaction with proteins is in line with the higher *s* factors for the halogenated carboxylic acids (e.g., $s = 1.33$ for iodoacetate; Table II).

β-Propiolactone was deduced to cause *r* mutations in 74 phage through GC→AT transitions (*120*), and these mutations may result from miscoding of O^6-alkylguanine following the hypothesis presented by Loveless (*10*). However, extensive studies of the in vitro reactions of β-propiolactone with DNA have so far not shown evidence for *O*-alkylation (*121*). The products detected (with their relative extents of formation in DNA) were 1-carboxyethyladenine (0.1–0.23), 3-carboxyethylcytosine (0.28–0.41), 7-carboxyethylguanine (1.00), and 3-carboxyethylthymine (0.29–0.39). The relative reactivities of the minor sites of alkylation appear to be somewhat higher than for the methylating agents (Table VI).

A further suggestion for the promutagenic base derived from β-propiolactone came from Chen et al. (*122*) who found a ring-closed derivative of 1-carboxyethyldeoxyadenosine, 3-(β-D-2-deoxyribosyl)-7,8-dihydropyrimido[2,1-*i*]purine-9-one (**18**) as a product from deoxyadenosine.

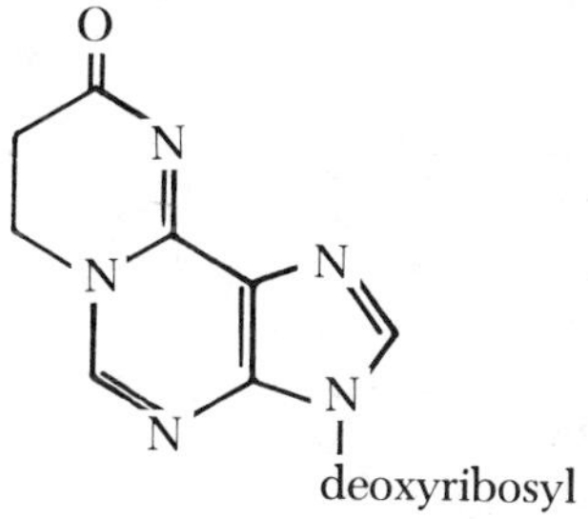

O
N
N
N
N
N
deoxyribosyl

18

In common with methylating agents (*69, 123, 124*) and chloroacetaldehyde (*125, 127*), β-propiolactone is able to modify synthetic deoxyribonucleotide templates and cause misincorporation of noncomplementary bases (in the Watson–Crick sense) in vitro (*128*). With the methylating carcinogens, miscoding induced in vitro can be attributed to mispairing of specific bases, particularly O^6-methylguanine and O^4-methylthymine, which were predicted (*10, 131*) to give the best steric fit in the Watson–Crick model for DNA replication, i.e., without much distortion of the double helix (*see* Figure 4). However, mispairing was not evident with β-propiolactone (*see* Table IX). Poly (dA) · oligo (dT) was used as template for DNA polymerase from avian myeloblastosis virus or from sea urchin, with up to one molecule of β-propiolactone bound per 180 template nucleotides, causing up to about one misincorporation of cytosine per normal incorporation of thymidine (*127*).

The provisional conclusion from the limited amount of work in this field is that *O*-alkylation of DNA bases is positively associated with miscoding in vitro for methylating agents, but for other carcinogens other types of miscoding may occur that so far do not fit in obvious fashion with the predictions from the Watson–Crick scheme.

Interesting suggestions for miscoding by arylated or aralkylated bases have been proposed by Kadlubar (*132, 133*).[1] A predominant reaction of metabolically activated 2-naphthylamine [a well-documented carcinogen in humans (Chapter 5)] occurs at the O-6 atom of guanine in DNA, but does not cause appreciable distortion of the double helix (*133*). With aralkylating metabolites of polycyclic aromatic hydrocarbons or with directly acting aralkylating agents, the predominant site of reaction in DNA is at N-2 of guanine (*see* Ref. 139 and Chapters 2 and 4), and Kadlubar (*132*) points out that a miscoding causing GC→CG transversions is a possibility if the attached aralkylated base rotates about its glycosidic linkage to the DNA macromolecular chain during replication.

Of the various miscoding possibilities illustrated in Figure 4, the ones that are likely to be involved in cancer-causative mutations are shown in Figure 5. The main factor that quantitatively influences the miscodings of O^6-methylguanine and O^4-methylthymine is the reactivity of the methylating agent; for example, *N*-methyl-*N*-nitrosoureas will be more effective than dimethyl sulfate or methyl methanesulfonate. This order accords with known mutagenic and carcinogenic potencies of these agents.

With aralkylating agents, the quantitative prediction becomes more subtle, and relative extents of attack on the extranuclear O-6 and N-2 atoms of guanine in DNA together with the frequency of miscoding of N^2-aralkylguanine or N^2-arylguanine would be significant factors.

With the metabolites of vinyl chloride, miscoding due to O^6-alkylation of guanine is possible in addition to the miscodings indicated in Table IX (*134*). The principal reaction product between deoxyguanosine and chloroethylene oxide, 7-(2-oxoethyl)guanine (**19a**), has been shown to be in equilibrium with the hemiacetal form (**19b**), which by elimination of water would yield the potentially miscoding base, O^6,N^7-ethenoguanine (**20**).

[1] These suggestions are also relevant to the discussions of aromatic hydrocarbons (Chapter 2), amines (Chapter 2), and activated metabolites thereof (Chapter 8) in this volume.

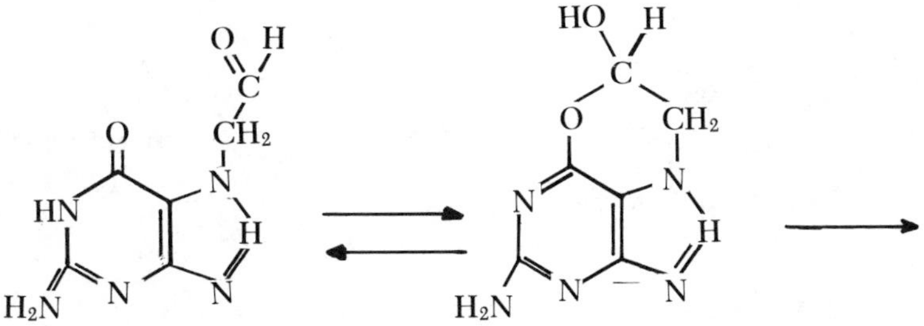

19a

19b

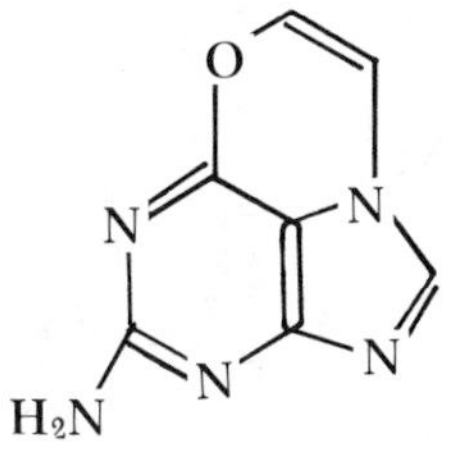

20

The research discussed can be used to amend and extend the original concepts of the theory that carcinogens act by inducing potentially miscoding bases in target DNA. The first proposal by Lawley and Brookes (*135*) that alkylation of DNA at the principal nucleophilic center, the N-7 of guanine, potentiated miscoding through the zwitterionic form of the 7,9-disubstituted guanine residue in DNA was contraindicated by comparative studies of methyl methanesulfonate and MNU as mutagens for T-even bacteriophage (*10, 129*). The much higher mutagenicity of MNU was associated with its ability to form a relatively higher proportion of O^6-methylguanine in the alkylation products of DNA, thus effectively "fixing" the previously proposed ionized miscoding form (*see* Figure 4b and c). Evidently the lack of miscoding by the zwitterionic form conforms with the suggestion that ionized forms of bases are not accepted by DNA polymerase enzymes (*136*).

The hypothesis from Loveless (*10*) that miscoding by *O*-alkylated bases is a powerful cause of mutation is supported by studies of miscoding in vitro (Table IX). Evidently O^6-methylguanine and O^4-methylthymine can act as adenine and cytosine respectively, in the Watson–Crick sense, by being accepted by polymerase enzymes as miscoding bases without distortion of the double helical structure of DNA; therefore, in terms of Equation 6, the presence of these bases in the template at the time of DNA replication will cause mutations with a high probability factor p_i. Removal of these bases by DNA repair mechanisms may intervene however, and this factor will be discussed in more detail subsequently.

In addition to their importance for directly acting alkylating agents, these miscodings are expected to result from alkylations of DNA that are mediated by

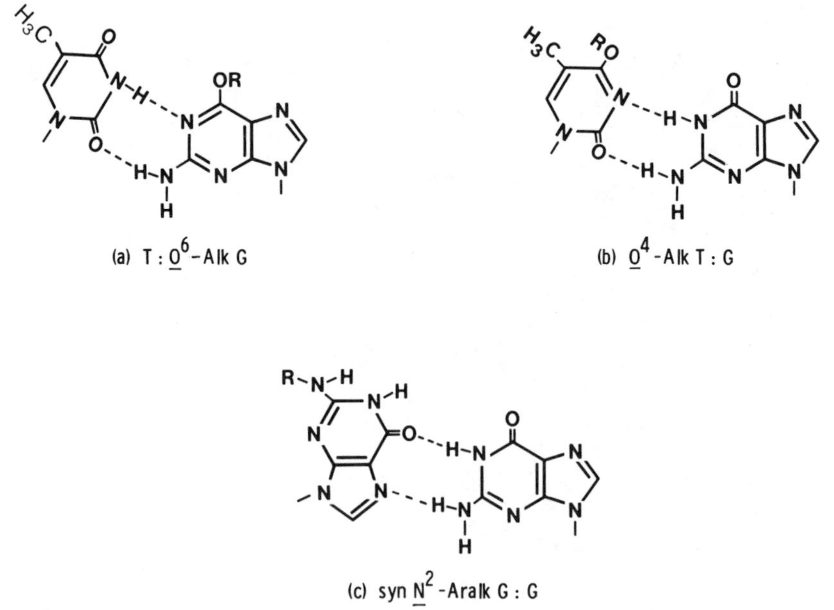

(a) T : $\underline{O}^6$-Alk G

(b) $\underline{O}^4$-Alk T : G

(c) syn $\underline{N}^2$-Aralk G : G

Carcinogens →	Chemical reaction →		Mispairing →		Mutation
Alkylating Agents & Dialkylnitrosamines	G–C	→ $\underline{O}^6$-AlkG–C	→	$\underline{O}^6$-AlkG–T	→ A–T
Aromatic Amines & Hydrocarbons	G–C	→ $\underline{N}^2$-ArG–C	→	Syn-$\underline{N}^2$-ArG–G	→ C–G

Figure 5. Miscoding of DNA bases suggested to be important in carcinogenesis.
(a) Miscoding of O^6-alkylguanine with thymine; (b) O^4-Alkylthymine with guanine (10, 131)*; (c) Miscoding of N^2-aralkylguanine with guanine* (132, 133)*; and (d) Mutations that are suggested to result from miscoding and are most likely to be important in carcinogenesis.* See also *the "Note Added in Proof."*

reactive metabolites of other carcinogens, such as *N*-nitrosodialkylamines and vinyl chloride, and from certain aromatic amines, notably 2-naphthylamine. The carcinogenic acylating agent dimethylcarbamoyl chloride can acylate DNA at the O-6 atom of guanine (*137*).

The aralkylating agents and metabolites of this type that are derived from polycyclic aromatic hydrocarbons react at the extranuclear N-2 atom of guanine in DNA (*138, 139*). Kadlubar's (*132*) suggestion for miscoding by N^2-guaninyl derivatives would invoke a certain probability for miscoding by these bases dependent on their confirmation at the time of DNA replication. O^6-Aralkylation of guanine in DNA has also been considered as a possible promutagenic reaction

Table IX

Miscoding by Alkylated Bases in Polydeoxyribonucleotide Templates in Vitro

Template	*Alkylating Mutagen*	*Polymerase Enzyme*	*Miscoding Base*	*Type of Miscoding*	*Efficiency of Miscoding*	*References*
Poly(dC-O^{6}MeG)	—[a]	RNA polymerase (*M. luteus*)	O^6-methylguanine	GC→GT(→AT)	~1	123
Poly(dC-dG)	dimethyl sulfate or *N*-methyl-*N*-nitrosourea	DNA polymerase I (*E. coli*)	O^6-methylguanine	GC→GT(→AT)	~0.5[b,c]	69
Poly(dA-dT)	dimethyl sulfate or *N*-methyl-*N*-nitrosourea	DNA polymerase I	O^4-methylthymine	AT→GT(→GC)	~1[d]	124,125
Poly(dA-dT)	chloroacetaldehyde[e]	DNA polymerase I	ethenoadenine	AT→AG(→CG)	~1/60	126
Poly(dC-dG)	chloroacetaldehyde	DNA polymerase I	ethenocytosine[f]	GC→AC(→AT)	~1/30	127

[a]Copolymer synthesized from deoxyribonucleotide precursors by using terminal deoxynucleotidyl transferase from calf thymus. O^6-Methyldeoxyguanosine was phosphorylated with carrot phosphotransferase.
[b]Dependent on amount of deoxycytidine triphosphate in medium; decreased amount of this precursor increased the efficiency.
[c]Significant miscoding by 3- or 7-methylguanines or 3-methylcytosine was contraindicated, a result that confirmed studies with bacteriophage (*128,129*).
[d]Significant miscoding by O^2-methylthymine, 1-,3-, and 7-methyladenines was contraindicated.

[e]Metabolite of vinyl chloride, $CH_2{=}CHCl \rightarrow \overset{\displaystyle O}{CH_2{-}CH}{-}Cl \rightarrow HCOCH_2Cl$ (epoxide: O bridging CH_2 and CH)
[f]Some miscoding by a guanine alkylation product; some misincorporation of thymine due to miscoding by ethenocytosine or the guanine product.

(*139*) as yet undetected, but for possibly explicable reasons. These topics are more fully discussed in Chapters 2 and 4.

The suggested miscodings that appear to be most important in mutations caused by carcinogens or chemical and physicochemical grounds are summarized in Figure 5.

The further possibility remains that miscoding "antimetabolites" generated by alkylation of DNA precursors could be accepted by polymerase enzymes, and thus incorporated into anomalous partner bases of DNA. This possible mode of action was suggested for cytotoxic alkylating agents by Timmis (*141*). The miscoding base O^6-methylguanine was not, however, incorporated into DNA in a detectable amount by bacterial or cultured mammalian cells (*142*), and the derived putative DNA precursor O^6-methyldeoxyguanosine is subject to demethylation by cytosol extracts from rat tissues (*143*), possibly by adenosine deaminase, a ubiquitous cellular enzyme. O^6-Ethyldeoxyguanosine was dealkylated at about only one-twentieth of the rate of the methyl analogue (*143*). A positive finding for incorporation of O^6-methylguanine into DNA of regenerating liver and intestine of rats (less than 1 fmol/mg of DNA) was reported by Pegg and Swann (*144*).

A small degree of incorporation of O^4-methylthymidine into DNA has been found for the cultured Chinese hamster cell line V79A (*145*). O^4-Methylthymidine (10^{-5} *M*) in growth medium caused substitution of about 1 per 10^6 thymidines in DNA, which was about the same level given by 0.5 m*M* MNU that resulted in 70% survival of cells. This finding is therefore consistent with the relatively weak action of cytosol extracts on this deoxyribonucleoside (*143*).

In summary, incorporation of miscoding bases into DNA of dividing cells remains an attractive possibility as a mechanism operative in carcinogenesis that is complementary to the miscoding by these bases that are induced into the template itself. So far evidence for this "antimetabolite" mechanism is lacking, and classical mutagens of this type, such as 5-bromodeoxyuridine, have not been found to act as carcinogens (*146, 147*). The miscoding probabilities of the classical mutagens, however, may well be quantitatively much less than for alkylated bases.

See also the "Note Added in Proof," page 468.

The alkylations of DNA that are expected to cause miscoding when alkylated cells divide will generally constitute only a minor fraction of the potential alkylation-induced damage to the template. Subsequent discussion will therefore deal with the related topics of alkylation reactions with DNA that are expected to cause inactivation of the template and the repair mechanisms that enable replication of the damaged DNA. As already noted, the net effect of these processes will depend on the nature of the alkylating agent, which affects the overall extent of alkylation and the relative extents of alkylation at various specific sites. The net effect also depends on subsequent processes: (1) further spontaneous chemical reactions such as cross-linking or hydrolytic removal (such as depurination) of alkylated bases, or (2) enzymically mediated removal of bases, with possibly the further stages of DNA strand breakage and reunion that complete repair processes.

The most conclusive evidence for mutagenesis induced by alkylating agents through the mechanism of direct miscoding so far available has come from the studies of Coulondre and Miller (*149*) with *E. coli.* A system was devised in which forward base substitution mutations could be analyzed at more than 80 possible sites of nonsense mutations (i.e., mutations that convert an amino acid codon to an amber- or ochre-chain termination codon) in the *lacI* gene of *E. coli.* This system enabled identification of mutations as transitions (GC→AT) and transversions (GT→TA; AT→TA; AT→CG; and GC→CG); the AT→GC transition could not be detected by forward mutations because of the nature of the genetic code, but could be determined by reversions and by conversions of ochre to amber mutants.

The action of two alkylating mutagens, *N*-methyl-*N*′-nitro-*N*-nitrosoguanidine and ethyl methanesulfonate, were compared with the action of UV radiation and nitroquinoline *N*-oxide. The alkylating agents induced base-substitution mutations with a remarkably high specificity of more than 99% for GC→AT transitions in forward mutations. The reversion studies showed that ethyl methanesulfonate induced AT→GC transitions at only about 0.01–0.02 of the frequency of GC→AT, while for *N*-methyl-*N*′-nitro-*N*-nitrosoguanidine, this factor was 0.01–0.10.

With regard to mechanisms, the first consideration was whether direct miscoding had occurred or whether action of error-prone repair mechanisms dependent on the *recA, lexA* system (*150*) was required. The second and related consideration was whether the results reflected the known chemistry of the action of the mutagens on DNA. If error-prone repair was the predominant cause of mutation, little if any correlation with initial chemical effects on DNA would be found, because any potentially cytotoxic modification of the template would stimulate this action. A third important factor was the distribution of the induced mutation frequency across the various sites. Very favored sites for mutation ("hotspots") were found for UV light and 2-aminopurine and were dependent on base sequence around the mutant site; no such hotspots were observed for the alkylating agents.

The results for the alkylating agents did conform to those expected for the direct miscoding mechanism. The spectra of mutation frequency vs. site of mutation were remarkably similar for both agents; therefore, the agents probably cause GC→AT transitions through the same process, despite their different reaction mechanisms. Ethyl methanesulfonate is classified as a "borderline" S_N1/S_N2 agent (*see* Table II), but *N*-methyl-*N*′-nitro-*N*-nitrosoguanidine methylates through the methyldiazonium ion (Scheme V) and therefore yields the same proportions of products in DNA as MNU. However, in aqueous media MNU reacts rapidly at pH 7 and 37 °C through an alkali-catalyzed decomposition, whereas the nitrosoguanidine reacts much more slowly unless thiols are present in the medium (*151*), and the thiol-catalyzed reaction appears to be its principal mode of methylation in cells. Evidently both the direct ethylation by the S_N1/S_N2 agent and the thiol-catalyzed methylations occur at the mutational sites with very similar relative frequencies. Although some dependence of reactivity of a given site in DNA on the neighboring base sequences would be expected and would be predicted to be more marked for S_N2 agents, the available evidence shows that this dependence is not very great. For example, McGhee and Felsenfeld (*152*) found that methylation by dimethyl sulfate of DNA in nucleosomes of rooster erythrocytes—which might be expected to show more variations in reactivity according to

$$\begin{matrix} CH_3 \\ \diagdown \\ N-NO \\ \diagup \\ CH_3 \end{matrix} \xrightarrow{[O]} \left[\begin{matrix} CH_2OH \\ \diagdown \\ N-NO \\ \diagup \\ CH_3 \end{matrix} \right] \rightarrow [CH_3 \cdot NH \cdot NO] \rightarrow [CH_3N{=}N{-}OH] \rightarrow [CH_3N_2^+] \rightarrow [CH_3^+]$$

N-Nitrosodimethylamine

$$CH_3N(NO)CONH_2 \xrightarrow{OH^-} [CH_3 \cdot NH \cdot NO] + NCO^- + H^+$$

N-Methyl-*N*-nitrosourea

$$CH_3N(NO)C(NH)NHNO_2 \xrightarrow{OH^-} [CH_3 \cdot NH \cdot NO] + NC \cdot \overline{N} \cdot NO_2 + H^+$$

N-Methyl-*N′*-nitro-*N*-nitrosoguanidine

$$CH_3N(NO)C(NH)NHNO_2 + HS \cdot CH_2 \cdot CH(NH_2)CO_2H$$

$$\rightarrow [CH_3 \cdot NH \cdot NO] + [HO_2C \cdot CH(NH_2) \cdot CH_2 \cdot S \cdot C(NH) \cdot NHNO_2]$$

$$\downarrow$$

$$\begin{matrix} HO_2C - & CH & - & N \\ & | & & \| \\ & H_2C & & C{-}NHNO_2 \\ & & \diagdown S \diagup & \end{matrix}$$

Scheme V. Activation of N-*nitrosodimethylamine (by metabolism) or of* N-*methyl*-N-*nitroso compounds (alkali- or thiol-catalyzed) to methylating agents.* N-*Methyl*-N-*nitrosourea is not activated by thiols in neutral aqueous solution.*

the position of the DNA in the nucleosome structure than would *E. coli* DNA—was remarkably random and similar to that of "naked" DNA, except for some enhanced reactivity at N-7 of guanine in a limited sequence.

The concept that the fairly evenly distributed spectrum of mutation could be ascribed to a random error-prone repair of alkylated sites was contraindicated by the comparative results for UV light as mutagen. This agent is virtually nonmutagenic in *lex*$^-$ strains of *E. coli,* unlike the alkylating agents used. Also, in contrast with the alkylating agents, UV light showed no specificity for GC→AT mutations and a markedly uneven distribution of frequency at specific mutational sites. Moreover, ethyl methanesulfonate, unlike the nitrosoguanidine, does not appear to induce error-prone repair in *E. coli.*

The miscoding O^6-alkylguanines induced by both agents is subject to repair removal from DNA of alkylated *E. coli* O^6-methylguanine by demethylation (*68*) (a quasi-enzymic process) and O^6-ethylguanine, at least in part, by the enzymic excision repair pathway that also repairs UV-induced damage (*153*). Deficiency in ability to remove O^6-methylguanine from DNA, as with the *E. coli ada* mutants of Jeggo (*154*), confers hypersensitivity (up to 6000-fold) to the mutagenic action of *N*-methyl-*N*′-nitro-*N*-nitrosoguanidine (*155*). This finding is in accord with the predominance of the GC→AT transition mechanism for this agent and the concept that the action is mediated by O^6-methylguanine as the promutagenic base. Some degree of difference between the methylating and ethylating agent might therefore be caused by the difference in the significant repair pathways for removal of promutagenic bases, but these differences are relatively small.

See also the "Note Added in Proof," page 468.

The further difference between the agents—the ability of *N*-methyl-*N*′-nitro-*N*-nitrosoguanidine to induce a significant (even though relatively small) proportion of AT→GC transitions—accords with the ability of this agent to induce the miscoding base O^4-methylthymine (Table VI), whereas its ethyl analog was not detected as a reaction product of DNA with ethyl methanesulfonate. Alternatively, according to Coulondre and Miller (*149*), this difference could be ascribed to error-prone repair.

A further possible mechanism is the induction of mutation by incorporation of alkylated DNA precursors, such as O^6-alkyldeoxyguanosine triphosphate, into DNA, which would be more likely to occur with the ethylating agent than the methylating agent, as noted earlier.

In summary, the miscoding of O^6-alkylguanine appears to be reasonably well established as the predominant mechanism for mutations induced by alkylating agents in *E. coli*. Such direct evidence is as yet not available for mutagenesis in mammalian cells, although the comparative mutagenicities in V79 cells of dimethyl sulfate and MNU, in relation to the methylation of cellular DNA, are consistent with this mechanism.

Apparently, in mammalian cell mutagenesis, miscoding mutagens such as *N*-methyl-*N*′-nitro-*N*-nitrosoguanidine and ethyl methanesulfonate can be distinguished by their ability to induce mutations to ouabain resistance, rather than to 8-azaguanine or thioguanine resistance (*156*). This distinction may well reflect the need for a functional enzyme (Na^+/K^+ ATPase) in the ouabain system, so that only structural changes in the ouabain-binding moiety of the proteins are scored as mutants, whereas grosser genetic damage can be detected in the other systems. An acridine mustard (ICR-191) (**4**) (a frameshift mutagen) and X-radiation did not induce ouabain mutations in S49 mouse lymphoma cells, but were effective inducers of thioguanine resistance (*156*). These comparative studies therefore show that the categorization of mutagens, in terms of their effects on DNA that account for their mechanisms of action in *E. coli*, can also apply to mutagenesis in mammalian cells.

A further deduction is that repair mechanisms that remove promutagenic groups from DNA of alkylated mammalian cells will also counteract mutagenesis, as with *E. coli*. The most extensively studied repair system of this type is the removal of O^6-methylguanine (*see* Figure 6) (reviewed in Ref. *157* and *159*).

The repair system was first shown for *E. coli* (*67*), subsequently for certain mammalian cells, e.g., rat liver (*160*), and more recently for cultured human fibroblasts (*161*) and human lymphocytes from peripheral blood (*162*). The technique used was to isolate DNA from cells or animals treated with [^{3}H]-or

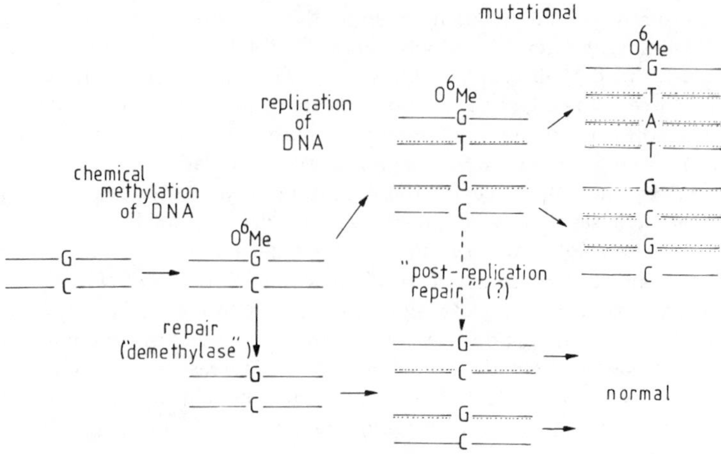

Figure 6. Suggested repair pathways for negation of the promutagenic effect of O⁶*-methylguanine in a DNA template.*

Demethylation of O⁶*-methylguanine in DNA with transfer of the methyl group to a cysteinyl residue of a protein occurs in* E. coli (68)*, mouse liver* (168)*, and human lymphocytes (V. M. Craddock, personal communication, 1981). Because organs of mice, other than liver, are deficient in this type of removal, some other pathway of repair or some form of post-replicative repair may occur.*

[^{14}C]methyl-labeled alkylating carcinogens. MNU or *N*-methyl-*N*′-nitro-*N*-nitrosoguanidine were usually used, because they give a reasonably high proportion of *O*⁶-methylguanine the ratio of this product to the principal product, 7-methylguanine, is 0.11 initially. If the repair removal of *O*⁶-methylguanine had occurred, then methylated DNA that is isolated after various times of incubation of the cells or after various times in vivo would show a decrease in the ratio of O-6 : N-7 methylation of guanine. The decrease results because 7-methylguanine is lost at a much slower rate from DNA, by spontaneous hydrolysis (half-life > 100 h) or even if subject to enzymatic removal.

This test has been applied to a fairly wide variety of cells, and some examples are shown in Table X. The principal findings are that the cells most proficient in removal of the promutagenic base are *E. coli* (except *ada*⁻ including *uvr*⁻), human cultured fibroblasts, human lymphocytes from peripheral blood, and liver of rats and mice (*163*). The cells that are relatively deficient in removal of *O*-6 methylguanine from DNA methylated by carcinogens are *E. coli* with inhibition of protein synthesis, *E. coli ada*⁻, mouse lymphocytes and cells of other organs except liver, and the Chinese hamster V79 lung cell line.

Following the concept that methylating carcinogens act through induction of mutations by miscoding, as discussed previously, the removal of promutagenic bases from the methylated template before its replication would be expected to counteract carcinogenesis. Conversely, deficiency in this respect would be expected to confer sensitivity to carcinogens, as shown by the hypersensitivity to mutagenesis of the *ada* mutants of *E. coli*. Furthermore, the occurrence of cell division before the repair process was complete would be expected to enhance the probability of carcinogenesis.

Table X

Removal of Methylpurines from DNA—Interspecies Comparison

Cells	*Extent of Methylation (µmol 7-MeGua)/ (mol DNA-P)*	*3-Methyladenine/ 7-Methylguanine*	*O⁶-Methylguanine/ 7-Methylguanine*
DNA methylated in vitro	21000	0.13	0.11*
E. coli AB1157	1502	~0.00	0.023
E. coli AB1886 (uvr^-)	100	~0.00	0.01
E. coli AB1157			
+ chloramphenicol	1838	~0.00	0.11*
Mouse (Balb/c,f)			
lymphocyte (thymus)	25	0.10	0.12*
Human (m)			
lymphocyte	25	0.090	0.054

NOTE: Ability of cells to remove from methylated DNA a promutagenic methylpurine (O^6-methylguanine) or a cytotoxic methylpurine (3-methyladenine), as indicated by the ratios (methylpurine : 7-methylguanine) in cellular DNA, 1 h (or 0.75 h for *E. coli*) after treatment of cells with *N*-methyl-*N*-nitrosourea at 37 °C. Significant lack of removal of O^6-methylguanine in this time is indicated by *.

These summaries are based on data from the following references: *E. coli, 153,154;* mouse in vivo, *11;* mouse in vitro, *162;* Chinese hamster V79 cells, *71;* and human cells in vitro, *161,162.*

Some evidence has been obtained in support of these concepts. Methylation of liver DNA in experimental animals is extensive following administration of *N*-nitrosodimethylamine, which reacts through the methyldiazonium ion generated by metabolic oxidation, as illustrated in Scheme V. Single doses of this methylating carcinogen to the rat are not carcinogenic, whereas multiple doses can be. The latter presumably enable sufficient O^6-methylguanine to remain in DNA while DNA synthesis is occurring in a reparative response to tissue damage by the carcinogen (reviewed in Ref. 157). If DNA synthesis is deliberately induced by partial hepatectomy, a single dose of the methylating carcinogens *N*-nitrosodimethylamine (*164*) or MNU (*165*) can cause liver cell tumorigenesis. Tumorigenesis does not result from parallel treatments with methyl methanesulfonate (*166*), which, at maximal dose levels not toxic to the whole animal, cannot give levels of O^6-methylation of guanine in DNA sufficient for carcinogenesis, unlike the nitroso compounds.

The general conclusion from studies of methylation-induced carcinogenesis in experimental animals (covered in more detail for nitroso compounds in Chapter 12 in Vol. 2 of this edition) is that persistent O^6-methylation of guanine in DNA of target cells is necessary but not sufficient for induction of cancer (*11, 167*).

Tissues that cannot remove O^6-methylguanine from DNA are not necessarily highly susceptible to the carcinogenic action of methylating carcinogens; strains of mice relatively resistant to the induction by MNU of lymphocytic lymphoma of thymus (the predominantly susceptible tissue in most strains) did not appear to be more proficient in removal of the promutagenic base from target DNA (*162*). Other factors must be sought to explain these differences in susceptibility of strains; these factors might include ability to counteract effects of methylation of cellular DNA by other repair mechanisms, such as those covered by the term "postreplicative." Unfortunately, detailed information on these mechanisms is lacking.

For *E. coli* (*68*) and mouse liver (*168*), the principal mechanism in cells by which the promutagenic O^6-methylguanine is reconverted to the normal base guanine in DNA is most likely direct demethylation. The methyl group is transferred to a thiol group of a protein and results in an *S*-methyl-L-cysteinyl residue. In *E. coli* this process is not truly enzymatic, because the receptor protein is unable to regenerate the active site (the thiol group of a cysteinyl residue), and new protein must be synthesized for further activity (*169*). In rat liver, the presumed demethylating protein is present in higher amounts after partial hepatectomy (*170*). The apparently constitutive levels of the protein in liver of rat (*171, 172*) and mouse (*11*) can be exhausted by single high doses of methylating carcinogens, such as *N*-nitrosodimethylamine or *N*-methyl-*N*-nitrosourea. The time-dependent effects of continuous treatments of rats by carcinogens on this activity are complex (*173, 174*) and are discussed in Chapter 12 in Vol. 2 of this edition.

Removal of O^6-ethylguanine in *E. coli* may occur by an analogous mechanism in part, but because *uvr*$^-$ strains appear to be deficient in this respect (although they remove O^6-methylguanine at the same rate as wild-type bacteria (*153*)), the excision repair enzymes that remove UV-light-induced lesions from DNA (pyrimidine dimers) are therefore indicated to remove O^6-ethylguanine.

Evidence regarding the removal of other promutagenic bases, such as O^4-alkylthymines, from DNA is as yet not as extensive as for O^6-alkylguanines. Saffhill and Fox (*145*) found that incorporated O^4-methylthymine was rapidly removed from DNA of V79 cells. Bodell et al. (*175*) reported evidence for enzymatic removal of O^4-ethylthymine, O^2-ethylated thymine, and cytosine from DNA of ethylated human fibroblast cell lines. A UV repair-deficient line derived from a patient with xeroderma pigmentosum was proficient in removal of these products, but showed some deficiency in removal of O^6-ethylguanine. In DNA of rat liver, O^2-ethylthymine appeared to be more persistent than O^4-ethylthymine (*176*).

Carcinogen-induced methylated bases that appear to be at most weakly promutagenic, such as 3-methyladenine and 7-methylguanine, were postulated to miscode through ionized forms (*66, 135*). They were also subject to removal from DNA by repair enzymes. 3-Methyladenine was deduced to be a cytotoxic lesion (*177*) in view of its rapid removal from all cells so far studied. For *E. coli*, enzymatic removal of 3-methyladenine and 3-methylguanine was indicated (*177*) by their disappearance from methylated DNA at rates much greater than those for spontaneous hydrolysis, whereas 7-methylguanine and 7-methyladenine appeared to be lost at about the same rates in cells as in solution. Enzymatic removal of 7-methylguanine had been indicated, however, for *Euglena* (*178*) and was subsequently deduced for liver of hamster (*163*), mice (*162*), and human fibroblasts (*161*).

An enzyme that effects removal of 3-methyladenine from methylated DNA has been isolated from *E. coli* (*179, 180*). This *N*-glycosylase releases the free base from methylated DNA. *E. coli tag* mutants deficient in this enzyme have been isolated (*181*). This type of enzyme has also been isolated from *Micrococcus luteus* (*182*) and a cultured human lymphoblast cell line (*183, 184*) and is present in extracts from rat and hamster liver (*185*). Extracts from *M. luteus* (*186*) and a human lymphoblast line (*184*) can also remove 3-methylguanine from methylated DNA.

Extracts that remove 7-methylguanine from methylated DNA have been obtained from *M. luteus* and *E. coli* (*187*), rat and hamster liver (*185*), and a human lymphoblast cell line (*184*). The *E. coli* extract was weak in this activity, which was also very labile, in contrast to the 3-methyladenine *N*-glycosylase.

A somewhat unexpected feature of the current knowledge of these enzymes is that methylation of adenine in DNA at N-1, which blocks one of the Watson–Crick hydrogen bonds between adenine and thymine, does not appear to stimulate a repair response either in mice in vivo (*11*) or in extracts of a human lymphoid cell line (*184*).

The formation of alkyl phosphotriesters in DNA did not appear per se to constitute a lethal lesion in bacteriophage (*188*) and did not appear to stimulate a repair response in mice in vivo (*11*), although it is expected that very slow hydrolysis of these groups could result under physiological conditions. Therefore, determinations of alkyl phosphotriesters in DNA could be used as an indication of damage to DNA in vivo by carcinogens (*189*). A physicochemical determination method has been devised (*190*) on the basis of the rate of hydrolysis of these groups in DNA with concomitant chain fission.

Repair mechanisms for removal of promutagenic bases from DNA would, as discussed, be expected to counteract mutagenesis and carcinogenesis, insofar as the latter results from miscoding of such bases. However, DNA repair has also been proposed to act in the opposite sense. It may enhance mutagenesis (*150*) and hence possibly carcinogenesis (*191*) while removing cytotoxic lesions from the damaged template by inducing an "error-prone repair" process. The principal evidence for this proposal came from studies on the action of UV radiation on *E. coli* (*192*), but parallel evidence for mammalian cells is lacking (*193*). DNA repair processes for DNA damage induced by most carcinogens in *E. coli* and mammalian cells involve excision repair, and deficiency in these processes often confers some degree of cross-sensitivity to cytotoxic action of both chemicals and radiation (*194*). Nevertheless, a reasonable assumption is that error-prone repair could be responsible for chemical carcinogen-induced somatic mutations. Evidence apparently in favor of this hypothesis has been found from studies with cells from patients with the rare inherited deficiency in excision repair for UV-induced damage associated with some forms of the disease xeroderma pigmentosum (*195, 196*). These cells are hypersensitive to both the cytotoxic and mutagenic actions of certain chemical carcinogens such as aromatic amines and polycyclic hydrocarbons.

Whereas there is ample evidence that this DNA repair deficiency confers hypersensitivity to induction of skin cancer by sunlight, evidence is so far lacking for an abnormally high incidence of internal tumors in xeroderma pigmentosum patients that would be expected to be caused by environmental chemical mutagens (*197*). Thus, the question of the significance of the hypersensitivity of cells to the cytotoxic and mutagenic action of carcinogens with regard to susceptibility of humans to cancer remains unresolved.

Those carcinogens that have been established to cause cancer in humans (discussed in more detail later) are more notable for cytotoxic action than for mutagenic potency; a classical example is mustard gas (*7*). Evidence from studies of the mutagenic action of the corresponding half mustard, 2-chloroethyl 2-ethyl sulfide, in *E. coli* (*198*) suggested that this mustard could induce miscoding through formation of an O^6-alkylguanine in DNA. Therefore, if the mustard gas-induced cross-linkage of DNA, a powerfully cytotoxic reaction (*199*), was repaired (*200, 201*), some mutagenic effects of residual monoalkylations might be expected. In addition to correlations with mutagenicity, the relationship between cytotoxic action of carcinogens and carcinogenesis has therefore also stimulated continuous interest. Berenblum's early work (*6*) on induction of skin cancer in mice showed mustard gas to be anticarcinogenic when applied to mouse skin together with an initiating agent. A possible explanation of the effect is that the cytotoxic action of mustard gas, unlike that of the classical promoting agents such as croton oil, reduced rather than increased the proliferation of initiated cells during subsequent tissue repair.

A novel concept to account for the apparent paradox of the carcinogenic potency of cytotoxic agents was proposed by Barrows and Shank (*202, 203*) as a result of studies of the effects of hepatotoxic carcinogens on biomethylation of DNA in liver of rats. A relevant example is the action of hydrazine (NH_2–NH_2), an inorganic hepatotoxin and principal metabolite of the antituberculosis drug isonicotinic acid hydrazide (**21**). Hydrazine is capable of inducing hepatocellular

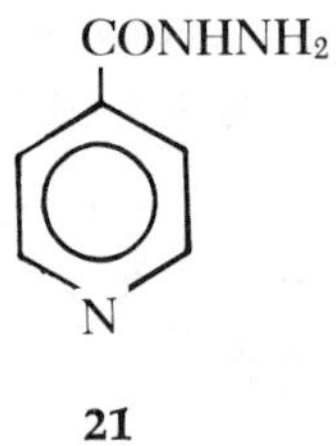

21

carcinoma and pulmonary adenocarcinoma in CBA/Cb/Se mice and hepatocarcinoma and spindle cell carcinoma of liver, lung adenocarcinoma, and breast fibroadenoma in Cb/Se rats (*204, 205*). Relatively large doses were required, e.g., 44 mg of hydrazine/kg by stomach tube daily for 36 weeks. Hydrazine gave positive results in short-term tests for mutagenesis (*116*), but its mode of action as a mutagen was not clarified.

When a dose of hydrazine (10 or 60 mg/kg, oral) was given to animals together with [^{3}H]methyl-labeled methionine (intraperitoneal), anomalous methylated bases (i.e., additional to the normal product of biomethylation of DNA, 5-methylcytosine) could be detected in DNA isolated from liver up to 20 h after hydrazine administration (*202*). These products included O^6- and 7-methylguanine, and this finding suggested that action of the hepatotoxin had reduced the specificity of the normally enzymically controlled biomethylation of DNA, which is confined to methylation at C-5 of cytosine, and that the methylating intermediate *S*-adenosylmethionine was acting as an alkylating mutagen under these conditions. The carcinogen had no significant effect on biomethylation of C-5 of cytosine in DNA.

An alternative theory of carcinogenesis mediated by carcinogen-induced anomalous biomethylation of DNA postulates that the significant effect is hypomethylation at C-5 of cytosine (*206*), with a consequent permanent effect on progeny of affected cells, following the concept that this activates gene expression (*207, 208*). Deficient biomethylation of DNA may occur during the process of DNA repair. Again, all genotoxic agents would be expected to cause this effect, with little quantitative correlation expected between carcinogenesis according to this mechanism and mutagenesis, except insofar as the latter involves deletion of genetic material.

The classical agents that cause hypomethylation of DNA are ethionine (**11**) (an antagonist of biomethylation through conversion to *S*-adenosylethionine, and a relatively weak carcinogen) and 5-azacytidine (**22**) (a nonmethylatable anti-

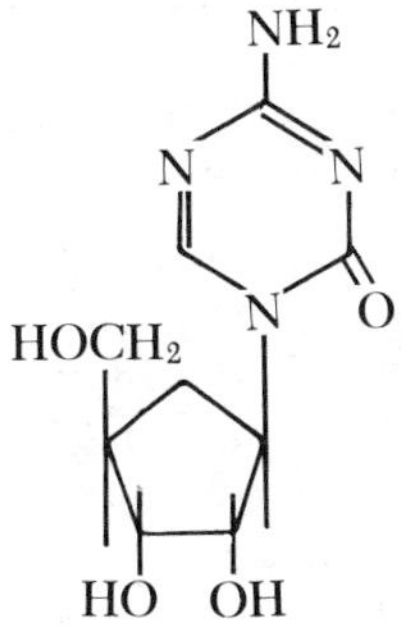

NH2

HOCH2

HO OH

22

metabolite analog of cytosine, and also at most a weak carcinogen). Therefore, hypomethylation of DNA probably is not a powerful cause of cancer but, as with the alternative mechanism based on anomalous biomethylation, it may apply to carcinogenesis induced by prolonged treatments with cytotoxic agents, which may be important for human cancer.

Overall, alkylation of DNA—whether direct or mediated by reactive alkylating metabolites of otherwise unreactive carcinogens—of the type that causes miscoding of the alkylated template is the most powerful cause of carcinogenesis by single administrations of carcinogens to experimental animals. Some contribution by an analogous mechanism involving incorporation of miscoding DNA precursors may also occur.

However, the significance of this mechanism may require further consideration with regard to carcinogenesis by multiple or continuous administration of cytotoxic carcinogens, which may not be alkylating agents themselves nor be metabolically converted to alkylating agents. Thus, cytotoxic action may disrupt the specificity of biomethylation of DNA by causing anomalous biomethylation to give miscoding bases in DNA. Induction of cancer in humans seems more likely to result from prolonged exposure to cytotoxic agents that are relatively weak carcinogens, rather than from single massive exposures to highly potent carcinogens. Therefore anomalous biomethylation of DNA may well prove to be particularly significant as a mechanism for induction of cancer in humans.

A significant factor of DNA repair processes in alkylation-induced carcinogenesis is the ability to remove promutagenic bases from alkylated DNA; a deficiency in this ability would cause relatively high susceptibility to mutagens, and therefore to carcinogens. Human cells so far examined seem more proficient in this respect than mouse cells, which are often used for testing carcinogens. Therefore, on these grounds, such animal tests will not underestimate the susceptibility of humans to relatively potent carcinogens. However, caution is clearly needed in extrapolating this deduction to the more likely causation of human cancer by prolonged exposures to relatively weak carcinogens, which may well be a more complex process. Also inherited deficiency in DNA repair no doubt confers enhanced susceptibility to carcinogenesis, but how this susceptibility results is far from clear.

In Vivo Dosimetry of Carcinogens Based on Alkylation of DNA

The previous sections discussed evidence implicating specific reactions of carcinogens with DNA as particularly powerful sources of mutations through miscoding. Therefore these reactions, according to the somatic mutation hypothesis, could also be important for carcinogenesis. In a given strain of mice, evidence was presented that extent of induction of miscoding bases, O^6-alkylguanines in target DNA, was positively associated with yield of tumors.

However, detailed analysis of extent and mode of alkylation of DNA is not practicable as an assessment of carcinogenic potency of a wide variety of carcinogens. Therefore, rapid screening methods have been sought for this purpose (*209, 210, 211*). The most widely used assay (*112, 113*), often denoted as the Ames test, is an indirect assessment of DNA damage expressed as reversion mutation in standard strains of bacteria.

A priori such tests seem quantitatively insufficient to reflect carcinogenic potency of chemicals, even if confined to directly acting alkylating agents. A more fundamental criticism is that "there may be whole classes of chemicals that are human carcinogens but which are not likely to be detected by any of today's short-term tests" (*210*).

Bartsch et al. (*211*) compared the mutagenic activity of a spectrum of alkylating carcinogens, as measured by an Ames test (reversion of *Salmonella typhimurium* TA100), with their carcinogenicity, as measured by a mean tumorigenic dose (TD_{50}). This dose is the daily dose of a carcinogen in milligrams per kilogram of body weight required to reduce by one-half the probability of rats or mice being tumor-free when administered over a standard lifetime. The compounds compared were, in order of decreasing mutagenicity according to the in vitro test, *N*-methyl-*N*′-nitro-*N*-nitrosoguanidine > glycidaldehyde ≅ 1,3-propanesultone > *β*-propiolactone, *N*-methyl-*N*-nitrosourea > epichlorohydrin > *N*-ethyl-*N*-nitrosourea; the range covered was approximately 1–10^3. The rank order of decreasing carcinogenicity, covering a range of about 1–500, was *N*-ethyl-*N*-nitrosourea > *N*-methyl-*N*-nitrosourea > *N*-methyl-*N*′-nitro-*N*-nitrosoguanidine ≅ 1,3-propanesultone > *β*-propiolactone > glycidaldehyde > epichlorohydrin. De-

Table XI

Correlation Between Mutagenicity (Induction of Small Chromosome Deletions in *Drosophila melanogaster*) and Carcinogenicity (Induction of Pulmonary Tumors in Strain A Mice)

Compound	*Mutagenicity*	*Carcinogenicity*
Triethylenemelamine	92	560[a]
Uracil mustard	9	10420
Naphthylamine mustard	3.5	8.3
Melphalan	1.5	2630
N,N-Bis(2-chloroethyl)-2,3-dimethoxyaniline	1.1	104
Butadiene dioxide	0.9	7.6
Mannitol myleran	0.08	3.3

NOTE: Compounds were administered by injection into adult male flies. Mutagenicity (*213*) denotes induced mutation frequency per 10^3 divided by concentration of agent (m*M*) at a dose less than the LD_{30} of adult males. Carcinogenicity (*215*) denotes 10^4 divided by positive response dose, i.e., dose (μmol/kg) at which one tumor per mouse was induced, as derived from a dose–response curve, log (no. of tumors per mouse) vs. log (dose).
[a]Calculated from data of Ref. 216.

spite the use of directly acting alkylating agents, which avoids any differences between metabolism in the different species, no quantitative correlation was obtained between mutagenicity and carcinogenicity as defined by these tests.

A comparative study by Fahmy and Fahmy (*213, 214*) of carcinogenicity and mutagenicity had given a convincing positive correlation. This study used, however, a limited series of alkylating agents that had similar chemical properties, and the eukaryote *Drosophila melanogaster* as test organism. The compounds chosen were 7 of 29 difunctional or trifunctional agents assessed for carcinogenic potency in mice (*215, 216*) and were typical of alkylating agents used in cancer chemotherapy, some of which are now regarded as carcinogenic for humans (*see* later, Table XIV) and which are all capable of exerting cytotoxic action through cross-linking of DNA. As shown in Table XI, ability to induce lung adenoma in strain A mice correlated positively with ability to induce small chromosomal deletions in *Drosophila melanogaster*. The deduction from this work and related studies was that carcinogenicity of alkylating agents did not correlate positively with ability of compounds to induce dominant lethal mutations or sex-linked recessive lethals, but a positive correlation was found with ability to induce small deletions, especially at the *Minute* and *bobbed* loci, i.e., those associated with RNA-forming genes.

As already noted, Fahmy and Fahmy's studies comparing carcinogenicity and mutagenicity in *Drosophila* were considered by them to favor an epigenetic mechanism of action of carcinogens (*102, 103*). This conclusion is at present subject to some controversy regarding interpretation of the significance of the data.

Table XII

Extent of Alkylation of DNA in Vivo at Short Times After Single Doses of Carcinogens—Representative Data for Liver DNA

Agent	*Animal*	*Route*	*Time (h)*	*Dose (mmol/kg)*	*Principal Products*	E/D[a]	*References*
			Methylating Agents				
Dimethyl sulfate	rat	iv	4	0.63	7-methylguanine[b]	28	218
Methyl methanesulfonate	mouse	ip	2–2.5	1.09		107	219
	rat	iv	16	1.09	7-methylguanine[b]	182	218
N-Methyl-*N*-nitrosourea	mouse	ip	1	0.04–0.78	7-methylguanine[c]	483	11,162
	rat	iv	4	0.87		264	218
N-Methyl-*N*′-nitro-*N*-nitrosoguanidine	mouse	ip	2	0.408	7-methylguanine[c]	118	219
			Ethylating Agents				
Ethyl methanesulfonate	mouse	ip	4	1.53	7-ethylguanine[d]	23	11
	rat	ip	17	2.16		46	220
N-Ethyl-*N*-nitrosourea	mouse	ip	1	2.09	7-ethylguanine[e]	13	11
	rat	iv	2	1.28		7	220
Ethionine	rat	ip	18	3.09	7-ethylguanine	0.2	221
Urethane (ethyl carbamate)	mouse	ip	12	3.0	ethyl phosphotriester(?)[f]	0.1	222
	mouse	ip	12	5.62	(?)	0.11[g] 0.02[h]	223

Cancer Chemotherapeutic Agents (mustards, etc.)							
Cyclophosphamide	rat	ip	24	0.43	n.d.[i]	62	224
Hemisulfur mustard	mouse	ip	1	0.178	7-hydroxyethythio-ethylguanine	674	225
Myleran (Bisulfan)	mouse	ip	5	0.163	n.d.[i]	25	225
	rat	ip	2	0.018		150	226
Nitrogen mustard (HN2)	rat	ip	6	0.019	n.d.[j]	42	227
Triethylenemelamine (TEM)	rat	ip	2	0.015	n.d.[i]	313	226
Alkyl Halides							
1,2-Dibromoethane[k] (ethylene dibromide)	rat	ip	24	0.015	n.d.[i]	180	228
Vinyl chloride[k]	rat	inhal.	5	0.185	7-oxoethylguanine	8	229

NOTE: For details of sex and strain of animals used, see the original references. In a comparative study with five strains of mice (*162*) no significant differences between strains were found.
[a]The extent of alkylation E measured in micromoles per mole of DNA-P; the dose D measured in millimoles per kilogram. Alkylation occurs at N-7 of guanine unless indicated otherwise.
[b]7-Methylguanine was about 80% of total products, O^6-methylguanine about 0.5%.
[c]7-Methylguanine was about 67% of total products, O^6-methylguanine about 7.5%.
[d]7-Ethylguanine was about 58% of total products, O^6-ethylguanine about 2%.
[e]7-Ethylguanine was about 11% of total products, O^6-ethylguanine about 7%.
[f]This suggested identification of products is in doubt according to Ref. 223.
[g]Female mice.
[h]Male mice.
[i]Products not isolated; results therefore could include incorporated radioactivity not in alkylation products.
[j]Products not identified, but were in DNA purine fraction; probably 7-alkylguanine mainly.
[k]Probably reacts in vivo through metabolism (to haloacetaldehyde?) not by direct alkylation.

These examples of comparative studies of mutagenicity and carcinogenicity illustrate that indirect means of estimation of damage to DNA in vivo by short-term mutagenicity tests may or may not correlate with carcinogenic potency according to the choice of data (for a review, *see* Ref. 209). However, the high range of quantitative values covered by these tests shows that weak carcinogens can have detectable biological activities of less than 10^{-3} of those of strong carcinogens, and that these differences most likely cannot be ascribed to any specific mode of alkylation of DNA. However, cytotoxic alkylating agents may cause cancer not by their direct action, but by some other mechanism, e.g., by causing anomalous biomethylation of DNA as a consequence of cytotoxic action.

The direct measurement of extent of alkylation of DNA by carcinogens in vivo, particularly in target organs, has therefore been suggested (*217*) to provide of itself a useful index of carcinogenic potency, albeit, like the rapid-screening tests, of approximate quantitative significance in this respect.

Representative values of extents of in vivo alkylation of DNA by carcinogens are shown in Table XII. The provisos necessary when correlating such data with carcinogenic potency have been discussed by Lutz (*217*); some considerations are as follows.

The influence of specific DNA alkylation reactions, such as ability to induce miscoding bases, has already been discussed. As an example, the "carcinogen binding index" (CBI) (or overall extent of alkylation) of DNA by methyl methanesulfonate would overestimate the carcinogenic potency of this methylating agent in comparison with that of *N*-methyl-*N*-nitrosourea. These compounds have similar binding indices, close to the value expected for even distribution of methylation throughout the tissues and their constituents (*see* Table XIII). For even distribution of alkylation (assumed to go to completion) the factor $K =$ extent of alkylation (micromoles of alkyl groups per gram of DNA) divided by dose (millimoles per kilogram of body weight) would be unity. The alternative expression used by Lutz (*217*) is given by

$$\text{CBI} = (\mu\text{mol of alkyl groups per mol of DNA–P})/(\text{dose, mmol/kg})$$
$$\text{CBI} = 336K$$

The numerical factor is the molecular weight of an average DNA nucleotide (Na salt, as normally isolated from animal tissues).

Some compounds react extensively near the site of injection and are not evenly distributed through the body. *N*-Methyl-*N*′-nitro-*N*-nitrosoguanidine, unlike methyl methanesulfonate or MNU, did not penetrate in appreciable amounts to bone marrow and thymus (*218*) after intraperitoneal injection into mice (*see* Table XIII). This finding was attributed to the mode of activation of the nitrosamidine to the proximate methylating species, methyldiazonium ion (Scheme V). Unlike MNU, which reacts through the same intermediate generated by alkali-catalyzed decomposition, *N*-methyl-*N*′-nitro-*N*-nitrosoguanidine hydrolyzes slowly at pH 7 and 37 °C, but more rapidly than thiol-catalyzed reactions. Apparently, thiol-catalyzed reactions predominate in cells (*151*).

As already noted, the majority of chemical carcinogens do not directly alkylate DNA in vivo, but require metabolic activation (*see* Chapter 8). In addition, several compounds usually classified as alkylating agents fell into this category (*230–32*),

Table XIII

Extent of Alkylation of DNA in Vivo: Ratio of Extent of Alkylation at N-7 of Guanine in Various Organs to That in Liver

Organ	*Dimethyl Sulfate,* *Rat*	*Methyl Methanesulfonate*		N-*Methyl*-N-*nitrosourea*		N-*Methyl*-N'-*nitro*-N-*nitrosoguanidine,* *Mouse*	*Ethyl Methanesulfonate*		N-*Ethyl*-N-*nitrosourea*	
		Mouse	*Rat*	*Mouse*	*Rat*		*Mouse*	*Rat*	*Mouse*	*Rat*
Bone marrow	—	0.84	—	0.38	—	<0.06	0.89	—	0.5	—
Brain	5.75	—	1.17	0.66	0.71	0.10	1.33	0.8	0.5	0.8
Kidney	1.75	—	1.07	0.60	0.92	0.44	—	0.9	—	0.8
Lung	6.5	—	1.00	0.52	0.79	0.67	1.33	1.0	0.7	0.8
Small bowel	—	1.00	—	0.72	0.60	1.92	1.09	—	0.8	—
Spleen	—	—	—	0.51	—	1.42	—	—	0.8	—
Testis	—	—	0.56	—	—	—	—	—	—	—
Thymus	—	0.94	—	0.43	—	0.10	0.94	—	0.5	—

NOTE: For details of dose, route of administration, and values determined for liver DNA, see Table XII.
— denotes not determined.

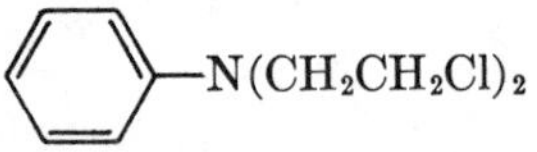

C_6H_5—$N(CH_2CH_2Cl)_2$

23

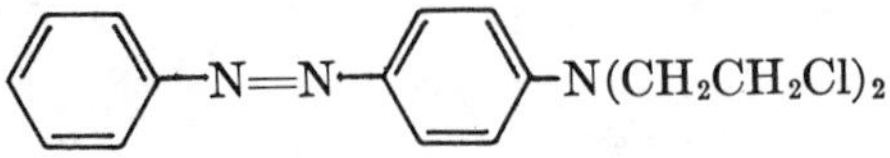

C_6H_5—N=N—C_6H_4—$N(CH_2CH_2Cl)_2$

24

$HO_2C(CH_2)_3$—C_6H_4—$N(CH_2CH_2Cl)_2$

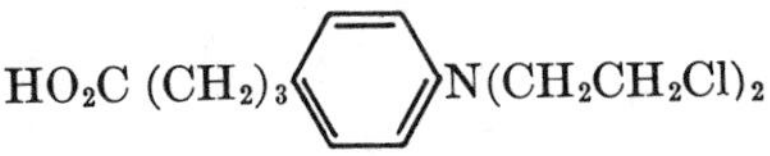

25

notably mitomycin C (**13**), cyclophosphamide (**8**), aniline mustard (**23**), azo mustard (**24**), and possibly chlorambucil (**25**). Mitomycin C, in addition to its known ability to cross-link DNA (*233*) after metabolic or extraneous chemical reduction, may also damage DNA through generation of free radicals (*234, 235*).

The generally more important function of metabolism of alkylating agents in vivo is to inactive them. The initial rate of reaction for rapidly hydrolyzed agents may be approximately the same as for in vitro hydrolysis. However, in some cases, such as for hemisulfur mustard (**1**), the initial rate in vivo can be slower than in vitro (*225*), probably because of some degree of sequestration of the fat-soluble alkylating agent in lipid compartments of the cells.

Some alkylating agents are activated by metabolism and react more rapidly in vivo than in a buffered neutral aqueous solution at 37 °C.

Alkylating agents that react relatively slowly in aqueous solution are generally expected to react within a more limited time in vivo because they are rapidly eliminated from the body by detoxifying enzymes. Glutathione transferase catalyzes their reaction with the thiol group of reduced glutathione (*236*). Thus, methyl methanesulfonate has a half-life of 9.5 h in aqueous solution at 37 °C (Table II), alkylates bacterial cells in suspension with a half-life of about 5 h (*237*), and is eliminated from the blood of rats within 1.5 h of its intravenous injection (*238*).

Another detoxification mechanism found for nitrogen mustard [HN2, bis(2-chloroethyl)methylamine] is *N*-dealkylation (*239*). This drug is largely converted to an inactive form by passage through the liver in the rat (*240*).

The net result of these factors of alkylation and detoxification is that the time course of alkylation of DNA (and other cellular constituents) in vivo consists of generally a fairly rapid initial phase, a maximal alkylation after at most a few hours, and then a decline. The decline is due to either turnover of alkylated constituents or to their selective removal (e.g., in the processes of DNA repair) (*225*). The level in DNA of some alkylation products that are apparently not subject to repair removal, such as phosphotriesters (*190*), reflects the amount of DNA synthesis subsequent to alkylation.

As noted by Lutz (*217*), the extents of alkylation of DNA in vivo, per unit dose administered, show a wide range of numerical values (*see* Table XII) and can be classified into three broad groups.

Some compounds, implicated in carcinogenesis as possible promoters (rather than as initiating agents or mutagens), such as saccharin, show very low values (< 0.1) of the covalent binding index. This result probably indicates that reaction does not occur through activated metabolites. Hormones such as estrone and diethylstilbestrol showed a low value (1–2) for binding to DNA of rat liver. This range is of the same order as found for ethylation of DNA by the weak liver carcinogen ethionine and by urethane (**26**). Although classified as ethylating

$$NH_2COOC_2H_5$$

26

agents in Table XII, the mechanisms of reaction of these carcinogens with DNA remain uncertain (*221–23*).

Among the alkylating agents of simple structure, methylating agents react more extensively with DNA in vivo than do ethylating agents (Table XII). The most extensively studied and most potent carcinogen of this type is *N*-methyl-*N*-nitrosourea, and the overall methylation of DNA in vivo, as well as the extent of formation of the promutagenic base O^6-methylguanine, is highest for this compound (*see also* Figure 1 and Table I).

The distribution of methylations by this carcinogen in nuclear DNA of liver, kidney, or brain of rats appears to be random (*241*), although a slight preference was found (*242*) for methylation of mitochondrial as opposed to nuclear DNA of liver (by a factor of 2.5). The extent of methylation of DNA in vivo was also closely proportional to dose up to about 60% of the LD_{50} (*11*).

Relatively few quantitative studies of in vivo DNA reactions have been made for other types of alkylating carcinogen, possibly because of the expense involved in obtaining isotopically labeled compounds. Developments in detection of alkylated bases in DNA by fluorescence measurements (*243, 244*) have made it possible to detect and quantify in vivo alkylation without the use of radiolabel, both in rat (*245*) and human (*246*) DNA.

Another factor is the lack of known alkylation products for determinations with alkylating agents of more complex structure. Brookes and Lawley (*247*) isolated 7-alkylguanines (**27, 28**) from reaction of nitrogen mustard with deoxyguanylic acid and DNA in vitro. Their work on products from Myleran has been extended by Tong and Ludlum (*248*). These advances should enable improve-

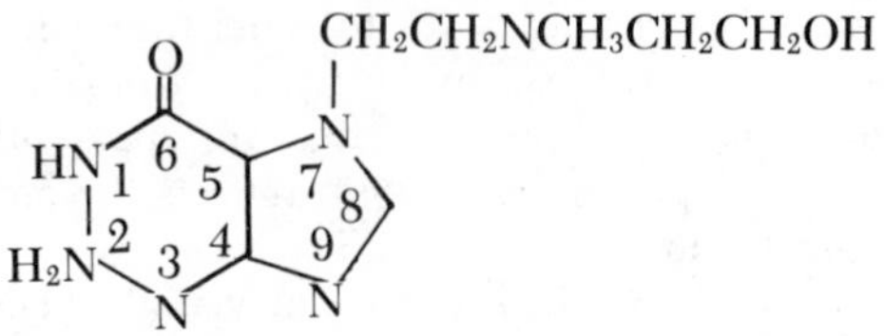

$CH_2CH_2NCH_3CH_2CH_2OH$

27

$CH_2CH_2NCH_3CH_2CH_2$

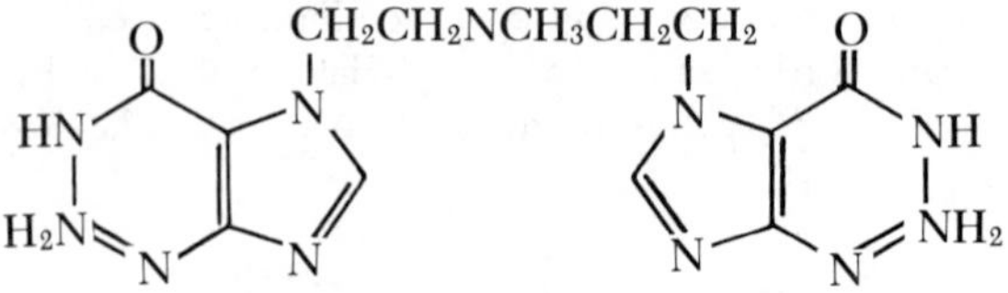

28

ments in the investigations of in vivo reactions of cancer chemotherapeutic agents that at present are rather sketchy (Table XII).

TEM, the most potent carcinogen of the series studied by Fahmy and Fahmy and Shimkin et al. (Table XI), had a relatively high binding index (Table XII). The highest set of values for this parameter were found for aflatoxin B_1 in liver of the rat. Swenson et al. (*249*) reported a value of 24,000 and Croy et al. (*250*) reported 31,000. *N*-Nitrosodimethylamine gave values around 7000 (reviewed in Ref. 217). Both these hepatocarcinogens require metabolic activation to enable their reactions with DNA (*see* Chapters 12 and 16 in Vol. 2 of this edition). This activation generally occurs more extensively in liver than in other tissues.

Very broadly, therefore, the correlation between ability to alkylate DNA in liver and carcinogenic potency reflects the very wide spectrum of values of the binding index, up to 30,000, and must be considered as a very crudely quantitative relationship. For example, vinyl chloride, a notable hepatocarcinogen both in experimental animals and humans (*251*), showed a low binding index (*229*) and would scarcely have been picked out as a dangerous carcinogen on this basis alone. However, the target cells for vinyl chloride are hemangioendothelial cells, not hepatocytes from which presumably the bulk of the DNA would originate in the binding index studies.

When other tissues are considered, little correlation is discernible between binding index and induction of tumors. Promutagenic alkylation of DNA may be considered as a necessary, but not sufficient, factor in tumorigenesis. Other factors appear to be at least equally important quantitatively, such as relative rates of proliferation, as opposed to differentiation or cell death of initiated cells.

A more subtle factor concerns synergistic effects, exemplified by the case of ethylene dibromide. Plotnick (*252*) reported that the hepatocarcinogenicity of this agent administered by inhalation in the rat (causing hemangiosarcoma) was enhanced by feeding disulfiram, a drug (Antabuse) used in alcoholism for aversion therapy. A possible explanation is that this synergistic drug acts by inhibiting detoxificative metabolism of the alkylating agent, thus effectively enhancing its metabolic activation to bromacetaldehyde (*253*), the mutagenic analog of the reactive intermediate derived from vinyl chloride.

The general conclusion from consideration of the available data on DNA alkylation in vivo is that further studies will be valuable in clarifying the mode of action of both potential industrial hazards, such as ethylene dibromide and vinyl chloride, and drugs such as mustards and Myleran used in cancer chemotherapy. However, the carcinogen binding index, defined as extent of alk lation of DNA in vivo relative to dose administered, must be judged as a very crude quantitative assessment of carcinogenic potential. As with other short-term tests for carcinogens, it is an indicator of potential initiation of cancer in the affected tissue.

The methods used to obtain data of the type shown in Tables XII and XIII are scarcely applicable to studies with humans to assess potential damage to DNA by carcinogens, because they involve administration of radioactive alkylating agents. However,the methylating drug DIC [4(5)-(3,3-dimethyl-1-triazeno)imidazole 5(4)-carboxamide] (*see* Scheme VI) was used in ^{14}C-methyl-labeled form for this purpose by Skibba and Bryan (*254*). The labeled drug was administered to two patients, and 7-[^{14}C]methylguanine was detected in the urine. This result indicates that nucleic acid methylation occurs in humans in vivo, as expected by analogy with results from animal experiments. However, urinary excretion of 7-methylguanine is quite normal and can not be used, without the use of radioactive label, to monitor methylation-induced in vivo DNA damage.

Excretion of 3-methyladenine, the principal minor DNA methylation product, could be used for this purpose because it does not appear to be a normal urinary purine (*255, 256*), is rapidly removed from DNA by repair enzymes, and is excreted unchanged.

Methylating and other alkylating carcinogens, in common with X-rays, also cause enhanced urinary excretion of DNA-derived thymidine and deoxycytidine and of 1-methylnicotinamide and its 6-pyridone (*256–59*). Relatively toxic doses appear to be required to enable quantitatively significant effects of this type.

Direct measurement of alkylation of DNA has been achieved in a victim of dimethylnitrosamine poisoning (*246*) by fluorometric detection of O^6-methylguanine in DNA. This method has considerable potential for dosimetry of carcinogen-induced damage in humans.

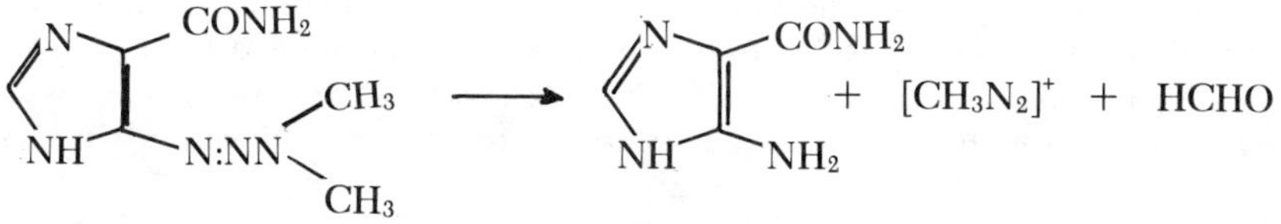

N CONNH2 CH3 NH N:NN CH3 ⟶ N CONH2 NH NH2 + $[CH_3N_2]^+$ + HCHO

Scheme VI. Metabolic oxidative demethylation of dacarbazine [5-(3,3-dimethyl-1-triazeno) imidazole-4-carboxamide].

Another alternative, already noted, is the assay of alkylphosphotriester groups in DNA (*190*). This method may not have sufficient sensitivity for human studies. DNA strand breakage and cross-linkage, either between DNA strands or between DNA and protein, can also be detected by the sensitive alkaline elution technique of Kohn et al. (*260, 261*). Current methods do not require isotopic prelabeling of the DNA and are adequate to monitor the low levels of alkylation expected to result from human exposures (e.g., as caused by 0.5 μM HN2) (*261*).

Ehrenberg et al. (*262–64*) developed a method for carcinogen dosimetry in vivo based on alkylation of hemoglobin, a relatively long-lived protein in blood, by using mass spectrometry to determine the content of *S*-alkylcysteine or *N*-alkylhistidines (*263*). This method has been applied to detect alkylation in vivo of humans exposed to the chemosterilant ethylene oxide (*262*).

Rate constants were determined for alkylation of hemoglobin cysteine and histidine in comparison with those for DNA guanine. These results showed that, for ethylene oxide, the rate of alkylation of cysteine and histidine was 0.5 and 0.2 of the rate for DNA guanine, respectively, and 1.0 and 0.2, respectively, for methyl methanesulfonate. The overall rate of alkylation of guanine by methyl methanesulfonate was six times as rapid as for ethylene oxide (*264*).

The general provisional conclusion to be drawn from this important work is that readily available techniques for monitoring extent of alkylation of hemoglobin in humans can be used as an estimate of the alkylation of DNA in vivo, provided, of course, that the alkylation is systemically and reasonably uniform. The results of Tables XII and XIII show that for water-soluble, nonlocally acting carcinogens, such as methyl methanesulfonate, this assumption appears to be valid.

However, many carcinogens may well react most extensively at the site of administration, e.g., in skin, or in the respiratory tract. They may also be chemically activated nonuniformly in various tissues (as with *N*-methyl-*N*′-nitro-*N*-nitrosoguanidine); or be metabolically activated nonuniformly (as with *N*-nitrosodimethylamine). Tests based on assays of blood cells may therefore underestimate nonsystemic in vivo alkylations. With regard to assays of methylation damage, another factor that may reduce the sensitivity of the method is the natural occurrence of *S*-methylcysteine in hemoglobins which has been reported for various species, including humans (*265*).

Dose–Response Relationships in Alkylation Carcinogenesis

Dose–response relationships can be obtained in experimental systems using animals to correlate induction of tumors and extent and mode of alkylation of target DNA in vivo. The extent of alkylation of DNA of humans can be determined in vivo, although at present the data are necessarily sparse. In principle, therefore, a rationale exists for extrapolation of experimental carcinogenesis data for chemical carcinogens from animals to humans. The crucial factor, of course, remains the relative susceptibility of animals and humans to the carcinogenic effect of a given dose of carcinogen measured in this way.

As an example of assessment of carcinogenic risk for humans based on animal data, one can quote the case of ethylene dibromide (1,2-dibromoethane).

The U.S. Environmental Protection Agency assumed a "single-hit" carcinogenic process recommended as appropriate by Crump et al. (*266*) for example, on theoretical grounds. This hypothesis is that the yield of tumors for low doses of a carcinogen is proportional to dose. From the known age-specific incidence of gastric tumors in rats due to administration of the carcinogen, at a dose level of 40 mg/kg/d, the assumed dose- and time-dependence was expressed as

$$-\ln(1 - p_t) = kD^m t^n$$

where p_t is the probability of tumor formation at time t and k is an empirically determined parameter relating this to dose (D) and time for rats. The exponent m was assumed to be unity (the "single-hit" assumption) and the exponent n from the age dependence of tumorigenesis in rats was 6.95.

These parameters led to the expectation that workers with exposure to ethylene dibromide at citrus fumigation centers (estimated at 3 ppm) would have an incidence of malignant neoplasms during their lifetime of as much as 55%. The observed level was 5%, although this was higher than that expected for a comparable nonexposed population (2%) (*267*).

It was concluded that the discrepancy could be ascribed to undetermined species-specific differences in response, particularly detoxification of the alkylating agent by conjugation with hepatic glutathione or DNA repair should detoxification be insufficient to prevent alkylation of DNA. Evidently knowledge of extent of DNA alkylation and of its repair would permit, as suggested, more rational dosimetry of carcinogens.

The salient factors involved in carcinogenesis have been embodied in a simple mathematical expression by Moolgavkar et al. (*268, 269*) These concepts appear to give a satisfactory basis for discussion of dose–response relationships in alkylation carcinogenesis and are derived from work on age-dependence of human tumors. This initial work was first interpreted (*270*) as indicating that human cancer is a "multi-stage" process; a later interpretation (*271, 272*) clarified it as a two-stage process.

The basic theory postulates that "initiation" of cancer is a rare event (a mutation in a stem cell), but that this initiation alone is not sufficient to produce a malignant tumor. It can result in a benign tumor (e.g., mouse skin papilloma), or premalignant state exemplified by polyposis coli. A second mutation (at the same site as the first on the homologous chromosome), or a homologous chromosomal exchange, is envisaged to be required to convert the "intermediate cell" to a malignant tumor stem cell (*see* Scheme VII).

The important factor is the rate of proliferation of the intermediate cells, expressed as the difference between the "birth rate" of intermediate cells and their "death rate" (incorporating their rate of terminal differentiation). Even a high rate of the initial mutation could be negated by failure of the mutant cells to divide and yield sufficient numbers to give an appreciable probability for the second mutation to occur. This explains immediately the conclusion reached from comparative studies of tumorigenesis vs. promutagenic DNA alkylation in various species, strains, and tissues, that such alkylation is necessary, but not sufficient, for carcinogenesis.

The equation deduced is

$$I(t) \approx \mu_1\mu_2 \int_0^t X(s)\exp[(\alpha_2-\beta_2)(t-s)]\,ds$$

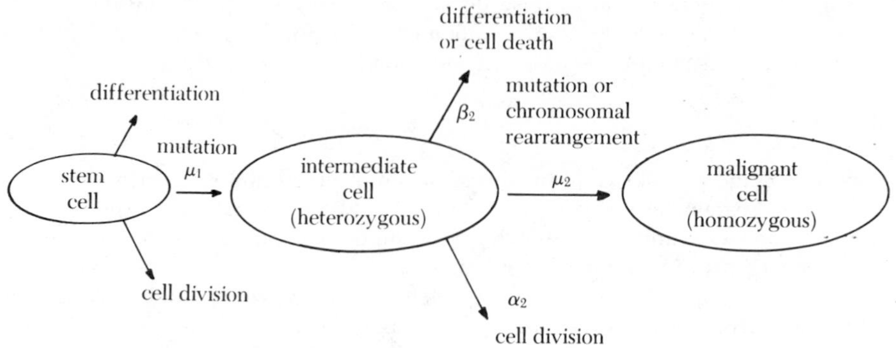

Scheme VII. Model for two-stage carcinogenesis [after Moolgavkar and Knudson (269)*].*

where μ_1 is the rate of conversion of a normal stem cell into an intermediate cell per cell per year, and μ_2 is the rate transition of intermediate cell into malignant cell per cell per year. These are the rates of mutation of normal to initiated and from initiated to malignant cells by using the somatic mutation hypothesis. The integral represents the number of intermediate cells available for the second process of mutation (or chromosomal rearrangement) to malignancy. The function $X(s)$ is the number of stem cells at time s; $\int_0^t X(s)ds$ is the number of cell divisions of stem cells up to time t; α_2 is the "birth rate" of intermediate cells per cell per year; and β_2 is the "death rate", including rate of terminal differentiation, of intermediate cells per cell per year.

Clearly the state of differentiation of the target tissue will determine the net value $(\alpha_2 - \beta_2)$, which may be positive or negative. Changes in this factor with age are expected. Thus for the case of human breast cancer, appropriate reasonable estimates of the parameters could account for the two-component, age-dependence curve of incidence often described as "Clemmesen's hook" (*268*). Maxima in such age-dependence curves, as seen for acute lymphocytic leukemia and retinoblastoma, can also be satisfactorily described by this equation, apart from the more general time-dependences approximating to the form $I(t) = kt^n$ where the exponent n is 5–10, according to the type of cancer. The exponent n, or apparent "hit number," is clearly greater than the number of sta ,es, which of course remains at 2.

With regard to experimental alkylation-induced carcinogenesis, the most extensively investigated and best quantified factor is the rate of mutation converting normal cells into initiated or intermediate cells. Admittedly the precise types of stem cell involved in cancer have yet to be isolated and studied. In view of the even distribution of alkylation, their extents of alkylation for systemically acting carcinogens in vivo can be reasonably approximated. The rate of mutation per alkylation can also be assessed, provided that the size of the target gene is assumed to be that of the target in the experimental mutation system used, i.e., about 300 guanine bases for the HGPRT gene.

The kinetics of induction of thymic lymphoma in mice after single injections of alkylating carcinogens, as analyzed by Frei and Lawley (*273*), showed two clear-cut stages. The first, reflecting dose-dependence on O^6-alkylation of DNA guanine, was a "2–3-hit" process for C57BL or RFM mice (*see* Figure 1), with a mean tumorigenic dose [i.e., giving a tumor yield of 63%; $-\ln(1-p_{250}) = 1$] of about 10 μmol of O^6-methylguanine per mol of DNA-P for C57BL(f) mice (corresponding to a rate of induced mutation of about 2×10^{-4} per cell per generation) and about 6 μmol for RFM(f) mice. The second was a single time-dependent hit with a latent period of about 70 d and the following expression was derived empirically

$$-\ln(1-p_{250}) = (kD)^n(t-t_0)$$

In relation to the Moolgavkar equation, this expression is a composite of the parameters involved. It can be reduced in part to these parameters by consideration of results from another experimental system, induction of papilloma in mouse skin.

For this system, the concepts of initiation and promotion were distinguished in the classical work of Mottram (*274, 275*) and Berenblum and Shubik (*276, 277*). Mottram (*278*) also showed that initiated cells, promoted to yield skin papillomas, could be converted into malignant cells through further treatment with an initiator.

The reinterpretation of these classical concepts by Moolgavkar and Knudson (*269*) is that initiators are mutagens, and promoters are quasi-hormonal stimulators of reparative hyperplasia or inhibitors of differentiation. Initiators increase the factor μ_1, and promoters increase the factor $(\alpha_2 - \beta_2)$.

The classical agents employed in the Berenblum–Mottram experiments were polycyclic aromatic hydrocarbons as initiators and croton oil (of which the active principal is phorbol ester) as promoter. The mutagenic potential of the hydrocarbon initiators was shown when Brookes and Lawley (*8*) demonstrated their in vivo reaction with mouse skin DNA. The mode of action of the promoters in general is certainly to stimulate reparative hyperplasia. This step can be done by purely mechanical abrasion of skin (*279*). Phorbol ester possibly could also act as a clastogen in mouse skin; it appears to do so in cultured human lymphocytes (*280*). If this occurred in mouse skin, it would imply that phorbol esters could also increase the factor μ_2 by causing chromosomal rearrangements.

As expected from their nature as mutagens, alkylating agents are initiators in mouse skin (*281, 282*). Furthermore, the kinetics of papilloma induction by *N*-methyl-*N*-nitrosourea applied to skin in a single dose followed by promotion with croton oil for 36 weeks showed that initiation was a single-hit process. For Balb/c mice, the empirical relationship was $-\ln(1-p_{36}) = kD$, and the mean tumorigenic dose $1/k$ was equal to 54 μmole of *N*-methyl-*N*-nitrosourea (data of Ref. 283 analyzed by P.D. Lawley).

The requirement for promutagenic DNA alkylation in papilloma induction is shown by the failure of relatively high doses of dimethyl sulfate (up to 162 μmol) to induce a significant yield of tumors in this system (*284*).

Therefore, as predicted by Moolgavkar and Knudson (*269*), the first stage of carcinogenesis by alkylation is a miscoding mutation (at rate μ_1), and this mutation leads to heterozygous mutant cell lines because it is a single-hit process and occurs in a single copy of a gene. To convert this into a homozygous mutation, a second mutation or chromosomal rearrangement (at rate μ_2) is required. This homozygous mutation may be the time-dependent single random event in the thymoma system.

The factors about which little is yet known quantitatively concern the relative rates of proliferation and cell death of initiated cell lines. Probably these factors are controlled by factors operative in differentiation, and the incorporation at specific sites into the cellular genome of proviral DNA of retroviruses seems a possible source of variation between strains of mice in this respect. This concept is supported by the observations by Frei (*285*) that AKR mice are hypersensitive to alkylation-induced thymoma, which in this strain shows 1–2 apparent dose-dependent hits as opposed to the apparently 2–3-hit process in other strains. The spontaneous thymoma that develops in aged AKR mice is attributed to the incorporation of proviral oncogenes of murine leukemia virus at a promoter site in the host cell DNA (*286*); it seems likely that this supplies one of the carcinogenic hits that is required to promote growth (or suppress differentiation) of initiated cells. The remaining dose-dependent hit may be a requirement for cytotoxicity of the alkylating agents to bone marrow (*287*) and may thus prevent the dilution of initiated stem cells in thymus by normal precursors from bone marrow. These possibilities remain for further investigation.

The classical studies of dose–response for alkylating carcinogens are those of Druckrey and coworkers (*288–90*) using mainly induction of liver cancer or sarcoma at the site of injection in rats. With alkylating agents, the latter method was generally used, and the results showed that sarcoma at the site of injection could be induced by relatively high doses of such agents as methyl methanesulfonate and dimethyl sulfate (*290*) (*see* Table XVIII for details), which have rarely shown positive results in other carcinogenesis test systems. The apparent hypersensitivity of this test has caused Grasso and Golberg (*291*) to cast doubt on its validity on the grounds that it may depend merely on a persistent toxic reaction of possibly physicochemical origin ("derangement of the process of connective tissue repair"). For example, hypertonic solutions of glucose caused local sarcoma by repeated injections into rats.

The work of Druckrey et al. (*290*) appears to negate this criticism. Not all the alkylating agents used gave positive results, and the relative potency of the agents, as expressed by an index derived by dividing the yield of tumors by the product of the average induction time and the dose, showed a wide range of values (*290*).

This relative index showed the following values: *n*-butyl *p*-toluenesulfonate and monomethyl sulfate, 0 (i.e., inactive); di-*n*-butyl sulfate, ethyl *p*-toluenesulfonate, ethylene sulfide, trimethylene oxide, about 10; methyl iodide, benzyl chloride, dimethyl sulfate, methyl methanesulfonate, 30–40; methyl-*p*-toluenesulfonate, 49; and diethyl sulfate, 63. These alkylating agents must be considered as relatively weak carcinogens, and have given few, if any, tumors in other types of test.

Among more potent carcinogens were 1,3-propanesultone, 130–210 with multiple injections and 470–800 with a single injection; *N*-methyl-*N*′-nitro-*N*-nitrosoguanidine, 200; β-propiolactone, 500; and TEM, 2000.

Most likely the rat is highly susceptible to induction of injection-site sarcoma by alkylating agents, but the factors deduced to be important for carcinogenesis in other systems, such as promutagenic alkylation of DNA, have yet to be determined in this system.

Another extensive comparative study of dose–response in alkylation carcinogenesis by Shimkin et al. (*215, 216*) used induction of lung tumors in strain A mice by intraperitoneal injections of agents. The data were presented as plots of logarithm of number of tumors found at 39 weeks vs. logarithm of dose. These plots were approximately straight lines of equal slope but different intercepts for the various agents; the value of the dose at the one-tumor-per-mouse level was taken as a measure of carcinogenic potency, expressed as 10,000/dose (for examples, *see* Table XI).

In their review of genetic toxicity of epoxides, Ehrenberg and Hussain (*264*) reinterpreted the data for butadiene dioxide (L-diepoxybutane) (12 thrice-weekly injections up to 2.5 mmol/kg) as conforming approximately to a "single-hit" relationship, with a mean tumorigenic dose of about 2 mmol/kg. They also superimposed the data for X-rays as carcinogen in the same system, but for RFM mice (*292*) (known to be highly sensitive to radiation) to obtain a "rad-equivalence" for the alkylating agent; on a "tentative" basis, 1 mmol/kg was equivalent to about 500 rad.

As with Druckrey's series, the carcinogenic index derived by Shimkin showed a wide range of numerical values (Table XI). The most potent alkylating agents were uracil mustard, HN2, Melphalan and TEM, with indices of over 500, and these achieved the same order of potency as the polycyclic aromatic hydrocarbons 3-methylcholanthrene and dibenz[*a,h*]anthracene. Therefore, the induction of lung tumors in strain A mice may be a more sensitive test for alkylating agents than induction of thymic lymphoma, because the cytotoxic disfunctional and trifunctional agents were not very potent in the latter system. Frei (*293*) furthermore found that ethyl methanesulfonate induced a significant yield of lung adenomas in the CFW/D inbred line of Swiss mice, but not a significant yield of thymoma.

Another system with potential as a sensitive test is the induction of skin tumors, including melanomas, in Syrian hamsters (*294*). Parish and Searle (*295*) showed that β-propiolactone was effective in this species.

To compare these various systems, which appear to be particularly sensitive tests for alkylating carcinogens, the relationships between tumor induction and dose expressed in terms of alkylation of target DNA should be determined. This study has as yet not been extensively attempted, except for the mouse thymoma system.

Alkylating Agents and Cancer in Humans

Exposure to Industrial Chemicals and Pesticides. The manufacture and use of what may be termed classical alkylating agents is obviously limited and expected to be severely controlled because of their generally high toxicity. It is perhaps surprising that any cases of cancer due to industrial exposure have been documented. More hazardous exposures might be expected for agents that are themselves relatively weakly reactive but that are possibly subject to metabolic activation to more reactive mutagens.

The classical case for directly acting agents remains that of mustard gas (**1**) (*7*). Its use as a war gas during 1914–1918 led to numerous exposures, but statistical analysis of data relating these exposures to deaths from cancer, chiefly of the respiratory tract, did not establish causality conclusively (*296, 297*). Possibly because of the lower, but more prolonged, levels of exposure, and no doubt because of the nonprevalence of cigarette smoking in Japan at the time, the outstanding case where respiratory neoplasia can be attributed to industrial exposure is that of the workers in a mustard gas plant in Okuno-jima, Japan, during 1929–1945. Among 322 males who had worked with mustard gas, 33 deaths from such neoplasms (30 of which were histologically confirmed) were reported between 1948 and 1966 (*7*). The expected number based on mortality rates for males with the same age distribution is 0.9. Neoplasms of the squamous or undifferentiated cell type occurred along the main airways of the respiratory tract: tongue, pharynx, sphenoidal sinus, larynx, trachea, and bronchi. No adenocarcinomas were found. The findings for mustard gas were similar to those for induced neoplasia in uranium miners, which are consistent with the known "radiomimetic" character of the alkylating agent.

The epidemiology of lung cancer was reviewed by Berg (*298*) who concluded that adenocarcinoma predominates in nonsmokers. This tumor may therefore be taken as the typical "spontaneous" type of tumor at this site. In cases attributed to industrial exposure, asbestos appeared to cause this type of tumor. This may support the concept that this agent is a promoting rather than an initiating agent. Otherwise, industrial exposure was associated with increased incidence of squamous cell and oat cell carcinoma, which is compatible with the observations for tumor induction by mustard gas.

Druckrey et al. (*299*) reported that one case of human cancer could plausibly be attributed to industrial exposure to another alkylating agent, dimethyl sulfate. The latent period was 11 years, and the age at death was 47 years. The carcinoma was characterized histologically as being of the oat cell type and was sited in the upper respiratory tract. Dimethyl sulfate has also proved carcinogenic in model experiments using an inhalation technique in the rat (*290*) by inducing squamous nasal carcinoma.

In the chemical industry, as in the research laboratory, many compounds in common use present possible carcinogenic hazards. In fact, any alkylating agent should be used under carefully controlled conditions where contact or ingestion is effectively ruled out. Alkyl halides and sulfates; diazomethane and its precursors, including *N*-methylnitrosamides; ethyleneimines; and reactive lactones, including β-propiolactone, are obvious examples. Extensive relevant surveys of the industrial use of alkylating agents are available, notably in the publications of Fishbein et al. (*300–302*). Recently the International Agency for Research in Cancer (IARC, Lyon, France) has summarized its invaluable and comprehensive surveys on the evaluation of the carcinogenic risk of chemicals to humans, and those aspects relevant to alkylating agents and some related compounds are summarized in Table XIV. The compounds are listed in Tables XV–XXXVII under the same classifications as used for the more comprehensive summaries of data from experimental animal studies.

Halogenated hydrocarbons, including several important industrial chemicals, are dealt with in more detail in Chapter 9, but mention may be made here of those alkyl halides that have occasioned particular biochemical interest.

The dihalides methylene chloride (*303*) and ethylene dibromide (*304*) have been categorized as potential in vivo alkylating agents on chemical grounds and are mutagenic in bacteria (*303*) and in *Drosophila melanogaster* (*304*). A related compound, the pesticide 1,2-dibromo-3-chloropropane, was found to cause aspermia in exposed workers (*305*). It is a well-established carcinogen for mice and rats and is considered by IARC to present a carcinogenic risk to humans. The well-established carcinogen ethylene dibromide probably acts in vivo at least in part through metabolic activation to either an analog of sulfur mustard, by conjugation with glutathione or cysteine (*304*), or by oxidation to bromacetaldehyde (reviewed in Ref. 253).

The vinyl halides are also known to act as mutagens through metabolic activation. Vinyl chloride is a major intermediate in the chemical industry as a monomer in plastics manufacture. Several studies of its mode of action as a mutagen have been reported. The relevant metabolites are chloracetaldehyde or chloroethylene oxide.

Alkyl phosphates are widely used in the pesticide and gasoline industries and elsewhere, but were possibly neglected in earlier studies of alkylation because of their relatively low reactivity, which generally involves transfer of a single alkyl group. For example, methylation of DNA in vitro by dichlorvos (**29**) was a relatively slow reaction with a half-life of 16 h at 37 °C in aqueous solution, and the ultimate extent of reaction was about 1/15 of that observed with the same concentration of methyl methanesulfonate (*306*). A detailed study of methylation of DNA bases by trimethyl phosphate was reported by Yamauchi et al. (*307*) who found evidence for reaction at the O-6 of guanine. This reaction occurred in DNA methylated by dichlorvos about the same relative proportion of products (about 0.4%) as by methyl methanesulfonate (*306*).

```
CH3O  O                    CH3O
    \ ||             Cl     \  O        OH   Cl
     \||            /        \ ||       |   /
      P—O—CH=C               P—O—CH—C—Cl
     /            \         /           \
CH3O               Cl   CH3O             Cl

        29                       30
```

The phosphotriester insecticides dichlorvos and trichlorphon (**30**) are mutagens in bacteria and *Drosophila* (reviewed in Ref. 308). Administration of ^{14}C-methyl-labeled dichlorvos (*309*) or trichlorphon (*310*) to rats resulted in urinary

Table XIV
Comprehensive Literature Surveys on Alkylating Agents and Related Compounds for Evaluation of the Carcinogenic Risk to Humans

Compound	Year, Volume, Page	Evaluation of Data: Experimental	Evaluation of Data: Humans
Alkyl Halides			
Methyl chloride	—	study in progress, using inhalation in mice	epidemiological study in progress
Methyl iodide	1977, 15, 245	carcinogenic in mice, rats	cases of poisoning reported; no epidemiological study
Methylene dichloride	1979, 20, 449	test in mice considered inadequate	widespread exposure, but no epidemiological study
Ethylene dibromide	1977, 15, 195	carcinogenic in mice, rats	case of poisoning reported; no epidemiological study, but *see* Ref. 267
Vinyl bromide	1979, 19, 367	test in mice considered inadequate	exposure known to have occurred; no epidemiological study
Vinyl chloride	1974, 7, 291	carcinogenic in rats, mice, hamsters (metabolically activated)	(1) causes angiosarcoma of liver, and tumors of brain, lung, and hematopoietic system
Vinylidene chloride	1979, 19, 439	carcinogenic in mice, rats	epidemiological study considered inadequate
Aralkyl Halides			
Benzyl chloride	1976, 11, 217	carcinogenic in rats	epidemiological study in progress
Alkyl Sulfates and Sulfonates (monofunctional)			
Dimethyl sulfate	1974, 4, 271	carcinogenic in rats	(2B) case reports of respiratory tract cancer, but so far not statistically significant in

			epidemiological study
Diethyl sulfate	1974, 4, 277	carcinogenic in rats	no epidemiological study
Methyl methanesulfonate	1974, 7, 253	carcinogenic in mice, rats	no epidemiological study
Ethyl methanesulfonate	1974, 7, 245	carcinogenic in mice, rats	no epidemiological study
Alkyl Phosphates			
Dichlorvos	1979, 20, 97	studies with mice, rats considered inconclusive	used as insecticide; no epidemiological study
Tris(2,3-dibromopropyl) phosphate	1979, 20, 575	carcinogenic in mice, rats	flame retardant, widespread exposure, regarded as possible carcinogenic risk
Miscellaneous Esters			
Ethyl acrylate	1979, 19, 57	reported negative in rats	no epidemiological study
Parasorbic acid	1976, 10, 199	carcinogenic in rats	occurs in berries of mountain ash; used in food products; no epidemiological study
Maleic hydrazide	1974, 4, 173	study with mice assessed as negative	used as herbicide; no epidemiological study
Aflatoxins	1972, 1, 145; 1976, 10, 51	carcinogenic in rats, rhesus monkeys, and other species	(2A) probably carcinogenic; dose–response estimates for liver cell cancer have been reported for aflatoxin B ingested from foodstuffs; other studies in progress
Sterigmatocystin	1972, 1, 175; 1976, 10, 245	carcinogenic in mice, rats, trout	biosynthesis precursor of aflatoxin B in molds; no epidemiological study
Griseofulvin	1976, 10, 153	carcinogenic in mice	used as antibiotic; epidemiological study in progress

Continued on next page

Table XIV Continued

Compound	Year, Volume, Page	Evaluation of Data: Experimental	Evaluation of Data: Humans
Cyclic Sulfides and Sultones			
Ethylene sulfide	1976, 11, 257	carcinogenic in rats	no epidemiological study
1,3-Propane sultone	1974, 4, 253	carcinogenic in mice, rats	industrial intermediate; no epidemiological study
Haloalkyl Ethers			
Chloromethyl methyl ether	1974, 4, 239	evaluation complicated by 1–8% of the potent carcinogen bis(chloromethyl) ether as contaminant	(1) technical grade, as used industrially, caused lung cancer
Bis(chloromethyl) ether	1974, 4, 231	carcinogenic in mice, rats	(1) two studies showed increased risk of lung cancer (mainly oat cell carcinoma); further epidemiology in progress.
1,2,3-Tris(chloro-methoxy)propane	1977, 15, 301	carcinogenic in mice	no epidemiological study
Sulfur Mustards			
Mustard gas	1975, 9, 181	carcinogenic in mice	(1) several studies showed respiratory tract cancers from both industrial and sporadic exposures
Nitrogen Mustards			
Aramite	1974, 5, 39	carcinogenic in dogs, mice, rats	formerly used as an acaricide; no epidemiological study
Nitrogen mustard, HN2	1975, 9, 193	carcinogenic in mice, rats	parent compound of several

			cytotoxic drugs; no epidemiological study
Chlorambucil	1975, 9, 125	carcinogenic in mice, rats	(2A) probably carcinogenic, on basis of incidence of leukemias and other tumors in treated patients; further studies in progress
Melphalan	1975, 9, 167	carcinogenic in mice, rats	(1) caused second primary malignancies (mainly acute leukemia) in treated patients
Chlornaphazin	1974, 4, 119	carcinogenic in mice, rats	(1) caused bladder cancer in patients treated for polycythemia vera
Mannomustine	1975, 9, 157	carcinogenic in mice	no epidemiological study
Uracil mustard	1975, 9, 235	carcinogenic in mice, rats	no epidemiological study
Epoxides (monofunctional)			
Ethylene oxide	1976, 11, 157	reported carcinogenic in mice after IARC survey	(2B) epidemiological study in progress; industrial exposure can cause in vivo alkylation
Propylene oxide	1976, 11, 191	carcinogenic in rats	epidemiological study in progress
Fusarenon-X	1976, 11, 169	studies with mice, rats considered inadequate	metabolite of fungus on grain; no epidemiological study
Epichlorhydrin	1976, 11, 131	carcinogenic in mice, rats	industrial intermediate; epidemiological study considered inadequate
cis-9,10-Epoxystearic acid	1976, 11, 153	study with mice considered inconclusive	no epidemiological study
Glycidaldehyde	1976, 11, 175	carcinogenic in mice, rats	no epidemiological study
Glycidyl oleate	1976, 11, 183	weakly positive in mice, insufficient data	no epidemiological study

Continued on next page

Table XIV Continued

Compound	Year, Volume, Page	Evaluation of Data: Experimental	Evaluation of Data: Humans
Glycidyl stearate	1976, 11, 187	negative in mice	no epidemiological study
Heptachlor epoxide	1979, 20, 129	carcinogenic in mice, rats	found in fat and body fluids, derived from heptachlor (an insecticide); epidemiological evidence considered inadequate
Styrene oxide	1976, 11, 201	negative in mice, carcinogenic in rats	skin irritant; no epidemiological study
Ethyleneimines (Aziridines) (monofunctional)			
Ethyleneimine	1975, 9, 37	carcinogenic in mice, rats	no epidemiological study
Aziridine ethanol	1975, 9, 47	carcinogenic in mice	no epidemiological study
Oxetanes, Lactones, etc.			
β-Propiolactone	1974, 4, 259	carcinogenic in mice, rats	industrial intermediate and chemosterilant; no epidemiological study
β-Butyrolactone	1976, 11, 225	carcinogenic in mice	no epidemiological study
γ-Butyrolactone	1976, 11, 231	reported inactive in mice, rats	no epidemiological study
Succinic anhydride	1977, 15, 265	study with rats considered inadequate	industrial chemical; no epidemiological study
Patulin	1976, 10, 205	carcinogenic in rats	metabolite of mold on apples; no epidemiological study
Penicillinic acid	1976, 10, 211	carcinogenic in mice, rats	no epidemiological study; study of related antibiotic (penicillin) in progress
Phenylbutazone	1977, 13, 183	no data available	used as anti-inflammatory drug;

			reports of toxicity; case reports of leukemia, but epidemiological study considered inadequate
Phenytoin	1977, 13, 201	carcinogenic in mice	used in epilepsy; epidemiological study in progress
Cyclophosphamide	1975, 9, 135 1981, 26, 165	carcinogenic in mice, rats	(1) case reports of acute myeloid leukemia, bladder cancer, and nonlymphocytic leukemia in treated patients; epidemiological study in progress
Difunctional Alkanesulfonates			
Myleran	1974, 4, 247	weakly positive in mice, rats, but studies considered inadequate	(2B) case reports of increased risk of leukemia and other tumors in treated patients; epidemiological study in progress
Treosulfan	1981, 26, 341	no animal data	(1) increased risk of acute nonlymphocytic leukemia in treated patients
Difunctional Epoxides			
Diepoxybutane	1976, 11, 115	carcinogenic in mice, rats	industrial cross-linking agent; no epidemiological study
1-Epoxy-3,4-epoxycyclohexane	1976, 11, 141	carcinogenic in mice	used in epoxy resin manufacture; no epidemiological study
3,4-Epoxy-6-methylcyclohexylmethyl-3,4-epoxy-6-methylcyclohexane carboxylate	1976, 11, 147	carcinogenic in mice	used in epoxy resin manufacture; no epidemiological study
Difunctional and Polyfunctional Ethyleneimines			
Triethylenemelamine	1975, 9, 95	carcinogenic in mice, rats	industrial chemical and cytotoxic drug; no epidemiological study

Continued on next page

Table XIV Continued

Compound	Year, Volume, Page	Evaluation of Data: Experimental	Evaluation of Data: Humans
Tris(aziridinyl)-*p*-benzoquinone	1975, 9, 67	carcinogenic in rats	antineoplastic cytotoxic drug; case reports available but considered inadequate for evaluation
Tris(aziridinyl)phosphine oxide(TEPA)	1975, 9, 75	study in rats considered inadequate	used as cytotoxic drug prior to introduction of thio-TEPA; no epidemiological study
Thio-TEPA	1975, 9, 85	carcinogenic in mice, rats	(2A) several studies suggest development of acute nonlymphocytic leukemia in treated patients

NOTE: As reported in IARC Monographs (published by the International Agency for Research in Cancer, Lyon, France) up to 1981. In the evaluation of data for humans, the numbers in parentheses indicate (1), carcinogenic for humans; (2A), probably carcinogenic for humans, group with stronger evidence; (2B), group with weaker evidence; the remainder could not be classified because of insufficient evidence.

excretion of 7-[^{14}C]methylguanine, a finding that indicates that methylation of nucleic acids might have occurred. However, exposure of rats to atmospheres containing ^{14}C-methyl-labeled dichlorvos at a "practical use concentration" of 0.007 ppm for 12 h (total inhaled dose of 0.136 μmol/kg) did not cause a detectable extent of methylation of DNA in various tissues, down to a limit of detection of 1.67 pmol/mol DNA–P (*311*). The binding index in the units of Table XII was less than about 12. Extensive detoxificative metabolism of dichlorvos by cholinesterase was expected to counteract its methylating ability in vivo. The mutagenic action of dichlorvos in *Escherichia coli* was shown by Bridges et al. (*312*) to resemble closely that of methyl methanesulfonate. This finding accords with its known reactivity towards DNA as a typical S_N2 alkylating agent (*306*). Thus it yields a low proportion of O^6-methylguanine in the DNA methylation products and has correspondingly low ability to induce mutations by direct miscoding.

Alternative modes of action as genotoxic agents not necessarily involving methylation were proposed for both dichlorvos and trichlorphon on the basis of data from tests with eukaryotic cells. Desmethyl trichlorphon, a nonalkylating metabolite of trichlorphon, was found to be mutagenic in the dominant lethal test in mice (*313*). Dichlorvos was reported to interfere with DNA repair induced by UV-light irradiation in human lymphocytes (*314*). Conventional mutagenesis tests in mammalian cell systems, however, hav eso far proved negative (*308*), a finding in line with the very weak in vivo methylating activity of these insecticides.

The available data from tests of carcinogenicity of dichlorvos were considered by IARC to be insufficient to permit evaluation. A relatively weak positive response from prolonged administration of trichlorphon to rats was found by Gibel et al. (*315, 316*), but this study was also categorized as inadequate for evaluation by IARC. Results of extensive prolonged tests using administration of trimethyl phosphate in drinking water to rats and mice have been presented (*317*), but no detailed evaluation by IARC has appeared.

Another phosphoric acid triester that became prominent as a potential carcinogen for humans (and as a result has been banned in the United States for treatment of children's clothing since 1977) is the flame retardant tris(2,3-dibromopropyl) phosphate (**31**). This compound may well become the classical case

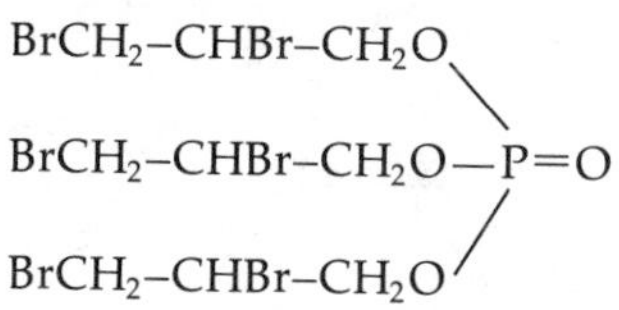

$$(BrCH_2\text{–}CHBr\text{–}CH_2O)_3P{=}O$$

31

where a potential carcinogenic hazard was deduced from (1) short-term bacterial mutagenesis tests (*318, 319*) (2), skin painting tests in mice (*320*), (3) and feeding studies in rats and mice (*321*). On the basis of these findings, its use was legally restricted (*321*). Deductions regarding the mode of action from mutagenesis tests were that direct action (perhaps as an alkylating agent) occurred at high concentrations. Perhaps surprisingly, metabolic activation appeared to be required at low concentrations (*319*); the mutations induced were base-pair substitutions.

The aliphatic epoxides constitute another large group of alkylating agents that are of considerable industrial importance. As with the phosphoric acid esters, their reactivity is comparatively low. This low reactivity may be contrasted with the high reactivity, particularly towards DNA, of the diol epoxide metabolites of carcinogenic polycyclic aromatic hydrocarbons.

With regard to industrial hazards of simple expoxides, the main interests have been directed toward the chemosterilant ethylene oxide (*264*) and styrene oxide (**32**), a metabolite of the industrial plastics monomer styrene (*322*). The details of correlations between alkylation of DNA and the mutagenicity of epoxides are discussed later. The detection of in vivo alkylation of hemoglobin in humans by ethylene oxide (*264*) will stimulate further interest in this area. It has recently been shown to cause injection-site sarcoma in mice (*323*). Styrene oxide induces sister chromatid exchange in human lymphocytes in culture (*322*) and is carcinogenic in rats (*324*), although previous studies with mice were considered inconclusive by IARC (*325*).

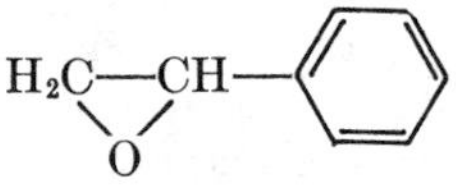

32

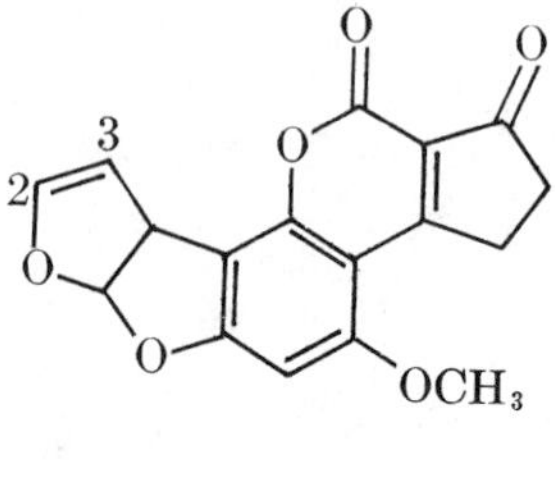

33

The carcinogenic lactones are a diverse group of compounds, among which *β*-propiolactone has been studied quite extensively. However, the best established human carcinogen in this group is aflatoxin B_1 (**33**), a mold product ingested in foodstuffs and beer, particularly in Africa. Some epidemiological evidence indicates that chronic hepatitis B virus infection is required as a cocarcinogen in this action (*326*). This compound had been classified as possibly directly acting, but in fact it is metabolically activated. The 8,9-epoxide reacts with DNA as the proximate mutagen and carcinogen (*327*). As already noted (Table XII), aflatoxin B_1 has probably the highest overall carcinogen binding index in rat liver of all carcinogens so far studied. Although well established to react at N-7 of guanine (for a review, *see* Ref. 327), no evidence suggests reaction at O-6, again possibly because of the relatively small proportion of reaction at this site. However, as already noted for β-propiolactone, bases other than O^6-alkylguanines have been suggested to be promutagenic.

Comparative studies of carcinogenicity of lactones were pioneered by Dickens (*328–30*), who commented on the possibility that they may be represented among the mutagens present in cigarette smoke. Dehydroacetic acid and an open-chain analog, sorbic acid (Table XXVI), used as fungistatic agents, were found to be carcinogenic in rats by subcutaneous injection but not by oral administration. Their hazard to humans is therefore in doubt (*331, 332*).

Ingestion of alkylating agents in the diet may be hazardous in some cases. Alcohol drinkers may be susceptible to esophageal cancer via diethyl epoxysuccinate (**34**) (*333*), and betel nut chewers are susceptible to cancer of the oropharynx via arecoline (**35**) (*334*).

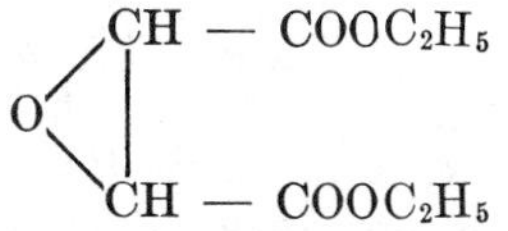

34

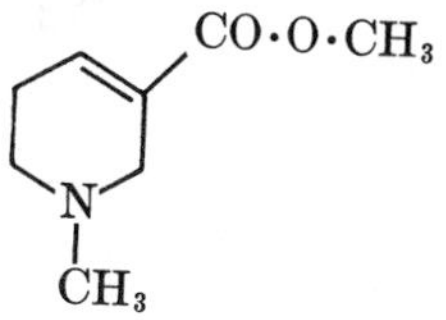

35

The possible contribution of pesticides in general to the causation of human cancer was discussed by Epstein in his book "The Politics of Cancer" (*335*). Some pesticides have been considered to fall into the category of lactones: the herbicide maleic hydrazide (**36**) (*336*), known alkylating agents such as the mutagen fungicide captan (**37**) (*337*), the acaricide Aramite (**38**), and the epoxide dieldrin

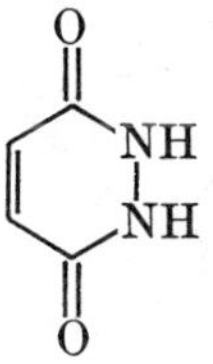

36

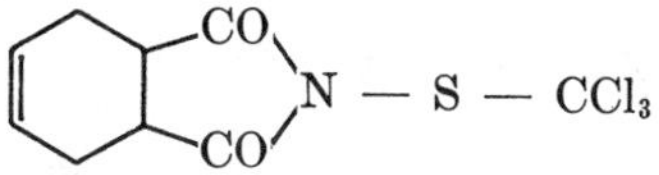

37

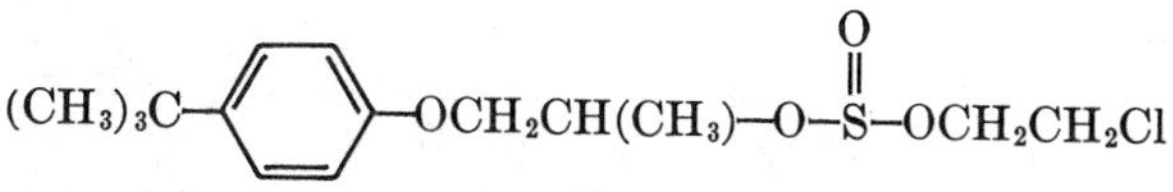

$(CH_3)_3C-C_6H_4-OCH_2CH(CH_3)-O-S(=O)-OCH_2CH_2Cl$

38

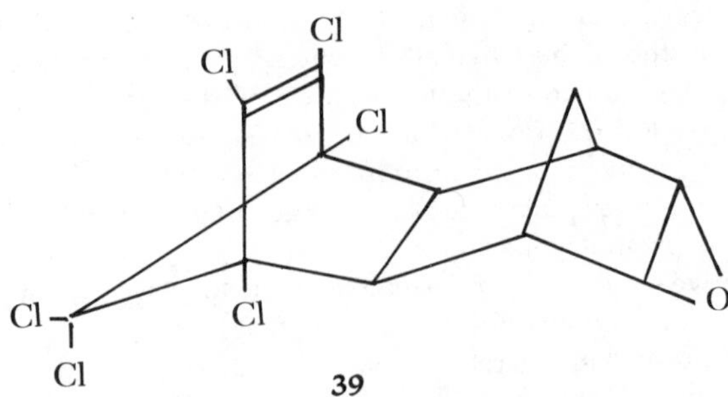

39

(**39**). During the period following the publication of Epstein's book, the magnitude of the carcinogenic hazard due to pesticides and other industrial chemicals became controversial. Peto (*338*) suggested that it had been exaggerated, but Epstein (*339*) maintained his original estimate that it could be a significant contributor to the totality of environmental carcinogenic hazards. Doll and Peto (*210*) later stated that at most 2% of cancer deaths in the United States are due to industrial products, compared with 35% attributed to diet and 30% to smoking.

Particular susceptibility of individuals to the environmental action of chemical carcinogens that are relatively weak mutagens might be expected to result from inherited impaired ability to repair DNA damage. Following the classical demonstration of susceptibility of xeroderma pigmentosum patients to UV-induced skin cancer (*195*), several other rare inherited syndromes have now been specified in which cancer susceptibility is associated with chromosomal instability and deficiency in DNA repair. These include Bloom's syndrome (*197*), ataxia telangiectasia (*340*), possibly Fanconi's anemia (*341*), and certain other inherited immunodeficiency states (*342*). The susceptibility of such individuals to radiation was generally the first indication of their proneness to cancer induced by specific agents, and the question of their susceptibility to chemicals is currently under intensive study (*197*).

Apart from mustard gas, the classical difunctional alkylating agents, including nitrogen mustards, are carcinogenic hazards mainly through their use in chemotherapy. However, an industrial cross-linking agent, bis(chloromethyl) ether, became prominent as an industrial carcinogen from a retrospective study among German workers for the period 1956–1962 (*343*) and from a Japanese report at around the same time (*344*). This agent now rivals mustard gas as a classical alkylating carcinogen for humans. Both agents are highly reactive in aqueous solution; bis(chloromethyl) ether has a half-life of less than 1 min (*345*). The monofunctional analog chloromethyl methyl ether was less active as a carcinogen in animal tests (*346*), and activity also decreased with increasing alkyl chain length in this series. In moist air, chloromethyl methyl ether is converted into the more carcinogenic difunctional agent (*35*).

Both chloromethyl methyl ether and bis(chloromethyl) ether are now regarded under U.S. health regulations as human carcinogens. Thirty cases of lung cancer attributed to industrial exposure to chloromethyl ethers were reported in the United States, six in Germany, and five in Japan (reviewed in Ref. *302*); like mustard gas, bis(chloromethyl) ether caused mainly oat cell carcinoma.

Interest in formaldehyde as a potential human carcinogen has been revived by the finding that its prolonged inhalation by rats caused squamous cell carcinoma of the nasal cavity (*347*). This finding parallels the action of bis(chloromethyl) ether in experimental inhalation carcinogenesis (*348*) and therefore raises the possibility that formaldehyde may be a lung carcinogen in humans. No epidemiological evidence for this possibility has yet been found, but this may reflect the inadequacy of the data (*347*).

Formaldehyde has been quoted as an example of a "noncarcinogenic mutagen" (*104, 349*), but it now appears that this view is no longer tenable. The products from its reactions with DNA include reversible methylol derivatives by reaction at amino groups, as well as a relatively small proportion of stable methylene-bridged cross-linked bases (*350, 351*). DNA–protein cross-linkage also occurs (*352*).

The industrial solvent hexamethylphosphoramide (**12**), also reported to cause squamous cell carcinoma of the nasal cavity of rats on inhalation (*353*), may act through metabolic oxidation to formaldehyde (*354*). Methylene dihalides and disulfonates may act the same way (*355*), although positive evidence for their carcinogenicity has not so far been found.

In summarizing the currently available data regarding alkylation-induced cancer in humans (apart from those due to chemotherapy), the evidence is clear that inhalation of the highly reactive and toxic agents mustard gas and the chloromethyl ethers has caused respiratory tract cancers. The dietary agent and powerful hepatotoxin aflatoxin B_1 appears to be a cause of liver cancer in specific areas, possibly in association with a hepatitis virus. Other agents, such as pesticides, are at present much less well defined as human carcinogens because of their weak chemical and biological activities. However, prolonged exposures to such weak carcinogens could add significantly to the totality of cancer causation. Some individuals, because of impaired DNA repair capability, could be particularly susceptible to cancer initiation by mutagens.

Chemotherapeutic Agents. The use of mutagenic and carcinogenic alkylating agents in industry is now under continuous scrutiny and control. However, such agents are extensively used in chemotherapy, particularly in cancer and allied diseases. This practice presents a carcinogenic hazard not only to the treated patients but also to those involved in administration of the drugs.

Evidence relevant to this problem has been reviewed from time to time (*356–62*) and only salient features from these extensive reports will be summarized here.

Haddow et al. (*363*) are credited with first raising the problems in using cancer chemotherapeutic drugs in 1948, and Shimkin et al. (*215, 216*) carried out the most extensive early study of carcinogenicity of cancer chemotherapeutic agents in the 1960s. The most clear-cut cases of human cancer caused by chemotherapy came from the use of chlornaphazin (2-naphthylamine mustard) (**40**) in polycythemia

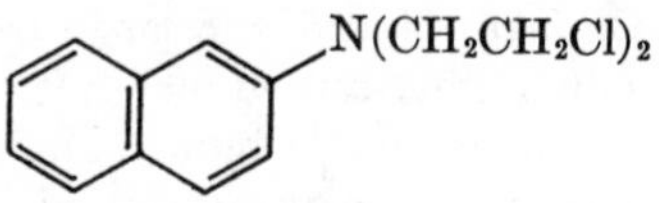

$$\text{(2-naphthyl)}-N(CH_2CH_2Cl)_2$$

40

vera (*364, 365*). However, direct action of the alkylating agent seems unlikely because the tumors induced were exclusively in the bladder, a known site of tumor induction in humans by 2-naphthylamine (*366*). Therefore metabolic activation of the mustard to yield this potent bladder carcinogen seemed the most likely explanation (*367, 368*).

However, the mutagenic, clastogenic, and carcinogenic effects of the alkylating agents demonstrated in animal tests indicate that they may act directly in humans as well. Hobbs (*369*) reviewed evidence that myeloma cells in patients treated with alkylating drugs could be mutated to drug-resistant forms and that benign tumors could be converted to malignant forms. To demonstrate early effects of cancer chemotherapeutic drugs, the detection of induced sister chromatid exchange in peripheral blood lymphocytes has proved to be a reasonably sensitive test (*370*). Nurses handling cytostatic drugs also showed a significantly higher degree of chromosomal damage than clerks in the same hospital (*371*). Mutagenicity of urine has also been used to show occupational exposure to mutagenic drugs for treated patients (*372*) and nursing staff (*373*).

The first report implicating a therapeutic agent as a leukemogenic agent came in 1945 from a study of polycythemia vera patients treated with ^{32}P (*374*). The subsequent use of chlorambucil (**25**) as a myelosuppressant in this disease prompted a study of its possible leukemogenic effect, which is now well established (*375*). The risk is 13.5 times as great for chlorambucil-treated patients (20% of the deaths were attributed to leukemia) as for those treated by phlebotomy alone, and 2.3 times as great as for those treated with ^{32}P.

Secondary acute nonlymphocytic leukemia now appears to be associated with alkylating agent therapy for a number of other conditions, including Hodgkin's disease; lymphosarcoma; chronic lymphocytic leukemia; cancers of ovary, lung, and breast; and malignant melanoma (*376*). In some cases a single cytostatic agent was implicated, as reported for Myleran (Busulfan) (**5**) (*377*) and Treosulfan (L-threitol 1,4-dimethane sulfonate, the dihydroxy derivative of Myleran) (**41**) (*376*).

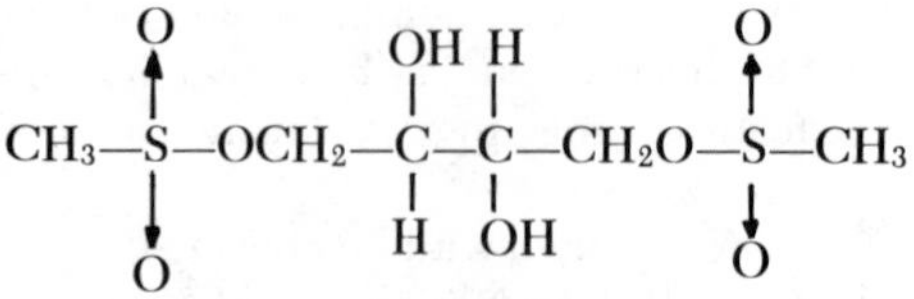

$$CH_3-S(\rightarrow O)_2-OCH_2-CH(OH)-CH(OH)-CH_2O-S(\rightarrow O)_2-CH_3$$

41

The second outstanding example of drug-induced neoplasia in humans is that of histiocytic lymphoma (formerly denoted reticulum cell sarcoma) in patients treated with immunosuppressive drugs, including alkylating agents such as cyclophosphamide (**8**) or chlorambucil (**25**) (*358, 378, 379*); antimetabolite drugs such as azathioprine (**42**) also appear to be causative agents. Skin cancer is also

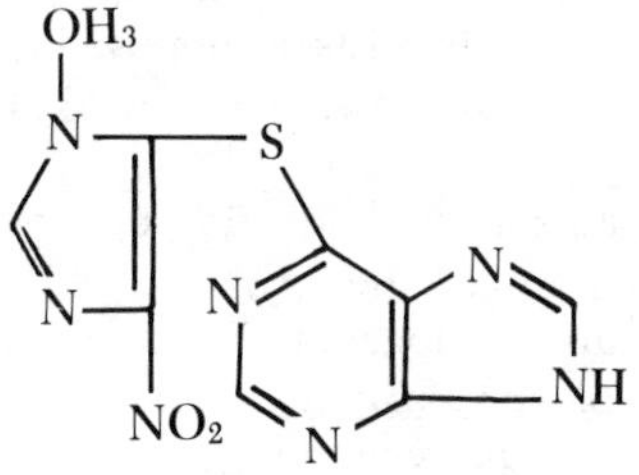

42

prominent, but to a lesser extent, in the spectrum of tumors associated with immunosuppression (*358*).

These observations have stimulated much interest in the etiology of drug-induced neoplasia in humans because it may give some indication of the etiology of cancer in general. The predominance of tumors of lymphoid tissues and leukemia shows some analogy with the predominance of such tumors, mainly thymic lymphoma, in the systemic action of the cytotoxic alkylating carcinogens (Myleran, TEM, and HN2) in mice (*380, 381*). A radiation-sensitive (and comparatively alkylation-sensitive) strain of mice (RFM) required multiple doses of these drugs to obtain significant yields of thymomas, and the yields of leukemia were not generally significantly greater than for controls. Thus, the carcinogenicity of the highly cytotoxic difunctional or polyfunctional alkylating agents appears to be much less than that of the potent mutagen *N*-methyl-*N*-nitrosourea (*cf.* Figure 1).

Louie and Schwartz (*382*) reviewed the problem of drug-induced human neoplasia and summarized the findings as follows. Immunosuppressants, principally azathioprine, appear to cause predominantly histiocytic lymphoma in humans. Azathioprine is not an alkylating agent and is at most a weak carcinogen (*383*), causing mainly thymoma in NZB or NZB × NZW mice by multiple injections. IARC considered that the available data for this compound could not be evaluated. Azathioprine-related tumors arose predominantly in younger people and could have extremely short latent periods, in some cases only a few months (*358, 379*). Some skin cancers, and a proportion of other epithelial tumors that was much less than that found for the general population, were also attributed to immunosuppression, but leukemia was rare. These results strongly suggest, therefore, that preselected groups of humans, like inbred strains of mice, can be particularly susceptible to systemically acting carcinogens.

The transplant patients who underwent immunosuppression appeared to resemble untreated patients with certain autoimmune diseases (e.g., autoimmune hemolytic anemia) who also show an excess of lymphomas compared with the general population. The mouse strains used for the test of azathioprine are also inherently susceptible to autoimmune disease. Louie and Schwartz (*382*) and Hoover (*358*) suggest that these induced lymphomas in humans may result from activation of a tumor virus, possibly the Epstein–Barr virus. The theory that the negation of immunosurveillance is the cause of human cancer in general (*384, 385*) is not supported by these data, however, because lymphoma is a minor contributor to the totality of human cancer; epithelial tumors predominate. A comparison of the cause of death of American chemists, as opposed to the population in general, showed that the most markedly excessive cancer in chemists was lymphoma (*386*).

The other striking feature of the induction of cancer in humans by cytotoxic drugs was that "aggressive chemotherapy," i.e., the use of cytotoxic alkylating agents, leads mainly to acute myelogenous (or nonlymphocytic) leukemia, not to lymphoma. This degree of specificity remains unexplained, but is stimulating continued investigation, particularly with regard to the chromosomal changes that appear to be associated with this type of leukemia (*376, 387–90*) and may be of diagnostic value and of etiologic significance.

With regard to the ethics of continuing to use carcinogenic alkylating drugs in treatment of patients, the general view is that this practice should continue. The benefits generally outweigh the risks, but such treatment should be reviewed continuously in the light of the type of study discussed here (*362, 379, 391*). These studies have already shown in some instances that relative carcinogenic risks of different agents can be assessed. Patients with autoimmune disorders appear to be particularly susceptible to these carcinogens, as well as to other immunosuppressants.

Representative Oncogenesis Tests with Alkylating Agents

In this section, data on animal tests are summarized in Tables XV–XXXVII for compounds classified according to chemical type. Sufficient detail has been given to enable fairly rapid comparisons to be made without reference to original literature. The literature must generally be consulted for details such as precise methods of dosimetry and administration, sex and age of animals, and any statistical evaluation of data.

The diversity of the chemical nature of the compounds and also of the type of test system used are obvious features of any attempted survey of this kind. This range prevents any overall quantitative comparison of carcinogenic potency of compounds. However, such comparisons can be valid when a single well-defined test system is used. For example, Shimkin et al. (*215*) (*see also* Ref. *392*) assigned numerical values for carcinogenic potency to 29 alkylating agents tested over a range of dose levels administered by intraperitoneal injection for ability to induce lung tumors in strain A/J mice. Druckrey et al. (*290*) assigned numerical tumorigenicity indices to 12 alkylating agents administered by subcutaneous injection to BD rats.

The general conclusion from these comparative studies was that most alkylating agents were not very potent carcinogens when compared with the classical polycyclic aromatic hydrocarbons such as 7,12-dimethylbenz[*a*]anthracene or benzo[*a*]pyrene. Graffi et al. (*393*) considered that the action of *N*-methyl-*N*-nitrosourea as a skin carcinogen in rodents was "not weaker than that of the strongest hydrocarbons."

Clayson (*394*) considered that "with few exceptions, it is difficult to accept that the carcinogenic activity of the biological alkylating agents has been firmly established, because so much of the evidence is concerned with the induction of subcutaneous sarcomas in the rat." He called for further tests using subcutaneous injection or skin painting in mice. The early tests with β-propiolactone (*329, 395*) appeared vulnerable to this criticism, although the results did show that in control animals, multiple injections of the vehicles used gave either no tumors during the test period or gave tumors after longer induction times than the tested compound. The use of subcutaneous injection tests was reviewed by Carter (*396*) and by Grasso and Goldberg (*291*).

In a succinct review of carcinogenesis tests in general, Roe and Tucker (*397*) noted some "discrepancies between the logical basis of routine carcinogenicity testing and current knowledge of mechanisms of carcinogenesis," with particular emphasis on the influence of diet, the immune status of animals, and the role of tumor viruses. The last two factors have been discussed in detail by Kouri et al. (*398*).

McDonald (*399*) found that nitrogen mustard, HN2, enhanced the rate of tumor appearance in female rats of the Holtzman strain, but tumors appeared in about the same numbers and of the same types in control animals kept for more than 1 year after the injections were started. The conclusion was that HN2 "was not in itself the carcinogenic agent," and "might have acted as a cocarcinogen in these groups of animals."

The concept of alkylating agents as cocarcinogens may appear to be at variance with the more generally accepted classification of these agents as initiators rather than promoting agents. In the classical two-stage carcinogenesis test using the mouse skin system, several alkylating agents were classified as initiating agents. Roe and Salaman (*281*) found TEM and β-propiolactone to be initiators in this system, and Salaman and Roe (*282*) found chlorambucil positive in this sense, but HN2, Myleran, and Melphalan were inactive.

Colburn and Boutwell (*400, 401*) used alkylation of DNA, RNA, or protein of mouse skin as an index of potency of several alkylating agents in this regard. They found a positive correlation between in vivo alkylation of DNA and initiating aiblity increasing in the following order: iodoacetic acid, 3-chloropropionic acid (noninitiators), 3-iodopropionic acid (weak initiator), and β-propiolactone (active initiator). With regard to promoting activity, they stated that "the binding data for β-propiolactone and iodoacetic acid are compatible with the theory that protein binding is important in promotion of skin tumorigenesis."

The situation may be envisaged to be of some complexity a priori, because in vivo alkylation of DNA, as discussed previously, can lead both to mutagenesis and to "reproductive cell death." The ability to initiate may be reasonably associated positively with mutagenic action. On the other hand, the cytotoxic action may be considered as "antipromotional" considering that promotion is associated with stimulation of target cell division. Therefore, alkylating agents can be both initiating agents and "anticarcinogenic" agents. This latter finding was reported for mustard gas (*6*) and for butadiene dioxide (*402, 403*), which inhibited tumor initiation in mouse skin by aromatic hydrocarbons. Furthermore, because alkylating agents are not specific reagents for DNA in vivo, but also react with proteins, the concept that alkylation of protein can play a role in promotion could accord with the activity of alkylating agents as complete carcinogens in some cases.

Slaga et al. (*404*) compared the effect of selected agents on macromolecular synthesis in target epidermal tissues of mouse skin with histological changes. The initiating agents urethane, 1,3-(γ)-propane sultone, β-propiolactone, and bis-(chloromethyl) ether all inhibited DNA synthesis immediately (up to about 1–2 d) after application, but subsequent recovery occurred after about 3 d and was associated with hyperplasia in the treated area of skin. These observations are consistent with the concept that initiation involves somatic mutation along with promoting action (the stimulation of cell division of mutant cells), as previously discussed in terms of the two-stage theory of carcinogenesis (*268, 269*).

The most comprehensive series of investigations of some alkylating agents of relatively simple structural types by several administration routes are those by Van Duuren et al. (*403*). β-Propiolactone and β-butyrolactone were classified as positive because they gave malignant tumors in long-term tests by four routes: application to skin of mice, subcutaneous injections in mice and rats, and gastric feeding to rats. The epoxides glycidaldehyde, *d,l*-1,2,3,4-diepoxybutane, and 1,2,5,6-diepoxyhexane gave tumors by the first three routes, but gastric tumors could not be induced. This result was ascribed to rapid acid-catalyzed hydrolysis of epoxides. At the estimated stomach pH of 1, β-lactones are not hydrolyzed.

Mice or rats were used in nearly all the tests recorded. In view of the supposition that alkylating agents act by direct reaction with target tissues, species-dependent differences reflecting different modes of metabolism should therefore not be expected to be very important. Parish and Searle (*295*) confirmed this assumption by showing that β-propiolactone can induce skin tumors in the guinea pig and golden hamster. The susceptibility of the latter species to melanotic tumor induction, noted for 7,12-dimethylbenz[*a*]anthracene and 4-nitroquinoline *N*-oxide, was also found with this alkylating agent.

In the overall assessment of alkylating agents as weak carcinogens, it was often necessary to use either relatively high doses, with the resulting complication of decreased survival of tested animals relative to controls, or multiple doses throughout a major part of the life span of the animals. In the search for more sensitive testing techniques, injection of neonatal animals has been a notable introduction. Walters et al. (*405*) used this method with ethyl methanesulfonate and in two strains of mice. Five daily subcutaneous injections during the first 5 d of life was a more effective administration method than a single injection within 1 d of birth. Five injections of 200 μg of ethyl methanesulfonate in 3% aqueous gelatin induced lung adenomas in all surviving Balb/c mice at 50 weeks, compared with 8.3% in the controls. The same procedure with arachis oil as the vehicle was ineffective, although a positive response was obtained in C57BL mice.

Chernozemski and Warwick (*406*) found that β-propiolactone was a potent hepatocarcinogen for male suckling mice (C57BL/6 × A)F_1, whereas treated baby females gave few hepatomas but had an enhanced incidence of malignant lymphomas. Adult mice were not susceptible to hepatocarcinogenesis by this agent.

Transplacental administration of alkylating agents was used, notably by Druckrey et al. (*290, 407*), by injection of single doses into pregnant rats at the 15th day of gestation. Dimethyl and diethyl sulfates and 1,3-propane sultone gave malignant tumors in the offspring, mainly in tissues of the nervous system.

Although tumors generally have been induced by alkylating agents at the application site, as expected from their ability to alkylate tissues in that vicinity [shown, for example, in Colburn and Boutwell's in vivo alkylation studies (*400, 401*)], many examples show tumor induction at distant sites. In some cases (*see* Table XIII) alkylation of cellular constituents was demonstrated at such sites. The apparent lack of simple positive correlation between extent of in vivo alkylation reactions and tumor yields has been noted already.

In view of the general assessment that alkylating carcinogens are initiators rather than promoters, the inability of alkylation to cause tumorigenesis in particular organs might be ascribed in part to lack of appropriate promotional stimulus. The applicability of the classical two-stage scheme of carcinogenesis to organs other than skin remains a problem for further study. The findings of Chernozemski and Warwick (*406*) for hepatocarcinogenic action of β-propiolactone illustrate the possible importance of hormonal status of the animal; male baby mice were much more susceptible than females.

An outstanding problem encountered throughout the work on experimental alkylation-induced carcinogenesis in animals that is possibly also reflected in human cancer attributed to alkylating agents is the apparent dichotomy between local and systemic action, with respect to dependence on the chemical reactivities of the alkylating agents.

Broadly, local carcinogenic action is often found with highly toxic, but not outstandingly mutagenic, agents. Thus in Druckrey's work (*290*) on induction of injection-site sarcoma in BD rats, agents such as dimethyl sulfate and methyl methanesulfonate were effective carcinogens. Previously these agents proved to be either weak carcinogens or, as assessed on results with a limited number of animals, effectively noncarcinogenic.

For example, methyl methanesulfonate, which is able to methylate DNA of target tissues following a single injection into C57BL mice, did not induce a significant yield of thymoma, in contrast with *N*-methyl-*N*-nitrosourea (*11*). However, Schneider et al. (*408*) obtained significant yields of brain tumors from multiple injections of methyl methanesulfonate into hooded rats, thus reinforcing the result based on relatively small numbers of brain tumors induced by single injections into Wistar rats by Swann and Magee (*218*). The relatively low yield of O^6-methylguanine in DNA methylation by methyl methanesulfonate appears to account for the low carcinogenicity of this agent. The relative lack of repair removal of this promutagenic base from DNA in brain (*158*) may enable detection of its carcinogenicity in this organ.

Injections into subcutaneous tissue of rats or mice may cause relatively high local levels of DNA methylation, but this result apparently has yet to be determined, as has the ability of this tissue to repair DNA methylation damage. The ability of initiated cells to multiply in this tissue with consequent promotional hyperplasia may also favor carcinogenesis.

Whatever the causative factors, the classification as carcinogens of a considerable proportion of the cytotoxic alkylating agents rests on evidence of local sarcoma induction from subcutaneous injections.

However, an approach to local carcinogenesis more relevant to human exposure for several alkylating carcinogens is to use administration by inhalation. Druckrey (*290*) showed that dimethyl sulfate, inhaled by rats, caused squamous carcinoma of the nasal cavity. Laskin and coworkers further developed the use of this method of administration and have shown that inhalation by rats of epichlorohydrin (1-chloro-2,3-epoxypropane) (**16**) (*409*) and of dimethyl carbamoyl chloride (*410*) also caused mainly this type of tumor. Bis(chloromethyl) ether gave both nasal and bronchial carcinomas; the nasal carcinomas were esthesioneuroepitheliomas (*410*). Formaldehyde has also been shown to induce squamous nasal carcinoma by Swenberg et al. (*347*) using a similar method.

Two established human respiratory carcinogens, mustard gas and bis(chloroethyl) ether, gave tumors throughout the respiratory tract, and therefore the tendency to localization of inhaled carcinogen-induced tumors in the nasal tract of rats has stimulated discussion (*347, 409*). Suggested factors are distribution of the carcinogen (*409*); the fact that rats, unlike humans, are obligatory nose breathers (*347*); and possibly cocarcinogenesis by sialodacryoadenitis virus (*347*). Therefore, humans may be particularly susceptible to cancer of the respiratory tract due to prolonged inhalation of relatively small doses of toxic alkylating carcinogens. Furthermore, inhalation studies with rats as a model for this process are useful, but are somewhat limited in that the upper respiratory tract of the rat may be specifically more susceptible.

With regard to a suitable animal model for systemic carcinogenesis by alkylating agents, the previous section discussed evidence that lymphoma and acute leukemia were predominant human tumors induced by chemotherapeutic agents. These findings are parallel to the predominant features of the systemic action of alkylating carcinogens in several strains of mice, notably AKR (*285*), NZB × NZW (F_1), RFM (*162*), CFW/D (*293*), and C57BL (*11, 273*), in which thymic lymphomas could be induced in high yields. The possible involvement of the C-type murine leukemic viruses as cocarcinogenic agents in this action is particularly indicated by Frei's work (*285*) showing the particular susceptibility of the AKR strain. The types of tumor induced are not identical for mouse and human, but most likely the systemic action of alkylating carcinogens in both species is basically due to the mutagenic action of the chemical agent on cells where the genome contains proviral DNA, and the specific types of tumor induced depend on the respective specific genetic backgrounds affected by this factor. EB virus is suggested to be involved for humans. Some parallelism was also noted between susceptibility of NZB × NZW (F_1) mice to alkylating carcinogens and their inherited susceptibility to autoimmune disease, and a similar association was noted for humans. Further comparative studies of the mode of action of alkylating carcinogens in mice as a model for carcinogenesis in humans appear to be warranted (*162*).

Oncogenesis Tests with Alkylating Agents in Relation to Their Chemical Structure and Reactivity

Simpler Alkyl Halides. Despite their extensive industrial use, the alkyl halides (Table XV) in general have not been subject to very extensive tests for carcinogenic

Table XV
Representative Oncogenesis Tests with Alkylating Agents and Some Related Compounds—Alkyl Halides

Compound	Animal	Strain or Type	Route	Dose (mg/kg)	Duration (d)	Tumors	Remarks	References
Methyl bromide	rat	white	inhal.	0.28–0.42[a]	176	none	probably inconclusive	416
Methyl iodide	rat	BD	sc	10,wkly × 50	580[b]	9/12 local sarcomas	a few tumors at other sites	290
				20,wkly × 45	620[b]	6/20 local sarcomas		
				50,single	610[b]	4/14 local sarcomas		
	mouse	—	inhal.	0.5[a] × 20	30	none	probably inconclusive	417
	rat	white	po	100–500,daily	71	none		
	mouse	A/He	ip	(8.5,21.3,44) (3 × wkly for 8 wks)	168	lung tumors 0.55 per mouse	sig ($P < 0.05$) only at highest dose, controls 0.22	14
Methylene dichloride[c]	mouse	NMRI,F_1 2–3 months old	skin	0.2 mL[c] × 25 (twice wkly)	675	2/50 tumors	one skin tumor	418
	mouse	A/St	ip	160,400,800 (3 × wkly for 16–17 wks)	168	lung tumors	not sig. different from controls	419
Chloroform	mouse	A	po (intragastric)	590 × 30 1180 × 30		3/5 hepatomas 4/5 hepatomas	tumors in females only; males died from renal necrosis	420
	mouse	C3H	inhal.	5[a]	540	0/72		421
	mouse	(C57 × DBA/2)	ac	200 μg[d] 200 μg × 8	519	not sig. greater than controls		422
	mouse	B6C3F1	po gavage	138–477 5 × wkly for 78 wks)	651	hepatocellular carcinomas	$P < 0.001$	412,423

Continued on next page

Table XV Continued

Compound	Animal	Strain or Type	Route	Dose (mg/kg)	Duration (d)	Tumors	Remarks	References
	rat	Osborne–Mendel	po gavage	100,200 (5 × wkly for 78 wks)	777	kidney epithelial tumors	$P = 0.0016$	412,423
Carbon tetrachloride[e]	mouse	A	po (intragastric)	160–2600	150	136/300 hepatomas	dose–response study	424
	mouse	B6C3F1	po gavage	1250,2500 (5 × wkly for 78 wks)	644	hepatocellular ca. 96/97(m), 83/85(f)		413,423,425
Ethylene chlorohydrin	rat	—	po	0.01–0.24%[d] in diet	up to 403	0/35		426
Ethylene dibromide	rat	—	inhal.	25 ppm[f] 7 h daily	213	0/40		427
	rat	Osborne–Mendel	po (intubation)	—[h]	378	31/31 gastric squamous carcinoma		428
	mouse	Ha:ICR	skin	25,50 mg (3 × wkly)	594	8/30 papillomas 3/30 carcinomas 26/30 lung tumors		429
				75 mg then promotion with phorbol ester		2/30 papillomas	not active as initiator	
	rat	Sprague–Dawley	inhal.	20 ppm	approx. 450	hemangiosarcoma of spleen 10/48(m) 6/48(f)	synergistic action of disulfiram in diet increased spleen tumors, also gave hepatocellular carcinoma	430

Ethylene dichloride	rat	Wistar	inhal.	200 ppm[f] 157 × 7 h exposures	212	0/30[i]		431
	mouse	Ha:ICR	skin	126 mg (3 × wkly)	594	26/30 lung tumors	no skin papillomas	429
Freon 112	mouse	Swiss S newborn	sc	not stated	365	1% sc sarcomas 5% hepatomas		432
Freon 113	rat	Wistar albino	inhal.	12000 ppm[f] 2 h/d 5d/wk	730	1/6 fibrangio-sarcoma	1/6 sc and 1/6 lung tumors; tumors in controls	433
Vinyl chloride[j]	rat	Wistar Ar/IRE (m)	inhal.	3%[f] 4 h/d 5 d/wk	380	15/26 skin (mostly epidermold ca.) 0/26 lung 3/26 osteo-chondroma		434
Vinylidene chloride	mouse	Ha:ICR	skin	121 mg then promotion with phorbol ester	594	8/30 papillomas	initiator but not complete carcinogen	429[j]
Allyl chloride	mouse	Ha:ICR	skin	94 mg then promotion with phorbol ester	594	7/30 papillomas	initiator but not complete carcinogen	429[j]

NOTE: Alkylnitroso compounds and dialkylnitrosamines or other carcinogens known to be metabolized to yield alkylating agents are not included in this compilation of data. Certain compounds generally classified as alkylating agents, although they are almost certainly converted to more reactive molecular species in vivo, such as cyclophosphamide, are included. Urethane and analogs (alkyl carbamates) are not included. Details about administration and histopathology are not given, and the original references should be consulted for this information. Generally only the principal types of tumor induced are listed. Tumor yields are expressed as number of tumors per number of animals used. For survival data, *see* original references.

[a] Inhalation dose, mg/L of air; 8 h/d, 5 d/wk.
[b] Average time of death.
[c] Inhalation tests over 6 months with various animal species have been reported (*435*), but no tumors were found.
[d] Amount given per dose, not mg/kg.
[e] Several other studies have been made; generally, inhalation or sc injection did not give tumors.
[f] Inhalation dose, ppm of air.
[g] Maximum tolerated dose; *see* reference for details. Also active in (C57B1 × C3H)F_1 mice by same route. Also active at half the maximum tolerated dose.
[h] Another study (*436*) also showed no carcinogenic effect by inhalation.
[i] For a review of other extensive tests *see* Ref. 415.
[j] This reference also reviews other tests and reports on tests with related compounds.

activity, but this deficiency has begun to be remedied. (*See also* Tables III and IV).

Tests with methyl chloride and methyl bromide are not yet adequate, according to IARC. Methyl iodine is carcinogenic in mice and rats, but the tests were not very extensive. Methylene dichloride has not so far proved to be significantly carcinogenic.

Chloroform (*412*) and carbon tetrachloride (*413*) have been more intensively studied, are accepted by IARC as proven carcinogens in animals, and are regarded as a carcinogenic risk to humans. Attempts to show that they react with DNA in vivo (through metabolic activation, since they are not directly reactive alkylating agents) were considered to be unconvincing by IARC (*412, 413*), although binding to proteins has been demonstrated. Rocchi et al. (*414*) found no binding of $^{14}CCl_4$ to DNA of liver of rats or mice 12 h after intraperitoneal injection. For mice only, pretreatment with 3-methylcholanthrene before $^{14}CCl_4$ injection gave an apparent DNA binding index of 51 (in the units of Table XII) from a dose of 0.367 mmol/kg. No products were characterized.

Ethylene dichloride and its fluoro-substituted derivatives were not significantly carcinogenic when administered to rats by inhalation. Ethylene dichloride and dibromide are carcinogenic to mice and rats when administered by gastric intubation, in the diet, or by repeated applications to skin, but were not active as initiators in a conventional test using skin application to mice (for a review, *see* Ref. 253). As previously discussed in connection with DNA binding of ethylene dibromide in vivo, metabolic conversions to sulfur mustard-type derivatives or to haloaldehydes may well be involved in their carcinogenic action. Haloaldehydes are also implicated for the well-established carcinogenic action of vinyl chloride. In view of its importance as a major industrial chemical intermediate, vinyl chloride has been very extensively studied (*415*), and molecular mechanisms of its action as a mutagen have been proposed.

β-Carbonyl-Substituted Alkyl Halides. These compounds (Table XVI) are classical S_N2 reagents and react principally with groups of high nucleophilicity, such as thiols. Although they are evidently feeble initiators, perhaps reflecting their lack of reactivity toward DNA, they may act as promoting agents by virtue of their ability to react with proteins in vivo (*400, 401*).

Aralkyl Halides. This group (Tables III and XVII) contains carcinogens of relatively high potency. They have been studied because of their relationship to carcinogenesis by polycyclic aromatic hydrocarbons and because they are suitable agents for structure–activity correlations.

Dipple et al. (*447*) reviewed the topic of selectivity of aralkylation of nucleic acid components and compared this with the reactions of simple alkylating agents. The classical factors of ionizing power of solvents and effects of substitution of the aryl moiety of the agents were used to rationalize reaction mechanisms. They concluded that increased delocalization of charge on the benzylic carbon of aralkylating agents favors their reaction at the exocyclic N-2 atom of guanine rather than at the O-6 atom, which is associated with S_N1 reaction of simple alkylating agents (for further discussion *see* Chapter 2). Aralkylation at N-2 of guanine in DNA has been suggested as promutagenic, leading to GC→CG transversions (*see* Figure 6), while O^6-alkylation would presumably lead to GC→AT transitions.

Table XVI

Representative Oncogenesis Tests—β-Carbonyl-Substituted Alkyl Halides

Compound	*Mouse Strain or Type*	*Route*	*Dose*	*Duration (d)*	*Tumors*	*Remarks*	*References*
Chloracetic acid	Ha:ICR	skin	2 mg,3 × wkly	580	none		284
Ethyl chloroacetate	Ha:ICR	skin	2 mg,3 × wkly	580	none		
Ethyl bromoacetate	Ha:ICR	skin	0.5 mg,3 × wkly	580	none		
			0.5 mg, promotion with phorbol ester, 2.5 μg, 3 × wkly	385	8/30 papilloma 1/30 carcinoma	3/30 papilloma in controls	
Chloracetone	stock	skin	—	133	none		
	albino	skin	0.2 mL 0.3% in acetone × 24[a]	365	44/19 papillomas	10/20 papillomas in controls	438
Iodoacetic acid[b]	rat hybrid	sc	multiple, total, 960 mg	596	1 inj. site fibroma, 1 inj. site fibrosarcoma, 1 plasma cell sarcoma		439
	Swiss	po	45 doses, total 36 mg	315	2/40 papillomas of forestomach	3/40 papillomas of forestomach in controls	440

Continued on next page

Table XVI Continued

Compound	*Mouse Strain or Type*	*Route*	*Dose*	*Duration (d)*	*Tumors*	*Remarks*	*References*
		skin	10 μmol × 6	210	none	with or without promotion by croton oil; alkylation of RNA, DNA, and protein studied	400,401
3-Bromopropionic acid	albino	skin	0.2 mL, 0.3% in acetone × 24[a]	365	78/20 papillomas	10/20 papillomas in controls	438
3-Iodopropionic acid		skin	120 μmol × 6	210	none	with or without croton oil	400,401

[a]Promotion with croton oil, 0.2 mL, 0.3% in acetone, 20 weeks. For details of time course and survival *see* original reference.
[b]Iodoacetic acid is a cocarcinogen in the mouse skin test system (*441*) and is a mitotic stimulator in this tissue (*442*).

Table XVII

Representative Oncogenesis Tests—Aralkyl Halides

Compound	*Animal*	*Strain or Type*	*Route*	*Dose*	*Duration (d)*	*Tumors*	*Remarks*	*References*
Benzyl chloride	rat	BD	sc	40 mg/kg wkly× 52 80 mg/kg wkly × 46	500 500	3/14 local sarcomas 6/8 local sarcomas		290
7-Bromomethylbenz-[*a*]anthracene	rat	CB-hooded	sc	0.025–0.25 mmol/kg	630	1-7/20 local sarcomas	13	
	mouse	Swiss S(f)	skin[a]	1 μmol[b] (321 μg)	112	4/25 papillomas[c]	1.2 papillomas/mouse	443
	mouse	Swiss S (f,new-born)	sc (is)[d]	266 μg × 3	up to 431	15/26 lung[c] 1/26 liver[c]		444
		Swiss S (m,new-born)	sc (is)[d]	266 μg × 3	up to 431	33/43 lung[c] 35/43 liver[c]	2 malignant lymphoma, 1 inj.-site sarcoma	
	mouse			5 μmol/kg	140	15/8 lung adenoma		448
7-Bromomethyl-12-methylbenz-[*a*]anthracene	rat	CB-hooded (f)	sc	0.0056–0.56 mmol/kg		1–15/20 local sarcomas		13
	mouse	Swiss S (f)	skin[a]	1 μmol[b]	112	22/25 papillomas[a]	4.1 papillomas/mouse	445
	mouse	Swiss S f,new-born)	sc (is)[d]	277 μg × 3	up to 431	16/17 lung[a] 3/17 liver		444
		Swiss S (m,new-born)	sc (is)[d]	277 μg × 3	up to 431	24/26 lung[c] 23/26 liver[c]		
	rat	Sprague–Dawley (f)	sc	0.1 mg × 20	200	6/12 inj.-site sarcomas	no mammary cancer	446
				1 mg × 20	200	3/5 inj.-site sarcomas		

Continued on next page

Table XVII Continued

Compound	Animal	Strain or Type	Route	Dose	Duration (d)	Tumors	Remarks	References
	mouse	A/He(f)		5–10 μmol/kg	140	25–47/6 lung adenoma		448
7-Chloromethyl-12-methylbenz-[a]anthracene	rat	Sprague–Dawley (f)	sc	1 mg × 20	200	9/9 inj.-site sarcomas	no mammary cancer	446
	mouse	A/He(f)		4 μmol/kg	140	34/12 lung adenoma		448
7-Iodomethyl-12-methylbenz-[a]anthracene	rat	Sprague–Dawley (f)	sc	0.1 mg × 20	200	5/5 inj.-site sarcomas	no mammary cancer	446
				1 mg × 20	200	4/11 inj.-site sarcomas		
9-Chloromethyl-anthracene	mouse	A/He(f)	iv	5 μmol/kg	140	3/8 lung adenoma	not sig. (controls 13/39)	448
9-Bromomethyl-anthracene				5 μmol/kg	140	9/8 lung adenoma		
10-Chloromethyl-9-methyl-anthracene				10,15 μmol/kg	140	9,31/8 lung adenoma		
10-Chloromethyl-9-chloro-anthracene				10 μmol/kg	140	15/8 lung adenoma		

[a]Promoted with Hecker's croton oil fraction A (10 μg, twice weekly, × 25).
[b]Single dose, as initiator.
[c]Refers to number of tumor-bearing animals; some had multiple tumors.
[d]Injection near root of tail to deliver to interscapular region.

The high potency of certain aralkyl halides was shown (*448*) in comparisons with the most potent polycyclic aromatic hydrocarbon, 7,12-dimethylbenz[*a*]anthracene, by using intravenous injection into strain A mice. As an example, 7-bromomethyl-12-methylbenz[*a*]anthracene gave a yield of lung adenomas about five times that of the parent hydrocarbon.

9-Chloromethylbenz[*a*]anthracene was not significantly carcinogenic when injected into strain A mice, but carcinogenicity (yielding multiple lung adenomas) was increased by either chloro- or methyl-substitution. On the grounds that the former decreases the rate of solvolysis of the parent aralkylating agent, whereas the latter increases it, solvolysis rate and carcinogenicity were not to be considered positively correlated. Further studies correlating in vivo alkylations, particularly of target DNA, appear warranted to clarify the relationship between reactivity and carcinogenicity for this group of agents.

Monofunctional Alkyl Sulfates and Sulfonates. This group includes chemically highly reactive compounds (Table XVIII). The methyl and ethyl esters of methanesulfonic acid in particular have been studied extensively as in vivo alkylating agents. These studies played an important part in the correlations between chemical reactivity and carcinogenicity of alkylating agents. The positive association between S_N1 reactivity and carcinogenicity predicts that carcinogenic potency should increase from methylating through ethylating to isopropylating agents. However, at a given concentration of agent, the overall extent of alkylation of DNA also decreases through this series. The net result is that the sulfates or sulfonates as a group are not highly potent carcinogens. Methyl and ethyl methanesulfonates can, however, induce tumors distant from the site of application. Ability to induce neurogenic tumors is associated with lack of DNA repair removal of O^6-alkylguanine from target tissues.

Wright (*450b*) suggested that diisopropyl sulfate may be the "hidden carcinogen" responsible for paranasal sinus tumors in workers engaged in manufacture of isopropylalcohol from propylene in the presence of sulfuric acid.

Alkyl Phosphates, Thiophosphonates, and Phosphonates. The outstanding carcinogen in this group (Table XIX) is tris (2,3-dibromopropyl) phosphate, used extensively as a flame retardant, and now regarded as a carcinogenic risk to humans because of extensive human exposures, particularly in children's sleepwear. It was reported as s directly acting mutagen at relatively high concentrations, but it required metabolic activation at low concentrations, so that its mode of action appears to warrant further study. Oral administration to mice and rats gave dose-dependent yields of tumors of forestomach, lung, kidney, and liver.

Somewhat in contrast, studies with other alkyl phosphates have not in general shown any marked carcinogenic activity, possibly reflecting their relatively weak chemical reactivity as alkylating agents. Trichlorphon gave liver carcinomas and papillomas of the forestomach, and diisopropyl fluorophosphate gave pituitary tumors. Assessment by IARC of the data for trichlorphon did not permit its evaluation as a carcinogenic hazard.

Miscellaneous Esters. Esters of fatty acids (Table XX) appear generally to be inactive. This conclusion is possibly consistent with their hydrolysis mainly at the

Table XVIII
Representative Oncogenesis Tests—Alkyl Sulfates and Sulfonates (Monofunctional)

Compound	*Animal*	*Strain or Type*	*Route*	*Dose (mg/kg) (or as stated)*	*Duration (d)*	*Tumors*	*Remarks*	*References*
Dimethyl sulfate	rat	BD	sc	8 wkly × 58	500[a]	7/12 local sarcoma 1/12 hepatocellular ca.		290
				16 wkly × 49	330[a]	4/6 local sarcoma		
				50 single		7/15 local sarcoma		
			iv	2–4, wkly		negative tumors		
			trans-placental iv	20		7/59 mostly of nervous system		
			inhal.	3–10 ppm 1 h, 5 × wkly		8/27 tumors, squamous ca. of nasal cavity, and others		
		Wistar	inhal.	0.5 ppm 6 h 2 × wkly		2/37 nasal ca. 1/37 lung ca.	no respiratory tract ca. in controls	449
				2 ppm 6 h every 2 wks		6/27 nasal ca. 1/27 lung ca.		
	mouse	(NMRI)	inhal.	0.5 ppm 6 h 2 × wkly		1/32 lung ca.	no nasal ca.	
				2 ppm 6 h every 2 wks		3/25 lung ca. (f, only)		
	hamster	Syrian Golden	inhal.	0.5 ppm 6 h 2 × wkly		no respiratory tract ca.		
				2 ppm 6 h every 2 wks				
	mouse	Ha:ICR	skin	0.1 mg 3 × wkly	475	none		284
				1 mg then promotion with phorbol ester 2.5 μg 3 × wkly	385	2/20 papillomas 0/20 carcinoma	3/30 papillomas in controls	
Diethyl sulfate	rat	BD	sc	25 wkly × 32	415[a]	6/12 local sarcoma	also active by transplacental route	290

				50 wkly × 32	350[a]	11/11 local sarcoma 1/11 adenocarcinoma		
Diisopropyl sulfate	rat	BD	sc	100 wkly × 15	604	14/15 local sarcoma		450
				300		8/15 local sarcoma 2/15 in remote organs		
Di-*n*-butyl sulfate	rat	BD	sc	500 wkly × 19	675[a]	2/7 local sarcoma		290
Glycol sulfate	mouse	Ha:ICR	skin	0.1 mg then promotion with phorbol ester	385	4/30 papilloma	3/30 in controls	284
			sc	0.5 mg, wkly	413	21/30 local sarcoma	glycol sulfite inactive	
Methyl methanesulfonate	rat	BD	sc	4 wkly × 46	635[a]	3/12 local sarcoma 1/12 nephroblastoma		290
				8 wkly × 46	490[a]	3/8 local sarcoma		218
	rat	Wistar albino	iv	72	—	1/20 spinal cord meningioma 2/20 brain astrocytoma		
				96	—	1/20 neurofibroma 1/20 brain oligodendroglioma		
				120	—	0/16		
		hooded	iv	100 wkly × 2 then 50 wkly × 13	684	14/28 brain tumors 3/28 bone marrow tumors 8/28 other	also 8/38 neurological tumors from transplacental administration in controls	408 451
	mouse	RF/Un (m, 1 wk old)	po	20 mg/100 mL in drinking water, ~30 mg/kg/d	550	2.1% stomach 4.2% liver 14.9% thymic lymphoma 70.2% lung adenoma 44.7% other (mainly retic. cell sarcoma) (% of 47 animals)	0 3.7% 3.7% 38.9% 60.5% (% of 162 animals)	
	mouse	CFW/D	ip	132	365	2/35 lymphoma	not statistically	293,452

Continued on next page

Table XVIII Continued

Compound	*Animal*	*Strain or Type*	*Route*	*Dose (mg/kg) (or as stated)*	*Duration (d)*	*Tumors*	*Remarks*	*References*
		inbred				8/35 lung adenoma	sig. greater than controls	
		C57BL/Cbi	ip	80–160	700	0/98		11
Ethyl methanesulfonate	mouse	CBA	ip	200×3^{b}	693^{a}	5% kidney, carcinoma 28% kidney, cystic papillary adenoma 89% lung, solid adenoma 11% lymphoma	3% kidney, 20% lung, 5% lymphoma in controls	453
	mouse	Balb/C (newborn)	sc	$200 \mu g^{c}$	280	9/45 lung adenoma	not sig. greater than controls	405
				$200\ \mu g \times 5^{c}$		8/51 lung adenoma		
			sc	$200\ \mu g \times 5^{d}$	280	31/31 lung adenoma	13.6 adenomas per survivor	
	mouse	C57B1 (newborn)	sc	$200\ \mu g \times 5^{c}$	420	5/39 lung adenoma	no tumors in controls	
	mouse	CFW/D inbred	ip	675	210	1/22 lymphoma 20/22 lung adenoma	not sig. sig.	293,452
		C57BL/Cbi	ip	200–400	700	5/133		11
	rat	Wistar albino	ip	275×3	—	12/24 kidney mesenchymal		220
				350	—	1/22 brain ependymoma		

	rat	Sprague–Dawley	ip	3 × 33 mg	365	various, 74% (f) 53% (m) 0% in controls	mainly anaplastic carcinoma of lung and especially in (f) adenocarcinoma of abdominal wall	454
		hooded	iv	110 wkly for 15 wks	684	39/28 brain tumors 7/28 bone marrow tumors 5 other	7/32 tumors by transplacental administration	408
n-Butyl methanesulfonate	mouse	albino "S"	skin	10 × 0.8 mg[e]	140	0/10		455
				10 × 8 mg[e]	140	0/10		
Methyl *p*-toluenesulfonate	rat	BD	sc	15 wkly × 53	470	7/10 local sarcoma 1 bronchial ca. 1 mammary ca. 1 ovarial ca.		290
Ethyl *p*-toluenesulfonate	rat	BD	sc	50 wkly × 65	600	3/11 local sarcoma		290
n-Butyl *p*-toluenesulfonate	rat	BD	sc	250 wkly × 34	up to 828	0/15		290
Allyl methanesulfonate	mouse	albino "S"	skin	10 × 1.35 mg[e]	140	12/20 papillomas	total of 42 papillomas	455
Propargyl methanesulfonate	mouse	albino "S"	skin	10 × 1.3 mg[e]	140	4/19 papillomas	1/20 papillomas in controls; not sig. (*t* test)	455

NOTE: In sc injections, compounds were administered in arachis oil unless otherwise stated.
[a]Mean survival time.
[b]At intervals of 3 weeks.
[c]Vehicle, arachis oil.
[d]Vehicle, 3% aqueous gelatine.
[e]Promotion with 18 weekly applications of 0.5% croton oil.

Table XIX

Representative Oncogenesis Tests—Alkyl Phosphates, Thiophosphates, and Phosphonates

Compound	*Animal*	*Strain or Type*	*Route*	*Dose (mg/kg)*	*Duration (d)*	*Tumors*	*Remarks*	*References*
Trimethyl phosphate	mouse	B6C3F1	intubation to stomach	50–500 3 × wkly	721		extensive results but not so far evaluated	317
	rat	Fischer F344						
Dimethyl-2,2-chloro-vinyl phosphate (Dichlorvos)	rat	White–Sherman	po (diet)	0.4–69.9	90		0/10	456
	rat	albino	po	10	42		0/?	457
	mouse	B6C3F1	po (diet)	average 318 and 635	630		differences from controls not sig.	458
	rat	Osborne–Mendel	po (diet)	average 150 and 326	735		differences from controls not sig.	
Dimethyl 1-hydroxy-2,2,2-trichloroethyl phosphonate (Trichlorphon)[a]	rat	Sprague–Dawley	ip	50–150, daily	60	0/15	reported inactive in mice, hamsters, by ip injection (Ref. 462)	459
	rat	BD	sc	50	800	2/24 i.site sarcoma		460
	rat	Wistar		30, 3 × wkly	up to 705	3/52 papilloma, forestomach		461[a]
	rat	Wistar	sc	30, 3 × wkly	up to 720	7/61 papilloma, forestomach		
	mouse	AB	skin	30, 3 × wkly	up to 790	1/16 liver carcinoma 1/16 papilloma, forestomach		
	mouse	AB	skin[b]	30, 3 × wkly	up to 781	1/9 liver carcinoma 2/19 papilloma, forestomach 1/19 local sarcoma		

Diethyl 2-chloro-vinyl phosphate	rat	Long–Evans	po (diet)	6.3–100 ppm	60	0/24		463
Dimethyl dithio-phosphate of diethyl mercap-tosuccinate	rat	—	po (diet)	100–5000 ppm	730	0/?		464
Diethyl *p*-nitrophenyl thiophosphate	rat	albino	po (diet)	10–50 ppm	365	1 sarcoma, mediastinum	considered not sig.	465
Diethyl *S*-ethyl-mercaptoethanol thiophosphate	rat	albino	po (diet)	1–50 ppm	112	0/90		466
Diethyl *S*-[2-ethylthio)-ethyl] phos-phorodithioate	rat	Sprague–Dawley	ip	0.25–1.5	60	0/25		467
Diisopropyl fluorophosphate	rat	Wistar	im	0.5 (every 75 h)	730	16/100 pituitary tumors (chromophobe adenoma)	spont. incidence "rare"	468
2-Ethylhexyl-diphenyl phosphate	rat	Carworth albino	po (diet)	0.625–5%	730	24/160 various	not sig. (9/40 in controls)	469
Tris(2,3-dibromo) phosphate	mouse	ICR/Ha	skin	10,30 mg, 3 × wkly	496	54/59 lung tumors	also tumors of forestomach, skin, oral cavity	320
	mouse	B6C3F1	po (diet)	500 1000	721	24/95 forestomach 35/92 squamous cell carcinomas and papillomas	also lung, kidney, liver tumors	
	rat	Fischer	po (diet)	50 100	721	69/216 kidney adenomas and adenocarcinomas		

[a]Several other results have been reported (*see* Refs. 315, 316, and 462), but IARC consider that the data for trichlorphon are not "adequate" by their criteria.
[b]Promotion with croton oil, weekly.

Table XX

Representative Oncogenesis Tests—Miscellaneous Compounds Including Esters, Alkyl Formates, Carbonates

Compound	*Animal*	*Strain or Type*	*Route*	*Dose*	*Duration (d)*	*Tumors*	*Remarks*	*References*
Ethyl formate	mouse	albino "S"	skin[a]	10 × 276 mg wkly	133	0/20		281
Diethyl carbonate	mouse	albino "S"	skin[a]	10 × 290 mg	210	2/25 papillomas	4/20 papillomas in controls	282
Tricaprylin	rat	albino	sc	0.1 mL	480	0/20	often used as a vehicle for carcinogens	420
	mouse	albino	sc	0.1 mL	400	0/57		
Tributyrin	rat	AES	po (diet)	15–25%	245	papillomatosis of forestomach		471
n-Butyl stearate	rat	Sprague–Dawley	po (diet)	0.01–6.25%	730	0/90		472
Ethyl acrylate	rat	Wistar	po (in water)	6–2000 ppm	730	0/50	"insufficient details" according to IARC	473,474

[a]Promotion with 18 weekly applications of croton oil (0.3 mL in acetone).

acyl–oxygen rather than at the alkyl–oxygen linkage, in contrast to the alkylating abilities of sulfate and phosphate esters.

Further tests with ethyl acrylate were considered desirable by IARC because this compound is produced industrially on a massive scale for use in paints and other products.

Monofunctional Epoxides. The parent compound, ethylene oxide, typifies the reactivity conferred by the strained three-membered ring (Tables XXI and XXII).

Early tests of ethylene oxide by skin painting (*475*) or by subcutaneous injection into rats (*476*) were negative. However, the use of the epoxide as a chemosterilant for bedding of a colony of albino mice for 150 d was suspected to have caused multiple tumors in 90% of exposed females compared with 0% in 83 controls not exposed to the treated bedding (*477*).

A subsequent test (*478*) used multiple subcutaneous injections of ethylene oxide (in 0.1 mL of tricaprylin) into mice. Dose-dependent induction of injection-site sarcoma was found at approximately the same incidence as that found in a parallel experiment with propylene oxide, which had been accepted previously as a carcinogen (*476*) because it gave injection-site sarcoma in rats. For both epoxides the yields of tumors at distant sites were not significantly different from those in control animals.

Epichlorohydrin, another epoxide of industrial importance, was first reported as inactive by skin painting of mice (*479*). It was subsequently found to be an initiator but not a complete carcinogen in this system (*284*) and was also found to be active by inhalation (*409*).

In extensive studies of epoxides, Van Duuren et al. (*480–82*) found other simple aliphatic epoxides generally to be inactive. It appears necessary to elongate the aliphatic chain of the molecule to enhance activity or to include other relatively hydrophobic groups conferring greater lipid solubility, but not all such modifications are effective in this respect (Table XXII).

An apparent exception to this generalization is glycidaldehyde. However, as shown by Van Duuren et al. (*542*), it can act as a difunctional agent in its reaction with guanosine, and difunctional epoxides are in general more potent carcinogens than monofunctional ones (*403*). Monofunctional agents with adjacent centers of unsaturation may be converted in vivo to difunctional agents (*480*).

Thus, epoxides can act as alkylating agents in neutral aqueous media and were shown to be mutagenic in numerous instances (*264, 300*). However, either the simpler monofunctional epoxides alkylate to an insufficient extent in vivo to cause carcinogenesis, or the types of reaction undergone do not lead to this effect. Propylene oxide reacts slowly with DNA in aqueous solution (*482*) introducing the $\cdot CH_2CH(OH)CH_3$ group by the S_N2 mechanism.

No studies of in vivo alkylation of DNA by epoxides appear to have been reported. However, active monofunctional epoxides such as styrene oxide and 1,2-epoxybut-3-ene (Table XXI) might react in part by the S_N1 mechanism with the derived carbonium ion being stabilized mesomerically. This reaction in turn might correlate with enhanced mutagenic, and therefore possibly tumor-initiating, activity according to the arguments discussed previously.

Some evidence has been presented (*483*) that ring-substituted styrene oxides are more mutagenic in a bacterial test system if they react with DNA in the

Table XXI

Representative Oncogenesis Tests—Epoxides (Monofunctional)

Compound	*Animal*	*Strain or Type*	*Route*	*Dose*	*Duration (d)*	*Tumors*	*Remarks*	*References*
Ethylene oxide	rat	albino	sc[a]	100[b]	—	0/12		476
	mouse	NMRI	sc	0.1–1 mg	637	6–12/100 i. site sarcoma	0/100 in controls	323,478
Propylene oxide	rat	albino	sc[a]	150[b]	739	8/12 local sarcomas	9/67 local sarcomas and 14/67 other neoplasms in analogous controls (*395*)	476
				150[c]	737	3/12 local sarcomas		
	mouse	NMRI	sc	0.1–2.5 mg wkly	637	3–15/100 i. site sarcoma	0/100 in controls	323
Glycidal-dehyde[d]	mouse	ICR/Ha Swiss	skin	10 mg, 3 × wkly in acetone	598	6/41 papillomas 3/41 squamous ca.		480
				3 mg, 3 × wkly in benzene		16/30 papillomas 8/30 squamous ca.		
			sc	0.1 mg, wkly	595	2/50 fibrosarcomas 1/50 squamous ca.		481
				3.3 mg, wkly	536	3/30 fibrosarcomas 2 squamous ca. 1 undiff. sarcoma		
	rat	Sprague–Dawley	po (intra-gastric)	33 mg, wkly	492	0/5		480
	rat	Sprague–Dawley	sc	1 mg, wkly	558	1/50 fibrosarcoma		480
				33 mg, wkly	539	5/20 local sarcomas		481
Glycidol	mouse	ICR/Ha Swiss	skin	5 mg, 3 × wkly in acetone	520	0/20		479
1,2-Epoxybutane	mouse	ICR/Ha Swiss	skin	10 mg, 3 × wkly in acetone	540	0/30		

1,2-Epoxy-3-butene	mouse	Swiss–Millerton	skin	100 mg, 3 × wkly no solvent	237[e]	3/30 papillomas 1/30 squamous ca.	considered active	482
1,2-Epoxy-hexadecane	mouse	ICR/Ha Swiss	skin	10 mg, 3 × wkly in acetone	427	2/41 papillomas 1/41 squamous	considered active; 1,2-epoxy-dodecane inactive	479
Epichlorohydrin	mouse	ICR/Ha	skin	2 mg, then promoted with phorbol ester	385	9/30 papillomas 1/30 carcinoma	3/30 in controls	284
			sc	1 mg, wkly		6/50 local sarcoma	1/50 in controls	346
	rat	Sprague–Dawley	inhal.	100 ppm 6 h × 30		15/140 nasal carcinoma	also dose–response and lifetime exposure data	409
Glycidal ester of hexanoic acid	rat	albino	sc[a]	200[b]	658	7/12 local sarcoma		476
Glycidal ester of dodecanoic acid	rat	albino	sc[a]	440[b]	626	6/12 local sarcoma		476
Glycidal ester of octadecanoic (stearic acid)	rat	albino	sc[a]	550[b]	608	4/12 local sarcoma		476
Styrene oxide	mouse	Swiss–Millerton	skin	10 mg, 3 × wkly in benzene	431[e]	3/30 papillomas 130 squamous ca.	considered active; sat. analog, ethyleneoxy-cyclohexane inactive	486
	rat	Sprague–Dawley	po	50,250 mg/kg, 4–5 × wkly	1092	stomach tumors (papillomas, carcinomas)	considered a very potent directly acting carcinogen	324

[a]Generally twice weekly.
[b]Total dose in arachis oil.
[c]Total dose in water.
[d]May be effectively difunctional, because both the aldehyde and epoxide groups react with guanosine (*482*).
[e]Median survival time.

Table XXII

Representative Oncogenesis Tests—Epoxides (Monofunctional) Reported to Be Inactive

Compound	*Test System*	*References*
Ethylene oxide[a]	mouse skin; rat sc	403,476
Glycidol	mouse skin	403
Epichlorhydrin[a]	mouse skin	479
Epibromohydrin	mouse skin	403
1,2-Epoxybutane	mouse skin	403
2,3-Epoxy-2-methylpropyl acrylate	mouse skin	479
9,10-Epoxystearic acid	mouse skin; mouse and rat sc	495
Glycidyl ester of stearic acid	rat sc	476
1,2-Epoxydodecane	mouse skin	403
Epoxycyclohexane	mouse skin; rat sc	403
1-Vinyl-3,4-epoxycyclohexane	mouse skin	403
Epoxycyclooctane	mouse skin	403
Indan epoxide	mouse skin	403
Limonene monoxide	mouse skin	403
Ethyleneoxycyclohexane	mouse skin	487
Dieldrin[b]	rat and dog po; rabbit skin	488
Andrin[c]	rabbit skin;	487
	rat po	489

[a]Subsequently reported positive, *see* Table XXI.
[b]*Endo, exo* isomer, hepatocarcinogen in mice (*485*).
[c]*Endo, endo* isomer of dieldrin.

"abnormal" fashion, i.e., by reaction at the C-atom of the epoxide ring that carries more substituents other than hydrogen (Scheme VIII). This mode of reaction has been associated with the S_N1 mechanism (*17*). However, as yet no evidence for alkylation of DNA at O-6, as opposed to N-7, of guanine by styrene oxide derivatives has been found.

Epoxides of particular interest as insecticides include the isomers dieldrin and endrin. Ingestion of these compounds in food has been considered as a potential carcinogenic hazard to humans (*484*), but no firm conclusion was reached. Dieldrin fed to mice in the diet caused hepatic tumors in a dose-dependent manner, but no evidence of positive carcinogenicity in other organs of mice was found. Tests with rats, dogs, and monkeys were also negative. Tests with endrin were not regarded as conclusive.

Monofunctional Ethyleneimines (Aziridines). Aziridines (Table XXIII) were first studied by Walpole (reviewed in Ref. 476), who was influenced by the view that substitution of long-chain alkyl groups into the aziridine nucleus enhanced the

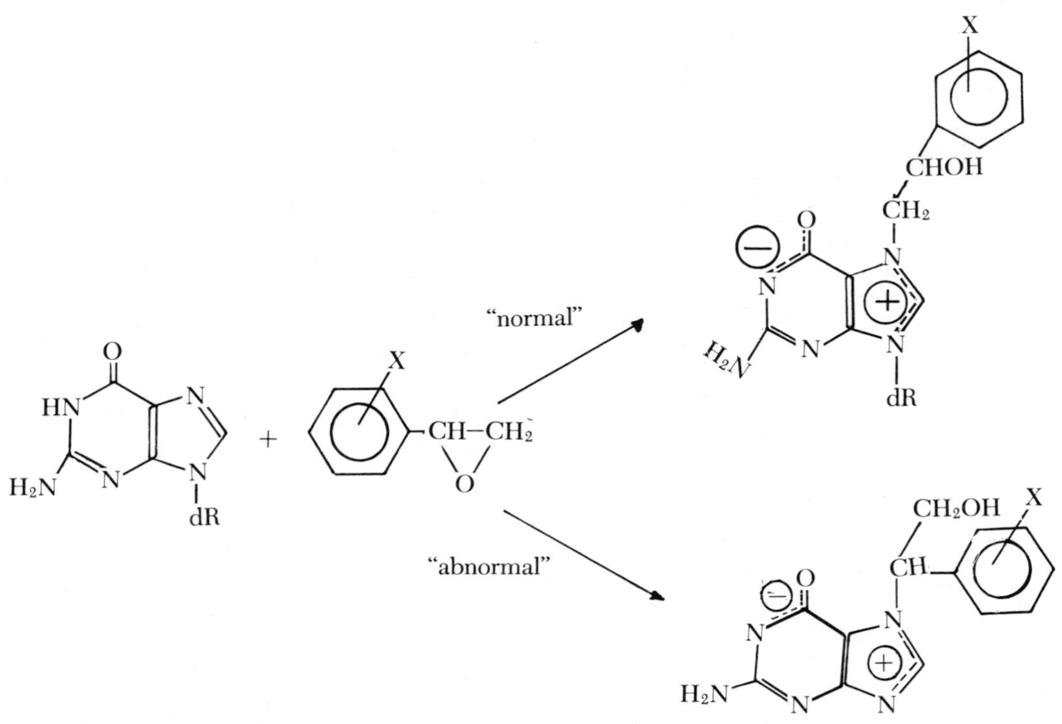

Scheme VIII. Reactions of substituted styrene oxides with deoxyguanosine [Sugiura and Goto (483)].

The "normal" reaction pathway, nucleophilic attack by N-7 of deoxyguanosine at CH_2 of a substituted styrene oxide, is proportionately higher than for styrene oxide ("normal" product 67%), if the substituents X are electron-withdrawing (e.g., X = m-Cl, "normal" product 90%). Nucleophilic attack is proportionately lower if X groups are electron-releasing (e.g., X = 3,4-dimethyl, "normal" product 53%). Mutagenicity of substituted styrene oxides correlated positively with "abnormal" reaction rate, rather than with overall reaction rate.

Table XXIII

Representative Oncogenesis Tests—Ethyleneimines (Monofunctional)

Compound	Animal	Strain or Type	Dose[a] (mg/kg)	Duration (d)	Tumors	Remarks	References
Ethyleneimine (aziridine)	rat	albino (m) albino (f)	20[b]	546	5/6 local sarcoma 1/6 local sarcoma	1/19 local sarcoma, 1/19 local fibroma, 4/19 other tumors in controls, but latent period generally longer in controls	395
		albino (m)	12[c]	540	0/6 local sarcoma 1/6 kidney carcinoma		
		albino (f)			2/6 local sarcoma		
	mouse	(C57BL XC3H)F_1	13, po	546	26/32 hepatomas 30/32 pulmonary tumors	similar result with two other strains, also i. site sarcoma by sc inj.	491
1,2-Propyleneimine	rat	CD	10×120,[d] gavage	420	20/26 breast 8/26 other in females 4/26 leukemia 4/26 glioma 9/26 other in males		492
N-Acetylethyleneimine	rat	albino	up to 210[b]	515	13/30 local sarcoma 3/30 other		
		albino (m)	160[c]	449	3/6 local sarcoma		
		albino (f)	80[c]		1/6 local sarcoma		
	mouse	C (m)	200[b]	371	6/20 local sarcoma		
		C3Hf (f)	180[b]		5/20 local sarcoma		
Aziridine ethanol	mouse	ICR/Ha Swiss	0.3 mg $\times$ 75[e]	525	10/30 local sarcoma		490
N-Butyrylethyleneimine	rat	albino	220[b]	489	11/12 local sarcoma 4/12 other		395
			225[c]	428	10/12 local sarcoma 1/12 other		
	mouse	C3Hf	488[b]	504	3/20 local sarcoma		

N-Diethylacetylethyleneimine	rat	albino	420–440[b]	314	9/12 local sarcoma 3/6 mammary ca. in (f) 2/6 other in (f)		
			225[c]	428	10/12 local sarcoma 1/12 other		
			400–460[d]	346	11/12 local sarcoma 5/6 mammary ca. in (f)		
	mouse	C3Hf(f)	488[b]	443	10/16 local sarcoma		
N-Caproylethyleneimine	rat	albino	49.5–51[b]	314	12/12 local sarcoma		
			52.5[d]	450	8/12 local sarcoma		
	mouse	C3Hf(m)	765[b]	385	5/16 local sarcoma		
		C3Hf(f)	360[b]		2/20 local sarcoma		
N-Nonanoylethyleneimine	rat	albino	760–860[b]	296	11/12 local sarcoma 3/12 other		
			720–740[d]	324	9/12 local sarcoma 5/12 other		
	mouse	C3Hf(m)	500[b]	504	4/20 local sarcoma		
N-Laurylethyleneimine	rat	albino	1000[b]	up to 741	1/12 local sarcoma 4/12 other		
N-Myristoylethyleneimine	rat	albino	3325[b]	229	8/12 local sarcoma		
	mouse	C3Hf(m)	1600[b]	395	13/20 local sarcoma		
N-Oleylethyleneimine	rat	albino	17[b]	178	11/12 local sarcoma		
N-Stearoylethyleneimine	rat	albino	27.5[b]	441	7/12 local sarcoma 2/12 other		395
Ethyleneiminosulfonylpropane	rat	albino	1250[b]	601	0/12		
Ethyleneiminosulfonylpentane	rat	albino	900[b]	601	0/12		
Ethyleneiminosulfonylheptane	rat	albino	1500[b]	601	0/12		
4-Chloro-6-ethyleneimino-2-phenylpyrimidine	rat	albino	960[b]	154	11/12 local sarcoma		
N-Cycloethyleneureidoazobenzene	rat	albino	1110–1140[b]	570	7/12 local sarcoma 1/12 other	corresponding *N*-dimethyl analog gave no local sarcomas, but did give 7/12 tumors at other sites	

[a]The route was sc, except where indicated otherwise. [b]Total dose; twice weekly injection in arachis oil. [c]Total dose; twice weekly injection in Carbowax 300. [e]Weekly injection in tricaprylin. [f]Twice weekly administration by gavage in water.

carcinogenic effectiveness of these agents. This factor may enhance the retention of the potential reactive compound in tissues near the injection site.

The commercial importance of some aziridines prompted some further studies by oral administration to mice (aziridine) and rats (2-methylaziridine) which proved positive.

The aziridines appear to be more powerfully carcinogenic than the epoxides, but this comparison must necessarily remain imprecise in view of the lack of comparative studies especially on in vivo alkylation.

Oxetanes, Lactones, and Related Compounds (Four-Membered Rings). Compounds of this group (Table XXIV), like the epoxides and ethyleneimines, embody strained-ring structures conferring reactivity toward nucleophiles (reviewed in Ref. 329) with cleavage of the CH_2–O bond.

The parent compound, oxetane (trimethylene oxide), and its β,β-dimethyl derivative are active but not very potent sarcomagens at the injection site. Druckrey et al. (*290*) derived a value of 19 for the carcinogenic index of trimethylene oxide.

The oxetanones, β-propiolactone and four-membered ring lactones, are fairly generally, but not always (Table XXVII), active carcinogens. The extensively investigated β-propiolactone is a "potent, though slow-acting carcinogen" (*290, 329*) with a carcinogenic index of 500. Substitution in the β-propiolactone ring weakens its activity.

Studies of the alkylation of DNA and its constituent nucleotides by β-propiolactone have not shown (*121, 122*) any clear-cut correlations with tumor-initiating activity. In vivo alkylation of DNA in mouse skin has been determined (*118, 119, 400, 401*) in a comparative study of β-propiolactone and β-carbonyl-substituted alkyl halides. Ability to alkylate DNA was positively associated with tumor-initiating ability.

Dickens and Jones (*499*) included penicillin in an early study of lactones and found that, at relatively high doses by subcutaneous injection, it gave injection-site sarcomas, suggesting possible alkylating activity (*329*). Longridge and Timms (*500*) pointed out that in reactions with nucleophiles, penicillin acts as an acylating agent, rather than as an alkylating agent (*see* Scheme IX). It was suggested that penicillinic acid (formed by oxidation of penicillin in aqueous media) was more likely to act as an alkylating agent (*500*). No evidence implicates penicillin as a carcinogen for humans (*328*).

Lactones and Related Compounds (Five-Membered Rings). Unlike the β-lactones, γ-lactones (Table XXV) are not inherently reactive because of their lack of ring strain. This lack of reactivity of γ-butyrolactone, therefore, is in accord with its inactivity as a carcinogen (*329, 403*).

However, certain modifications of the five-membered ring structure, notably the presence of ethylenic bonds, can enhance both chemical reactivity (which has so far been studied principally with regard to reactions with thiols) and sometimes carcinogenicity. The relationship between reactivity toward thiols and carcinogenic potency is not a simple positive correlation (*501*). For example, the α,β-unsaturated γ-lactones (*e.g.*, 4-hydroxypent-2-enoic acid lactone, Scheme X) react with thiols in neutral aqueous solution, with the β-carbon atom as the electrophilic

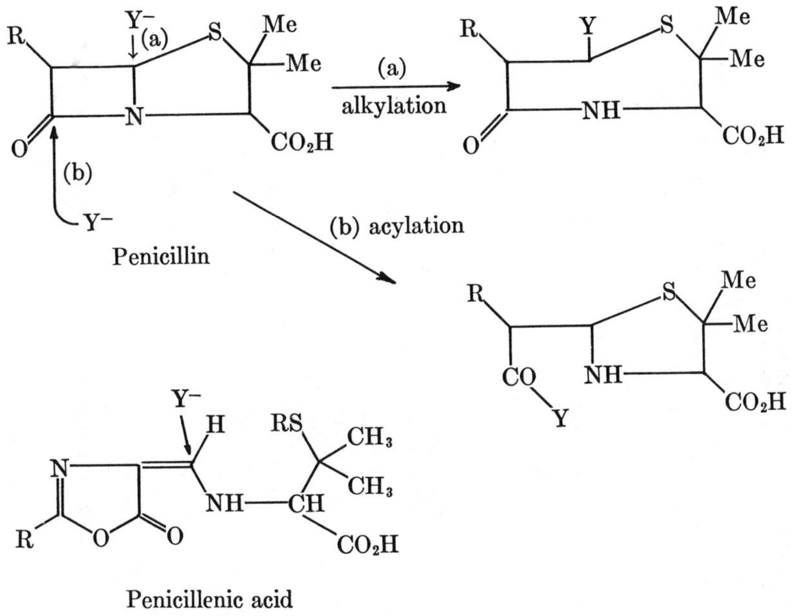

Scheme IX. Possible reactions of penicillin and penicillenic acid (500).

center, to give alkylation products. Several lactones of this type are carcinogenic (*329*). Thiols also react with the noncarcinogenic, 4-hydroxypent-3-enoic acid lactone, but the products are derived by *S*-acylation, rather than by *S*-alkylation, and are unstable; the product with cysteine rearranges rapidly to yield an *N*-acylated cysteine. Jones and Young (*501*) point out that this latter reaction in vivo would be reparable by proteolytic enzymes, whereas alkylation would be irreversible. The alkylation products can also undergo further nucleophilic attack at the carbonyl group, thus introducing the possibility of in vivo cross-linking reactions.

Dickens (*329*) has shown further that inclusion of an external double bond at the 4-position of the γ-lactones, as in methylprotoanemonin, conferred carcinogenic activity and also enhanced that of the α,β-unsaturated lactones.

With regard to vinylene carbonate, Jones and Young (*501*) found no cysteine reaction products and suggested that an in vivo hydrolysis product was probably the ultimate carcinogen. Dickens (*329*) noted that several natural products embody the structural features of the reactive γ-lactones and suggested that compounds of this type might occur as endogenous carcinogens.

Lactones and Related Compounds (Six-Membered Rings). With respect to chemical reactivity, this group of compounds (Tables XXVI and XXVII) may be considered analogous to the five-membered ring lactones, i.e., α,β-ethylenic bonds are necessary for activity, and the results of oncogenesis tests are generally also parallel (*329*). Sorbic acid, an open-chain analog of α,β-unsaturated lactones, also proved active in one test, but this activity was not confirmed subsequently (*332*).

Table XXIV

Representative Oncogenesis Tests—Oxetanes, Lactones, and Related Compounds (Four-Membered Rings)

Compound	*Animal*	*Strain or Type*	*Route*	*Dose (mg/kg)*	*Duration (d)*	*Tumors*	*Remarks*	*References*
Trimethylene oxide	rat	BD	sc	40 × 56, wkly	550[a]	6/14 local sarcomas		290
				80 × 56, wkly	550	5/6 local sarcomas 1/6 vaginal carcinoma		
β,β-Dimethyltri-methylene oxide	rat	Wistar	sc	1 mg × 102[b]	742	2/4 local sarcomas	493	
3,3-Dimethyl-2-oxetanone	mouse	B6C3F1	stomach tube	75,150,3 × wkly	721	numerous		494
	rat	Fischer	stomach tube	150,300,3 × wkly	735	numerous		
β-Propiolactone	rat	albino	sc	440–480[c]	508	9/12 local sarcomas		476
	rat	Wistar	sc	0.1 mg × 68[d]	238	4/4 local sarcomas	1/11 thoracic tumor in controls	
				1.0 mg × 88[e]	308	10/10 local sarcomas		
				2.0 mg × 66[f]	385	2/4 local sarcomas		
	mouse	albino "S"	skin	155 mg[d]	133	160/19 papillomas		281
			skin	7.5 mg, wkly × 52	385	5/10 papillomas	2 malignant ca.	495
			iv, tail	1–10 mg[e]	183	inj. site papillomas	no lung tumors	
	mouse	albino	skin	7.5 mg × 70[g]	322	1/25 squamous carcinoma	weak response attributed to hydrolysis in impure acetone	496
				7.5 mg × 120[g]	420	20/45 squamous ca. and others		
	mouse	Swiss	skin	5 mg, 3 × wkly[g]	ca. 250	21/30 papillomas 11/30 cancers	dose–response study, *see* original ref.	497
	mouse	Swiss ICR/Ha	sc	0.73 mg, wkly[h]	503	9/30 fibrosarcomas 3/30 adenoca.		481

					6/30 squamous cell ca.		
guinea pig	—	skin	12.5 mg, 2 × wkly[g]	up to 1176	3/9 keratoacanthomas 1/9 melanoma 1/9 hepatoma 1/9 lacrimal gland tumor	also pigmented naevi	295
golden hamster	—	skin	12.5 mg, 2 × wkly[g]	up to 700	8/17 keratoacanthomas 4/17 melanomas 5/17 papillomas 2/17 squamous cell ca.		265
mouse	"susceptible" (f)		120 μmol × 6[d]	210	97% papillomas 11% carcinomas	binding to DNA, RNA, and protein studied	400
mouse	B6AF$_1$, neonates (m)	ip	0.5 mg (~100 mg/kg)[i]	476	65% hepatomas 47% lung tumors 9% lymphomas	controls 4% hepatomas, 49% lung tumors, nil lymphomas	406
	neonates (f)	ip	0.5 mg[i]		nil hepatomas 27% lung tumors 20% lymphomas	controls nil hepatomas, 24% lung tumors, nil lymphomas	
	neonates (m)	skin	3 mg[i]	476	19% hepatomas 44% lung tumors nil lymphomas		
	neonates (f)	skin	3 mg[i]	476	3% hepatomas 55% lung tumors 3% lymphomas		
	adults (m)	ip	80 mg/kg[i]	546	9% hepatomas 55% lung tumors 14% lymphomas	controls, 6.7% hepatomas, 44% lung tumors, nil lymphomas	
	adults (f)	ip	80 mg/kg[i]	546	nil hepatomas 40% lung tumors	controls, 1% hepatomas,	

Continued on next page

Table XXIV Continued

Compound	Animal	Strain or Type	Route	Dose (mg/kg)	Duration (d)	Tumors	Remarks	References
						17% lymphomas	34% lung tumors, 5% lymphomas	
β-Butyrolactone	mouse	Swiss ICR/Ha	skin	10 mg, 3 × wkly[j]	466	4/30 papillomas 21/30 carcinomas		498
				1 mg, single	468	0/20 papillomas 0/20 carcinomas		
	mouse	Swiss ICR/Ha	skin	1 mg, single, then croton resin promotion	468	3/20 papillomas 1/20 carcinomas		
				10 mg, 3 × wkly[j]	598	1/40 papillomas 1/40 cancer		480
				10 mg, 3 × wkly[k]	467	20/30 papillomas 16/30 cancers		
4,5-Epoxy-3-hydroxyvaleric acid β-lactone	mouse	Swiss ICR/Ha	skin	10 mg, 3 × wkly[k]	514	5/30 papillomas	benign tumors only; considered negative as carcinogen	498

α-Carboxy-β-phenyl-β-propiolactone	rat	Wistar	sc	2 mg × 128[b]	735	1/4 local sarcoma	499
α,α-Diphenyl-β-propiolactone	rat	Wistar	sc	1 mg × 38[b]	735	1/3 local sarcoma	
Penicillin G	rat	Wistar	sc	2 mg × 92[b]	700	1/4 local sarcoma 1/4 remote fibroma 1/4 thyroid alveolar carcinoma	499
				2 mg × 104[b]	735	1/4 local sarcoma	493
				2 mg × 130[b]	742	2/4 local fibrosarcoma	

[a] Mean time of death of tumor-bearing animals.
[b] Twice weekly injection in arachis oil.
[c] Twice weekly injection in arachis oil, total dose stated.
[d] Multiple doses in acetone, total dose stated, promotion with croton oil.
[e] Multiple doses in Ringer solution, total dose stated.
[f] Twice weekly injection in water.
[g] Applied in acetone solution (generally twice weekly).
[h] In tricaprylin (octanoin).
[i] In arachis oil.
[j] In acetone.
[k] In benzene.

Table XXV

Representative Oncogenesis Tests—Lactones and Related Compounds (Five-Membered Rings)

Compound	*Dose*	*Duration (d)*	*Tumors*	*Remarks*	*References*
γ-Butyrolactone	2 mg × 122[a]	700	0/5	considered	499
mouse, ICR/Ha, skin	10 mg, 3 × wkly[b]	292	2/30 papillomas 1/30 cancer	negative	486
Maleic anhydride	1 mg × 122[a]	742	2/3 local fibrosarcomas		493
α,β-Dimethyl maleic anhydride	2 mg × 130[a]	728	3/5 local sarcomas		502
Succinic anhydride	2 mg × 130[a]	742	3/3 local sarcomas		502
4-Hydroxyhex-2-enoic acid lactone	2 mg × 128[a]	714	2/4 local fibrosarcomas	isomeric-3-enoic lactone inactive	499

Methyl protoanemonin	2 mg × 128[a]	735	3/5 local fibrosarcomas		499
4-Hydroxyhex-4-enoic acid lactone	1 mg × 116[a]	693	3/5 local sarcomas		499
Patulin (Clavacin)	0.2 mg × 122[a]	483	4/4 local sarcomas		499
Penicillic acid	1 mg × 128[a]	469	4/4 local sarcomas		499
	0.1 mg × 122[a]	742	1/4 local sarcomas		
	2 mg × 104[c]	723	4/5 local sarcomas		493
mouse	0.2 mg × 76[a]	588	6/19 local sarcomas		502
Bovolide	2 mg × 130[a]	742	5/5 local sarcomas		502
α-Methyltetronic acid	2 mg × 130[a]	693	2/4 local sarcomas	not transplantable	502
Vinylene carbonate	2 mg × 130[a]	588	6/6 local sarcomas		
Sarkomycin	2 mg × 84[a]	742	1/6 local myxosarcoma		

NOTE: Except where indicated, the species tested was the Wistar rat, and the route was sc.
[a]In arachis oil.
[b]In benzene.
[c]In water.

α,β-unsaturated γ-lactones,

e.g. 4-hydroxypent-2-enoic acid lactone

RSH; RS

β,γ-unsaturated γ-lactones,

e.g. 4-hydroxypent-3-enoic acid lactone

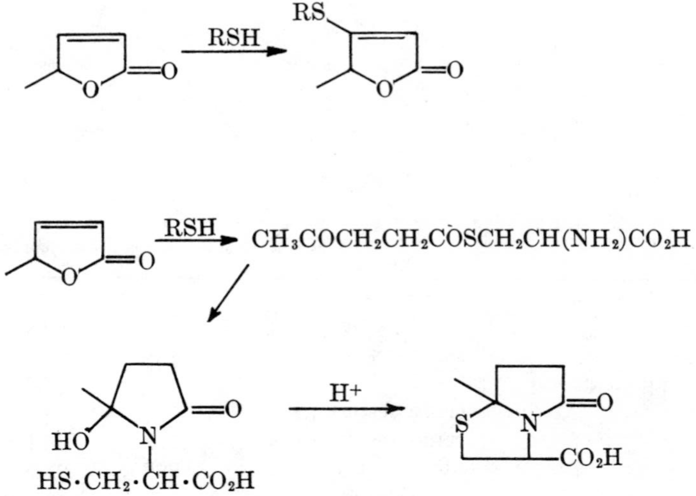

RSH; $CH_3COCH_2CH_2COSCH_2CH(NH_2)CO_2H$

HO; N; $HS \cdot CH_2 \cdot CH \cdot CO_2H$

H^+

S; N; CO_2H

Scheme X. Reactions of unsaturated γ-lactones with cysteine [(RSH; $R = CH_2CH(NH_2)\ CO_2H$)] at pH 7 (501).

Table XXVI

Representative Oncogenesis Tests—Lactones and Related Compounds (Six-Membered Rings)

Compound	*Animal*	*Strain or Type*	*Dose*[a]	*Duration (d)*	*Tumors*	*Remarks*	*References*
(+) Parasorbic acid	rat	Wistar	0.2 mg × 64[b]	665	4/6 local sarcomas		493
			2 mg × 64[b]	742	4/5 local sarcomas		
Maleic hydrazide	rat	Wistar	2 mg × 130[b]	742	3/6 local sarcomas 1/6 hepatoma		502
	mouse	Swiss (infant male)	55 mg[c]	343	65% hepatomas	8% in controls	503
		(C57BL × C3H)F	3000 ppm in diet	540	no sig. increase over controls		491
Sorbic acid	rat	Wistar	2 mg × 130[b]	679	5/6 local sarcomas	reactive open-chain analog of lactones; reported inactive by Ref. 332	331
Dehydroacetic acid			2 mg × 130[b]	595	5/6 local sarcomas		

[a]The route was sc, except where indicated otherwise.
[b]Twice weekly injection in arachis oil.
[c]During first 3 weeks of life; in water or tricaprylin; contaminated with 0.4% hydrazine (*see* Ref. 504).

Table XXVII

Representative Oncogenesis Tests—Lactones and Related Compounds Reported Inactive

Compound	*Animal*	*Route*	*References*
Four-Membered Rings			
Diketene	mouse	skin	475,486
	mouse	sc	
	rat	sc	
4,5-Epoxy-3-hydroxyvaleric acid β-lactone	mouse	skin	
3-Hydroxy-2,2-dimethylbutyric acid β-lactone	mouse	skin	475
3-Hydroxy-2,2-dimethyl-4,4,4-trichlorobutyric acid β-lactone	mouse	skin	475
2,2,4-Trimethyl-3-hydroxy-3-pentenoic acid β-lactone[a]	mouse	skin	475
	mouse	sc	
3-Hydroxy-2,2,4-trimethyl-heptanoic acid β-lactone	mouse	skin	475
Five-Membered Rings			
γ-Butyrolactone	mouse	skin	486
	rat	sc	499
β-Angelicalactone	mouse	skin	499,475
	rat	sc	
α-Angelicalactone	mouse	skin	480
	rat	sc	499
4-Hydroxyhex-3-enoic acid lactone	rat	sc	499
N-Ethylmaleimide	rat	sc	502
Six-Membered Rings			
Coumarin	rat	sc	502
6-Acetamidocoumarin	rat	ig	505

[a]Reported positive for rat with sc injection by Van Duuren et al. (*481*).

The aflatoxins (Chapter 16 in Vol. 2 of this edition) fall into the structural class of six-membered ring lactones, but their carcinogenic potency can be both quantitatively higher than and qualitatively different from typical lactones. They are highly active by oral and intratracheal administration. Both in rats and humans, their carcinogenicity is due to metabolic activation.

Maleic hydrazide is also unlikely to act by direct in vivo alkylation, but its mode of action is as yet uncertain. It failed to cause tumors in mice or rats by oral administration (*491*). The findings of Epstein et al. (*336, 503*) that injection of maleic hydrazide into newborn mice caused hepatomas (in males only) "could not be assessed" (*504*) because 0.4% hydrazine (a hepatocarcinogen) was present as an impurity in the sample used.

Cyclic Sulfides and Sultones. (*See* Table XXVIII.) Ethylene sulfide, the analog of ethylene oxide, is a sarcomagen at the injection site in the rat, although not of high potency. The value of the carcinogenic index derived by Druckrey et al. (*290*) was 9, compared with 500 for β-propiolactone.

1,3-Propane sultone is "highly reactive" and "a potent carcinogen" with an index of 130–210 by multiple injection and 470–800 by single injection (*407*). The next higher homolog, 1,4-butane sultone, was much less carcinogenic. The reactivity towards nucleophiles presumably involves fission of the CH_2-O bond, as with β-propiolactone; the enhanced reactivity relative to that of saturated γ-lactones has been ascribed to the greater electron-withdrawing power of the OSO_2 group compared with that of the OCO group. No studies of in vivo alkylation by sultones have been reported.

Haloalkyl Ethers. This group of compounds (Table XXIX) has found wide industrial use and exhibits cytotoxic and irritant properties associated with the chemical reactivity of alkylating types of agents (*403*). Bis(chloromethyl) ether is now classified by the IARC as a human carcinogen. Its monofunctional analog, chloromethyl ethyl ether, is at most a much weaker carcinogen (*475*), but the industrial product under this name was sufficiently contaminated with the more potent difunctional agent to be considered as a carcinogenic hazard. As already noted, inhalation tests of bis(chloromethyl) ether with rats gave bronchial carcinomas, and therefore resembled the effect on humans more closely than did tests of other locally acting directly reactive potentially difunctional alkylating agents such as epichlorohydrin and formaldehyde.

Nitrogen Mustards (Monofunctional and 2-Chloroethylsulfonic Acid Derivatives). Monofunctional aliphatic 2-chloroethylamines (Table XXX) yield relatively stable cyclic imonium ions in aqueous solution. Detailed studies with 2-(chloroethyl)diethylamine suggested that reaction of these ions with nucleophiles proceeds by the S_N2 mechanism (*21*). As previously discussed, this mechanism may not be correct for 2-chloroethylarylamines, which may react in part through the S_N1 mechanism. No studies of in vivo alkylation by monofunctional nitrogen mustards have been made. The sulfur mustard analog, 2-chloroethyl 2-hydroxyethyl sulfide, alkylated tissue constituents in vivo, including DNA, but has not been tested as a carcinogen.

A plant growth regulator used on food crops, (2-chloroethyl)trimethylammonium chloride, was tested extensively by prolonged oral administration to F344 Fischer rats and B6C3F1 mice. It was evaluated as not carcinogenic for either sex of either strain of animal (*509*).

Schoental and Bensted (*513*) found significant carcinogenic activity with *N*-(2-chloroethyl)-*N*-nitrosourethane, and attributed this to its "mixed difunctionality" as a mustard and nitroso compound. Such compounds have found wide application as cancer chemotherapeutic agents, notably the monofunctional nitrogen mustard CCNU, which so far appears to be a rather weak carcinogen (*515*).

Monofunctional nitrogen mustards derived from heterocyclic amines prepared by the Institute for Cancer Research (Philadelphia) have become widely known as the "ICR" series of potential antitumor agents. They showed remarkable specificity as fluorochrome stains (*514*), a result indicating specific interaction with

Table XXVIII

Representative Oncogenesis Tests—Cyclic Sulfides and Sultones

Animal	Strain or Type	Route	Dose (mg/kg)	Duration (d)	Tumors	References
			Ethylene Sulfide			
rat	BD	sc	8 × 50[a]	500[b]	1/15 local sarcomas	290
			16 × 50		4/12 local Sarcomas	
			1,3-Propane Sultone			
rat	BD	sc	15 × 14[a]	295[b]	7/12 local sarcomas	290
					1/12 tumor of nervous tissue	
					1/12 other	
			30 × 13[a]	270[b]	11/11 local sarcomas	
			15 × 15[c]	280[b]	18/18 local sarcomas	
			10[d]	500[b]	4/15 local sarcomas	
			30[d]	400[b]	12/18 local sarcomas	
			100[d]	285[b]	18/18 local sarcomas	
		po	30[e]	340[b]	2/10 nervous tissue	
					2/10 other	
		iv	10–40, wkly[e]	492	5/29 nervous tissue	
					4/29 other	
		iv	150[e]	350[b]	3/32 nervous tissue	
					6/32 other	
		transplacental	20		3/25 nervous tissue	
			60		2/25 nervous tissue	
					2/25 other	

rat	Charles River CD	ig	28 × 120[f]	420	in males, 12/26 glioma, 11/26 other; in females, 7/26 breast, 15/26 glioma, 10/26 other	506
mouse	ICR/Ha Swiss	sc	0.3 mg × 63	371[g]	12/30 local sarcomas; 9/30 other	490
mouse	CDI	skin	50 μmol[h]	210	73/28	404
			100 μmol	210	96/30 papillomas	
			1,4-Butane Sultone			
rat	BD	sc	30 × 76[e]	610[b]	1/12 local sarcoma	290
		iv	30 × 84		0/16	
		po	30[e]	708	2/16 adeno ca.; 6/16 other	
mouse	ICR/Ha	sc	1 mg, wkly	580	3/30 local sarcoma; 1/30 squamous carcinoma	284

[a]Weekly injection in arachis oil.
[b]Mean induction time.
[c]Injection in aqueous buffer solution.
[d]Single injection in oil.
[e]Weekly injection or fed in aqueous solution.
[f]Twice weekly, by gavage in water. Similar results were found with 56 mg/kg for 32 weeks.
[g]Weekly injection in tricaprylin.
[h]Promotion with 0.5 mg croton oil, twice wkly.

Table XXIX
Representative Oncogenesis Tests—Haloalkyl Ethers

Compound	*Animal*	*Strain or Type*	*Route*	*Dose*	*Duration (d)*[a]	*Tumors*	*Remarks*	*References*
Chloromethyl methyl ether	mouse	ICR/Ha Swiss	skin	0.1–1 mg[b]	540	0/60	active as initiator[c]	475
				0.1 mg[d]	496	7/20 papillomas 4/20 carcinomas	(activity due to contamination with bis(chloro-methyl)ether?)	
				1 mg[b]	488	5/20 papillomas 1/20 carcinoma		
	rat	Sprague–Dawley	sc	3 mg × 45[e]	515	1/20 fibrosarcoma	considered inactive	
	mouse	ICR Swiss (newborn)	sc	125 μL/kg[f]	183	17/99 adenomas	7/50 in controls	507
Bis(chloromethyl) ether	mouse	ICR/Ha	skin	2 mg × 129[b]	313	13/20 papillomas 12/20 carcinomas	active carcinogen	475
			skin	1 mg[b]	474	5/20 papillomas 2/20 carcinomas	active as initiator	
	rat	Sprague–Dawley	sc	3 mg × 16 then 1 mg wkly		5/20 fibrosarcoma		
	mouse	ICR Swiss (newborn)	sc	12.5 μL/kg[f]	183	45/100 adenomas	7/50 in controls	507
	mouse	A/Heston	inhal.	1 ppm, 6th/d 82 d	196	55% lung tumors	statistically sig. rel. to controls; analogous expt. with chloro-methyl methyl ether not sig. positive	508

	rat	Sprague–Dawley (m)	inhal.	0.1 ppm 6 h/d 5 d/wk	up to 900	17/200 nasal esthesioneuro-epitheliomo 9/200 other nasal tumors 13/200 lung squamous cell carcinoma 1/200 lung adeno-carcinoma	dose–response study	348
	hamster	Golden Syrian	inhal.	0.1 ppm 6 h/d 5 d/wk	up to 560	1/100 lung carcinoma		
Octachlorodi-*n*-propyl ether	mouse	ICR/Ha Swiss	skin	1 mg[f]	450	3/20 papillomas 1/20 carcinoma	active as initiator	475
α,α-Dichloro-methyl ether	mouse	ICR/Ha Swiss	skin	1 mg[f]	450	3/20 papillomas 1/20 carcinoma	active as initiator	
Monochloro-acetaldehyde diethyl acetal	mouse	ICR/Ha Swiss	skin	1 mg[f]	450	1/20 papillomas	considered inactive	

[a]Median survival time.
[b]In benzene.
[c]Activity possibly due to contamination with bis(chloromethyl) ether (?).
[d]Promotion with phorbol ester.
[e]In nujol.
[f]In arachis oil.

Table XXX

Representative Oncogenesis Tests—Nitrogen Mustards (Monofunctional) and 2-Chloroethylsulfonic Acid Derivatives

Compound	*Animal*	*Strain or Type*	*Route*	*Dose*	*Duration (d)*	*Tumors*	*Remarks*	*References*
(2-Chloroethyl)-trimethylammonium chloride	mouse	(C57-BL/6 × C3H/Anf) F_1	ig po	21.5 mg/kg × 21 then 65 ppm in diet	540	lymphomas, pulmonary and liver tumors	in "uncertain range" statistically also evaluated as noncarcinogenic for F344 rats	491, 509
N-(2-Chloroethyl)aminoazobenzene	rat	Wistar	po	0.07% in diet	240	0/14		510
Methanesulfonic acid 2-chloroethyl ester (CB 1506)	mouse	A/J	ip	380 μmol/kg[a]	273	pulmonary, rel. potency[b] 26	"borderline activity"	215
Aramite [2-(4,-*t*-butylphenoxy) isopropyl-2-chloroethyl sulfite]	rat	Wistar	po	400 ppm in diet	730	2/100 hepatic carcinomas 5/100 cholangeal adenomas		511
	dog	mongrel	po	500–1429 ppm in diet	1280	20/19 adenocarcinomas and other tumors		512
	mouse	(C57-BL/6 × C3H/Anf) F_1	ig then po	1112 ppm in diet	567	sig. yield of lymphomas, hepatomas, and pulmonary tumors		496

N-(2-Chloroethyl)-*N*-nitrosourethane	rat	white, Porton	intragastric	6–100 mg/kg	up to 400	4/10 stomach carcinomas 2/10 other carcinomas	"mixed difunctional" agent-mustard and nitroso compound	513
1-(Chloroethyl)-3-cyclohexyl-1-nitrosourea (CCNU, Lomustine)	mouse	Swiss-Webster	ip	1.25–5 mg/kg 3 × wkly for 6 mos.	540	66% in (f), 54% in (m) mainly lymphosarcoma		516, 517
	rat	Wistar	iv	1.5–20 mg/kg every 6 wks (7–10 injections)	7600	lung adenomas interim report		515, 518
		Sprague–Dawley	po (gavage)	5 mg	180	"inconclusive"		519
			ip	3,6 mg/kg 3 × wkly for 6 mos.	540	lung tumors: 46% (f) and 46% (m); sig. greater than controls: 0.5% (f) and 2% (m)		516, 517
"Quinacrine ethyl half mustard," [ICR-125, 9-(2-(2-chloroethyl)amino)-ethylamino)-6-chloro-2-methoxyacridine]	mouse	A/J	ip	1280 μmol/kg[a]	273	pulmonary, rel. potency[b] 7.8	"borderline activity"	215
ICR-170 [9-(3-(ethyl-2-chloroethyl)aminoethylamino)-6-chloro-2-methoxyacridine]	mouse	A/J	ip				inactive by ip route	215

Continued on next page

Table XXX Continued

Compound	Animal	Strain or Type	Route	Dose	Duration (d)	Tumors	Remarks	References
		A/He (f)	iv	5 μmol/kg × 2	140	lung adenomas	active by iv route	448[d]
			iv	6 μmol/kg × 2		15/7	partial protective effect of immunization	
			iv (pre-immunized)			129/29		
						58/29[e]		
						39/26[f]		
ICR-191[2-methoxy-6-chloro-9[3-(chloroethyl)aminopropylamino]-acridine]		A/He (f)	iv	up to 120 μmol/kg	140	0.47 lung adenomas per mouse	not sig. different from controls (0.36)	

[a]Range of dose levels used; "positive response dose," giving one tumor/mouse shown, was deduced from data.
[b]Denotes (10,000/positive response dose), *see* footnote *a*.
[c]Range of dose levels used; highest level did not give "positive response" of statistical significance relative to controls.
[d]Reports data for eight other heterocyclic mustard compounds.
[e]Mice preimmunized using human serum albumin.
[f]Preimmunization with ICR-170-alkylated human serum albumin.

chromosomes. Earlier tests for carcinogenicity in strain A mice by Shimkin et al. (*215*) did not show any marked activity, but Peck et al. (*448*) attributed this result to the use of the intraperitoneal route of administration. When the intravenous route was used, some of these compounds proved to be highly active inducers of lung adenomas, a finding that indicated lack of penetration of the drugs to the target tissues in the earlier experiments.

Not all the heterocyclic mustards have proved active, however, and some positive correlation with their antitumor activity was discerned. A degree of protection against induction by ICR-170 of lung adenomas was obtained by preimmunization of the mice by using human serum albumen and Freund's adjuvant. This protective action was not enhanced by using an ICR-170-alkylated antigen.

The pesticide Aramite contains a chloroethyl group and was found to be carcinogenic in three animal species. Whether it acts as an alkylating agent is unknown.

The somewhat analogous 2-chloroethylphosphonic acid (**43**), a plant growth regulator, was remarkable in that not only did it prove negative in Shimkin's test system using strain A mice (*520*) but, in a dose-dependent fashion, it reduced the incidence of lung adenomas from the spontaneous level of 0.36 per mouse to 0.11 at 20 mg/kg (by intraperitoneal injection, three times weekly for 24 weeks) and to 0 at 80 mg/kg. Furthermore, it reduced the carcinogenic effect of urethane in this system. This inhibitory effect on carcinogenesis was attributed to its breakdown in vivo to yield ethylene, an inhibitor of DNA synthesis.

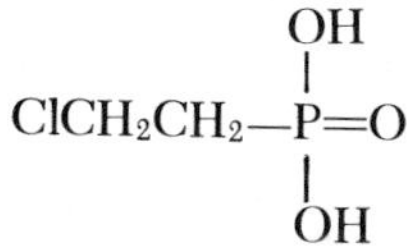

$$ClCH_2CH_2{-}P(=O)(OH)_2$$

43

Difunctional and Polyfunctional Nitrogen and Sulfur Mustards and Some Related Cytotoxic Agents (Tables XXXI, XXXII, and XXXIII). Mustard gas, although a carcinogen in humans, was relatively difficult to establish as a carcinogen by testing in animals (Table XXXI). Somewhat similarly, only the more recent tests with the nitrogen mustard HN2 have been entirely convincing. Both these compounds and the potentially trifunctional HN3 are potent cytotoxic agents. The difunctional agents have been extensively studied with regard to the concept that their cytotoxic action arises principally from their ability to inactivate template DNA by cross-linking. Considerable attention has also been devoted to their related effects in stimulating DNA repair mechanisms.

Formation of diguaninyl alkylation-induced cross-linked bases in DNA was first shown by chemical analytical methods for mustard gas (*1, 536, 537*), and interstrand cross-linkage was shown by physicochemical methods for the

Table XXXI
Representative Oncogenesis Tests—Sulfur and Nitrogen Mustards

Compound	Animal Strain or Type[a]	Route	Dose	Duration (d)	Tumors	Remarks	References
Mustard gas	A	iv	0.25 mL of sat. aq. soln. (0.065% × 4)	112	93% lung adenomas	61% in controls	5
				112	68% lung adenomas	13% in controls	4
	A	sc	0.05 mL of 0.05% soln. in olive oil × 5	450	13/26 lung adenomas 3/26 other	15/30 lung adenomas 7/30 other in controls	
Di-(2-chloroethyl) methylamine, HN2	C3H	sc	as above × 6	600	8/16 mammary 5/16 other	7/16 mammary in controls 10/16 other	
	A	inhalation	15-min exposure to vapor	520	44% lung adenomas	27% in controls	521
	—	sc	1 mg/kg wkly × 50	580	3/20 lung carcinoma 2/20 lung adenoma 2/20 other		522
	C3H	sc	0.025 mg × 6	~360	21/37 pulmonary 17/37 hepatoma and some other	6/39 pulmonary 18/39 hepatoma in controls	4
	Swiss	iv, ip, sc	0.5 mg/kg wkly	up to 270	15–20% sarcomas and adenocarcinoma	no tumors in controls	523
	albino	sc	0.3–0.4 mg/kg wkly × 64	448	1/138 lymphoma	strain with no spont. lung adenoma	524
	albino	skin	0.1 mg × 15[b]	133	4/10 skin tumors		281
	albino	sc, ip	0.4 mg/kg monthly × 9	600	15.6% tumors, mostly sarcomas	13.2% in controls, but mustard inj. animals showed tumors earlier	399

			0.4 mg/kg single	600	13.3% tumors		
			1 mg/kg × 9,	600	17.2% tumors		
			1 mg/kg single	600	13.3% tumors		
	RF	iv	2.4 mg/kg × 4	554	21% thymic lymphoma	8% in controls	380, 381
	A/J	ip	3 μmol/kg[c]	273	lung tumors rel. potency[c] of mustard—3300	"highly potent" inj. in water, "barely active" in tricaprylin	215
	A/J	iv	0.5 μmol/kg[c]	294	lung tumors rel. potency[d]—20,000		215
	BR46 rat	iv	0.11 mg/kg, total 5.72 mg/kg	480[e]	26% malignant tumors 18% benign[f]	dose of 7% of LD_{50} to simulate chemotherapy; 6% malignant tumors in controls, 5% benign; statistically sig. positive	525
Tris(2-chloroethyl)amine	—	sc	1 mg/kg wkly × 10	567	2/4 lung carcinoma 1/4 local sarcoma 1/4 lung adenoma		522

[a]Except where indicated, the animal tested was the mouse.
[b]In acetone; promotion with croton oil.
[c]Injection in water, 3 × weekly; range of dose levels, "positive response dose," shown, giving one lung tumor/mouse.
[d]Denotes (10,000/positive response dose), *see* footnote *b*.
[e]Average induction time.
[f]Variety of tumor types, *see* original reference for histopathology.

Table XXXII

Representative Oncogenesis Tests—Nitrogen Mustards (Difunctional)

Compound	*Animal*	*Strain or Type*	*Route*	*Dose*	*Duration (d)*	*Tumors*	*Remarks*	*References*
Nitrogen mustard *N*-oxide	rat	BD	sc	15 mg/kg × 16	730	2/36 sarcomas 1/36 carcinoma	a few tumors also by iv or ip	525
	mouse	dd/I (7-d old)	sc	650 mg/kg × 4	180	57% thymic lymphomas 43% lung adenomas 21% lung cancer 16% Harderian gland adenomas	22% lung adenomas, no other tumors in controls	526
	rat	BR46	iv	4.2 mg/kg, multiple, total 218 mg/kg	480[a]	27% malignant, 7% benign tumors[b]	statistically sig. positive; dose simulates chemotherapy	527
Chlorambucil	mouse	albino S	skin	0.27 mg × 10[c]	224	30/25 papillomas		282
	mouse	A/J	ip	60 μmol/kg[d]	273	rel. potency[e] 170		215
	mouse	Swiss Webster	ip	1.5–3 3 × wkly for 6 mos.	540	lung tumors 22/35 (m) 20/28 (f) lymphosarcomas 6/35 (m) 4/28 (f) ovarian tumors 10/28	in controls, lung tumors 10/101 (m), 21/153 (f); lympho-sarcomas 3/101 (m), 4/153 (f) ovarian tumors 6/153	516
	rat	Sprague–Dawley	ip	2.2–4.5 3 × wkly for 6 mos.	540	lymphomas 8/33 (m)		
Melphalan	mouse	albino S	skin	0.144 mg × 10[c]	224	7/25 papillomas	D-enantiomer of equal activity	282
	mouse	A/J	ip	3.8 μmol/kg[d]	273	rel. potency[e] 2630		215
	mouse	Swiss Webster	ip	0.75–1.5 3 × wkly for 6 mos.	540	lung tumors, 11/44 (m) 10/23 (f)		516

						lymphosarcomas 13/44 (m)		
	rat	Sprague–Dawley	ip	0.9–1.8 3 × wkly for 6 mos.	540	peritoneal sarcomas 11/20 (m), 10/23 (f)		
Aniline mustard	mouse	A/J	ip	96 μmol/kg[d]	273	rel. potency[e] 104		215
	rat	—	sc	2 mg/kg wkly × 20	400[f]	5/12[g]	mitotic abnormalities observed in primary tumors	528
	mouse	—	sc	1 mg/kg, wkly × 20	400[f]	1/12[g]		
p-Toluidine mustard	rat	—	sc	2 mg/kg, wkly × 20	365[f]	5/12[g]		528
	mouse	—	sc	1 mg/kg, wkly × 20	330[f]	2/12[g]		
α-Naphthylamine mustard	rat	—	sc	2 mg/kg, wkly × 20	270[f]	6/12[g]		528
	mouse	—	sc	1 mg/kg, wkly × 20	400[f]	2/12[g]		
β-Naphthylamine mustard	rat	—	sc	2 mg/kg, wkly × 20	240[f]	12/12[g]		528
	mouse	—	sc	1 mg/kg, wkly × 20	300[f]	2/12[g]		
	mouse	A/J	ip	1200 μmol/kg[d]	273	rel. potency[e] 8.3		215
Hydroquinone mustard	mouse	A/J	ip	66 μmol/kg[d]	273	rel. potency[e] 150		215
Mannomustine	mouse	A/J	ip	60 μmol/kg[b]	273	rel. potency[e] 280		215
	rat	BR46	iv	4 mg/kg, multiple, total 208 mg/kg	450[a]	11% malignant, 5% benign tumors[b]	statistically sig. positive; dose simulates chemotherapy	527
Dibromomannitol	mouse	Swiss–Webster	ip	90–180 3 × wkly for 6 mos.	540	lung tumors, 8/41 (m) 19/40 (f)	weakly active in mice, negative in rats	516
Dibromodulcitol	mouse	Swiss–Webster	ip	45–90 3 × wkly for 6 mos.	540	lung tumors, 8/41 (m), 14/30 (f)	weakly active in mice, negative in rats	516
1,3-Bis(2-chloroethyl)-1-nitrosourea	rat	Sprague–Dawley	ip	0.7–1.5	540	14/40 lung tumors (m) 18/40 various malignant tumors	weaker activity in (f)	517

Continued on next page

Table XXXII Continued

Compound	*Animal*	*Strain or Type*	*Route*	*Dose*	*Duration (d)*	*Tumors*	*Remarks*	*References*
	mouse	Swiss–Webster	ip	1.25	540	8/21 various malignant tumors (f)	weaker activity in (m)	
Cisplatin	mouse	A/Jax (f)	ip	3.25 wkly × 10 1.62 wkly × 19	240	14.2 lung adenomas per 15.8	0.8 adenomas per mouse in controls	529
		CD-1 (f)	ip	1.62 wkly × 16 skin promotion with croton oil	364	15/30, 3.2 papillomas per mouse		

[a]Mean induction time.
[b]Various types, *see* original reference for histopathology.
[c]Applied in acetone; promotion with croton oil.
[d]Twelve 3 × weekly injection in water over a range of dose levels; "positive response dose" quoted gave one lung tumor/mouse.
[e]Relative potency denotes (10,000/positive response dose), *see* footnote *b*.
[f]Latent period.
[g]"Mostly sarcomas at site of injection".

Table XXXIII

Representative Oncogenesis Tests—Nitrogen Mustards Derived from Heterocyclic Compounds

Compound	Animal Strain or Type[a]	Route	Dose	Duration (d)	Tumors	Remarks	References
Uracil mustard	A/J	ip	0.96 μmol/kg[b]	273	lung, rel. potency[c] 10,420		215
Chloroquine mustard	A/J	ip	18 μmol/kg[b]	273	lung, rel. potency[c] 560	active as hydro-chloride, inactive as pamoate (salt of CH_2 (C_{10}-$H_5OHCO_2H)_2$)	215
Quinacrine ethyl mustard	A/J	ip	30 μmol/kg[b]	273	lung, rel. potency[c] 330		215
Benzimidazole mustard	A/J	ip	36 μmol/kg[b]	273	lung, rel. potency[c] 280		215
Cytoxan	A/J	ip	360 μmol/kg[b]	273	lung, rel. potency[c] 28		215
	A	ip	0.02 mg × 5		pulmonary adenomas		530
	A	ip	5 mg/kg × 30	294	37.5% various[d]	18% in controls, $p = 0.263$	531
			5 mg/kg × 30	336	55% various	30% in controls, $p = 0.183$	
	dd	ip	13 mg/kg, multiple		11% benign	statistically sig. positive	527
	BR 46 rat	iv	676 mg/kg, total		17% malignant[d]		
	NZB/NZW(f)	sc	5.7 daily	up to 560	15/15 mostly mammary carcinoma 17/19	cyclophospha-mide increased lifespan from 46 to 80 wks.	532
	Sprague–Dawley rat	po in water	5 × wkly	up to 985		malignant tumors "wide spectrum" but organ-specific effect on bladder, as with humans	533
			0.31		37/73		
			0.63		27/73		
			1.25		26/67		
			2.5		22/58		

Continued on next page

Table XXXIII Continued

Compound	Animal Strain or Type[a]	Route	Dose	Duration (d)	Tumors	Remarks	References
Isophosphamide	A/He	po in water	24 × 18.8		12/20 lung tumors	19/60 in controls, sig. increase in all treated groups	534
			24 × 47		13/20		
			5 × 260		10/20		
						other tests "inconclusive"	535
5-Chloroquine mustard	A/J	ip	25 μmol/kg[e]	273	rel. potency nil		215
Benzalpurine mustard	A/J	ip	36 μmol/kg[e]	273	rel. potency nil		215

[a] Except where indicated, the animal tested was the mouse.
[b] Range of dose levels used; "positive response dose" giving one lung tumor/mouse quoted.
[c] Relative potency denotes 10,000/"positive response dose," *see* footnote *a*.
[d] For details of histopathology, *see* original reference.
[e] Highest dose, negative response relative to controls.

nitrogen mustard HN2 (*538–43*). Intrastrand linkages also result from alkylation of DNA by difunctional and polyfunctional agents (*544–46*), as shown by combined application of both chemical analytical and physicochemical determinations.

Monofunctional agents cannot cross-link by direct alkylation. They can cause cross-linking to a much lesser extent than difunctional agents, possibly through hydrolytic depurination of alkylpurines, a reaction subsequent to initial alkylation of DNA (*547*). They have also been shown to cause DNA–protein cross-linkage (*548–50*).

Sensitive tests for DNA interstrand cross-linking and for DNA–protein cross-linking are now available (*51, 260, 551*). Comparative studies correlating the two types of cross-linking with cytotoxic action by using platinum diammines suggest that the "biologically important lesions are most likely interstrand and/or intrastrand cross-links" in DNA rather than the DNA–protein cross-links (*551*). Carcinogenic action on the other hand most likely does not depend on cross-linking, because monofunctional alkylating agents can be at least as potent as difunctional ones. The main difficulty in demonstrating carcinogenic action of difunctional agents seems to be due to their high cytotoxicity, which limits the doses that can be administered. Multiple administrations of relatively low doses of these agents are often required to cause significant yields of tumors.

Apart from mustard gas, HN2, and *cis*-platinum diammines, DNA cross-linking has been shown for triethylene melamine (*552, 553*), thio-TEPA (*543*), butadiene dioxide, mitomycin C (*555*), and 1,2:5,6-dianhydrogalactitol (*556, 557*), as representative of the various types of difunctional and polyfunctional alkylating agents. The *D*- and *L*- forms of butadiene oxide cross-link DNA of T7 phage, but not the *meso* form (*554*), although both *DL*- and *meso* forms are carcinogenic (*30*).

The extensive series of mustards used by Shimkin et al. (*215*) showed no clear correlation between carcinogenicity and tumor growth inhibitory properties, but Fahmy and Fahmy (*213*) found correlations with mutagenicity for certain mustards. Specifically, ability to induce mutations at certain loci (RNA-forming genes) in *Drosophila* was positively correlated with carcinogenicity, not overall mutagenicity.

As with monofunctional agents, the mustards are initiators in two-stage carcinogenesis in mouse skin (*282*); HN2 was reported to have only "borderline" activity in this system, but chlorambucil and melphalan were unequivocally active.

Systemic carcinogenic action of mustards has been shown for induction of lung tumors in strain A mice (*215*) and thymic lymphoma in RFM mice (*380, 381*).

Statistically significant yields of tumors at various sites were obtained by Schmähl and Osswald (*527*) by using intravenous administration in rats according to a dose schedule designed to mimic the use of mustards as chemotherapeutic agents. The *N*-oxide of HN2 appears to be more carcinogenic than HN2 itself.

According to the evaluations by IARC, the mustards used clinically as cytostatic agents should be regarded as carcinogenic hazards to humans. An extensively documented example is cyclophosphamide (Cytoxan), which is metabolically activated to phosphoramide mustard as the reactive alkylating

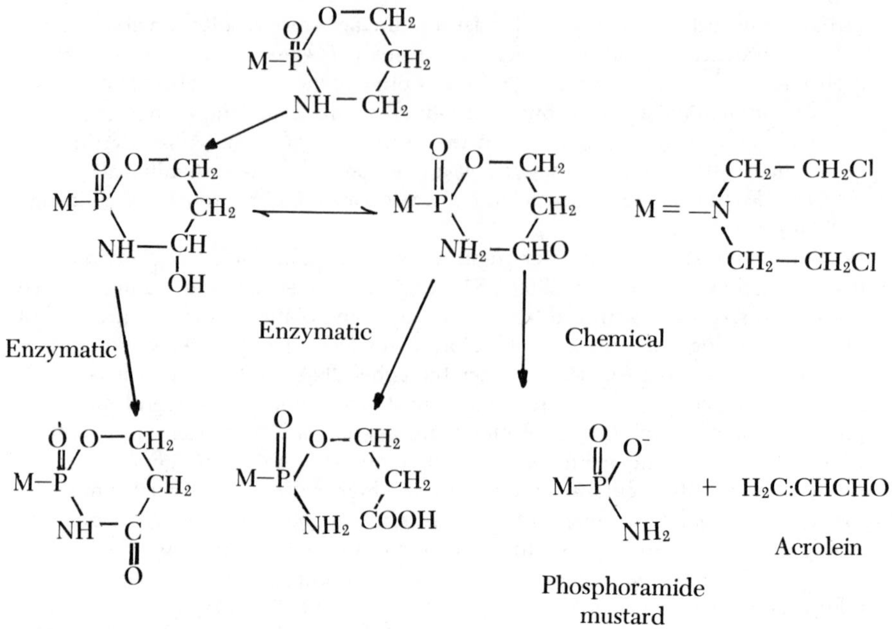

$$M = -N(CH_2-CH_2Cl)_2$$

Enzymatic — Enzymatic — Chemical

Phosphoramide mustard + $H_2C{:}CHCHO$ Acrolein

Scheme XI. Metabolism of cyclophosphamide (558). *Phosphoramide mustard is believed to be the principal cytotoxically active metabolite of the mustard type, but acrolein is responsible for cytotoxicity and concomitant tumor-promoting activity in bladder* (559).

species in vivo. Another metabolite, acrolein (*see* Scheme XI) (*558*), is held responsible for the toxic action of the drug on the bladder (*559*). As reviewed by the IARC (*560*), numerous researchers reported malignancy in patients following cyclophosphamide therapy, principally bladder cancers and acute nonlymphocytic leukemias. In an experimental model system for induction of bladder cancer in Balb/c mice, synergism was demonstrated between cyclophosphamide and the known bladder carcinogen 2-naphthylamine (*561*). As already discussed, acute nonlymphocytic leukemias appear to be the most general secondary malignancy resulting from use of cytotoxic alkylating drugs in humans, but cancers have been reported to be induced at several other sites.

Difunctional Sulfonates. The carcinogenicity of compounds falling into this category (Table XXXIV) has not been very extensively studied, in contrast to their cytotoxicity. The straight-chain dimethanesulfonoxyalkanes of the type CH_3SO_2O-$(CH_2)_nOSO_2CH_3$ have been of considerable interest as cytotoxic agents, particularly in chronic myeloid leukemia (*563*). The specific action as depressants of circulating neutrophils of a homologous series ($n = 2$–10) showed that activity was maximal at $n = 4$, i.e., with Myleran (Busulfan). Chemical reactivity as measured by solvolysis increased from $n = 2$–4, but for $n = 4$–10 it was approximately the same. Introduction of methyl substituents to the terminal C-atoms of the alkyl chain was expected to change the mechanism of alkylation from "largely S_N2 to an S_N1 type"

Table XXXIV

Representative Oncogenesis Tests—Alkanesulfonates (Difunctional)

Compound	*Animal*	*Strain or Type*	*Route*	*Dose*	*Duration (d)*	*Tumors*	*Remarks*	*References*
Myleran	mouse	albino	skin	2–6 mg total[a]	154	1/33	inactive as initiator at highest tolerated dose	281
	mouse	RF	iv	12 mg/kg × 4	614	35% thymic lymphomas	8% in controls	380, 381
	rat	BR46	po	0.13 mg/kg multiple, 6.76 mg/kg total	670[b]	6% benign,[c] 11% malignant	statistical sig. in doubt	527
	rat	—	sc	2 mg/kg × 20	240[b]	5/10 local sarcomas		528
	mouse	B6C3F1	ip	250,500 ppm 3 × wkly	365	"completed, data inconclusive"		562
	rat	Sprague–Dawley	ip	600 ppm 3 × wkly	365	"completed, data inconclusive"		562
1,6-Dimethane-sulfonoxy-hexane	mouse	—	sc	1 mg/kg × 20	450[b]	1/10		
	rat	—	sc	2 mg/kg × 20	365[b]	4/10		
				1 mg/kg × 20	300[b]	2/10		528
1,8-Dimethane-sulfonoxy-octane	mouse	—	sc	2 mg/kg × 20	365[b]	4/10		528
	rat	—	sc					
Mannitol myleran	mouse	—	sc	1 mg/kg × 20	430[b]	1/10		
	mouse	A/J	ip	3000 μmol/kg[d]	273	rel. potency[e] 3.3		215

[a]Multiple application in acetone; promotion with croton oil.
[b]Average induction time.
[c]For details of histopathology, *see* original reference.
[d]Range of doses used; "positive response dose" giving one lung tumor/mouse quoted.
[e]Denotes (10,000/"positive response dose").

(*564*) (*cf.* the change in mechanisms through methyl, ethyl, and isopropyl halides). In the resulting series, $CH_3SO_2OCH(CH_3)(CH_2)_{n-2}CH(CH_3)OSO_2CH_3$, the cytotoxic action was again maximal at $n = 4$, but overall it was lower than that of the nonmethylated series.

Various suggestions have been made to explain the rather specific cytotoxic action of Myleran and its homologs, but as yet none appear to be convincing. Although too few studies of carcinogenicity have been made to enable any useful assessment of the relevance of these hypotheses in this area, it may be useful to mention some of them briefly, with regard to any future work.

The principal in vivo reactions of Myleran and its monofunctional analog ethyl methanesulfonate are with thiol groups. The ability of Myleran to form cyclic sulfonium ions (derivatives of tetrahydrothiophene, *see* Scheme XII) was demon-

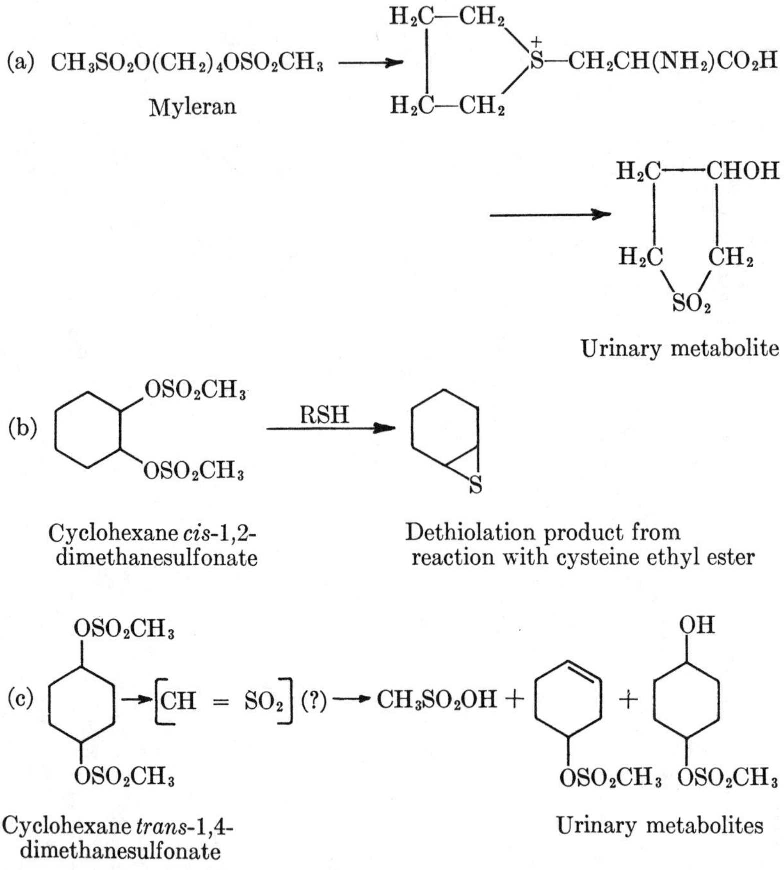

(a) $CH_3SO_2O(CH_2)_4OSO_2CH_3$ → (H_2C—CH_2 / H_2C—CH_2 ring) $\overset{+}{S}$—$CH_2CH(NH_2)CO_2H$

Myleran

→ (H_2C—CHOH / H_2C CH_2 / SO_2 ring)

Urinary metabolite

(b) OSO_2CH_3 / OSO_2CH_3 —RSH→ S

Cyclohexane *cis*-1,2-dimethanesulfonate

Dethiolation product from reaction with cysteine ethyl ester

(c) (OSO_2CH_3 / OSO_2CH_3 cyclohexane) → [CH = SO_2] (?) → CH_3SO_2OH + (cyclohexene, OSO_2CH_3) + (OH cyclohexane, OSO_2CH_3)

Cyclohexane *trans*-1,4-dimethanesulfonate

Urinary metabolites

Scheme XII. Reactions and metabolism of Myleran and cyclohexane dimethane sulfonates. Key: (a) (582) *and (b)* (583)*, reactions with cysteine or derivatives—"dethiolation"; and (c)* (583)*, elimination reaction.*

strated by Roberts and Warwick (*565*). Clearly this type of reaction could account for the dependence of cytotoxicity on chain length, since cycloalkylation would be favored at around $n = 4$ or 5, as previously noted by Timmis and Hudson (*564*). The products of cycloalkylation are unstable and decompose in vivo to yield tetrahydrothiophene derivatives, i.e., "dethiolation" of cysteinyl groups results (*566*).

The possible importance of cycloalkylation for cytotoxicity has been questioned, notably by Jones and coworkers (*567*), who found that the homolog 1,3-bis(methanesulfonyloxy)propane ($n = 3$) resembles Myleran in its effects on hemopoiesis and spermatogenesis but does not cycloalkylate in vitro or in vivo (*568*). Furthermore, studies with dimethanesulfonates of cyclohexane showed that noncycloalkylating isomers (1,3- and 1,4-derivatives, Scheme XII) are cytotoxic, but the 1,2-derivative is inactive, although able to dethiolate cysteine ethyl ester (*567*).

The 1,3- and 1,4-dimethanesulfonates undergo S_N1 elimination reactions with this cysteine derivative, and elimination reaction products were found in rat urine after administration of ^{35}S-labeled *trans*-1,4-dimethanesulfonate. Cycloalkylation and dethiolation were thought to represent detoxification processes, whereas the significant cytotoxic action of the methanesulfonates may involve cleavage of the methanesulfonyloxy group to yield sulfene ($CH_2{=}SO_2$). Sulfene is a highly reactive electrophile that Jones and Campbell (*567*) suggest may be liberated in vivo by a base-activated reaction.

Further evidence contraindicating a conventional alkylation mechanism for Myleran was obtained by Addison and Berenbaum (*569*), who found that exogenous cysteine potentiated rather than diminished the immunosuppressive action of Myleran in mice.

As these authors also point out, whereas Myleran can react with DNA, albeit to a small extent even in vitro, it inactivates phage T7 in the manner characteristic of a monofunctional agent, and interstrand cross-linkage could not be detected (*541*). However, Tong and Ludlum (*248*) reinvestigated alkylation of DNA by Myleran and confirmed that in vitro this agent does yield the cross-linked product 1,4-di(7-guaninyl)butane. It does not yet appear to be known whether this product is formed in vivo, or whether it results from interstrand as opposed to intrastrand cross-linking of DNA.

Whatever molecular mechanisms contribute to the biological action of Myleran, they evidently do not confer marked carcinogenic potency, since most investigators using this agent found no significantly positive results (Table XXXIV). Koller (*528*) briefly reported the induction of sarcomas at the injection site in mice and rats by Myleran and two homologs. Shimkin et al. (*31*) found Mannitol Myleran a relatively weak inducer of lung adenomas in strain A/J mice (relative potency of 3.3, compared with 280 for the analogous mannitol mustard) and expected that Myleran (not tested) would behave similarly.

Another report (*562*) has been briefly stated to yield "inconclusive data" from prolonged administration to mice or rats by intraperitoneal injections.

Despite the apparent failure to demonstrate any marked carcinogenicity of Myleran by conventional animal tests, it must now be considered as a carcinogenic hazard to humans. For example, from the study of long-term effects on patients given cytotoxic therapy with Myleran, Stott et al. (*377*) concluded that their "findings suggest that Busulfan (Myleran) is leukemogenic though its mode of action is uncertain." A similar conclusion was reached for the dihydroxy derivative of Myleran, Treosulfan (1,2,3,4-butanetetrol, 1,4-dimethanesulfonate) (*376*) although as yet no animal carcinogenicity data are available for this drug.

Difunctional Epoxides. The relationship between structure and activity for this group of compounds (Table XXXV) has been discussed in some detail by Van Duuren (*403*). He considered that three monoepoxides found to be active might be converted in vivo to difunctional agents.

The importance of the ability of carcinogenic epoxides to react with two nucleophilic centers was stressed, although not all difunctional epoxides are active (Table XXXVI). Van Duuren (*403*) pointed out that the distance between the reactive groups in the difunctional epoxides could range from about 0.4 nm (diepoxybutane) to about 1.0 nm. Cross-linking between nucleic acid molecules or between DNA and nucleohistones was considered more likely to be important for carcinogenicity than cross-linking between the strands of the DNA double helix. If this last reaction occurred between the most reactive nucleophilic sites in DNA at N-7, atoms of guanine residues would be required to span a distance of about 0.8 nm.

The ability of *D*- and *L*- forms of diepoxybutane to induce interstrand cross-linking in DNA of T7 phage has been demonstrated (*554*). Cross-linking by the *meso* form was not detected, and it was the least efficient isomer in the inactivation of the phage. *d,l*-Diepoxybutane was a somewhat more effective initiator than the *meso* form in two-stage carcinogenesis in mouse skin (*403*). The alkylation sites in DNA that are involved in interstrand cross-linking by diepoxybutane have not been specified as yet.

Difunctional and Polyfunctional Ethyleneimines. All the compounds tested (Table XXXVII) have been classed as positive, except the chemosterilant Apholate. They are all mutagens and chromosome-breaking agents (for a comprehensive review, *see* Ref. 300). TEM (*553*) and Mitomycin C (*555*) are powerful cross-linking agents for DNA, although the latter requires metabolic or chemical reduction for activation. The induction of lymphoma in mice by TEM may involve some form of activation of tumor virus (*381*).

Summary and Conclusions

The alkylating agents include carcinogens of particular chemical interest. Their reactions in vivo will often, but not always, be the same as those in vitro because in some cases metabolic activation may intervene. This situation stimulates interest in their mode of action, not only as active compounds, but also as models for reactive metabolites of other carcinogens.

The initial hopes that the relative simplicity of in vivo alkylation reactions would enable specification of the essential cellular receptors of chemical carcinogens were not fulfilled. Alkylating agents did not appear to react specifically with any cellular target. In fact, the major type of reaction that generally occurs in vivo with thiols is now regarded fairly widely as mainly detoxificative in nature. However, protein alkylation does play a part in carcinogenesis. As Colburn and

Table XXXV

Representative Oncogenesis Tests—Epoxides (Difunctional)

Compound	*Animal Strain or Type*[a]	*Route*	*Dose*	*Duration (d)*	*Tumors*	*Remarks*	*References*
Butadiene dioxide (*d,l*-form)	albino rat	ip	1–2 mg/kg × 12	540	1/14 sarcoma	reported inactive on mouse skin	570
	ICR/Ha Swiss	skin	3 mg, 3 × wkly	475[b]	6/30 carcinomas	weakly active	
		skin	1 mg, single[c]	137[d]	7/20 papillomas 2/20 carcinomas	active as initiator, in promotion tests an active inhibitor	475
Butadiene dioxide (meso form)	Sprague–Dawley rat	sc	1.1 mg, wkly[e]	589	5/30 local malignant sarcomas	inactive by gastric feeding	481
		sc	1 mg, wkly[e]	550	9/50 local malignant sarcomas 1/50 adenocarcinoma		
	ICR/Ha Swiss	skin	10 mg, 3 × wkly	357[b]	4/30 carcinomas		498
		skin	1 mg, single[c]	163[d]	4/20 papillomas 0/20 carcinomas	less active as initiator than *d,l*-form	475
	C3H	skin	continuous painting	450	1/4 cancer 2/4 papillomas		479
	A	ip	1320 μmol/kg[f]	273	lung, rel. potency[f] 7.6		
1,2,4,5-Diepoxypentane	ICR/Ha Swiss	skin	10 mg, 3 × wkly	490[b]	10/30 papillomas 3/30 carcinomas		215
1,2,5,6-Diepoxyhexane	ICR/Ha	skin	2 mg, 3 × wkly	427[b]	13/30 papillomas 10/30 carcinomas		480
		sc	1 mg, wkly[e]	533	2/30 fibrosarcomas 1/30 adenocarcinoma		481
	Sprague–Dawley rat	sc	1 mg, wkly[e]	552	1/50 fibrosarcoma		

Continued on next page

Table XXXV Continued

Compound	Animal Strain or Type[a]	Route	Dose	Duration (d)	Tumors	Remarks	References
1,2,6,7-Diepoxyheptane	ICR/Ha	skin	1 mg, 3 × wkly	464[b]	9/30 papillomas 1/30 carcinomas		498
1,2,7,8-Diepoxyoctane	ICR/Ha	skin	1 mg, 3 × wkly	385[d]	7/30 keratoacanthomas 4/30 carcinomas		480
1-Ethyleneoxy-3,4-epoxycyclohexane, "Vinylcyclohexene dioxide"	Swiss	skin	10 mg, 3 × wkly	326[b]	14/30 papillomas 9/30 carcinomas	first studied in Ref. 586	
	C3H	skin	continuous painting	520	3/17 papillomas 1/17 cancer	weakly positive in rats	479
2,5-Dimethyl-1,2,5,6-diepoxyhex-3-yne	ICR/Ha	sc	0.5–1 mg wkly	665	9/60 local sarcomas	inactive by skin painting	284
1,2,4,5,9,10-triepoxydecane	ICR/Ha	sc	1 mg wkly	635	11/60 local sarcomas		284
3,4-Epoxy-6-methylcyclohexylmethyl-3,4-epoxy-6-methylcyclohexanecarboxylate	ICR/Ha	skin	1 mg, 3 × wkly	392[d]	11/30 keratoacanthomas 11/30 carcinomas	first studied in Ref. 479 and reported positive	480
Modified bis-phenol diglycidyl ethers	C3H	skin	continuous painting	700	6/28 papillomas 3/28 cancers		479
Triethylene glycol, diglycidyl ether, "Epodyl"	A	ip	14.400 μmol/kg[f]	273	lung, rel. potency 0.7		215

[a]Except where indicated, the animal studied was the mouse. [b]Median survival time. [c]Promotion with phorbol esters. [d]Appearance of first papilloma, duration generally about 550 d. [e]About 65 mg total dose. [f]Range of doses; "positive response dose" giving one lung tumor/mouse quoted. [g]Relative potency denotes (10,000/positive response dose). [h]In skin painting applications, acetone was generally used as solvent.

Table XXXVI

Representative Oncogenesis Tests—Epoxides (Difunctional) Reported Inactive

Compound	*Route*[a]	*References*
Bis(2,3-epoxy-2-methylpropyl) ether	skin	479
Ethylene glycol bis(2,3-epoxy-2-methylpropyl) ether	skin	479
Bis(3,4-epoxy-6-methylcyclohexylmethyl) adipate	skin	479
Limonene dioxide	skin	479
1,2,3,4-Diepoxycyclohexane	skin	403
1,2,5,6-Diepoxycyclooctane	skin	
9,10,12,13-Diepoxystearic acid	skin	403
Resorcinoldiglycidyl ether	skin	
Hexaepoxysqualene	skin	
1,4-Bis(2,3-epoxypropyl) piperazine	ip	215
1,1′-Bis(2,3-epoxypropyl)-4,4′-bipiperidine	ip	

NOTE: Ref. 479 also reported 10 other compounds of this type inactive.
[a]In all cases, the animal studied was the mouse.

Boutwell (*400, 401*) have pointed out, this process is particularly likely to be significant in the promotion stage of the two-stage mechanisms of carcinogenesis.

Historically, the alkylating agents emerged as the classical carcinogenic mutagens. With aromatic hydrocarbons and amines, demonstration of carcinogenicity preceded that of mutagenicity. With the alkylating agents, the reverse has often been true. This situation, of course, is understandable because many test organisms in chemical mutagenesis do not metabolize many carcinogens at all or inappropriately to yield the ultimate reactive forms. Generally, there are no effective barriers to reactions of alkylating agents with DNA in vivo.

Considerable attention has been devoted to this group of compounds in the area of detection of chemical modifications of DNA as an index of potential mutagenic action. The question remains whether this approach is relevant for assessment of a carcinogenic hazard. Probably few researchers would now doubt the equation of the initiation stage in carcinogenesis with some type of somatic mutation.

As yet, demonstration of the nature of the required mutation(s) has not been achieved, although several suggestions have been made, including ones that mutations cause instability of the structure of chromosomes or of the cell surface or cause deletions of RNA-forming genes. The key problems in this area are doubtless those concerned with the control of cell division. In a comprehensive model for two-stage carcinogenesis, a first initiating event has been equated with a mutation, and promotion has been equated with proliferation of initiated cells to give sufficient numbers to permit a significant chance that a second event of a mutational type could occur to give a malignant cell. Alkylating agents can now be

Table XXXVII

Representative Oncogenesis Tests—Ethyleneimines (Difuctional and Polyfunctional)

Compound	Animal	Strain or Type	Route	Dose	Duration (d)	Tumors	Remarks	References
Triethylene melamine	mouse	A	ip	7.5 µg × 10	100	8/10 pulmonary adenomas	2/15 in controls	571
	mouse	A	ip	50 µg × 2	126	24/30 animals with pulmonary tumors	2.64 tumors/ mouse	
	mouse	albino S	skin	240 µg	154	0/10		281
				240 µg[a]	154	18/10	active initiator	
	mouse	RF	ip	1.5 mg/kg × 4	563	33% thymic lymphoma	8% in controls; myeloid leukemia incidence accelerated but no overall increase	380, 381
	rat	—	sc	10 mg/kg[b], total	450	11/12 local sarcomas		395, 476
	rat	Wistar	sc	10 mg/kg[b], total	506	5/12 local sarcomas		
1,3-Bis(ethyleneiminosulfonyl)propane	rat	Wistar	sc	8 mg/kg[b], total		6/12 local sarcomas		476
Trenimon	rat	BR46	iv	0.03 mg/kg, total	450	11% benign[c]	considered positive	527
				1.56 mg/kg		24% malignant		
Tris(1-aziridinyl) phosphine oxide	rat	Fischer	po	1–300 µg per d × 260	up to 565	33/58 neoplastic[c] lesions	part of detailed methodological study; classed as weakly carcinogenic	572

2,2,4,4,6,6-Hexakis (1-aziridinyl)-2,2,4,4,6,6-hexahydro-1,3,5,2,4,-6-triazatriphosphorine	rat	Fischer	po	3–300 μg per d $\times$ 260	up to 565	18/60 neoplastic[c] lesions	detailed study; tumor distribution similar to that of controls	572
Bis(1-aziridinyl) morpholinophosphine sulfide	mouse	A/J	ip	120 μmol/kg[d]	273	lung, rel. potency[e] 83		215
Tris(1-aziridinyl) phosphine sulfide	mouse	A/J	ip	60 μmol/kg[d]	273	lung, rel. potency[c] 170		215
	rat	BR46	iv	1 mg/kg, total 52 mg/kg	450	17% benign[c] 30% malignant	considered positive	527
Mitomycin C[f]	rat	BR46	iv	0.52 mg/kg $\times$ 5	540	4% benign 34% malignant	5% benign, 6% malignant in controls	527
	rat	Sprague–Dawley	ip	0.038–0.15 mg/kg	540	peritoneal sarcomas 27/29 (m) 30/31 (f)		516

[a]Applied in acetone; followed by promotion with croton oil.
[b]Repeated injection in arachis oil of 1 mg/kg.
[c]For details *see* original reference.
[d]Range of doses used; "positive response dose" giving one lung tumor/mouse quoted.
[e]Denotes (10,000/positive response dose).
[f]Although strictly a monofunctional ethyleneimine, behaves as difunctional agent in vivo.

classified beyond doubt as initiating mutagens, but their role in promotion, which is a balance between cytotoxic action and reparative cell division, is not yet easy to define.

A survey of the carcinogenic action of the wide variety of alkylating agents in various strains and species of animal shows a correspondingly wide spectrum of response, and generalizations are not obvious.

Some fruitful comparisons between experimental and human carcinogenesis by alkylating agents are beginning to emerge. Systemic action of these carcinogens in mice can give high yields of tumors of the lymphoid system (mainly thymic lymphoma) with a considerable dependence of the strain of mouse. In humans, the use of alkylating agents in cytotoxic chemotherapy, or as immunosuppressants, has also given malignant lymphomas, although these are histiocytic rather than lymphocytic as in mice. Synergism between chemical carcinogens and tumor viruses is strongly indicated for lymphoma induction in mice and is also suspected in humans. Acute nonlymphocytic leukemia is the predominant (but not the only) secondary malignancy induced following cancer chemotherapy by alkylating agents. The use of cyclophosphamide or of naphthylamine mustard can cause bladder cancer; metabolic conversions of cyclophosphamide to acrolein (as a cytotoxic promoter) and of naphthylamine mustard to 2-naphthylamine (a potent bladder carcinogen) are believed to be involved in these cases.

Local carcinogenic action has often been used in experimental studies with alkylating agents, chiefly by subcutaneous injections yielding local sarcomas. Inhalation studies have been used in view of the findings that certain industrial alkylating agents have caused respiratory tract tumors in humans. In the rat it has been possible to induce mainly nasal tumors by this route of administration, but it appears to be more difficult to cause tumors of bronchus and lung. These organs are more susceptible in humans.

Apart from their use in establishing animal models for human carcinogenesis, alkylating agents have proved particularly useful for fundamental studies on the molecular mechanisms of carcinogenesis.

The ability of alkylating agents to induce significant chemical lesions in cellular DNA, and thus to cause appropriate DNA repair mechanisms to operate, has been demonstrated with mammalian cells both in vitro and to some extent in vivo. Three principal mechanisms by which tumor initiation could result have thus been suggested: (1) mutation induction by the replication of DNA containing promutagenic alkylated bases, (2) mutation induction by replication of misrepaired alkylated DNA, and (3) tumor virus activation by derepression of provirus.

Some attention has been devoted to the question of whether certain types of alkylation damage may be more effective than others in causing various biological effects. The cross-linking action of difunctional alkylating agents appears to be reasonably well established as conferring cytotoxicity by interference with replication of DNA. With respect to mutagenesis, current interest concerns the indication that alkylating agents reacting through the S_N1 mechanism may be more powerful mutagens, because they are able to attack a wider range of nucleophiles than S_N2 reagents. These sites include ones in nucleic acids, O-atoms, and in some cases amino groups, in addition to the ring N-atoms that are generally the most nucleophilic centers. Specific suggestions have been made concerning the nature of the induced promutagenic groups, notably the O^6-alkylguanines (*10*).

Detailed studies in vitro using alkylated polydeoxyribonucleotide templates and in vivo using *E. coli* have confirmed the importance of this mode of alkylation of DNA. However, O^6-alkylation of guanine in DNA is not, of course, the only promutagenic reaction of carcinogens, and other candidates for this role are under investigation.

A modifying factor of major importance in mutagenesis, and therefore in tumor initiation, is enzymatic repair of alkylated cellular DNA. One outstanding example is the demethylation of O^6-methylguanine, and considerable variation in ability of cells to effect this removal of a promutagenic group have been revealed. So far, human cells appear to be remarkably proficient in this respect, and this may indicate comparative resistance of the human species to carcinogenesis insofar as it can be ascribed to action of alkylating mutagens. Inherited or acquired deficiency in DNA repair may thus be a major factor enhancing carcinogenic risk for a given level of exposure to such mutagens, and this area of research will no doubt continue to be developed as contributory to our knowledge of the etiology of cancer.

Note Added in Proof

Regarding page 341 and Scheme IV. The mechanism of reaction of the *n*-propyldiazonium ion has been investigated in more detail by Scribner and Ford (*573*). As predicted in the present review of the previous work of Park et al. (*40, 41*), the new findings confirm the expectation that the isomerization resulting in isopropylation occurs more extensively when O-6 atoms, as opposed to N-7 atoms, of guanine in RNA are alkylated. The mechanism preferred by Scribner and Ford is not identical with the classical S_N1 concept due to Ingold. They suggest that a transition complex is formed between the diazonium ion and both nucleophiles, but that the transition state for reaction at O-6 of guanine is much "looser" than that for reaction at N-7, thus permitting rearrangement to occur with greater facility.

Regarding page 351. A notable advance has been reported in the search for the target genes for chemical mutagens in transformation (the "oncogenes"). Two groups (*574, 575*) have found that DNA of a human bladder carcinoma cell line, capable of transforming NIH-3T3 cells by transfection, can be distinguished from "normal" human bladder cell DNA in that it possesses a single alteration in base sequence. This alteration causes the affected codon to code for the amino acid valine instead of the "normal" glycine in a protein constituent of the cell membrane denoted p21. Transfecting DNA derived from two strains of rat sarcoma virus also showed alterations at the same codon, with the substituted amino acids being arginine and serine.

These precisely defined "point" mutations (in the literal sense that they involve alteration of a single specific base pair in DNA) correspond to GC $\rightarrow$ TA transversions (glycine to valine), or GC $\rightarrow$ AT transitions (glycine to arginine or serine). They are therefore consistent with the concept that oncogenes can be generated from normal genes by single base-pair changes, as postulated for alkylating agents. However, the precise significance of these mutations in the two-stage mechanism of carcinogenesis was admitted to be as yet unclear (*575*).

The diversity of the various possible base-pair changes in mutations according to the nature of the promutagenic alteration of DNA by alkylating carcinogens has recently been reviewed comprehensively (*576, 577*).

Regarding pages 352–59 and Figures 4 and 5. Studies of the specificity of carcinogen-induced mutagenesis in the *lac* I gene of *E. coli* [as previously reported for alkylating carcinogens (*149*)] have been extended (*578*) to an aralkylating agent. This agent is the benzo[*a*]pyrene diol epoxide that was deduced to be the principal metabolite of the parent hydrocarbon and that mediates in its initiation of cancer. The principal type of mutation induced was found to be a single base-pair change, the GC → TA transversion, rather than the GC → CG transversion suggested on theoretical grounds by Kadlubar (*132*). The observed transversion may result from a type of "error-prone" repair in which an adenine base is inserted opposite to a chemically altered base. The altered base serves as a block to DNA polymerase (as typified by the thymine dimer induced by UV radiation) (*578*).

Regarding page 361. Further studies on the mechanism of repair of O^6-methylguanine have been carried out by using liver of mice (*580*) and rats (*581*) and a human lymphoid cell line (*581*). In both cases demethylation of O^6-methylguanine to guanine was found to be the principal pathway, with transfer of the methyl group to a cysteinyl moiety of a receptor protein.

This compound may well be the quasi-enzyme that also removes the methyl group, if mammalian cells are analogous to *E. coli* in this respect. The relevant protein has been isolated from *E. coli* (*582*); it has a molecular weight of 18,400 and contains four or five cysteine residues. It reacts stoichiometrically with O^6-methylguanine in DNA (*583*) (preferring the double-stranded form), and is not therefore a truly catalytic enzyme.

Investigations of this type of DNA repair in human lymphocytes in relation to disease states have been started (*584, 585*). In one report, patients with chronic lymphocytic leukemia were stated to be more proficient in removal of O^6-methylguanine than were normal subjects (*584*). The method used was assay of the demethylase quasi-enzyme.

Another study (*585*), using analyses of methylated DNA, reported relative deficiency in patients suffering from certain autoimmune diseases, such as Behçet's disease and systemic lupus erythematosus, but not scleroderma.

Both studies reported a spectrum of repair capability in normal healthy subjects; some such subjects were relatively deficient, analogous to that found previously for repair of UV-induced DNA damage as assessed by unscheduled DNA synthesis (*586*). The relative repair deficiency found in the autoimmune diseases was suggested to be a possible factor determining susceptibility to these diseases, provided that some other genetic predisposition was present. This suggestion was based on the hypothesis that somatic mutations may be involved in their etiology. The findings of supernormal repair proficiency in the leukemic lymphocytes, on the other hand, may appear at first sight somewhat unexpected, and may have implications for treatment of the disease by alkylating cytotoxic drugs.

It can be expected, however, that studies of this type relating ability to repair chemical carcinogen-induced DNA damage and etiology will be extended to other forms of leukemia and cancer.

Literature Cited

1. Brookes, P.; Lawley, P.D. *Biochem. J.* **1960**, *77*, 478.
2. Auerbach, C.; Robson, J.M. *Nature* (*London*) **1946**, *157*, 302.
3. Strong, L.C. *Br. J. Cancer* **1949**, *3*, 97.
4. Heston, W.E. *JNCI, J. Natl. Cancer Inst.* **1953**, *14*, 131.
5. Heston, W.E. *JNCI, J. Natl. Cancer Inst.* **1950**, *11*, 415.
6. Berenblum, I. *J. Pathol. Bacteriol.* **1931**, *34*, 731.
7. Wada, S.; Miyanishi, M.; Nishimoto, Y.; Kambe, S.; Miller, R.W. *Lancet* **1968**, *i*, 1611.
8. Brookes, P.; Lawley, P.D. *Nature* (*London*) **1964**, *202*, 781.
9. Sims, P.; Grover, P.L.; Swaisland, A.; Pal, K.; Hewer, A. *Nature* (*London*) **1974**, *252*, 326.
10. Loveless, A. *Nature* (*London*) **1969**, *223*, 206.
11. Frei, J.V.; Swenson, D.H.; Warren, W.; Lawley, P.D. *Biochem. J.* **1978**, *174*, 1031.
12. Osterman-Golkar, S.; Ehrenberg, L.; Wachtmeister, C.A. *Radiat. Bot.* **1970**, *10*, 303.
13. Dipple, A.; Levy, L.S.; Lawley, P.D. *Carcinogenesis* **1981**, *2*, 103.
14. Poirier, L.A.; Stoner, G.D.; Shimkin, M.B. *Cancer Res.* **1975**, *35*, 1411.
15. Ingold, C.K. "Structure and Mechanism in Organic Chemistry," 2nd ed.; Cornell Univ.: New York, 1969; Chap. VII.
16. Streitweiser, A. *Chem. Rev.* **1956**, *56*, 571.
17. Wells, P.R. *Chem. Rev.* **1963**, *63*, 171.
18. Warwick, G.P. *Cancer Res.* **1963**, *23*, 315.
19. Ross, W.C.J. In "Biological Alkylating Agents"; Butterworths: London, 1962.
20. Price, C.C. *Ann. N.Y. Acad. Sci.* **1958**, *68*, 663.
21. Price, C.C.; Gaucher, G.M.; Koneru, P.; Shibakawa, R.; Sowa, J.R.; Yamaguchi, M. *Ann. N.Y. Acad. Sci.* **1969**, *163*, 593.
22. Bardos, R.J.; Datta-Gupta, N.; Hebborn, P.; Triggle, D.J. *J. Med. Chem.* **1965**, *8*, 167.
23. Bardos, T.J.; Chmielewicz, Z.F.; Hebborn, P. *Ann. N.Y. Acad. Sci.* **1969**, *163*, 1006.
24. Price, C.C. *Handb. Exp. Pharmacol.* **1975**, *38* (2), 1.
25. Sneen, R.A.: Larsen, J.W. *J. Am. Chem. Soc.* **1969**, *91*, 362.
26. Swain, C.G.; Scott, C.B. *J. Am. Chem. Soc.* **1953**, *75*, 141.
27. Petty, W.L.; Nichols, P.L., Jr. *J. Am. Chem. Soc.* **1954**, *76*, 4385.
28. Ross, W.C.J. *Adv. Cancer Res.* **1953**, *1*, 397.
29. Hudson, R.F. "Structure and Mechanism in Organo-Phosphorus Chemistry"; Academic: London, 1965; p. 110.
30. Van Duuren, B.L.; Goldschmidt, B.M. *J. Med. Chem.* **1966**, *9*, 77.
31. Barnard, P.W.C.; Robertson, R.E. *Can. J. Chem.* **1961**, *39*, 881.
32. Garrett, E.R.; Goto, S.; Stubbins, J.F. *J. Pharm Sci.* **1965**, *54*, 119.
33. Veleminsky, J.; Osterman-Golkar, S.; Ehrenberg, L. *Mutat. Res.* **1970**, *10*, 169.
34. Pearson, R.G.: Langer, S.H.; Williams, R.V.; McGuire, W.J. *J. Am. Chem. Soc.* **1952**, *74*, 5130.
35. Parker, R.E.; Isaacs, N.S. *Chem. Rev.* **1959**, *59*, 737.
36. Ogston, A.G. *Trans. Faraday Soc.* **1948**, *44*, 45.

37. Hudson, R.F.: Withey, R.J. *J. Chem. Soc.* **1964**, 3513.
38. March, J. "Advanced Organic Chemistry: Reactions, Mechanisms and Structure"; McGraw-Hill: New York, 1968; Chap. 10.
39. Kirmse, W. *Angew. Chem.* **1976**, *15*, 251.
40. Park, K.K.; Archer, M.C. *Chem.-Biol. Interact.* **1977**, *18*, 349.
41. Park, K.K.; Archer, M.C.; Wishnok, J.S. *Chem.-Biol. Interact.* **1980**, *29*, 139.
42. Pearson, R.G.; Songstad, J. *J. Am. Chem. Soc.* **1967**, *89*, 1827.
43. Sykes, P. "Guidebook to Mechanism in Organic Chemistry"; Longmans: London, 1961; Chap. 3.
44. Swain, G.C.; Scott, C.B.; Lohmann, K.H. *J. Am. Chem. Soc.* **1953**, *75*, 136.
45. Ludlum, D.B. *Biochim. Biophys. Acta* **1967**, *142*, 282.
46. Shooter, K.V. *Chem.-Biol. Interact.* **1975**, *11*, 575.
47. Turtoczky, I.; Ehrenberg, L. *Mutat. Res.* **1969**, *8*, 229.
48. Neale, S. *Mutat. Res.* **1972**, *14*, 155.
49. Burnet, F.M. "Auto-immunity and Auto-immune Disease"; MTP: Lancaster, 1972.
50. Burch, P.R.J. "Biology of Cancer: A New Approach"; MTP: Lancaster, 1976.
51. Kohn, K.W. "Molecular Actions and Targets for Cancer Chemotherapeutic Agents"; Sartorelli, A.C.; Lazo, J.S.; Bertino, J.R., Eds.; Academic: New York, 1981; Chap. 1.
52. Tong, W.P.; Ludlum, D.B. *Cancer Res.* **1981**, *41*, 380.
53. Lawley, P.D. "Molecular and Environmental Aspects of Mutagenesis"; Prakash, L.; Sherman, F.; Miller, M.W.; Lawrence, C.W.; Taber, H.W., Eds.; C.C. Thomas: Springfield, IL, 1974; Chap. 2.
54. Swenson, D.H.: Lawley, P.D. *Biochem. J.* **1978**, *171*, 575.
55. Walles, S.; Ehrenberg, L. *Acta Chem. Scand.* **1969**, *23*, 1080.
56. Lawley, P.D.; Orr, D.J.; Jarman, M. *Biochem. J.* **1975**, *145*, 73.
57. Olah, G.A. *Chem. Brit.* **1972**, *8*, 281.
58. Beranek, D.T.; Weis, C.C.; Swenson, D.H. *Carcinogenesis* **1980**, *1*, 595.
59. Lawley, P.D.; Shah, S.A. *Chem.-Biol. Interact.* **1973**, *7*, 115.
60. Lawley, P.D. "Screening Tests in Chemical Carcinogenesis"; Montesano, R.; Bartsch, H.; Tomatis, L., Eds.; World Health: Albany, 1976; pp. 181–210.
61. Singer, B. *JNCI, J. Natl. Cancer Inst.* **1979**, *62*, 1329.
62. Drake, J.W.; Baltz, R.H. *Annu. Rev. Biochem.* **1976**, *45*, 907.
63. Drinkwater, H.R.; Miller, E.C.; Miller, J.A. *Biochemistry* **1980**, 5087.
64. Shearman, C.W.; Loeb, L.A. *J. Mol. Biol.* **1979**, *128*, 197.
65. Lawley, P.D.; Martin, C.N. *Biochem. J.* **1975**, *145*, 85.
66. Krieg, D.R. *Prog. Nucleic Acid Res. Mol. Biol.* **1963**, *2*, 125.
67. Lawley, P.D.; Orr, D.J. *Chem.-Biol. Interact.* **1970**, *2*, 154.
68. Olsson, M.; Lindahl, T. *J. Biol. Chem.* **1980**, *255*, 10569.
69. Abbott, P.J.; Saffhill, R. *Biochim. Biophys. Acta* **1979**, *562*, 51.
70. Newbold, R.F.; Warren, W.; Medcalf, A.S.C.; Amos, J. *Nature (London)* **1980**, *283*, 596.
71. Warren, W.; Crathorn, A.R.; Shooter, K.V. *Biochim. Biophys. Acta* **1979**, *563*, 82.
72. Olsen, A.S.; Milman, G. *J. Biol. Chem.* **1974**, *249*, 4038.
73. Sega, G.A.; Wolfe, K.W.; Owens, J.G. *Chem.-Biol. Interact.* **1981**, *33*, 253.
74. Ehling, U.H.; Cumming, R.B.; Malling, H.V. *Mutat. Res.* **1968**, *5*, 417.
75. Partington, M.; Bateman, A.J. *Heredity* **1964**, *19*, 191.
76. Partington, M.; Jackson, H. *Genet. Res.* **1963**, *4*, 333.
77. Ehling, U.H. "Chemical Mutagenesis in Mammals and Man"; Vogel, F.; Rohrborn, G., Eds.; Springer-Verlag: Berlin, 1970; Chap. 5.
78. Epstein, S.S.; Bass, W.; Arnold, E.; Bishop, Y. *Science (Washington, D.C.)* **1970**, *168*, 584.

79. Epstein, S.S.; Shafner, H. *Nature (London)* **1968**, *219*, 385.
80. Moutschen, J. *Genetics* **1961**, *46*, 291.
81. Cattanach, B.M. *Z. Vererbungsl.* **1959**, *90*, 1.
82. Röhrborn, G. *Humangenetik* **1965**, *1*, 576.
83. Brittinger, D. *Humangenetik* **1966**, *3*, 156.
84. "DNA Repair and Mutagenesis in Eukaryotes"; Generoso, W.M.; Shelby, M.D.; de Serres, F.J., Eds.; Plenum: New York, 1980.
85. "Methods in Mammalian Mutagenesis"; Roderick, T.H.; Sheridan, W., Eds.; *Genetics* **1979**, *92*, Suppl., pp. S1–S209.
86. Russell, W.L.; Kelly, E.M.; Hunsicker, P.R.; Bangham, J.W.; Maddux, S.C.: Phipps, E.L. *Proc. Natl. Acad. Sci. U.S.A.* **1979**, *76*, 5818.
87. Perry, P.; Evans, H.J. *Nature (London)* **1975**, *258*, 121.
88. Sasaki, M.S., in Ref. 84, Ch. 19.
89. Wolff, S.; Rodin, B.; Cleaver, J.E. *Nature (London)* **1977**, *265*, 347.
90. Swenson, D.H.; Harbach, P.R.; Trzos, R.J. *Carcinogenesis* **1980**, *1*, 931.
91. "Mammalian Cell Transformation by Chemical Carcinogens"; Mishra, N.; Dunkel, V.; Mehlman, M., Eds.; Senate: Princeton Junction, NJ, 1980.
92. Styles, J.A., in Ref. 91, Chap. 5.
93. Price, P.J.; Mishra, N.K., in Ref. 91, Chap. 8.
94. Casto, B.C., in Ref. 91, Chap. 9.
95. DiPaolo, J.A.; Casto, B.C. "Screening Tests in Chemical Carcinogenesis"; Montesano, R.; Bartsch, H.; Tomatis, L., Eds.; I.A.R.C.: Lyon, 1976; pp. 415–32.
96. Heidelberger, C., in Ref. 91, Chap. 1.
97. Kakunaga, T. *Int. J. Cancer* **1973**, *12*, 463.
98. Shih, C.; Shilo, B.-Z.; Goldfarb, M.P.; Dannenberg, A.; Weinberg, R.A. *Proc. Natl. Acad. Sci. U.S.A.* **1979**, *76*, 5714.
99. Favera, R.D.; Gelmann, E.P.; Gallo, R.C.; Wong-Staai, F. *Nature (London)* **1981**, *292*, 31.
100. "Neoplastic Transformation in Differentiated Epithelial Cell Systems in Vitro"; Franks, L.M.; Wigley, C.B., Eds.; Academic: New York, 1979.
101. Rasmuson, B.; Svahlin, H.; Rasmuson, Å.; Montell, I.; Olofsson, H. *Mutat. Res.* **1978**, *54*, 33.
102. Fahmy, M.J.; Fahmy, O.G. *Cancer Res.* **1980**, *40*, 3374.
103. Fahmy, M.J.; Fahmy, O.G. *Mutat. Res.* **1980**, *72*, 165.
104. Auerbach, C. *Mutat. Res.* **1981**, *81*, 257.
105. Teich, N.; Lowy, D.R.; Hartley, J.W.; Rowe, W.P. *Virology* **1973**, *51*, 163.
106. Lwoff, A. *Bacteriol. Rev.* **1953**, *17*, 269.
107. Loveless, A. "Genetic and Allied Effects of Alkylating Agents"; Butterworths: London, 1966.
108. Heinemann, B. "Chemical Mutagens: Principles and Methods for Their Detection"; Hollaender, Alexander; De Serres, Frederick J., Eds.; Plenum: New York, 1971; Vol. 1, Chap. 8.
109. Loveless, A.; Shields, G. *Virology* **1964**, *24*, 668.
110. Moreau, P.; Bailone, A.; Devoret, R. *Proc. Natl. Acad. Sci. U.S.A.* **1976**, *73*, 3700.
111. Speck, W.T.; Santella, R.M.; Rosenkranz, H.S. *Mutat. Res.* **1978**, *54*, 101.
112. Ames, B.N.; McCann, J.; Yamasaki, E. *Mutat. Res.* **1975**, *31*, 347.
113. McCann, J.; Choi, E.; Yamasaki, E.; Ames, B.N. *Proc. Natl. Acad. Sci. U.S.A.* **1975**, *72*, 5135.
114. "Evaluation of Short Term Tests for Carcinogens"; de Serres, F.J.; Ashby, J., Eds.; Elsevier: New York, 1981.
115. Thomson, J.A., in Ref. 114, Chap. 18.

116. Ashby, J., in Ref. 114, Chap. 11.
117. Roberts, J.J.; Warwick, G.P. *Biochem. Pharmacol.* **1963**, *12*, 1441.
118. Colburn, N.H.; Boutwell, R.K. *Cancer Res.* **1966**, *26*, 1701.
119. Boutwell, R.K.; Colburn, N.H.; Muckerman, C.C. *Ann. N.Y. Acad. Sci.* **1969**, *163*, 751.
120. Corbett, T.H.; Heidelberger, C.; Dove, W.F. *Mol. Pharmacol.* **1970**, *6*, 667.
121. Segal, A.; Solomon, J.J.; Mignano, J.; Dino, J. *Chem.-Biol. Interact.* **1981**, *35*, 349.
122. Chen, R.; Mieyal, J.J.; Goldthwait, D.A. *Carcinogenesis* **1981**, *2*, 73.
123. Mehta, J.R.: Ludlum, D.B. *Biochim. Biophys. Acta* **1978**, *521*, 770.
124. Saffhill, R.; Abbott, P.J. *Nucleic Acids Res.* **1978**, *5*, 1971.
125. Abbott, P.J.; Saffhill, R. *Nucleic Acids Res.* **1977**, *4*, 761.
126. Hall, J.A.; Saffhill, R.; Green, T.; Hathway, D.E. *Carcinogenesis* **1981**, *2*, 141.
127. Barbin, A.; Bartsch, H.; Leconte, P.; Radman, M. *Nucleic Acids Res.* **1981**, *9*, 375.
128. Sirover, M.A.; Loeb, L.A. *Nature (London)* **1974**, *252*, 414.
129. Loveless, A.; Hampton, C.L. *Mutat. Res.* **1969**, *7*, 1.
130. Smith, B.J. *Chem.-Biol. Interact.* **1977**, *16*, 275.
131. Lawley, P.D.; Orr, D.J.; Shah, S.A.; Farmer, P.B.; Jarman, M. *Biochem. J.* **1973**, *135*, 193.
132. Kadlubar, F.F. *Chem.-Biol. Interact.* **1980**, *31*, 255.
133. Kadlubar, F.F.; Melchior, W.B., Jr.; Flammang, T.J.; Gagliano, A.G.; Yoshida, H.; Geacintor, N.W. *Cancer Res.* **1981**, *41*, 2168.
134. Scherer, E.; Van der Laken, C.J.; Gwinner, L.M.; Laib, R.J.; Emmelot, P. *Carcinogenesis* **1981**, *2*, 671.
135. Lawley, P.D.; Brookes, P. *Nature (London)* **1962**, *192*, 1081.
136. Koch, A.L.; Miller, C. *J. Theor. Biol.* **1965**, *8*, 71.
137. Segal, A.; Maté, U.; Solomon, J.J.; Van Duuren, B.L. *Proc. Am. Assoc. Cancer Res.* **1981**, *22*, 84.
138. Dipple, A.; Brookes, P.; Mackintosh, D.S.; Rayman, M.P. *Biochemistry* **1971**, *10*, 4323.
139. Osborne, M.R. *Trends Biochem. Sci. (Pers. Ed.)* **1979**, *4*, 213.
140. Moschel, R.C.; Hudgins, W.R.; Dipple, A. *J. Am. Chem. Soc.* **1981**, in press.
141. Timmis, G.M. *Biochem. Pharmacol.* **1960**, *4*, 49.
142. Miller, C.T.; Lawley, P.D.; Shah, S.A. *Biochem. J.* **1973**, *136*, 389.
143. O'Connor, P.J.; Saffhill, R. *Chem.-Biol. Interact.* **1979**, *26*, 91.
144. Pegg, A.E.; Swann, P.F. *Biochim. Biophys. Acta* **1979**, *565*, 241.
145. Saffhill, R.; Fox, M. *Carcinogenesis* **1980**, *1*, 487.
146. Craddock, V.M. *Chem.-Biol. Interact.* **1981**, *35*, 139.
147. Trainin, M.; Kaye, A.M.; Berenblum, I. *Biochem. Pharmacol.* **1964**, *13*, 263.
148. Tong, W.P.; Ludlum, D.B. *Proc. Am. Assoc. Cancer Res.* **1981**, *22*, 117.
149. Coulondre, C.; Miller, J.H. *J. Mol. Biol.* **1977**, *117*, 577.
150. Witkin, E. *Bacteriol. Rev.* **1976**, *40*, 869.
151. Lawley, P.D.; Thatcher, C.J. *Biochem. J.* **1970**, *116*, 693.
152. McGhee, J.D.; Felsenfeld, G. *Proc. Natl. Acad. Sci. U.S.A.* **1979**, *76*, 2133.
153. Warren, W.; Lawley, P.D. *Carcinogenesis* **1980**, *1*, 67.
154. Jeggo, P. *J. Bacteriol.* **1979**, *139*, 783.
155. Cairns, J. *Nature (London)* **1980**, *286*, 176.
156. Friedrich, U.; Coffino, P. *Proc. Natl. Acad. Sci. U.S.A.* **1977**, *74*, 679.
157. Craddock, V.M. "Liver Cell Cancer"; Cameron, H.M.; Linsell, D.A.; Warwick, G.P., Eds.; Elsevier: Amsterdam, 1976; Chap. 8.
158. Kleihues, P.; Cooper, H.K.; Buecheler, J. "Primary Liver Tumors"; Remmer, H.; Bolt, H.M.; Bannasch, P.; Popper, H., Eds.; MTP: Lancaster, 1978; pp. 313–26.
159. Margison, G.P.; O'Connor, P.J. "Chemical Carcinogens and DNA"; Grover, P.L., Ed.; CRC: Boca Raton, FL, 1979; Vol. 1, Chap. 5.

160. O'Connor, P.J.; Capps, M.J.; Craig, A.W. *Br. J. Cancer* **1973**, *27*, 153.
161. Medcalf, A.S.C.; Lawley, P.D. *Nature (London)* **1981**, *289*, 796.
162. Harris, G.; Lawley, P.D.; Olsen, I. *Carcinogenesis* **1981**, *2*, 403.
163. Margison, G.P.; Swindell, J.A.; Ockey, C.H.; Craig, A.W. *Carcinogenesis* **1980**, *1*, 91.
164. Craddock, V.M. *JNCI, J. Natl. Cancer Inst.* **1971**, *47*, 889.
165. Craddock, V.M.; Frei, J.V. *Br. J. Cancer* **1974**, *30*, 503.
166. Craddock, V.M. *Chem.-Biol. Interact.* **1975**, *10*, 313, 323.
167. Kleihues, P.; Bamborschke, S.; Doerjer, G. *Carcinogenesis* **1980**, *1*, 111.
168. Bogden, J.M.; Eastman, A.; Bresnick, E. *Nucleic Acids Res.* **1981**, *9*, 3089.
169. Robins, P.; Cairns, J. *Nature (London)* **1980**, *280*, 74.
170. Pegg, A.E.; Perry, W.; Bennett, R.A. *Biochem. J.* **1981**, *197*, 195.
171. Kleihues, P.; Margison, G.P. *JNCI, J. Natl. Cancer Inst.* **1974**, *53*, 1839.
172. Nicoll, J.W.; Swann, P.F.; Pegg, A.E. *Nature (London)* **1975**, *254*, 261.
173. Swann, P.F.; Mace, R. *Chem.-Biol. Interact.* **1980**, *31*, 235.
174. Margison, G.P. *Carcinogenesis* **1981**, *2*, 431.
175. Bodell, W.J.; Singer, B.; Thomas, G.H.; Cleaver, J.E. *Nucleic Acids Res.* **1979**, *6*, 2819.
176. Steward, A.P.; Scherer, E.; Emmelot, P. *FEBS Lett.* **1979**, *100*, 191.
177. Lawley, P.D.; Warren, W. *Chem.-Biol. Interact.* **1976**, *12*, 211.
178. Olson, A.O.; McCalla, D.R. *Biochim. Biophys. Acta* **1969**, *186*, 229.
179. Kirtikar, D.M.; Goldthwait, D.A. *Proc. Natl. Acad. Sci. U.S.A.* **1974**, *71*, 2022.
180. Riazuddin, S.; Lindahl, T. *Biochemistry* **1978**, *17*, 2110.
181. Karran, P.; Lindahl, T.; Øfsteng, I.; Evensen, G.B.; Seeberg, E. *J. Mol. Biol.* **1980**, *140*, 101.
182. Laval, J. *Nature (London)* **1977**, *269*, 829.
183. Brent, T.P. *Biochemistry* **1979**, *18*, 911.
184. Singer, B.; Brent, T.P. *Proc. Natl. Acad. Sci. U.S.A.* **1981**, *78*, 856.
185. Margison, G.P.; Pegg, A.E. *Proc. Natl. Acad. Sci. U.S.A.* **1981**, *78*, 861.
186. Shackleton, J.; Warren, W.; Roberts, J.J. *Eur. J. Biochem.* **1979**, *97*, 425.
187. Laval, J.; Pierre, J.; Laval, F. *Proc. Natl. Acad. Sci. U.S.A.* **1981**, *78*, 852.
188. Shooter, K.V.; Howse, R.; Merrifield, R.K. *Biochem. J.* **1974**, *137*, 313.
189. Shooter, K.V. *Nature (London)* **1978**, *274*, 612.
190. Shooter, K.V.; Merrifield, R.K. *Anal. Biochem.* **1980**, *103*, 110.
191. Radman, M.; Caillet-Fauquet, P.; Defais, M.; Villani, G. "Screening Tests in Chemical Carcinogenesis"; Montesano, R.; Bartsch, H.; Tomatis, L., Eds.; IARC: Lyon, 1976; pp. 537–48.
192. Witkin, E.M. *Proc. Natl. Acad. Sci. U.S.A.* **1974**, *71*, 1930.
193. Cleaver, J.E. *Mutat. Res.* **1977**, *44*, 291.
194. McCormick, J.J.; Maher, V.M. "DNA Repair and Mutagenesis in Eukaryotes"; Generoso, W.M.; Shelby, M.D.; de Serres, F.J., Eds.; Plenum: New York, 1980; Chap. 20.
195. Cleaver, J.E. *Proc. Natl. Acad. Sci. U.S.A.*. **1969**, *63*, 428.
196. Robbins, J.H.; Kraemer, K.H.; Lutzner, M.A. *Ann. Intern. Med.* **1974**, *80*, 221.
197. German, J. "DNA Repair and Mutagenesis in Eukaryotes"; Generoso, W.M.; Shelby, M.D.; de Serres, F.J., Eds.; Plenum: New York, 1980; Chap. 30.
198. Gilbert, R.M.; Rowland, S.; Davison, C.L.; Papirmeister, B. *Mutat. Res.* **1975**, *28*, 257.
199. Lawley, P.D.; Brookes, P. *Nature (London)* **1965**, *206*, 480.
200. Reid, B.D.; Walker, I.G. *Biochim. Biophys. Acta* **1969**, *179*, 179.
201. Roberts, J.J.; Brent, T.P.; Crathorn, A.R. *Eur. J. Cancer* **1971**, *7*, 515.
202. Barrows, L.R.; Shank, R.C. *Proc. Am. Assoc. Cancer Res.* **1980**, *21*, 110.
203. Becker, R.A.; Barrows, L.R.; Shank, R.C. *Carcinogenesis* **1981**, *2*, 1181.
204. Biancifiori, C.; Ribacchi, R. *Nature (London)* **1962**, *194*, 488.

205. Severi, L.; Biancifiori, C. *JNCI, J. Natl. Cancer Inst.* **1968**, *41*, 331.
206. Holliday, R. *Br. J. Cancer* **1979**, *40*, 513.
207. Holliday, R.; Pugh, J.E. *Science (Washington, D.C.)* **1975**, *187*, 226.
208. Razin, A.; Riggs, A.D. *Science (Washington, D.C.)* **1980**, *210*, 604.
209. Venitt, S. *Br. Med. Bull.* **1980**, *36*, 57.
210. Doll, R.; Peto, R. *JNCI, J. Natl. Cancer Inst.* **1981**, *66*, 1191.
211. "Long- and Short-Term Screening Assays for Carcinogens: A Critical Appraisal"; IARC: Lyon, 1980.
212. Bartsch, H.; Malaveille, C.; Camus, A.M.; Martel-Planche, G.; Brun, G.; Hautefeuille, A.; Sabadie, N.; Barbin, A.; Kuroki, T.; Drevon, C.; Piccoli, C.; Montesano, R. "Molecular and Cellular Aspects of Carcinogen Screening Tests"; Montesano, R.; Bartsch, H.; Tomatis, L., Eds.; IARC: Lyon, 1980; pp. 179–241.
213. Fahmy, O.G.; Fahmy, M.J. *Cancer Res.* **1970**, *30*, 195.
214. *Ibid.* **1972**, *32*, 550.
215. Shimkin, M.B.; Weisburger, J.H.; Weisburger, E.K.; Gubareff, N.; Suntzeff, V. *JNCI, J. Natl. Cancer Inst.* **1966**, *36*, 915.
216. Shimkin, M.B. *Adv. Cancer Res.* **1955**, *3*, 223.
217. Lutz, W.K. *Mutat. Res.* **1979**, *65*, 289.
218. Swann, P.F.; Magee, P.N. *Biochem. J.* **1968**, *110*, 39.
219. Frei, J.V.; Lawley, P.D. *Chem.-Biol. Interact.* **1976**, *13*, 215.
220. Swann, P.F.; Magee, P.N. *Biochem. J.* **1971**, *125*, 841.
221. Swann, P.F.; Pegg, A.E.; Hawks, A.; Farber, E.; Magee, P.N. *Biochem. J.* **1971**, *123*, 175.
222. Pound, A.W.; Franke, F.; Lawson, T.A. *Chem.-Biol. Interact.* **1976**, *14*, 149.
223. Dahl, G.A.; Miller, J.A.; Miller, E.C. *Cancer Res.* **1978**, *38*, 3793.
224. Harbers, E.; Warnecke, P.; Hollandt, H.; Kruse, K. *Z. Krebsforsch.* **1977**, *88*, 237.
225. Brookes, P.; Lawley, P.D. "Isotopes in Experimental Pharmacology"; Roth, L.J., Ed.; Univ. of Chicago: Chicago, 1965; Chap. 31.
226. Trams, E.G.; Nadkarni, M.V.; Smith, P.K. *Cancer Res.* **1961**, *21*, 560.
227. Wheeler, G.P.; Skipper, H.E. *Arch. Biochem. Biophys.* **1957**, *72*, 465.
228. Hill, D.L.; Shih, T.W.; Johnston, T.P.; Struck, R.F. *Cancer Res.* **1978**, *38*, 2438.
229. Bolt, H.M.; Filser, J.G.; Laib, R.J.; Ottenwälder, H. *Arch. Toxicol. Suppl. 3* **1980**, 129.
230. Jarman, M.; Foster, A.B. *Adv. Pharmacol. Ther. Proc. Int. Congr. Pharmacol., 7th* **1978**, *7*, 225.
231. Farmer, P.D.; Cox, P.J.; Jarman, M. In "Characterization and Treatment of Human Tumors"; Davis, W.; Harrap, K.R., Eds.; *Int. Congr. Ser.—Excerpta Med.* **1978**, *420*, 281.
232. Roboz, J. *Adv. Cancer Res.* **1978**, *27*, 201.
233. Szybalski, W.; Iyer, V.N. *Fed. Proc. Fed. Am. Soc. Exp. Biol.* **1964**, *23*, 946.
234. Murakami, H. *J. Theor. Biol.* **1966**, *10*, 236.
235. Cerutti, P.A. In "DNA Repair: A Laboratory Manual of Research Procedures"; Friedberg, E.C.; Hanawalt, P.C., Eds.; Dekker: New York, 1981; Vol. 1, Part A, Chap. 6.
236. Jollow, D.J. *Arch. Toxicol. Suppl. 3* **1980**, 95.
237. Lawley, P.D.; Brookes, P. *Biochem. J.* **1968**, *109*, 433.
238. Swann, P.F. *Biochem. J.* **1968**, *110*, 49.
239. Trams, E.G.; Nadkarni, M.V. *Cancer Res.* **1956**, *16*, 1059.
240. Cobb, L.M. *Int. J. Cancer* **1966**, *1*, 329.
241. Chang, M.J.W.; Webb, T.E.; Koestner, A. *Cancer Lett.* **1979**, *6*, 123.
242. Wunderlich, V.; Schütt, M.; Böttger, M.; Graffi, A. *Biochem. J.* **1970**, *118*, 99.
243. Hemminki, K. *Chem.-Biol. Interact.* **1979**, *28*, 269.
244. Hemminki, K. *Carcinogenesis* **1980**, *1*, 311.

245. Herron, D.C.; Shank, R.C. *Anal. Biochem.* **1979**, *100*, 58.
246. Herron, D.C.; Shank, R.C. *Cancer Res.* **1980**, *40*, 3116.
247. Brookes, P.; Lawley, P.D. *J. Chem. Soc.* **1961**, 3923.
248. Tong, W.P.; Ludlum, D.B. *Biochim. Biophys. Acta* **1980**, *608*, 174.
249. Swenson, D.H.; Lin, J.K.; Miller, E.C.; Miller, J.A. *Cancer Res.* **1977**, *37*, 172.
250. Croy, J.G.; Essigmann, J.M.; Reinhold, V.N.; Wogan, G.N. *Proc. Natl. Acad. Sci. U.S.A.* **1978**, *75*, 1745.
251. "The Evaluation of Carcinogenic Risk of Chemicals to Humans," IARC Monograph, IARC: Lyon, 1974, 1979; Vol. 7, p. 291; Vol. 19, p. 377.
252. Plotnick, H.B. *J. Am. Med. Assoc.* **1978**, *239*, 1609.
253. Rannug, U. *Mutat. Res.* **1980**, *76*, 269.
254. Skibba, J.L.; Bryan, G.T. *Toxicol. Appl. Pharmacol.* **1971**, *18*, 707.
255. Löfroth, G.; Osterman-Golkar, S.; Wennerberg, R. *Experientia* **1974**, *15*, 641.
256. Shaikh, B.; Huang, S.-K.S.; Pontzer, N.J. *Chem.-Biol. Interact.* **1980**, *30*, 253.
257. Chu, B.C.F.; Lawley, P.D. *Chem.-Biol. Interact.* **1974**, *8*, 65.
258. *Ibid.* **1975**, *10*, 333.
259. *Ibid.* **1975**, *10*, 407.
260. Kohn, K.W.; Ewig, R.A.G.; Erickson, L.C.; Zwelling, L.A. In "DNA Repair, a Laboratory Manual of Research Procedures"; Friedberg, E.C.; Hanawalt, P.C., Eds.; Dekker: New York, 1981; Vol. 1, Part B, Chap. 29.
261. Erickson, L.C.; Osieka, R.; Sharkey, N.A.; Kohn, K.W. *Anal. Biochem.* **1980**, *106*, 169.
262. Calleman, C.J.; Ehrenberg, L.; Jansson, B.; Osterman-Golkar, S.; Segerbäck, D.; Svensson, K.; Wachtmeister, C.A. *J. Environ. Pathol. Toxicol.* **1978**, *2*, 427.
263. Ehrenberg, L.; Osterman-Golkar, S. *Teratogen. Carcinogen. Mutagen.* **1980**, *1*, 105.
264. Ehrenberg, L.; Hussain, S. *Mutat. Res.* **1981**, *86*, 1.
265. Bailey, E.; Connors, T.A.; Farmer, P.B.; Gorf, S.M.; Rickard, J. *Cancer Res.* **1981**, *41*, 2514.
266. Crump, K.S.; Hoel, D.G.; Langley, C.H.; Peto, R. *Cancer Res.* **1976**, *36*, 2973.
267. Ramsey, J.C.; Park, C.N.; Ott, M.; Gehring, P.J. *Toxicol. Appl. Pharmacol.* **1979**, *47*, 411.
268. Moolgavkar, S.H.; Day, N.E.; Stevens, R.G. *J. Natl. Cancer Inst.* **1980**, *65*, 559.
269. Moolgavkar, S.H.; Knudson, A.G., Jr. *JNCI, J. Natl. Cancer Inst.* **1981**, *66*, 1037.
270. Nordling, C.O. *Br. J. Cancer* **1953**, *7*, 68.
271. Armitage, P.; Doll, R. *Br. J. Cancer* **1957**, *11*, 161.
272. Knudson, A.G., Jr.; Hethcote, H.W.; Brown, B.W. *Proc. Natl. Acad. Sci. U.S.A.* **1975**, *72*, 5116.
273. Frei, J.V.; Lawley, P.D. *JNCI, J. Natl. Cancer Inst.* **1980**, *64*, 845.
274. Mottram, J.C. *J. Pathol. Bacteriol.* **1944**, *56*, 181.
275. *Ibid.* **1944**, *56*, 391.
276. Berenblum, I.; Shubik, P. *Br. J. Cancer* **1947**, *1*, 379.
277. *Ibid.* **1949**, *3*, 109.
278. Mottram, J.C. *Br. J. Exp. Pathol.* **1945**, *26*, 1.
279. Argyris, T. *J. Invest. Dermatol.* **1980**, *75*, 360.
280. Emerit, I.; Cerutti, P. *Nature (London)* **1981**, *144*.
281. Roe, F.J.C.; Salaman, M.H. *Br. J. Cancer* **1955**, *9*, 177.
282. Salaman, M.H.; Roe, F.J.C. *Br. J. Cancer* **1956**, *10*, 363.
283. Waynforth, H.B.; Magee, P.N. *Gann Monogr. Cancer Res.* **1975**, *17*, 439.
284. Van Duuren, B.L.; Goldschmidt, B.M.; Katz, C.; Seidman, J.; Paul, J.S. *JNCI, J. Natl. Cancer Inst.* **1974**, *53*, 695.
285. Frei, J.V. *Carcinogenesis* **1980**, *1*, 721.
286. Steffen, D.; Bird, S.; Rowe, W.P.; Weinberg, R.A. *Proc. Natl. Acad. Sci. U.S.A.* **1979**, *76*, 4554.

287. Frei, J.V.; Maitra, S.C. *Chem.-Biol. Interact.* **1974**, *9*, 65.
288. Druckrey, H. *UICC Monograph No. 7*, Truhaut, R., Ed.; Springer–Verlag: Heidelberg, 1967; p. 60.
289. Port, R.; Schmähl, D.; Wahrendorf, J. *Oncology* **1976**, *33*, 66.
290. Druckrey, H.; Kruse, H.; Preussmann, R.: Ivankovic, S.; Landschütz, C. *Z. Krebsforsch.* **1970**, *74*, 241.
291. Grasso, P.; Golberg, L. *Food Cosmet. Toxicol.* **1966**, *4*, 269, 297.
292. Yuhas, J.M.; Walker, A.E. *Radiation Res.* **1973**, *54*, 261.
293. Frei, J.V. *Chem.-Biol. Interact.* **1971**, *3*, 117.
294. Goerttler, K.; Loehrke, H.; Schweizer, J.; Hesse, B. *Cancer Res.* **1980**, *40*, 155.
295. Parish, D.J.; Searle, C.E. *Br. J. Cancer* **1966**, *20*, 200, 206.
296. Case, R.A.M.; Lea, A.J. *Br. J. Prev. Soc. Med.* **1955**, *9*, 62.
297. Beebe, G.W. *JNCI, J. Natl. Cancer Inst.* **1960**, *25*, 1231.
298. Berg, J.W. "Morphology of Experimental Respiratory Carcinogenesis: Proceedings"; Nettesheim, P.; Hanna, M.G., Jr.; Deatherage, J.W., Jr., Eds.; DOE: Oak Ridge, TN, 1970; p. 93.
299. Druckrey, H.; Preussmann, R.; Nashed, N.; Ivankovic, S. *Z. Krebsforsch.* **1966**, *68*, 103.
300. Fishbein, L.; Flamm, W.G.; Falk, H.L. "Chemical Mutagens, Environmental Effects on Biological Systems"; Academic: New York, 1970; Chap. 7 and 8.
301. Fishbein, L. "Chromatography of Environmental Hazards, Carcinogens, Mutagens and Teratogens"; Elsevier: Amsterdam, 1972; Vol. 1.
302. Fishbein, L. "Potential Industrial Carcinogens and Mutagens"; *Stud. Environ. Sci.* Elsevier: Amsterdam, 1979, Vol. 4.
303. "The Evaluation of Carcinogenic Risk of Chemicals to Humans"; IARC Monograph, IARC: Lyon, 1979; Vol. 20, p. 458.
304. Vogel, E.; Chandler, J.L.R. Experientia **1974**, *30*, 621.
305. "The Evaluation of Carcinogenesis Risk of Chemicals to Humans"; IARC Monograph, IARC: Lyon, 1979; Vol. 20, pp. 83–96.
306. Lawley, P.D.; Shah, J.A.; Orr, D.J. *Chem.-Biol. Interact.* **1974**, *8*, 171.
307. Yamauchi, K.; Tanabe, T.; Kinoshita, M. *J. Org. Chem.* **1976**, *41*, 3691.
308. Wild, D. *Mutat. Res.* **1975**, *32*, 133.
309. Wennerberg, R.; Löfroth, G. *Chem.-Biol. Interact.* **1974**, *8*, 339.
310. Dedek, W.; Lohs, K.; Fischer, G.W.; Schmidt, R. *Pestic. Biochem. Physiol.* **1976**, *6*, 101.
311. Wooder, M.F.; Wright, A.S.; King, L.J. *Chem.-Biol. Interact.* **1977**, *19*, 25.
312. Bridges, B.A.; Mottershead, R.P.; Green, M.H.L.; Gray, W.J.H. *Mutat. Res.* **1973**, *19*, 295.
313. Dedek, W.; Scheufler, H.; Fischer, G.W. *Arch. Toxicol.* **1975**, *33*, 163.
314. Perocco, P.; Fini, A. *Tumori* **1980**, *66*, 425.
315. Gibel, W.; Lohs, K.; Wildner, G.P.; Ziebarth, D. *Arch. Geschwulstforsch.* **1971**, *37*, 303.
316. Gibel, W.; Lohs, K.; Wildner, G.P.; Ziebarth, D.; Stieglitz, R. *Arch. Geschwulstforsch.* **1973**, *41*, 311.
317. NIH Publication No. 80–453 U.S. Dept.of Health, Education, and Welfare, Public Health Service, National Inst. of Health, 1978, pp. 238–43.
318. Blum, A.; Ames, B.N. *Science* (*Washington, D.C.*) **1977**, *195*, 17.
319. Prival, M.J.; McCoy, E.C.; Gutter, B.; Rosenkranz, H.S. *Science* (*Washington, D.C.*) **1977**, *195*, 76.
320. Van Duuren, B.L.; Loewengart, G.; Seidman, I.; Smith, A.C.; Melchionne, S. *Cancer Res.* **1978**, *38*, 3236.
321. "The Evaluation of Carcinogenic Risk of Chemicals to Humans"; IARC Monograph, IARC: Lyon, **1979**; Vol. 20, pp. 575–88.

322. Norppa, H.; Sorsa, M.; Pfäffli, P.; Vainio, H. *Carcinogenesis* **1980**, *1*, 357.
323. Dunkelberg, H. *Br. J. Cancer* **1979**, *39*, 588.
324. Maltoni, C.; Failla, G.; Kassapidis, G. *Med. Lav.* **1979**, *5*, 358.
325. *IARC Monograph* "The Evaluation of Carcinogenic Risk of Chemicals to Humans"; IARC: Lyon, **1979**; Vol. 19, pp. 278–80.
326. Kew, M.C. "Primary Liver Tumors"; Remmer, H.; Bolt, H.M.; Bannasch, P.; Popper, H., Eds.; MTP: Lancaster, 1978; Chap. 14.
327. Garner, R.C.; Martin, C.N. "Chemical Carcinogens and DNA"; Grover, P.L., Ed.; CRC: Boca Raton, FL, 1979; Vol. 1, Chap. 7.
328. Dickens, F. "UICC Monograph No. 7" Truhaut, R., Ed.; Springer–Verlag: Berlin, 1967; p. 144.
329. Dickens, F. *Br. Med. Bull.* **1964**, *20*, 96.
330. Dickens, F. *Annu. Symp. Fundam. Cancer Res. [Proc.], 20th* **1967**, 447.
331. Dickens, F.; Jones, H.E.H.; Waynforth, H.B. *Br. J. Cancer* **1966**, *20*, 134.
332. *Ibid.* **1968**, *22*, 762.
333. Boyland, E.; Down, W.H. *Eur. J. Cancer* **1971**, *7*, 495.
334. Boyland, E.; Nery, R. *Biochem. J.* **1969**, *113*, 123.
335. Epstein, S. S. "The Politics of Cancer"; Sierra: San Francisco, 1978.
336. Epstein, S.S.; Andrea, J.; Jaffe, H.; Joshi, S.; Falk, H.; Mantel, N. *Nature (London)* **1967**, *215*, 1388.
337. Bridges, B.A.; Mottershead, R.P.; Rothwell, M.A.; Green, M.A.; Green, M.H.L. *Chem.-Biol. Interact.* **1972**, *5*, 77.
338. Peto, R. *Nature (London)* **1980**, *284*, 297.
339. Epstein, S.S.; Swartz, J.B. *Nature (London)* **1981**, *289*, 127.
340. Paterson, M.C.; Smith, P.J. *Annu. Rev. Genet.* **1979**, *13*, 291.
341. Swift, M. *Nature (London)* **1971**, *230*, 370.
342. Berg, K. "Genetic Damage in Man Caused by Environmental Agents"; Berg, K., Ed.; Academic: New York, 1979. pp. 1–24.
343. Thiess, A.M.; Hey, W.; Zeller, H. *Zbl. Arbeits Med.* **1973**, *23*, 97.
344. Sakabe, H. *Ind. Health* **1973**, *11*, 145.
345. Tou, J.C.; Westover, L.B.; Sonnabend, L.F. *J. Phys. Chem.* **1974**, *78*, 1096.
346. Van Duuren, B.L.; Katz, C.; Goldschmidt, B.M.; Frenkel, K.; Sivak, A. *JNCI, J. Natl. Cancer Inst.* **1972**, *48*, 1431.
347. Swenberg, J.A.; Kerns, W.D.; Mitchell, R.I.; Gralla, E.J.; Pavkov, K.L. *Cancer Res.* **1980**, *40*, 3398.
348. Kuschner, M.; Laskin, S.; Drew, R.T.; Capiello, V.; Nelson, N. *Arch. Environ. Health* **1975**, *30*, 73.
349. Burdette, W.J. *Cancer Res.* **1955**, *15*, 201.
350. Feldman, M.Y. *Prog. Nucleic Acid Res. Mol. Biol.* **1975**, *13*, 1.
351. Chan, Y.F.M.; Crane, L.E.; Lange, P.; Shapiro, R. *Biochemistry* **1980**, *19*, 5525.
352. Ross, W.E.; Shipley, N. *Mutat. Res.* **1980**, *79*, 277.
353. Zapp, J.A., Jr. *Science (Washington, D.C.)* **1975**, *190*, 422.
354. Jones, A.R.; Jackson, H. *Biochem. Pharmacol.* **1968**, *17*, 2247.
355. Edwards, K.; Jackson, H.; Jones, A.R. *Biochem. Pharmacol.* **1970**, *19*, 1791.
356. Sieber, S.M.; Adamson, R.H. *Adv. Cancer Res.* **1975**, *22*, 57.
357. Harris, C.C. *Cancer* **1976**, *37*, 1014.
358. Hoover, R. "Origins of Human Cancer: Cold Spring Harbor Conferences on Cell Proliferation"; Hiatt, H.H.; Watson, J.D.; Winsten, J.A., Eds.; Cold Spring Harbor: Cold Spring Harbor, N.Y., 1977; pp. 368–79.
359. Adamson, R.H.; Sieber, S.M. *Ibid.* pp. 429–43.
360. Editorial *Lancet* **1977** *i*, 519.
361. Auclerc, G.; Jacquillat, C.; Auclerc, M.F.; Weil, M.; Bernard, J. *Cancer* **1979**, *44*, 2017.

362. Geary, C.G. *Br. J. Hosp. Med.* **1980**, 538.
363. Haddow, A.; Harris, R.J.C.; Kon, G.A.R.; Roe, E.M.F. *Philos. Trans. Soc. London, Ser. A* **1948**, *241*, 167.
364. Videbaek, A. *Acta Med. Scand.* **1964**, *176*, 45.
365. Thiede, T.; Chievitz, E.; Christensen, B.C. *Acta Med. Scand.* **1964**, *175*, 721.
366. Case, R.A.M.; Hosker, M.E.; McDonald, D.B.; Pearson, J.T. *Br.J. Ind. Med.* **1954**, *11*, 75.
367. Boyland, E. UICC Monograph No. 7; Truhaut, R., Ed.; Springer–Verlag: Berlin, 1967; p. 204.
368. Boyland, E. *Prog. Exp. Tumor Res.* **1969**, *11*, 222.
369. Hobbs, J.R. *Br. Med. J.* **1971**, *2*, 67.
370. Lambert, B.; Ringborg, U.; Harper, E.; Lindblad, A. *Cancer Treat. Rep.* **1978**, *62*, 1413.
371. Waksvik, H.; Klepp, O.; Brøgger, A. *Cancer Treat. Rep.* **1981**.
372. Siebert, D.; Simon, V. *Mutat. Res.* **1973**, *19*, 65.
373. Falck, K.; Gröhn, P.; Sorsa, M.; Vainio, H.; Heinonen, E.; Holsti, L.R. *Lancet* **1979**, *i*, 1250.
374. Tinney, W.S.; Polley, H.F.; Hall, B.E.; Griffen, H.Z. *Mayo Clin. Proc.* **1945**, *20*, 49.
375. Berk, P.D.; Golberg, J.D.; Silverstein, M.N.; Weinfeld, A.; Donovan, P.B.; Ellis, J.T.; Landaw, S.A.; Laszlo, J.; Najean, Y.; Pisciotta, A.V.; Wasserman, L.R. *N. Engl. J. Med.* **1981**, *304*, 441.
376. Pedersen-Bjergaard, J.; Nissen, N.I.; Sørensen, H.M.; Hou-Jensen, K.; Larsen, M.S.; Ernst, P.; Ersbøl, J.; Knudtzon, S.; Rose, C. *Cancer* **1980**, *45*, 19.
377. Stott, H.; Fox, W.; Girling, D.J.; Stephens, R.J.; Galton, D.A.G. *Br. Med. J.* **1977**, *2*, 1513.
378. Kinlen, L.J.; Sheil, A.G.R.; Peto, J.; Doll, R. *Br. Med. J.* **1979**, *2*, 1461.
379. Penn, I. "Strategies in Clinical Hematology" Gross, R.; Hellriegel, K.P., Eds.; Springer–Verlag: New York, 1979.
380. Conklin, J.W.; Upton, A.C.; Christenberry, K.W. *Cancer Res.* **1965**, *25*, 20.
381. Upton, A.C.; Jenkins, V. K.; Walburg, H.E., Jr.; Tyndall, R.L.; Conklin, W.L.; Wald, N. *Natl. Cancer Inst. Monogr.* **1966**, *22*, 329.
382. Louie, S.; Schwartz, R.S. *Semin. Hematol.* **1978**, *15*, 117.
383. Casey, T.P. *Blood* **1968**, *31*, 396.
384. Thomas, L. "Cellular and Humoral Aspects of Hypersensitive States"; Lawrence, H.W., Ed.; Hoeber-Harper: New York, 1961; p. 529.
385. Burnet, F.M. *Transplant Rev.* **1971**, *7*, 3.
386. Li, F.P.; Fraumeni, J.F.; Mantel, N.; Miller, R.W. *JNCI, J. Natl. Cancer Inst.* **1969**, *43*, 1159.
387. Rowley, J.D.; Golomb, H.M.; Vardiman, J. *Blood* **1977**, *50*, 759.
388. Yunis, J.J.; Bloomfield, C.S.; Ensrud, K. *N. Engl. J. Med.* **1981**, *305*, 135.
389. Pedersen-Bjergaard, J.; Philip, P. *Ibid.* 342.
390. Berk, P.D.; Wasserman, L.R. *Ibid.* 343.
391. Shimkin, M.R. *Cancer* **1954**, *7*, 410.
392. Zweifel, J.R. *JNCI, J. Natl. Cancer Inst.* **1966**, *36*, 937.
393. Graffi, A.; Hoffmann, F.; Schütt, M. *Nature* (*London*) **1967**, *214*, 611.
394. Clayson, D.B. "Chemical Carcinogenesis"; Churchill: London, 1962.
395. Walpole, A.L.; Roberts, D.C.; Rose, F.L.; Hendry, J.A.; Homer, R.F. *Br. J. Pharmacol.* **1954**, *9*, 306.
396. Carter, R.L. "Metabolic Aspects of Food Safety"; Roe, F.J.C., Ed.; Blackwells: Oxford, 1970; p. 569.
397. Roe, F.J.C.; Tucker, M.J. *Int. Congr. Ser.—Excerpta Med.* Duncan, W.A.; Ed.; **1974**, *311*, 171.

398. Kunjuraman, T.N.; O'Neill, B.; Kouri, R.E. In "Genetic Differences in Chemical Carcinogenesis"; Kouri, R.E., Ed.; CRC: Boca Raton, 1980; Chap. 4.
399. McDonald, G.O. "Dissemination of Cancer, Prevention and Therapy"; Cole, W.H.; McDonald, G.O.; Roberts, S.S.; Southwick, H.W., Eds.; Appleton Century Crofts, Inc. New York, 1961.
400. Colburn, N.H.; Boutwell, R.K. *Cancer Res.* **1968**, *28*, 642.
401. *Ibid.* 653.
402. Van Duuren, B.L. *Prog. Exp. Tumor Res.* **1969**, *11*, 31.
403. Van Duuren, B.L. *Ann. N.Y. Acad. Sci.* **1969**, *163*, 633.
404. Slaga, T.J.; Bowden, G.T.; Shapas, B.G.; Boutwell, R.K. *Cancer Res.* **1973**, *33*, 769.
405. Walters, M.A.; Roe, F.J.C.; Mitchley, B.C.V.; Walsh, A. *Br. J. Cancer* **1967**, *21*, 367.
406. Chernozemski, I.N.; Warwick, G.P. *JNCI, J. Natl. Cancer Inst.* **1970**, *45*, 709.
407. Druckrey, H.; Kruse, H.; Preussmann, R.; Ivankovic, S.; Landschütz, C.; Gimmy, J. *Z. Krebsforsch.* **1970**, *75*, 69.
408. Schneider, J.; Warzot, R.; Schreiber, D.; Heiderstadt, R. *Exp. Pathol.* **1978**, *16*, 157.
409. Laskin, S.; Sellakumar, A.R.; Kuschner, M.; Nelson, N.; La Mendola, S.; Rusch, G.M.; Katz, G.V.; Dulak, N.C.; Albert, R.E. *JNCI, J. Natl. Cancer Inst.* **1980**, *65*, 751.
410. Laskin, S.; Kuschner, M.; Katz, G.V. *J. Environ. Pathol. Toxicol.* **1981** in press.
411. Laskin, S.; Kuschner, J.; Drew, R.T.; Cappiello, V.P.; Nelson, N. *Arch. Environ. Health* **1971**, *23*, 135.
412. "The Evaluation of Carcinogenic Risk of Chemicals to Humans"; IARC Monograph, IARC: Lyon, 1979; Vol. 20, p. 401.
413. *Ibid.* p. 371.
414. Rocchi, P.; Prodi, G.; Grilli, S.; Ferreri, A.M. *Int. J. Cancer* **1973**, *11*, 419.
415. "The Evaluation of Carcinogenic Risk of Chemicals to Humans"; IARC Monograph, IARC: Lyon, 1979; Vol. 19, p. 377.
416. Irish, D.D.; Adams, E.M.; Spencer, H.C.; Rowe, V.K. *J. Ind. Hyg. Toxicol.* **1940**, *22*, 218.
417. Buckell, M. *Br. J. Ind. Med.* **1950**, *7*, 122.
418. Muller, E. *Arch. Hyg. Bakteriol.* **1968**, *152*, 23.
419. Theiss, J.C.; Stoner, G.D.; Shimkin, M.B.; Weisburger, E.K. *Cancer Res.* **1977**, *37*, 2717
420. Eschenbrenner, A.B.; Miller, E. *JNCI, J. Natl. Cancer Inst.* **1945**, *5*, 251.
421. Deringer, M.K.; Dunn, T.B.; Heston, W.E. *Proc. Soc. Exp. Biol. Med.* **1953**, 83, 474.
422. Roe, F.J.C.; Carter, R.L.; Mitchley, B.C.V. *Annu. Rep., Cancer Res. Campaign* **1968**, *46*, 13.
423. "Report on Carcinogenesis Bioassay of Chloroform", DHEW/PUB/NIH–76–1279, NCI, Bethesda, MD, 1976.
424. Eschenbrenner, A.B. *JNCI, J. Natl. Cancer Inst.* **1944**, *4*, 385.
425. Weisburger, E.K. *EHP, Environ. Health Perspect.* **1977**, *21*, 7.
426. Ambrose, A.M. *Arch. Ind. Hyg.* **1950**, *2*, 591.
427. Rowe, V.K.; Spencer, H.C.; McCollister, D.D.; Hollingsworth, R.L.; Adams, E.M. *Arch. Ind. Hyg. Occup. Med.* **1952**, *6*, 158.
428. Olson, W.A.; Habermann, R.T.; Weisburger, E.K.; Ward, J.M.; Weisburger, J.H. *JNCI, J. Natl. Cancer Inst.* **1973**, *51*, 1993.
429. Van Duuren, B.L.; Goldschmidt, B.M.; Loewengart, G.; Smith, A.C.; Melchionne, S.; Seidman, I.; Roth, D. *JNCI, J. Natl. Cancer Inst.* **1979**, *63*, 1433.
430. Plotnick, H.B.; Weigel, W.W.; Richards, D.E.; Cheever, K.L.; Kommineni, C. "Ethylene Dichloride: Economic Importance and Potential Health Risks"; McElheny, V.K., Ed.; Cold Spring Harbor: Cold Spring Harbor, NY, 1980; Banbury Report No. 5, pp. 279–86.

431. Spencer, H.C.; Rowe, V.K.; Adams, E.M.; McCollister, D.D.; Irish, D.D. *Arch. Ind. Hyg. Occup. med.* **1951**, *4*, 482.
432. Fujii, K.; Epstein, S.S. *Toxicol. Appl. Pharmacol.* **1969**, *14*, 613.
433. Desoille, H.; Truffert, L.; Bourguignon, A.; Delavierre, P.; Philbert, M.; Girard-Wallon, C. *Arch. Mal. Prof. Med. Trav. Secur. Soc.* **1968**, *29*, 381.
434. Viola, P.L.; Bigotti, A.; Caputo, A. *Cancer Res.* **1971**, *31*, 516.
435. Heppel, L.A.; Neal, P.A.; Perrin, T.L.; Orr, M.L.; Porterfield, V.T. *J. Ind. Hyg. Toxicol.* **1944**, *26*, 8.
436. Maltoni, C.; Valgimigli, L.; Scarnato, C. "Ethylene Dichloride: Economic Importance and Potential Health Risks"; Cold Spring Harbor: Cold Spring Harbor, NY, 1980; Banbury Report No. 5, pp. 3–33.
437. Crabtree, H.B. *J. Pathol. Bacteriol.* **1940**, *51*, 303.
438. Searle, C.E. *Cancer Res.* **1966**, *26*, 12.
439. Tagashira, Y. *Gann* **1954**, *45*, 601.
440. Berenblum, I.; Haran-Ghera, N. *Cancer Res.* **1957**, *17*, 329.
441. Gwynn, R.H.; Salaman, M.H. *Br. J. Cancer* **1953**, *7*, 482.
442. Rusch, H.P.; Bosch, D.; Boutwell, R.K. *Acta Unio Int. Cancrum* **1955**, *11*, 699.
443. Dipple, A.; Slade, T.A. *Eur. J. Cancer* **1970**, *6*, 417.
444. Roe, F.J.C.; Dipple, A.; Mitchley, B.C.V. *Br. J. Cancer* **1972**, *26*, 461.
445. Dipple, A.; Slade, T.A. *Eur. J. Cancer* **1971**, *7*, 473.
446. Flesher, J.W.; Sydnor, K.L. *Cancer Res.* **1971**, *31*, 1951.
447. Dipple, A.; Moschel, R.C.; Hudgins, W.R. *Drug Metab. Rev.* **1981**, in press.
448. Peck, R.M.; Tan, T.K.; Peck, E.B. *Cancer Res.* **1976**, *36*, 2423.
449. Schlögel, F.A.; Bannasch, P. *Naunyn-Schmiedebergs Arch. Pharmakol.* **1970**, *266*, 441.
450a. Druckrey, H.; Gimmy, J.; Landschütz, C. *Z. Krebsforsch.* **1973**, *79*, 135.
450b. Wright, U. in "Toxicology in Occupational Medicine" Deichmann, W.B., Ed., Elsevier: Amsterdam, 1979, p. 93.
451. Clapp, N.K.; Craig, A.W.; Toya, R.E., Sr. *Science* (*Washington, D.C.*) **1968**, *161*, 913.
452. Frei, J.V. *Chem.-Biol. Interact.* **1971**, *7*, 436.
453. Alexander, P.; Connell, D.I. "Cellular Basis and Etiology of Late Somatic Effects of Ionizing Radiation" Harris, R.J.C., Ed.; Academic: London, 1962; p. 259.
454. Hruschesky, W.; Sampson, D.; Murphy, G.P. *JNCI, J. Natl. Cancer Inst.* **1972**, *49*, 1077.
455. Roe, F.J.C. *Cancer Res,* **1957**, *17*, 64.
456. Durham, W.F.; Gaines, T.B.; McCanley, R.H.; Sedlak, B.S.; Mattson, A.M.; Hayes, W.J. *Arch. Ind. Health* **1957**, *15*, 340.
457. Klotsche, C. *Z. Angew. Zool.* **1956**, 87.
458. "Bioassay of Dichlorvos for Possible Carcinogenicity," DHEW Publication NIH 77–810, 1977, US Govt. Printing Office,; Washington, D.C.
459. Du Bois, K.P.; Cotter, G.J. *Arch. Ind. Health* **1955**, *11*, 53.
460. Preussmann, R. *Food Cosmet. Toxicol.* **1968**, *6*, 576.
461. Gibel, W.; Lohs, K.; Wildner, G.P.; Ziebarth, D. *Arch. Geschwulstforsch.* **1971**, *37*, 303.
462. Teichmman, G.; Hauschild, F. *Arch. Geschwulstforsch.* **1978**, *48*, 301, 718.
463. Kodama, J.K.; Morse, M.S.; Anderson, H.H.; Dunlap, M.K.; Kine, C.H. *Arch. Ind. Hyg.* **1954**, *9*, 45.
464. Hazleton, I.W.; Holland, E.G. *Arch. Ind. Hyg.* **1953**, *8*, 399.
465. Barnes, J.M.; Denz, F.A. *J. Hyg.* **1951**, *49*, 430.
466. Barnes, J.M.; Denz, F.A. *Br. J. Ind. Med.* **1954**, *11*, 11.
467. Bembinski, T.J.; du Bois, K.P. *Arch. Ind. Health* **1958**, *17*, 192.
468. Glow, P.H. *Nature* (*London*) **1969**, *221*, 1265.
469. Treon, J.E.; Dutra, F.M.; Cleveland, F.P. *Arch. Ind. Hyg.* **1953**, *8*, 170.

470. Miller, E.C.; Miller, J.A. *Cancer Res.* **1960**, *20*, 133.
471. Salmon, W.D.; Copeland, D.H. *JNCI, J. Natl. Cancer Inst.* **1949**, *10*, 361.
472. Smith, C.C. *Arch. Ind. Hyg.* **1953**, *7*, 310.
473. Borzecella, J.F.; Larson, P.S.; Hennigar, G.R., Jr.; Huf, E.G.; Crawford, E.M.; Blackwell Smith, R., Jr. *Toxicol. Appl. Pharmacol.* **1964**, *6*, 29.
474. "The Evaluation of Carcinogenic Risk of Chemicals to Humans"; IARC Monograph, IARC: Lyon, 1979; Vol. 19, pp. 57–71.
475. Van Duuren, B.L.; Sivak, A.; Goldschmidt, B.M.; Katz, C.; Melchionne, S. *JNCI, J. Natl. Cancer Inst.* **1969**, *43*, 481.
476. Walpole, A.L. *Ann. N.Y. Acad. Sci.* **1958**, *68*, 750.
477. Reyniers, J.A.; Sacksteder, M.R.; Ashburn, L.L. *JNCI, J. Natl. Cancer Inst.* **1964**, *32*, 1045.
478. Dunkelberg, H. *Br. J. Cancer* **1982**, *46*, 924.
479. Weil, C.S.; Condra, N.; Haun, C.; Striegel, J.A. *Am. Ind. Hyg. Assoc. J.* **1963**, *24*, 305.
480. Van Duuren, B.L.; Langseth, L.; Goldschmidt, B.M.; Orris, L. *JNCI, J. Natl. Cancer Inst.* **1967**, *39*, 1217.
481. Van Duuren, B.L.; Langseth, L.; Orris, L.; Teebor, G.; Nelson, N.; Kuschner, M. *JNCI, J. Natl. Cancer Inst.* **1966**, *37*, 825.
482. Lawley, P.D.; Jarman, M. *Biochem. J.* **1972**, *126*, 893.
483. Sugiura, K.; Goto, M. *Chem.-Biol. Interact.* **1981**, *35*, 71.
484. "The Evaluation of Carcinogenic Risk of Chemicals to Man," IARC Monograph, IARC: Lyon, 1974; Vol. 5, pp. 125–56.
485. Walker, A.I.T.; Thorpe, E.; Stevenson, D.E. *Food Cosmet. Toxicol.* **1973**, *11*, 415.
486. Van Duuren, B.L.; Nelson, N.; Orris, L.; Palmes, E.D.; Schmitt, F.L. *JNCI, J. Natl. Cancer Inst.* **1963**, *31*, 41.
487. Treon, J.F.; Cleveland, F.P. *J. Agric. Food Chem.* **1955**, *3*, 402.
488. Ortega, P.; Wayland, J.H.; Durham, W.F. *Arch. Pathol.* **1957**, *64*, 614.
489. Speck, L.B.; Maaske, C.A. *Arch. Ind. Health* **1958**, *18*, 268.
490. Van Duuren, B.L.; Melchionne, S.; Blair, R.; Goldschmidt, B.M.: Katz, C. *JNCI, J. Natl. Cancer Inst.* **1971**, *46*, 143.
491. Innes, J.R.M.; Ulland, B.M.; Valerio, M.G.; Petrucelli, L.; Fishbein, L.; Hart, E.R.; Pallotta, A.J.; Bates, R.R.; Falk, H.L.; Gart, J.J.; Klein, M.; Mitchell, L.; Peters, J. *JNCI, J. Natl. Cancer Inst.* **1969**, *42*, 1101.
492. Ulland, B.; Finkelstein, M.; Weisburger, E.K.; Rice, J.M.; Weisburger, J.H. *Nature (London)* **1971**, *230*, 460.
493. Dickens, F.; Jones, H.E.H. *Br. J. Cancer* **1963**, *17*, 100.
494. NIH Publication No. 80–453, U.S. Dept. of Health, Education, and Welfare, National Inst. of Health, 1978; pp. 790–94.
495. Roe, F.J.C.; Glendenning, O.M. *Br. J. Cancer* **1956**, *10*, 357.
496. Searle, C.E. *Br. J. Cancer* **1961**, *15*, 804.
497. Palmes, E.D.; Orris, L.; Nelson, N. *Am. Ind. Hyg. Assoc. J.* **1962**, *23*, 257.
498. Van Duuren, B.L.; Orris, L.; Nelson, J. *JNCI, J. Natl. Cancer Inst.* **1965**, *35*, 707.
499. Dickens, F.; Jones, H.E.H. *Br. J. Cancer* **1961**, *15*, 85.
500. Longridge, J.L.; Timms, D. *J. Chem. Soc. (B)* **1971**, 848.
501. Jones, J.B.; Young, J.M. *J. Med. Chem.* **1968**, *11*, 1176.
502. Dickens, F.; Jones, H.E.H. *Br. J. Cancer* **1965**, *19*, 392.
503. Epstein, S.S.; Mantel, N. *Int. J. Cancer* **1968**, *3*, 325.
504. "The Evaluation of Carcinogenic Risk of Chemicals to Man"; IARC Monograph, IARC: Lyon, 1974; Vol. 4, p. 177.
505. Griswold, D.P., Jr.; Casey, A.E.; Weisburger, E.K.; Weisburger, J.H. *Cancer Res,* **1968**, *28*, 924.

506. Ulland, B.; Finkelstein, M.; Weisburger, E.K.; Rice, J.M.; Weisburger, J.H. *Nature* **1971**, *230*, 460.
507. Gargus, J.L.; Reese, W.H., Jr.; Rutter, H.A. *Toxicol. Appl. Pharmacol.* **1969**, *15*, 92.
508. Leong, B.K.J.; Macfarland, H.N.; Reese, W.H., Jr. *Arch. Environ. Health* **1971**, *22*, 663.
509. "Bioassay of (2-Chloroethyl)trimethylammonium Chloride for Possible Carcinogenicity", NCI Tech. Rep. Ser. No. 158, DHEW Pub. No. (NIH) 79–1714, **1979**.
510. Kensler, C.J.; Shubik, P.; Hartwell, J.L. In "PHS Publication No. 149, Suppl. 1," U.S. Dept. of Health, Education, and Welfare, Washington, D.C., 1957.
511. Popper, H.; Sternberg, S.S.; Oser, B.L.; Oser, M. *Cancer* **1960**, *13*, 1035.
512. Sternberg, S.S.; Popper, H.; Oser, B.L.; Oser, M. *Cancer* **1960**, *13*, 780.
513. Schoental, R.; Bensted, J.P.M. *Cancer Res.* **1971**, *31*, 573.
514. Caspersson, T.; Zech, L.; Modest, E.J.; Foley, G.E.; Wagh, U.; Simonsson, E. *Exp. Cell Res.* **1969**, *58*, 128.
515. "The Evaluation of Carcinogenic Risk of Chemicals to Humans"; IARC Monograph, IARC: Lyon, 1981; Vol. 26, pp. 137–49.
516. Weisburger, J.H.; Griswold, D.P.; Prejean, J.D.; Casey, A.E.; Wood, H.B.; Weisburger, E.K. *Recent Results Cancer Res.* **1975**, *52*, 1.
517. Weisburger, E.K. *Cancer* **1977**, *40*, 1935.
518. Eisenbrand, G.; Habs, M.; Zeller, W.J.; Frebig, H.; Berger, M.; Zelesny, O.; Schmähl, D. In "Proceedings International Symposium on Nitrosoureas in Cancer Treatment", Imbach, J.L.; Serrou, B.; Schein, P., Eds.; Elsevier: Amsterdam, in press **1981**.
519. Griswold, D.P., Jr.; Casey, A.E.; Weisburger, E.K.; Weisburger, J.H.; Schabel, F.M., Jr. *Cancer Res.* **1966**, *26*, 619.
520. Theiss, J.C.; Shimkin, M.B. *Food Cosmet. Toxicol.* **1980**, *18*, 129.
521. Heston, W.E.; Levallain, W.D. *Proc. Soc. Exp. Biol. Med.* **1953**, *82*, 457.
522. Boyland, E.; Horning, E.S. *Br. J. Cancer* **1949**, *3*, 118.
523. Griffin, A.C.; Brandt, E.L.; Tatum, E.L. *J. Am. Med. Assoc.* **1950**, *144*, 571.
524. Narpozzi, A. *Boll. Soc. Ital. Biol. Sper.* **1954**, *29*, 1168.
525. Steinhoff, D.; Kuk, B.T. *Z. Krebsforsch.* **1957**, *62*, 112.
526. Matsuyama, M.; Suzuki, H.; Nakamura, T. *Br. J. Cancer* **1969**, *23*, 167.
527. Schmähl, D.; Osswald, H. *Arzneimittelforsch.* **1970**, *20*, 1461.
528. Koller, P.C. *Mutat. Res.* **1969**, *8*, 207.
529. Leopold, W.R.; Miller, E.C.; Miller, J.A. *Cancer Res.* **1979**, *39*, 913.
530. Duhig, J.T. *Arch. Pathol.* **1965**, *79*, 177.
531. Tokuoka, S. *Gann* **1965**, *56*, 537.
532. Walker, S.E.; Bole, G.G., Jr. *J. Lab. Clin. Med.* **1973**, *82*, 619.
533. Schmähl, D.; Habs, M. *Int. J. Cancer* **1979**, *23*, 706.
534. Stoner, G.D.; Shimkin, M.B.; Kniazeff, A.J.; Weisburger, J.H.; Weisburger, E.K.; Gori, G.B. *Cancer Res.* **1973**, *33*, 3069.
535. "The Evaluation of Carcinogenic Risk of Chemicals to Humans"; IARC Monograph, IARC: Lyon, 1981; Vol. 26, pp. 237–47.
536. Lawley, P.D.; Brookes, P. *Exp. Cell. Res., Suppl.* **1963**, *9*, 512.
537. Brookes, P.; Lawley, P.D. *J. Cell Comp. Physiol. Suppl. 1* **1964**, *64*, 111.
538. Geiduschek, E.P. *Proc. Natl. Acad. Sci. U.S.A.* **1961**, *47*, 950.
539. Doskočil, J.; Šormova, Z. *Collect. Czech. Chem. Commun.* **1965**, *30*, 481.
540. Kohn, K.W.; Spears, C.L.; Doty, P. *J. Mol. Biol.* **1966**, *19*, 266.
541. Verly, W.G.; Brakier, L. *Biochim. Biophys. Acta* **1969**, *174*, 674.
542. Chun, E.H.L.; Gonzales, L.; Lewis, F.S.; Jones, J.; Rutman, R.J. *Cancer Res.* **1969**, *29*, 1184.
543. McCann, J.J.; Lo, T.M.; Webster, D.A. *Cancer Res.* **1971**, *31*, 1573.

544. Lawley, P.D.; Lethbridge, J.H.; Edwards, P.A.; Shooter, K.V. *J. Mol. Biol.* **1969**, *39*, 181.
545. Walker, I.G. *Can. J. Biochem.* **1971**, *49*, 332.
546. Edwards, P.A.; Shooter, K.V. *Biopolymers* **1971**, *10*, 2079.
547. Burnotte, J.; Verly, W.G. *Biochim. Biophys. Acta* **1972**, *262*, 449.
548. Steele, W.J. *Proc. Am. Assoc. Cancer Res.* **1962**, *3*, 364.
549. Grunicke, H.; Bock, K.W.; Becher, H.; Gäng, V.; Schnierda, J.; Puschendorf, B. *Cancer Res.* **1973**, *33*, 1048.
550. Nietert, W.C.; Kellicutt, L.M.; Kubinski, H. *Cancer Res.* **1974**, *34*, 859.
551. Zwelling, L.A.; Kohn, K.W. *Cancer Treat. Rep.* **1979**, *63*, 1439.
552. Lawley, P.D.; Brookes, P. *J. Mol. Biol.* **1967**, *25*, 143.
553. Doskočil, J. *Collect. Czech. Chem. Commun.* **1965**, *30*, 479.
554. Verly, W.G.; Brakier, L.; Feit, P.W. *Biochim. Biophys. Acta* **1971**, *228*, 400.
555. Iyer, V.N.; Szybalski, W. *Science (Washington, D.C.)* **1964**, *145*, 55.
556. Institoris, E.; Fox, B.W. *Chem. Biol. Interact.* **1978**, *22*, 99.
557. Institoris, E.; Tamás, J. *Biochem. J.* **1980**, *185*, 659.
558. Connors, T.A. "Cancer Chemotherapy, 1979"; Pinedo, H.M., Ed.; Elsevier: Amsterdam, **1979**; pp. 25–55.
559. Cox, P.J. *Biochem. Pharmacol.* **1979**, *28*, 2045.
560. "The Evaluation of Carcinogenic Risk of Chemicals to Humans"; IARC Monograph, IARC: Lyon, 1981; Vol. 26, pp. 182–85.
561. Yoshida, M.; Numoto, S.; Otsuka, H. *Gann* **1979**, *70*, 645.
562. Griswold, D.; Prejean, J.D.; quoted in "Information Bulletin on Survey of Chemicals Being Tested for Carcinogenicity"; IARC: Lyon, 1981; p. 114.
563. Haddow, A.; Timmis, G.M. *Lancet* **1953**, *i*, 207.
564. Timmis, G.M.; Hudson, R.F. *Ann. N.Y. Acad. Sci.* **1958**, *68*, 727.
565. Roberts, J.J.; Warwick, G.P. *Biochem. Pharmacol.* **1961**, *6*, 217.
566. Roberts, J.J.; Warwick, G.P. *Nature (London)* **1959**, *183*, 1509.
567. Jones, A.R.; Campbell, I.S.C. *Biochem. Pharmacol.* **1972**, *21*, 2811.
568. Edwards, K.; Jones, A.R. *Biochem. Pharmacol.* **1971**, *20*, 1781.
569. Addison, I.; Berenbaum, M.C. *Br. J. Cancer* **1971**, *25*, 172.
570. Hendry, J.A.; Homer, R.F.; Rose, F.L.; Walpole, A.L. *Br. J. Pharmacol* **1951**, *6*, 235.
571. *Ibid.* 201.
572. Hadidian, Z.; Fredrickson, T.N.; Weisburger, E.K.; Weisburger, J.H.; Glass, R.M.; Mantel, N. *JNCI, J. Natl. Cancer Inst.* **1968**, *41*, 985.
573. Scribner, J.D.; Ford, G.P. *Cancer Lett.* **1982**, *16*, 51.
574. Tabin, C.J.; Bradley, S.M.; Bargmann, C.I.; Weinberg, R.A.; Papageorge, A.G.; Scolnick, E.M.; Dhar, R.; Lowy, D.R.; Chang, E.H. *Nature (London)* **1982**, *300*, 143.
575. Reddy, E.P.; Reynolds, R.K.; Santos, E.; Barbacid, M. *Nature (London)* **1982**, *300*, 149.
576. Swenson, D.H.; Kadlubar, F.F. In "Microbial Testers Probing Carcinogenesis"; Falkner, I.C., Ed.; Dekker: New York, 1981; p. 3.
577. Singer, B.; Kusmierek, T. *Annu. Rev. Biochem.* **1982**, *52*, 655.
578. Eisenstadt, E.; Warren, A.J.; Porter, J.; Atkins, D.; Miller, J.H. *Proc. Natl. Acad. Sci., U.S.A.* **1982**, *79*, 1945.
579. Strauss, B.S., personal communication.
580. Bogden, J.M.; Eastman, A.; Bresnick, E. *Nucleic Acids Res.* **1981**, *9*, 3089.
581. Craddock, V.M.; Henderson, A.R.; Gash, S. *Biochem. Biophys. Res. Commun.* **1982**, in press.
582. Demple, B.; Jacobsson, A.; Olsson, M.; Robins, P.; Lindahl, T. *J. Biol. Chem.* **1982**, in press.
583. Lindahl, T.; Demple, B.; Robins, P. *EMBO J.* **1982**, *1*, in press.

584. Waldstein, E.A.; CaO, E.-H.; Miller, M.E.; Cronkite, E.P.; Setlow, R.B. *Proc. Natl. Acad. Sci., U.S.A.* **1982**, *79*, 4786.

585. Harris, G.; Asbery, L.; Lawley, P.D.; Denman, A.M.; Hylton, W. *Lancet* **1982**, *ii*, 952.

586. Madden, J.J.; Falek, A.; Shafer, D.A.; Glick, J.H. *Proc. Natl. Acad. Sci., U.S.A.* **1979**, *76*, 5769.

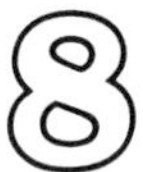

DNA Interactions of Reactive Intermediates Derived from Carcinogens

M. R. OSBORNE

Pollards Wood Research Station, Chester Beatty Research Institute, Institute of Cancer Research: Royal Cancer Hospital, Nightingales Lane, Chalfont St. Giles, Bucks HP8 4SP England

CARCINOGENIC ALKYLATING (MAINLY METHYLATING) AGENTS were described in Chapter 7, and the carcinogenic potency of a series of agents was related to the agent's ability to alkylate DNA in mammalian cells and to the structure and properties of the products formed. This chapter examines other agents that alkylate DNA, and describes how the theory of carcinogenesis by simple alkylating agents can be extended to cover a wider range of compounds.

The carcinogens that have been found to alkylate DNA include natural products, pollutants, solvents, drugs, and organic intermediates of diverse chemical structures. The compounds have little in common except their ability to bind to cellular macromolecules. Miller (*1*) pointed out that each one is an electrophile or can be converted to one by metabolic activation within the cell; the resulting electrophilic (mostly alkylating) agents then attack cellular proteins and nucleic acids. This general mechanism of action has been corroborated in recent years, notably by the discovery that polycyclic hydrocarbons can also be converted to alkylating agents by metabolism. During the same time, studies have indicated the increasing probability that DNA, rather than RNA or protein, is the most important target for carcinogenesis by alkylating agents (*2*), and the major research effort in chemical carcinogenesis in recent years has revolved around the interaction of these agents with DNA.

The detailed mechanisms by which carcinogens are metabolized and converted to alkylating agents and the mutagenic and carcinogenic potency of the various agents are discussed elsewhere in this book. Our present purpose is to examine the agents from the point of view of a DNA molecule and try to answer the following questions:

- For which carcinogens is there evidence that the compound or one of its metabolites alkylates DNA in vivo? How good is the evidence?
- Does the carcinogenicity of general alkylating agents correlate with their reactivity to DNA or with their S_N1 character as found for the methylating agents (Chapter 7)?

0065-7719/84/0182-0485$11.00/1

- At what site on DNA do the agents bind? Is carcinogenic activity associated with any particular reaction site?
- Does attack take place randomly over the whole genome, or are some agents highly carcinogenic because they attack some specific region of the genome that is crucial for carcinogenesis?

Several things can happen to an alkyl group bound to DNA in vivo. All of these, except the first, could conceivably lead to the killing, mutation, or carcinogenic transformation of the cell:

- Loss of alkyl group, spontaneously or by enzymic dealkylation, without damage to the DNA
- Loss of alkylated base leaving an apurinic (or apyrimidinic) site
- Repair by enzymes possibly leading to incorporation of errors
- Strand breakage
- Reaction of the alkyl group at a second site causing cross-linkage of the DNA to itself or to protein
- DNA or RNA synthesis using the alkylated DNA as a template and resulting in inhibition of nucleic acid synthesis and possibly in errors through mispairing of modified bases

The extent to which these processes occur and their possible biological effects will be briefly reviewed.

Carcinogens That Alkylate DNA

The ability to react with DNA in vivo is well established for the compounds listed in Table I, and if the compound requires metabolic activation, the reactive intermediate is also listed. The reaction products of the presumed ultimate carcinogen and DNA have been characterized, and the positions of substitution on DNA are given beginning with the site most heavily attacked. Proving that the suggested intermediates given in Table I are the most important is difficult, and for certain compounds, other reactive metabolites are being investigated. For instance, metabolism of benzo[*a*]pyrene yields not only the diol epoxide as shown in Table I, but also benzo[*a*]pyrene 4,5-oxide and 9-hydroxybenzo[*a*]pyrene 4,5-oxide which are also alkylating agents and may account for some of the observed binding of benzo[*a*]pyrene to DNA in vivo (*152*). Mechanisms involving free-radical intermediates that arise by metabolism or by photo-oxidation of carcinogens have also been suggested (*153,154*), but the products of such reactions with DNA have not been characterized, and such mechanisms will not be discussed in this chapter.

The compounds listed in Table II are also believed to bind to DNA in vivo, but the structures of the products are unknown. Most of the compounds require metabolic activation, and in some cases a reactive metabolite is known. Activation of the benzanthracene derivatives, dibenzanthracenes, and methylchrysene gives a terminal ring diol epoxide in each case; it is likely that these metabolites alkylate DNA to give products similar to those from benzopyrene diol epoxide and DNA.

The mechanism by which nitrosamines are converted to alkylating agents by metabolism is still unclear. In the case of *N*-nitrosodimethylamine, the enzymic oxidation of one methyl group was thought to lead to its loss as formaldehyde, leaving *N*-nitrosomethylamine. This compound would then rearrange to yield methyldiazonium ion, diazomethane, or free methyl cations:

$$CH_3 \cdot N\,(NO) \cdot CH_3 \rightarrow CH_2O + CH_3 \cdot NH \cdot NO \rightarrow CH_3 \cdot N{:}N^+ \rightarrow CH_2{:}N{:}N \text{ or } CH_3^+$$

The intermediacy of diazomethane has been disproved by experiments with labeled nitrosodimethylamine that showed that the methyl group was transferred intact in the methylation of guanine (*155*). Little evidence for the above pathway exists, and evidence against it was discussed by Olah (*156*) who suggested the methylmethyleneimmonium ion $CH_3 \cdot NH^+{:}CH_2$ as a reactive intermediate. With other alkyl nitrosamines, the situation is even less clear. Alkylation of DNA in vivo by nitrosodi-*n*-propylamine leads to both 7-*n*-propylguanine and 7-methylguanine residues. On the basis of the mechanism outlined above, one would expect the alkylating agent to be the propyl carbonium ion $CH_3 \cdot CH_2 \cdot CH_2^+$, which readily rearranges to the isopropyl ion $CH_3 \cdot CH^+ \cdot CH_3$. The absence of 7-isopropylguanine from the alkylated DNA indicates that alkylation at the 7-position does not proceed via the carbonium ion (*17*), but O^6-isopropylguanine is obtained as a minor product, probably by *n*-propylation followed by rearrangement (*19*). The formation of 7-methylguanine probably results from β-oxidation of one side chain (*157*):

$$Pr_2NNO \rightarrow CH_3 \cdot CHOH \cdot CH_2 \cdot NPr \cdot NO \rightarrow CH_3 \cdot CHO + CH_3 \cdot NPr \cdot NO \rightarrow CH_3N_2^+$$

Cyclic nitrosamines such as *N*-nitrosopiperidine and *N*-nitrosomorpholine probably alkylate DNA by a similar mechanism, but the resulting alkylguanines have not been identified, except for one product from nitrosomorpholine that appears to be 7-hydroxyethylguanine. The metabolism of nitrosamines and the formation of alkylating agents from them have been more fully discussed by Magee (*155*), Lijinsky (*95*), and Margison (*158*). An alternative hypothesis, that nitrosamines can act as nitrosating rather than alkylating agents, was offered by Buglass (*159*) and by Singer (*160*).

Most of the compounds of Table II have been tested by treating rats or mice with radioactive material and then demonstrating that DNA isolated from these animals was radioactively labeled. In many cases it has not been proven that this label represents carcinogens covalently bound to DNA. Most carcinogens bind to proteins to a higher extent than to DNA, and the activity may have resulted from protein contamination of the isolated DNA. Labeling of DNA could also arise from degradation of the carcinogen that results in the release of tritium or single-carbon fragments that are then incorporated into newly synthesized DNA (*161*). Apparently, carcinogens may also cause methylation of DNA by an indirect mechanism. For example, 7-methylguanine was detected in the liver DNA of rats fed *N*-nitrosopyrrolidine, but the methyl group was not derived from the nitrosamine (*150*).

The binding of compounds marked with footnote *b* in the reference column in Table II to the DNA of animals has not been proven; the evidence rests on the binding to DNA in vitro, which usually requires an enzymic activation system, along with the indirect evidence that the compounds are cytotoxic, mutagenic, and

Table I

Carcinogens that Alkylate DNA: Position of Attack Known

Agent	*Formula*	*Active Metabolite*[a]	*Reaction Site*	*References*[b]
Dimethyl sulfate	$(CH_3)_2SO_4$	*	7G,3A,1A,3C,7A	3[c]
Methyl methanesulfonate	$CH_3O \cdot O_2SCH_3$	*	7G,3A,1A,3C	4[c]
1-Methyl-1-nitrosourea	$CH_3 \cdot N(NO) \cdot CONH_2$	*	7G,3A,O6G[d]	5[c]
Streptozotocin	$HOCH_2$; O; OH; OH; HO; $CH_3N(NO)CONH$	*	7G,O6G,3A,7A	6
Methylnitrosourethane (Ethyl N-methyl-N-nitroso-carbamate)	$CH_3 \cdot N(NO) \cdot COOCH_2CH_3$	*	7G	7[c]
1-Methyl-3-nitro-1-nitroso-guanidine	$CH_3 \cdot N(NO) \cdot C(NH) \cdot NH \cdot NO_2$	*	7G,3A,O6G	8[c]
N-Nitrosodimethylamine	$(CH_3)_2N \cdot NO$	see text	7G,3A	[c]
1,2-Dimethylhydrazine	$CH_3NH \cdot NHCH_3$	possibly $CH_3 \cdot NO{:}N \cdot CH_2OH$	7G,3A,O6G	9
Dichlorvos (Dimethyl-2,2-dichlorovinyl phosphate)	$(CH_3O)_2PO \cdot O \cdot CH{:}CCl_2$	?	7G,3G[e]	10, 11
1-Methyl-3-phenyltriazene	$CH_3NHN{=}N-C_6H_5$		7G,O6G	12
1,1-Dimethyl-3-phenyltriazene	$(CH_3)_2NN{=}N-C_6H_5$		7G,O6G,3A	13
Dacarbazine (5-(3,3-Dimethyl-1-triazeno)imidazole-4-carboxamide)	NH_2CO; $(CH_3)_2NN{=}N-$; N; NH		7G	14
Diethyl sulfate	$(CH_3CH_2)_2SO_4$	*	7G,3A,O6G,3C,7A	5
Ethyl methanesulfonate	$CH_3CH_2O \cdot O_2SCH_3$	*	7G,3A,1A[d]	5[c]
Ethionine	$CH_3CH_2S \cdot CH_2 \cdot CH_2 \cdot CH(NH_2) \cdot COOH$		7G	15
Urethane (Ethyl carbamate)	$CH_3CH_2O \cdot CO \cdot NH_2$		1,N6A†,3,N4C†,7G	16[f]
1-Ethyl-1-nitrosourea	$CH_3CH_2 \cdot N(NO) \cdot CONH_2$	*	O6G,7G[d]	5[c,g]

N-Nitrosodiethylamine	$(CH_3CH_2)_2N \cdot NO$	see text	7G,O6G	[c]
N-Nitrosodipropylamine	$(CH_3 \cdot CH_2 \cdot CH_2)_2N \cdot NO$	see text	7G,O6G	17,18,19
N-Nitroso-(2-oxopropyl)propylamine	$CH_3CO \cdot CH_2 \cdot N(NO) \cdot CH_2CH_2CH_3$		7G,O6G	20
N-Nitrosodibutylamine	$(CH_3CH_2CH_2CH_2)N \cdot NO$	see text	7G	18
N-Nitrosobenzylmethylamine	$CH_3N(NO)CH_2$–(benzene ring)		7G,O6G	21,22
Propanesultone (1,2-Oxathiolane-2,2-dioxide)	(five-membered ring: O, SO_2)	*	7G,1A	23
N-Nitrosocyclohexylmethylamine	$CH_3N(NO)$–(cyclohexane ring)		7G	24
Vinyl chloride	$CH_2{:}CHCl$	$CH_2Cl \cdot CHO$ or CH_2—$CHCl$ (epoxide, O bridge)	3,N4C†,1,N6A†, 3,N2G† [h]	25–28
Dianhydrogalactitol	CH_2—$CH \cdot CHOH \cdot CHOH \cdot CH$—$CH_2$ (two epoxide O bridges)	*	7G[i]	29
Propiolactone	CH_2—CH_2 / CO—O (four-membered ring)	*	7G,1A,3C	30–32
Formaldehyde	CH_2O	*	N2G,N6A,N4C[i]	33,34
Mustard gas (Bis-2-chloroethyl sulfide)	$S(CH_2 \cdot CH_2Cl)_2$	*	7G[i]	[c]
Half-mustard (2-Chloroethyl ethyl sulfide)	$CH_3CH_2 \cdot S \cdot CH_2 \cdot CH_2Cl$	*	7G,3A	[c]
Nitrogen mustard (Bis(2-chloroethyl)-methylamine)	$CH_3 \cdot N(CH_2 \cdot CH_2Cl)_2$	*	7G[i]	[c]
2-Chloroethyldiethylamine	$(C_2H_5)_2N \cdot CH_2 \cdot CH_2Cl$	*	7G,N6A	35
Busulfan (Myleran; 1,4-Bis(methanesulfonyloxy)butane	$CH_3SO_2 \cdot O \cdot CH_2CH_2CH_2CH_2 \cdot O \cdot O_2SCH_3$	*	7G,N6A,N4C,O6G[i]	36
BCNU (1,3-Di(2-chloroethyl)-1-nitrosourea)	$ClCH_2 \cdot CH_2 \cdot N(NO) \cdot CO \cdot NH \cdot CH_2 \cdot CH_2Cl$	*	7G,1,N6A†,3C,3, N4C†,O6G[i]	37–40
CCNU (1-(2-Chloroethyl)-3-cyclohexyl-1-nitrosourea)	$ClCH_2CH_2N(NO)CONH$–(cyclohexane ring)	*	7G,3C,3,N4C† [i]	40

Continued on next page

Table I Continued

Agent	*Formula*	*Active Metabolite*[a]	*Reaction Site*	*References*[b]
Triethylenemelamine (2,4,6-Tri(aziridin-1-yl)-1,3,5-triazene)	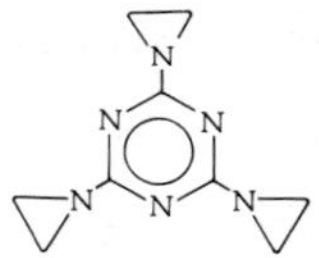 (structure: triazine ring with three aziridin-1-yl N groups)	*	7G[i]	41,42
1′-Hydroxyestragole	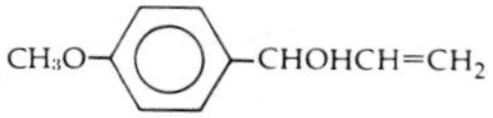 CH_3O–C₆H₄–$CHOHCH{=}CH_2$	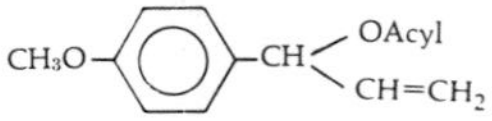 CH_3O–C₆H₄–CH(OAcyl)$CH{=}CH_2$	N2G,N6A	43
1′-Hydroxysafrole	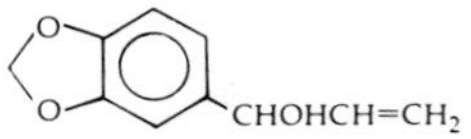 (methylenedioxyphenyl)–$CHOHCH{=}CH_2$	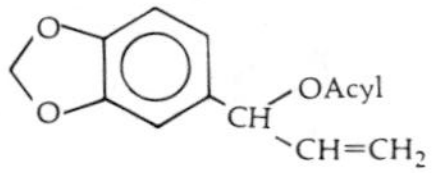 (methylenedioxyphenyl)–CH(OAcyl)$CH{=}CH_2$	N2G,N6A	44
Azaserine (O-Diazoacetyl-L-serine)	$N_2CH \cdot CO \cdot O \cdot CH_2 \cdot CH(NH_2) \cdot COOH$	*	7G	45
4-Nitroquinoline 1-oxide	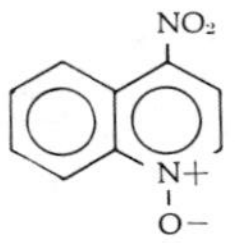 4-NO_2-quinoline N^+–O^-	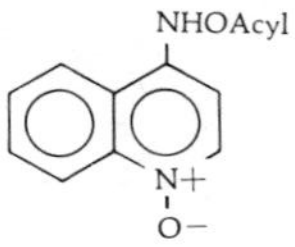 4-NHOAcyl-quinoline N^+–O^-	8G,O6G,N6A[j]	46–48
p-Methylaminoazobenzene	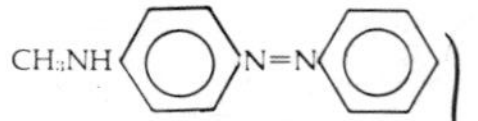 CH_3NH–C₆H₄–N=N–C₆H₅	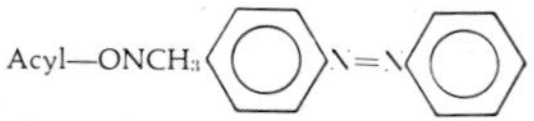 Acyl—$ONCH_3$–C₆H₄–N=N–C₆H₅	8G[k],N2G	49–51
p-Dimethylaminoazobenzene	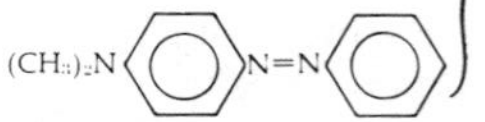 $(CH_3)_2N$–C₆H₄–N=N–C₆H₅			

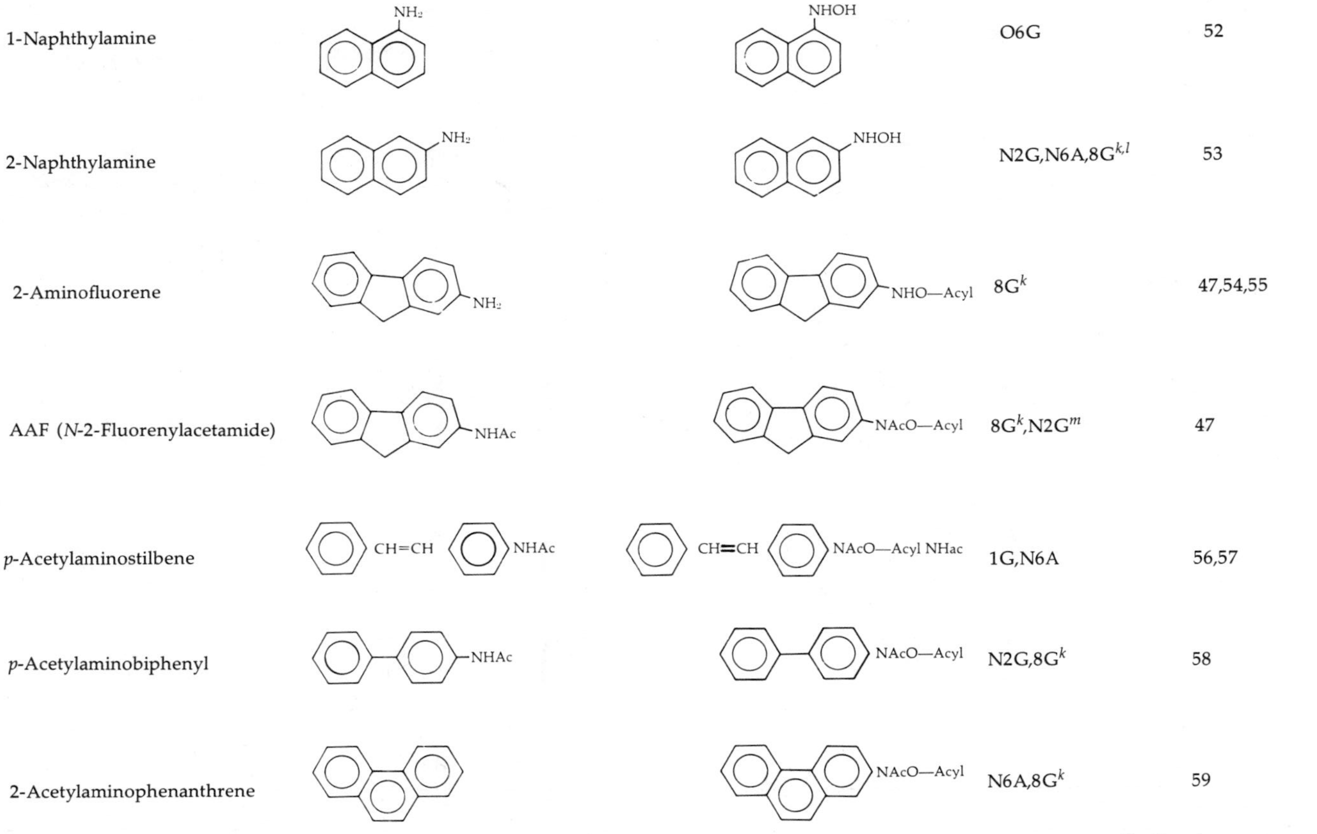

1-Naphthylamine	O6G	52
2-Naphthylamine	N2G,N6A,8G[k,l]	53
2-Aminofluorene	8G[k]	47,54,55
AAF (*N*-2-Fluorenylacetamide)	8G[k],N2G[m]	47
p-Acetylaminostilbene	1G,N6A	56,57
p-Acetylaminobiphenyl	N2G,8G[k]	58
2-Acetylaminophenanthrene	N6A,8G[k]	59

Continued on next page

Table I Continued

Agent	*Formula*	*Active Metabolite*[a]	*Reaction Site*	*References*[b]
Aflatoxin B_1			$7G^l$,3A or 7A	60^n
Aflatoxin B_2			$7G^l$	61
Sterigmatocystin			$7G^l$	62,63
7-Bromomethylbenzanthracene		*	N2G,N6A,C	64
7-Bromomethyl-12-methylbenzanthracene		*	N2G,N6A,C	65

Benzanthracene		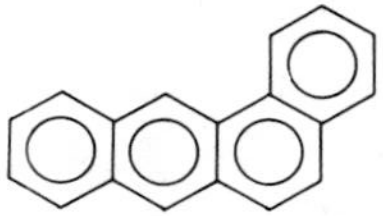 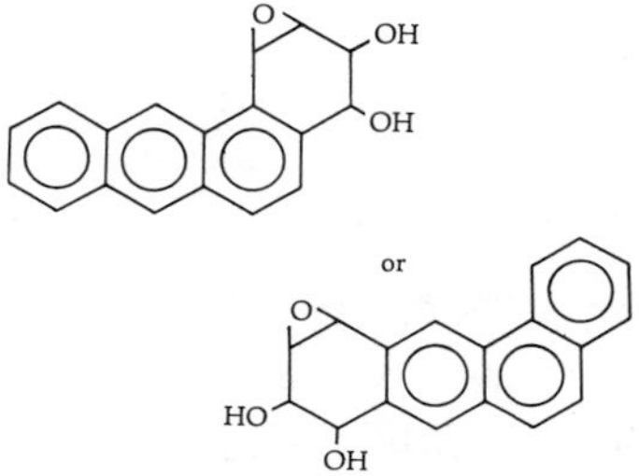 N2G	66
Benzo[*a*]pyrene		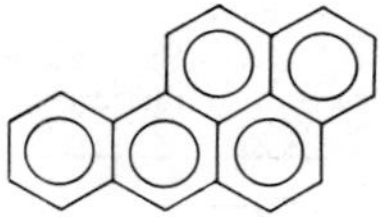 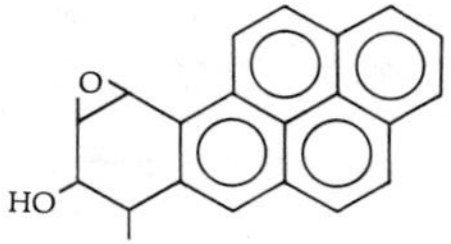 N2G,N6A[o]	67–72
7,12-Dimethylbenzanthracene 5,6-oxide	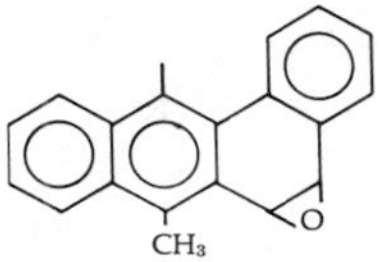 *	N2G,8G[p]	73–74
11-Methyl-15,16-dihydro-cyclopenta[*a*]phenanthren-17-one		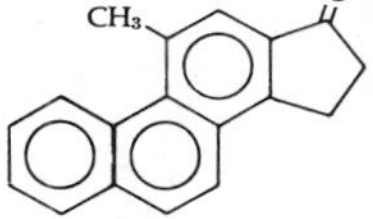 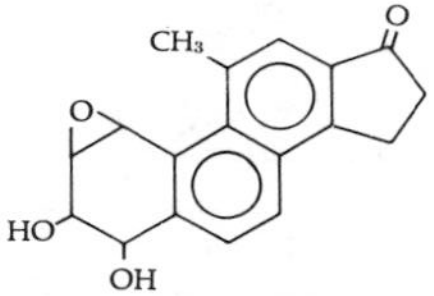 N2G	75,76

Continued on next page

Table I Continued

Agent	*Formula*	*Active Metabolite*[a]	*Reaction Site*	*References*[b]
3-Amino-1-methyl-5*H*-pyrido(4,3-*b*)indole	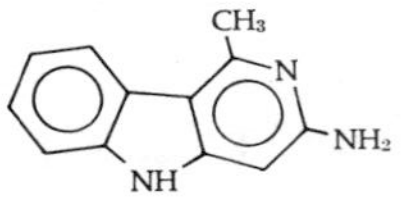	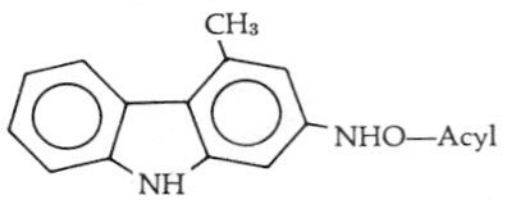	8G	77,78
2-Amino-6-methyl-dipyrido(1,2-*a*,3′,2′-*d*)imidazole	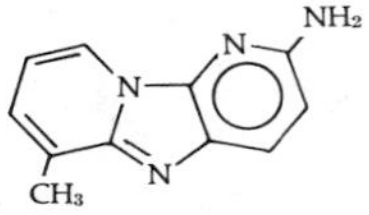	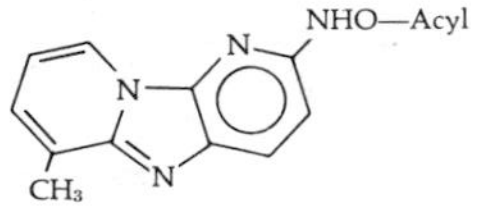	8G	77,79

[a]Key: *, direct-acting agent; †, reacts at two positions and forms a new ring.
[b]References are for the determination of the structure of the adducts. For further evidence of DNA alkylation in vivo see Ref. 80.
[c]*See* Chapter 7 in this volume.
[d]Also to a smaller extent: attack at 7A, 1A, 3C, 3G, and the pyrimidine oxygens, and considerable alkylation of the phosphate groups.
[e]Considered here as a methylating agent, but Segerbäck (*82*) found the extent of methylation of DNA in vivo to be very small and suggested that release of dichloroacetaldehyde was a more important mode of action.
[f]The *N*-methyl and *N*-ethyl derivatives also bind (*84*). Only the ethyl group of urethane is transferred to the DNA. The observation that tritium was lost from the ethyl group during binding led Dahl (*85*) to suggest that vinyl carbamate was an intermediate. Pound (*86*) claimed that the phosphate groups were major sites of alkylation, but Floot (*87*) found that phosphotriesters were not a significant product.
[g]Butylnitrosourea reacts with DNA in vitro at 3A, 7G, and 06G (*80*).
[h]Reaction products from chloroacetaldehyde and DNA in vitro. The other likely reactive metabolite chloroethylene oxide gives a 7-substituted guanine that forms a labile tricyclic base (*26*).
[i]Also cross-linked derivatives joined at these positions.
[j]The relative proportions are unknown.
[k]8-Arylaminopurines are formed by attack of the nitrogen atom, not alkylation products.
[l]Along with opening of the imidazole ring.
[m]Along with loss of one or both acyl groups. Possible reaction at 7G in vitro (*81*). *See* Chapter 4 for details.
[n]*See* Chapter 16 in Vol. 2 of this edition.
[o]Attack at 7G, O6G, N4C, and phosphate have also been detected in vitro.
[p]Reaction sites on RNA; presumably also on DNA.

Table II

Carcinogens and Other Agents that Alkylate DNA: Position of Attack Unknown

Agent	*Formula*	*References*[a]
Aniline mustard (Bis-*N*-2-chloroethylaniline)	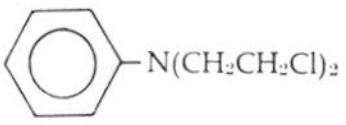 $-N(CH_2CH_2Cl)_2$	88
Chlorambucil	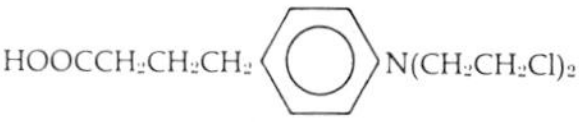 $HOOCCH_2CH_2CH_2$ $N(CH_2CH_2Cl)_2$	89
Cyclophosphamide	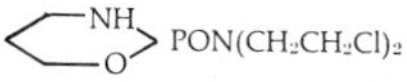 NH, O $PON(CH_2CH_2Cl)_2$	90,91
Triaziquone (Tri(aziridin-1-yl)benzoquinone)	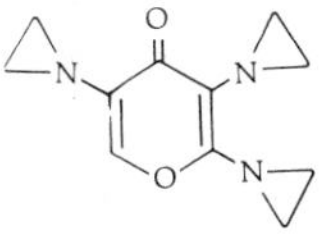 O, N, N, O, N	80
ThioTepa (Tri(aziridin-1-yl)phosphine sulfide)	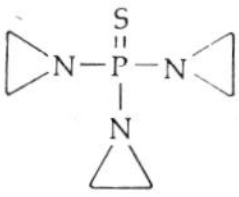 S, N–P–N, N	92
Apholate (Hexaaziridino-triphosphazene)	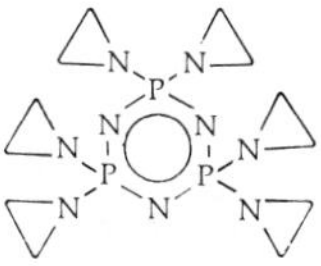 N, P, N, N, N, N, N, P, P, N, N, N	93[b]
Mitomycin C	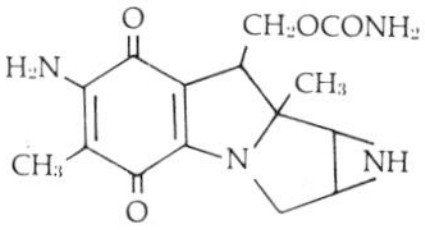 O, CH_2OCONH_2, H_2N, CH_3, CH_3, N, NH, O	41,42[b,c]
3-Aziridin-1-yl-4,6-dinitrobenzamide	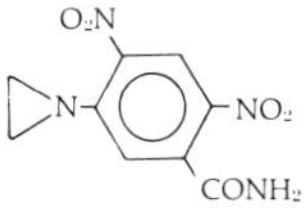 O_2N, N, NO_2, $CONH_2$	94
N-Nitroso-*N*-methylaniline	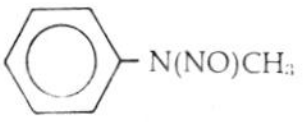 $N(NO)CH_3$	95
Nitrosocarbaryl (Naphth-1-yl-*N*-methyl-*N*-nitrosocarbamate)	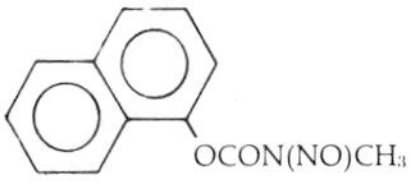 $OCON(NO)CH_3$	96
N-Nitroazetidine	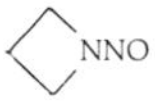 NNO	95
N-Nitrosopyrrolidine	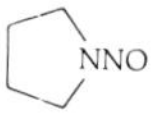 NNO	95,97[d]
N-Nitrosopiperidine	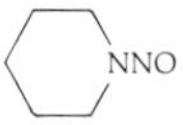 NNO	95

Continued on next page

Table II Continued

Agent	*Formula*	*References*[a]
N-Nitrosoperhydroazepine	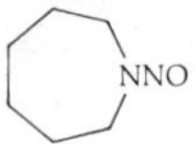 NNO	95,97
N-Nitrosomorpholine	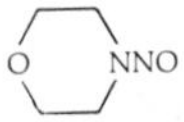 O NNO	95
3,5-Dimethyl-4-nitrosomorpholine	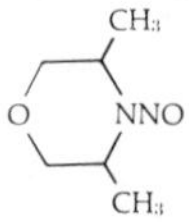 CH_3 O NNO CH_3	98
1,4-Dinitrosopiperazine	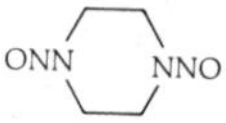 ONN NNO	95
N-Nitrosobis(2-oxopropylamine)	$(CH_3COCH_2)_2NNO$	99
Nitrosocimetidine	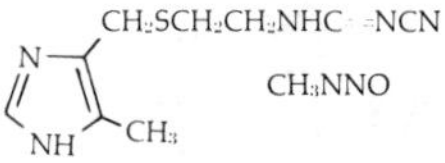 $CH_2SCH_2CH_2NHC{=}NCN$ CH_3NNO N NH CH_3	100,101
Aniline	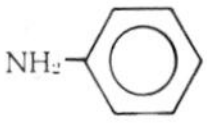 NH_2	102[e]
Quinoline	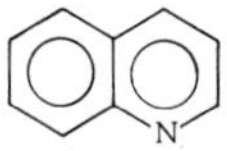 N	103[b]
Benzidine	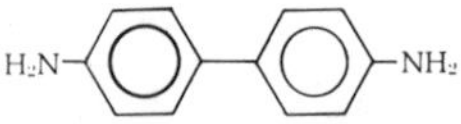 H_2N NH_2	104,105[b]
Dehydroheliotridine	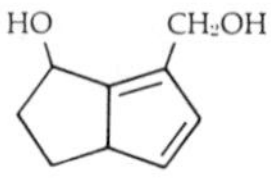 HO CH_2OH	106[b]
p-Aminoazobenzene	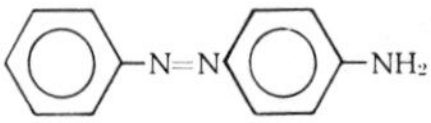 N=N NH_2	107
Methylazoxymethanol acetate or glucoside (Cycasin)	O $CH_3N{=}NCH_2OR$	108
N-Acetoxybenzamide	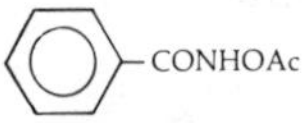 CONHOAc	109[b]
Michler's ketone (4,4′-Bis-dimethylaminobenzophenone)	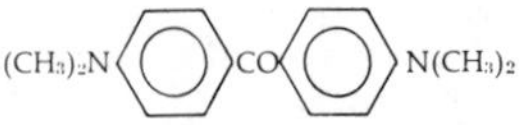 $(CH_3)_2N$ CO $N(CH_3)_2$	110[e]
Nitracrine (1-nitro-9-(3-dimethylaminopropyl)acridine)	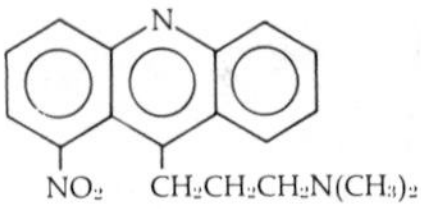 N NO_2 $CH_2CH_2CH_2N(CH_3)_2$	111

Agent	*Formula*	*References*[a]
1-Nitropyrene	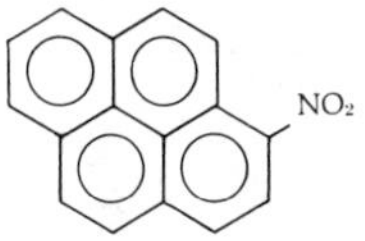 NO_2	112
Nitrofurans	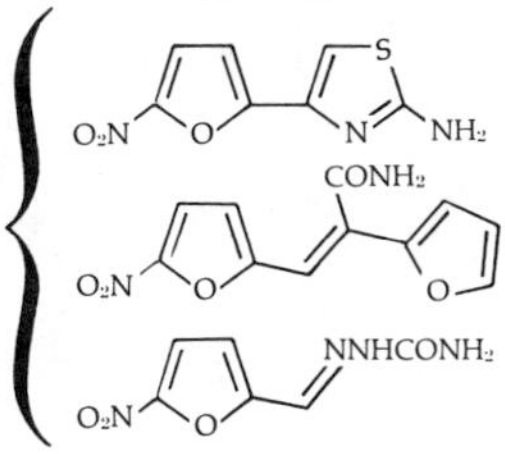 O_2N, S, N, NH_2; $CONH_2$, O_2N, O; O_2N, $NNHCONH_2$	113
2-*N*-Ethylcarbamoxymethylfuran	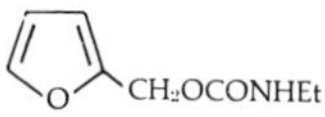 $CH_2OCONHEt$	114[e]
Methyl carbamate	CH_3OCONH_2	82
Propyl carbamate	$CH_3CH_2CH_2OCONH_2$	82
Acrolein	$CH_2{=}CHCHO$	115[e]
Mycophenolic acid	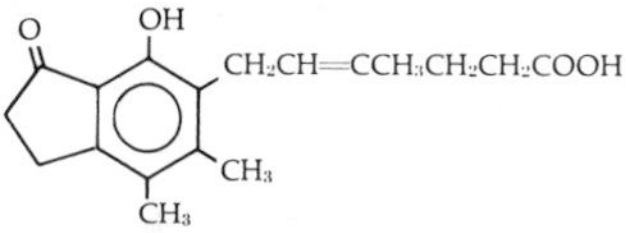 O, OH, $CH_2CH{=}CCH_3CH_2CH_2COOH$, CH_3, CH_3	116
Butylated hydroxytoluene (2,6-Di-t-butyl-4-methylphenol)	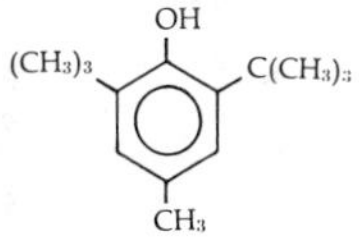 OH, $(CH_3)_3$, $C(CH_3)_3$, CH_3	117[e]
Benzene	C_6H_6	118,119
Anthracene	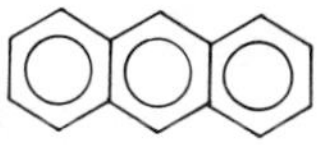	120[e]
Dibenz[*a,c*]anthracene	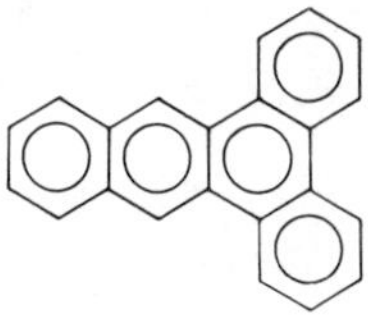	121
Dibenz[*a,h*]anthracene	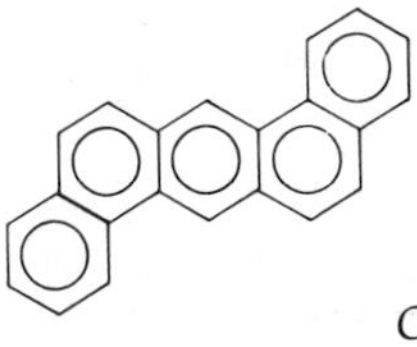	121

Continued on next page

Table II Continued

Agent	*Formula*	*References*[a]
7-Methylbenzanthracene	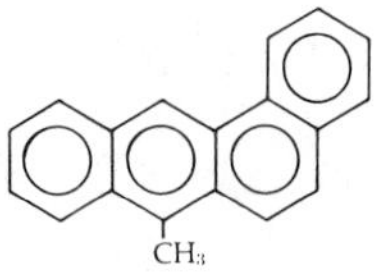 CH₃	122,123[f]
7,12-Dimethylbenzanthracene	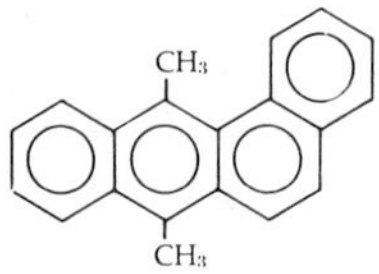 CH_3, CH_3	124[f]
3-Methylcholanthrene	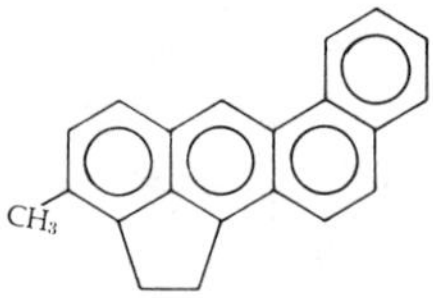 CH_3	125[f]
5-Methylchrysene	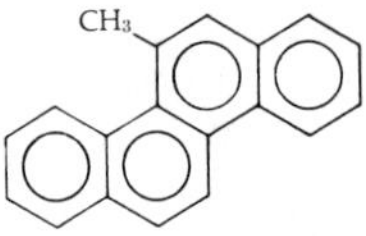 CH_3	126
Hydroxybenzopyrenes (2-, 3-, and 9-)	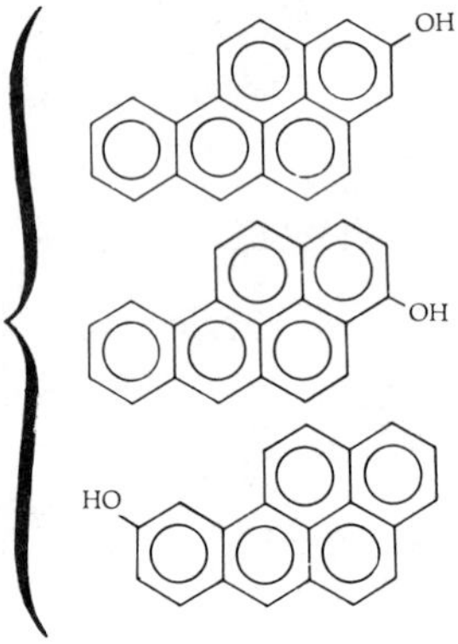 OH; OH; HO	127–129[b]
6-Acetoxymethyl-benzo[*a*]pyrene	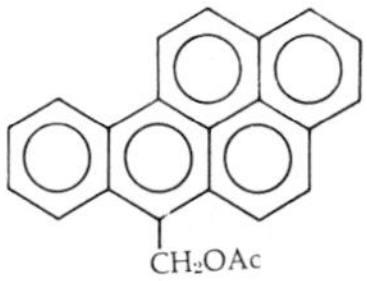 CH_2OAc	130[b]
Benzo[*a*]pyrene 4,5-oxide	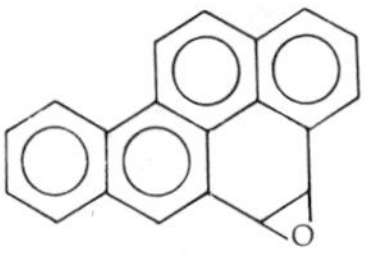 O	131[b]

Table II Continued

Agent	*Formula*	*References*[a]
Dibenzo[*a,e*]fluoranthene	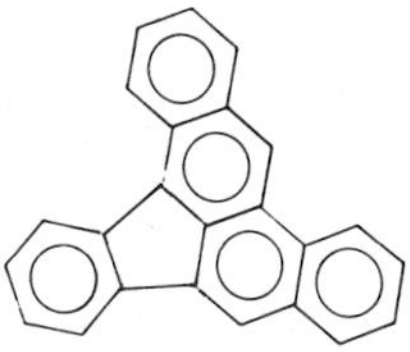	132
Cholesterol	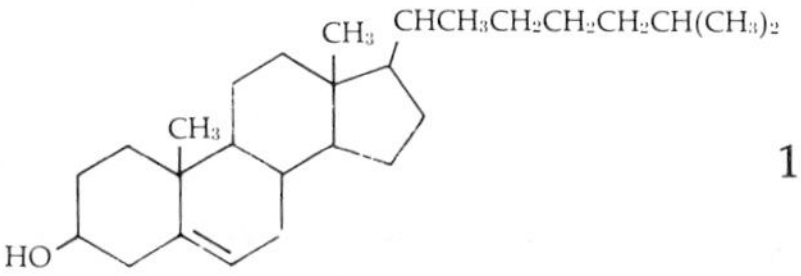 CH_3 $CHCH_3CH_2CH_2CH_2CH(CH_3)_2$; CH_3; HO	133[b]
Cholic acid	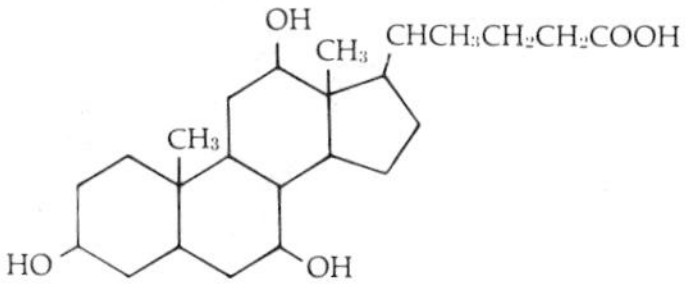 OH; CH_3 $CHCH_3CH_2CH_2COOH$; CH_3; HO; OH	133[b]
Estrone; Estradiol	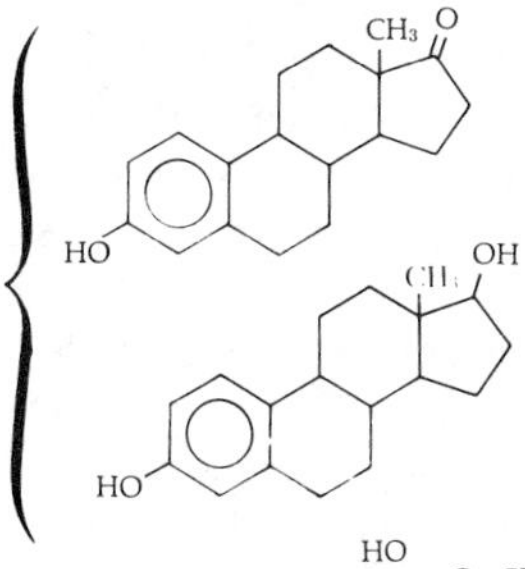 CH_3 O; HO; CH_3 OH; HO	134–138
17-Ethinylestradiol	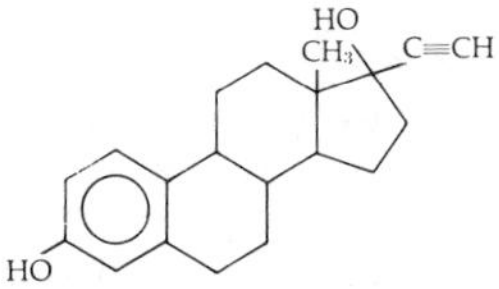 HO CH_3 C≡CH; HO	134,139[c]
Diethylstilbestrol	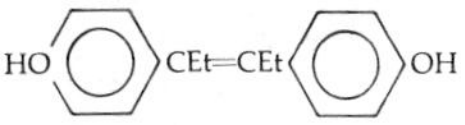 HO–⟨⟩–CEt=CEt–⟨⟩–OH	140a
Aflatoxin G_1	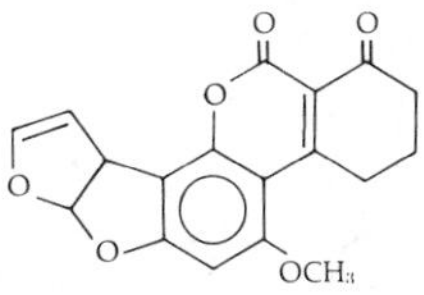 O O; O; O; O; OCH_3	140b
Aflatoxin M_1	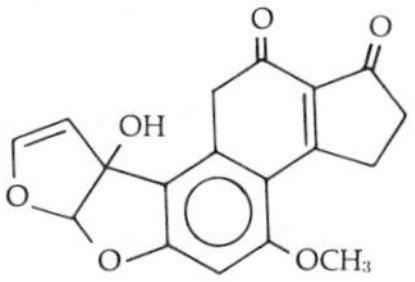 O O; OH; O; O; OCH_3	62[e]

Continued on next page

Table II Continued

Agent	*Formula*	*References*[a]
Methyl bromide	CH_3Br	141
Carbon tetrachloride	CCl_4	142,143[e]
Trichloroethylene	$Cl_2C{:}CHCl$	144[b]
1,2-Dichloroethane	$ClCH_2 \cdot CH_2Cl$	145[b]
1,2-Dibromoethane	$BrCH_2 \cdot CH_2Br$	146[e]
Hexachlorobiphenyl	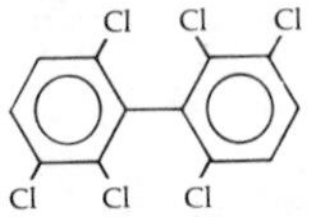	147,148

[a]For more details, *see* references given or the review by Lutz (*80*).
[b]Binds to DNA in vitro; indirect evidence of binding in vivo.
[c]Activated by reduction to a DNA-binding agent (*42, 149*); does not bind at 7-guanine (*42*).
[d]Mechanism of binding to DNA obscure. May cause methylation of DNA (*150*), cross-linking (*97*), or reaction with guanine residues to give a 1,N^2-cyclic adduct (*151*).
[e]Binding to DNA in vivo reported, but not confirmed.
[f]Derivatives hydroxylated in the sidechains also bind to cellular DNA; also dihydrodiol and diol epoxide metabolites are the principal intermediates in the binding of the hydrocarbons to DNA.

carcinogenic. In general, compounds that can bind to DNA following microsomal activation also can bind to the DNA of mammalian cells in culture and to the DNA of whole animals; in the case of polycyclic hydrocarbons, though, the relative proportions of different products differ considerably (*161,162*).

Compounds marked (c) in the reference column of Table II have been reported to bind to DNA in vivo only once. Benzene, anthracene, and aniline bind only to a very small extent if at all, as would be expected from their low or zero mutagenic and carcinogenic potency.

The literature contains conflicting reports of the ability of steroids to bind to DNA. Zachariah (*133*) showed that bacteria are able to metabolize cholesterol and cholic acid to unknown metabolites that attack DNA; Blackburn (*163*) showed that cholesterol oxide is a possible intermediate in this reaction. It has been reported that estrone binds to rat liver DNA in vivo (*134*) and that estrone and estradiol, but not cholesterol, are bound to DNA by microsomal activation (*135–37*). The intermediate was believed to be an epoxide based on the 1,2,3,4-ring, but Duncan (*138*) found that the amount of binding is insignificant.

Chlorinated hydrocarbons are not potent carcinogens, but it is of great importance to know whether they are carcinogenic at all because of their widespread use as solvents, organic synthetic intermediates, and pesticides. If they bind to DNA in vivo, it is only to a very low extent. The binding of carbon tetrachloride to DNA (*142,143*) was thought to occur through oxidation to CCl_3 radicals (*164*). Chloroform, $CHCl_3$, did not bind to rat or mouse liver nucleic acids (*165*). 2,2′,3,3′,6,6′-Hexachlorobiphenyl bound to mouse liver DNA (*147*); the reactive intermediate was thought to be the 4,5-oxide. The insecticide DDT is metabolized in part to an α-chloro epoxide, which is an alkylating agent (*166, 167*); this may attack DNA as does the epoxide of vinyl chloride. The highly toxic pollutant 2,3,7,8-tetrachlorodibenzo-*p*-dioxin (TCDD) did not bind to rat liver

DNA to any significant extent (*168*) so its toxic and possible carcinogenic properties must be through a different mechanism.

A few other carcinogens might be metabolized to yield alkylating agents, but no proof of binding to nucleic acids in vivo could be found in the literature. These agents include a number of plant products (*169*). The pyrrolizidine alkaloids are oxidized to epoxides (*170*) or to 3-acyloxymethylpyrroles (*169*), both of which could alkylate cellular DNA. Dehydroretronecine was found to alkylate the amino group of deoxyguanosine in vitro (*171*). Many fungal products bind physically to DNA in vitro, and some may also bind covalently. Hurley (*172*) suggested a mechanism for the binding of anthramycin, sibiromycin, or tomamycin to DNA in vitro. The antitumor agent CC-1065 may bind to DNA through its cyclopropane group (*173, 174*). The suspected carcinogen acrylonitrile, $CH_2{:}CH \cdot CN$, is converted by metabolism to an epoxide that reacts with DNA (*175*).

Carcinogenicity and Reactivity

In general, correlation of carcinogenic potency with parameters of reactivity for alkylating agents has not been possible, but it has been done for the methylating agents (Chapter 7). The only other series for which such correlations look promising is the aralkylating agents. According to Dipple (*176*), 7-bromomethyl-12-methylbenzanthracene (BrMBA) reacted with a model nucleophile, 4-*p*-nitrobenzylpyridine, with a half-life of 1 min; related compounds that reacted faster or slower were less carcinogenic, and this finding suggested an optimum chemical reactivity for carcinogenic activity. For polycyclic diol epoxides, many of which have not yet been synthesized, the theoretically calculated reactivity of the diol epoxide correlated with the carcinogenic potency of the hydrocarbon from which it could be derived (*177–79*). But Hsu (*180*) found that the carcinogenic potency of a polycyclic diol epoxide correlated poorly with the extent to which it alkylated bacteriophage DNA.

Position of Substitution

The positions of alkylation of DNA by direct-acting methylating and ethylating agents are discussed elsewhere (Chapter 7); in brief, the simple "S_N2" agents attack 7-guanine first and 3-adenine second. The nitrosamides attack these sites as well as the oxygen atoms of guanine and the phosphate group. The other agents in Table I may be divided into four classes: other alkylating agents, aralkylating agents, arylnitreniums, and cross-linking agents.

The other alkylating agents (propiolactone, half-mustards, and aflatoxin epoxide) react at the ring nitrogens of DNA bases as does methyl methanesulfonate; the preponderant product is again the 7-alkylguanine.

The ultimate carcinogens derived from estragole, safrole, and the polycyclic hydrocarbons are aralkylating agents, i.e., $Ar \cdot CH_2^+$ or $Ar \cdot CHR^+$. These agents attack DNA at the amino groups of the bases in order of quantity: $N^2G > N^6A > N^4C$. This behavior was somewhat unexpected because these amino groups are not positions of high electron density in DNA. A feature that has caused some confusion is that reaction with nucleoside monomers often gave different products from those found with DNA. Benzo[*a*]pyrene diol epoxide reacted with DNA principally at N^2-guanine, but it reacted with deoxyguanosine to a greater extent at other positions including the O^6- and 7-positions (*68*). The same may be true of the *K*-region oxides of polycyclic hydrocarbons; 7,12-dimethylbenzanthracene 5,6-oxide attacked RNA at N^2-guanine (*73*), but attacked guanylic acid at the 7-position (*181*). Attacks at the 8-position of guanosine and at the sugar hydroxyls have also been reported (*74, 182, 183*).

Two attempts have been made to rationalize the pattern of substitution of aralkylating agents on DNA. Moschel (*184*) studied benzylating agents as model compounds. He showed that substitution was favored at the amino group by a reagent of S_N1 character and at O^6-guanine by a reagent having a "hard" leaving group. Pullman (*185*) calculated the electronegativity of various positions on the purines and pyrimidines and showed that although the amino groups were unfavorable sites for attack by comparison with the ring nitrogens, this difference in reactivity was reduced in the double helix. The order of reactivity found, $N^2G > N^6A > N^4C$, was to be expected.

The arylhydroxylamines of Table I arise either by reduction of a carcinogenic nitro compound or by oxidation of an aromatic amine. Loss of hydroxide or acylate ion then leaves an electron-deficient nitrogen atom. These compounds are therefore not alkylating agents, but are considered in this chapter because some of the observed products with DNA involve arylation rather than substitution by nitrogen:

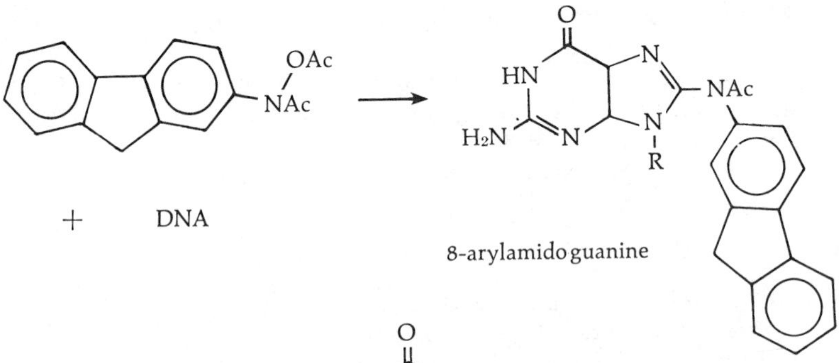

OAc
NAc
+ DNA
O
HN
N
NAc
H_2N
N
N
R

8-arylamidoguanine

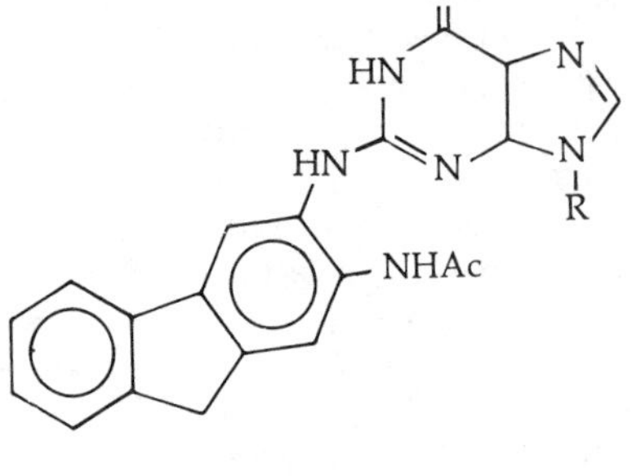

O
HN
N
HN
N
N
R
NHAc

N^2-arylguanine

The arylamines of Table I attack several different positions of guanine, and the choice depends on the nature of the aryl group. These differences have been rationalized by Scribner and Fisk (*186*) who showed that some of the results could have been predicted by molecular orbital theory. A different theoretical approach was taken by Ornstein and Rein (*187*) who examined the reaction of hydroxylaminoquinoline oxide with DNA; they concluded that the adenine residues should be at least as reactive as the guanine residues, but that the adenine adducts were lost by depurination.

The results of Table I show that carcinogens attack DNA at a large variety of sites and consequently do not encourage the belief that carcinogenesis depends on the substitution of one particular site (such as the O^6-position of guanine). It has been postulated that substitution at 7-guanine is ineffective at causing mutation or initiation of tumors and that a site involved in base-pairing, such as N^2- or O^6-guanine, must be involved in carcinogenesis. If this postulate is true, one must then explain how aflatoxin, which binds almost exclusively at 7-guanine, is such a potent carcinogen. Two explanations have been offered: (1) the major product is not the 7-guanine adduct, but it rearranges to give 7-substituted guanines during its isolation and characterization (*188*); and (2) minor but still unidentified products are responsible for the biological effects. A second product present in 1/30 the amount of the major product might be sufficient to account for the mutagenicity of aflatoxin B_1 (*189, 190*).

Regional Specificity

Another explanation for the different carcinogenic potencies of alkylating agents with similar ability to alkylate DNA is that the more carcinogenic agents may have a specific ability to alkylate the region of the genome that determines malignant transformation. The idea that an agent may attack some parts of the genome more than others comes from genetics; certain "hot spots" are known to be much more mutable by a chemical agent than others. It is possible that there is such a "hot spot" corresponding to malignant transformation. Fahmy (*191*) showed that carcinogenic alkylating agents are more potent than noncarcinogens of similar mutagenicity at causing "Minute" and "bobbed" mutations in *Drosophila* and suggested that specific mutations at similar RNA-forming genes in mammalian cells may be important in carcinogenesis.

Several attempts have been made to demonstrate by chemical means that alkylating agents attack certain regions of DNA more than others. In most of these studies, animals or mammalian cells grown in culture were treated with the agent; their chromatin was then isolated and fractionated to find whether one fraction of the DNA had a higher level of bound carcinogen than another. The results of such experiments are listed in Table III. Six ways of fractionating the DNA have been used.

Nuclear and Mitochondrial DNA. Several studies have shown that mitochondrial DNA is modified by alkylating agents to a much higher level than is nuclear DNA. Because the mitochondrion accounts for only about 1% of the total DNA of the cell, the nucleus still contains a greater proportion of the total number of DNA adducts. A probable explanation for the higher binding level in mitochondria is that the DNA there is in close contact with lipids that contain the ultimate carcinogens in solution and that help to protect the carcinogens from hydrolysis (*193, 196*). In the

Table III

Regional Specificity in Alkylation of DNA

Agent[a]	*Tissue*	*Result*	*Reference*
MNU	Rat	Mitochondrial > nuclear	*192*
DMN	Rat and hamster	Mitochondrial > nuclear	*193*
MMS, DMN	Rat liver	Mitochondrial = nuclear	*194*
DMBA, BP[b]	Mouse cells	Mitochondrial > nuclear	*195*
BPDE	Mouse cells	Mitochondrial > nuclear	*196*
Aflatoxin B_1	Rat liver	Mitochondrial > nuclear	*197*
Mustard gas	Mouse cells	Satellite = main band	*198*
DMBA	Mouse skin	Satellite = main band	*199*
MMS	Mouse	Satellite = main band	*200*
BP	Rat lung	Matrix fraction primarily	*201*
MNNG	Human cells	Nascent DNA = remainder	*202*
3MC[c]	Mouse cells	Euchromatin > heterochromatin	*203*
HAAF	Rat liver	Euchromatin > heterochromatin[d]	*204,205*
AAF	Rat liver	Euchromatin > heterochromatin	*206*
HAAF	Rat liver	Euchromatin = heterochromatin	*207*
HAAF	Rat liver	Euchromatin > heterochromatin	*208*
DMN, MNU	Rat liver	Euchromatin > heterochromatin	*209*
DMN	Rat liver	DNase 1 sensitive regions	*210,211*
DMN	Rat liver	DNase 1 sensitive regions[d]	*212*
HAAF	Rat liver	DNase 1 resistant regions[d]	*213*
HAAF	Rat liver	DNase 1 resistant regions	*214*
BP/microsomes	Nuclei	DNase 1 sensitive regions[e]	*215*
BP/microsomes	Nuclei	DNase 1 resistant regions	*216*
DMN	Rat liver	DNase 1—no distinction	*217*
MNU	Rat brain	DNase 1 sensitive regions	*218*
MNU	Nuclei	DNase 1 sensitive regions	*219*
BP	Human cells	DNase 1 sensitive regions	*220*
CCNU	Human cells	DNase 1 sensitive regions	*221*
NQO	Human cells	DNase 1—no distinction	*222*
AAAF	Chromatin	Staph. nuclease sensitive regions	*223*
HAAF	Rat liver	Staph. nuclease sensitive regions	*214*
AAAF	Human cells	Micr. nuclease sensitive regions[d]	*224*
HAAF	Rat liver	Micr. nuclease—no distinction	*207*
Trioxsalen/UV	Nuclei	Micr. nuclease sensitive regions	*225,226*
BP/microsomes	Nuclei	Staph. nuclease sensitive regions	*215,216*
BP	Hamster cells	Micr. nuclease—no distinction	*227*
BP	Human cells	Micr. nuclease—no distinction	*228*
BP	Mouse cells	Micr. nuclease—no distinction	*229*
BPDE	Chromatin	Staph. nuclease sensitive regions	*230*
BPDE	Nuclei	Micr. nuclease sensitive regions	*231,232*
BPDE	Mouse cells	Micr. nuclease sensitive regions[d]	*229*
BPDE/BP oxide	Human cells	Micr. nuclease sensitive regions	*233*
BrMBA	Human cells	Staph. nuclease resistant regions	*234*
CCNU	Human cells	Micr. nuclease resistant regions	*221*

Table III Continued

Agent[a]	*Tissue*	*Result*	*Reference*
NQO	Human cells	Micr. nuclease sensitive regions	*222*
DMN	Rat liver	Micr. nuclease—no distinction	*217*
MNU	Nuclei	Micr. nuclease sensitive regions	*219*
Aflatoxin B_1	Trout liver	Micr. nuclease sensitive regions	*235*
DMN	Rat liver	Repetitive = single-copy	*236*
MNU	Rat (three tissues)	Repetitive > single-copy	*237*
DMBA	Mouse skin	Repetitive > single-copy	*238*
BP	Hamster cells	Repetitive > single-copy	*239*
BPDE	DNA	GC- or AT-rich regions primarily	*240*
DMS	Nucleosomes	No specificity or periodicity	*241*
BPDE	DNA	Restriction enzymes; no specificity	*242*
BPDE	DNA	Restriction enzyme; no specificity[f]	*243*
AAAF	SV40 virus	Restriction enzymes; one fragment more	*244*
AAAF	Nucleosomes	Immunoelectron microscopy; not random	245

[a]The carcinogens used were AAAF, *N*-acetoxy-*N*-2-fluorenylacetamide; AAF, *N*-2-fluorenylacetamide; BP, benzo[*a*]pyrene; BPDE, 7,8-dihydroxy-9,10-epoxy-7,8,9,10-tetrahydrobenzo[*a*]pyrene; BrMBA, 7-bromomethylbenzanthracene; CCNU, 1-(2-chloroethyl)-3-cyclohexyl-1-nitrosourea; DMBA, 7,12-dimethylbenzanthracene; DMN, *N*-nitrosodimethylamine; DMS, dimethyl sulfate; HAAF, *N*-hydroxy-*N*-2-fluorenylacetamide; 3MC, 3-methylcholanthrene; MMS, methyl methanesulfonate; MNNG, 1-methyl-3-nitro-1-nitrosoguanidine; MNU, 1-methyl-1-nitrosourea; and NQO, 4-nitroquinoline 1-oxide.
[b]Also 3MC, benzanthracene, and methylcyclopentaphenanthrenone.
[c]Also dibenz[*a,h*]anthracene; no difference observed with dibenz[*a,c*]anthracene.
[d]However the lesions were removed faster from those regions initially having the most bound carcinogen.
[e]New data in Ref. 216.
[f]The extent of modification depended only on the guanine content of the fragment.

case of aflatoxin, the mitochondrion contains enzymes that are capable of binding the carcinogen to DNA (*246*).

The postulate that cancer could result from an alteration in the properties of the mitochondrion (*247*) is consistent with the fact that carcinogens bind to mitochondrial DNA to a great extent.

Main and Satellite DNA. Mouse DNA may be separated by centrifugation into a main band and a small satellite band; the function of this satellite DNA is unknown. It appears to be highly repetitive in sequence (*248*). Mustard gas, methyl methanesulfonate, and dimethylbenzanthracene have been found to bind to the same extent in both fractions.

Euchromatin and Heterochromatin. Two methods have been used to separate the two fractions: by shearing and centrifugation or by partial digestion with DNase II. The euchromatin band is believed to represent DNA that is being transcribed (active chromatin), and the heterochromatin band is believed to represent inactive or repressed DNA, but the evidence is not conclusive. Most researchers found that a significantly higher level of carcinogens became bound in the euchromatin fraction.

Partial Digestion with Other Enzymes. DNase I appears to digest active chromatin faster than inactive chromatin (*249*), and results with this enzyme should therefore be similar to those with DNase II. Micrococcal (staphylococcal) nuclease digests the "linker" DNA of chromatin before attacking the nucleosomes. Several groups have demonstrated that the fraction of chromatin that is more rapidly digested by these enzymes has a larger amount of carcinogen bound to it. However, some of these reports contradict each other and show that such experiments are difficult to interpret. In some cases, it is not clear whether binding to DNA alone was measured, or whether binding to protein was included. Another possible source of confusion is that the presence of bound carcinogen may catalyze or inhibit digestion of chromatin by the enzyme, though one study has shown that digestion is not affected by the binding of benzopyrene (*216*). If the cell DNA repair system first removes carcinogens bound to the most accessible regions of chromatin, the distribution of bound carcinogen will change with time. Thus cells exposed to *N*-acetoxy-*N*-2-fluorenylacetamide (AAAF) initially contained a higher level of *N*-2-fluorenylacetamide (AAF) in the linker region, but after incubation ultimately more was found in the nucleosome core region (*224*). Another possible complication is that the nucleosome structure may not be static, but instead may rearrange while the lesion is being repaired (*234*); Kaneko (*224*) gives evidence that this rearrangement does not happen.

Repetitive and Single-Copy DNA. In the technique of Cot analysis, DNA is fractionated according to the speed with which single-stranded fragments are reannealed to the complementary strand. The fast-annealing fraction contains highly repetitive DNA whose function is unknown; it does not appear to code for proteins. The few studies that have been carried out (*236–39*) indicated that this fraction contained a slightly higher level of bound carcinogen than did DNA of unique sequence.

Restriction Enzyme Analysis and DNA Sequencing. The foregoing methods examine the whole genome and separate the DNA into crude fractions. Recently single sites or particular fragments of DNA have been examined. One study has shown that while AAAF attacks isolated simian virus DNA randomly, treatment of the same virus within a cell leads to modification of one particular fragment of its DNA more than the other fragments (*244*); perhaps certain DNA sequences are more readily attacked than others for steric reasons. Using synthetic polymers, Gotoh (*250*) showed that guanine in the sequence CGC was attacked by hydroxylaminoquinoline oxide more readily than guanine in GGG. Aflatoxin, however, caused more modification of doublet guanines than two single guanines in a piece of bacterial DNA of known sequence (*251*). Nitrogen mustard attacked guanine residues in human DNA without regard for sequence (*252*). Both AAAF and benzo[*a*]pyrene diol epoxide attacked all the guanine residues of a bacteriophage DNA (*253*).

Conclusion. The most striking result of the experiments described in this section, which may have consequences for the theory of carcinogenesis, is the effect on mitochondrial DNA. The other experiments have yielded disappointing results. In the case of the methylating agents, there is little convincing evidence that any directed alkylation occurs in the genome. The larger alkylating agents appear to cause more modification of the more accessible regions of DNA, but the significance of this observation to the mechanism of carcinogenesis is still unclear.

Spontaneous Loss of Alkyl Group

Spontaneous loss is known to occur in only a few cases. Formaldehyde alkylates DNA to give hydroxymethyl adducts that are so labile that it is difficult to prove their existence (*34*). The bound form of aflatoxin B_1 has an RO·CHR′·N group that is more stable, but it is still subject to slow hydrolysis; after 24 h under physiological conditions, most of the bound aflatoxin is released again as aflatoxin 2,3-dihydrodiol (*188*; see following section). The polycyclic hydrocarbon oxides and diol epoxides give adducts that are in effect substituted 2-hydroxyethylpurines, and as expected these products are stable under normal conditions. However, the reaction of benzo[*a*]pyrene 4,5-oxide or diol epoxide must also give some labile products, because nucleic acids are known to catalyze the decomposition of these agents into BP-4-phenol (*254*) and BP-tetraol (*255*), respectively. Benzo[*a*]pyrene diol epoxide is believed to attack the phosphate groups of nucleic acids (*69*), but the reaction appears to cause no chain breakage (*256*) so if phosphotriesters are formed, they must hydrolyze again with release of the hydrocarbon as BP-tetraol.

Depurination or Depyrimidination

Alkylation of the bases of DNA increases the rate at which they are spontaneously lost by hydrolysis of the base–sugar bond. The rate of loss of methylated purines from DNA has been found to be in the order 7-Me-A > 3-Me-A > 7-Me-G > 3-Me-G (*3*). Methylated pyrimidine nucleosides may also be lost; O^2-ethyldeoxycytidine and O^2-ethylthymidine lost deoxyribose on incubation at pH 7 (*257*). These compounds are very minor products of DNA alkylation, so depyrimidination is unlikely to be a significant biological event.

Apart from the methylating and ethylating agents, several other carcinogens attack DNA at 7-guanine and 3-adenine (Table I) and would therefore be expected to cause depurination. The aflatoxin–DNA adduct suffers three modes of decay in vitro: (1) loss of aflatoxin as already mentioned; (2) depurination to yield a free aflatoxin–guanine adduct; and (3) imidazole ring-opening to give a stable aflatoxin–pyrimidine adduct (*188, 258, 259*; *see* Chapter 4 in this volume):

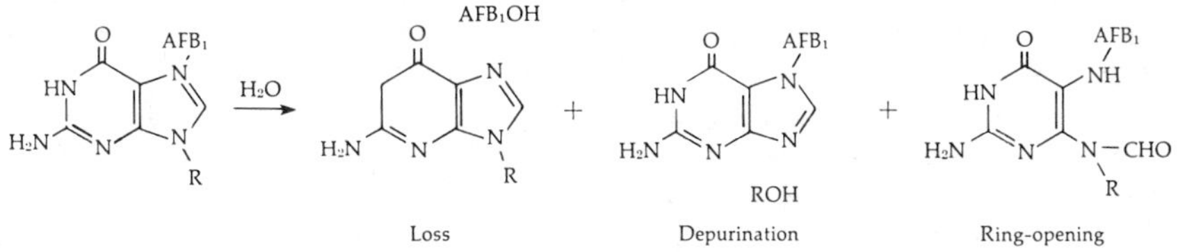

H_2O → AFB_1OH + ROH + N–CHO

Loss Depurination Ring-opening

The adducts in which guanine is substituted at O-6 or N-2 are relatively stable to breakage of the purine–sugar bond. Thus the benzo[*a*]pyrene diol epoxide–N^2-deoxyguanosine adduct has a half-life of about a year (Osborne, unpublished data). Depurination has been detected in DNA treated with this diol epoxide (*256*), but this resulted from a minor reaction at 7-guanine; the 7-guanine adduct was lost from the DNA with a half-life of 3 h (*260*). DNA reacted with AAAF, or *N*-benzoylmethylaminoazobenzene also suffers loss of purines because of previously undetected attack at 7-guanine (*87*).

Whether depurination of its DNA is harmful to the organism is not clear. DNA loses purines at a slow but measurable rate in the absence of bound carcinogens, and the resulting apurinic sites are efficiently repaired. Three mechanisms have been formulated by which an apurinic site could lead to more permanent damage:

1. Strand breakage. The 3′-phosphate group adjacent to an apurinic site in DNA is subject to ready removal by acid or alkali (*261*). How frequently apurinic sites yield single-strand breaks in vivo is not clear. Lindahl (*262*) estimated the half-life for this process at physiological pH to be 190 h, but the reaction is known to be catalyzed by amines and may be faster in vivo.
2. Mutation. Errors in repair of an apurinic site or attempts to replicate DNA on a depurinated template may lead to mutation. Shearman (*263–65*) showed that a 10% depurinated sample of DNA was replicated in vitro with an error rate of 1 in 4000. Kunkel (*265*) found that apurinic sites in bacteriophage DNA were read during replication with an increase in guanine→adenine reversion frequency; the observed rate of mutation may be sufficient to account for the mutagenicity of aflatoxin by this mechanism (*266*).
3. Cross-linkage. Depurination yields free aldehyde groups that may attack amino groups elsewhere on the DNA or on nearby proteins and result in a stable cross-link. Only 1 in 140 of the depurinations caused by methyl methanesulfonate resulted in such cross-linkage (*267*).

Removal by Enzymes

Many studies have established that alkylation products of DNA in vivo disappear faster than would be expected from their stabilities in vitro, presumably as a result of enzyme action. The absolute rates of enzymic removal are difficult to measure in vivo because (1) it is difficult to ascertain that radioactivity lost from the DNA represents truly covalently bound carcinogen; (2) some activity is lost as a result of cell death and multiplication; (3) uncertainty about intracellular conditions leads to uncertainty about the spontaneous rate of loss of alkylated bases from DNA in the absence of enzymes; and (4) rates of loss are unpredictably dose-dependent because the agent may either induce or inactivate the repair systems. For these reasons, studies of the loss of bound carcinogens from DNA have usually involved comparisons of different animals, different cell lines, different tissues, or different base adducts in order to gain some insight into the mechanism of carcinogen loss and its significance to carcinogenesis. The subject has been extensively reviewed by Roberts (*268*). Most studies have been of the loss of methyl groups from DNA. Because this work has already been well reviewed (*see* Chapter 7 in this volume and Refs. 158, 268–70), it will not be described here.

The loss from DNA of substituents other than methyl groups is not as well understood. Table IV lists papers that describe the disappearance of such adducts with time. The following general features of this research may be noted.

All the agents were subject to excision from DNA in vivo despite their diversity of structure. In experiments where animals or cells in culture were treated with an agent requiring metabolic activation, the DNA binding level followed a bell-shaped curve. The level reached a maximum several hours after application when the rate of binding was balanced by the rate of excision; the exact time after application that this maximum was reached varied for different carcinogens (*65, 300*).

Most of the adducts were excised from the DNA of mammalian cells in culture fairly rapidly at first; typically half the maximum binding level was observed after 24 h. The loss of DMBA, however, appeared to be very slow at first (*283*).

The initial rate of loss decreased with increasing dose of carcinogen, probably because the repair systems were themselves inactivated by the agent.

The loss of carcinogen adducts seldom followed first-order kinetics; the process appeared to slow down with time. In some cases, this behavior has been related to the presence of two or more adducts in the DNA which are excised at different rates. There was evidence that the disappearance of cross-links formed by sulfur and nitrogen mustards was faster than the loss of monoadducts (*275–77, 280*); these links were probably cut out at one end leaving a 7-guanylethyl group attached to the DNA. Cells treated with 7-bromomethylbenzanthracene had hydrocarbon attached to both adenine and guanine in their DNA; mammalian cells lost the adenine derivatives first (*286, 287*), but bacteria lost the guanine adducts more rapidly (*282*). Cells treated with benzo[*a*]pyrene contained adducts that resulted from alkylation of the DNA by both *anti* and *syn* isomers of benzo[*a*]-pyrene diol epoxide. Some workers found that the adducts derived from the *syn* isomer were more quickly removed (*228, 290, 291*), while other researchers, who fractionated the products still further, found that this simple conclusion was not justified (*292, 294*). Eastman (*293*) found that mammalian cells lost benzo[*a*]-pyrene–adenine products more rapidly than the guanine products.

The kinetics of removal of AAF (acetylaminofluorene; fluorenylacetamide) adducts from DNA were complex. The guanine–8-AAF adduct was lost first with a half-life of 10 h in rats (*306*). The deacetylated guanine–8-fluorenamine adduct and the guanine–N^2-AAF adduct remained longer and for this reason were presumed to have more biological importance (*47, 306*). Aflatoxin adducts are lost from the DNA spontaneously, as has already been noted. Whether the process in vivo is assisted by enzymes is not clear. The ring-opened form of the adduct is stable in DNA in vitro, and more stable than the initial adducts in vivo; it disappears slowly, presumably by enzymic excision. Again, this stability has suggested greater biological importance.

In most cases some activity was still associated with the DNA at the end of the experiment. Some alkyl groups obviously persisted in the DNA of animals for a long time, for several weeks in the case of urethane in mouse liver (*281*), DMBA in mammary tissue (*298*), dimethylaminoazobenzene in rat liver (*302*), and

Table IV

Loss of Bound Carcinogens from DNA

Carcinogen[a]	*Tissue*	*% Loss in 24 h*[b]	*Reference*
ENU	*E. coli*		*271*
ENU	Rat liver, brain	10	*272*
ENU	Hamster cells	50	*273*
ENU	Human cells	60	*274*
Mustard gas	*E. coli*	[c]	*275*
Mustard gas	Mouse cells	[c]	*276*
Mustard gas	Mouse cells	60[c]	*277*
Mustard gas	Rat cells	50	*278*
Mustard gas	Human cells	40[c]	*279*
MNM	Mouse cells	60[c]	*280*
ADNB	*E. coli*		*94*
Ethyl carbamate	Mouse liver		*281*
Ethyl carbamate	Mouse skin	60	*82*
BrMBA	*E. coli*	[d]	*282*
BrMBA	Mouse cells	50	*283, 284*
BrMBA	Mouse skin		*65*
BrMBA	Hamster cells	50	*285*
BrMBA	Hamster & human cells	70[d,e]	*286*
BrMBA	Human cells	20[d]	*287*
BrMBA	Human cells	[e]	*288*
BP	Mouse skin		*289*
BP	Mouse skin	15[d]	*121*
BP	Mouse & hamster cells	40[d]	*290*
BP	Hamster cells	[d]	*227, 291–93*
BP	Human cells	40[d]	*228*
BP/BPDE	Mouse cells	20	*294*
BPDE	Human cells	20[c]	*295*
BPDE	Human cells	50[c]	*296*
BPDE	Human cells	50	*233*
BP oxide	Human cells	80[d]	*233*
DMBA	Mouse cells	0	*284*
DMBA	Mouse skin		*289*
DMBA	Mouse skin	0[d]	*121*
DMBA	Rat intestine	0	*297*
DMBA	Rat mammary gland	0	*298*
DMBA	Rat cells	20	*299*
3MC/DBA	Mouse skin		*289, 300*
MeCPPO	Mouse		*301*
DAB	Rat liver		*302*
NQO	*E. coli*		*303*
NQO	Human cells	80	*304*
NQO	Human cells	70[c]	*305*
Nitrofurans	*E. coli*	[d]	*113*
AAF[f]	Rat cells	50[d]	*306*
AAF[f]	Rat liver	10–15	*307, 308*
AAF[f]	Rat liver	10[d]	*46, 309*

Table IV Continued

Carcinogen[a]	*Tissue*	*% Loss in 24 h*[b]	*Reference*
AAF[f]	Rat liver	70	*310*
AAF[f]	Rat liver and kidney		*311, 312*
AAF[f]	Several cells	30[e]	*313, 314*
AAF[f]	Human cells		*315, 316*
AAF[f]	Human cells	20[e]	*317*
AAAP	Rat liver		*318*
AAAP	Human cells	40[e]	*317*
Aflatoxin B_1	Trout and eggs	15	*319*
Aflatoxin B_1	Rat		*61, 140, 320*
Aflatoxin B_1	Rat and hamster	60	*321*
Aflatoxin B_1	Rat liver	50–70[d]	*322, 323*
Aflatoxin B_1	Human cells	60	*188, 324*

[a]The carcinogens used were ENU, 1-ethyl-1-nitrosourea; MNM, di(2-chloroethyl)methylamine; ADNB,5-(1-aziridino)-2,4-dinitrobenzamide; BrMBA, 7-bromomethylbenzanthracene; BP, benzo[*a*]-pyrene; BPDE, 7,8-dihydroxy-9,10-epoxy-7,8,9,10-tetrahydrobenzo[*a*]pyrene; DMBA, 7,12-dimethylbenzanthracene; 3MC, 3-methylcholanthrene; DBA, dibenzanthracene; MeCPPO, 11-methyl-15,16-dihydrocyclopenta[*a*]phenanthren-17-one; DAB, *p*-dimethylaminoazobenzene; NQO, 4-nitroquinoline 1-oxide; AAF, *N*-2-fluorenylacetamide; and AAAP, *N*-acetoxy-*N*-2-phenanthrylacetamide.
[b]Typical loss observed in the first 24 h; approximate values only.
[c]Except in Ref. 279 there was evidence that the cross-linked diguanylethane was removed faster than the rest of the bound carcinogen.
[d]Different adducts were removed at different rates. See text.
[e]Cells from xeroderma pigmentosum patients were unable to excise.
[f]AAF and its hydroxy and acetoxy derivatives. For further examples see Table III, entries marked with footnote *d*.

O^6-ethylguanine in rat brain (*272*). How this residual material differed from that which was more rapidly excised was not clear. This material may have been bound to another site on DNA, or to another region of DNA that is inaccessible to repair enzymes. Phosphotriesters resulting from alkylation of the phosphate group are stable, and their presence may be used as an assay for long-term exposure to alkylating agents (*325*). On the other hand, Feldman (*233*) and Yang (*295*) suggested that the residual activity might represent carcinogen bound to inaccessible areas of the chromatin; this suggestion is corroborated by some experiments listed in Table III that demonstrate that "active" or nuclease-accessible regions of DNA are repaired faster than "inactive" or inaccessible regions.

When mammalian cells in culture were treated with a carcinogen, removal of carcinogen adducts from the DNA was accompanied by uptake of thymidine from the medium. This finding indicated "unscheduled" DNA synthesis. Also, recovery of the viability of the cells demonstrated that the repair mechanism was essentially error-free (*295, 317*). The ability of carcinogens to stimulate DNA synthesis and the mechanisms of repair are discussed by Roberts (*268*).

Cells from patients with some variants of the disease xeroderma pigmentosum—a deficient ability to repair DNA damage caused by UV light—also lacked the ability to remove large alkyl groups from their DNA. This finding implied some commonality in the mechanisms of removal of thymine dimers caused by radiation and removal of adducts of BrMBA (*288*), benzo[*a*]pyrene (*296*), nitroquinoline oxide (*305*), or AAF (*314, 315*).

Another question is whether the carcinogenic potency of an alkylating agent depends on the ability of repair systems to remove the adducts from DNA. Adducts that survive the longest would be the most likely to cause mutation or other forms of biological damage. On the whole, the results of Table IV support this hypothesis; mammalian cells appear to be quite capable of excising the most potent carcinogens known. Individual instances have been reported in which a potent carcinogen was excised more slowly than a less potent carcinogen. The highly carcinogenic hydrocarbon DMBA remained bound to mouse cell DNA much longer than the less carcinogenic 3-methylcholanthrene or BrMBA; adducts containing dimethylbenzanthracene were postulated to be resistant to enzymic excision because of steric crowding around its point of attachment to DNA (*284*). Adducts derived from 7-bromomethyl-12-methylbenzanthracene and the less potent BrMBA were, however, lost from DNA at the same rate (*283*). The observation that adducts derived from the *syn* isomer of benzopyrene diol epoxide were lost from cellular DNA faster than those from the *anti* isomer may help to explain its lower carcinogenic potency, but the difference in rate would seem insufficient to explain the difference in potency completely. The carcinogen dibenz[*a,h*]anthracene persisted longer in mouse skin DNA than the weak or noncarcinogen dibenz[*a,c*]anthracene (*121*).

DNA Breakage

Two ways have been established to determine the ability of carcinogens to cause single-strand breakage of DNA: The first is to separate the carcinogen-bound DNA strands in alkali and then estimate the molecular weight of the single strands by ultracentrifugation or by chromatography. Any lesions in the DNA that give rise to chain breakage in alkaline solution will also be detected by this method, and the induction of strand breaks and such alkali-labile sites are therefore considered together. The other method is to treat supercoiled circular DNA with the carcinogen and observe its conversion to a relaxed open circular form that results on breakage of one strand. This technique measures the extent of single-strand breakage in the absence of alkali (*326*).

The many observations of single-strand breakage of cellular DNA following administration of carcinogens have been listed by Roberts (*268*) and Kohn (*327*). Four known mechanisms for this type of breakage are known:

1. Phosphotriesters. Alkylation at the phosphate group creates a phosphotriester that is stable at neutral pH but is readily cleaved in alkaline solution. Cleavage may either result in loss of the alkyl group or a break in the sugar–phosphate chain:

```
  nucleoside                    nucleoside                                       nucleoside
      |                             |                  O^1                           |
      O                             O                   |                            O
      |            OH^1             |                   |                            |
Alkyl—O—P=O      ------>          O—P=O     +    Alkyl—O—P=O          +     Alkyl—O—P=O
      |                             |                   |                            |
      O                             O                   O                            O^1
      |                             |                   |
  nucleoside                    nucleoside          nucleoside
                                   Loss                      Single-strand breakage
```

Table V

Induction of Breaks or Alkali-Labile Sites in DNA by Carcinogens in Vitro

Compound	*Reference*
Dimethyl sulfate	*329, 330*
Methyl methanesulfonate	*326, 330–32*
1-Methyl-1-nitrosourea	*326, 329, 333*
1-Methyl-3-nitro-1-nitrosoguanidine	*334*
Ethyl methanesulfonate	*326, 329–32*
Nitrogen mustard	*252*
N-Acetoxy-AAF	*326, 333, 335*
4-Hydroxylaminoquinoline 1-oxide	*336*
Aflatoxin B_1	*251*
7-Bromomethylbenzanthracene	*333*
Benzopyrene-diolepoxide[a]	*256, 326, 337–39*
Bleomycin	*340, 341*
1,1-Dichloroethane	*342*
1-(2-Chloroethyl)-3-*p*-cyanophenyltriazene	*343*

Note: Drinkwater (*326*) also showed that 1-ethyl-1-nitrosourea, propiolactone, 1′-acetoxyestragole and *N*-benzoyloxy-*N*-methyl-4-aminoazobenzene induced alkali-labile sites in DNA. A number of other agents, including *N*-nitrosodimethylamine, formaldehyde, bis (2-chloroethyl)urea, campothecin, mitomycin, and nitrofurans are known to induce breaks or alkali-labile sites in DNA in vivo (*268*).
[a] 7*r*,8*t*-Dihydroxy-9*t*,10*t*-epoxy-7,8,9,10-tetrahydrobenzo[*a*]pyrene.

2. Depurination. (*See* previous section. ***Depurination or Depyrimidination.***)
3. Excision. Single-strand breakage in vivo may result from enzyme action; either the chain is cut by an endonuclease preparatory to the excision of a sequence containing an alkylated base, or the alkylated base is removed by a specific glycosylase leaving an apurinic site, which may be then excised by a phosphodiesterase specific for apurinic sites (*328*).
4. Replication. In multiplying cells, gaps may be left in new DNA synthesized on an alkylated DNA template.

Table V lists alkylating agents that have been found to induce breaks or alkali-labile sites in vitro. These agents must act via phosphotriesters or depurination. The simple alkylating agents methyl and ethyl methanesulfonate acted by both mechanisms at comparable rates (*330, 331*). Shooter (*329*) showed how to distinguish the two pathways in the breakage of DNA treated with dimethyl sulfate or methyl or ethyl nitrosourea; each agent caused breaks via depurination, and the nitrosoureas also caused breaks via phosphotriester formation. DNA treated with nitrogen mustard or with derivatives such as cyclophosphamide suffers breakage in alkali; the breaks were mainly at guanine residues; therefore, depurination, rather than phosphotriester formation, was a probable mechanism (*252*).

The reactive metabolite of aflatoxin B_1 also induced cleavage of DNA at sites adjacent to guanine (*251*), as would be expected in view of the induced depurination already mentioned. The mechanism of breakage by AAF (*335*), bromomethylbenzanthracene (*333*), or benzo[*a*]pyrene diol epoxide (*256*) is less clear, because the major products from the action of these agents on DNA are not subject to ready loss. In the case of benzo[*a*]pyrene diol epoxide, the kinetics (*256*) and predominant cleavage at guanine (*339*) have indicated that loss of 7-alkylguanine, a minor product, creates alkali-labile sites, but detailed examination suggested that other mechanisms may also be operating (*337*). The strand breaks induced in DNA on incubation with 4-hydroxylaminoquinoline oxide were believed to result from free-radical reactions (*336*). Drinkwater (*326*) treated viral DNA with a wide range of alkylating carcinogens and showed that the number of alkali-labile sites induced was equal to the number of apurinic sites, except with the nitrosoureas, which acted by the phosphotriester pathway to some extent. Bleomycin (*340, 341*) causes breakage of DNA in vitro, but the mechanism is as yet unclear.

The agents listed in Table V also induce DNA single-strand breakage or the induction of alkali-labile sites in vivo. (For lists of references *see* Kohn (*327*) or Roberts (*268*).)

The presence of single-strand breaks in cellular DNA is less serious for the organism than might be imagined, because these lesions are efficiently repaired. Damjanov (*344*) found that the time needed to repair such DNA damage depended on the agent that caused the damage, but the reasons for this relation were not clear. A large number of single-strand breaks may cause permanent damage if their repair is prone to error, or if the coincidental breakage of complementary DNA strands at nearby sites results in an irreparable scission of the molecule.

Cross-linkage

If the alkyl group attached to DNA has a second reactive group, it can attack another site on DNA or on a neighboring protein and result in a DNA–DNA or DNA–protein cross-link. Of the alkylating agents listed in Tables I and II, the sulfur and nitrogen mustards, the chlorethylnitrosoureas, and formaldehyde are bifunctional and cause cross-linking in vivo (*see* Chapter 7). A number of monofunctional agents, including propiolactone and propanesultone (1,2-oxathiolane 2,2-dioxide), were also shown to cause some cross-linkage of DNA in vitro (*345*), which may occur through depurination (*see* previous section). AAAF also caused some linkage of DNA to protein; Metzger (*346*) suggested a possible mechanism for this linkage. Polycyclic aromatic groups attached to DNA may cause cross-linkage by being partially oxidized to reactive radical intermediates. It is, however, doubtful that any of these reactions play a part in the mechanism of carcinogenesis.

Template Activity In Vitro

Some understanding of the way alkylating agents can act as mutagens can be gained by study of DNA synthesis (replication) or RNA synthesis (transcription) in vitro using alkylated DNA as a template. For instance, the presence of an alkylated guanine (1) may stop synthesis (template inactivation); (2) may direct the incorporation of cytidylic acid (nonmutagenic), the incorporation of thymidylic or uridylic acid (causing a base-pair transition), or the incorporation of adenylic or guanylic acid (causing a transversion); or (3) may cause synthesis to continue elsewhere on the DNA template (producing DNA with gaps or deletions).

The evidence that methylated bases in template DNA can cause point mutations has been reviewed elsewhere (*see* Chapter 7 and Refs. 347, 348). Briefly, it appears that 7-methylguanine and N^6-methyladenine residues are nonmutagenic; that O^6-methylguanine directs the incorporation of both cytidylic and thymidylic acid; and that 3-methylcytosine and N^2-methylguanine cause random incorporation of nucleotides into the daughter nucleic acid.

Little is known about the template properties of DNA that contains other simple alkyl groups. Propiolactone-reacted DNA, which contains 7-carboxyethylguanine residues, was a poor template for RNA polymerase (*349*), and evidence that both RNA (*349*) and DNA (*350*) incorporated noncomplementary nucleotides on such a template was reported. Modification of DNA with the presumed ultimate carcinogen derived from vinyl chloride produced ethenoadenine and ethenocytosine residues; these residues directed both RNA polymerase (*351*) and DNA polymerase (*352*) to incorporate adenylic for cytidylic acid and cytidylic for adenylic acid, and thus caused transversions.

The template activity of DNA modified by large alkyl groups has been reviewed by Grunberger (*353, 354*). The presence of AAF (*355–57*), aflatoxin (*358*), or benzo[*a*]pyrene diol epoxide (*359–61*) adducts greatly diminished or abolished the priming activity of DNA.

In general, initiation of RNA or DNA synthesis is not affected by AAF (*355, 362, 363*) or benzopyrene diol epoxide (*359–61*) lesions on the template, but elongation is inhibited, and the newly synthesized nucleic acid is shorter than that produced on an unmodified template. Presumably the enzyme stops when it reaches a modified site on the template, and the new chain is spontaneously terminated. By using a primer of known sequence, Moore (*253*) has shown that termination of synthesis on both AAF and benzo[*a*]pyrene diol epoxide-modified DNA primers occurs mainly at guanine residues, as would be expected because these residues are the major sites of modification. However, Schwartz (*206*) found that DNA isolated from rats treated with AAF was not equally affected in its priming activity; one chromatin fraction was unchanged in its activity as a template for RNA polymerase.

Some evidence indicates that benzo[*a*]pyrene residues on DNA do not completely block replication or transcription at that point. Yamaura (*364*) and Leffler (*353, 360*) found that the daughter nucleic acids were longer than would be expected if each lesion caused termination of synthesis; they concluded that the enzymes had some ability to "read through" the lesion. Whether this process is error-free or causes deletions or point mutations remains to be determined; Yamaura (*364*) found no evidence that the wrong base was incorporated.

The evidence cited seems to indicate that although mutation by methylating agents may be explained on the basis of errors in replication of methylated DNA as observed in vitro, mutation by larger alkylating agents requires the intermediacy of repair systems to restore the template activity of the DNA. The process may be observed in cells in culture (*353, 354*) but is then confused by the effects of the carcinogen on the repair and replication systems as well as on the DNA itself.

Acknowledgments

The author is supported by Grant RO1 CA2580701 from the U.S. National Cancer Institute, and the Institute of Cancer Research is supported by the Medical Research Council and Cancer Research Campaign.

Literature Cited

1. Miller, J.A. *Cancer Res.* **1970**, *30*, 559.
2. Brookes, P. In "Biological Reactive Intermediates"; Jollow, D.J.; Kocsis, J.J.; Snyder, R.; Vainio, H., Eds.; Plenum: New York, 1977; p. 470.
3. Lawley, P.D.; Warren, W. *Chem.-Biol. Interact.* **1976**, *12*, 211.
4. Lawley, P.D.; Brookes, P. *Biochem. J.* **1963**, *89*, 127.
5. Singer, B. *Prog. Nucleic Acid Res. Mol. Biol.* **1975**, *15*, 219.
6. Bennett, R.A.; Pegg, A.E. *Cancer Res.* **1981**, *41*, 2786.
7. Schoental, R. *Biochem. J.* **1969**, *114*, 55P.
8. Gichner, T.; Veleminsky, J. *Mutat. Res.* **1982**, *99*, 129.
9. Rogers, K.J.; Pegg, A.E. *Cancer Res.* **1977**, *37*, 4082.
10. Lawley, P.D.; Shah, S.A.; Orr, D.J. *Chem.-Biol. Interact.* **1974**, *8*, 171.
11. Wennerberg, R.; Löfroth, G. *Chem.-Biol. Interact.* **1974**, *8*, 339.
12. Margison, G.P.; Likhachev, A.J.; Kolar, G.F. *Chem.-Biol. Interact.* **1979**, *25*, 345.
13. Kleihues, P.; Kolar, G.F.; Margison, G.P. *Cancer Res.* **1976**, *36*, 2189.
14. Skibba, J.L.; Bryan, G.T. *Toxicol. Appl. Pharmacol.* **1971**, *18*, 707.
15. Swann, P.F.; Pegg, A.E.; Hawks, A.; Farber, E.; Magee, P.N. *Biochem. J.* **1971**, *123*, 175.
16. Ribovich, M.L.; Miller, J.A.; Miller, E.C.; Timmins, L.G. *Carcinogenesis* **1982**, *3*, 539.
17. Park, K.K.; Archer, M.C.; Wishnok, J.S. *Chem.-Biol. Interact.* **1980**, *29*, 139.
18. Krüger, F.W. *Z. Krebsforsch.* **1971**, *76*, 145.
19. Scribner, J.D.; Ford, J.P. *Cancer Lett.* **1982**, *16*, 51.
20. Leung, K.H.; Park, K.K.; Archer, M.C. *Toxicol. Appl. Pharmacol.* **1980**, *53*, 29.
21. Kleihues, P.; Veit, C.; Wiessler, M.; Hodgson, R.M. *Carcinogenesis* **1981**, *2*, 897.
22. Hodgson, R.M.; Wiessler, M.; Kleihues, P. *Carcinogenesis* **1980**, *1*, 861.
23. Goldschmidt, B.M.; Frenkel, K.; Van Duuren, B.L. *J. Heterocycl. Chem.* **1974**, *11*, 719.
24. Lijinsky, W.; Keefer, L.; Loo, J.; Ross, A.E. *Cancer Res.* **1973**, *33*, 1634.
25. Green, T.; Hathway, D.E. *Chem.-Biol. Interact.* **1978**, *22*, 211.
26. Scherer, E.; Van der Laken, C.J.; Gwinner, L.M.; Laib, R.J.; Emmelot, P. *Carcinogenesis* **1981**, *2*, 671.
27. Laib, R.J.; Gwinner, L.M.; Bolt, H.M. *Chem.-Biol. Interact.* **1981**, *37*, 219.
28. Oesch, F.; Doerjer, G. *Carcinogenesis* **1982**, *3*, 663.
29. Institoris, E. *Chem.-Biol. Interact.* **1981**, *35*, 207.
30. Chen, R.; Mieyal, J.J.; Goldthwait, D.A. *Carcinogenesis* **1981**, *2*, 73.
31. Hemminki, K. *Chem.-Biol. Interact.* **1981**, *34*, 323.
32. Segal, A.; Solomon, J.J.; Mignano, J.; Dino, J. *Chem.-Biol. Interact.* **1981**, *35*, 349.
33. Chaw, Y.F.M.; Crane, L.E.; Lange, P.; Shapiro, R. *Biochemistry* **1980**, *19*, 5525.
34. Feldman, M.Y. *Prog. Nucleic Acid Res. Mol. Biol.* **1973**, *13*, 1.
35. Price, C.C.; Gaucher, G.M.; Koneru, P.; Shibakawa, R.; Sowa, J.R.; Yamaguchi, M. *Biochim. Biophys. Acta* **1968**, *166*, 327.
36. Tong, W.P.; Ludlum D.B. *Biochim. Biophys. Acta* **1980**, *608*, 174.
37. Tong, W.P.; Ludlum, D.B. *Cancer Res.* **1981**, *41*, 380.
38. Tong, W.P.; Kirk, M.C.; Ludlum, D.B. *Biochem. Biophys. Res. Commun.* **1981**, *100*, 351.
39. Gombar, C.T.; Tong, W.P.; Ludlum, D.B. *Biochem. Pharmacol.* **1980**, *29*, 2639.
40. Tong, W.P.; Kirk, M.C.; Ludlum, D.B. *Cancer Res.* **1982**, *42*, 3102.
41. Brookes, P.; Lawley, P.D. *J. Mol. Biol.* **1967**, *25*, 143.

42. Tomasz, M. *Biochim. Biophys. Acta* **1970**, *213*, 288.
43. Phillips, D.H.; Miller, J.A.; Miller, E.C.; Adams, B. *Cancer Res.* **1981**, *41*, 176.
44. Phillips, D.H.; Miller, J.A.; Miller, E.C.; Adams, B. *Cancer Res.* **1981**, *41*, 2664.
45. Zurlo, J.; Curphey, T.J.; Hiley, R.; Longnecker, D.S. *Cancer Res.* **1982**, *42*, 1286.
46. Kawazoe, Y.; Araki, M.; Huang, G.F.; Okamoto, T.; Tada, M.; Tada, M. *Chem. Pharm. Bull.* **1975**, *23*, 3041.
47. Kriek, E. In "Carcinogenesis: Fundamental Mechanisms and Environmental Effects"; Pullman, Bernard, Ts'O, P.O.P., Gelboin, H., Eds.; Reidel: Dordrecht, Netherlands, 1980; p. 103.
48. Bailleul, B.; Galiègue, S.; Loucheux-Lefebvre, M.H. *Cancer Res.* **1981**, *41*, 4559.
49. Lin, J.K.; Miller, J.A.; Miller, E.C. *Cancer Res.* **1975**, *35*, 844.
50. Beland, F.A.; Tullis, D.L.; Kadlubar, F.F.; Straub, K.M.; Evans, F.E. *Chem.-Biol. Interact.* **1980**, *31*, 1.
51. Tarpley, W.G.; Miller, J.A.; Miller, E.C. *Cancer Res.* **1980**, *40*, 2493.
52. Kadlubar, F.F.; Miller, J.A.; Miller, E.C. *Cancer Res.* **1978**, *38*, 3628.
53. Kadlubar, F.F.; Unruh, L.E.; Beland, F.A.; Straub, K.M.; Evans, F.E. *Carcinogenesis* **1980**, *1*, 139.
54. Kriek, E.; Westra, J.G. *Carcinogenesis* **1980**, *1*, 459.
55. Beland, F.A.; Allaben, W.T.; Evans, F.E. *Cancer Res.* **1980**, *40*, 834.
56. Scribner, N.K.; Scribner, J.D.; Smith, D.L.; Schram, K.H.; McCloskey, J.A. *Chem.-Biol. Interact.* **1979**, *26*, 27, 47.
57. Gaugler, B.J.M.; Neumann, H.G.; Scribner, N.K.; Scribner, J.D. *Chem.-Biol. Interact.* **1979**, *27*, 335.
58. Kriek, E. *Cancer Lett.* **1979**, *7*, 141.
59. Scribner, J.D.; Naimy, N.K. *Cancer Res.* **1975**, *35*, 1416.
60. Garner, R.C. *Br. Med. Bull.* **1980**, *36*, 47.
61. Swenson, D.H.; Lin, J.K.; Miller, E.C.; Miller, J.A. *Cancer Res.* **1977**, *37*, 172.
62. Essigmann, J.M.; Donahue, P.R.; Story, D.L.; Wogan, G.N.; Brunengraber, H. *Cancer Res.* **1980**, *40*, 4085.
63. Essigmann, J.M.; Barker, L.J.; Fowler, K.W.; Francisco, M.A.; Reinhold, V.N.; Wogan, G.N. *Proc. Natl. Acad. Sci. U.S.A.* **1979**, *76*, 179.
64. Dipple, A.; Brookes, P.; Mackintosh, D.S.; Rayman, M.P. *Biochemistry* **1971**, *10*, 4323.
65. Rayman, M.P.; Dipple, A. *Biochemistry* **1973**, *12*, 1202, 1538.
66. Hemminki, K.; Cooper, C.S.; Ribeiro, O.; Grover, P.L.; Sims, P. *Carcinogenesis* **1980**, *1*, 277, 505.
67. Osborne, M.R.; Beland, F.A.; Harvey, R.G.; Brookes, P. *Int. J. Cancer* **1976**, *18*, 362.
68. Osborne, M.R.; Jacobs, S.; Harvey, R.G.; Brookes, P. *Carcinogenesis* **1981**, *2*, 553.
69. Koreeda, M.; Moore, P.D.; Yagi, H.; Yeh, H.J.C.; Jerina, D.M. *J. Am. Chem. Soc.* **1976**, *98*, 6720.
70. Straub, K.M.; Meehan, T.; Burlingame, A.L.; Calvin, M. *Proc. Natl. Acad. Sci. U.S.A.* **1977**, *74*, 5285.
71. Ashurst, S.W.; Cohen, G.M. *Int. J. Cancer* **1981**, *27*, 357.
72. Jeffrey, A.M.; Weinstein, I.B.; Jennette, K.W.; Grzeskowiak, K.; Nakanishi, K.; Harvey, R.G.; Autrup, H.; Harris, C. *Nature (London)* **1977**, *269*, 348.
73. Jeffrey, A.M.; Blobstein, S.H.; Weinstein, I.B.; Beland, F.A.; Harvey, R.G.; Kasai, H.; Nakanishi, K. *Proc. Natl. Acad. Sci. U.S.A.* **1976**, *73*, 2311.
74. Frenkel, K.; Grunberger, D.; Kasai, H.; Komura, H.; Nakanishi, K. *Biochemistry* **1981**, *20*, 4377.
75. Abbott, P.J.; Coombs, M.M. *Carcinogenesis* **1981**, *2*, 629.
76. Wiebers, J.L.; Abbott, P.J.; Coombs, M.M.; Livingston, D.C. *Carcinogenesis* **1981**, *2*, 637.
77. Hashimoto, Y.; Shudo, K.; Okamoto, T. *Mutat. Res.* **1982**, *105*, 9.
78. Pezzuto, J.M.; Moore, P.D.; Hecht, S.M. *Biochemistry* **1981**, *20*, 298.

79. Mita, S.; Ishii, K.; Yamazoe, Y.; Kamataki, T.; Kato, R.; Sugimura, T. *Cancer Res.* **1981**, *41*, 3610.
80. Lutz, W. *Mutat. Res.* **1979**, *65*, 289.
81. Segerbäck, D. *Hereditas* **1981**, *94*, 73.
82. Pound, A.W.; Lawson, T.A. *Cancer Res.* **1976**, *36*, 1101.
83. Dahl, G.A.; Miller, J.A.; Miller, E.C. *Cancer Res.* **1978**, *38*, 3793.
84. Pound, A.W.; Franke, F.; Lawson, T.A. *Chem.-Biol. Interact.* **1976**, *14*, 149.
85. Floot, B.G.J.; Phillipus, E.J.; Scherer, E.; den Engelse, L. *Chem.-Biol. Interact.* **1978**, *21*, 331.
86. Ortlieb, H.; Kleihues, P. *Carcinogenesis* **1980**, *1*, 849.
87. Tarpley, W.G.; Miller, J.A.; Miller, E.C. *Carcinogenesis* **1982**, *3*, 81.
88. Poynter, R.W. *Biochem. Pharmacol.* **1970**, *19*, 1387.
89. Trams, E.G.; Nadkarni, M.V.; Smith, P.K. *Cancer Res.* **1961**, *21*, 560.
90. Harbers, E.; Warnecke, P.; Hollandt, H.; Kruse, K. *Z. Krebsforsch.* **1977**, *88*, 237.
91. Tew, K.D.; Taylor, D.M. *JNCI, J. Natl. Cancer Inst.* **1977**, *58*, 1413.
92. Wheeler, G.P.; Alexander, J.A. *Arch. Biochem. Biophys.* **1957**, *72*, 476.
93. Manfait, M.; Alix, A.J.P.; Butour, J.L.; Labarre, J.F.; Sournies, F. *J. Mol. Struct.* **1981**, *71*, 39.
94. Venitt, S. *Chem.-Biol. Interact.* **1971**, *3*, 177.
95. Lijinsky, W. *Prog. Nucleic Acid Res. Mol. Biol.* **1976**, *17*, 247.
96. Regan, J.D.; Setlow, R.B.; Francis, A.A.; Lijinsky, W. *Mutat. Res.* **1976**, *38*, 293.
97. Ross, A.E.; Lawson, T. *Cancer Lett.* **1982**, *15*, 329.
98. Rao, M.S.; Scarpelli, D.G., Lijinsky, W. *Carcinogenesis* **1981**, *2*, 731.
99. Lawson, T.A.; Gingell, R.; Nagel, D.; Hines, L.A.; Ross, A. *Cancer Lett.* **1981**, *11*, 251.
100. Jensen, D.E.; Magee, P.N. *Cancer Res.* **1981**, *41*, 230.
101. Gombar, C.T.; Magee, P.N. *Chem.-Biol. Interact.* **1982**, *40*, 149.
102. Roberts, J.J.; Warwick, G.P. *Int. J. Cancer* **1966**, *1*, 179.
103. Tada, M.; Takahashi, K.; Kawazoe, Y.; Ito, N. *Chem.-Biol. Interact.* **1980**, *29*, 257.
104. Martin, C.N., Eckers, S.F. *Carcinogenesis* **1980**, *1*, 101.
105. Zenser, T.V.; Mattammal, M.B.; Armbrecht, H.J.; Davis, B.B. *Cancer Res.* **1980**, *40*, 2839.
106. Black, D.N.; Jago, M.V. *Biochem. J.* **1970**, *118*, 347.
107. Sonnenbichler, J.; Reichhart, F. *Z. Krebsforsch.* **1978**, *91*, 55.
108. Zedeck, M.S.; Brown, G.B. *Cancer* **1977**, *40*, 2580.
109. Skipper, P.L.; Tannenbaum, S.R.; Thilly, W.G.; Furth, E.E.; Bishop, W.W. *Cancer Res.* **1980**, *40*, 4704.
110. Scribner, J.D.; Koponen, G.; Fisk, S.R.; Woodworth, B. *Cancer Lett.* **1980**, *9*, 117.
111. Gniazdowski, M.; Ciesielska, E.; Szmigiero, L. *Chem.-Biol. Interact.* **1981**, *34*, 355.
112. Messier, F.; Lu, C.; Andrews, P.; McCarry, B.E.; Quilliam, M.A.; McCalla, D.R. *Carcinogenesis* **1981**, *2*, 1007.
113. Wentzell, B.; McCalla, D.R. *Chem.-Biol. Interact.* **1980**, *31*, 133.
114. Guengerich, P.F. *Biochem. Pharmacol.* **1977**, *26*, 1909.
115. Munsch, N.; Marano, F.; Frayssinet, C. *Biochimie* **1974**, *56*, 1433.
116. Nery, R.; Nice, E. *J. Pharm. Pharmacol.* **1971**, *23*, 842.
117. Nagawa, Y.; Hiraga, K.; Suga, T. *Biochem. Pharmacol.* **1980**, *29*, 1304.
118. Lutz, W.K.; Schlatter, C. *Chem.-Biol. Interact.* **1977**, 18, *241*.
119. Gill, D.P.; Ahmed, A.E. *Biochem. Pharmacol.* **1981**, *30*, 1127.
120. Lin, S.S.; Dao, T.L. *Proc. Soc. Exp. Biol. Med.* **1971**, *138*, 814.
121. Phillips, D.H.; Grover, P.L.; Sims, P. *Int. J. Cancer* **1978**, *22*, 487.
122. Baird, W.M.; Dipple, A.; Grover, P.L.; Sims, P.; Brookes, P. *Cancer Res.* **1973**, *33*, 2386.

123. Tierney, B.; Hewer, A.; Walsh, C.; Grover, P.L.; Sims, P. *Chem.-Biol. Interact.* **1977**, *18*, 179.
124. Cooper, C.S.; Ribeiro, O.; Hewer, A.; Walsh, C.; Grover, P.L.; Sims, P. *Chem.-Biol. Interact.* **1980**, *29*, 357.
125. King, H.W.S.; Osborne, M.R.; Brookes, P. *Int. J. Cancer* **1977**, *20*, 564.
126. Melikian, A.A.; LaVoie, E.J.; Hecht, S.S.; Hoffmann, D.; Wynder, E.L. *Proc. Am. Assoc. Cancer Res.* **1981** abstr. 333.
127. Dock, L.; Undeman, O.; Graslund, A.; Jernstrom, B. *Biochem. Biophys. Res. Commun.* **1978**, *85*, 1275.
128. Owens, I.S.; Legraverend, C.; Pelkonen, O. *Biochem. Pharmacol.* **1979**, *28*, 1623.
129. King, H.W.S.; Thompson, M.H.; Brookes, P. *Int. J. Cancer* **1976**, *18*, 339.
130. Tay, L.K.; Sydnor, K.L.; Flesher, J.W. *Chem.-Biol. Interact.* **1979**, *25*, 35.
131. Baird, W.M.; Harvey, R.G.; Brookes, P. *Cancer Res.* **1975**, *35*, 54.
132. Perin-Roussel, O.; Ekert, B.; Zajdela, F.; Jacquignon, P. *Cancer Res.* **1978**, *38*, 3499.
133. Zachariah, P.K.; Slaga, T.; Berry, D.L.; Bracken, W.M.; Buty, S.G.; Martinsen, C.M.; Juchau, M.R. *Cancer Lett.* **1977**, *3*, 99.
134. Jaggi, W.; Lutz, W.K.; Schlatter, C. *Chem.-Biol. Interact.* **1978**, *23*, 13.
135. Blackburn, G.M.; Orgee, L.; Williams, G.M. *J. Chem. Soc., Chem. Commun.* **1977**, 386.
136. Tsibris, J.C.M.; McGuire, P.M. *Biochem. Biophys. Res. Commun.* **1977**, *78*, 411.
137. Pelkonen, O.; Boobis, A.R.; Nebert, D.W. "Polynuclear aromatic hydrocarbons"; Jones, Peter W.; Freudenthal, Ralph I., Eds.; Raven: New York, 1978; p. 383.
138. Duncan, S.j.; Brookes, P.; *Cancer Lett.* **1979**, *6*, 351.
139. Bolt, H.M.; Kappus, H. *J. Steroid Biochem.* **1974**, *5*, 179.
140a. Blackburn, G.M., Thompson, M.H., King, H.W.S. *Biochem. J.* **1976**, *158*, 643.
140b. Lijinsky, W.; Lee, K.Y.; Gallagher, C.H. *Cancer Res.* **1970**, *30*, 2280.
141. Djalali-Behzad, G.; Hussain, S.; Osterman-Golkar, S.; Segerback, D. *Mutat. Res.* **1981**, *84*, 1.
142. Rocchi, P.; Prodi, G.; Grilli, S.; Ferreri, A.M. *Int. J. Cancer* **1973**, *11*, 419.
143. Gomez, M.I.D.; Castro, J.A. *Toxicol. Appl. Pharmacol.* **1980**, *56*, 199.
144. Banerjee, S.; Van Duuren, B.L. *Cancer Res.* **1978**, *38*, 776.
145. Banerjee, S.; Van Duuren, B.L.; Oruambo, F.I. *Cancer Res.* **1980**, *40*, 2170.
146. Hill, D.L.; Shih, T.W.; Johnston, T.P.; Struck, R.F. *Cancer Res.* **1978**, *38*, 2438.
147. Morales, N.M.; Matthews, H.B. *Chem.-Biol. Interact.* **1979**, *27*, 99.
148. Narbonne, J.F.; Daubeze, M. *Toxicology* **1980**, *16*, 173.
149. Tomasz, M.; Lipman, R. *Biochemistry* **1981**, *20*, 5056.
150. Hunt, E.J.; Shank, R.C. *Biochem. Biophys. Res. Commun.* **1982**, *104*, 1343.
151. Chung, F.L.; Hecht, S.S. *Proc. Am. Assoc. Cancer Res.* **1982**, *23*, 249.
152. Ashurst, S.W.; Cohen, G.M. *Carcinogenesis* **1982**, *3*, 267.
153. Nagata, C.; Kodama, M.; Kimura, T.; Aida, M. In "Carcinogenesis: Fundamental Mechanisms and Environmental Effects"; Pullman, B.; Ts'o, P.O.P.; Gelboin, H., Eds.; Reidel: Dordrecht, Netherlands, 1980; p. 43.
154. Demopoulos, H.B.; Pietronigro, D.D.; Flamm, E.S.; Seligman, M.L. *J. Environ. Pathol. Toxicol.* **1980**, *3*, 273.
155. Magee, P.N.; Montesano, R.; Preussmann, R. "Chemical Carcinogens," Searle, C.E., Ed.; ACS MONOGRAPH SERIES No. 173, ACS: Washington, D.C., 1976; p. 491.
156. Olah, G.A.; Donovan, D.J.; Keefer, L.K. *JNCI, J. Natl. Cancer Inst.* **1975**, *54*, 465.
157. Loeppky, R.N.; Christiansen, R. In "Environmental Aspects of N-Nitroso Compounds"; Walker, E.A.; Castegnaro, M.; Griciute, L.; Lyle, R.E., Eds.; IARC: Lyon, 1978; p. 117.
158. Margison, G.P.; O'Connor, P.J. In "Chemical Carcinogens and DNA"; Grover, P.L., Ed.; CRC: Boca Raton, 1979; Vol. 1, p. 111.
159. Buglass, A.J.; Challis, B.C.; Osborne, M.R. In "N-Nitroso Compounds in the Environ-

ment"; Bogovski, P.; Walker, E.A., Eds.; International Agency for Research on Cancer: Lyon, 1974; p. 94.
160. Singer, S.S.; Lijinsky, W.; Singer, G.M. In "Environmental Aspects of N-Nitroso Compounds"; Walker, E.A.; Castegnaro, M.; Griciute, L.; Lyle, R.E., Eds.; IARC: Lyon, 1978; p. 175.
161. Thompson, M.H.; Osborne, M.R.; King, H.W.S.; Brookes, P. *Chem.-Biol. Interact.* **1976**, *14*, 13.
162. King, H.W.S.; Thompson, M.H.; Brookes, P. *Cancer Res.* **1975**, *35*, 1263.
163. Blackburn, G.M.; Rashid, A.; Thompson, M.H. *J. Chem. Soc., Chem. Commun.* **1979**, 420.
164. Shah, H.; Hartman, S.P.; Weinhouse, S. *Cancer Res.* **1979**, *39*, 3942.
165. Gomez, M.I.D.; Castro, J.A. *Cancer Lett.* **1980**, *9*, 213.
166. Gold, B.; Leuchen, T.; Brunk, G.; Gingell, R. *Chem.-Biol. Interact.* **1981**, *35*, 159.
167. Planche, G.; Croisy, A.; Malaveille, C.; Tomatis, L.; Bartsch, H. *Chem.-Biol. Interact.* **1979**, *25*, 157.
168. Poland, A.; Glover, E. *Cancer Res.* **1979**, *39*, 3341.
169. Culvenor, C.C.J.; Jago, M.V. In "Chemical Carcinogens and DNA"; Grover, P.L., Ed.; Chemical Rubber Company: Boca Raton, FL, 1979; Vol. 1, p. 161.
170. Schoental, R. *Nature (London)* **1970**, *227*, 401.
171. Robertson, K.A. *Cancer Res.* **1982**, *42*, 8.
172. Hurley, L.H.; Gairola, C.; Zmijewsky, M. *Biochem. Biophys. Acta* **1977**, *475*, 521.
173. Chidester, C.G.; Krueger, W.C.; Mizsak, S.A.; Duchamp, D.J.; Martin, D.G. *J. Am. Shem. Soc.* **1981**, *103*, 7629.
174. Li, L.H.; Swenson, D.H.; Schpok, S.L.F.; Kuentzel, S.L.; Dayton, B.D.; Krueger, W.C. *Cancer Res.* **1982**, *42*, 999.
175. Guengerich, F.P.; Geiger, L.E.; Hogy, L.L.; Wright, P.L. *Cancer Res.***1981**, *41*, 4925.
176. Dipple, A.; Levy, L.S.; Lawley, P.D. *Carcinogenesis* **1981**, *2*, 103.
177. Smith, I.A.; Berger, G.D.; Seybold, P.G.; Servé, M.P. *Cancer Res.* **1978**, *38*, 2968.
178. Osborne, M.R. *Cancer Res.* **1979**, *39*, 4760.
179. Loew, G.; Poulsen, M.; Ferrell, J.; Chaet, D. *Chem.-Biol. Interact.* **1980**, *31*, 319.
180. Hsu, W.T.; Lin, E.J.; Fu, P.P.; Harvey, R.G.; Weiss, S.B. *Biochem. Biophys. Res. Commun.* **1979**, *88*, 251.
181. Blobstein, S.H.; Weinstein, B.; Grunberger, D.; Weisgras, J.; Harvey, R.G. *Biochemistry* **1975**, *14*, 3451.
182. Kasai, H.; Nakanishi, K.; Frenkel, K.; Grunberger, D. *J. Am. Chem. Soc.* **1977**, *99*, 8500.
183. Nakanishi, K.; Komura, H.; Miura, I.; Kasai, H.; Frenkel, K.; Grunberger, D. *J. Chem. Soc., Chem. Commun.* **1980**, 82.
184. Moschel, R.C.; Hudgins, W.R.; Dipple, A. *J. Org. Chem.* **1979**, *44*, 3324.
185. Pullman, B.; Pullman, A. In "Carcinogenesis: Fundamental Mechanisms and Environmental Effects"; Pullman, B.; Ts'o, P.O.P.; Gelboin, H., Eds.; Reidel: Dordrecht, Netherlands, 1980; p. 55.
186. Scribner, J.D.; Fisk, S.R. *Tetrahedron Lett.* **1978**, *48*, 4759.
187. Ornstein, R.L.; Rein, R. *Chem.-Biol. Interact.* **1980**, *30*, 87.
188. Cerutti, P.A.; Wang, V.T.; Amstad, P. In "Carcinogenesis: Fundamental Mechanisms and Environmental Effects"; Pullman, B.; Ts'o, P.O.P.; Gelboin, H., Eds.; Reidel: Dordrecht, Netherlands, 1980; p. 465.
189. Stark, A.A.; Essigmann, J.M.; Demain, A.L.; Skopek, T.R.; Wogan, G.N. *Proc. Natl. Acad. Sci. U.S.A.* **1979**, *76*, 1343.
190. Stark, A.A. *Annu. Rev. Microbiol.* **1980**, *34*, 235.
191. Fahmy, O.G., Fahmy, M.J. *Cancer Res.* **1972**, *32*, 550.
192. Wunderlich, V.; Schütt, M.; Böttger, M.; Graffi, A. *Biochem. J.* **1970**, *118*, 99.

193. Wunderlich, V.; Tetzlaff, I.; Graffi, A. *Chem.-Biol. Interact.* **1971**, *4*, 81.
194. Wilkinson, R.; Hawks, A.; Pegg, A.E. *Chem.-Biol. Interact.* **1975**, *10*, 157.
195. Allen, J.A.; Coombs, M.M. *Nature (London)* **1980**, *287*, 244.
196. Backer, J.M.; Weinstein, I.B. *Science (Washington, D.C.)* **1980**, *209*, 297.
197. Niranjan, B.G.; Bhat, N.; Avadhani, N.G. *Science (Washington, D.C.)* **1982**, *215*, 73.
198. Flamm, W.G.; Bernheim, N.J.; Spalding, J. *Biochim. Biophys. Acta* **1969**, *195*, 273.
199. Zeiger, R.S.; Salomon, R.; Kinoshita, N.; Peacock, A.C. *Cancer Res.* **1972**, *32*, 643.
200. Bodell, W.J.; Banerjee, M.R. *Nucleic Acids Res.* **1976**, *3*, 1689.
201. Emminki, K.; Vainio, H. *Cancer Lett.* **1979**, *6*, 167.
202. Scudiero, D.; Strauss, B. *Mutat. Res.* **1976**, *35*, 311.
203. Moses, H.L.; Webster, R.A.; Martin, G.D.; Spelsberg, T.C. *Cancer Res.* **1976**, *36*, 2905.
204. Moyer, G.H.; Gumbiner, B.; Austin, G.E. *Cancer Lett.* **1977**, *2*, 259.
205. Schwartz, E.L.; Goodman, J.I. *Chem.-Biol. Interact.* **1979**, *26*, 287.
206. Schwartz, E.L.; Goodman, J.I. *Chem.-Biol. Interact.* **1979**, *27*, 1.
207. Walker, M.S.; Becker, F.F.; Rodriguez, L.V. *Chem.-Biol. Interact.* **1979**, *27*, 177.
208. Schwartz, E.L.; Braselton, W.E.; Goodman, J.I. *JNCI, J. Natl. Cancer Inst.* **1981**, *66*, 667.
209. Faustman, E.M.; Goodman, J.I. *Toxicol. Appl. Pharmacol.* **1981**, *58*, 379.
210. Cooper, H.K.; Margison, G.P.; O'Connor, P.J.; Itzhaki, R.F. *Chem.-Biol. Interact.* **1975**, *11*, 483.
211. Galbraith, A.; Barker, M.; Itzhaki, R.F. *Biochim. Biophys. Acta* **1979**, *561*, 334.
212. Ramanathan, R.; Rajalakshmi, S.; Sarma, D.S.R.; Farber, E. *Cancer Res.* **1976**, *36*, 2073.
213. Ramanathan, R.; Rajalakshmi, S.; Sarma, D.S.R. *Chem.-Biol. Interact.* **1976**, *14*, 375.
214. Metzger, G.; Wilhelm, F.X.; Wilhelm, M.L. *Biochem. Biophys. Res. Commun.* **1977**, *75*, 703.
215. Jahn, C.L.; Litman, G.W. *Biochem. Biophys. Res. Commun.* **1977**, *76*, 534.
216. Jahn, C.L.; Litman, G.W. *Biochemistry* **1979**, *18*, 1442.
217. Pegg, A.E.; Hui, G. *Cancer Res.* **1978**, *38*, 2011.
218. Cox, R. *Cancer Res.* **1979**, *39*, 2675.
219. Berkowitz, E.M.L.; Silk, H. *Cancer Lett.* **1981**, *12*, 311.
220. Arrand, J.E.; Murray, A.M. *Nucleic Acids Res.* **1982**, *10*, 1547.
221. Tew, K.D.; Sudhakar, S.; Schein, P.S.; Smulson, M.E. *Cancer Res.* **1978**, *38*, 3371.
222. Nose, K. *Cancer Lett.* **1981**, *14*, 205.
223. Metzger, G.; Wilhelm, F.X.; Wilhelm, M.L. *Chem.-Biol. Interact.* **1976**, *15*, 257.
224. Kaneko, M.; Cerutti, P.A. *Cancer Res.* **1980**, *40*, 4313.
225. Wiesehahn, G.P.; Hyde, J.E.; Hearst, J.E. *Biochemistry* **1977**, *16*, 925.
226. Cech, T.; Pardue, M.L. *Cell* **1977**, *11*, 631.
227. Baird, W.M.; Dumaswala, R.U. In "Polynuclear Aromatic Hydrocarbons: Chemistry and Biological Effects"; Bjorseth, A.; Dennis, A.J., Eds.; Battelle: Columbus, 1980; p. 471.
228. Feldman, G.; Remsen, J.; Shinohara, K.; Cerutti, P. *Nature (London)* **1978**, *274*, 796.
229. Jack, P.L.; Brookes, P. *Nucleic Acids Res.* **1981**, *9*, 5533.
230. Yamasaki, H.; Roush, T.W.; Weinstein, I.B. *Chem.-Biol. Interact.* **1978**, *23*, 201.
231. Kootstra, A.; Slaga, T.J.; Olins, D.E. *Chem.-Biol. Interact.* **1979**, *28*, 225.
232. Kootstra, A.; Slaga, T.J. *Biochem. Biophys. Res. Commun.* **1980**, *93*, 954.
233. Feldman, G.; Remsen, J.; Wang, T.V.; Cerutti, P. *Biochemistry* **1980**, *19*, 1095.
234. Oleson, F.B.; Mitchell, B.L.; Dipple, A.; Lieberman, M.W. *Nucleic Acids Res.* **1979**, *7*, 1343.
235. Bailey, G.S.; Nixon, J.E.; Hendricks, J.D.; Sinnhuber, R.O.; Van Holde, K.E. *Biochemistry* **1980**, *19*, 5836.
236. Galbraith, A.I.; Chapleo, M.R.: Itzhaki, R.F. *Nucleic Acids Res.* **1978**, *5*, 3357.
237. Chang, M.J.W.; Webb, T.E.; Koestner, A. *Cancer Lett.* **1979**, *6*, 123.
238. Shoyab, M. *Proc. Natl. Acad. Sci. U.S.A.* **1978**, *75*, 5841.

239. Jack, P.L.; Brookes, P. *Int. J. Cancer* **1980**, *25*, 789.
240. Iyer, R.; Triplett, L.L.; Slaga, T.J.; Papaconstaninou, J. "Abstracts of Papers," 176th Natl. Meeting, ACS, 1978, Biol. 103.
241. McGhee, J.D.; Felsenfeld, G. *Proc. Natl. Acad. Sci. U.S.A.* **1979**, *76*, 2133.
242. Pulkrabek, P.; Leffler, S.; Grunberger, D.; Weinstein, I.B. *Biochemistry* **1979**, *18*, 5128.
243. Mengle, L.; Gamper, H.; Bartholomew, J. *Cancer Lett.* **1978**, *5*, 131.
244. Beard, P.; Kaneko, M.; Cerutti, P.A. *Nature (London)* **1981**, *291*, 84.
245. Lang, M.C.; Murcia, G.; Mazen, A.; Fuchs, R.P.P., Leng, M.; Daune, M. *Chem.-Biol. Interact.* **1982**, *41*, 83.
246. Niranjan, B.G.; Avadhani, N.G. *J. Biol. Chem.* **1980**, *255*, 6575.
247. Wilkie, D.; Egilsson, V.; Evans, I.H. *Lancet* **1975**, *i*, 697.
248. John, B.; Miklos, G.L.G. *Int. Rev. Cytol.* **1979**, *58*, 1.
249. Garel, A.; Axel, R. *Proc. Natl. Acad. Sci. U.S.A.* **1976**, *73*, 3966.
250. Gotoh, O.; Wada, A.; Tada, M.; Tada, M. *Gann* **1978**, *69*, 61.
251. D'Andrea, A.D.; Haseltine, W.A. *Proc. Natl. Acad. Sci. U.S.A.* **1978**, *75*, 4120.
252. Grunberg, S.M.; Haseltine, W.A. *Proc. Natl. Acad. Sci. U.S.A.* **1980**, *77*, 6546.
253. Moore, P.; Strauss, B.S. *Nature (London)* **1979**, *278*, 664.
254. Murray, A.W.; Grover, P.L.; Sims, P. *Chem.-Biol. Interact.* **1976**, *13*, 57.
255. Geacintov, N.E.; Ibanez, V.; Gagliano, A.G.; Yoshida, H.; Harvey, R.G. *Biochem. Biophys. Res. Commun.* **1980**, *92*, 1335.
256. Shooter, K.V.; Osborne, M.R.; Harvey, R.G. *Chem.-Biol. Interact.* **1977**, *19*, 215.
257. Singer, B.; Kröger, M.; Carrano, M. *Biochemistry* **1978**, *17*, 1246.
258. Wang, T.V.; Cerutti, P. *Biochemistry* **1980**, *19*, 1692.
259. Groopman, J.D.; Croy, R.G.; Wogan, G.N. *Proc. Nat. Acad. Sci. U.S.A.* **1981**, *78*, 5445.
260. King, H.W.S.; Osborne, M.R.: Brookes, P. *Chem.-Biol. Interact.* **1979**, *24*, 345.
261. Lawley, P.D. *Prog. Nucleic Acid Res. Mol. Biol.* **1966**, *5*, 89.
262. Lindahl, T.; Andersson, A. *Biochemistry* **1972**, *11*, 3618.
263. Shearman, C.W.; Loeb, L.A. *Nature (London)* **1977**, *270*, 537.
264. Shearman, C.W.; Loeb, L.A. *J. Mol. Biol.* **1979**, *128*, 197.
265. Kunkel, T.A.; Shearman, C.W.; Loeb, L.A. *Nature (London)* **1981**, *291*, 349.
266. Schaaper, R.M.; Loeb, L.A. *Proc. Natl. Acad. Sci. U.S.A.* **1981**, *78*, 1773.
267. Burnotte, J.; Verly, W.G. *Biochim. Biophys. Acta* **1972**, *262*, 449.
268. Roberts, J.J. *Adv. Radiat. Biol.* **1978**, *7*, 211.
269. Pegg, A.E. *Adv. Cancer Res.* **1977**, *25*, 195.
270. Laval, J.; Laval, F. In "Molecular and Cellular Aspects of Carcinogen Screening Tests"; Montesano, R.; Bartsch, H.; Tomatis, L., Eds.; IARC: Lyon, 1980; p. 55.
271. Lawley, P.D.; Warren, W. *Chem.-Biol. Interact.* **1975**, *11*, 55.
272. Goth, R.; Rajewsky, M.F. *Proc. Natl. Acad. Sci. U.S.A.* **1974**, *71*, 639.
273. Goth-Goldstein, R. *Cancer Res.* **1980**, *40*, 2623.
274. Goth-Goldstein, R. *Nature (London)* **1977**, *267*, 81.
275. Lawley, P.D.; Brookes, P. *Nature (London)* **1965**, *206*, 480.
276. Walker, I.G. *Can. J. Biochem.* **1971**, *49*, 332.
277. Reid, B.D.; Walker, I.G. *Biochim. Biophys. Acta* **1969**, *179*, 179.
278. Ball, C.R.; Roberts, J.J. *Chem.-Biol. Interact.* **1970**, *2*, 321.
279. Crathorn, A.R.; Roberts, J.J. *Nature (London)* **1966**, *211*, 150.
280. Yin, L.; Chun, E.H.L.; Rutman, R.J. *Biochim. Biophys. Acata* **1973**, *324*, 472.
281. Lawson, T.A.; Pound, A.W. *Eur. J. Cancer* **1973**, *9*, 491.
282. Venitt, S.; Tarmy, E.M. *Biochim. Biophys. Acta* **1972**, *287*, 38.
283. Dipple, A.; Schultz, E. *Cancer Lett.* **1979**, *7*, 103.
284. Dipple, A.; Hayes, M.E. *Biochem. Biophys. Res. Commun.* **1979**, *91*, 1225.
285. Friedlos, F.; Roberts, J.J. *Nucleic Acids Res.* **1978**, *5*, 4795.
286. McCaw, B.A.: Dipple, A.; Young, S.; Roberts, J.J. *Chem.-Biol. Interact.* **1978**, *22*, 139.

287. Lieberman, M.W.; Dipple, A. *Cancer Res.* **1972**, *32*, 1855.
288. Slor, H. *Mutat. Res.* **1973**, *19*, 231.
289. Brookes, P.; Lawley, P.D. *Nature (London)* **1964**, *202*, 781.
290. Shinohara, K.; Cerutti, P.A. *Proc. Natl. Acad. Sci. U.S.A.* **1977**, *74*, 979.
291. Baird, W.M.; Diamond, L. *Biochem. Biophys. Res. Commun.* **1977**, *77*, 162.
292. Ivanovic, V.; Geacintov, N.E.: Yamasaki, H.; Weinstein, I.B. *Biochemistry* **1978**, *17*, 1597.
293. Eastman, A.; Mossman, B.T.; Bresnick, E. *Cancer Res.* **1981**, *41*, 2605.
294. Brown, H.S.; Jeffrey, A.M.; Weinstein, I.B. *Cancer Res.* **1979**, *39*, 1673.
295. Yang, L.L.; Maher, V.M.; McCormick, J.J. *Proc. Natl. Acad. Sci. U.S.A.* **1980**, *77*, 5933.
296. Day, R.S.; Scudiero, D.; Dimattina, M. *Mutat. Res.* **1978**, *50*, 383.
297. Marquardt, H.; Phillips, F.S.; Bendich, A. *Cancer Res.* **1972**, *32*, 1810.
298. Janss, D.H.; Moon, R.C.; Irving, C.C. *Cancer Res.* **1972**, *32*, 254.
299. Tay, L.K.; Russo, J. *Carcinogenesis* **1981**, *2*, 1327.
300. Phillips, D.H.; Grover, P.L.; Sims, P. *Int. J. Cancer* **1979**, *23*, 201.
301. Abbott, P.J.; Crew, F. *Cancer Res.* **1981**, *41*, 4115.
302. Warwick, G.P.; Roberts, J.J. *Nature (London)* **1967**, *213*, 1206.
303. Ikenaga, M.; Ichikawa-Ryo, H.; Kondo, S. *J. Mol. Biol.* **1975**, *92*, 341.
304. Watanabe, M.; Horikawa, M. *Mutat. Res.* **1975**, *28*, 295.
305. Ikenaga, M.; Takebe, H.; Ishii, Y. *Mutat. Res.* **1977**, *43*, 415.
306. Howard, P.C.; Casciano, D.A.: Beland, F.A.; Shaddock, J.G. *Carcinogenesis* **1981**, *2*, 97.
307. Irving, C.C.; Veazey, R.A. *Cancer Res.* **1969**, *29*, 1799.
308. Witschi, H.; Epstein, S.M.; Farber, E. *Cancer Res.* **1971**, *31*, 270.
309. Kriek, E. *Cancer Res.* **1972**, *32*, 2042.
310. Szafarz, D.; Weisburger, J.H. *Cancer Res.* **1969**, *29*, 962.
311. Poirier, M.C.; True, B.A.; Laishes, B.A. *Cancer Res.* **1982**, *42*, 1317.
312. Beland, F.A.; Dooley, K.L.; Jackson, C.D. *Cancer Res.* **1982**, *42*, 1348.
313. Amacher, D.E.; Lieberman, M.W. *Biochem. Biophys. Res. Commun.* **1977**, *74*, 285.
314. Amacher, D.E.; Elliott, J.A.; Lieberman, M.W. *Proc. Natl. Acad. Sci. U.S.A.* **1977**, *74*, 1553.
315. Ahmed, F.E.; Setlow, R.B. *Proc. Natl. Acad. Sci. U.S.A.* **1977**, *74*, 1548.
316. Scudiero, D.; Norin, A.; Karran, P.; Strauss, B. *Cancer Res.* **1976**, *36*, 1397.
317. Heflich, R.H.; Hazard, R.M.; Lommel, L.; Scribner, J.D.; Maher, V.M.; McCormick, J.J. *Chem.-Biol. Interact.* **1980**, *29*, 43.
318. Scribner, J.D.; Koponen, G. *Chem.-Biol. Interact.* **1979**, *28*, 201.
319. Croy, R.G.; Nixon, J.E.: Sinnhuber, R.O.; Wogan, G.N. *Carcinogenesis* **1980**, *1*, 903.
320. Bennett, R.A.; Essigmann, J.M.; Wogan, G.N. *Cancer Res.* **1981**, *41*, 650.
321. Garner, R.C.; Wright, C.M. *Chem.-Biol. Interact.* **1975**, *11*, 123.
322. Croy, R.G.; Wogan, G.N. *Cancer Res.* **1981**, *41*, 197.
323. Hertzog, P.J.; Smith, J.R.L.; Garner, R.C. *Carcinogenesis* **1980**, *1*, 787.
324. Wang, T.V.; Cerutti, P.A. *Cancer Res.* **1979**, *39*, 5165.
325. Shooter, K.V. *Nature (London)* **1978**, *274*, 612.
326. Drinkwater, N.R.; Miller, E.C.; Miller, J.A. *Biochemistry* **1980**, *19*, 5087.
327. Kohn, K.W. *Methods Cancer Res.* **1975**, *16*, 291.
328. Kirtikar, D.M.; Goldthwait, D.A. *Proc. Natl. Acad. Sci. U.S.A.* **1974**, *71*, 2022.
329. Shooter, K.V.; Merrifield, R.K. *Chem.-Biol. Interact.* **1976**, *13*, 223.
330. Strauss, B.; Hill, T. *Biochim. Biophys. Acta* **1970**, *213*, 14.
331. Rhaese, H.J.; Freese, E. *Biochim. Biophys. Acta* **1969**, *190*, 418.
332. Snyder, R.D.; Regan, J.D. *Mutat. Res.* **1981**, *91*, 307.
333. Thielmann, H.W. *Z. Krebsforsch.* **1977**, *90*, 37.
334. Mizusawa, H.; Tanaka, S.; Kobayashi, M.; Koike, K. *Biochem. Biophys. Res. Commun.* **1977**, *74*, 570.

335. Deering, R.A.; Taylor, W.D.; Burns, L.R. *Biophys. J.* **1975**, *15*, 181.
336. Nagao, M.; Sugimura, T. *Adv. Cancer Res.* **1976**, *23*, 131.
337. Gamper, H.B.: Straub, K.; Calvin, M.; Bartholomew, J.C. *Proc. Natl. Acad. Sci. U.S.A.* **1980**, *77*, 2000.
338. Kakefuda, T.; Mizusawa, H.; Lee, C.H.R.; Madigan, P.; Feldman, R.J. In "Carcinogenesis: Fundamental Mechanisms and Environmental Effects"; Pullman, B.; Ts'o, P.O.P.; Gelboin, H., Eds.; Reidel: Dordrecht, Netherlands, 1980; p. 389.
339. Haseltine, W.A.; Lo, K.M.; d'Andrea, A.D. *Science (Washington, D.C.)* **1980**, *209*, 929.
340. "Fundamental and Clinical Studies of Bleomycin"; Carter, S.K.; Ichikawa, T.; Mathé, G.; Umezawa, H., Eds.; Univ. of Tokyo: Tokyo, 1976.
341. Garner, R.C.; Martin, C.N. In "Chemical Carcinogens and DNA"; Grover, P.L., Ed.; Chemical Rubber Co.: Boca Raton, 1979; Vol. 1, p. 187.
342. Waskell, L. *Mutat. Res.* **1978**, *57*, 141.
343. Lown, J.W.; Singh, R. *Biochem. Pharmacol.* **1982**, *31*, 1257.
344. Damjanov, I.; Cox, R.; Sarma, D.S.R.; Farber, E. *Cancer Res.* **1973**, *33*, 2122.
345. Morin, N.R.; Zeldin, P.E.; Kubinski, Z.O.; Bhattacharya, P.K.; Kubinski, H. *Cancer Res.* **1977**, *37*, 3802.
346. Metzger, G.; Werbin, H. *Biochemistry* **1979**, *18*, 655.
347. Singer, B.; Kröger, M. *Prog. Nucleic Acid Res. Mol. Biol.* **1979**, *23*, 151.
348. Singer, B. In "Carcinogenesis: Fundamental Mechanisms and Environmental Effects"; Pullman, B.; Ts's, P.O.P.; Gelboin, H., Eds.; Reidel: Dordrecht, Netherlands, 1980; p. 91.
349. Troll, W.; Rinde, E.; Day, P. *Biochim. Biophys. Acta* **1969**, *174*, 211.
350. Sirover, M.A.; Loeb, L.A. *Nature (London)* **1974**, *252*, 414.
351. Spengler, S.; Singer, B. *Nucleic Acids Res.* **1981**, *9*, 365.
352. Barbin, A.; Bartsch, H.; Leconte, P.; Radman, M. *Nucleic Acids Res.* **1981**, *9*, 375.
353. Grunberger, D.; Weinstein, I.B. *Prog. Nucleic Acid Res. Mol. Biol.* **1979**, *23*, 105.
354. Grunberger, D.; Weinstein, I.B. In "Chemical Carcinogens and DNA"; Grover, P.L., Ed.; Chemical Rubber Co.: Boca Raton, 1979; Vol. 2, p. 59.
355. Millette, R.L.; Fink, L.M. *Biochemistry* **1975**, *14*, 1426.
356. Guzzo, G.G.; Glazer, R.I. *Cancer Res.* **1976**, *36*, 1041.
357. Berthold, V.; Thielmann, H.W.; Geider, K. *FEBS Lett.* **1978**, *86*, 81.
358. Edwards, G.S.; Wogan, G.N. *Biochim. Biophys. Acta* **1970**, *24*, 597.
359. Hsu, W.T.; Lin, E.J.S.; Harvey, R.G.; Weiss, S.B. *Proc. Natl. Acad. Sci. U.S.A.* **1977**, *74*, 3335.
360. Leffler, S.; Pulkrabek, P.; Grunberger, D.; Weinstein, I.B. *Biochemistry* **1977**, *16*, 3133.
361. Mizusawa, H.; Kakefuda, T. *Nature (London)* **1979**, *279*, 75.
362. Glazer, R.I. *Cancer Res.* **1976**, *36*, 2282.
363. Yu, F.L.; Feigelson, P. *Proc. Natl. Acad. Sci. U.S.A.* **1972**, *69*, 2833.
364. Yamaura, I.; Marquardt, H.; Cavalieri, L.F. *Chem.-Biol. Interact.* **1978**, *23*, 399.

Carcinogenicity of Organic Halogenated Compounds

9

HELMUT GREIM and THOMAS WOLFF

Gesellschaft für Strahlen- und Umweltforschung München,
Institut Toxikologie und Biochemie, D-8042 Neuherberg, Germany

HALOGENATED HYDROCARBONS ARE ENCOUNTERED in numerous occupational and nonoccupational situations; therefore, their carcinogenic potential is a critical concern. They are starting materials, intermediates, and by-products for organic syntheses. They are used as fire retardants, solvents, and pesticides, and can be found in many commercial products.

More than 50 of these chemicals have produced tumors in one or more animal species or have been mutagenic in either animals or in vitro test systems. However, the evaluation of animal data for estimation of risks to humans is still a matter of great controversy. So far, only two substances, bis(chloromethyl) ether and vinyl chloride, have been shown to be carcinogenic to humans by epidemiological evidence, in addition to their tumorigenic effect in animals. Obviously, the lack of epidemiological evidence does not mean that a chemical is not carcinogenic to humans. Only a few studies have been carried out on humans exposed to these chemicals. If cohort studies or case–control studies are available, the evidence for tumorigenicity is frequently weakened by incomplete epidemiological data, insufficient periods of observation, and exposure to more than one chemical (e.g., another industrial chemical or the chemicals in cigarette smoke).

Although the exact mechanism of chemical carcinogenesis is not clear, two major categories of carcinogens can be distinguished: those acting by genotoxic mechanisms and those acting by epigenetic mechanisms. The genotoxic agents usually bind covalently to DNA and generally are mutagenic. Chemicals acting by epigenetic mechanisms do not directly damage the genome but exert their effects by interfering with the hormonal status, by immunosuppression, by chronic tissue injury, or by promotion. This classification implies substantial differences in the risk evaluation. Genotoxic carcinogens are believed to be effective after a single or low-dose exposure. In contrast, the epigenetic carcinogens have to be applied repeatedly or at relatively high doses to cause, for example, cytotoxic effects, which are the prerequisites for their carcinogenicity. Generally, the effective doses by far exceed the levels observed in the human environment. Epigenetically acting carcinogens may have quantifiable levels below which no appreciable hazard to humans exists. The differentiation between genotoxic and epigenetic carcinogens requires information on their metabolism; tissue distribution; route and rate of excretion; mutagenicity, especially in the various in vitro systems; interaction with

0065-7719/84/0182-0525$13.65/1

cellular macromolecules, such as proteins or nucleic acids; organ-specificity of cytotoxic effects; and promoting activity. We have included the information available on these parameters in this chapter in view of their importance for risk estimation.

The halogenated hydrocarbons used as pesticides will be discussed separately, because they constitute a relatively homogeneous group with many similarities in their pharmacokinetics and biological effects. Generally, they are slowly metabolized and persist in the mammalian organism. Furthermore, many of these compounds induce the enzymes involved in the metabolism of xenobiotics, enhance the proliferation of cells, or cause a hypertrophy; thus, all indications are that they function as tumor promoters rather than as genotoxic agents.

A vast amount of literature is available on the chemicals presented in this chapter. Only the major aspects of the recent data could be described.

Agents for Organic Synthesis

Monomers and Polymers. *trans*-1,4-DICHLOROBUTENE (1,4-DICHLORO-2-BUTENE). This chemical is manufactured by the chlorination of butadiene via 3,4-dichloro-1-butene and is used as an intermediate in the production of hexamethylenediamine and chloroprene (*1*).

It has produced mutations in *Salmonella typhimurium* TA 100, and this effect was enhanced by liver microsomes from mice or humans (*2*). In analogy to other open-chain β-chloroethers (*3*), the enhancing effect indicates that *trans*-1,4-dichlorobutene is metabolized to an epoxide intermediate that may represent the ultimate alkylating carcinogen. The chemical has also induced mutations in *Escherichia coli* and *Streptomyces cerevisiae* (*4, 5*). A weak carcinogenic effect was observed in mice. In a group of 30 female ICR/Ha Swiss mice receiving a weekly subcutaneous injection of 0.05 mg, 3 mice developed local sarcomas during the 77-week study (*3*). In a similar study, no tumors appeared either after interperitoneal application or after three 1-mg applications to the skin (*3*). When phorbol myristyl acetate was used concomitantly as a promoting agent, 1 out of 30 female rats developed a skin papilloma, whereas the promoter alone induced three papillomas and one skin carcinoma. No case reports or epidemiological data are available.

CHLOROPRENE (2-CHLORO-1,3-BUTADIENE) AND POLYCHLOROPRENE. Chloroprene is the monomer for the elastomer neoprene. It is produced by two routes: (1) the dimerization of acetylene and the addition of hydrogen chloride; or (2) the chlorination of butadiene and dehydrochlorination of a resultant dichlorobutene, 3,4-dichloro-1-butene (*1*). The total world production of chloroprene in 1977 was estimated at 3×10^8 kg (*6*).

The toxicology of chloroprene has been recently reviewed by Haley (*7*) and Clary et al. (*8*). It is highly toxic by inhalation, ingestion, and skin absorption. In humans, acutely high exposure has caused conjunctivitis, corneal necrosis, dermatitis, depilation, pulmonary edema, lack of appetite, indigestion, nervousness, hypotension, and shortness of breath. The results of long-term studies on exposed workers are contradictory. In one investigation, excesses of lung and skin cancer were reported (*9, 10*). However, several inconsistencies in this study have been recognized (*6*). Two other studies, which also had limitations, did not show excess rates of lung and skin cancer (*11, 12*).

The chemical has been tested for carcinogenicity in rats by oral, subcutaneous, and intratracheal administration and in mice by skin application (*13*). No carcinogenic effect was detected. In a single-generation study, 100 mg/kg of chloroprene was given to female rats by stomach tube on the 17th day of gestation. Their offspring were treated weekly with 50 mg/kg by stomach tube from the time of weaning until their natural death, and no increased tumor incidence was seen in the treated animals (*14*). However, Bartsch et al. (*15, 16*) reported weak mutagenicity to *Sal. typhimurium* strains that was enhanced in the presence of a metabolically active liver fraction, and Sanotskii (*17*) reported cytogenetic effects on human lymphocytes.

By analogy to vinyl chloride and 1,1-dichloroethylene, the metabolic formation of an epoxide, which is considered the ultimate mutagen, has been suggested (*18, 19*). The apparent discrepancy between mutagenicity in an in vitro test system and lack of carcinogenic effect in animals may be explained by a potent inactivation of the reactive intermediate in the intact animal (*7*). In the case of the intact animal, chloroprene or its metabolites are conjugated with glutathione (*20*) and excreted as mercapturic acids in the urine (*21*), whereas insufficient glutathione is available for conjugation in the in vitro mutagenicity test systems (*22*).

Polychloroprene is derived from chloroprene by polymerization. It is a white-to-amber, rubbery solid with a molecular weight of 80,000–200,000 (*23*). It softens above 80 °C and liberates hydrogen chloride and chlorine when combusted (*24*). No data on toxic effects in animals or humans are available.

TETRAFLUOROETHYLENE AND POLYTETRAFLUOROETHYLENE. Tetrafluoroethylene is produced commercially by the pyrolysis of chlorodifluoromethane at high temperatures, and the highly purified product is used in the production of Teflon and several resins (*25*). The total world production of tetrafluoroethylene in 1977 was estimated to be 1.5–2.0 $\times 10^7$ kg.

Only limited chronic toxicity studies have been performed with the monomer. When male rats were exposed to 3500 ppm for 30 min, no gross pathology was noted in the organs after 14 d. The animals did excrete small amounts of fluoride in their urine, and this result indicates the metabolism of tetrafluoroethylene (*26*).

In humans, acute exposure induces irritation of the eyes and respiratory system, fever, pain, weakness, nausea, and vomiting (*27*). In contrast, polytetrafluoroethylene discs, squares, fragments, or powder implanted subcutaneously or intraperitoneally in mice or rats induces local sarcomas (*28–31*). However, relevance of such data is debatable; local sarcomas from implants are considered to result from constant irritation rather than from the chemical itself (*32*). One case of a local fibrosarcoma has been reported in a patient 10.5 years after implantation of a polytetrafluoroethylene–dacron arterial prosthesis.

VINYL CHLORIDE (CHLOROETHYLENE) AND ITS POLYMERS. Vinyl chloride (VC) is almost exclusively (96–97%) used for polyvinyl chloride (PVC) production. The annual world production is approximately 12 $\times 10^9$ kg (*33*). Limited amounts of vinyl chloride have been used as aerosol propellant and as an anesthetic (*34*).

Metabolism, mutagenicity, macromolecular binding, and carcinogenicity in humans have recently been reviewed by Hopkins (*35, 36*). Microsomal mixed-function oxidase plays an active and possibly the major role in the metabolism of the monomer, especially at low doses, to chloroethylene oxide and 2-chloroacetaldehyde. In the rat this pathway is saturable; at increased doses, a greater portion escapes metabolism and is expired unchanged (*37*). In the urine, glutathione conjugates of the chloroethylene oxide or 2-chloroacetaldehyde appear as mercapturic acids.

Mutagenicity to *E. coli* and *Sal. typhimurium*, as in other mutagenicity test systems, most likely results from metabolic formation of the oxide (*38–40*). Chloroethylene oxide and chloroacetaldehyde bind to cellular macromolecules and, in particular, alkylate the nucleic acids (*41*). N^7-Hydroxyethylguanine; 1,N^6-ethenoadenosine; ethenodeoxycytidine; and ethenodeoxyadenosine have been isolated from rats and mice exposed to [^{14}C]-labeled VC (*42*).

Health hazards of VC were not established until 1966. The first toxicological lesion observed was acroosteolysis in reactor cleaners in a PVC production plant (*33*). Acroosteolysis is a combination of lytic lesions of the bones (usually the terminal phalanges), Raynaud's syndrome, and a sclerodermatous skin change. As a result of these clinical findings, experimental work was undertaken to induce acroosteolysis in animals. These studies revealed a high incidence of carcinoma in animals exposed to VC at a concentration of 250 ppm (*43*). The results to date show that VC administered by inhalation produces angiosarcoma of the liver and other organs in rats, mice, and hamsters. Moreover, Zymbal gland carcinoma in the external auditory meatus (rats); breast cancer (mice); nephroblastoma (rats); lung adenoma (mice); skin trichoepithelioma, lymphoma, and forestomach papilloma (hamsters) have all been observed (*44, 45*). Exposure at 50 ppm for 5 h/d, 5 d/week for 6 months did not significantly increase tumor incidence in rats and mice, except for mammary gland tumors in female mice up to 12 months following exposure (*46*).

Approximately 50 cases of angiosarcoma of the liver in humans have been reported. In addition, the increased incidence of brain cancer and lung cancer in approximately the same number of cases indicates that these sites are also target organs (*33, 47–49*). The degree of risk involved in low-level exposures up to 5 ppm has not been established. However, years ago individuals were exposed to concentrations of 1000 ppm and more (*50*), and recent careful reviews do not substantiate the reports that occupational or environmental VC exposure induced mutagenic effects (*36, 51*).

There are concerns specifically related to occupational exposure to the polymer PVC: (1) Altered pulmonary function and fibrotic lung changes that have occurred in workers exposed to PVC dust (*52*); and (2) the hazards of the carbon monoxide, hydrochloric acid, and phosgene released in the combustion of PVC plastics (*53*).

VINYLDENE CHLORIDE (1,1-DICHLOROETHYLENE) AND THE 1,2-DICHLOROETHYLENES. Vinylidene chloride is almost exclusively used in the production of copolymers, primarily with vinyl chloride. Approximately 10% of total production is used for the manufacture of modacrylic fibers (*54*).

Biotransformation of vinylidene chloride, recently reviewed by Cooper (*55*), results in the exhalation of CO_2 together with the unchanged product (*56*). Thiodihydroxyacetic acid and *N*-acetyl-*S*-cysteinylacetyl derivatives, together with chloroacetic acid, dithiohydroxyacetic acid, and thiohydroxyacetic acid, have been isolated in urine (*57, 58*); this finding indicates that glutathione conjugation is a major mechanism of inactivation (*59*). The initiating stage in metabolism is the monooxygenase-dependent formation of an epoxide that rearranges to the corresponding acyl chloride (*57, 60, 61*). This epoxide has been proposed to be the ultimate mutagenic species that induces mutations in *E. coli* K12, and *Sal. typhimurium* strains in the presence of a liver microsomal fraction (*16, 38, 39, 60, 61*). The carcinogenicity of vinylidene chloride is surprisingly specific in respect to species, organ, and sex. In male mice, exposure of 25 ppm preferentially induced adenocarcinoma in the kidneys (*62–64*). Another study revealed bronchioloalveolar adenomas and angiosarcoma of low frequency in the livers (*65, 66*). In the rat, low incidences of angiosarcoma, mammary fibroadenomas, and carcinomas occurred with no dose dependence (*63, 65*). No tumors were found in the Chinese hamster (*64*). In a National Cancer Institute carcinogenesis bioassay, vinylidine chloride was administered by gavage to rats at doses of 1 or 5 mg/kg. Mice received 2 or 10 mg/kg. The 104-week chronic exposure was not carcinogenic (*66*). No data on the carcinogenicity or mutagenicity of vinylidene chloride–vinyl chloride copolymers are available.

The *cis*- and *trans*-1,2-dichloroethylenes are widely used as solvents for fats, oils, waxes, and particularly rubber. Hepatotoxic effects have been observed in rodents (*67*). Although the 1,2-dichloroethylenes are metabolized by microsomal monooxygenases via an epoxide, they are not mutagenic in the presence or absence of liver-activating enzymes (*38, 68*). So far, no data on carcinogenesis bioassays are available.

VINYLIDENE FLUORIDE (1,1-DIFLUOROETHYLENE) AND POLYVINYLIDENE FLUORIDE. Vinylidene fluoride is used exclusively for the manufacture of its polymer. Although approximately 2×10^6 kg is produced annually, little information on its toxicity is available. Bartsch et al. (*17*) observed a marginal mutagenicity in the *Salmonella* microsome assay in which the bacteria were exposed for 24 h to an atmosphere containing 50% of the chemical in the air.

Subcutaneous skin application tests in mice did not conclusively demonstrate carcinogenic activity (*69*). More information was derived from a long-term study performed by Maltoni et al. (*69*): Rats were given 4.12 or 8.25 mg/kg/d by gavage for 4–5 d/week for 141 weeks. Nearly 9% of the treated animals had tumors of the adipose tissue compared with 4% of control males and 0.5% of control females. However, no statistical analysis of the data was provided.

Intermediates. BENZYL CHLORIDE (α-CHLOROTOLUENE) AND RELATED COMPOUNDS. Benzyl chloride is made by chlorination of toluene. It is used for manufacturing the vinyl resin plasticizer butylbenzyl phthalate, in the vulcanization of fluororubbers, and in the benzylation of disinfectant phenol derivatives (*70*).

Benzyl chloride is a direct alkylating agent. It is a weak mutagen on *Sal. typhimurium* (*71*) and is active in the transformation of mammalian cell cultures (*72*). Local sarcomas at the site of subcutaneous injections have been found in rats (*73*). In a skin-painting study on mice, 2, 3, and 10 μL of benzyl chloride were applied to the dorsal skin once or twice a week for 7.2 to 11.7 months (*74*). The chemical had a strong locally irritating effect. Squamous cell carcinomas of the skin were seen in the low-dose group with an incidence of 15%, but no carcinomas were observed in the high-dose group. No tumors in other organs have been observed. A lung tumorigenicity test in mice after intraperitoneal administration was negative (*75*). When benzyl chloride was given intravenously to male mice, alkylation of hemoglobin and of the N^7-guanine of DNA occurred in brain, testis, and liver; within 24 h, N^7-alkylation decreased, but hemoglobin alkylation increased (*76*).

Among the workers in a small plant that produced benzoyl chloride, three lung cancers and one maxillary malignant lymphoma were found (*77*). Two lung cancer deaths occurred in another factory where approximately 20 workers were employed regularly in benzoyl chloride manufacture (*78*). In a skin-painting study in mice, 2 and 3 μL of benzoyl chloride administered twice a week for 50 weeks produced a skin tumor incidence of 10% within 560 d (*74*). The same dosage schedule of benzotrichloride induced a 68% incidence of skin cancers and a 58% incidence of pulmonary tumors within 399 d.

BIS(CHLOROMETHYL) ETHER. This chemical is widely used for chloromethylation in organic synthesis. It is produced by saturating a solution of paraformaldehyde in cold sulfuric acid with hydrogen chloride. Formation increases in both air and liquid in the presence of formaldehyde and chloride (*79*), and it is stable in moist air (*80*). Spontaneous formation of bis(chloromethyl) ether in the air in textile plants has been reported by some researchers and refuted by others (*80*).

Bis(chloromethyl) ether is a human carcinogen (*81*). Epidemiological studies in workers exposed to the chemical for 6 to 15 years showed an increased incidence of lung cancers (*82–86*). A genetic risk of occupational exposure has also been reported (*87*). Inhalation studies in rats confirmed the high risk of lung cancer (*88*). In a recent inhalation study, rats and mice were exposed to 1, 10, and 100 ppb for 6 h/d, 5 d/week, for 6 months and subsequently were observed for the duration of their natural life span (*89*). Of the rats exposed to 100 ppb, 86.5% developed nasal tumors and 4% developed pulmonary adenomas. No tumors were seen in the lower dose groups. In mice, the high dose induced pulmonary adenomas. Because of its alkylating properties bis(chloromethyl) ether is a directly acting mutagen in the *Salmonella* test (*90*).

BIS(2-CHLOROISOPROPYL) ETHER [BIS(2-CHLORO-1-METHYLETHYL) ETHER]. This ether, together with bis(2-chloroethyl) ether, is a by-product in the synthesis of propylene oxide and ethylene oxide and has been found as an outfall of this production in rivers and drinking water (*91*). The chemical is mutagenic to *Sal. typhimurium,* and microsomal activation enhances the mutagenic activity significantly (*92*). However, a carcinogenesis bioassay in which rats were given 100 and 200 mg/kg by gavage 5 d/week for 103 weeks was negative (*93*).

3,3′-DICHLOROBENZIDINE (4,4′-DIAMINO-3,3′-DICHLOROBIPHENYL). This chemical and its hydrochloride and sulfate salts are used principally as intermediates for dyestuffs synthesis (*94*) and less often as a curing agent in the production of polyurethane foams. The occupational hazards of dichlorobenzidine production are difficult to determine from epidemiological evidence, because its production is frequently associated with the production of the bladder carcinogen benzidine (*95*).

In rats and hamsters it produced a high incidence of adenomas and carcinomas of the Zymbal gland, the bladder, and other organs (*96–98*). It is mutagenic even without metabolic activation in *Sal. typhimurium,* and its mutagenicity increases greatly in the presence of a microsomal activating system; under this condition, dichlorobenzidine is more active than benzidine (*99*). Very little is known about the metabolism of dichlorobenzidine. One beneficial investigation would be to determine whether benzidine derivatives, such as *o*-substituents, are formed and excreted in the urine as is found with *o*-toluidine- and dianisidine-derived dyes (*100*). After oral administration, the ^{14}C-labeled chemical was well absorbed and distributed in the tissues 24 h after administration; the highest levels were found in the liver, followed by the kidneys, lungs, and spleen (*101*). Approximately half of the total ^{14}C-radioactivity measured in the liver and kidneys was covalently bound to cellular macromolecules. In vitro studies on the interaction of 3,3′-dichlorobenzidine with polyribonucleotides indicate that guanine is the main site for binding of the chemical or its microsome-mediated metabolites (*102*). The major route of excretion is in the feces (60%) and less via the kidneys (30%). In bile, 60% of 3,3′-dichlorobenzidine is excreted as conjugates.

DIMETHYLCARBAMOYL CHLORIDE. This chemical has been reported as an intermediate in the production of several carbamate pesticides, such as tandex, dimetilan, and primicarb, as well as in the synthesis of a few anticholinesterase agents: neostigmine bromide, its methyl sulfate, and pyridostigmine bromide (*103*). It is also used for the synthesis of dyes and the rocket fuel dimethylhydrazine (*104*).

The carcinogenic potency of dimethylcarbamoyl chloride was first reported by Van Duuren (*105*). In mice, skin application induced skin tumors; subcutaneous injection induced subcutaneous sarcomas; and intraperitoneal application induced local sarcomas and papillary tumors of the lungs. In rats, lifetime inhalation of 1 ppm for 6 h/d, 5 d/week induced nasal cancer in almost 100% of the treated animals (*106*). The chemical is a direct mutagen in *Sal. typhimurium* (*71*). No cancer deaths or indication of lung cancer have been detected in 107 workers who had been exposed to dimethycarbamoyl chloride for 6 months to 12 years (*107*).

EPICHLOROHYDRIN (1-CHLORO-2,3-EPOXYPROPANE). Epichlorohydrin is widely used as a solvent for resins, gums, cellulose esters, paints, and lacquers and as a raw material in the manufacture of epoxy resins. Its use and biological activities have been thoroughly reviewed (*108*).

It induced squamous cell carcinomas of the nasal epithelium in rats following daily inhalation of 100 ppm for 6 h; forestomach tumors in rats after administration of 375, 750, or 1500 ppm in the drinking water for 81 weeks (*109*); and local sarcomas in mice after subcutaneous or intramuscular application (*105, 108*). Being an alkylating agent, epichlorohydrin is a direct mutagen to bacteria and in mouse lymphoma cells (*110, 111*); it also induced mutations in *Drosophila melanogaster* (*111*). Negative results have been obtained in the dominant lethal assay with ICR/Ha Swiss mice after a single intraperitoneal injection of 150 mg/kg (*112*). Addition of epichlorohydrin to human lymphocytes in culture induced a dose-dependent increase in chromosomal aberrations (*113*). These data stimulated further testing, but cytogenetic analysis in exposed workers yielded equivocal evidence for clastogenic effects on the lymphocytes (*114*). Currently available case–control studies do not provide evidence for carcinogenicity of epichlorohydrin in humans (*109, 115*).

HEXACHLOROBUTADIENE (PERCHLOROBUTADIENE). This chemical is obtained as a by-product in a number of industrial reactions, such as the synthesis of tetrachloroethylene, trichloroethylene, and carbon tetrachloride (*5*). It is preferentially used as a recovery agent for chlorine-containing gas in chlorine plants, as an intermediate to produce lubricants or rubber compounds, as a solvent for elastomers, as a heat-transfer liquid, as a hydraulic fluid, and as a fumigant in vineyards (*116*).

The kidney is the major target organ where hexachlorobutadiene produces necrosis of the proximal tubulus (*117, 118*). Renal necrosis was also seen in rats following inhalation exposure (25 ppm, 15 times in 6 h) (*119*), dermal application (*120*), and oral administration [150 and 450 ppm in the diet for 90 d (*121*)]. Possibly as a result of the renal necrosis, approximately 23% of male rats and 25% of female rats developed renal adenoma and adenosarcomas after 2 years of being fed the high dose of 20 mg/kg/d. At the intermediate dose of 2 mg/kg/d, the effects were limited to an increased hyperplasia of renal tubular epithelium but no neoplasms; females also exhibited increased excretion of coproporphyrins. The lowest dose of 0.2 mg/kg caused no discernible ill effects in this study (*117*).

Reproductive performance of rats given a daily dose of 20 mg/kg for 90 d was not affected (*122*). No sound data on metabolism or mutagenicity are available, nor are there case reports or epidemiological evaluation of human exposure.

By-Products. HALOGENATED DIBENZODIOXINS. *2,3,7,8-Tetrachlorodibenzodioxin (TCDD)* (**I**). TCDD is the best known of the chlorodibenzo-*p*-dioxins. It is a relatively low-concentration by-product in the synthesis of trichlorophenol, which is the industrial precursor of the antiseptic hexachlorophene and the defoliant (2,4,5-trichlorophenoxy)acetic acid (2,4,5-T).

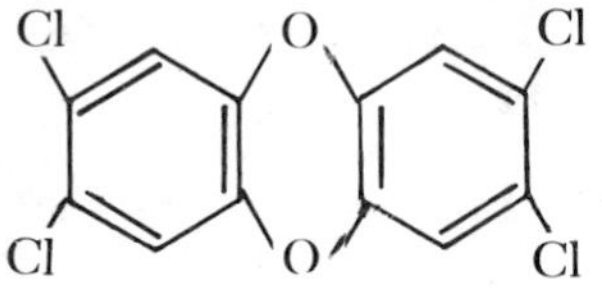

Cl O Cl

Cl O Cl

I

Its toxicity to animals and humans, as well as the accidents that resulted in human exposure, have been reviewed (*123*). Of the 75 possible chlorine-substituted dibenzo-*p*-dioxin isomers, TCDD is the most comprehensively studied. To date, 22 accidents have been reported in which more than 1100 people were exposed. The most prevalent results of exposure were chloracne, polyneuritis, sensory impairments, and liver damage. Unfortunately few epidemiologic studies have been conducted on these events regarding carcinogenicity. In Germany, 6 out of 25 exposed workers died of cancer 25 years after an accident; the expected number of cancer deaths in the control population was four (*124*). Although its effect on reproduction is known in animals (*125–28*), neither the Seveso accident investigation nor the Oregon study has demonstrated similar effects on human reproduction (*129*).

In Sweden, TCDD contamination of 2,4,5-T has also been connected with an almost sixfold increase in soft tissue carcinoma in workers using herbicides (*130*). No increased tumor rate occurred in a long-term study of mice given 2,4,5-T contaminated with a level of TCDD sufficient to supply approximately 0.27 μg of TCDD/kg/d (*131*). However, in a lifetime study of rats ingesting 0.1 μg of TCDD daily in their diets, the incidence of hepatocellular carcinomas and squamous cell carcinoma of the lung, hard palate/nasal turbinates, or tongue increased compared with controls, whereas the incidence of tumors of the pituitary gland, uterus, mammary gland, pancreas, and adrenal gland decreased (*132*). The primary hepatic ultrastructural change at this high-dose level was proliferation of the rough endoplasmatic reticulum. Other toxic effects included increased mortality, decreased body weight gain, increased urinary excretion of porphyrins and δ-aminolevulinic acid, slightly depressed erythroid parameters, and increased activities of hepatic serum enzymes. Rats treated with 0.01 μg/kg/d showed a lesser degree of toxicity. No effects were seen at 0.001 μg/kg/d.

In a carcinogenesis bioassay, TCDD was administered by gavage 2 d/week for 104 weeks at doses of 0.01, 0.05, or 0.5 μg/kg/week to rats and male mice and at doses of 0.04, 0.2, or 2.0 μg/kg/week to female mice (*133*). Among the high-dose groups the following was observed: rats and mice, toxic hepatitis; rats, increased incidences of thyroid adenomas; female rats, liver neoplasms; mice, dose-dependent hepatocellular carcinomas; and female mice, thyroid tumors.

In a dermal carcinogenicity study, female mice received 0.005 μg of TCDD 3 d/week for 99–104 weeks; males received 0.001 μg (*134*). In the females, a significantly higher incidence of fibrosarcoma in the skin integumentary system occurred than in the males.

When ^{14}C-labelled TCDD is ingested by rats, the radioactivity is stored primarily in the liver and to a lesser extent in the fat. Continuous administration to rats leads to a 40% accumulation in the liver, but a steady state is reached within several months. The major route of elimination is the feces and, to a lesser extent, the urine (*135*). The whole-body half-life of TCDD was estimated to be approximately 4 weeks in the rat (*135*), 3–6 weeks in the guinea pig (*136*), and less than 2 weeks in the hamster (*137*). In the bile of dogs, 2-hydroxy-TCDD, 2-hydroxy-triCDD, and dihydroxy-triCDD have been isolated; these derivatives also undergo biliary secretion in rats (*138*).

One of the most prominent effects of TCDD is its strong inducing capability on enzymes, such as δ-aminolevulinic acid synthetase, the microsomal monooxygenases, arylhydrocarbon hydroxylase (*139–41*), glucuronosyltransferase (*142, 143*), DT-diaphorase, aldehyde dehydrogenase, and ornithine decarboxylase (*144*). Several authors propose that this effect is the main mechanism of the carcinogenic, embryotoxic, hypothyroid, hepatotoxic, porphyrinogenic, or immunosuppressive activity of TCDD (*145–48*). The chemical may also impair the metabolism of other xenobiotics (e.g., pentachlorophenol) and thus impair its detoxification (*149*). Hussain et al. (*150*) found TCDD to be mutagenic in bacterial systems, whereas no tumor-initiating or tumor-promoting effect was observed in mouse skin when the two-stage initiating system of carcinogenesis was applied (*151, 152*).

Other Halogenated Dibenzodioxins and Dibenzofurans (**II**). Little information is available on the mutagenic or carcinogenic potential of the highly toxic dibenzodioxins.

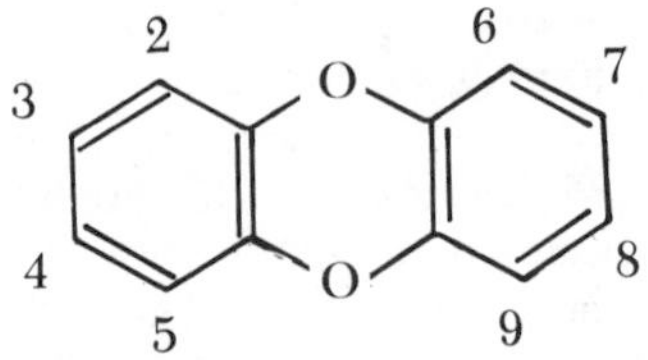

2 6 7 3 O 4 O 8 5 9

II

Poland et al. recently established a correlation between structure and biological activity for their arylhydrocarbon hydroxylase-inducing effect and for their binding ability to a presumed cytosolic receptor (*145*). The biologically active derivatives have three common denominators: (1) halogen atoms in at least three of the lateral ring positions (positions 2, 3, 7, and 8), (2) an order of potency of substitution of Br < Cl < F < NO_2, and (3) at least one unsubstituted ring position.

A similar structure–activity relationship is reported for the halogenated dibenzofurans (*153*), which are highly toxic in animals and humans (*154, 155*). They are environmental contaminants associated with the polychlorinated biphenyls (*156, 157*) and have been found in the livers and blood of patients with Yusho, the poisoning that occurred in Japan as a result of high exposure to polychlorinated biphenyls (*158, 159*). Transfer across the placenta to fetuses and to offspring has been reported in mice (*160*).

Mutagenicity tests of 2,9-dichlorodibenzofuran, 3,6-dichlorodibenzofuran, 2,3,7,8-tetrachlorodibenzofuran, and octachlorodibenzofuran were negative for *Salmonella* strains TA 98 and TA 100 with and without microsomal extracts (*161*). There are no experimental indications of carcinogenicity for these compounds to date.

Fire Retardants

Approximately 1×10^9 kg of flame retardants is currently produced, mainly for use in fabrics, plastics, and carpets. Nearly two-thirds of these products are inorganics, such as alumina trihydrate and antimony oxide; the remaining one-third consist of a large number of brominated and chlorinated organic derivatives (*162*).

Polybrominated Biphenyls (PBBs). PBBs are mixtures of brominated biphenyls with 4–8 bromine atoms/molecule and are used as fire retardants in thermoplastic resins (*163*). One such mixture, mainly hexabromobiphenyl and heptabromobiphenyl, caused widespread contamination of livestock in Michigan during 1973 (*164*). Although it is toxic to animals and affects the liver, endocrine, skin, kidney, and lymphatic system (*165, 166*), no relevant clinical symptoms have been observed in the Michigan farm families who were exposed to the chemical (*167, 168*). In the contaminated livestock, high rates of deaths, stillbirths, and spontaneous abortions were reported (*166*). Subsequent studies in laboratory animals revealed that a daily intake of PBBs in the feed (25 mg/kg or 100 ppm) very early in pregnancy can lead to resorption of the fetuses, while administration later in pregnancy can give rise to offspring with lower birth weight and some malformations (*166, 169*).

Exposure to high doses of PBBs has induced liver cancer in rats and mice. Rats given a single oral dose of 1000 mg of PBB/kg developed neoplastic nodules in their livers within 6 months after dosing (*170*). Similar atypical liver nodules are observed after 6 months in rats exposed to multiple doses of PBBs (*171*). When rats were given a single oral dose of 1000 mg/kg or 1 oral dose of 100 mg/kg every 3 weeks for 36 weeks, the incidence of hepatocellular carcinomas was 41% in the single-dose group and 63% in the multiple-dose group at 26 months of age (*172*). After a single oral dose of 200 mg/kg, the incidence of neoplastic nodules 18–22 months later was 31%, but no liver cancers were observed (*172*). Similar results have been observed in an oral carcinogenesis bioassay conducted in rats and mice: Over a period of 6 months, 0.1, 0.3, 1.0, and 10 mg/kg/d, 5 d/week, were given; 23 months after the end of exposure different types of liver tumors were noticed in all rats that received doses above 0.1 mg/kg/d and in all female rats at doses above 1 mg/kg/d. In mice similar results were reported (*173*).

Tris(2,3-dibromopropyl) Phosphate (Tris-BP) (III). Tris-BP was used as a flame retardant in polyurethane foams, plastics, and children's sleepwear until 1977. By that time approximately 1×10^9 kg of the compound had been produced (*174, 175*).

$$
\begin{array}{l}
\qquad OCH_2\text{—}CHBr\text{—}CH_2Br \\
\quad / \\
O{=}P\text{—}OCH_2\text{—}CHBr\text{—}CH_2Br \\
\quad \backslash \\
\qquad OCH_2\text{—}CHBr\text{—}CH_2Br
\end{array}
$$

III

The chemical is activated to a potent mutagen in the *Sal. typhimurium* assay (*176, 177*). It also decreased the size of DNA in monolayers of human cells (*178*) and induced sister chromatid exchanges in Chinese hamster cells, but no chromosomal aberrations were observed (*179*). Long-term feeding studies in rats and mice induced renal tubular cell adenomas and carcinomas in 55% of the animals. Preneoplastic lesions and severe toxic nephrosis were seen in 98% of the animals (*180, 181*). To achieve these comparable results, the rats received 50 and 100 ppm, while the mice received 500 and 1000 ppm. This species difference seems to be due to the higher capability of the rat to convert tris-BP to reactive intermediates, presumably bis(2,3-dibromopropyl) phosphate and 2,3-dibromopropyl phosphate (*174*). Both of these derivatives are less mutagenic than tris-BP when tested on the *Sal. typhimurium* TA 100 strain, but more nephrotoxic to rats after single intraperitoneal doses of 10–200 mg/kg (*174*). When male rats were given 100 mg of tris-BP/kg via stomach tube, 5 d/week for 4–52 weeks, toxic tubular nephrosis developed from tubular lesions and adenocarcinomas developed from hyperplastic areas at these sites. At 52 weeks, three of five survivors were found to have adenomas of the descending colon (*182*). Dermal administration three times weekly to mice for 420–96 d induced benign and malignant tumors of the skin, forestomach, and oral cavity (*183*).

After the withdrawal of tris-BP in 1977, tetrakis(hydroxymethyl) phosphonium chloride has been used as a substitute, but it also has been shown to be carcinogenic in animals after skin application (*183*).

Vinyl Bromide and Polyvinyl Bromide. Vinyl bromide is a flame retardant added in small amounts to modacrylic fibers which are used in clothing, home furnishings, and industry (*184*). The polymer is unstable even at room temperature and is of little use (*185*).

Vinyl bromide is debrominated in rats exposed to the chemical (*186*), and pretreatment with phenobarbital enhances the debromination. It is the reactive metabolite formed during metabolism that seems to be hepatotoxic, because concomitant pretreatment of the rats with Arochlor 1254 and phenobarbital increased serum D-ketoglutarate transaminase and serum sorbitol dehydrogenase (*187, 188*). Bartsch et al. (*17*) presented strong evidence that the reactive intermediate formed by microsomal metabolism is bromoethylene oxide. They also suggested that this intermediate is the ultimate mutagen in the *Salmonella* microsome test. In animals, glutathione seems to be involved in the metabolic inactivation of the metabolite; vinyl bromide administration to rats decreases hepatic glutathione content (*188*).

In the mouse, vinyl bromide or polyvinyl bromide did not induce skin tumors after topical application for 420 d, whereas 48 weekly subcutaneous injections of the polymer induced sarcomas at the site of injection (*189*). An inhalation study in male and female rats which were exposed to 10, 50, 250, and 1250 ppm resulted in an increased incidence of liver angiosarcomas at the three highest dose levels (*190*).

Solvents

Bis(2-chloroethyl) Ether. This ether is used as a solvent for many resins, rubber, and cellulose esters in the paint and varnish industry, as an extracting agent in the petroleum industry, and in the textile industry (*191*).

Bis(2-chloroethyl)ether is a weak mutagen in the standard *Salmonella* assay (*100, 192*) but highly mutagenic when assayed in a desiccator or in suspension (*100*). Its mutagenicity was not enhanced in the presence of a metabolic activating system. It was not mutagenic in the host-mediated assay (*100*), nor did it induce heritable translocation in mice (*193*). Only weak carcinogenic effects, if any, have been observed. In one older study hepatomas occurred in mice after dietary application (*131*). Marginal effects have been seen after subcutaneous administration (*89*).

A major step in the biotransformation of bis(2-chloroethyl) ether in rats is the cleavage of the ether linkage, which results in the urinary excretion of thiodiglycolic acid and, to a lesser degree, the 2-chloroethanol-β-D-glucuronide (*194*). Comparison of the metabolic rates of bis(2-chloroethyl) ether and bis(2-chloroisopropyl) ether indicates that the possible greater mutagenic and carcinogenic properties of the ethyl ether may result from the greater ease with which it is cleaved in vivo at the ether linkage to form reactive intermediates (*195*).

Carbon Tetrachloride (Tetrachloromethane). Carbon tetrachloride is primarily used in the production of fluorocarbons. It is also used as a solvent (approximately 10% of its use), as a grain fumigant, and as a treatment for cattle and sheep infected with hookworm and liver fluke (*196*). It is present in the atmosphere, probably via the photodecomposition of haloalkanes (*197*), as well as in food, drinking water, and human tissue (*198*).

The toxicity of CCl_4 results from its biotransformation, and a reasonably substantial relationship exists between its toxicity, especially to the liver, and lipid peroxidation (*199*). Most likely the microsomal monooxygenase splits the molecule and forms the trichloromethyl and monoatomic chlorine free radicals (*200, 201*).

Although CCl_4 reactants bind irreversibly to macromolecules, including DNA (*202, 203*), no mutagenicity has been observed in *E. coli* or *Sal. typhimurium* (*97, 203*). In various strains of rats it induced liver tumors, including hepatocellular carcinomas, after inhalation, subcutaneous, and intramuscular administration (*204–7, 212*). Weak embryotoxicity has been observed in rats (*211*), mice (*208, 209*), and hamsters (*210*). In humans, one case of liver cell carcinoma has been described (*205*), and it occurred 7 years after acute poisoning.

Chloroform (Trichloromethane). The estimated world production of this chemical in 1973 was 2.45×10^8 kg (*213*). It is used for the production of chlorodifluoromethane; as a solvent for the extraction and purification of antibiotics, vitamins, and flavors; as a general solvent for adhesives, resins, and pesticides; and as a fumigant (*214*). Until its use in human drug products was banned by the U.S. Food and Drug Administration in 1976, approximately 1900 human drugs contained chloroform (*215*). It is found in the air, surface water, drinking water, food, and human tissue (*198, 216–18*). In water, the main source of chloroform is formed primarily by chlorination of organic matter (*219*).

The molecular basis for the toxicity of chloroform to animals and humans has been investigated for decades and has been reviewed thoroughly (*220*). Chloroform is easily absorbed by inhalation, oral ingestion, and topical application. It is metabolized to CO_2, which is exhaled together with the unaltered chemical. Metabolism by microsomal enzymes forms the alkylating agent phosgene (*220, 221*), which might be responsible for the toxic effects. The reactive intermediate covalently binds to tissue macromolecules (*213, 222*), and a correlation between binding and the extent of renal and hepatic necrosis has been observed (*223, 224*). However, there are species differences in the rate of metabolism; it is highest in the mouse, lower in the rat, and lowest in the rhesus monkey (*225*) and humans (*226*). These differences, as well as the extremely high concentrations required to induce tumors in laboratory animals, have to be considered in the risk evaluation of human exposure (*227, 228*). Chloroform was tested by oral administration in three experiments using mice and one using rats. At daily doses exceeding 150 mg/kg, it produced hepatomas and hepatocellular carcinomas in mice, malignant kidney tumors in male rats, and tumors of the thyroid in female rats (*229, 230*).

Chloroform is not mutagenic to bacteria (*100, 203, 231*); it failed to induce chromosome damage or sister chromatid exchanges in cultured human lymphocytes (*231*); and it is not teratogenic in mice (*232*). Fetotoxicity in rats occurred in an air concentration of 20 g/m^3, which was also toxic to the mothers (*233*).

Chloromethyl Methyl Ether. Like bis(chloromethyl) ether, this chemical is widely used as a chloromethylation agent and as a solvent for polymerization reactions (*234*). Commercial products can be contaminated with 1–8% bis(chloromethyl) ether (*235, 236*). Skin application to mice, subcutaneous application to mice and rats, and intraperitoneal injection of newborn mice induced carcinomas and lung adenomas (*89, 237, 238*). Inhalation induced carcinoma of the lung in rats (*239*).

The investigations of Van Duuren (*237, 240, 241*) and Nelson (*89*) imply that the γ-haloethers should be classified with the biologically active alkylating agents. In general, bifunctional γ-haloethers have been found to be more active than the monofunctional analogs. As the chain length increases and the chlorine moves further away from the ether oxygen, reactivity and carcinogenicity decrease. Because of its high reactivity, chloromethyl methyl ether is a direct mutagen in bacterial test systems (*97*).

Occupational exposure has been clearly associated with an increased risk of lung cancer (*89, 91, 235, 236, 242*). However, recent findings indicate that the risk may be due to contamination with bis(chloromethyl) ether, which is present at up to 7% in industrial chloromethyl methyl ether.

Dihalomethanes: Dichloromethane, Dibromomethane, and Diiodomethane. Of the three dihalomethanes, dichloromethane has the greatest commercial importance. Several hundred million kilograms are produced annually and are used mainly as paint removers, degreasing solvents, and aerosal propellants (*243*). Dibromomethane is a by-product in the synthesis of bromochloromethane (*244*). Because of its instability, its former use as a fire retardant has been discontinued. Diiodomethane is of no commercial importance.

Dichloromethane was mutagenic in the *Salmonella* test in the presence and absence of a liver microsomal activation system (*245*). It did not show genotoxicity in the DNA repair test with freshly isolated hepatocytes (*246*). No increased rate of lung tumors was seen in mice (*247*). A 2-year inhalation study with rats and hamsters exposed to 0, 500, 1500, and 3500 ppm for 6 h/d, 5 d/week, gave no evidence of an increased tumor rate (*248*). The 11 salivary gland tumors among the 124 male rats at 3500 ppm as compared with 1 among 124 male controls is explained by a combination of viral salivary infection with the high exposure to the chemical.

The metabolism of dihalomethanes in mammals, including humans, has been thoroughly investigated, and the studies indicate at least two major pathways: (1) oxidation by microsomal monooxygenase yielding carbon monoxide (*249*), which then initiates carboxyhemoglobin formation (*250*), and (2) conjugation to glutathione ultimately yielding formaldehyde (*251*). The thioether formed during dihalomethane metabolism is highly mutagenic on *Sal. typhimurium* (*252*). The thioethers that are formed with dibromomethane and diiodomethane in the presence of postmitochondrial supernatant containing glutathione S-transferase and glutathione are also highly mutagenic to *Sal. typhimurium* (*253*). Because the rate of dihalomethane metabolism follows the halide order I > Br > Cl, thioether formation from dichloromethane is expected to be slowest (*254*). In rats, the metabolic rate of inhaled dichloromethane was shown to reach a maximum at 50 ppm (*250*). This saturation effect must be considered when evaluating dose–effect curves for this chemical.

1,2-Dichloroethane (Ethylene Dichloride). This chemical is produced in quantities of 4–6 $\times 10^9$ kg/year. It is mainly used for the production of vinyl chloride and, to a lesser degree, for the production of haloalkenes and elastomers. Other miscellaneous applications include its use as a solvent and as a fumigant (*255*). It has been found in surface water, air, and exhaled air of humans (*256, 257*).

As has been described for the dihalomethanes, 1,2-dichloroethane is metabolically activated by microsomal dechlorination and subsequent glutathione conjugation that results in the formation of the thioether (*24*). Accordingly, 1,2-dichloroethane was weakly mutagenic in *Sal. typhimurium* (*258, 259*). Addition of microsomal enzymes, cytoplasm, and NADP enhanced this effect; a further increase was observed after adding glutathione (*260*). The existence of this metabolic system in *Drosophila melanogaster* is indicated by the high frequency of mutation induced by 1,2-dichloroethane in this species (*264–66*).

In the rat 1,2-dichloroethane is metabolized to chloroacetic acid possibly via 2-chloroethanol (*261*), which is also a mutagen (*262*). Chloroacetic acid, *S*-carboxymethylcysteine, and thiodiacetic acid are all excreted in the urine of rats (*261*). Little in vitro dechlorination of 1,2-dichloroethane has been observed in rabbit liver preparations (*263*).

In a National Cancer Institute (NCI) study, rats and mice received 47 and 95 mg/kg/d of 1,2-dichloroethane by gavage for 78 weeks; the following observation period was 32 and 23 weeks for the low- and high-dose rats, respectively, and 12–13 weeks for the mice (*267*). In the rats, squamous cell carcinomas of the forestomach and hemangiosarcomas were seen in both sexes; subcutaneous fibromas were specific to males, and mammary adenocarcinomas were specific to females. Mice of both sexes showed alveolar/bronchiolar adenomas; females also had mammary adenocarcinomas and endometrial tumors.

In humans, many instances of acute poisoning have been observed (*268, 269*); documented cases include dysfunction of liver, kidney, and the hemopoietic system that were preceded by anorexia, nausea, and abdominal pain. However, no epidemiological studies or case reports on carcinogenicity are available.

1,2-Dibromoethane (Ethylene Dibromide). Several hundred million kilograms of this chemical is produced annually for use as a lead scavenger in antiknock gasolines, as a soil and grain fumigant, as a solvent, and in syntheses of dyes and pharmaceuticals (*270*). It has been found in air, water, and soil (*271*), although a decreasing amount in the environment is expected due to the decreasing use of leaded gasoline.

Biotransformation in the rat, mouse, and guinea pig leads to urinary excretion of *S*-(2-hydroxyethyl)cysteine, *N*-acetyl-*S*-(2-hydroxyethyl)cysteine, and its *S*-oxide (*272*); the involvement of glutathione conjugation in vivo and in vitro has been described (*273*). As with 1,2-dichloroethane, a glutathione conjugate, specifically the 2-halothioether, seems to be the ultimate mutagen in *Sal. typhimurium* (*274*).

1,2-Dibromoethane is a weak mutagen without metabolic activation (*81, 258, 259*), and no mutagenicity has been observed in the *Salmonella* host-mediated assay (*275*) or in the dominant lethal assay in mice (*119*).

1,2-Dibromoethane induced squamous cell carcinomas in the stomach of rats and mice after daily oral intubation (*276*); this result indicates a direct alkylating effect at the site of contact (*277*). Rats and mice developed carcinoma, adenocarcinoma, and adenoma of the nasal cavities following 78–103 weeks of exposure at concentrations of 10 and 40 ppm. In addition, hemangiosarcoma and fibrosarcoma in the circulatory system and alveolar/bronchiolar carcinoma and adenoma were found in these animals (*278*). Rats fed 20 ppm of 1,2-dibromoethane for 18 months experienced high mortality and increased tumor incidences in one or both sexes of the mammary gland, spleen, adrenal, liver, kidney, and subcutaneous tissue. Neoplasms were seen earlier and occurred with a higher incidence in rats concomitantly receiving 0.05% disulfiram (*279*). In rats disulfiram was found to increase radioactivity in main organs after oral administration of ^{14}C-labeled 1,2-dibromoethane (*280*).

Findings of malignant neoplasms in respiratory and gastrointestinal tracts in 161 workers exposed in chemical plants are found equivocal because of the small population and the exposure to numerous other chemicals (*281*).

Hexachloroethane (Perchloroethane). This chemical is used for many applications, for example, as a plasticizer, as an accelerator in rubber, as a fermentation retardant, as an insecticide, in the formulation of extreme pressure lubricants, and for cellulose esters (*282*).

Very little is known on its biological effects. At least 10 metabolites are present in the urine or are exhaled after dosing of rabbits; the exhaled metabolites are possibly due to dehydrochlorination and dehalogenation without oxidation (*283*). Recently, hexachloroethane was reported to be carcinogenic in mice, because it induces hepatocellular carcinoma after oral administration. No tumors were seen in rats (*284*).

Pentachloroethane (Pentalin). Pentachloroethane (PCE) is a solvent for fats and oils in metal cleaning. A technical-grade formulation, in which the major contaminant is hexachloroethane (4.2%), has been assayed in a carcinogenicity study (*285*). In this study, PCE was administered by gavage at levels of 75 or 100 mg/kg/d to rats, and 250 or 500 mg/kg/d to mice. In the rats, no increased tumor incidence was seen. In the mice, survival time was shortened in both groups. Increased incidence of hepatocellular carcinoma and adenoma occurred in all treated mice, but no other increases in primary tumor incidence were seen. Pentachloroethane has been shown to be metabolized in mice to trichloroethylene (18–48%) and tetrachloroethylene (12–31%) (*286*). Both of these chloroethylenes produce hepatocellular carcinomas in mice but not in rats.

1,1,2,2-Tetrachloroethane (Acetylene Tetrachloride). This substance is mainly used as an intermediate in the production of trichloroethylene; its application as an insecticide or a solvent is of minor importance (*282*).

In mice it is subject to sequential loss of chlorine atoms that terminates in the formation of CO_2; the CO_2 is then exhaled with minute amounts of tri- and tetrachloroethylene (*286*). Incubation with rat liver microsomes or the reconstituted monoxygenase system produces dichloroacetyl chloride, which can bind covalently to various nucleophiles or hydrolyze to dichloroacetic acid (*287*). Mutagenicity has been observed in *E. coli* and in the *Salmonella* test (*258, 288*). It induced hepatocellular carcinoma in mice but not in rats (*289*). Embryonic effects and a low incidence of malformation were found in offspring after high dosage to female mice (*290*).

Tetrachloroethylene (Perchloroethylene). An estimated 6×10^9 kg of this chemical was produced in 1972 mainly for use as a solvent in the textile industry, as an industrial metal cleaner, and as an intermediate in the production of fluorocarbons (*291*). Because of its wide use and relative stability, it is found in air, water, food, marine organisms, and human tissues (*198, 257, 291*).

The chemical is readily absorbed through the lungs and, to some extent, in the gastrointestinal tract and the skin (*292*). Metabolism occurs via an epoxide (*293*) to form trichloroacetic acid, which has been detected in the urine of rats. Both trichloroacetic acid and trichloroethanol have been detected in the urine of exposed human volunteers and in the rat liver perfusate (*294, 295*). Toxic effects in humans include irritation of the skin and mucous membranes, lung edema, gastrointestinal symptoms, and neurological effects (*292*).

Reports on the mutagenicity and carcinogenicity of tetrachloroethylene remain debatable. There is one unconfirmed positive result reported in bacteria (*296*), but it is not mutagenic in the *Salmonella* microsome assay (*17*) or in *E. coli* (*45*), whereas trichloroethylene, 1,1-dichloroethylene, and vinyl chloride were. This variation has been explained by metabolic differences: the symmetrically halogenated tetrachloroethylene and the *cis*- and *trans*-1,2-dichloroethylene form relatively stable oxiranes during metabolic activation, whereas the nonsymmetrically halogenated ethylenes mentioned form less stable oxiranes and other degradation products that have mutagenic activities (*45, 293*). Tetrachloroethylene did not induce chromosomal aberrations in mice (*296*), and no embryotoxicity or teratogenicity was observed in rats and mice at nontoxic doses (*297*).

The carcinogenicity bioassay conducted by NCI indicated that mice but not rats exposed by gavage to 500 or 1000 mg/kg throughout their lifetime showed an increased incidence of hepatocellular carcinoma (*298*). In a chronic inhalation study, exposure to 300 and 600 ppm/d for 1 year with a subsequent 18-month observation period did not prove to be carcinogenic in rats (*299*). A dose–response study in mice and studies in four strains of rats at NCI are near completion.

The species differences in the carcinogenic effect so far detected seem to be due to quantitative differences in the metabolic activation process (*300*). Mice metabolized tetrachloroethylene 8.5 times faster than rats; the amount of irreversible binding of the ^{14}C-labeled compound to macromolecules was sevenfold in mice, as was cytotoxicity, at equal doses. However, no radioactivity was bound to liver DNA in either species. These results indicate an epigenetic effect of tetrachloroethylene; it induces hepatocellular carcinoma in mice on the basis of a recurrent hepatotoxicity during lifetime exposure of high cytotoxic doses.

1,1,1-Trichloroethane (Methylchloroform). Only one report in the literature describes a weak mutagenic effect in the *Salmonella* microsome assay (*100*). Studies with rats and mice for male and female reproductive function, embryo development, and teratogenicity gave negative results (*297, 301*).

In a carcinogenesis bioassay, rats received 750 or 1500 mg/kg orally by gavage for 78 weeks and mice received 2000 or 4000 mg/kg increasing to 3000 and 6000 mg/kg at week 10 for a total of 96 weeks (*302*). The neoplasms observed were not attributable to 1,1,1-trichloroethane exposure. Because of the shortened life spans of both the rats and the mice, the data are equivocal and a second study is now underway.

Metabolism of the chemical seems to be slow in rats and mice (*303*). After inhalation of 1500 ppm, more than 90% of the parent chemical was eliminated by exhalation in both species. The remaining radioactivity was recovered as CO_2 in the expired air and as nonvolatile radioactivity in the urine, feces, carcass, and cage wash. No change was seen in the pharmacokinetics after 16-month exposure to 1500 ppm for 6 h/d, 5 d/week.

Technical grade 1,1,1-trichloroethane contains impurities that might be responsible for adverse effects (*304*). Of 22 samples, 18 contained 30–900 μg of vinylidene chloride/mL. Further contaminants were 1,1-dichloroethane, trichloroethylene, and 1,1,2-trichloroethane; nitromethane, 1,2-epoxybutane, *t*-butyl alcohol, and dioxane were present as stabilizers.

1,1,2-Trichloroethane (Vinyl Trichloride). Approximately 1×10^9 kg of this chemical is produced annually to be used mainly in the production of 1,1-dichloroethylene and as an industrial solvent (*282*). It is one of the 72 compounds that have been detected in drinking water and is a sea water pollutant (*305*).

1,1,2-Trichloroethane is readily absorbed through the skin (*306, 307*) and induces hepatotoxicity and kidney damage (*308*). Oral application to mice resulted in urinary excretion of chloroacetic acid, *S*-carboxymethylcysteine, thiodiacetic acid and small amounts of glycolic acid, 2,2-dichloroethanol, 2,2,2-trichloroethanol, oxalic acid, and trichloroacetic acid. These products suggest that metabolism is via chloroacetaldehyde (*309*).

In a carcinogenesis bioassay, 1,1,2-trichloroethane was administered by gavage for a period of 78 weeks at time-weighted average doses of 46 and 92 mg/kg/d to rats and 195 and 390 mg/kg/d to mice. Hepatocellular carcinoma and adrenal pheochromocytomas were observed in the mice but not the rats (*310*). No mutagenicity has been found in the *Salmonella* test (*260*).

Trichloroethylene (Acetylene Trichloride). Annual production of this chemical is several hundred million kilograms for use mainly as a solvent for degreasing, in the textile industry, in food processing (decaffeinated coffee), and in many consumer products such as automobile cleansers, buffing solutions, spot removers, rug cleaners, disinfectants, and deodorants (*311*). The loss of trichloroethylene to the environment was estimated to be over 1×10^6 tons in 1972 (*198*).

Because of its widespread use, its metabolism and toxicity have been studied extensively. However, great variations in impurities and manufacturing processes produce inconsistencies in the experimental results. Exposure to 100–400 ppm in the air for 7 h/d, 5 d/week, for 6 months was tolerated without toxic effects by rats, rabbits, guinea pigs, and monkeys (*312*). Cirrhosis and portal hypertension occurred after repeated bouts of acute hepatotoxicity caused by trichloroethylene (*313*).

Metabolism of trichloroethylene proceeds via an oxirane that, by a Lewis acid catalytic type, rearranges to the nonreactive chloral hydrate in microsomes of mammals (*314*). Bacteria may not express this enzymatic mechanism, and this plausible difference could account for the weak mutagenic effects found in *E. coli* and *Sal. typhimurium* in the presence of a metabolic activation system (*45, 99*). Observations of mutagenicity to *Salmonella* without metabolic activation (*296*) most likely stem from impurities, such as epichlorohydrin and 1,2-epoxybutane (*117*) that are added as stabilizers. Because rats possess a higher epoxide hydrolase activity than mice (*315*), a higher detoxication of these epoxides in the rat is suggested. This metabolic difference would explain the occurrence of hepatocellular tumors and lung tumors in mice but not in rats when nonpurified trichloroethylene was used (*316*). However, in an 18-month inhalation study of trichloroethylene stabilized with an amine base (100 and 500 ppm 6 h/d, 5 d/week; 30 males and 30 females per dose), no indication of carcinogenic potential was found in mice, rats, or Syrian hamsters (*317*). More recently, NCI conducted a carcinogenesis bioassay of epichlorohydrin-free trichloroethylene in rats and mice. Rats and mice received gavage doses of 500 and 1000 mg/kg and 1000 mg/kg, respectively, five times a week for 2 years (*318*). Both doses exceeded the maximum tolerated dose for male rats. Dose-related toxic changes in the kidneys were produced in both sexes of rats and mice. In rats, incidence of renal tubular adenocarcinoma increased only in the high-dose males. In mice, hepatocellular carcinoma was found in both sexes.

Studies on pharmacokinetics and macromolecular interaction revealed a higher metabolic rate, hepatic macromolecular binding, cytotoxicity, and regenerative processes in livers of mice than in rats, as well as a very low DNA interaction even in mice (*319–21*). When coupled with the weak or negative mutagenic effects in vitro and the toxic effects in livers and kidneys observed in the carcinogenesis bioassays, these data suggest an epigenetic mechanism in tumor formation that would only occur on chronic administration of high cytotoxic doses of trichloroethylene.

The chemical was neither embryotoxic nor teratogenic in rats and mice (*299, 321*); it was negative in the dominant lethal assay in mice (*322*); and it did not induce chromosomal aberrations in mice (*296*) or premalignant lesions in rats after inhalation of 2000 ppm for 3 months, 8 h/d, for 5 d/week (*323*).

No statistically significant excess of cancer was observed in an epidemiological study (*324*). Due to the small sample size and the relatively short duration of exposure, no assessment of carcinogenicity could be made (*311*). In highly exposed degreasers, hypodiploid cells were seen in peripheral lymphocytes, but no chromosomal aberrations (*325*). Sister chromatid exchanges have been found to be increased in lymphocytes of six chronically exposed workers who had elevated blood levels of trichloroethanol and trichloroacetic acid (*326*).

Besides the microsomal oxidation via 2,2,3-trichlorooxirane—suggested because of the spectral changes of the microsomal cytochrome P-450 (*327*)—to chloral hydrate (*314*), trichloroethylene is reduced to trichloroethanol and formation of trichloroacetic acid is observed in vivo and in vitro (*328*). Involvement of cytochrome P-450 in the chlorine migration without formation of the oxirane has also been reported (*329*).

Miscellaneous Agents

3,3′-Dichlorobenzidine [4,4′-Methylenebis(2-chloroaniline) or 4,4′-Diamino-3,3′-dichlorodiphenylmethane] (IV). About 5×10^6 kg of this substance is produced annually, mainly for use as a curing agent for isocyanate-containing polymers (*330*). It was mutagenic in the *Salmonella* test (*97*). The chemical induces carcinoma of the liver and lung in rats and mice (*331–33*). Urinary tract tumors were reported in dogs (*334*). The target variance might be due to species difference in the metabolism and excretion of the chemical, but no information on its metabolism is available.

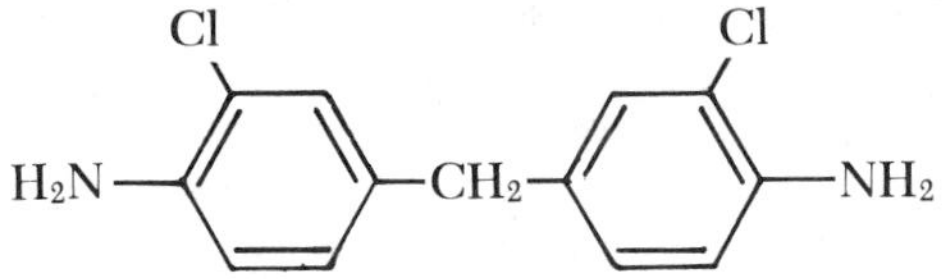

Cl Cl

H_2N—⟨ring⟩—CH_2—⟨ring⟩—NH_2

IV

Allyl Chloride (3-Chloro-1-propene). This chemical is used as a monomer in the synthesis of various plastics, resins, and allyl-substituted pharmaceuticals or incorporated into surface coating adhesives. The U.S. annual production is approximately 1×10^9 kg (*335*).

Metabolism of allyl chloride was studied by Kaye et al. (*336*). In rats, it is conjugated with glutathione and excreted in the urine as mercapturic acids. *S*-Allyl glutathione and *S*-allyl-2-cysteine were also detected in the bile. Epoxidation to form epichlorohydrin has been suggested as another metabolic pathway (*335*).

Allyl chloride is a direct-acting mutagen in the *Salmonella* test and in *E. coli* when sufficient measures are taken to prevent evaporation (*337, 338*). In an early study, no increases in tumor rates were observed in rats, guinea pigs, and rabbits after inhalation of 3 ppm of allyl chloride for 6 months (*339*). A more recent NCI study (*340*) reported that the compound, when administered by gavage, caused a low incidence of squamous cell carcinomas and papillomas of the forestomach in both male and female mice; the study was considered inadequate to detect a possible carcinogenic effect in rats due to the poor survival of these animals. It is tempting to suggest that the chemical is sufficiently inactivated in the intact animal by glutathione conjugation; this inactivation mechanism has already been proposed for 1,1-dichloroethylene (*20, 67*) and chloroprene (*21*).

4-Chloromethylbiphenyl (4-CMB) (V). In *Sal. typhimurium* and *E. coli*, 4-CMB is a direct-acting mutagen. Additions of a microsomal mix reduced this potency in the *Salmonella* test (*341*). It induced sister chromatid exchanges and chromosomal aberrations in cultured rat liver epithelial cells, but no chromosomal aberrations in cultured human lymphocytes and V79 cells. Minimal chromosomal aberrations were seen in the Chinese hamster bone marrow test; no effect was observed on mouse genocytes (*342*). In a skin painting test, 100 μL of 4-CMB was applied to the dorsal region of mice twice weekly. After 7 months of treatment, not one of the 20 animals appeared to have been affected by the chemical (*341*). A weak positive effect has been shown in the sebaceous gland suppression test (*343*).

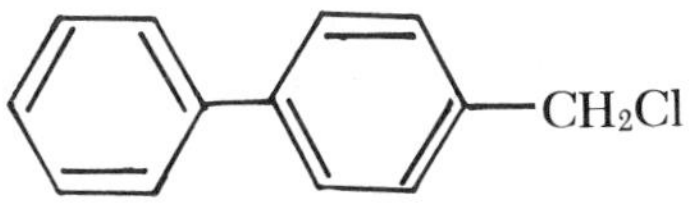

CH_2Cl

V

Polychlorinated Biphenyls (PCBs)

PCBs are liquid mixtures of about 50 to 100 single isomers and congeners that vary widely in the amount and position of the chlorine substituents in the biphenyl molecule. These products have gained extensive use in industry, predominantly in capacitors and transformers or as hydraulic and heat-transfer fluids. Usage in open systems (e.g., as a plasticizer), improper disposal, and leakage of discharged materials appear to be the major sources of environmental contamination by PCBs (*344*). Two extensive reviews are available on the chemistry, metabolism, animal toxicology, and human exposure of PCBs (*344, 345*). The carcinogenic potential of PCBs has also been discussed in detail (*346–49*).

Because of their poor metabolism, PCBs—particularly those with a higher degree of chlorination—tend to accumulate in wildlife (*349*) and, via the food chain, in humans (*350*). At present, fish consumption seems to be the main source of PCB uptake by humans (*345*). Although the general intake of the population is assumed to be very low, questions about long-term health effects, particularly carcinogenic effects, were raised when some 2000 Japanese were poisoned in 1968. They ingested rice oil contaminated with PCBs, polychlorinated terphenyls (PCTs), and polychlorinated dibenzofurans (PCDFs) (*351, 352*).

These "Yusho" patients suffered from dermal symptoms, including chloracne and pigmentation, and exhibited signs of ocular, neurological, and endocrine disorders. The total average intake was estimated to be 0.6 g of PCBs and PCTs and 3 mg of PCDFs during a period of 10 weeks. A decade after the exposure, the incidence of neoplasias in Yusho patients was examined: neoplasms accounted for 35% of the 31 deaths; the mortality rate from neoplasms of the nonpoisoned population was 21% (*353*). Autopsy of 10 patients revealed 2 cases of liver carcinoma and 1 of lung carcinoma (*354*).

The carcinogenic potential of PCBs for humans had been suspected prior to these two studies in 1976 when an increased incidence of malignant melanomas was reported for a group of 72 petrochemical workers who had been exposed to Aroclor 1254 from 1941 to 1950 (*355*). Another 1976 epidemiological study among 300 former PCB workers initiated by the PCB producer Monsanto could not link the incidence of melanomas and other tumors to PCB exposure (*356*).

A number of long-term studies in mice and rats given commercial PCB mixtures orally revealed neoplastic nodules and, in some cases, carcinomas of the liver, but no tumors in other organs. Kanechlor 500 induced hepatocellular carcinomas and nodular hyperplasia in male mice from the dd strain given a dietary dose of 500 ppm/d for 1 year (*357*). The less chlorinated products Kanechlor 300 and 400 were inactive. Neoplastic liver nodules were observed when male mice of the BALBc/J strain were fed 300 ppm of Aroclor 1254, which is similar to Kanechlor 500 in chlorine content (*358*). In the rat, high-chlorinated biphenyls also showed stronger effects than the less chlorinated products. After a feeding period of 2 years at a dietary level of 100 ppm, Aroclor 1260 and Clophen A-60 both produced hepatocellular carcinomas in female Sherman and in male Wistar rats, respectively (*359, 360*). The low-chlorinated product Clophen A-30 was ineffective in the Wistar rats (*360*). Nodular hyperplasia, hepatomas, and cholangiohepatomas were diagnosed in Charles River rats of both sexes that were fed 100 ppm of Aroclor 1242, 1254, and 1260 for 2 years (*361*). Female rats from the Donryu strain developed multiple adenomatous nodules following a 400-d treatment with Kanechlor 400 at doses varying between 38 and 616 ppm (*362*). Apparently the stronger tumorigenic potential of the high-chlorinated biphenyls observed in these studies parallels the stronger biological activity, such as liver toxicity (363), and the greater capability to induce hepatic monooxygenases (*364*).

In contrast to the high doses applied to mice and rats, rhesus monkeys showed hypertrophic and hyperplastic changes of the gastric mucosa, a result that suggests preneoplastic alterations, at dietary doses of 25 ppm after only 2 months of exposure (*365*).

In addition to the carcinogenic and tumorigenic effects, PCBs were also shown to increase the incidence of liver tumors induced by other carcinogens. For example, Kanechlor 500 enhanced the formation of liver tumors in mice that received α- or β-isomers of benzene hexachloride (*357*). Strong tumor-promoting effects of PCBs were also observed in rats exposed primarily to diethylnitrosamine (*366*), *N*-2-fluorenylacetamide (*367*), and 3′-methyl-4-dimethylaminoazobenzene (*368*). The moderate response observed in the carcinogenicity studies with PCBs might result from a high potential to promote but a low potential to initiate preneoplastic lesions.

Pesticides

From the large group of halogenated pesticides, only a few have been tested in long-term studies. We have subdivided these pesticides into several subgroups. The first group, summarized in Table I, contains pesticides that are carcinogenic in two or more animal species. In the second group, summarized in Table II, are chemicals proven to be carcinogenic in mice; studies with these compounds in rats showed either negative or inconclusive results. The third group comprises pesticides that have been labeled noncarcinogens.

Extensive reviews on carcinogenic and toxic effects by Sternberg (*369*), Burchfild and Storrs (*370*), Metcalf (*371a*), and Falk (*371b*) are available.

Substances That Are Carcinogenic in Two or More Species. Organochlorine Pesticides. Organochlorine pesticides have been widely used in agriculture for several decades and are now ubiquitous contaminants of the environment. Except for hexachlorobenzene, which is a fungicide, all compounds are used as

Table I
Pesticides That Are Carcinogenic in Two or More Species

Compound	*Species, Strain*	*Dietary Concentration (Duration of Treatment)*[a]	*Type of Tumor*	*Reference*
Chlordecone (Kepone) (**VI**)	mouse, B6C3F1 hybrid	T1 ♂: 20,23 ppm T1 ♀: 20,40 ppm (80/90 w)	well-differentiated hepatocellular carcinoma	*373*
	rat, albino	10, 25 ppm (2 y)	hepatocellular carcinoma	*375*
	rat, Osborne–Mendel	T1 ♂: 26 ppm T1 ♀: 24 ppm (80/112 w)	heptocellular carcinoma	*373*
1,2-Dibromo-3-chloropropane	mouse, (C57BL×C3H)F1	♂: ~200 mg/kg/d ♀: ~100 mg/kg/d (54 w)	squamous cell carcinoma	*374*
	mouse, B6C3F1 hybrids	T2 ♂: 114, 219 mg/kg/d T2 ♀: 110, 209 mg/kg/d (47/60 w)	squamous cell carcinoma of forestomach, frequent metastases in abdominal viscera and lungs	*376*
	mouse, Swiss	sc: 35 mg/mouse; 3 times/w (440/495 d)	lung and stomach tumors	*377*
	mouse, Swiss	inh: 0.6 and 3.0 ppm (104 w)	lung tumors	*378*
	rat, Osborne–Mendel	24–30 mg/kg/d	squamous cell carcinoma of forestomach, adenocarcinoma of the mammary gland	*374*
		T2: 15, 29 mg/kg/d (64/78 w)	squamous cell carcinoma of forestomach, adenocarcinoma of the mammary gland	*376*
Heptachlor (**VII**) and heptachlor epoxide (**VIII**)	mouse, C3H	10 ppm (heptachlor, heptachlor epoxide) (2 y)	hepatoma, hepatic carcinoma	*379*
	mouse, Charles River CD1	5, 10 ppm 75:25 heptachlor epoxide–heptachlor) (18 m)	liver carcinoma	reported in *379*
	mouse, B6C3F1	T1 ♂: 14 ppm T1 ♀: 18 ppm (technical-grade heptachlor) (80 w)	liver carcinoma	*380*

Continued on next page

Table I Continued

Compound	Species, Strain	Dietary Concentration (Duration of Treatment)[a]	Type of Tumor	Reference
	rat, Carsworth Farm–Nelson	5, 10 ppm heptachlor epoxide (100 w)	hepatic carcinoma in females	reported in *379*
	rat, Osborne–Mendel	T1: 51 ppm technical-grade heptachlor (80 w)	follicular cell thyroid neoplasms	*380*
Hexachlorobenzene	mouse, Swiss	100, 200, 300 ppm (120 w)	liver cell tumors	*381*
	hamster, Syrian	50, 100, 200 ppm (life span)	hepatoma, hemangioendothelioma, thyroid adenoma	*382*
1,2,3,4,5,6-Hexachlorocyclohexane (HCH) (technical mixture of isomers, predominantly α-HCH)	mouse, dd (♂)	660 ppm (24 w)	hepatomas	*383*
	mouse, ICR–JCL	600 ppm (26 w)	liver nodules	*384*
	mouse, dd	300, 600 ppm (32 w)	hepatomas	*385*
α-HCH	mouse, ICR–JCL	600 ppm (26 w)	liver nodules (frequently malignant)	*384*
	mouse, dd	300, 600 ppm (32 w)	hepatomas	*385*
		250, 500 ppm (24 w)	hepatocellular carcinoma, liver nodular hyperplasia	*386, 387*
	mouse, DDY ICR DBA/2 C3H/He	500 ppm (24 w)	hepatocellular carcinoma, nodular hyperplasia	*388*
	mouse, C57BL/6	500 ppm (24 w)	nodular hyperplasia	*388*
	rat, Wistar	♂: 1000, 15000 ppm (72 w)	hyperplastic nodules, hepatocellular carcinoma	*391*a
		800 ppm (104 w/life span)	hyperplastic nodules, carcinomas, and malignant neoplasms in females	*392, 404,* as reported in *393*

Table I Continued

Compound	*Species, Strain*	*Dietary Concentration (Duration of Treatment)*[a]	*Type of Tumor*	*Reference*
β-HCH	mouse, ICR–JCL	600 ppm (26 w)	benign liver tumors	*384*
	mouse, CF1	200, 400 ppm (110 w)	benign and malignant liver tumors	*389*
Lindane (γ-HCH)	mouse, ICR–JCL	600 ppm (26 w)	liver nodules	*384*
	mouse, dd	600 ppm (32 w)	hepatomas, cellular carcinomas	*385*
	mouse, CF1	400 ppm (110 w)	benign and malignant liver tumors, lung metastases	*389*
	rat, Osborne–Mendel	T1 ♂: 236, 472 ppm T1 ♀: 135, 275 ppm (80 w)	carcinomas and adenomas of endocrine organs (pituitary, thyroid, adrenal, ovary), neoplastic nodules, and liver carcinoma	*395*
Methoxychlor (**IX**)	mouse, B6C3F1	T1 ♂: 1746, 3491 ppm T1 ♀: 997, 1994 ppm (77/92 w)	bone hemangiosarcoma in females	*398*
	mouse, C3H	750 ppm (2 y)	hepatocellular carcinoma in males	*399* (as reported in 429a)
	mouse, BALB/c	750 ppm (2 y)	testis carcinoma, malignant liver neoplasms	*400*
	rat, Osborne–Mendel	100, 200, 500, 2000 ppm (104 w)	hyperplastic nodules, hepatocellular carcinomas (2000 ppm), ovary carcinoma (500 ppm)	*401* (as reported in 429a)
		T2 ♂: 448, 750 ppm T2 ♀: 845, 1385 ppm (78/111 w)	hyperplastic nodules and carcinomas of the liver, ovary (1385 ppm), hemangiosarcoma in spleen of males	*398*
Mirex (**X**)	mouse, (C57BL/6×C3HAnf)F1 (C57BL/6×AKR)F1 hybrids	10 mg/kg bw (d 7–28) and 26 ppm (66 w)	hepatoma	*131, 396*

Continued on next page

Table I ***Continued***

Compound	Species, Strain	Dietary Concentration (Duration of Treatment)[a]	Type of Tumor	Reference
		sc: 1000 mg/kg (single injection)	reticulum cell sarcomas	*396*
	rat, CD	50, 100 ppm (2 y)	neoplastic liver nodules, liver cell carcinoma, fibrosarcoma, squamous cell carcinoma	*397*
Toxaphene (polychlorinated camphenes)	mouse, B6C3F1	T1: 99, 198 ppm (80 w)	hepatocellular carcinomas, neoplastic nodules	*402*
	rat, Osborne–Mendel	T1: 550, 1100 ppm (80/108 w)	follicular cell carcinomas, thyroid adenomas	*402*
2,4,6-Trichlorophenol	mouse, B6C3F1	♂: 5000, 10,000 ppm (105 w) T1 ♀: 5214, 10,428 ppm	hepatocellular carcinomas or adenomas	*403*
	rat, Fischer 344	5000, 10,000 ppm (106/107 w)	lymphoma, leukemia in males	*403*

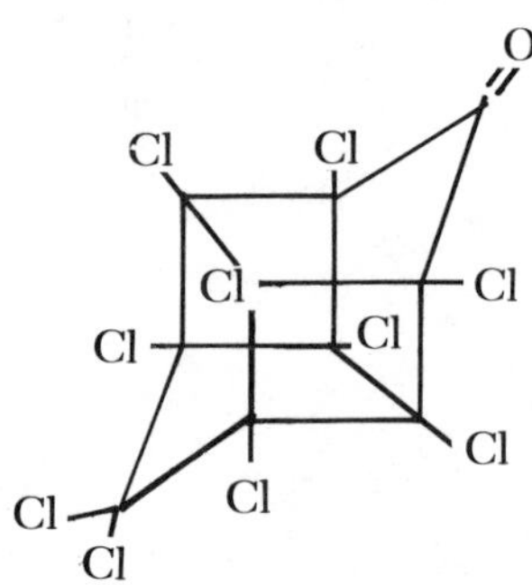

VI

VII

VIII

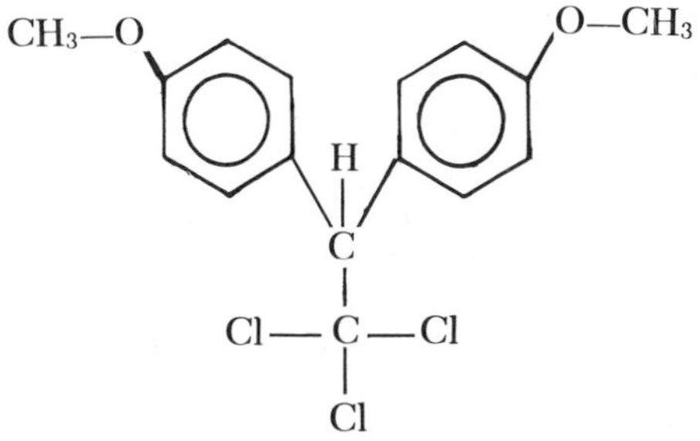

IX

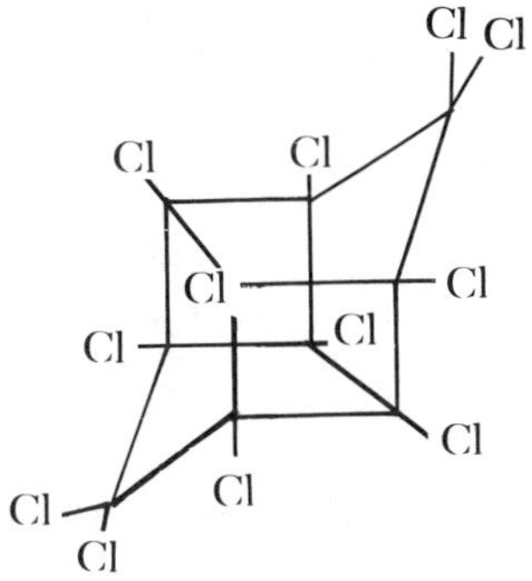

X

[a]T1 indicates time weight average of dietary concentration; T2 indicates time weight average of dose. Only doses and experiments that caused a significant increase of tumor incidence over controls are given. If not mentioned, animals of both sexes were used. Concentration is given in parts per million (milligrams of compound per kilogram of diet) when administered in the diet or in milligrams of compound per kilogram of body weight when administered by gavage. Subcutaneous injection is indicated by sc; inhalation is indicated in inh. First number in parentheses indicates the duration of treatment; second number indicates total experimental period.

insecticides. Two products are mixtures of isomers or congeners: technical-grade hexachlorocyclohexane (HCH) contains a varying amount of α-, γ-, and δ-isomers; and toxaphene is a complex product consisting of more than 150 different compounds with 4–12 different chlorine atoms/molecule, and it is manufactured by chlorination of camphenes (*372*).

During the past decade, the application of these chemicals was restricted or questioned. In the United States, the use of chlordecone (kepone) and mirex was cancelled by the Environmental Protection Agency (EPA) in 1976. Hexachlorobenzene, HCH, and toxaphene were made subjects of rebuttable presumption by the EPA. Since 1983, the only approved use for heptachlor is for underground termite control. In Japan, the use of lindane and heptachlor was discontinued in 1971 and 1972, respectively (*372*).

The types of tumor most frequently observed in the carcinogenicity studies listed in Table I were tumorigenic and carcinogenic alterations of the hepatobiliary system. These alterations are typified as hepatoma, cholangioma, liver carcinoma, bile duct adenoma, neo- or hyperplastic nodules, and cancer of the biliary system. Among the hepatocarcinogenic compounds are the chlorinated hydrocarbons chlordecone, heptachlor and its epoxide, hexachlorobenzene, hexachlorocyclohexane, mirex, and toxaphene. The results of the numerous long-term feeding studies in various strains of mice and rats are summarized in Table I.

Chlordecone increased the incidence of well-differentiated hepatocellular carcinomas in mice and rats of both sexes (*373*). An earlier study gave similar results; the number of survivors, however, was very low (*375*).

Heptachlor and its epoxide both increased the incidence of hepatomas and hepatic carcinomas in male and female C3H mice (*379*). This study was confirmed by other studies that used technical-grade heptachlor (*380*) or heptachlor epoxide

(*379*). Heptachlor epoxide induced an excess of hepatocarcinoma in female CFN rats. The incidence in males of this strain was only significant when hepatocarcinomas and hyperplastic nodules were combined (*379*). Female Osborne–Mendel rats fed with technical-grade heptachlor developed follicular cell thyroid neoplasms. No liver tumors were reported (*380*).

Hexachlorobenzene of high purity was administered to Swiss mice at doses of 50, 100, 200, and 300 ppm in the diet. Both sexes in the groups treated with the three highest doses developed liver tumors (*381*). Another study was performed with Syrian golden hamsters that received 50, 100, and 200 ppm of the pure compound for their lifetime. Hepatomas occurred in all treated groups compared with none in the controls. Hemangioendotheliomas were found in the highest dose group only. Alveolar thyroid adenomas were also observed (*382*).

Hexachlorocyclohexane (HCH) represents one of the most important and widely used insecticides. It is produced in large amounts in many countries. The insecticidal activity of HCH is due to the γ-isomer lindane that is extracted from technical-grade HCH by organic solvents. Numerous studies have been undertaken to evaluate tumorigenic effects, predominantly in mice. As stated in Table I, all HCH isomers tested were liver carcinogens. Technical-grade HCH, which contains about 60% α-HCH (*383*), showed moderate effects compared with 100% α-HCH and lindane. The severity of the response further appeared to depend on the duration of treatment. β-HCH did not induce any tumors in two strains of mice after about 6 months of treatment (*385–87*) but did induce benign and malignant liver tumors after 2 years of treatment (*389*). Similarly, liver carcinomas induced by lindane were not detected after 6 months of feeding (*384–87*), but they appeared after prolonged treatment for 110 weeks (*389*). In mice treated with α-HCH, the proportion of tumor-bearing animals increased to almost 100% between 20 and 36 weeks of treatment (*390*). In Wistar rats, α-HCH induced hyperplastic nodules in a high proportion of animals in both the 1000- and 1500-ppm dose groups and carcinomas in 3 of 13 animals in the high-dose group. No tumors were found in controls (*391a, 391b*). A lower dose of 800 ppm of α-HCH induced hyperplastic nodules (5/10) and carcinomas (3/10) in females only (*392, 404*). β-HCH given to Osborne–Mendel rats produced liver carcinomas in 3 of 8 survivors. Although no controls were available, the accepted incidence of spontaneous liver carcinoma in this strain is 1 in 50 (*393*). In an NCI study that was evaluated by Reuber (*394*), neoplasms were detected at various sites in Osborne–Mendel rats that were fed lindane at doses between 135 and 472 ppm for 80 weeks.

In addition to neoplastic nodules and carcinomas of the liver, there was a striking induction of tumors and carcinomas, especially in females, in endocrine organs, including the thyroid, pituitary, and adrenal gland, as well as the ovary (*395*). The evaluation of this study is controversial. The IARC registered only a slight excess of thyroid C-cell tumors in females and no significant incidence of other tumors (*372*).

A response in rats differing from that in mice was reported for the insecticides mirex and toxaphene. Mice that received dietary treatment or a single subcutaneous injection with mirex developed hepatomas and reticulum cell sarcomas (*131, 396*). In rats treated with mirex for 2 years, fibrosarcomas, fibromas, and squamous cell sarcomas of the ear duct were found, in addition to hepatocellular carcinomas and large-sized hepatomas (*397*). Technical-grade toxaphene induced hepatocellular carcinomas and neoplastic nodules in mice (*402*). However Osborne–Mendel rats that were given this product for 80 weeks followed by an observation period of 30 weeks showed follicular cell carcinomas and adenomas of the thyroid in both sexes and neoplasms of the pituitary in females. No liver tumors were reported (*402*).

The organochlorines, in contrast to the carcinogenic effect, showed negative results in bacterial and mammalian mutagenicity test systems. Chlordecone was negative in the dominant lethal assay in rats after repeated administration of 3.6 and 11.4 mg/kg of body weight (*405*). Mirex was negative in the hepatocyte DNA repair assay (*406*).

Hexachlorobenzene was ineffective in the dominant lethal test with rats at doses up to 60 mg/kg of body weight (*407*) and in an in vitro test system with *Sacch. cerevisiae* (*408*). Heptachlor and its expoxide were not mutagenic in the *Salmonella* assay with and without liver microsomes (*409*) and did not induce recessive lethals in *Drosophila* (*410*). Negative results were also obtained in the dominant lethal assay performed with rats that were fed 1 and 5 ppm of heptachlor (*411*) and with mice that received single doses of 7.5 and 15 mg/kg of body weight of a 25:75 heptachlor–heptachlor epoxide mixture (*412*). However, the frequency of chromosomal aberrations in bone marrow cells increased 21 h after injection of heptachlor in mice (*413*). In transformed human cells (VA-4) in vitro, heptachlor and heptachlor epoxide induced unscheduled DNA synthesis in the presence of a rat liver microsomal activation system (*414*); the validity of this human test system has been questioned, because heptachlor did not induce DNA repair in primary hepatocyte cultures of mice, rats, and hamsters (*406*). HCH and its isomers were ineffective in both systems. Negative results were obtained for lindane in VA-4 cells (*414*), bacteria (*415*), and *Drosophila* (*410*). α-HCH did not produce mutations in yeast (*416*), and technical HCH was negative in bacteria (*417*). Toxaphene showed mutagenic activity in vitro in the Ames assay without an activation system (*418*), but it did not induce dominant lethal mutations in mice treated once intraperitoneally with 36 and 180 mg/kg or five times orally with 40 and 80 mg/kg (*112*).

The data that show negative or marginal mutagenic activity indicate that organochlorine pesticides exert their carcinogenic effects by a mechanism that does not require a direct interaction with the DNA.

In line with the lack of mutagenicity even in the presence of a metabolically activating system is the poor metabolic rate of these compounds. There was no evidence of an electrophilic metabolism. Heptachlor forms the only epoxide in this series. This metabolite, although rapidly formed by liver monooxygenases (*419*), is a relatively stable compound and is found to be stored in human adipose tissue (*420*). Toxaphene is somewhat exceptional because it is considerably dechlorinated during metabolism in vivo; almost 50% of the chlorine substituents were excreted as chloride ions in the urine within 2 weeks (*421*).

1,2-DIBROMO-3-CHLOROPROPANE (DBCP). DBCP has been widely used in the United States, Europe, the Soviet Union, and Japan as a soil fumigant for the control of nematodes in a variety of fruits and crops. It was first produced in the United States in 1955. In 1977, the presence of DBCP in pesticides was found to pose an "imminent hazard" to humans, and the registration by the EPA was suspended.

Increased sterility (*422*) and aspermia (*423*) was observed in several groups of industrial workers exposed to DBCP. Depression of sperm count seems to develop quickly after exposure and seems to be reversible when exposure is removed (*424*).

DBCP was carcinogenic in mice and rats. The pattern of response clearly differed from that observed with organochlorine pesticides. In a feeding experiment, mice developed squamous cell carcinomas of the forestomach (*374*). Frequent metastases in adjacent tissues, such as lung and abdominal viscera, and gastric carcinomas were observed in another study. Animals bearing tumors died as early as 27 weeks after the beginning of treatment (*376*). Repeated application to mouse skin induced lung and stomach tumors (*377*). Only lung tumors were found in a long-term inhalation study with mice. In rats fed DBCP by gavage, a high amount of gastric carcinomas was induced in the survivors; females developed mammary adenocarcinomas (*374, 376*). Furthermore, DBCP initiated skin tumors in mice in a two-stage initiation promotion experiment (*377*). Apparently, DBCP is readily activated to the ultimate carcinogen at specific sites of the organism such as forestomach and lung, and the site affected depends on the route of administration. DBCP has been identified as a bacterial (*176, 425, 426*) and mammalian (*427*) mutagen. Metabolic activation was essential because DBCP was only mutagenic in the presence of the postmitochondrial supernatant (*425*).

METHOXYCHLOR. Methoxychlor is a structural analog of dichlorodiphenyltrichloroethane (DDT) that contains a methoxy group instead of the *p*-chlorine atom in the phenyl ring. It is similar to DDT in that it has a low toxicity and is used as an insecticide against a wide range of insects on fruit, crops, and cattle. It is generally applied by ground and aerial spraying. In contrast to DDT, methoxychlor is rapidly metabolized, predominantly by *O*-demethylation, to the corresponding phenolic metabolites and excreted (*428*).

Controversial evaluations have been published on the carcinogenicity of this compound. In 1979, the IARC concluded from one long-term study in mice and four studies in rats that the available data did not provide sufficient evidence of its carcinogenicity in animals (*372*). Subsequently, a review by Reuber stated carcinogenic effects in the liver of both mice and rats (*399*), in the testes (*400*) and bone (*398*) of mice, and in several endocrine organs of female rats (*398*) (*reported in* Ref. 429a). This evaluation was based on unpublished studies of the U.S. Food and Drug Administration (FDA), which were not included in the IARC evaluation, and on a divergent interpretation of the data of the NCI rat study (*398*).

It is possible that some of the carcinogenic effects, such as the neoplastic lesions in the sex organs, are related to the estrogenic activity of methoxychlor or its metabolites (*429b*).

2,4,6-TRICHLOROPHENOL (TCP). TCP has been used as a wood preservative, bactericide, and antimildew agent. TCP was administered in a long-term feeding study with high doses to B6C3F1 mice and F344 rats (*403*): Mice that received a diet containing 5000 and 10,000 ppm for 2 years showed a dose-related incidence of hepatocellular carcinomas or adenomas. Male rats revealed a dose-related incidence of lymphomas or leukemias.

Substances Carcinogenic in Mice. Table II shows compounds that have established carcinogenic effects in various strains of mice when given orally. The tumors were principally of the liver and included benign and malignant neoplasms. In a few studies, tumors of lung or lymph tissues were also diagnosed. Two compounds, diallate and quintozene, induced skin tumors or systemic reticulum cell sarcomas after subcutaneous administration.

When the pesticides of Table II were tested in rats, the results were either inconclusive or inadequate. Two pesticides, aldrin and its primary metabolite dieldrin, did not produce tumors in rats at dietary doses between 5 and 60 ppm of aldrin or 10 and 50 ppm/kg of bodyweight dieldrin fed over 2 years (*391a, 391b, 430, 431, 456a*).

The other compounds, when administered at high doses to rats, showed effects that might be considered inconclusive. With chlordane, 10 of 75 and 7 of 65 rats developed thyroid neoplasms vs. 3 of 58 and 5 of 51 thyroid tumors in pooled controls (*457*). The incidence of histiocytomas in treated males was 8 of 88 vs. 2 of 58 in pooled controls.

Several studies with rats were undertaken to test for the carcinogenicity of DDT. The results, however, were equivocal. In an early experiment with the Osborne–Mendel strain, 11 of 81 rats surviving after 18 months had nodular adenomatoid hyperplasia, which is reported to be rare in this strain (*391b*). Another study revealed undifferentiated bronchogenic carcinomas in 8 of 60 rats fed 80 ppm compared with 2 of 60 in controls; no incidence was seen in the group fed 200 ppm (*430, 432*).

A study by Reuber (*433*) reported hepatocellular carcinomas in Osborne–Mendel rats fed with 200–800 ppm of DDT for 2 years (*433*). In contrast, a study performed with B6C3F1 mice and Osborne–Mendel rats given 22–175 ppm and 210–642 ppm, respectively, in the diet resulted in the conclusion that DDT was not carcinogenic to rats and mice under these conditions (*434*).

Hamsters tolerated higher doses than did mice and did not develop tumors in excess over controls (*435*); this result indicates that the high doses alone may not be the cause of the carcinogenic response in mice.

Most of the compounds of this group were not mutagenic in bacteria. The exceptions were diallate, which was mutagenic after metabolic activation, and strobane, which showed a slight mutagenicity in the absence of the activation system (*436*).

These results and the weak mutagenic activity of halogenated cyclodienes point to a marginal, if any, interaction with genetic material. In contrast to these findings, a study by Ahmed et al. (*414*) suggests a direct interaction of these compounds with cellular DNA. Chlordane, aldrin, and dieldrin, as well as 2,4-dichlorophenoxyacetic acid (2,4-D) and captan, induced unscheduled DNA synthesis in human fibroblast cultures. The significance of this study, however, has been questioned (*406*).

Results show that this group of compounds possesses a marginal carcinogenicity, if any, in other species than mice.

Table II

Pesticides That Are Carcinogenic in Mice

Compound	*Mouse Strain*	*Dietary Concentration (duration of treatment)[a]*	*Type of Tumor*	*Reference*
Aldrin (**XI**)	B6C3F1	♂: 4, 8 ppm ♀: 3, 6 ppm (80/93 w)	hepatocellular carcinoma	*456a*
Captan (**XII**)	B6C3F1	8000, 16,000 ppm (80/91 w)	polypoid carcinoma	*456b*
Chlordane (**XIII**)	Charles River CD-1	25, 50 ppm (18 m)	hepatocellular carcinoma	*379*
	B6C3F1	T1 ♂: 30, 56 ppm T1 ♀: 30, 64 ppm (80 w)	hepatocellular carcinoma	*457*
Chlordimeform (**XIV**)	MAG	100, 500 ppm (2 y)	hemangioendothelioma	*458*
Chlorobenzilate (**XV**)	(C57BL/6×C3HAnf)F1 (C57BL/6×AKR)F1	215 mg/kg (d 7–28) and 603 ppm (80 w)	hepatoma in males	*131*
Dieldrin (**XVI**)	CF1	1, 2.5, 5.0, 10 ppm (132 w)	liver cell tumors	*389, 460*
	not specified	2.5, 5.0 ppm (80 w)	hepatocellular carcinoma	*456a*
Diallate (**XVII**) (Avadex)	(C57BL/6×C3HAnf)F1 and (C57BL/6×AKR)F1	215 mg/kg (d 7–28) and 560 ppm (74 w)	hepatomas, lung adenoma in males	*131*
	(C57BL/6×C3HAnf)F1 and (C57BL/6×AKR)F1	sc: 1000 mg/kg (single injection at d 28)	systemic reticulum cell sarcomas	*461*
Dichlorodiphenyltrichloroethane (DDT) (**XVIII**)	(C57BL/6×C3HAnf)F1 and (C57BL/6×AKR)F1	46 mg/kg (d 7–28) and 140 ppm (77 w)	hepatomas, malignant lymphomas in females	*131*
	BALB/c	3 ppm (5-generation study)	lung carcinoma, lymphoma, leukemia	*462*
	BALB/c	250 ppm (2-generation study)	liver cell tumors	*463, 464*
	CF1	2, 10, 50, 250 ppm (2-generation study)	liver cell tumors, some metastases	*465, 466*

Table II Continued

Compound	*Mouse Strain*	*Dietary Concentration (duration of treatment)*[a]	*Type of Tumor*	*Reference*
	"A-strain"	10 ppm (5-generation study)	lung adenomas	*467*
	CF1	50, 100 ppm (2 y)	liver tumors	*460*
	CF1	100 ppm (26 m)	liver tumors	*389*
Dichlorodiphenyl-dichloroethane (DDD) (**XIX**)	CF1	250 ppm (life span)	hepatomas	*468*
Dichlorodiphenyl-dichloroethylene (DDE) (**XX**)	CF1	250 ppm (life span)	hepatomas	*468*
Strobane (polychlorinated terpenes)	(C57BL/ 6×C3HAnf)F1 and (C57BL/ 6×AKR)F1	4.6 mg/kg (d 7–28) and 11 ppm (76 w)	hepatomas in males, malignant lymphomas	*131*
Tetrachlorvinphos (**XXI**)	B6C3F1	8000, 16,000 ppm (80/92 w)	hepatocellular carcinomas	*469*

[a]T1 indicates time weight average of dietary concentration; T2 indicates time weight average of dose. Only doses and experiments which caused a significant increase of tumor incidence over controls are given. If not mentioned, animals of both sexes were used. Concentration is given in parts per million (milligrams of compound per kilogram of diet) when administered in the diet or in milligrams of compound per kilogram of body weight when administered by gavage. Subcutaneous injection is indicated by sc. First number in parentheses indicates the duration of treatment; second number indicates total experimental period.

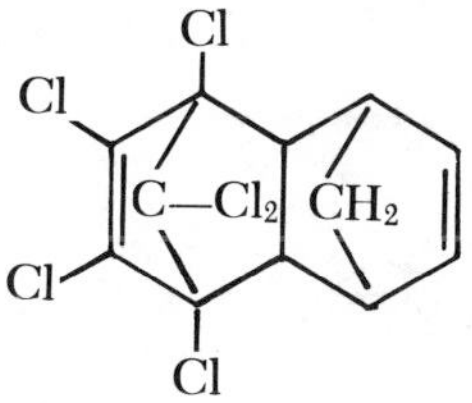

XI

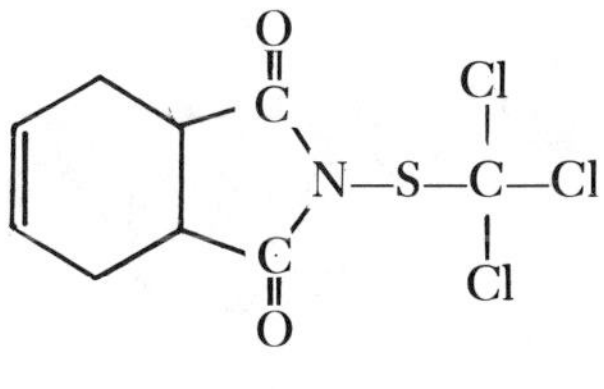

XII

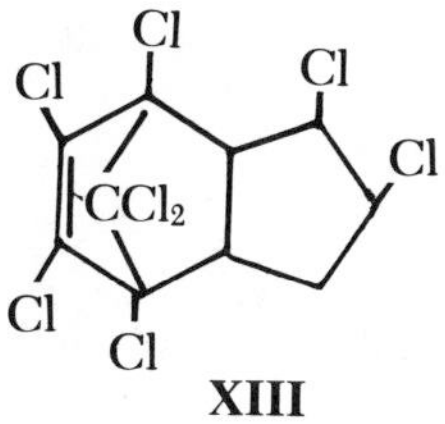

XIII

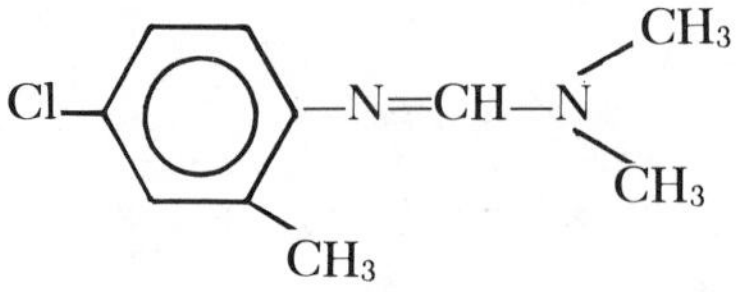

XIV

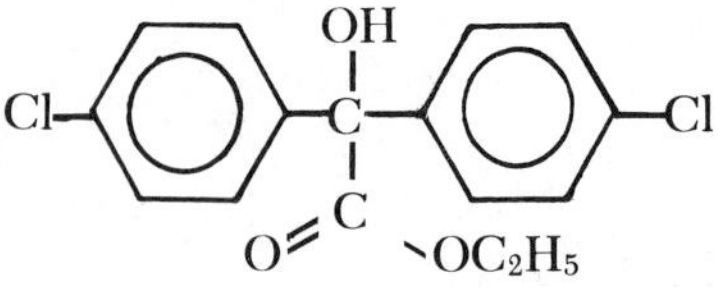

XV

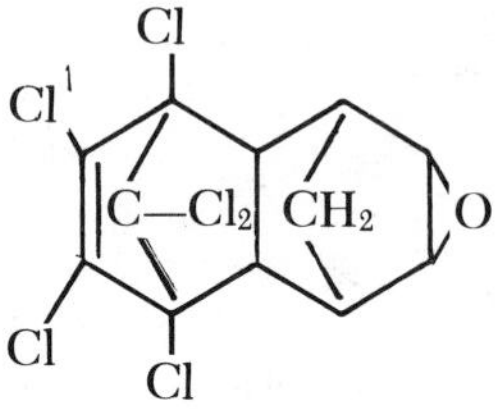

XVI

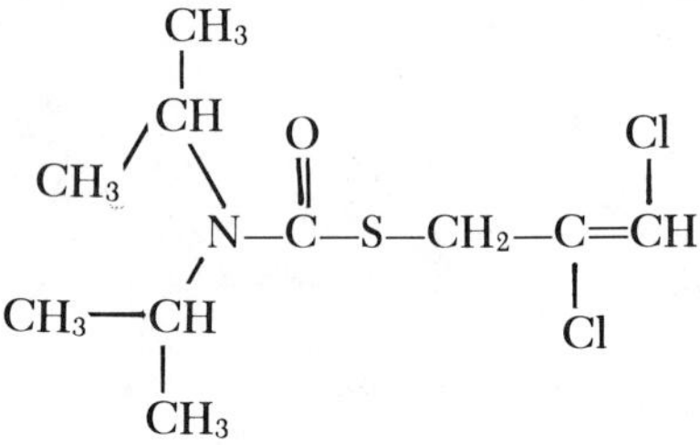

XVII

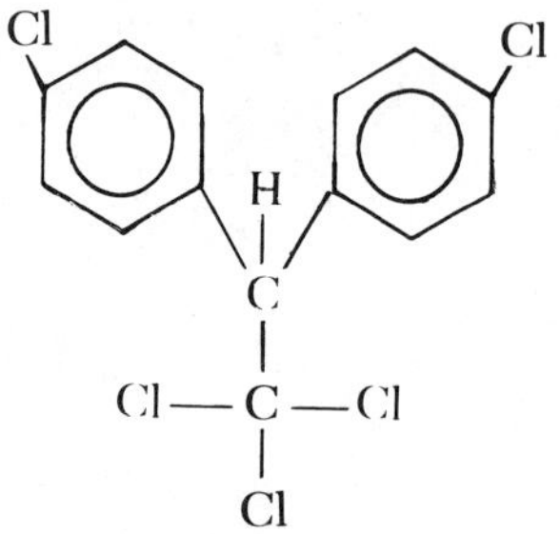

XVIII

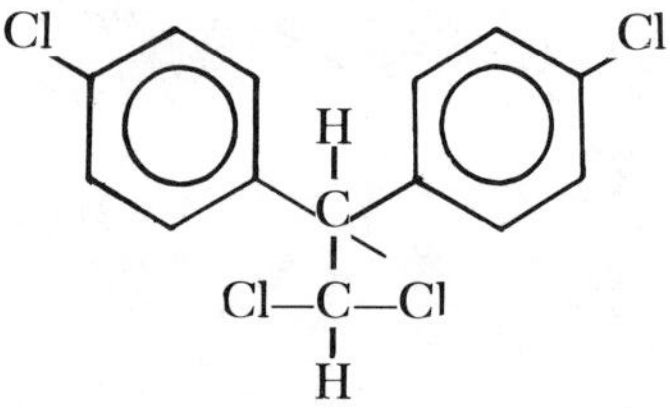

XIX

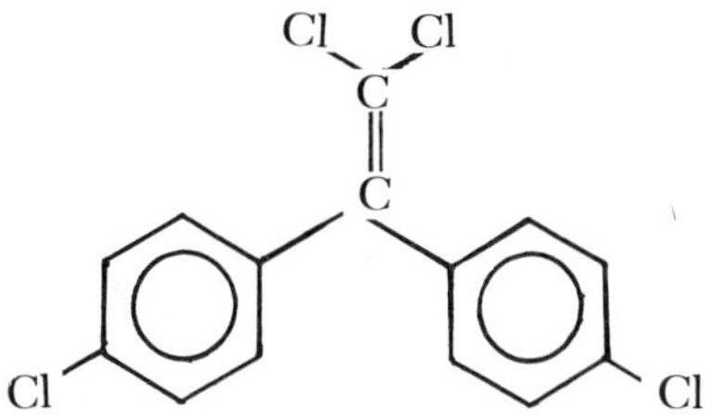

XX

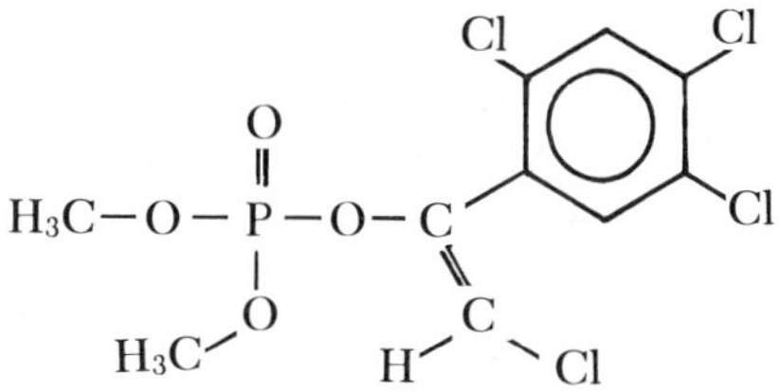

XXI

"Noncarcinogenic" Compounds. The compounds discussed in this section have all been labeled noncarcinogenic, at least in mice. Chloropropham is also considered negative in rats and hamsters (*438*). Anilazin, coumaphos, endosulfan, and endrin are in this category on the basis of NCI studies (*437, 439–41*).

Other chlorinated pesticides have been tested by Innes et al. (*131*) and were assigned to be negative in mice after oral administration for 18 months. Among these were simazine, propazine, 2,4-D and its commercial esters, 2,4,5-trichlorophenoxyacetic acid (2,4,5-T), dichlone, dicryl, folpet, botran, ovex, 2-(2,4-dichlorophenoxy)propionic acid, tetrafidon, telodrin, genite R-99, and endosulfan. 2,4-D and several of its esters as well as 2,4,5-T were also tested in mice and rats (*442*). Although some signs of increased tumor incidence were noted these studies were not evaluated by the IARC because of limitations due to inadequate reporting or to small sample size.

Conflicting results on the carcinogenic effect in mice are known for quintozene. Innes et al. (*131*) observed hepatomas in one feeding study; 7-day-old hybrid mice were fed 464 mg/kg of body weight for the first 3 weeks, then 1206 ppm for an additional 71 weeks. However, Wedig et al. (*443*) found no significant increase in the incidence of malignant tumors when males and females were fed high doses of 3000 and 9000 ppm for 78 weeks. This result was confirmed by an NCI study in mice that received similarly high doses of quintozene (*444*). No increased incidence of tumors was seen in rats that were given dichlorvos (*445*).

Table III
Storage of Pesticides in Humans

	Concentration		
Compound	*Adipose Tissue (ppm)*	*Milk (ppm on fat basis)*	*Blood (µg/mL)*
Aldrin/dieldrin	0.1–0.5	0.01–0.6	—
Chlordecone	—	—	0.17–0.26[a]
DDT, DDE	2–30	0.1–16	—
Heptachlor epoxide	0.01–0.13	0.01–0.6	—
Hexachlorobenzene	—	0.01–10.1	—
Lindane (γ-HCH)	0.1–1.7	0.01–1.2	—

SOURCE: Data were compiled from the IARC Monographs on "Evaluation of Carcinogenic Risk of Chemicals to Humans," Lyon, Vol. 5 (1974) and Vol. 20 (1979).
[a]Concentration in workers manufacturing chlordecone.

Trichlorfon was found to be tumorigenic in the mammary gland of the rat at dietary doses of 250, 500, and 1000 ppm sustained for 2 years (*446, 447*). Other authors noted that the incidence of mammary tumors was not increased in trichlorfon-fed rats (*448, 449*). No data on long-term studies with mice are available.

Toxicity and Carcinogenicity of Pesticides in Humans. The populations of many countries have been exposed to various agricultural chemicals for 15–40 years. Residues of these chemicals or their metabolites have been detected in small quantities in nearly all foods. Furthermore, a considerable number of pesticides, particularly those that are poorly metabolized, have been found in human body fluids and tissues (Table III). To our knowledge, no systematic studies have been undertaken to monitor the uptake and residue levels of highly exposed persons, such as pesticide manufacturing workers or farmers exposed during application of the chemicals. However, there are a number of cases of occupational intoxication caused by misuse.

Industrial workers exposed to chlordecone by inhalation, ingestion, and skin contact showed several symptoms of neurotoxicity, abnormal liver function, and dermatitis. The severity of the symptoms was correlated with blood levels of chlordecone. High concentrations of this insecticide were found in the liver and body fat of exposed workers (*450*). The serum half-life was between 63 and 148 d (*451*). Sterility after occupational exposure to 1,2-dibromo-3-chloropropane has already been described in this chapter. Eight women exposed to toxaphene by aircraft spraying exhibited a higher incidence of chromosome aberrations than did control individuals (*452*). A relationship between blood dyscrasia and exposure to heptachlor and/or chlordane was suggested by case reports from Italy (*453*).

The most severe case of intoxication by a pesticide occurred in Turkey between 1955 and 1959. Over 4000 individuals developed porphyria cutanea tarda after they consumed grain contaminated by hexachlorobenzene. The majority of the patients were 4–14-year-old boys who ingested an estimated 50–200 mg of this chemical daily. Abnormal porphyrin metabolism persisted for 20 years after ingestion, but no data on carcinogenic effects have been reported so far (*454*).

Only one epidemiological study exists that reports carcinogenic effects among pesticide workers exposed to a variety of substances, including 2-4-D, 2-methyl-4-chlorophenoxyacetic acid (MCPA), DDT, HCH, toxaphene, methylparathion, 4,6-dinitro-*o*-cresol (DNOC), thiocarbamate, and some copper-containing fungicides (*455*). Some workers had also been exposed to arsenic-containing agents at an earlier time. The time of exposure varied between 6 and 23 years. Eleven of 316 individuals developed lung cancer, which is a 20-fold higher incidence than expected from the age-specific general population. Although these findings do not permit conclusions to be drawn on the carcinogenic potential of individual pesticides in humans, the report does indicate that a high risk may exist for the specific group of pesticide appliers.

Conclusion

The organic halogenated compounds discussed in this chapter comprise a large and heterogeneous group of chemicals that differ greatly in structure, metabolism, and biological activity. It is therefore fitting that they also differ in their mode of carcinogenic action. Some of the compounds clearly are initiators of tumor formation, i.e., genotoxic agents, whereas others apparently work by epigenetic mechanisms, such as recurrent organ-specific cytotoxicity. For some compounds, both mechanisms might be operative. For others the data are lacking to make a distinction.

When extracting the present data from the literature, we were frequently confronted with contradictory statements on the carcinogenicity of the various chemicals. This dissension was most striking for the evaluation of the neoplastic lesions in rodents and for the compounds that could not clearly be identified as tumor initiators. The reasons for the discrepancies are to be sought less in differences in the experimental designs or the identification and classification of tumors than in the interpretation of the data.

The problems of interpreting carcinogenicity data are obviously not specific for the organic halogenated compounds; however, they are particularly pressing for this group of substances. Many of them do not exert their effects by overtly attacking DNA but by some other poorly specified mechanism. Furthermore, this group contains a large number of chemicals that are widely distributed in the environment and are of great economical value. A particular problem arises from the evaluation of positive results that could only be obtained at very high doses of the test compounds. Although there is a need and a scientific basis for using the maximum tolerable dose (MTD) in bioassays for carcinogenicity, one has to realize that at high concentrations these chemicals may exert effects profoundly different from those at low concentrations. For example, massive doses may saturate or exhaust the pathways of metabolic inactivation or the processes of elimination. By these mechanisms they may become cocarcinogens or may indirectly function as tumor promoters. Clearly, in such cases the knowledge of the mechanistic aspects precludes a simple extrapolation from high to low doses. For all of these reasons, we support the general plea for intensifying the examination of the pharmacokinetics and toxicity of the chemicals in conjunction with the carcinogenesis bioassays. This information may be the key for the evaluation of data on the carcinogenicity of chemicals that apparently act through nongenetic mechanisms, such as chloroform, carbon tetrachloride, and perchloroethylene.

Aside from this point, the major issue remains the clarification of the mechanism of chemical carcinogenesis. Significant progress would be made if the distinction between genotoxic and epigenetic modes of action could be verified and if the existence of threshold levels for any of these processes could be established. These advances would provide a more solid basis for the evaluation of the carcinogenesis bioassay data and would allow a closer approximation of the human risk.

Acknowledgment

The authors wish to thank Judy Byers, Elisabeth Pilarski, and Ursula Welscher for expert assistance in the preparation of the manuscript.

Literature Cited

1. Bauchwitz, P.S. In "Encyclopedia of Chemical Technology," 2nd ed.; Kirk, R.E.; Othmer, D.F., Eds.; Wiley: New York, 1964; pp. 215–31.
2. Bartsch, H.; Malaveille, C.; Barbin, A.; Planche, G.; Montesano, R.; *Proc. Am. Assoc. Cancer Res.* **1976**, *17*, 17.
3. Van Duuren, B.L.; Goldschmidt, B.M.; Seidman, J.; *Cancer Res.* **1975**, *35*, 2553–57.
4. Mukai, F.H.; Hawryluk, J. *Mutat. Res.* **1973**, *21*, 228.
5. Loprieno, N. Second Meeting of the Scientific Committee of the Carlo Erba Foundation, Dec. 12, 1975, pp. 129–40.
6. "Monographs on the Evaluation of Carcinogenic Risk of Chemicals to Humans" IARC: Lyon, 1979; Vol. 19, pp. 131–56.
7. Haley, T.J. *Clin. Toxicol.* **1978**, *13*, 153–70.
8. Clary, J.J.; Feron, V.J.; Renzel, P.G.J. *Toxicol. Appl. Pharmacol.* **1978**, *46*, 375–84.
9. Khachatryan, E.A. *Vopr. Onkol.* **1972**, *18*, 85–86.
10. Khachatryan, E.A. *Gig. Tr. Prof. Zabol.* **1972**, *18*, 54–55.
11. Pell, S. *J. Occup. Med.* **1978**, *20*, 21.
12. Infante, P.F. *EHP, Environ. Health Perspect.* **1977**, *21*, 251.
13. Zil'Fyan, V.N.; Fichidzhyan, B.S.; Garibyan, D.K.; Pogosova, A.M. *Vopr. Onkol.* **1977**, *23*, 61–65.
14. Ponomarkov, V.; Tomatis, L. *Oncology* **1980**, *37*, 136–41.
15. Bartsch, H.; Malaveille, C.; Montesano, R.; Tomatis, L. *Nature (London)* **1975**, *255*, 641–43.
16. Bartsch, H.; Malaveille, C.; Barbin, A.; Planche, G. *Arch. Toxicol.* **1979**, *41*, 249–77.
17. Sanotskii, I.V. *Environ. Health Perspect.* **1976**, *17*, 85–93.
18. Haley, T.J. *J. Toxicol. Environ. Health* **1975**, *1*, 47–73.
19. Haley, T.J. *Clin. Toxicol.* **1975**, *8*, 633–43.
20. Plugge, H.; Jaeger, R. *Toxicol. Appl. Pharmacol.* **1979**, *50*, 565–72.
21. Summer, K.H.; Greim, H. *Biochem. Biophys. Res. Commun.* **1980**, *96*, 566–73.
22. Summer, K.-H.; Göggelmann, W.; Greim, H. *Mutat. Res.* **1980**, *70*, 269–78.
23. "Merck Index, Ninth ed.; Merck and Co.: Rahway, NJ, Windholz, M.; Ed.; 1976; p. 840.
24. Csonev, B. *Banyasz. Kut. Intez. Kozl.* **1969**, *13*, 125.
25. McCane, D.J. In "Encyclopedia of Polymer Science and Technology, Plastics, Resins, Rubbers and Fibers"; Bikales, N.M., Ed.; Interscience: New York, 1970; Vol. 13, pp. 623–24, 626–627.

26. Dilley, J.V.; Carter, V.L.; Harris, E.S. *Toxicol. Appl. Pharmacol.* **1974**, *27*, 582–90.
27. "Toxic and Hazardous Industrial Chemicals Safety Manual," International Technical Safety Institute, Tokyo, 1979, pp. 509–10.
28. Tomatis, L.; Shubik, P. *Nature* (*London*) **1963**, *198*, 600–601.
29. Oppenheimer, B.S.; Oppenheimer, E.T.; Danishefsky, J.; Stout, A.P.; Eirich, F.R. *Cancer Res.* **1963**, *15*, 333–40.
30. Bryson, G.; Bischoff, F. *Prog. Exp. Tumor Res.* **1969**, *11*, 100–33.
31. Simmers, M.H.; Agnew, W.F.; Pudenz, R.H. *Bol. Inst. Estud. Med. Biol.* [*Univ. Nac. Auton. Mex.*] **1963**, *21*, 1–13.
32. Gangolli, S.D.; Grasso, P.; Golberg, L. *Food Cosmet. Toxicol.* **1967**, *5*, 601–21.
33. Walker, A.E. *Br. J. Dermatol.* **1981**, *105*, Suppl. 21, 19–21.
34. "Toxikologie und Hygiene der technischen Lösungsmittel"; Lehmann, K.B.; Flury, F., Eds.; Verlag-Springer: Berlin, 1938; p. 130.
35. Hopkins, J. *Food Cosmet. Toxicol.* **1979**, *17*, 403–405, 542–44, 681–82.
36. Hopkins, J. *Food Cosmet. Toxicol.* **1980**, *18*, 94–96, 200–201.
37. Bolt, H.M.; Filser, J.G.; Laib, R.J.; Ottenwälder, H. *Arch. Toxicol.* **1980**, Suppl. 3, 129–42.
38. Greim, H.; Bonse, G.; Radwan, Z.; Reichert, D.; Henschler, D. *Biochem. Pharmacol.* **1975**, *24*, 2013–17.
39. Bartsch, H.; Malaveille, C.; Montesano, R. *Int. J. Cancer* **1975**, *15*, 429–37.
40. Hubermann, E.; Bartsch, H.; Sachs, L. *Int. J. Cancer* **1975**, *16*, 639–44.
41. Guengerich, F.P.; Mason, P.S.; Stott, W.T.; Fox, T.R.; Watanabe, P.G. *Cancer Res.* **1981**, *41*, 4391–98.
42. Hathway, D.E. *Br. J. Cancer* **1981**, *44*, 597–600.
43. Maltoni, C.; Le Femine, G. *Ann. N.Y. Acad. Sci.* **1975**, *246*, 195–218.
44. Maltoni, C.; Le Femine G.; Ciliberti, A.; Cotti, G.; Caretti, D. *Environ. Health Perspect.* **1981**, *41*, 3–29.
45. Suzuki, Y. *Environ. Health Perspect.* **1981**, *41*, 31–52.
46. Hong, C.B.; Winston, J.M.; Thornbury, L.P.; Lee, C.C. *J. Toxicol. Environ. Health* **1981**, *7*, 909–24.
47. Bartsch, H.; Montesano, R. *Mutat. Res.* **1975**, *32*, 93–144.
48. Infante, P.F. *Environ. Health Perspect.* **1981**, *41*, 89–94.
49. Beaumont, J.J.; Brelow, N.E. *Am. J. Epidemiol.* **1981**, *114*, 725–34.
50. Emmerich, K.H.; Norpoth, K. *J. Cancer Res. Clin. Oncol.* **1981**, *102*, 1–11.
51. Clemmessen, J. *Mutat. Res.* **1982**, *98*, 97–100.
52. Lilis, R. *Environ. Health Perspect.* **1981**, *41*, 167–69.
53. Froneberg, B.; Johnson, P.L.; Landrigan, P.J. *Br. J. Ind. Med.* **1982**, *39*, 239–43.
54. Fishbein, L. "Potential Industrial Carcinogens and Mutagens"; Elsevier: Amsterdam, 1979; p. 178.
55. Cooper, P. *Food Cosmet. Toxicol.* **1980**, *18*, 435.
56. Norris, J.M. "Technical Association Pulp and Paper Industry," Paper Synthesis Conference, Chicago, IL, 1977.
57. Jones, B.K.; Hathway, D.E. *Chem.-Biol. Interact.* **1978**, *20*, 27–41.
58. Reichert, D.; Werner, W.; Metzler, M.; Henschler, D. *Arch. Toxicol.* **1979**, *42*, 159–69.
59. Jaeger, R.J.; Conolly, R.B.; Murphy, S.D. *Exp. Mol. Pathol.* **1974**, *20*, 187–98.
60. Henschler, D. *Environ. Health Perspect.* **1978**, *21*, 61–64.
61. Kosta, A.K.; Ivanetich, K.M. *Biochem. Pharmacol.* **1982**, *31*, 2083–92.
62. Jones, B.K.; Hathway, D.E. *Cancer Lett.* **1978**, *5*, 1–11.
63. Maltoni, C. *Environ. Health Perspect.* **1977**, *21*, 1–5.
64. Maltoni, C.; Cotti, G.; Morisi, L.; Chieco, P. *Med. Lav.* **1977**, *68*, 241–62.
65. Lee, C.C., Bhandari, J.C.; Winston, J.M.; House, W.B.; Dixon, R.L.; Woods, J.S. *J. Toxicol. Environ. Health* **1978**, *4*, 15–30.

66. National Institutes of Health, CAS No. 75–35–4, 1981, DHHS Publ. No. 82–1784, NTP 81–82.
67. Jenkins, L.J.; Traubulus, M.J.; Murphy, S.D. *Toxicol. Appl. Pharmacol.* **1972**, *23*, 501.
68. Costa, A.K.; Ivanetich, K.M. *Biochem. Pharmacol.* **1982**, *31*, 2093–102.
69. Maltoni, C.; Tivoli, D. *Med. Lav.* **1979**, *5*, 363.
70. "Monographs on the Evaluation of Carcinogenic Risk of Chemicals to Humans"; IARC: Lyon, 1976; Vol. 11, p. 217.
71. McCann, J.; Spingarn, N.E.; Kobori, J.; Ames, B. *Proc. Natl. Acad. Sci. U.S.A.* **1975**, *72*, 979–83.
72. Dunkel, V.C.; Wolff, J.S.; Pienta, R.J. *Cancer Bull.* **1977**, *29*, 167–74.
73. Druckrey, H.; Kruse, H.; Preussmann, R.; Ivankovic, S.; Landschütz, C. *Z. Krebsforsch.* **1970**, *74*, 241–70.
74. Fukuda, K.; Matsushita, H.; Sakabe, H.; Takemoto, K. *Gann* **1981**, *72*, 655–64.
75. Poirier, L.A.; Stoner, G.D.; Shimkin, M. *Cancer Res.* **1975**, *35*, 1411–15.
76. Walles, S.A.S. *Toxicol. Lett.* **1981**, *9*, 379–87.
77. Sakabe, H.; Matsushita, H.; Koshi, S. *Ann. N.Y. Acad. Sci.* **1976**, *271*, 67–70.
78. Sakabe, H.; Fukuda, K. *Ind. Health* **1977**, *15*, 173–74.
79. Kallos, G.J.; Solomon, R.A. *Am. Ind. Hyg. Assoc.* **1973**, 34, 469–73.
80. Collier, L. *Environ. Sci. Technol.* **1972**, *6*, 930.
81. OSHA, Occupational Safety and Health Standards, Carcinogens. Fed. Reg. (1974), *39*, 3768–3773.
82. Nelson, N. *Ann. N.Y. Acad. Sci.* **1976**, *271*, 81–90.
83. Sakabe, H. *Ind. Health* **1973**, *11*, 145–48.
84. Thiess, A.M.; Hey, W.; Zeller, H. *Zentralbl. Arbeitsmed., Arbeitsschutz. Prophyl.* **1973**, *23*, 97–102.
85. Reznik, G.; Wagner, H.H.; Atay, Z. *J. Environ. Pathol. Toxicol.* **1977**, *1*, 105–11.
86. Bettendorf, U. *Verh. Dtsch. Ges. Pathol.* **1976**, *60*, 457.
87. Zudova, Z.; Landa, K. *Mutat. Res.* **1977**, *46*, 242–43.
88. Kuschner, M.; Laskins, S.; Drew, R.T.; Capiello, V.; Nelson, N. *Arch. Environ. Health* **1975**, *30*, 73–77.
89. Lelong, B.K.J.; Kociba, R.J.; Jersey, G.C. *Toxicol. Appl. Pharmacol.* **1981**, *58*, 269–81.
90. McCann, J.; Choi, E.; Yamasaki, E.; Ames, B.N. *Proc. Natl. Acad. Sci. U.S.A.* **1975**, *72*, 5135–39.
91. Kleupfer, R.D.; Fairless, B.J. *Environ. Sci. Technol.* **1972**, *6*, 1062–63.
92. Simmon, V.F.; Kauhanen, K.; Tardiff, R.G. In "Progress in Genetic Toxicology"; Scott, D.; Bridges, B.A.; Sobels, F.H., Eds.; Elsevier: Amsterdam, 1977; pp. 249–56.
93. National Cancer Institute, Technical Report Series, CAS No. 108–60–1, 1979, NCJ–CG–Tr–191.
94. The Society of Dyes and Colourists, Colour Index, 3rd ed. *4*, 1971.
95. "Monographs on the Evaluation of Carcinogenic Risk of Chemicals to Humans"; IARC: Lyon, 1972; Vol. 1., p. 80.
96. Pliss, G.B. *Vopr. Onkol.* **1959**, *5*, 524.
97. Stula, E.F.; Sherman, H.; Zapp, J.A. *Toxicol. Appl. Pharmacol.* **1971**, *19*, 380–86.
98. Sellakumar, A.R.; Montesano, R.; Saffiotti, U. *Proc. Am. Assoc. Cancer Res.* **1969**, *10*, 78.
99. Garner, R.C.; Walpole, A.C.; Rose, F.L. *Cancer Lett.* **1975**, *1*, 39–42.
100. Rinde, E.; Troll, W. *JNCI, J. Natl. Cancer Inst.* **1975**, *55*, 181–82.
101. Hsu, R.S.; Sikka, H.C. *Toxicol. Appl. Pharmacol.* **1982**, *84*, 306–16.
102. Bratcherd, S.C.; Sikka, H.C. *Chem.-Biol. Interact.* **1982**, *38*, 369–75.
103. "Monographs on the Evaluation of Carcinogenic Risk of Chemicals to Humans"; IARC: Lyon, 1976; Vol. 12, pp. 77–84.
104. Anonymous, "Occupational Health Safety Letter," **1976**, *6*, 7.

105. Van Duuren, B.L.; Goldschmidt, B.M.; Katz, C.; Seidman, I.; Paul, T.S. *JNCI, J. Natl. Cancer Inst.* **1974**, *53*, 695–700.
106. Sellakumar, A.R.; Laskin, S.; Kuschner, M.; Rusch, G.; Katz, G.V.; Snyder, C.A.; Albert, R.E. *J. Environ. Pathol. Toxicol.* **1980**, *4*, 107–15.
107. von Hey, W.; Thiess, A.M.; Zeller, H. *Zentralbl. Arbeits-med., Arbeitschutz. Prophyl.* **1974**, *24*, 71–77.
108. Sram, R.J.; Tomatis, L.; Clemmesen, J.; Bridges, B.A. *Mutat. Res.* **1981**, *87*, 299–319.
109. Konishi, Y.; Kawabata, A.; Denda, A.; Ikeda, T.; Katada, H.; Maruyama, H.; Higashgushi, R. *Gann* **1980**, 922–23.
110. Henschler, D.; Eder, E.; Neudecker, T.; Metzler, M. *Arch. Toxicol.* **1977**, *37*, 233–36.
111. Knaap, A.G.A.C.; Voogd, C.E.; Kramers, P.G.N. *Mutat. Res.* **1982**, *101*, 199–208.
112. Epstein, S.S.; Arnold, E.; Andrea, J.; Bass, W.; Bishop, Y. *Toxicol. Appl. Pharmacol.* **1972**, *23*, 288–325.
113. Kucerova, M.; Polivkova, Z.; Sram, R.; Matousek, V. *Mutat. Res.* **1976**, *34*, 271–78.
114. Sram, R.J.; Zudova, Z.; Kuleshow, N.P. *Mutat. Res.* **1980**, *70*, 115–20.
115. Enterline, P.E. *Ann. N.Y. Acad. Sci.* **1981**, *381*, 344–49.
116. "Monographs on the Evaluation of Carcinogenic Risk of Chemicals to Humans"; IARC: Lyon, 1979; Vol. 20, pp. 179–93.
117. Kociba, R.J.; Keyes, D.G.; Jersey, G.C.; Ballard, J.J.; DiMenber, D.A.; Quast, J.F.; Wade, C.E.; Humiston, C.G.; Schwetz, B.A. *Am. Ind. Hyg. Assoc. J.* **1977**, *38*, 589–602.
118. Lock, E.A.; Ishmael, J. *Toxicol. Appl. Pharmacol.* **1981**, *57*, 79–87.
119. Gage, J.C. *Br. J. Ind. Med.* **1970**, *17*, 1–18124.
120. Duprat, P.; Gradiski, D. *Acta Pharmacol. Toxicol.* **1978**, *43*, 346–53.
121. Harleman, J.M.; Seinen, W. *Toxicol. Appl. Pharmacol.* **1979**, *47*, 1–14.
122. Schwetz, B.A.; Smith, F.A.; Humiston, C.G.; Quast, J.F.; Kocib, R.J. *Toxicol. Appl. Pharmacol.* **1977**, *42*, 387–98.
123. Poland, A.; Knutson, J.C. *Annu. Rev. Pharmacol. Toxicol.* **1982**, *22*, 517–54.
124. Thiess, A.M.; Frentzel-Beyme, R. 5th International Medichem Congress, San Francisco, Nov. 5–9, 1977.
125. Courtney, K.D.; Moore, J.A. *Toxicol. Appl. Pharmacol.* **1971**, *20*, 396–403.
126. Murray, F.J.; Smith, F.A.; Nitschke, K.D.; Humiston, C.G.; Kociba, R.J.; Schwetz, B.A. *Toxicol. Appl. Pharmacol.* **1977**, *41*, 200–201.
127. Neubert, D.; Zens, P.; Rothenwallner, A.; Merker, H.J. *EHP, Environ. Health Perspect.* **1973**, *5*, 67–79.
128. Sparschu, G.L.; Dunn, F.L.; Lisowe, R.W.; Rowe, V.K. *Food Cosmet. Toxicol.* **1971**, *9*, 527–30.
129. *Fed. Regist.* **1979**, *44*, 15874. *Nature* (*London*) **1980**, *284*, 111.
130. Hardell, L.; Sandström, A. *Br. J. Cancer* **1979**, *39*, 711–17.
131. Innes, J.R.M.; Ulland, B.M.; Valerio, M.G.; Petrucelli, L.; Fishbein, L.; Hart, E.R.; Pallotta, A.J.; Bates, R.R.; Falk, H.L.; Gart, J.J.; Klein, M.; Mitchell, I.; Peters, J. *JNCI, J. Natl. Cancer Inst.* **1969**, *42*, 1101–14.
132. Kociba, R.J.; Keyes, D.G.; Beyes, J.E.; Carreon, R.M.; Wade, C.E.; Dittenber, D.A.; Kalnins, R.P.; Franson, L.E.; Park, N.C.; Barnarad, S.D.; Hummel, R.A.; Humiston, C.G. *Toxicol. Appl. Pharmacol.* **1978**, *46*, 279–303.
133. National Institutes of Health, CAS No. 1746–01–6, Technical Report Series No. 209.
134. National Institutes of Health, CAS No. 1746–01–6, Technical Report Series No. 201.
135. Rose, J.Q.; Ramsey, J.C.; Wentzler, T.H.; Hummel, R.A.; Gehring, P.J. *Toxicol. Appl. Pharmacol.* **1976**, *36*, 209–26.
136. Gasiewicz, T.A.; Neal, R.A. *Toxicol. Appl. Pharmacol.* **1979**, *51*, 329–39.

137. Olson, J.R.; Gasiewicz, T.A.; Neal, R.A. *Toxicol. Appl. Pharmacol.* **1980**, *56*, 78–85.
138. Weber, H; Poiger, H.; Schlatter, C. *Xenobiotica* **1982**, *12*, 353–57.
139. Poland, A.; Glover, E. *Mol. Pharmacol.* **1974**, *10*, 349–59.
140. Greig, J.B.; De Matteis, F. *Environ. Health Perspect.* **1973**, *5*, 211–19.
141. Lucier, G.W.; McDaniel, O.S.; Hook, G.E.R.; Fowler, B.A.; SonaWane, B.R.; Faeder, E. *Environ. Health Perspect.* **1973**, *5*, 199–209.
142. Lucier, G.W.; McDaniel, O.S.; Hook, G.E.R. *Biochem. Pharmacol.* **1975**, *24*, 325–34.
143. Hook, G.E.R.; Haseman, J.K.; Lucier, G.W. *Chem.-Biol. Interact.* **1975**, *10*, 199–214.
144. Neal, R.A.; Beatty, P.W.; Gasiweicz, T.A. *Ann. N.Y. Acad. Sci.* **1979**, *320*, 204–13.
145. Poland, A.; Greenlee, W.F.; Kende, F. *Ann. N.Y. Acad. Sci.* **1979**, *320*, 214–30.
146. Thunberg, T.; Ahlborg, U.G.; Johnsson, H. *Arch. Toxicol.* **1980**, *42*, 265–74.
147. Barsotti, D.A.; Abrahamson, L.J.; Allen, J.R. *Bull. Environ. Contam. Toxicol.* **1979**, *21*, 463–69.
148. Goldstein, J.A.; Linko, P.; Bergman, H. *Biochem. Pharmacol.* **1982**, *31*, 1607–13.
149. Ahlborg, U.G.; Thunberg, T. *Arch. Toxicol.* **1978**, *40*, 55–61.
150. Hussain, S.; Ehrenberg, L.; Lofroth, G.; Gejvall, T. *Ambio* **1972**, *1*, 32–33.
151. Berry, D.L.; DiGiovanni, J.; Juchau, M.R.; Bracken, W.M.; Gleason, G.L.; Slaga, T.J. *Res. Commun. Chem. Pathol. Pharmacol.* **1978**, *20*, 101–107.
152. DiGiovanni, J.; Viaje, A.; Berry, D.L.; Slaga, T.J.; Juchau, M.R. *JNCI, J. Natl. Cancer Inst.* **1978**, *61*, 135–40.
153. Poland, A.; Glover, E.; Kende, A.S. *J. Biol. Chem.* **1976**, *251*, 4936–46.
154. Vos, J.G.; Kowman, J.H.; van der Maas, H.L.; ten Noever de Brauw, M.C.; de Vos, R.H. *Food Cosmet. Toxicol.* **1969**, *8*, 625–33.
155. Bauer, H.; Schulz, K.H.; Spiegelberg, U. *Arch. Gewerbepathol. Gewerbehyg.* **1961**, *18*, 538–55.
156. Bowes, G.M.; Mulvihill, M.J.; Simoneit, B.R.; Burlingame, A.L.; Risebrough, R.W. *Nature (London)*, **1975**, *256*, 305–307.
157. Nagayama, J.; Kuratsune, M.; Masuda, Y. *Bull. Environ. Contam. Toxicol.* **1976**, *15*, 9–13.
158. Nagayama, J.; Masuda, Y.; Kuratsune, M. *Food Cosmet. Toxicol.* **1977**, *15*, 195–98.
159. Kashimoto, T.; Miyata, H.; Kunita, S.; Tung, T.C.; Hsu, S.T.; Chang, K.J.; Tang, S.Y.; Ohi, G.; Nakagawa, J.; Yamamoto, S.I. *Arch. Environ. Health* **1981**, *36*, 312–29.
160. Nagayama, J.; Tokudome, S.; Kuratsune, M.; Masuda, Y. *Food Cosmet. Toxicol.* **1980**, *18*, 153–57.
161. Schoeny, R. *Mutat. Res.* **1982**, *101*, 45–56.
162. Hutzinger, O.; Sandstrom, G.; Safe, S. *Chemosphere* **1976**, *1*, 3–10.
163. Norström, A.; Anderson, K.; Rappe, C. *Chemosphere* **1976**, *4*, 255–61.
164. Carter, L.J. *Science (Washington, D.C.)* **1976**, *192*, 240–43.
165. Gupta, B.N.; McConnell, E.E.; Harris, M.W.; Moore, J.A. *Toxicol. Appl. Pharmacol.* **1981**, *57*, 99–118.
166. Damstra, T.; Jurgelski, W.; Posner, H.S.; Vouk, V.B.; Bernheim, N.J.; Guthrie, J.; Luster, M.; Falk, H.L. *Environ. Health Perspect.* **1982**, *44*, 175–88.
167. Anderson, H.A.; Wolff, M.S.; Lilis, R.; Holstein, E.C.; Valciukas, J.A.; Anderson, E.K.; Petrocci, M.; Sarkozi, L.; Selikoff, J. *Ann. N.Y. Acad. Sci.* **1979**, *320*, 684–792.
168. Stross, J.Y.; Smokler, J.A.; Isbister, J.; Wilcox, K.R. *Toxicol. Appl. Pharmacol.* **1981**, *58*, 145–50.
169. Harris, S.J.; Cecil, H.C.; Bitman, J. *Environ. Health Perspect.* **1978**, *23*, 295–300.
170. Kimbrough, R.D.; Burse, V.W.; Liddle, J.A. *Environ. Health Perspect.* **1978**, *23*, 265–73.
171. Gupta, B.N.; Moore, J.A. *Am. J. Vet. Res.* **1979**, *40*, 1458–68.
172. Kimbrough, R.D.; Groce, D.G.; Korver, M.P.; Burse, V.W. *JNCI, J. Natl. Cancer Inst.* **1981**, *66*, 535–42.
173. "National Toxicology Program Technical Report on the Toxicology and Carcino-

genesis Bioassay of Polybrominated Biphenyl Mixture;" Research Triange Park, NC, 1982.

174. Søderlund, E.J.; Nelson, S.D.; von Bahr, C.; Dybing, E. *Fundam. Appl. Toxicol.* **1982**, *2*, 187–94.
175. Seabaugh, T.F.; Collins, X.; Hoheisel, C.A.; Bierbower, G.W.; McLaughlin, J. *Food Cosmet. Toxicol.* **1981**, *19*, 67–72.
176. Prival, M.J.; McCoy, E.C.; Gutter, B.; Rosenkranz, H.S. *Science (Washington, D.C.)* **1977**, *195*, 76–78.
177. Søderlund, E.; Nelson, S.D.; Dybing, E. *Acta Pharmacol. Toxicol.* **1982**, *51*, 78–80.
178. Gutter, B.; Rosenkranz, H.S. *Mutat. Res.* **1977**, *56*, 89–90.
179. Furukawa, M.; Sirianni, S.R.; Tan, J.C.; Huang, C.C. *JNCI, J. Natl. Cancer Inst.* **1978**, *60*, 1179–81.
180. National Cancer Institute, Technical Report Series CAS No 126–72–7, NCJ–CG–TR 76, 1978.
181. Reznik, G.; Hardisty, J.M.; Russefield, A. *JNCI, J. Natl. Cancer Inst.* **1979**, *63*, 205–12.
182. Reznik, G.; Reznik-Schüller, H.; Rice, J.M.; Hague, B.F. *Lab. Invest.* **1981**, *44*, 74–83.
183. Van Duuren, B.L.; Loewengart, G.; Seidman, I.; Smith, A.C.; Macchionne, S. *Cancer Res.* **1978**, *38*, 3236–40.
184. LeBlanc, R.B. *Fiber Prod.* **1977**, 10, 12, 16, 65.
185. Ramey, K.C.; Lini, D.C. In "Encyclopedia of Polymer Science and Technology, Plastics, Resins, Rubbers, Fibers"; Bikales, N.M., Ed.; Interscience: New York, 1971; Vol. 14, pp. 273–81.
186. VanStee, E.W.; Patel, J.M.; Gupta, B.N.; Drew, R.T. *Toxicol. Appl. Pharmacol.* **1975**, *41*, 175.
187. Conolly, R.B.; Jaeger, R. *Environ. Health Perspect.* **1977**, *21*, 131–35.
188. Drew, R.T.; Patel, J.W.; VanStee, E.W. *Toxicol. Appl. Pharmacol.* **1976**, *37*, 176–77.
189. Van Duuren, B.L. *Environ. Health Perspect.* **1977**, *21*, 17–23.
190. Huntington Research Center, Project 7511–253, 1978.
191. "Potential Industrial Carcinogens and Mutagens"; Fishbein, L., Ed.; Elsevier: Amsterdam, 1979; pp. 256–57.
192. Norpoth, K.; Reisch, A.; Heinecke, A. In "Short-Term Test Systems for Detecting Carcinogens"; Norpoth, K.H.; Garner, R.C., Eds.; Springer Verlag: Berlin, 1980; pp. 312–22.
193. Jorgenson, T.A.; Rushbrook, C.J.; Newell, G.W.; Tardiff, R.G. *Mutat. Res.* **1978**, *53*, 124.
194. Lingg, R.D.; Kaylor, W.H.; Glass, J.H.; Pyle, S.M.; Tardiff, R.G. *Toxicol. Appl. Pharmacol.* **1978**, *45*, 248–49.
195. Ling, R.D.; Kaylor, W.H.; Pyle, S.M.; Domino, M.M.; Smith, C.C.; Wolfe, G.F. *Arch. Environ. Contam. Toxicol.* **1982**, *11*, 173–83.
196. "Monograph on the Evaluation of the Carcinogenic Risk of Chemicals to Humans"; IARC: Lyon, 1979; Vol. 20, pp. 371–99.
197. Lillian, D.; Singh, H.B.; Appleby, L.; Lobban, R.; Arnts, R.; Bumpert, R.; Hague, R.; Toumey, J.; Kasazis, J.; Antell, M.; Hansen, D.; Scott, B. *Environ. Sci. Technol.* **1975**, *9*, 1042–48.
198. Dowty, B.; Carlosle, D.; Laseter, J.L.; Storer, J. *Science (Washington, D.C.)*, **1975**, *187*, 75–77.
199. Plaa, G.L.; Witschi, H. *Annu. Rev. Pharmacol. Toxicol.* **1976**, *16*, 125–41.
200. Frank, H.; Haussmann, H.J.; Remmer, H. *Chem.-Biol. Interact.* **1982**, *40*, 193–208.
201. Noguchi, T.; Fong, K.L.; Lai, E.P.; Alexander, S.S.; King, M.M.; Olson, L.; Poyer, J.L.; McCay, P.B. *Biochem. Pharmacol.* **1982**, *31*, 615–24.
202. Rocchi, P.; Prodi, G.; Grilli, S.; Ferreri, A.M. *Int. J. Cancer* **1973**, *11*, 419–25.
203. Uehleke, H.; Werner, T.; Greim, H.; Krämer, M. *Xenobiotica* **1977**, *7*, 393–400.

204. Eschenbrenner, A.B.; Miller, E. *JNCI, J. Natl. Cancer Inst.* **1944**, *4*, 385–88.
205. Costa, A.; Weber, G.; Bartoloni, S.T.; Omer, F.; Campana, G. *Arch. "De Vecchi" Anat. Patol. Med. Clin.* **1963**, *39*, 303–56.
206. Kawasaki, H. *Kurume Med. J.* **1965**, *12*, 37–42.
207. Reuber, M.D.; Glover, E.L. *JNCI, J. Natl. Cancer Inst.* **1970**, *44*, 419–27.
208. Kiplinger, G.F.; Kensler, C.J. *JNCI, J. Natl. Cancer Inst.* **1963**, *30*, 837–43.
209. Weisburger, E.K. *Environ. Health Perspect.* **1977**, *21*, 7–16.
210. Della Porta, G.; Terracini, B.; Shubik, P. *JNCI, J. Natl. Cancer Inst.* **1961**, *26*, 855–63.
211. Schwetz, B.A.; Leong, B.K.J.; Gehring, P.J. *Toxicol. Appl. Pharmacol.* **1974**, *28*, 452–64.
212. Tracey, J.P.; Sherlock, P. *N.Y. State J. Med.* **1968**, *68*, 2202–2204.
213. Pearson, C.R.; McConnell, G. *Proc. R. Soc. London, Ser. B* **1975**, *18*, 305–32.
214. "Monograph on the Evaluation of the Carcinogenic Risk of Chemicals to Humans"; IARC: Lyon, 1979, Vol. 20, pp. 401–24.
215. U.S. Food and Drug Administration, Fed. Register, 1976, *41*, 26842–26845.
216. Russel, J.W.; Schadoff, L.A. *J. Chromatogr.* **1977**, *134*, 375–84.
217. Schackelford, W.M.; Keith, L.H. EPA 600/4–76–062, U.S. EPA, 1976, 165–68.
218. Kleopfer, R.D. In "Identification and Analysis of Organic Pollutants of Water"; Keith, L.H., Ed.; Ann Arbor Science: Ann Arbor, MI, 1976; pp. 391–416.
219. Rook, J.J. Water Treat. Exam. **1974**, *23*, 234–37.
220. Pohl, L.R. In "Reviews in Biochemical Toxicology"; Hodgson, Bend, Philpot, Eds.; Elsevier: North Holland, 1979; pp. 79–107.
221. Pohl, L.R.; Martin, J.L.; George, J.W. *Biochem. Pharmacol.* **1980**, *99*, 3271–76.
222. Pereira, M.A.; Chang, L.W. *Chem.-Biol. Interact.* **1982**, *39*, 89–99.
223. Ilett, K.F.; Reid, W.D.; Sipes, I.G.; Krishna, G. *Exp. Mol. Pathol.* **1973**, *19*, 215–29.
224. Vesell, E.S.; Lang, C.M.; White, W.J.; Passanti, G.T.; Hill, R.N.; Clemens, T.L.; Liu, D.K.; Johnson, W.D. *Fed. Proc. Fed. Am. Soc. Exp. Biol.* **1976**, *35*, 1125–32.
225. Brown, D.M.; Langley, P.F.; Smith, D.; Taylor, D.C. *Xenobiotica* **1974**, *4*, 151–63.
226. Fry, B.J.; Taylor, T.; Hathway, D.E. *Arch. Int. Pharmacodyn. Ther.* **1972**, *196*, 98–111.
227. Reitz, R.H.; Gehring, P.J.; Park, C.N. *Food Cosmet. Toxicol.* **1978**, *16*, 511–14.
228. Uehleke, H. *Vom Wasser* **1980**, *54*, 171–78.
229. Eschenbrenner, A.B.; Miller, E. *JNCI, J. Natl. Cancer Inst.* **1945**, *5*, 251–55.
230. National Cancer Institute, 1976, PB–264–018.
231. Kirkland, D.J.; Smith, K.L.; Van Abbe, N.J. *Food Cosmet. Toxicol.* **1981**, *19*, 651–56.
232. Thompson, D.J.; Warner, S.D.; Robinson, V.B. *Toxicol. Appl. Pharmacol.* **1974**, *29*, 348–57.
233. Dilley, J.V.; Chernoff, N.; Kay, D.; Winslow, N.; Newell, G.M. *Toxicol. Appl. Pharmacol.* **1977**, *41*, 196.
234. "Monographs on the Evaluation of the Carcinogenic Risk of Chemicals to Humans"; IARC: Lyon, 1974; Vol. 4, pp. 239–45.
235. Figuera, W.G.; Raszkowski, R.; Weiss, W. *N. Engl. J. Med.* **1973**, *288*, 1094–96.
236. Albert, R.E.; Pasternack, B.S.; Shore, R.E.; Lippmann, M.; Nelson, N.; Ferris, B. *Environ. Health Perspect.* **1975**, *11*, 209–14.
237. Van Duuren, B.L.; Goldschmidt, B.M.; Katz, C.; Langseth, L.; Mercado, C.; Sivak, A. *Arch. Environ. Health* **1968**, *16*, 472–76.
238. Gargus, J.L.; Reese, W.H.; Rutter, H.A. *Toxicol. Appl. Pharmacol.* **1969**, *15*, 92–96.
239. Leong, B.K.; MacFarland, H.N.; Reese, W.H. *Arch. Environ. Health* **1971**, *22*, 663–66.
240. Van Duuren, B.L.; Katz, C.; Goldschmidt, B.M.; Frenkel, K.; Sivak, A. *JNCI, J. Natl. Cancer Inst.* **1972**, *48*, 1431–39.
241. Van Duuren, B.L. *Ann. N.Y. Acad. Sci.* **1969**, *163*, 828–36.
242. Nelson, N. *N. Engl. J. Med.* **1973**, *288*, 1123–24.

243. "Monographs on the Evaluation of the Carcinogenic Risk of Chemicals to Humans"; IARC: Lyon, 1979; Vol. 20, pp. 449–65.
244. "The Merck Index," Ninth Ed.; Merck and Co.: Rahway, NJ, 1976; p. 5930.
245. Jongon, W.M.F.; Alink, G.M.; Koeman, J.H. *Mutat. Res.* **1978**, *56*, 245–48.
246. Andrae, U.; Wolff, T. *Arch. Toxicol.* **1983**, *52*, 287–90.
247. Theiss, J.C.; Stoner, G.D.; Shimkin, M.B.; Weisburger, E.K. *Cancer Res.* **1977**, *37*, 2717–20.
248. Dow Chemical Corp., Midland, MI, 1980.
249. Kubic, V.L.; Anders, M.W. *Biochem. Pharmacol.* **1978**, *27*, 2349–55.
250. McKenna, M.J.; Zempel, J.A.; Braun, W.H.J. *Toxicol. Appl. Pharmacol.* **1982**, *65*, 1–10.
251. Ahmed, A.E.; Anders, M.W. *Biochem. Pharmacol.* **1978**, *27*, 2021–25.
252. van Bladeren, P.J.; Breimer, D.D.; Rotteveel-Smijs, G.M.T.; Jong, R.A.W.; Buis, W.; van der Gen, A.; Mohn, G.R. *Biochem. Pharmacol.* **1980**, *29*, 2975–87.
253. Jongen, W.M.F.; Harmsen, E.G.M.; Alink, G.M.; Koeman, J.H. *Mutat. Res.* **1982**, *95*, 183–89.
254. van Bladeren, P.J.; Breimer, D.D.; Rotteveel-Smijs, G.M.T.; Mohn, G.R. *Mutat. Res.* **1980**, *74*, 341–46.
255. "Monographs on the Evaluation of the Carcinogenic Risk of Chemicals to Humans"; IARC: Lyon, 1979; Vol. 20, pp. 429–48.
256. Ewing, B.B.; Chain, E.S.K.; Cook, J.C.; Evans, C.A.; Hopke, P.K.; Perkins, E.G. EPA-560/6–77–015, Washington, DC, U.S. Environmental Protection Agency, 1977, 63–64, 73.
257. Conkle, J.P.; Camp, B.J.; Welch, B.E. *Arch. Environ. Health* **1975**, *30*, 290–95.
258. Brem, H.; Stein, A.B.; Rosenkranz, H.S. *Cancer Res.* **1974**, *34*, 2576–79.
259. McCann, J.; Simmon, V.; Streitwieser, D.; Ames, B.N. *Proc. Natl. Acad. Sci. U.S.A.* **1975**, *72*, 3190–93.
260. Rannung, U.; Sundval, A.; Ramel, C. *Chem.-Biol. Interact.* **1978**, *20*, 1–16.
261. Yllner, S. *Acta Pharmacol. Toxicol.* **1971**, *30*, 257–65.
262. Rannung, U.; Göthe, R.; Wachtmeister, C.A. *Chem.-Biol. Interact.* **1976**, *12*, 251–63.
263. Van Dyke, R.A.; Wineman, C.G. *Biochem. Pharmacol.* **1971**, *20*, 463–70.
264. Shakarnis, V.F. *Genetika* **1969**, *5*, 89–95.
265. Nylander, P.-O.; Olofsson, H.; Rasmuson, B.; Svahlin, H. *Mutat. Res.* **1978**, *57*, 163–67.
266. National Cancer Institute, DHEW Publication No. (NIH) 78–1361, U.S. Dept. of Health, Education and Welfare, 1978.
267. National Cancer Institute, Technical Report Series, 1978, CAS No. 107–06–2, NCJ–CG–TR–55.
268. Delplace, Y.; Cavigneaux, A.; Cabasson, G. *Arch. Mal. Prof. Med. Trav. Secur. Soc.* **1962**, *23*, 816–17.
269. Martin, G.; Knorpp, K.; Huth, K.; Heinrich, F.; Mittermayer, D. *Dtsch. Med. Wochenschr.* **1968**, *93*, 2002–10.
270. Fishbein, L. In "Potential Industrial Carcinogens and Mutagens"; Elsevier: Amsterdam, 1979; pp. 241–45.
271. Anonymous, *Toxic Materials News* **1976**, *3*, 2–3.
272. Plotnick, H.B.; Conner, W.L. *Res. Commun. Chem. Pathol. Pharmacol.* **1976**, *13*, 251–58.
273. Nachtomi, E. *Biochem. Pharmacol.* **1970**, *19*, 2853–60.
274. van Bladeren, P.J.; van der Gen, A.; Breimer, D.D.; Mohn, G.R. *Biochem. Pharmacol.* **1979**, *28*, 2521–24.
275. Buselmaier, W.; Röhrborn, G.; Proppin, P. *Mutat. Res.* **1973**, *21*, 25–26.

276. Powers, M.B.; Voelker, R.W.; Page, N.P.; Weisburger, E.K.; Kraybill, H.F. *Toxicol. Appl. Pharmacol.* **1975**, *33*, 171–72.
277. Jones, A.R.; Edwards, K. *Experientia* **1968**, *24*, 1100–1101.
278. National Cancer Institute, Washington D.C., 1980, Technical Report Series, CAS No. 106–93–4, NCJ–CG–TR 210.
279. Wong, L.C.K.; Winston, J.M.; Hong, C.B.; Plotnick, H. *Toxicol. Appl. Pharmacol.* **1982**, *63*, 155–65.
280. Plotnick, H.B.; Weigel, N.N.; Richards, D.E.; Chever, K.L. *Res. Commun. Chem. Pathol. Pharmacol.* **1979**, *26*, 535–45.
281. Ott, M.G.; Scharnweber, H.C.; Langner, R.R. Dow Chemical Co., Midland, MI, 1977.
282. Hardin, D.W.F. In "Kirk-Othmer Encyclopedia of Chemical Technology," 2nd ed.; Interscience: New York, 1964; Vol. 5, pp. 154–70.
283. Jondorf, W.R.; Parke, D.V.; Williams, R.T. *Biochem. J.* **1957**, *65*, 14P.
284. National Cancer Institute, DHEW Publication No. (NIH) 78–1318, National Institutes of Health, 1978.
285. Mennear, J.H.; Haseman, J.K.; Sullivan, D.J.; Bernal, E.; Hildebrandt, P.K. *Fundam. Appl. Toxicol.* **1982**, *2*, 82–87.
286. Yllner, S. *Acta Pharmacol. Toxicol.* **1971**, *29*, 499–512.
287. Halpert, J. Drug Metab. Dispos. **1982**, *10*, 465–68.
288. Callen, D.F.; Wolf, C.R.; Philpot, R.M. *Mutat. Res.* **1980**, *77*, 55–63.
289. National Cancer Institute, Technical Report Series, CAS No. 79–34–5, NCJ–CG–TR–27, 1978.
290. Schmidt, R. *Biol. Rundsch.* **1976**, *14*, 220–23.
291. "Monographs on the Evaluation of the Carcinogenic Risk of Chemicals to Humans"; IARC: Lyon, 1979; Vol. 20, pp. 491–514.
292. Patel, R.; Janakiraman, N.; Towne, W.D. *Environ. Health Perspect.* **1977**, *21*, 247–49.
293. Henschler, D.; Bonse, G. *Arch. Toxicol.* **1977**, *39*, 7–12.
294. Bonse, G.; Urban, T.; Reichert, D.; Henschler, D. *Biochem. Pharmacol.* **1975**, *24*, 1829–34.
295. Ikeda, M. *Environ. Health Perspect.* **1977**, *21*, 239–45.
296. Cerna, M.; Kypenova, H. *Mutat. Res.* **1977**, *46*, 214–15.
297. Schwetz, B.A.; Leong, B.K.J.; Gehring, P.J. *Toxicol. Appl. Pharmacol.* **1975**, *32*, 84–96.
298. National Cancer Institute, Technical Report Series, CAS No. 127–18–4, NCI–CG–TR–13, 1977.
299. Rampy, L.W.; Quast, J.F.; Leong, B.K.J.; Gehring, P.J. In "Proceedings of the First International Congress on Toxicology"; Plaa, G.L.; Duncan, W.A.M., Eds.; Academic: New York, 1978; p. 562.
300. Schuhmann, A.M.; Watanabe, P.G.; Reitz, R.H.; Gehring, P.J. In "Toxicology of the Liver"; Plaa, G.; Hewitt, W.R., Eds.; Raven: New York, 1982; p. 311.
301. Lane, H.W.; Riddle, B.L.; Borzelleca, J.F. *Toxicol. Appl. Pharmacol.* **1982**, *63*, 409–21.
302. National Cancer Institute, Technical Report Series, CAS No. 71–55–6, NCJ–CG–TR–3, 1977.
303. Schumann, A.M.; Fox, T.R.; Watanabe, P.G. *Fundam. Appl. Toxicol.* **1982**, *2*, 27–34.
304. Henschler, D.; Reichert, D.; Metzler, M. *Int. J. Occup. Health Saf.* **1980**, *47*, 263–68.
305. Coleman, W.E.; Lingg, R.D.; Melton, R.G.; Kopfler, F.C. In "Identification and Analysis of Organic Pollutants in Water"; Keith, L.H., Ed.; Ann Arbor Science; Ann Arbor, MI, 1976; pp. 305–27.
306. Kronevi, T.; Wahlberg, J.; Holmberg, B. *Acta Pharmacol. Toxicol.* **1977**, *41*, 298–305.
307. Jakobson, J.; Holmberg, B.; Wahlberg, J.E. *Acta Pharmacol. Toxicol.* **1977**, *41*, 497–506.
308. Klaassen, C.D.; Plaa, G.L. *Toxicol. Appl. Pharmacol.* **1966**, *9*, 139–51.
309. Yllner, S. *Acta Pharmacol. Toxicol.* **1971**, *30*, 248–56.
310. National Cancer Institute, Technical Report Series, CAS No. 79–00–5, NCJ–CG–TR–74, 1978.

311. "Monographs on the Evaluation of the Carcinogenic Risk of Chemicals to Humans"; IARC: Lyon, 1979; Vol. 20, pp. 545–72.
312. Adams, E.M.; Spencer, H.C.; Rove, V.K.; McCollister, D.D.; Irish, D.D. *AMA Arch. Ind. Hyg. Occup. Med.* **1951**, *4*, 469–81.
313. Thiele, D.L.; Eigenbrodt, E.J.; Ware, A.J. *Gastroenterology* **1982**, *83*, 926–29.
314. Bonse, G.; Henschler, D. *CRC Crit. Rev. Toxicol.* **1976**, *4*, 395–409.
315. Oesch, F. *Xenobiotica* **1973**, *3*, 305–40.
316. National Cancer Institute, DHEW Publ. No. (NIH) 76–802, 1976.
317. Henschler, D.; Romen, W.; Elsässer, H.M.; Reichert, D.; Eder, E. *Arch. Toxicol.* **1980**, *43*, 237–48.
318. National Institute of Health, NTP–81–84, CAS No. 79–01–6, NIH Publ. No. 82–1799, 1982.
319. Stott, T.; Quast, J.F.; Watanabe, P.G. *Toxicol. Appl. Pharmacol.* **1982**, *62*, 137–51.
320. Parchman, L.G.; Magee, P.N. *J. Toxicol. Environ. Health* **1982**, *9*, 797–813.
321. Healy, T.E.J.; Poole, T.R.; Hopper, A. *Br. J. Anaesth.* **1982**, *54*, 337–40.
322. Slacik-Erben, R.; Roll, R.; Franke, G.; Uehleke, H. *Arch. Toxicol.* **1980**, *45*, 37–44.
323. Laib, R.J.; Stöckle, G.; Bolt, H.M. *Arch. Toxicol.* **1977**, Suppl. 2, 463.
324. Axelson, O.; Andersson, K.; Hogstedt, C.; Holmberg, B.; Molina, G.; de Verdier, A. *JOM, J. Occup. Med.* **1978**, *20*, 194–96.
325. Konietzko, H.; Haberlandt, W.; Heilbronner, H.; Reill, G.; Weichardt, H. *Arch. Toxicol.* **1978**, *40*, 201–206.
326. Gu, Z.W.; Sele, B.; Chmara, D.; Jalbert, P.; Vincent, M.; Vincent, F.; Marka, C.; Faure, J. *Ann. Genet.* **1981**, *24*, 105.
327. Uehleke, H.; Tabarelli-Poplawski, S.; Bonse, G.; Henschler, D. *Arch. Toxicol.* **1977**, *37*, 95–105.
328. Ikeda, M.; Miyake, Y.; Ogata, M.; Ohmori, S. *Biochem. Pharmacol.* **1980**, *29*, 2983–92.
329. Miller, R.E.; Guengerich, F.P. *Biochemistry* **1982**, *21*, 1090–95.
330. "Monographs on the Evaluation of the Carcinogenic Risk of Chemicals to Humans"; IARC: Lyon, 1974; Vol. 4, pp. 65–71, 73–77, 79–85.
331. Grundmann, E.; Steinhoff, D. *Z. Krebsforsch.* **1970**, *74*, 28–39.
332. Russfield, A.B.; Homburger, F.; Boger, E.; Weisburger, E.K.; Weisburger, J.H. *Toxicol. Appl. Pharmacol.* **1975**, *31*, 47–54.
333. Stula, E.F.; Sherman, H.; Zapp, J.A.; Clayton, J.W. *Toxicol. Appl. Pharmacol.* **1975**, *31*, 159–76.
334. Stula, E.F.; Barnes, J.R.; Sherman, H.; Reinhardt, C.F.; Zapp, J.A. *J. Environ. Pathol. Toxicol.* **1977**, *1*, 31–50.
335. Fishbein, L. In "Potential Industrial Carcinogens and Mutagens"; Fishbein, L., Ed.; Elsevier: Amsterdam, 1979; pp. 194–96.
336. Kaye, C.M.; Clapp, J.J.; Young, L. *Xenobiotica* **1972**, *2*, 129–39.
337. McCoy, E.C.; Burrows, L.; Rosenkranz, H.S. *Mutat. Res.* **1978**, *57*, 11–15.
338. Eder, E.; Neudecker, T. *Naunyn-Schmiederbergs Arch. Pharmakol.* **1978**, Suppl. 302, 83.
339. Torkelson, T.R.; Wolf, M.A.; Oyen, F.; Rowe, V.K. *Am. Ind. Hyg. Assoc. J.* **1959**, *20*, 217–23.
340. National Cancer Institute, Technical Report Series, CAS No. 107–05–1, NCI–CG–TR–73, 1978.
341. Ashby, J.; Trueman, R.W.; Stylor, J.A.; Penman, M.G.; Paton, D. *Carcinogenesis* **1981**, *2*, 33–39.
342. Scott, D. *Mutat. Res.* **1982**, *100*, 313–31.
343. Ashby, J.; Gaunt, C.; Robinson, M. *Mutat. Res.* **1982**, *100*, 391–93.
344. "Halogenated Biphenyls, Terphenyls, Naphtalenes, Dibenzodioxins and Related Products"; Kimbrough, R.D. Ed.; Elsevier: Amsterdam, 1980.
345. *Environ. Health Perspect.* **1978**, *24*, 133–89.
346. Allen, J.R.; Norback, D.H. In "Origins of Human Cancer"; Hiatt, H.H.; Watson, J.D.;

Winsten, J.A., Eds.; Cold Spring Harbor Laboratory: Cold Spring Harbor, NY, 1977; pp. 173–86.

347. "Monographs on the Evaluation of the Carcinogenic Risk of Chemicals to Humans: Polychlorinated Biphenyls and Polybrominated Biphenyls"; IARC: Lyon, 1978; Vol. 18.
348. Kimbrough, R.D. *Ann. N.Y. Acad. Sci.* **1979**, *320*, 415–18.
349. Risebrough R.W.; Rieche, P.; Peakall, D.B.; Herman, S.G.; Kirven, N. *Nature (London)* **1968**, *220*, 1098–102.
350. Biros, F.J.; Walker, A.C.; Medberry, A. *Bull. Environ. Contam. Toxicol.* **1970**, *5*, 317–23.
351. Kuratsune, M. et al. *Environ. Health Perspect.* **1972**, *1*, 119.
352. Kuratsune, M. In "Halogenated Biphenyls, Terphenyls, Naphtalenes, Dibenzo-dioxins and Related Products"; Kimbrough, R.D., Ed.; Elsevier: Amsterdam, 1980; p. 287–92. 92.
353. Urabe, H.; Koda, H.; Asahi, M. *Ann. N.Y. Acad. Sci.* **1979**, *320*, 273–76.
354. Kikuchi, M.; Shigematsu, N.; Umeda, G. *Fukuoka Igaku Zasshi* **1979**, *70*, 215–22.
355. Bahn, A.K.; Rosenwaike, I.; Herman, H.; Grover, P.; Stellman, J.; O'Leary, K. *N. Engl. J. Med.* **1976**, *295*, 450.
356. "Preliminary Information from Ongoing PCB Study," released by Monsanto Industrial Chemicals Co., Public Relations Department, 800 N. Lingbergh Boulevard, St. Louis, MO 63166, 1976.
357. Ito, N. et al. *JNCI, J. Natl. Cancer Inst.* **1973**, *51*, 1637–46.
358. Kimbrough, R.D.; Linder, R.E. *JNCI, J. Natl. Cancer Inst.* **1974**, *53*, 547–52.
359. Kimbrough, R.D.; Squire, R.A.; Linder, R.E.; Strandberg, J.D.; Montali, R.J.; Burse, V.W. *JNCI, J. Natl. Cancer Inst.* **1975**, *55*, 1453–59.
360. Schäffer, E.; Greim, H.; Baumann, M. *Berl. Muench. Tieraerztl. Wochenschr.* **1982**, *95*, 18.
361. Wheeler, E.P. Monsanto Co., St. Louis, Nov. 17, 1971.
362. Kimura, N.T.; Baba, T. *Gann* **1973** *64*, 105–8.
363. McConnell, E.E. In "Halogenated Biphenyls, Terphenyls, Naphtalenes, Dibenzodioxins and Related Products"; Kimbrough, R.D., Ed.; Elsevier: Amsterdam, 1980; p. 109–36.
364. Goldstein, J.A. In "Halogenated Biphenyls, Terphenyls, Naphthalenes, Dibenzodioxins and Related Products"; Kimbrough, R.D., Ed.; Elsevier: Amsterdam, 1980; p. 169.
365. Allen, J.R.; Carstens, C.A.; Barsotti, D.A. *Toxicol. Appl. Pharmacol.* **1974**, *30*, 440–51.
366. Nishizumi, M. *Gann* **1979**, *70*, 835–37.
367. Tatematsu, M.; Nakanishi, K.; Murasaki, G.; Miyata, Y.; Hirose, M.; Ito, N. *JNCI, J. Natl. Cancer Inst.* **1979**, *63*, 1411–16.
368. Kimura, N.T.; Kanematsu, T.; Baba, T. *Z. Krebsforsch. Klin. Onkol.* **1976**, *87*, 257–66.
369. Sternberg, S.S. *Pharmacol. Ther.* **1979**, *6*, 147–o6.
370. Burchfield, H.P.; Storrs, E.E. In Kraybill, H.F.; Mehlman, M.A., Eds. "Environmental Cancer, Advances in Modern Toxicology"; Wiley: New York, 1977; Vol. III, 38, pp. 319–71.
371a. Metcalf, R.L. In "The Future for Insecticides: Needs and Prospects"; Metcalf, R.L.; McKelvey, J.J., Jr., Eds.; Wiley: New York, 1974; pp. 223–85.
371b. Falk, H.L.; Thompson, S.J.; Kotin, P. *Arch. Environ. Health* **1965**, *10*, 847–58.
372. "Monographs on the Evaluation of the Carcinogenic Risk of Chemicals to Humans"; IARC: Lyon, 1979; Vol. 20.
373. National Cancer Institute, Carcinogenesis Program, Division of Cancer Cause & Prevention, 1976.
374. Olson, W.A.; Habermann, R.T.; Weisburger, E.K.; Ward, J.M.; Weisburger, J.H. *JNCI, J. Natl. Cancer Inst.* **1973**, *51*, 1993–95.

375. Epstein, S.S. *Sci. Total Environ.* **1978**, *9*, 1–62.
376. National Cancer Institute, Carcinogenesis Technical Report Series, No. 28, 78–828, 1978.
377. Van Duuren, B.L.; Goldschmidt, B.M.; Loewengart, G.; Smith, A.C.; Melchionne, S.; Seidman, J.; Roth, D. *JNCI, J. Natl. Cancer Inst.* **1979**, *63*, 1433–39.
378. Reznik, G.; Stinson, S.F.; Ward, J.M. *Cancer Lett.* **1980**, *10*, 339–42.
379. Epstein, S.S. Sci. Total Environ. **1976**, *6*, 103–54.
380. National Cancer Institute, Carcinogenesis Technical Report Series No. 9, 1977.
381. Cabral, J.R.P.; Mollner, T.; Raitano, F.; Shubik, P. *Int. J. Cancer* **1979**, *23*, 47–51.
382. Cabral, J.R.P.; Shubik, P.; Mollner, T.; Raitano, F. *Nature (London)* **1979**, *269*, 510–11.
383. Nagasaki, H.; Tomii, S.; Mega, T.; Marugami, M.; Ito, N. *Gann* **1971**, *62*, 431.
384. Goto, M.; Hattori, M.; Miyagawa, T.; Enomoto, M. *Chemosphere* **1972**, *6*, 279–82.
385. Hanada, M.; Yutani, C.; Miyaji, T. *Gann* **1973**, *64*, 511–13.
386. Ito, N.; Nagasaki, H.; Arai, M. In "New Methods in Environmental Chemistry and Ecological Chemistry"; Coulston, F.; Korte, F.; Goto, M., Eds.; International Academic: Tokyo, 1973; pp. 141–47.
387. Ito, N.; Nagasaki, H.; Arai, M.; Sugihara, S.; Makiura, S. *JNCI, J. Natl. Cancer Inst.* **1973**, *51*, 817–26.
388. Nagasaki, H.; Kawabata, H.; Miyata, Y.; Inoue, K.; Hirao, K.; Aoe, H.; Ito, N. *Gann* **1975**, *66*, 185–91.
389. Thorpe, E.; Walker, A.I.T. *Food Cosmet. Toxicol.* **1973**, *11*, 433–522.
390. Ito, N.; Hananouchi, M.; Sugihara, S.; Shirai, T.; Tsuda, H.; Fukushima, S.; Nagasaki, H. *Cancer Res.* **1976**, *36*, 2227–34.
391a. Ito, N.; Nagasaki, H.; Aoe, H.; Sugihara, S.; Miayta, Y.; Arai, M.; Shirai, T. *JNCI, J. Natl. Cancer Inst.* **1975**, *54*, 801–805.
391b. Fitzhugh, O.G.; Nelson, A.A. *J. Pharmacol. Exp. Ther.* **1947**, *89*, 18–30.
392. Fitzhugh, O.G.; Nelson, A.A.; Frawley, J.P. *J. Pharmacol. Exp. Ther.* **1950**, *100*, 59–66.
393. Reuber, M.D. *J. Environ. Pathol. Toxicol.* **1980**, *4*, 355–72.
394. Reuber, M.D. *Environ. Res.* **1979**, *19*, 460–81.
395. National Cancer Institute, Carcinogenesis Technical Report Series No. 14, 1977.
396. National Technical Information Service, "Evaluation of Carcinogenic, Teratogenic and Mutagenic Activities of Selected Pesticides and Industrial Chemicals," Vol. 1, Carcinogenic Study, Washington D.C., U.S. Dept. of Commerce, 1968.
397. Ulland, B.M.; Page, N.P.; Squire, R.A.; Weisburger, E.K.; Cypher, R.L. *JNCI, J. Natl. Cancer Inst.* **1977**, *58*, 133–40.
398. National Cancer Institute, Carcinogenesis Technical Report Series No. 35, 1978.
399. Davis, K.J. memorandum to Hansen, W., Food and Drug Administration, Washington, D.C., January 30, 1969.
400. Reuber, M.D. *J. Cancer Res. Clin. Oncol.* **1979**, *93*, 173–79.
401. Nelson, A.A. memorandum to Lehman, A.J., Food and Drug Administration, Washington, D.C., October 23, 1951.
402. National Cancer Institute, DHEW Publ. No. (NIH) 79–837, Carcinogenesis Testing Program, Division of Cancer Cause & Prevention, 1979.
403. National Cancer Institute, Carcinogenesis Technical Report Series No. 155, 1979.
404. Nelson, A.A. FDA memorandum: "Pathological Changes Produced in Wistar Rats by Feeding Technical Benzene Hexachloride and the Pure Isomers at Levels of 5 to 1600 ppm in the Diet for 2 Years," January 30, 1950.
405. Simon, G.S.; Kopps, B.R.; Tardiff, R.G.; Borzelleca, J.F. *Toxicol. Appl. Pharmacol.* **1978**, *45*, 330–31.
406. Maslansky, D.J.; Williams, G.M. *J. Toxicol. Environ. Health* **1981**, *8*, 121–30.
407. Khera, K.S. *Food Cosmet. Toxicol.* **1974**, *12*, 471–77.
408. Guerzoni, M.E.; Del Cupolo, L.; Ponti, I. *Riv. Sci. Tecnol. Alimenti. Nutr. Um.* **1976**, *6*, 161–65.

409. Marshall, T.C.; Dorough, H.W.; Swim, H.E. *J. Agric. Food Chem.* **1976**, *24*, 560–63.
410. Benes, V.; Sram, R. *Ind. Med.* **1969**, *38*, 50–52.
411. Cerey, K.; Izakovic, V.; Ruttkay-Nedecka, J. *Mutat. Res.* **1973**, *21*, 26.
412. Arnold, D.W.; Kennedy, G.L., Jr.; Kerlinger, M.L.; Calandra, J.C.; Calo, C.J. *J. Toxicol. Environ. Health* **1977**, *2*, 547–55.
413. Markarjan, D.S. *Genetika (Moscow)* **1966**, *1*, 132–37.
414. Ahmed, F.E.; Hart, R.W.; Lewis, J.J. *Mutat. Res.* **1977**, *42*, 161–74.
415. Buselmaier, W.; Röhrborn, G.; Propping, P. *Biol. Zentralbl.* **1972**, *91*, 311–25.
416. Shahin, M.M.; van Borstel, R.C. *Mutat. Res.* **1977**, *48*, 173–80.
417. Shirasu, Y.; Moriya, M.; Kato, K.; Furuhashi, A.; Kada, R. *Mutat. Res.* **1976**, *40*, 19–30.
418. Hooper, N.K.; Ames, B.N.; Saleh, M.A.; Casida, J.E. *Science (Washington, D.C.)* **1979**, *205*, 591–93.
419. Wong, D.; Terriere, L. *Biochem. Pharmacol.* **1965**, *14*, 375–77.
420. Curley, A.; Burse, V.W.; Jennings, R.W.; Villanueva, E.C.; Tomatis, L.; Akazaki, K. *Nature (London)* **1973**, *272*, 338–40.
421. Ohsawa, T.; Knox, J.R.; Khalifa, S.; Casida, J.E. *J. Agric. Food Chem.* **1975**, *23*, 98–106.
422. Whorton, D.; Milby, T.H.; Krauss, R.M.; Stubbs, H.A. *J. Occup. Med.* **1979**, *21*, 161–66.
423. U.S. Occupational Safety and Health Administration Federal Register, *42*, 45536–49, 1977.
424. Glass, R.I.; Lyness, R.N.; Mengle, D.C.; Powell, K.E.; Kahn, E. *Am. J. Epidemiol.* **1979**, *109*, 346–51.
425. Stolzenberg, S.J.; Hine, C.H. *J. Toxicol. Environ. Health* **1979**, *5*, 1149–58.
426. Blum, A.; Ames, B.N. *Science (Washington, D.C.)* **1977**, *195*, 17–23.
427. Teramoto, S.; Saito, R.; Aoyama, H.; Shirasu, Y. *Mutat. Res.* **1980**, *77*, 71–78.
428. Kapoor, I.P.; Metcalf, R.L.; Nystrom, R.F.; Sangha, G.K. *J. Agric. Food Chem.* **1970**, *18*, 1145–52.
429a. Reuber, M.D. *Environ. Health Perspect.* **1980**, *36*, 205–19.
429b. Nelson, J.A.; Struck, P.F.; James, R. *J. Toxicol. Environ. Health* **1977**, *3*, 366–67.
430. Deichmann, W.B.; Keplinger, M.; Sala, F.; Glass, E. *Toxicol. Appl. Pharmacol.* **1967**, *11*, 88–103.
431. Deichmann, W.B.; MacDonald, W.E.; Blum, E.; Bevilacqua, M.; Radomski, J.L.; Keplinger, M.; Balkus, M. *Ind. Med. Surg.* **1970**, *39*, 426–34.
432. Radomski, J.L.; Deichmann, W.B.; MacDonald, W.E.; Glass, E.M. *Toxicol. Appl. Pharmacol.* **1965**, *7*, 652–56.
433. Reuber, M.D. *Tumori* **1978**, *64*, 571–77.
434. National Cancer Institute, Carcinogenesis Technical Report Series No. 131, 1978.
435. Agthe, C.; Carcia, H.; Shubik, P.; Tomatis, L.; Wenyon, E. *Proc. Soc. Exp. Biol. Med.* **1970**, *134*, 113–16.
436. Rinkus, S.J.; Legator, M.S. *Cancer Res.* **1979**, *39*, 3289–318.
437. National Cancer Institute, Technical Report Series, NCI–CG–TR–104, 1978.
438. Larson, P.S.; Crawford, E.M.; Blackwell Smith, R., Jr.; Hennigar, G.R.; Haag, H.B.; Finnegan, J.K. *Toxicol. Appl. Pharmacol.* **1960**, *2*, 659–73.
439. National Cancer Institute, Carcinogenesis Technical Report Series No. 96, 1979.
440. National Cancer Institute, Carcinogenesis Technical Report Series No. 62, 1977.
441. National Cancer Institute, Carcinogenesis Technical Report Series No. 12, 1979.
442. "Monographs on the Evaluation of the Carcinogenic Risk of Chemicals to Humans"; IARC: Lyon, 1977; Vol. 15.
443. Wedig, J.H.; Sperling, F.; Miller, R. Olin Corporation, unpublished report of an analysis of data submitted by the National Cancer Institute, 1976.
444. National Cancer Institute, Carcinogenesis Technical Report Series No. 61, 1978.

445. Blair, D.; Dix, K.M.; Hunt, P.F.; Thorpe, E.; Stevenson, D.E.; Walker, A.I.T. *Arch. Toxicol.* **1976**, *35*, 281–94.
446. Doull, J.; Vesselinovitch, D.; Root, M.; Cowan, J.; Meskauskas, J.; Fitch, F. unpublished report by Department of Pharmacology, University of Chicago.
447. Doull, J.; Vesselinovitch, D.; Fitch, F.; Meskauskas, J.; Root, M.; Cowan, J. unpublished report by Department of Pharmacology, University of Chicago.
448. Grundmann, E.; Hobik, H.P. unpublished report submitted by Farbenfabriken Bayer A.G., Federal Republic of Germany.
449. Lorke, D.; Loser, E. unpublished report submitted by Farbenfabriken Bayer A.G., Federal Republic of Germany.
450. Cohn, W.J.; Boylan, J.J.; Blanke, R.V.; Fariss, M.W.; Howell, J.R.; Guzelian P.S. *N. Engl. J. Med.* **1978**, *298*, 243–48.
451. Adir, J.; Caplan, Y.H.; Thompson, B.C. *Life Sci.* **1978**, *22*, 699–702.
452. Samosh, L.V. *Tsitol. Genet.* **1974**, *8*, 24–27.
453. Infante, P.F.; Epstein, S.S.; Newton, W.A., Jr. *Scand. J. Work Environ. Health* **1978**, *4*, 137–50.
454. Peters, H.A. *Fed. Proc, Fed. Am. Soc. Exp. Biol.* **1976**, *35*, 2400–2403.
455. Barthel, E. *Z. Erkr. Atmungsorgane* **1976**, *146*, 266–74.
456a. National Cancer Institute, Carcinogenesis Technical Report Series No. 21, 1978.
456b. National Cancer Institute, Carcinogenesis Technical Report Series, CAS. No. 133–06–2, Washington, D.C.
457. National Cancer Institute, Carcinogenesis Technical Report Series No. 8, 77–808, 1977.
458. Suter, P.; Zak, F.; Sachsse, K.; Hess, R. unpublished report from Toxicology/Pathology, Ciby-Geigy, Ltd., Basel, Switzerland, submitted by Ciba-Geigy, Ltd. to WHO, reported in Pesticide Residues in Food, Evaluations, FAO, 1978.
459. Walker, A.I.T.; Stevenson, D.E.; Robinson, J.; Thorpe, E.; Roberts, M. *Toxicol. Appl. Pharmacol.* **1969**, *15*, 345–73.
460. Walker, A.I.T.; Thorpe, E.; Stevenson, D.E. *Food Cosmet. Toxicol.* **1973**, *11*, 415–32.
461. National Technical Information Service, (1968) "Evaluation of Carcinogenic, Teratogenic and Mutagenic Activities of selected Pesticides and Industrial Chemicals" Carcinogenic Study, Washington D.C., U.S. Department of Commerce, Vol. 1.
462. Tarjan, R.; Kemény, T. *Food Cosmet. Toxicol.* **1969**, *7*, 215–22.
463. Terracini, B.; Testa, M.C.; Cabral, J.R.; Day, N. *Int. J. Cancer* **1973**, *11*, 747–64.
464. Terracini, B.; Cabral, R.J.; Testa, M.C. In "Proceedings of the 8th Inter-American Conference on Toxicology: Pesticides and the Environment, a Continuous Controversy", Miami, FL, 1973. Deichmann, W.B., Ed.; Intercontinental Medical: New York, 1973; p. 77.
465. Tomatis, L.; Turusov, V.; Day, N.; Charles, R.T. *Int. J. Cancer* **1972**, *10*, 489–506.
466. Turusov, V.S.; Day, N.E.; Tomatis, L.; Gati, E.; Charles, R.T. *JNCI, J. Natl. Cancer Inst.* **1973**, *51*, 983–97.
467. Shabad, L.M.; Kolesnichenko, T.S.; Nikonova, T.V. *Int. J. Cancer* **1973**, *11*, 688, and **1972**, *9*, 365–73.
468. Tomatis, L.; Turusov, V.; Charles, R.T.; Boiocchi, M. *JNCI, J. Natl. Cancer Inst.* **1974**, *52*, 883–91.
469. National Cancer Institute, Carcinogenesis Technical Report Series No. 33, 1978.

10

Inorganic Carcinogenesis

JOHN P. W. GILMAN[1]

University of Guelph, Guelph, Ontario, Canada

SABINE H. H. SWIERENGA

Health and Welfare Canada, Ottawa, Ontario, Canada

THE PRIMARY CARCINOGEN IN ENVIRONMENTAL CARCINOGENESIS can be either a chemical or a physical agent. Chemicals in particular also play major synergistic roles in subsequent tumor development. Some workers believe that as much as 50–90% of human cancer may be attributable to chemical exposure (*1*). This high estimate has, however, been countered by more conservative estimates, as low as 5%, of other authorities (*2*). At this juncture, the general view among scientists is that one-third to two-thirds of all cancers are causally related to the innumerable exogenous chemicals present in our modern day environment (*3, 4*). A majority of identified chemical carcinogens are organic or radioactive elements; however, a number of inorganic compounds, particularly metals and metalloid pollutants, have been causally implicated in occupational and environmental cancers (*5–9*).

Inorganic chemicals with carcinogenic properties may be divided into the following four groups: (1) metals and metalloids and their compounds; (2) minerals; (3) radioactive metals; and (4) other inorganic elements. This chapter only examines groups 1 and 4; minerals, such as asbestos, are discussed in Chapter 11.

Metals as Environmental and Occupational Carcinogens

Metals and metal compounds make up the majority of potentially carcinogenic inorganic chemicals that do not contain a radioisotope. Rather surprisingly, little information on the carcinogenic potential of metals in animals or humans was published before 1945 (*10, 11*). The two exceptions are (1) claims for a causal relationship between As and skin cancer dating back to early in the 19th century

[1]Current address: Gilman and Associates, Consultants, P.O. Box 1738, Summerland, British Columbia, Canada VOH 1Z0

0065-7719/84/0182-0577$14.10/1

and (2) an uncontrolled report on the carcinogenicity of metallic As, Cr, and Co in rabbits (*12*).

The concentrations of naturally occurring metals in the environment probably are far too low to constitute a carcinogenic risk. Exceptions to this comforting generalization though have always existed within the work environment and are appearing with increasing frequency in both general urban (industrial) and rural (agricultural) environments. The burning of fossil fuels in internal combustion engines and coal-fired power plants creates a constant source of pollution, particularly in urban environments. Particles of As, Be, Cd, Pb, and Ni released into the atmosphere through these processes are, if absorbed in more than trace amounts, metabolic poisons with either an effective or suspected carcinogenic potential to humans (*13*).

Natural and man-made exposure levels of the principal metallic pollutants in the environment have been extensively reviewed with emphasis on atmosphere (*7, 13*), water (*6*), and foods (*14*) as the major agents of dispersion.

Several metals that are widely recognized as constituting a carcinogenic risk to humans, such as As, Be, Cr, and Ni have been the subject of numerous epidemiological and experimental studies directed toward the assessment of human risk, confirmation of carcinogenicity, and elucidation of mechanisms of action. Recent reviews have examined occupational (*5, 15, 16*), general environmental (*8, 9, 17, 18*), and iatrogenic (*19*) exposure to these metals. To relate metal carcinogenesis with human exposure, Flessel et al. (*9*) have attempted to devise an index of carcinogenicity of various metals based on the relative importance of human, animal, and short-term studies.

Assessment of Carcinogenesis

Epidemiology. Studies on metal carcinogenesis, primarily on workers in heavy industry, are essential for the final assessment of carcinogenic risk to humans. However, as methods of detection, these studies suffer from inherent limitations in sensitivity and interpretability. Even under industrial conditions where the concentration of the element under study is likely to be high, cancers will not occur in statistically meaningful numbers until after many years of exposure. Such studies are essentially retrospective and imply a prolonged build-up of harmful effects in the population at risk. Time from first exposure to neoplasia in humans in metal carcinogenesis is often extremely long; latencies of over 30 years are by no means exceptional. When the population in an epidemiological study is small or the chemical is a weak carcinogen, even a 50% increase in incidence could go undetected (*20*). Finally, because of exposure to other possibly carcinogenic chemicals and varied genotypes and life-styles (e.g., smoking habits) of the population under study, it is all too easy to argue that epidemiological findings are inconclusive and that further study is necessary to confirm a suspected causal correlation.

Dose–Response Relationships. Identification of a chemical as an environmental or industrial carcinogen is based on its dose–effect (qualitative) response. Evaluation of risk will, in addition, be influenced by the frequency of effect at various exposure levels (dose–response).

Dose of a chemical carcinogen from the environment can never be expressed in precise metric terms; instead it must be stated in terms of sampled concentrations in air, food, and water; duration of exposure; measurements from the excreta of exposed individuals; and so forth.

The principles of risk assessment, the problems associated with classifying an element as an industrial carcinogen, and the difficulties involved in establishing permissible exposure levels have been thoroughly reviewed by Norseth (*21*). In regard to the work place, he concludes that "minimizing exposure to a 'suspected' carcinogen should not be postponed because of difficulties in assessing the actual risk." This principle should apply equally to suspected environmental carcinogens even though the so-called safe exposure levels based on epidemiological evidence are even harder to determine with certainty. Threshold limit values (TLVs), published and regularly revised by the American Conference of Governmental Industrial Hygienists (*22*), provide a useful guideline on permissible exposure levels applicable to the workplace.

Animal Studies. The early identification of carcinogenic agents and the initiation of preventive measures require experimental studies either to support epidemiological findings or to indicate which compounds deserve epidemiological studies. Positive results from long-term animal tests in more than one species constitute a strong indication that a chemical may be a real carcinogenic risk to humans. Many chemical compounds have been shown to be carcinogenic in experimental animals that have not been established as human carcinogens. Such a situation might reflect either insufficient epidemiological study and/or levels of environmental exposure that are too low to induce a statistically significant cancer incidence (*23*). With the possible exception of As, all established human chemical carcinogens also induce neoplastic disease in animals; the patterns of development and metabolic pathways are frequently similar (*18, 23*). Nonetheless, extrapolations from experimental animals to humans must be made with caution and should be supported by epidemiological evidence. Dosage in animal carcinogenesis experiments is usually much more massive than in human exposure; the large doses may increase the sensitivity of the bioassay, but then the results are not necessarily applicable to human risk assessment (*16*). The cost and time involved in long-term animal tests are further limitations to their use as preliminary toxicity-screening assays.

Short-Term Assays. The rapid development of a variety of short-term assays for toxicity testing during the past decade has facilitated the otherwise insurmountable task of screening vast numbers of chemical compounds for mutagenicity and possible carcinogenicity. The results of these assays provide a rational basis for decisions and priorities in regard to long-term animal testing and epidemiological studies.

A wide variety of short-term in vitro assays has been applied to metal toxicity testing. Detailed description of some of these assays and their application to the testing of metals can be found in a review by Stout and Rawson (*24*). Generally, the tests can be divided into four categories: (1) mutation assays with prokaryotic organisms, such as *Bacilus subtilis, Salmonella typhimurium* (usually the Ames test), and *Escherichia coli*; (2) mutation and chromosome damage assays with eukaryotic organisms, such as yeast and plants; (3) cell-free biochemical assays using synthetic polynucleotides or purified DNA polymerases to assess fidelity of DNA synthesis, and (4) mutation, cell transformation, DNA damage and repair, and cytogenetic end point assays using mammalian cell systems.

Microbial assays have not been as successful as mammalian cell tests in validating and predicting carcinogenicity of metal compounds. For example, Hollstein and McCann (*25*) state that the standard Ames test is not suitable for metals because of the large amounts of Mg salts (citrate, sulfate, and phosphate) in the basic reaction mixture. Mammalian cells provide more efficient systems for metabolizing the metals to active carcinogens, as well as greater quantities of the primary target DNA and chromosomes. The most frequently reported metal toxicity has been as chromosome aberrations in a variety of cell types, for instance, in human lymphocytes following industrial in vivo exposure. Lead compounds, for example, are active chromosome-damaging agents in this assay (*26*). Several short-term assays appear to be particularly sensitive to metal toxicity and have been used to correlate large numbers of metal compounds with known carcinogenicity. These tests include the cell-free "fidelity of DNA synthesis" assay of Sirover and Loeb (*27*) that uses purified DNA polymerase, the "enhancement of viral transformation" assay of Casto et al. (*28*), a mutation assay at the hypoxanthine–guanine phosphoribosyltransferase (HGPRT) locus in Chinese hamster ovary cells (*29*), and the Syrian hamster embryo cell transformation assay of Di Paolo et al (*30*). Other assay systems may be equally sensitive but need further validation. All of these systems are discussed further in the section on established carcinogens.

Because short-term carcinogenicity assays can be performed rapidly, a much broader range of inorganic compounds has been tested with these than with animal experiments. Thus, in some cases, compounds that were positive in short-term studies have no other adequate carcinogenic data to validate the findings. Such compounds should receive high priorities for further study, particularly in cases of extensive human exposure; the convincing correlations that have already been obtained between positive short-term assay results and substances of known carcinogenicity support such directed study (*25*).

Metal Carcinogens

Classification Criteria. Standard criteria for classifying carcinogens in terms of their potential risk to humans have not been firmly established. In this review, potentially carcinogenic metal compounds have been classified in terms of (1) short-term tests for carcinogenicity, (2) long-term animal test results, and (3) epidemiological findings:

- *Established carcinogens* are substances for which the epidemiologic evidence of carcinogenicity is considered conclusive. In most instances these data have been corroborated by positive results in long-term animal tests and several short-term assay systems. (*21, 31*).
- *Suspected carcinogens* are substances for which the epidemiological data to date are insufficient or inconclusive, but which have proven to be carcinogenic in animal bioassays in at least two mammalian species (*21*) and have tested positively in at least two short-term assay systems.
- *Possible carcinogens* are chemicals for which no firm epidemiological evidence of carcinogenicity exists at the present time. Evidence suggestive of a

primary carcinogenic action is usually limited to inconclusive animal tests and positive results in two or more short-term test systems.

- *Carcinogenic cofactors* fall into two categories: (1) compounds that are not necessarily primary carcinogens, but appear to have a promoting, enhancing, or inhibitory effect and have been shown in animal experiments to act synergistically in the carcinogenic process; and (2) chemicals that exert an anticarcinogenic influence in certain animal models.

Metals that may be classified as carcinogens or carcinogenic cofactors in terms of the above criteria may and often do exist in noncarcinogenic forms.

Established Carcinogens. Table I lists the four metals classified as established human carcinogens and summarizes the epidemiological and animal evidence on which the classification has been based. Short-term assay results for these metals are listed in Table II.

ARSENIC. *Short-Term Assays.* Leonard (*32*) reported As toxicity following in vivo exposure in several short-term assays, such as the dominant lethal test in mice and chromosome aberrations in human lymphoctyes. Further, As compounds appear to be powerful chromosome-damaging agents in vitro in a wide variety of species incluing humans (Table II).

Leonard (*32*) also noted that most studies performed on the mutagenic activity of As have provided positive results; however, these studies have been exclusively bacterial assays, in some cases with repair-deficient bacteria. Mammalian cell mutagenesis data are curiously very limited. Similarly, only a few studies of cell transformation following As exposure have been reported, and all of these assays used the same system: Syrian hamster embryo cells (Table II).

Thus, As compounds appear to be potent clastogens in a wide variety of cells, but mutagenic only in bacterial systems. Both arsenite and arsenate compounds are active in short-term assays, although the former are generally more active (*33*). Arsenate is thought to be reduced in biological systems to the active arsenite form (*32*). However, Oguni et al. (*34*) reported a plant toxicity assay involving enzyme induction in which arsenate, but not arsenite, was positive.

Animal Experiments. Repeated attempts at tumor induction with arsenicals in experimental animals over a 60-year period have consistently resulted in either negative or equivocal results (*see* reviews in Refs. 5, 35, 36). Almost all of these studies have utilized either mouse or rat models with skin painting or oral administration (*37–39*). A more recent long-term inhalation study gave no increased evidence of respiratory tumors in a tumor-susceptible strain of mice (*40*).

Several studies seem to suggest that As may have an inhibiting rather than a promoting action on the carcinogenicity of dimethylbenzanthracene (DMBA), urethane (*41*), and methylcholanthrene (*42*) in mice. Kroes (*43*) failed to demonstrate any synergism between diethylnitrosamine and lead or sodium arsenate in rats.

A study involving oral administration of As to dogs over a 2-year period gave negative results (*44*); however, a 2-year observation period is too short in the dog to determine negative results in metal carcinogenesis (*36*).

A rare positive tumor response to As has been reported by Oswald (*45*). Lymphomas were induced in 11 of 19 mice after 20 weekly intravenous injections

Table I

Established Carcinogens

	Human Risk			Experimental Tumorigenesis		
Element	*Route*[a]	*Class*[b]	*Target*	*Species*	*Route*[a]	*Target/Type*
As	ingest inhal dermal	iat occ env	skin lung lymph(?)	mouse	iv	lymphomas
Bordeaux mix (As, Cu, Ca)	inhal dermal	occ	lung skin	rat	it	resp. carcinomas
Be (low-fired BeO)	inhal	occ env	lung	rabbit mouse rat monkey	imed iv it inhal	osteosarcomas lung carcinomas
Cr(VI) (low-solubility)	inhal ingest	occ	lung GI tract	rat mouse	sc, im it inhal	resp. carcinomas sarcomas at site renal carcinomas
Ni	inhal	occ	upper resp. tract, lung	rat mouse rabbit cat	sc, im inhal iren isin	rhabdomyosarcomas fibrosarcomas leiomyosarcomas resp. carcinomas

[a] im, intramuscular; imed, intramedullary (bone); ingest, ingestion; inhal, inhalation; iren, intrarenal; isin, intrasinus implant; it, intratracheal; iv, intravenous; and sc, subcutaneous.
[b] iat, iatrogenic; occ, occupational; and env, general environmental.

of 0.5 mg of sodium arsenate. Postnatal injections of arsenic increased this tumor incidence.

Ishinishi (*46*) reported that As_2O_3, As containing copper ore, and flue dust had cocarcinogenic or enhancing action with benzo[*a*]pyrene when instilled intratracheally into rats in 15 weekly doses. In the same experiment, rats were also comparably treated with the arsenicals alone; mortality was high, and the two adenomas and one adenocarcinoma observed in the 25 survivors cannot be considered firm evidence of a primary carcinogenic effect of As.

A single intratracheal instillation of a simulated As-containing spray—a Bordeaux mixture with $CuSO_4$, $Ca(OH)_2$, and $Ca_3(AsO_4)_2$—in rats resulted in broncheogenic adenocarcinomas and alveolar cell carcinomas in 9 of 15 survivors. This report experimentally confirms the increased risk of lung tumors seen among vineyard workers who were exposed to this pesticide mixture, but it only suggests the causal involvement of As, because the compounds were not tested individually (*47*).

Epidemiological Studies. The accumulation of epidemiological reports over 150 years that appear to link As causally with cancer of the skin, lung, and more recently, the lymphatic system and internal organs is generally considered sufficient evidence for its carcinogenic risk to humans, despite the lack of firm experimental evidence (*3, 7*).

Cancers associated with As in humans usually involve either occupational or iatrogenic exposure through the oral or respiratory routes (*15, 19, 32, 35*). Population exposures that are neither occupational nor iatrogenic have been related to (1) arsenic in the water supply resulting in an excess of precancerous dermatoses and skin cancer (*48*) and (2) chronic regional arsenic contamination resulting in cancers at various sites (*49–51*).

Excessive cancer incidences, particularly of epidermoid lung cancer, have been frequently reported among workers exposed to As in combination with Pb, Zn, Au, Cu, and other metals in the mining, smelting, and chemical insecticide industries (*49, 52–55*). Agricultural workers using arsenical preparations also seem to be at excessive risk for lung (*56*) and skin (*57*) cancer.

The medicinal use of arsenicals has been causally linked to bronchial carcinoma, skin cancers, and angiosarcoma of the liver (*19, 32, 58–60*). Persons with arsenical keratosis and multiple basal cell carcinoma linked to prior As ingestion may also develop internal malignant neoplasms (*61*).

Conclusions. Arsenic is generally accepted as an established carcinogen for humans on the basis of the epidemiological evidence for its carcinogenicity alone. This view has gained some support, although inconclusive, from short-term bioassays showing As to be a strong chromosome-damaging agent both in vivo and in vitro. Mammalian cell mutagenesis and transformation have been investigated by using the Syrian hamster embryo cell model, but studies using other models are needed on these processes.

Essentially no evidence exists in support of the carcinogenicity of As in experimental animals. A few studies suggest cofactor effects; some are inhibitory and others are cocarcinogenic. Several reviewers have been hesitant to endorse unequivocally the carcinogenicity of As and have urged that further studies, both experimental and epidemiological, should be undertaken (*32, 35, 36*). The existing

Table II

Genotoxicity of Established Metal Carcinogens: Short-Term Assays

Assay		*As*		*Be*		*Cr*		*Ni*
In vivo tests[a]	+*	review (*32*)	+	mouse (*336*), hamster (*66*)	+*	mouse (*82, 83*), hamster (*66*), human (*26, 84, 369*), chick embryo (*370*), *Drosophila* (*371*)	+	review (*90*), mouse dominant lethal test (*389*)
Cytotoxicity	+	plant cells (*34*)			+/−	plant cells (*34*)		
DNA effects								
biochemical assays[b]	+	(*355*)	+	(*27, 63, 64*)	+	(*27, 63, 355*)	+	(*27, 63, 65*)
Rec assay[c]	+	(*33, 113, 114*)	+	(*113, 114*)	+	(*33, 113, 114, 372*)	−	(*33, 113, 114*)
Pol A assay[d]			−	(*367*)	+	(*367*)		
DNA damage[e]	+*	strand breaks (*111*)			+*	strand breaks (*111*), fragmentation (*179*), DNA binding (*373*)	−*	strand breaks (*111, 112*)
inhibition of DNA synthesis							+	rodent cells (*126, 379*), in vivo exposure (*112*)
DNA repair assay[f]	+*	(*356*)			+*	(*85, 179*)		
Chromosome aberrations	+*	human leukocytes (*69, 357, 358, 359*), Chinese hamster cells (*359, 360*), mouse fibroblasts (*361*), *Zea mais* (*362*), LEP cells (*363*)	−* +	(*69*) pig cells (*70*)	+*	human cells (*372, 374*), Chinese hamster cells (*375–78*), mouse cells (*85, 379*), *Vicia faba* (*117*), Syrian hamster cells (*380*)	+	rat cells (*116*), *Vicia faba* (*117*), *Pisum* (*118*), *Allium cepa* (*119*)
Sister chromatid exchange[g]	+*	(*359, 364*)			+*	human leukocytes (*381*), Chinese hamster cells (*376, 378, 381*)	+*	human leukocytes (*120, 121*)

Mutation bacteria[h]	 +	*E. coli* (*33*) *Sal. typhimurium* (*344, 365*)	+/−	*Sal. typhimurium* (*25*)	+ 	review (*5*), *E. coli* (*23, 275, 372, 382, 383*) *Sal. typhimurium* (*33, 85, 275, 344, 382–85*)	+/− +	*Sal. typhimurium* (*25*) *Sal. typhimurium* (*115*)
yeast and plant cells			+	*S. cerevisiae* (*366*)	+	*S. pombe* (*386*)	+	*Vicia faba* (*117*)
mammalian cells	+	mouse lymphoma cells (*86*)	+	Chinese hamster cells (*29, 65*)	+	Chinese hamster cells (*375, 387*) mouse tumor cells (*86, 122*)	+ −	Chinese hamster (*29, 65, 124*), Syrian hamster (*127*), and mouse tumor cells (*122*)
Mammalian cell transformation[i]	+	Syrian hamster embryo cells (*66, 68*)	+	Syrian hamster embryo cells (*66, 67*)	+	Syrian hamster embryo cells (*66–68, 99, 380*), hamster kidney (*388*), mouse embryo (*85*)	+	Syrian hamster embryo cells (*66–68, 99, 127*), rat embryo cells (*125*), mouse embryo cells (*121*)
Enhanced virus transformation[j]	+	(*28*)	+	(*28*)	+	(*28*)	+	(*28*)

Key: +, positive test result; −, negative test result; +/−, weakly positive test result; *, includes data for human cells.
[a]Analysis following in vivo exposure that includes teratogenesis, host-mediated assay (*368*), dominant lethal test (*417*), cytogenetic tests, such as chromosome aberrations, and micronucleus test (*82*).
[b]Infidelity of DNA structure or replication in cell-free systems (*27*).
[c]Differential growth sensitivities of wild-type and DNA repair-deficient strains of *B. subtilis.*
[d]Differential growth sensitivities of wild-type and DNA repair-deficient strains of *E. coli.*
[e]Single-strand breaks of target cell DNA quantified by alkaline elution (*112*), or ethidium bromide fluorescence technique (*111*). Usually assayed in mammalian cells.
[f]Assayed in mammalian cells by ^{3}H-thymidine incorporation as "unscheduled DNA synthesis."
[g]Ref. 378.
[h]Includes Ames test for *Sal. typhimurium* mutagenesis.
[i]Measured by altered growth in vitro and tumor induction in appropriate hosts.
[j]Enhancement of virus-induced malignant transformation of Syrian hamster embryo cells (*28*).

evidence indicates that more stringent study is also needed on the pharmacokinetics and cofactor role of As (*62*).

Arsenic is invariably mixed with other toxic inorganic, organic, and physical substances in environmental and occupational settings, and its possible synergistic role could be critically important. Animal experiments have mostly investigated skin or dietary exposure of rats and mice to specific compounds of As. These studies are far from sufficient to evaluate human risk. Other species should be studied, and, more importantly, exposure conditions should more closely simulate the human occupational experience.

BERYLLIUM. *Short-Term Assays.* Results for Be toxicity in short-term assays are shown in Table II. Beryllium compounds have consistently decreased fidelity of DNA and RNA synthesis (*27, 63, 64*). They have been significantly positive in mammalian cell mutagenesis (*29, 65*) and transformation assays (*66–68*), as well as in the metal-sensitive enhancement of viral transformation (*28*) All of these mammalian cell assays have used hamster cell systems. Data for chromosome damage are limited and conflicting: Paton and Allison (*69*) reported Be as inactive in human white blood cells, whereas Talluri and Guiggiani (*70*) reported chromosome aberrations in cultured pig lymphocytes and kidney cells.

Animal Experiments. Evidence of the carcinogenicity of Be to experimental animals was first reported by Gardner and Heslington (*71*). Both zinc beryllium silicate and beryllium oxide given intravenously to rabbits induced osteosarcomas, but the comparable Zn compounds and silicic acid did not. Osteosarcoma induction has since been reported in mice and rabbits after intratracheal, intramedullary, and intravenous administration of various Be compounds, primarily BeO in relatively massive doses (reviewed in Refs. 5, 13, 72). Dutra et al. (*73*) also reported osteosarcomas along with osseous metastases after inhalation of BeO.

Primary lung tumor induction in rats by Be inhalation was first reported by Vorwald (*74*). Pulmonary carcinomas in rats and in monkeys from the inhalation of several Be compounds have since been recorded.

Low-fired BeO is a potent experimental carcinogen, probably due to its greater in vivo solubility, while high-fired BeO rarely induces tumors (*75, 76*).

Epidemiology. While reviewing the evidence for carcinogenicity of metals for humans, Sunderman (*77*) refers to conflicting reports on the association between increased cancer risk and occupational exposure to Be. Recent epidemiological studies (*78–80*) clearly show a consistent excess risk of lung cancer among workers occupationally exposed to Be. These significant increases proved to be independent of variables such as age, study group selection, and personal characteristics of workers, even those with unstable employment patterns. It was also shown to be improbable that the excess risk could be attributed to cigarette smoking.

BeO is probably the common human exposure form of Be. Other than under occupational conditions, dangerous exposure levels of BeO and other experimentally carcinogenic Be compounds are not generally encountered by the public. However, the increasing use of coal as an energy source may significantly enhance atmospheric exposure to this element, because Be is associated with the organic components of coal. On combustion, these components disseminate as small particles of oxides (*13*). A new gas lantern mantle is a little known source of excessive Be exposure; approximately 600 μg of volatilized Be metal is released from it within the first 15 min of lighting (*81*). Such sources of Be aerosols constitute a nonoccupational environmental hazard in view of the published U.S. and Canadian air quality safety guidelines: 1 $\mu g/m^3$ over an 8-h period and 0.01 $\mu g/m^3$ over a 24-h period, respectively (*13*).

Conclusions. Beryllium and certain Be compounds have in the past been classified as being only probably carcinogenic to humans (*3*) on the basis of suggestive human epidemiological evidence. However, more recent epidemiological reports on Be in industry and in neighborhood studies of large population groups in the United States (*78, 80*) are considered sufficiently conclusive to indict Be as an established lung carcinogen in humans.

The classification of Be as an established carcinogen is further supported by the positive short-term assay results (Table II) and by the numerous positive reports of lung tumor induction in several species of experimental animals. The U.S. National Toxicology Program has now included Be and certain Be compounds in its list of carcinogens (*4*).

CHROMIUM. *Short-Term Assays.* Of all the metals, Cr is the most active in short-term tests (Table II). It causes DNA and chromosome damage following in vivo exposure (teratogenicity review, *26*; micronucleus test, *82–84*) and is positive in all DNA and chromosome damage, mutation, and cell transformation assays in a wide variety of organisms. Hexavalent Cr is a much more potent genotoxic agent than is trivalent Cr. However, trivalent Cr has been reported as positive in a few tests, such as chromosome aberrations in mouse embryo cells (*85*), mutagenesis in L51784 mouse lymphoma cells (*86*), and malignant transformation in mouse embryo cells (*85*). The carcinogenicity and mutagenicity of this element have been reviewed by Leonard and Lauwerys (*87*).

Animal Experiments. The carcinogenicity of hexavalent Cr(VI) following parenteral injection by several routes into rats is firmly established for a number of compounds (*26, 88*). The most carcinogenically potent Cr(VI) compounds are the slightly soluble salts, particularly $CaCrO_4$, $PbCrO_4$, and $ZnCrO_4$. The more soluble Na_2CrO_4 and K_2CrO_4 have exhibited little or no tumorigenic activity (*89, 90*).

Respiratory cancers have been induced in rats by intrabroncheal implantation and by inhalation (*91, 92*).

Intramuscular injection of lead chromate induced tumors in 37 of 50 rats; 31 were sarcomas and 3 were renal carcinomas (*93*). The renal tumors are of interest because the association of lead with kidney carcinoma in the rat suggests the possibility of Pb and Cr interaction.

Evidence for the carcinogenicity of Cr compounds in other laboratory species is much less convincing than for the rat. Numerous experiments in mice using Cr(VI) compounds have given negative or questionably positive results (*26, 94*). In one instance a $CaCrO_4$-inhalation study produced negative results in mice (*94*); however a later study reported the induction of lung tumors (*92*). The carcinogenicity of Cr(VI) compounds has not been sufficiently investigated in hamsters, guinea pigs, or rabbits. The limited published information suggests that both the guinea pig and the hamster may prove useful models for inhalation tests (*95*).

Trivalent Cr compounds and chromite ores have shown little or no carcinogenic activity in experimental animals. The occasional tumors that have been attributed to Cr(III) treatment very probably reflect the traces of Cr(VI) that may contaminate even reagent grade Cr(III) compounds (*96*).

Epidemiology. Numerous epidemiological studies have investigated the occupational hazard of Cr (reviewed in Refs. 13, 26, 77, 97, 98). The lung has been the primary target organ in all studies in which the selective risk of cancer was significantly elevated. The slightly soluble members of hexavalent Cr(VI) compounds (e.g., $CaCrO_4$ and $ZnCrO_4$) appear to present the greatest risk (*90, 99*).

Epidemiologically inconclusive evidence of increases in gastrointestinal cancers among workers in various chromate-producing industries was included in a number of the reports on lung cancer risk (*100–102*)

In contrast to the numerous and detailed epidemiological studies on cancer in the chromate-producing industries, little information exists on the risk to workers involved in the use of chromates. Studies have shown increased mortality from respiratory and gastrointestinal cancer in chromeplaters, and the increase is attributed to excessive chromic acid exposure (*100*). A recent report (*103*) documents significant increases in tumors of the respiratory tract, but not of other sites, among aircraft spray painters who had been exposed to $ZnCrO_4$ at least 20 years prior to the study. The same study, however, found no excess of cancer among electroplaters exposed to chromic acid.

Reports on cancer among metal polishers and electroplaters, as well as inhabitants in the vicinity of such work, showed significant increases in cancer of the esophagus, liver, and larynx, but not of the lung (*104, 105*). A report on workers in the iron–chromium alloy industry, in which benzo[*a*]pyrene exposure was also noted, indicated a significantly increased incidence of esophageal and lung cancer (*106*). It is difficult to conclusively attribute such findings to the Cr exposure even though the risk is associated with the chromate industry. Such inexact and inadequately characterized exposure patterns are common in epidemiological studies on metal carcinogenesis; consequently it is much easier to implicate an industrial process as a cancer hazard than a specific element or compound (*90*).

Conclusion. Several hexavalant Cr salts are considered established carcinogens. Short-term test findings, along with the experimental animal evidence, clearly indicate that a number of low-solubility Cr compounds are carcinogenic. In humans, the epidemiological evidence convincingly supports a causal relationship to respiratory cancers among chromate-production workers. A similar risk appears to exist for those exposed through user occupations, such as electropainting and spray painting. The relative risk associated with the solubility and oxidation state of Cr compounds under conditions of human exposure has yet to be determined.

NICKEL. *Short-Term Assays.* Norseth (*90*) has reviewed teratogenic effects of nickel, especially the embryotoxicity of soluble Ni salts in experimental animals. Sunderman et al. (*107, 108*) have reported teratogenic effects in rat and hamster fetuses following exposure of dams to $Ni(CO)_4$ inhalation.

The genotoxicity of Ni compounds is shown in Table II and has been reviewed in depth by Sunderman (*109*). Ni is reported to be active in cell-free DNA damage assays (*27, 63, 110*), although it did not induce DNA single-strand breaks in human blood cells and animal tissues (*68, 111*). Ni compounds have persistently proven negative in the microbial Rec assay (*33, 113, 114*), but have proven positive in the standard Ames test (*25*), in a *Sal. typhimurium* fluctuation test (*115*), and in all assays with higher organisms. Ni compounds caused aberrant mitoses in rat embryo cultures (*116*) and aberrant chromosomes in *Vicia faba* (*117*), *Pisum* (*118*), and *Allium cepa* (*119*) cells. Induction of sister chromatid exchanges was shown in human lymphocytes (*120, 121*). Ni compounds were positive in mammalian cell mutation assays (*29, 65, 122–24*; Swierenga, unpublished) and in cell transformation assays (*28, 66–68, 121, 125–27*). Rivedal and Sanner (*127*) showed enhanced benzo[*a*]pyrene-induced cell transformation when Syrian hamster embryo cells were also treated with $NiSO_4$ and other metal salts. These authors suggest that the metals may be more potent as promoters than as initiators in the transformation process.

Hui and Sunderman (*112*) showed that prior injection of $Ni(CO)_4$ in partially hepatectomized rats resulted in approximately a 50% inhibition of [^3H]thymidine uptake in the liver and kidney. Similar treatment with $NiCl_2$ significantly inhibited DNA synthesis in the kidney but not in the liver. Hui and Sunderman's observations of ^{63}Ni binding to DNA confirmed an earlier study by Webb et al. (*128*).

Animal Experiments. A reported excess in the incidence of cancers of the nasal sinuses and lungs among workers in a Canadian Ni refinery (*129*) prompted extensive experimental studies on the tumorigenicity of dust and its metallic components from the sintering plant. Nickel subsulfide (Ni_3S_2) and NiO proved to be highly carcinogenic to both rats and mice and had a marked affinity for striated muscle, whereas the amorphous NiS failed to induce any tumors under similar conditions (*130–32*). These findings have since been confirmed by numerous studies (reviewed in Ref. 15). The degree of carcinogenic potency has been related to the cellular uptake of nickel sulfide compounds in vitro (*133, 134*); these studies also demonstrated that nonpotent amorphous NiS particles were not actively phagocytosed by CHO cells unless chemically reduced.

A dose–response relationship has been established for Ni_3S_2. Mn, Al, and Co are known to have an anticarcinogenic effect on the incidence of certain types of chemically induced tumors. Mn, but not Al, Cu, or Co, inhibited the tumorigenic action of Ni_3S_2 (*77*). Ni_3S_2 in white skeletal muscle of rabbits has induced either rhabdomyosarcomas or leiomyosarcomas from the myoblastic mesenchymal cells adjacent to the implanted metal (*135*).

Early investigations on the carcinogenicity of inhaled metallic Ni (*136*) and gaseous $Ni(CO)_4$ (*137*) reported the induction of epidermoid tumors and adenocarcinomas in the lungs of rats (*138*). Ni_3S_2 inhalation (6 h/d, 5 d/week for 78 weeks) caused a 14% incidence of bronchial and bronchoalveolar neoplasms in 226 exposed rats compared with 1% of the 241 controls (*139*). Under similar exposure to a refinery dust containing NiO, NiS, and metallic Ni, two of five surviving rats developed pulmonary squamous cell carcinomas, while the 47 controls were tumor-free (*140*).

Implants of Ni_3S_2 into one frontal sinus of eight cats induced invasive upper respiratory tract epidermoid and adenocarcinomas in two animals, while the comparable implants of FeO in the opposite sinus had no effect (*141*). Heterotropic tracheal transplants treated with Ni_3S_2 resulted in 7 carcinomas and 47 sarcomas in 124 transplanted tracheas, whereas no tumors developed in the 10 controls (*142*).

Ni in combination with either benzo[*a*]pyrene or 20-methylcholanthrene injected intratracheally in the rat resulted in a marked enhancement of lung tumor incidence over results obtained with each agent alone (*143, 144*). The possibility of a similar synergistic interaction with Ni and V has been hypothesized and is under investigation (F. S. LaBella, personal communication).

Ni_3S_2 has also induced malignant sarcomas in 16 of 19 intratesticularly injected rats. Although four of these tumors were rhabdomyosarcomas, none of them involved the specific genital cells (*145*). Of particular interest are the reports of Ni_3S_2-induced intrarenal tumorigenesis, which leads to polycythemia and an enhanced production and/or release of erythropoietin (*146*).

Epidemiology. Various cancer causes of death in different occupational subgroups were studied in 54,000 Canadian male employees from the International Nickel Company plants at Port Colborne and in the Sudbury area of Ontario (*147, 148*). Cancer mortality was significantly elevated among the sintering subgroup of workers at both locations ($P < 0.001$). Ni cancer target sites that have been identified are the nasal sinuses, lung, larynx, and kidney (*149*). An analysis of data for each of these sites showed a 14-fold and an 80-fold increase of nasal tumors among workers employed in sintering occupations at Sudbury and Port Colborne, respectively, compared with other refinery workers. There was a fourfold and a threefold increase in lung cancer incidence among workers at Sudbury and Port Colborne, respectively. Statistical evidence did not demonstrate an increased risk of laryngeal or kidney cancer death at either location, although three deaths from kidney cancer were recorded at Port Colborne versus an expected incidence of 1.59 (*148*).

An increased nasal cancer risk has also been demonstrated among U.S. refinery employees. In a U.S. combined refinery and Ni alloy manufacturing plant, employees showed a dose–response relationship between Ni exposure and slightly increased incidences of lung, stomach, and prostate cancers (*150*). The observation on stomach cancers is of interest in view of the occurrence of gastric cancer and sarcomas among Ni refinery workers in Russia (*151*).

A Norwegian Ni refinery study showed significantly increased nasal, lung, and larynx cancer deaths in a cohort of 2241 workers; the highest incidence occurred in the roasting, smelting, and electrolysis departments (*152, 153*). A threefold increase in nasal tumor deaths was also noted in the urban population adjacent to the refinery compared with Norway as a whole. Similarly, the respiratory cancer incidence in the New Caledonia population as a whole was higher than that of other South Pacific Islands and was highest in the urban area near the island's Ni refinery; Ni workers exhibited a threefold increase in lung cancer, after adjustment for age and smoking, over that of other workers (*154*).

Clinical investigations on workers with 8 or more years exposure in a Norwegian refinery showed that 43% had pathological changes in nasal biopsy materials versus 26% in the control group; 13 of the 318 nickel workers biopsied had nasal polyps, two of which were considered carcinomatous. Length of employment and tobacco consumption both showed statistically significant correlations with the rhinoscopical findings; hand-rolled cigarettes specifically were shown to be highly contaminated with Ni (*155*).

A sputum-screening study on 268 asymptomatic sintering plant workers employed in a Canadian Ni refinery revealed 11 lung and 1 larynx cancer cases; all of the cases except one were smokers (*156*).

Although Ni_3S_2 is almost certainly the most common active agent in Ni carcinogenesis, undoubtedly other Ni salts, such as $NiCl_2$ and $NiSO_4$, should be implicated in cancers from exposure to the electrolytic processes; $Ni(CO)_4$ is probably much less important in the induction of occupational cancer than originally thought (*90*).

Conclusion. The short-term, animal, and epidemiological evidence all clearly identify certain Ni compounds as established carcinogens. The relatively insoluble compounds such as Ni_3S_2 appear to be the most active. These views conform to those expressed by the expert panels for the evaluation of carcinogenic risk established by the U.S. National Toxicology Program (*4*) and the International Agency for Research on Cancer (*157*).

Suspected Carcinogens. Table III summarizes the epidemiological and experimental animal evidence for classifying Cd and some Fe compounds as suspected human carcinogens. Short-term assay results for these compounds are shown in Table IV.

CADMIUM. *Short-Term Assays.* Cd was teratogenic in rats, hamsters, and mice (reviewed in Ref. 158). Cd compounds also caused dominant lethals in vivo in *Drosophila* (*159*), transformation of Syrian hamster embryo cells in vitro after transplacental exposure, and chromosome aberrations in human lymphocytes (*160*). Micronucleus tests were negative (reviewed in Ref. 82).

Cd toxicity reported in short-term in vitro assays is shown in Table IV. Positive results were reported in all types of assays, including DNA damage tests, mutation assays in prokaryotic and eukaryotic organisms, and mammalian cell transformation assays. Cd induced chromosome aberrations in several species including humans; however, one study (*69*) reported negative results. Cd-induced sister chromatid exchanges in Chinese hamster ovary cells were dependent on the type of serum used in the cell cultures (*161*). These short-term assay data indicate that Cd compounds are genotoxic.

Animal Experiments. Fibrosarcomas may be induced at the site of injection of soluble inorganic Cd salts in the rat, but not in the mouse (*162, 163*). Rhabdomyosarcomas and fibrosarcomas with numerous metastases developed after single injections of powdered Cd (*164, 165*).

Testicular atrophy, interstitial cell hyperplasia, and neoplasia occurred in both rats and mice after single subcutaneous injections of soluble Cd salts (*157, 166–68*).

Zn injected subcutaneously afforded partial protection for rats against Cd induction of local fibrosarcoma and interstitial cell tumors (*167*) and afforded complete protection for mice against testicular tumors (*169*). Mesotheliomas were induced in the pleural cavity of rats from combined intrathoracic implantation of Cd and Zn but not from either metal alone (*170*).

Table III
Suspected Carcinogens

	Human Risk			*Experimental Tumorigenesis*		
Element	*Route*[a]	*Class*[b]	*Target*	*Species*	*Route*[a]	*Results*
Cd	inhal	occ	prostate	rat	sc, im	sarc. at site
			kidney	mouse, rat	sc	IC tumors[c]
			lung	rat	prostate	prostate tumors
Iron–carbohydrate complexes	im	iat	buttocks	rat, mouse, hamster, rabbit	im	sarc. at site
Fe_2O_3 dust (hematite mining)	inhal	occ	lung	mouse	inhal	lung[d]
				rat, mouse	sc, im	negative
			gastric	mouse hamster	it	cocarcinogen[e]

[a] im, intramuscular; inhal, inhalation; it, intratracheal; and sc, subcutaneous.
[b] occ, occupational; and iat, iatrogenic.
[c] IC tumors are intestinal cell tumors in testes.
[d] Unconfirmed report (*191*); all other attempts negative.
[e] Physical and chemical cofactor in organic chemical carcinogenesis.

Table IV

Genotoxicity of Suspected Metal Carcinogens: Short-Term Assays

Assay[a]		*Cd*		*Fe*
In vivo tests	+*	teratogenic in rodents (review, *158*), transplacental cell transformation in Syrian hamsters (*66*), chromosome effects in humans (*160*), dominant lethal in *Drosophila* (*159, 390*)		
	−	mouse micronucleus test (review, *82*)		
Cytotoxicity	+	plant cells (*34*), chick hepatocytes (*391*)		
DNA effects				
biochemical assays	+	(*27, 63, 211, 274*)	−	(*27, 63*)
Rec assay	+	(*33, 113, 114*)	−	(*33, 113, 114*)
DNA damage	+	strand breaks (*392*)		
	−*	strand breaks (*111*)		
Chromosome aberrations	+*	human leukocytes (*277, 393*), Chinese hamster cells (*161, 360*), *Vicia faba* (*117*)	+	ferritin, Chinese hamster cells (*179*), *Pisum* (*118*), *Allium cepa* (*119*), *Vicia faba* (*117*)
	−*	(*69*)	−*	iron dextran (*69*)
Sister chromatid exchange	−	Chinese hamster cells (*161*)		
Mutation				
bacteria	+	*E. coli* (*394*), *Sal. typhimurium* (*276, 395*)	+	*Sal. typhimurium* (*180*)
	−	*E. coli* (*275*)		
plant cells	+	rice, *Cv. sona* (*181*)	+	rice, *Cv. sona* (*181*), *Vicia faba* (*117*)
mammalian cells	+	Chinese hamster cells (*124*), mouse lymphoma (*86*)	+	Chinese hamster cells (*29, 124*)
	−	mouse mammary carcinoma (*122*)		

Continued on next page

Table IV Continued

Assay[a]		*Cd*		*Fe*
Mammalian cell transformation	+	Syrian hamster embryo cells (*66, 68*)	−	Syrian hamster embryo cells (*66*)

Key: +, positive test result; −, negative test result; *, includes data for human cells.
[a]Explanation of assays given in Table II footnotes.

When $CdSO_4$ was administered orally to mice and rats at three dose levels, the tumor yield was equivalent to that in the controls; no neoplastic changes were observed in the prostate glands (*171, 172*). Direct injection of a $CdCl_2$ solution into the rat prostate induced tumors (*173*), but subcutaneous injections proved inconclusive; histological changes, including castrate regression, were noted in both groups. Methylcholanthrene injected into the prostate induced a similar spectrum of tumors and histological changes except for castrate regression (*173*).

Epidemiology. Several reviews examine the possible association between occupational exposure to Cd and an increased risk of cancer of the prostate, kidney, and lung (*7, 77, 174*).

Of 70 men who were exposed to CdO for more than 10 years in the production of alkaline batteries, three of five cancer deaths were from prostate cancer (*175*). Of 248 men in the same industry with at least 1 year of exposure, the prostate cancer incidence was 4 versus the 0.58 expected (*176*); 3 of these cases were ones referred to previously by Potts (*157*). At least three other studies failed to show an excess of any types of cancer among Cd-exposed workers, but all of these studies examined small samples with insufficient exposure time (*7, 157*).

CdO exposure among 292 smelter workers was associated with 4 prostate cancers versus the 1.5 expected. When adjusted for a 20-year interval from onset of exposure, the difference of 4 versus 0.88 expected would be significant (*157*). This study also showed a significantly increased risk of lung carcinoma apparently in the absence of any appreciable exposure to other potentially carcinogenic metals (*177*).

A report on 64 cases of renal cancer showed a significant association with occupational exposure to Cd. A synergistic role for cigarette smoking was suggested because the relative risk to smokers exposed to Cd was over four times that of nonsmokers who were not occupationally exposed (*178*).

Conclusions. Cadmium is teratogenic in rodents and genotoxic in short-term assays, and these findings suggest that it is carcinogenic to mammals.

Although the well-established local carcinogenicity of Cd, as well as its indirect effect on the testes of rats and mice, may seem more or less irrelevant to the assessment of cancer risk in humans, the same cannot be said for the reported induction of prostate tumors in rats. Several epidemiological studies have suggested the association of Cd with an increased risk of prostate, lung, and kidney cancers, but in all cases the data are insufficient to be conclusive.

Despite the contrary view expressed in one review (*98*), more animal experimentation and epidemiological studies should be conducted, especially ones to evaluate further the prostatic cancer hazard. In the meantime, as concluded by the IARC committee, Cd and certain Cd compounds should be considered potentially carcinogenic and therefore classified as suspected carcinogens.

IRON AND ORGANIC AND INORGANIC IRON COMPOUNDS. *Short-Term Assays.* Short-term assay results for Fe are shown in Table IV. Most investigators tested inorganic Fe salts. Whiting et al. (*179*) assayed the Fe complex ferritin in CHO cells and reported chromosome aberrations.

Little evidence for the genotoxicity of inorganic Fe compounds was found. Negative data were reported for cell-free (*27, 63*) and microbial (*33, 113, 114*) assays, except for a positive response for Fe(II) in the Ames test (*180*). However, Fe compounds were mutagenic in several plant and animal assays (*29, 117, 124, 181*); chromosome damage was reported in plant cells (*117–19*) and Chinese hamster cells (*182*), but not in human lymphocytes (*69*). Fe compounds were negative in a Syrian hamster embryo cell transformation assay (*66*), and only weakly positive in the enhanced virus transformation assay (*28*).

Animal Experiments—Iron–Carbohydrate Complexes. Large amounts of iron dextran have produced sarcomas at the injection site in rats, mice, hamsters, and rabbits (*183*, reviewed in Refs. 5 and 184). Iron dextran has not induced tumors in dogs or guinea pigs (*185*). Dextran alone is generally considered noncarcinogenic (*186*), although some carcinogenic effects have been reported in rodents (*187*). An iron sorbitol–citric acid complex was also not carcinogenic (*188*). Some rather equivocal evidence exists that dextran and other iron carbohydrate complexes may enhance the incidence of neoplasms at sites remote from the injection point (*189, 190*).

Animal Experiments—Iron Dusts. The long-suspected causal association between lung cancer and the mining of hematite ores (Fe_2O_3) has stimulated numerous attempts to demonstrate the carcinogenicity of iron dust in experimental animals. An isolated early report (*191*) that daily exposure of mice to Fe_2O_3 increased the incidence of lung tumors has never been confirmed. Indeed, there is ample evidence that these dusts alone do not act as primary carcinogens when administered parenterally (*131, 192, 193*) or when introduced into the respiratory tract (*194–98*).

Fe_2O_3 particles have played a synergistic or cocarcinogenic role with carcinogens such as benzo[*a*]pyrene (BP) and diethylnitrosamine (DEN) in respiratory tumorigenesis, most notably in the hamster model (*194, 196, 198*). As a cofactor, Fe_2O_3 may act in a largely nonspecific manner through irritation and impaired clearance or as a mechanical carrier of the primary carcinogenic hydrocarbons (*196, 199, 200*). However, two observations suggest that Fe_2O_3 must also act on the respiratory epithelium as a specific chemical cocarcinogen (*201*): (1) Fe_2O_3 induced severe basal cell hyperplasia of the tracheobronchial epithelium (*202*) and (2) subcutaneous DEN followed by intratracheal Fe_2O_3 resulted in many more tumors than did DEN alone (*195*). Fe_2O_3, when administered after DEN injection, was a more effective cocarcinogen than inhaled smog (*203*).

Epidemiology—Iron–Carbohydrate Complexes. Intramuscular injections of Fe as a possible cause of sarcomata in humans has been reviewed (*5, 19, 185*); the general consensus is that insufficient evidence exists to confirm a causal relationship. Of 196 cases of sarcoma of the buttocks, 90 had reviewable drug histories; of these 90, 4 had received intramuscular injections of Fe, and the intervals between injection and appearance of tumors were relatively short (*19*).

Solid-state (foreign body) carcinogenesis, following the formation of an insoluble Fe compound at the injection site, has been reviewed as a possible mechanism in experimental sarcoma induction by iron polysaccharide complexes (*184*).

Epidemiology—Iron Oxide Dust. Underground hematite mining, as an occupation, is classified as a Group I carcinogenic risk to humans by the IARC (*3*). This view is based on the usually moderate but consistent increases in lung cancer incidence among hematite miners in Sweden, England, France, the United States, and other countries. The role of Fe_2O_3 dust in this process remains unclear because of the concomitant exposure of the populations at risk to other potential carcinogens, such as radon daughters and diesel exhaust (*7, 77, 204*). A report on 270 cases of bronchial cancer among French iron miners showed that the incidence was 2.3 times as great as that previously recorded among metallurgists with comparable smoking habits (*205*).

Exposure to Fe dust among foundry workers and smelters was also associated with elevated lung cancer mortality (*97, 206, 207*). A proportional mortality study on 3013 white male foundry workers in the United States showed 208 lung cancer deaths as opposed to the 142 expected (*208*). Another study on foundry workers, who were employed for more than 5 years prior to 1938, showed a twofold increase in the incidence of both lung and digestive tract cancer (*209*). The observation of an increased gastric cancer incidence supports earlier reports that Fe dust may be linked to gastric cancer (*184, 210*). These studies also serve to emphasize the prolonged latency that must be expected in most metal carcinogenesis.

Conclusion. Iron dextran was listed as a carcinogen in a recent report by the U.S. Toxicology Program (*4*). Nevertheless, iron dextran should probably be considered a suspected carcinogen until more data on the association between Fe injections and sarcoma of the buttocks in humans are accumulated and analyzed.

There is no evidence that Fe_2O_3 alone is carcinogenic. However, its established role as a mechanical carcinogenic cofactor and its probable role as a chemical cocarcinogen in experimental animals strongly suggest that Fe_2O_3 might exert synergistic action in the occurrence of occupational lung cancer among hematite miners and foundry workers (*202*).

Possible Carcinogens. Table V summarizes the epidemiological and animal experimental evidence used to classify Co, Cu, Pb, Li, Sn, and Zn as possible human carcinogens. Short-term assay results for these compounds are shown in Table VI.

COBALT. *Short-Term Assays.* Co toxicity studies in vitro are summarized in Table VI. DNA damage, including decreased fidelity of DNA and RNA synthesis in cell-free

Table V

Possible Carcinogens

	Experimental Animal Tumorigenesis			Human Risk
Element	*Species*	*Route*[a]	*Results*	*Class*[b]
Co	rabbit	ios	osteosarcomas	iat
	rat	sc, im	rhabdomyosarcomas	occ
Cu	mice	itest	testicular tumors	env (IUD)
(Cu–As mix, Bordeaux mix)	rats	it	resp. carcinomas	occ
Pb	rats	sc, oral	renal tumors and	occ
		im, oral	sarcomas	env
Li				iat
Zn	fowl	itest	teratomas	occ
	rats			
	mice			

[a]im, intramuscular, ios, intraosseous; it, intratracheal; itest, intratesticular; sc, subcutaneous.
[b]iat, iatrogenic; occ, occupational; env, general environmental (IUD, intrauterine device).

systems (*27, 63, 211*) and single-strand breaks (*111*) in human lymphocytes, has been reported.

Other assays with both lower and higher organisms have given conflicting results: in the Rec assay, Co compounds were positive in two studies (*113, 114*) and negative in a third study (*33*). Co was mutagenic in *Vicia faba* (*117*), Chinese hamster V79 (*65*), and CHO (*29*) cells, but not in mouse lymphoma cells (*123*). Chromosome alterations were found in plant cells (*117, 119*) but not in human lymphocytes (*69*). However, Co compounds were positive in two mammalian cell transformation assays (*28, 99*).

Animal Experiments. The development of sarcomata after intraosseous injection of metallic Co in rabbits was reported over 40 years ago (*212*). Since then local sarcomas from the injection of Co powder and several Co salts by various routes have been reported in rabbits (*213*) and rats (*131, 214*). Mice, however, failed to develop malignant tumors even when double the dose that induced a 50% incidence in rats was administered (*130*).

Co has a particular affinity for striated muscle in tumorigenesis (*128, 132*). This observation is interesting in view of (1) the Co-related fatal myopathies in humans after excessive consumption of Co-fortified beer (*215*); and (2) the cardiotoxic effects of orally administered Co salts in rabbits and rats (*216*).

Intratracheal injections of Co dust resulted in severe bronchial hyperplasia in hamsters (*217*). Inhalation of aerosols of cobaltous oxide resulted in pneumoconiosis but failed to induce tumors or to enhance the carcinogenic effects of cigarette smoke in hamsters (*218*).

Cobaltous chloride and sodium cobaltinitrite, when administered intraperitoneally, showed a significant antitumorigenic effect on the incidence of skin carcinoma from painting with methylcholanthrene (*77, 219*).

Epidemiology. There is no epidemiological evidence that occupational exposure to Co enhances the risk of neoplasia in humans (*5*), but very few studies have been conducted. Somewhat conflicting opinions exist on the toxicity of Co in relation to occupational interstitial lung disease and pneumoconiosis among tungsten carbide workers (*220, 221*). Industrial carbides may contain 5–12% Co, as well as other potentially pathogenic metals such as V and Ti.

Metal alloys are widely used in medical prostheses. Over time and/or under certain conditions, Co and other alloying metals may be leached from stainless steels and enter surrounding tissues (*222*). Scattered case reports from human and veterinary medicine suggest that, on occasion, these ions may be carcinogenic (*223–25*). Wear particles from Co–Cr alloy prostheses induce tumors on injection into rats (*226, 227*).

The potential toxicity, including carcinogenicity, associated with the medical use of Co is controversial (*228*). Co stimulates erythropoietin production and has been used successfully on cases of aplastic anemia in renal failure when other measures have failed (*229*). However, in view of its many side effects, including potential carcinogenicity, the general consensus is that cobalt should be used with great circumspection (*19, 228*).

Conclusions. More extensive epidemiological studies are needed to clarify the role, if any, of Co as an industrial or an iatrogenic cancer hazard.

The tumorigenicity of Co is firmly established in two species of experimental animals; its anticarcinogenic action is established in a third species. The considerable accumulation of short-term assay evidence implicates Co as a potential hazard. On the basis of these data, Co is considered to constitute a possible carcinogenic risk to humans.

COPPER. *Short-Term Assays.* Cu has not been tested extensively in short-term assays; available data are shown in Table VI. Cu compounds were active in all assays undertaken on higher organisms, including mutation, cell transformation, and enhanced virus transformation (*28, 99, 124*). Cu compounds caused chromosome aberrations in various plant species (*117–19*). They were positive in cell-free DNA and RNA damage assays (*27, 63, 211*), but not in the microbial Rec assay (*33, 113, 114*).

Animal Experiments. A number of reports have examined the protective role of Cu against organic chemical carcinogenesis induction and in Cu–Zn serum homeostasis during cancer development (*77, 202*). However only a few, often incidental, references have appeared on the carcinogenicity of Cu alone.

Parenterally implanted pellets of $CuSO_4$ failed to induce tumors in rats (*131*). No tumors were found in 50 Fischer-344 rats 470 d after intramuscular injection of pure Cu powder (*230*). Intertesticular Cu implants resulted in sarcomas, seminomas, and chorioepitheliomas in mice (*231*). Bordeaux mixture (1-–2% of $CuSO_4$) and copper oxychloride have successfully reproduced the Cu-containing granulomatous interstitial pulmonary lesions of the so-called "vineyard sprayers lung" (*232*).

One study recorded the induction of lung carcinomas in 9 of 15 rats from an intratracheal injection of a synthetic Bordeaux mixture (*47*). The authors attributed this response to the presence of 0.07 mg of As $[Cu_3(A_sO_4)_2 \cdot 3H_2O]$ in their mix but also commented on the unknown influence of $(CuSO_4 \cdot 5H_2O)$–(CuO) interactions on the carcinogenic response. The numerous negative attempts to demonstrate the carcinogenicity of As compounds in animals along with the histopathological response of guinea pig pulmonary tissues to a Ca–Cu (Bordeaux) mixture strongly suggests a synergistic if not a primary role for Cu.

Hepatoma incidence in rats from dietary ethionine may be suppressed by the simultaneous oral administration of Cu (*233*). The possible mechanisms involved have been reviewed (*77*).

Epidemiology. Industrial and environmental exposure to Cu is always associated with concomitant insult from other toxic elements, particularly As, Pb, and SO_2. Several epidemiological studies of Cu smelter workers have shown significant excesses of lung cancer deaths (*53, 234, 235*) that have been tentatively attributed to As; Cu was not considered to be causally implicated.

Epidemiological reports from Germany and France on enhanced cancer incidences in agricultural workers exposed to $CuSO_4$-, CaO-, and $Ca_3(AsO_4)_2$-containing sprays also have usually attributed the excesses of lung, liver, and skin cancer to the As moiety (*236, 237*). Reports from Portugal however have consistently linked the liver and lung lesions of vineyard sprayers with inhaled and ingested Cu, which the Portuguese investigators consider a potential cancer-stimulating substance (*232, 238*).

Metallic Cu induces free radicals and possibly malonaldehyde; for this reason it may be considered a potential carcinogenic hazard. Its wide use since 1969 in intrauterine devices (IUDs) has raised concern about a possible endometrial and cervical cancer risk (*19*). In view of the frequently long latent periods for metal-induced cancers, cytological monitoring of women with Cu IUDs for cervical cancer lesions should continue (*239*).

Conclusion. Because of its activity in short-term assays and the difficulties in interpreting much of the limited experimental and epidemiological information, Cu is classified as a possible carcinogen. The data reviewed suggest that Cu might act as a cofactor with As in the induction of certain occupational cancers. Concern over the carcinogenicity of Cu is further supported by (1) similarities between its chemistry and the chemistry of known carcinogenic metals and (2) its tendency to form tightly bound complexes and chelates (*184*), For these reasons, the possible carcinogenic role of Cu deserves much more attention than it has been given to date.

LEAD. *Short-Term Assays.* Pb was active in several short-term in vivo assays. Simmon et al. (*368*) reported a fourfold increase in mutation frequency of *Sal. typhimurium* after in vivo exposure to lead acetate in mice; according to the authors, this intraperitoneal host-mediated assay is generally insensitive for screening purposes. Pb was active in several *Drosophila* assays (*82, 240*). Chromosome damage in humans exposed to Pb compounds has been reviewed (*26, 241*). The IARC (*26*) reported on 11 positive studies, as well as on teratogenic effects (*241*). Negative results were reported in a dominant lethal (*242*) and a micronucleus (*82*) test.

Toxicity of Pb in short-term in vitro assays is shown in Table VI. Pb compounds were notably inactive in assays using lower organisms: *B. subtilis, E. coli, Sal. typhimurium*, yeast, and green algae. However, they were active in cell-free biochemical tests and in plant and mammalian cell assays, including chromosome

Table VI

Genotoxicity of Possible Metal Carcinogens: Short-Term Assays

Assay[a]	*Co*	*Cu*	*Pb*	*Li*	*Sn*	*Zn*
In vivo tests	+ teratogenic chick embryo (*370, 396*)		+* chromosome effects in humans (*26, 241*), teratogenic (*26, 370*), genetic effects in mice, (*398*) and *Drosophila* (*240*) − genetic effects in mice (*82, 242*)		+ chromosome effects in rats (*432*) and *Drosophila* (*240, 268*), enzyme inhibition, rat liver (*405*) − host-mediated and dominant lethal test in rats (*406*)	+ chromosome effects in rats (*277*)
Cytotoxicity		+ plant cells (*34*)	+ plant cells (*34*)		+/− plant cells (*34*)	
DNA effects						
biochemical assays	+ (*27, 63, 211*)	+ (*27, 63, 211*)	+ (*27, 63, 211*)			+/− (*27*) − (*63, 211, 274*)
Rec assay	+ (*114*) +/− (*113*) − (*33*)	− (*33, 113, 114*)	− (*33, 113, 114*)	− (*113, 114*)	− (*33, 113, 114*)	− (*33*)
Pol A assay			− (*367*)			
DNA damage	+* strand breaks (*111*)				+* strand breaks (*111*)	−* strand breaks (*111*)
inhibition of DNA synthesis					+ (*269*, McLean and Swierenga, unpublished)	
Chromosome aberrations	+ *Vicia faba* (*117*) *Allium cepa* (*119*)	+ *Vicia faba* (*117*), *Allium cepa* (*119*), *Pisum* (*118*)	+* *Allium cepa* (*399*) Chinese hamster (*400*), human leukocytes (*401, 402*)	+ *Allium cepa* (*119*)	+/− *Pisum* (*118*)	+* human leukocytes (*277, 278*)

	−* human leukocytes (*69*)			+/− *Pisum* (*118*)	−* human cells (*406*)	+/− *Pisum* (*118*)
Sister chromatid exchange			+* human leukocytes (*120*) −* human leukocytes (*403*)			
Mutation bacteria			− *Sal. typhimurium* (*367, 382*)			+ *Sal. typhimurium* (*276*) +/− *Sal. typhimurium* (*25*) − *E. coli* (*275*)
yeast and plants	+ *Vicia faba* (*117*)	+ rice (*181*)	+ rice (*181*)			+ *Vicia faba* (*117*)
			− *S. cerevisiae* (*366*), algae (*404*)			
mammalian cells	+ Chinese hamster cells (*29, 65*)	+ Chinese hamster cells (*124*)	+ Chinese hamster cells (*124*), mouse lymphoma (*86*)		+ rat liver cells (Swierenga and McLean, unpublished)	+ Chinese hamster cells (*124*)
	− mouse lymphoma (*123*)		− mouse lymphoma (*123*)			− mouse lymphoma (*123*)
Mammalian cell transformation	+* Syrian hamster embryo (*99*), human fibroblasts (*60, 397*)	+ Syrian hamster embryo (*99*)	+ Syrian hamster embryo (*30, 67, 68*)	+ enhanced NiS carcinogenesis in Syrian hamster embryo cells (*134*)		− Syrian hamster embryo (*66*)
Enhanced virus transformation	+ (*76*)	+ (*28*)	+ (*28*)	− (*28*)		+ (*28*)

Key: +, positive test result; −, negative test result; +/−, weakly positive test result; and *, includes data for human cells.
[a]Explanation of assays given in Table II footnotes.

aberration tests in onion cells, hamster cells, and human lymphocytes, as well as in mutagenesis and transformation assays in various mammalian cell systems.

Animal Experiments. The carcinogenicity of Pb was first shown experimentally almost 30 years ago when renal tumors, including carcinoma of the cortex, were induced in 19 of 29 rats that received repeated weekly 20-mg subcutaneous injections of lead phosphate (*243*).

Several reviews (*5, 26, 244*) have detailed the numerous reports of renal tumor induction in rats and mice from chronic oral and parenteral exposure to high levels of various Pb compounds. The dose dependence noted in renal tumor induction (*245*) might account for the negative effects reported from very low doses (*246*). Kidney tumors did not develop in either dogs or hamsters from chronic dietary exposure to Pb (*247, 248*).

Less well-documented reports have linked Pb compounds to the induction of tumors in rats at the site of injection and in a variety of organs, including testis, lung, adrenals, pituitary, cerebrum, and thyroid (*249, 250*). Oral and intramuscular injections of Pb powder in rats (*93*) and subcutaneous injections of tetraethyllead in mice (*251*) both gave inconclusive indications of lymphoma induction. An incompletely reported study suggests that diets low in both Pb and Mg may significantly increase the incidence of malignant lymphomas in rats, whereas an excess of lead (high Pb and low Mg) prevents this leukemogenic response (*252*).

Lung tumors were induced by combined intratracheal injections of benzo[*a*] pyrene (BP) and lead oxides but not with either substance alone (*253*). Hepatoma development was accelerated when lead acetate and 3-methyl-4-dimethylamino-azobenzene were combined (*254*). A study on possible synergism between lead arsenate and diethylnitrosamine (*43*) gave equivocal results. The possibility of a synergistic or cocarcinogenic interaction between Pb and potential respiratory carcinogens deserves further study.

Epidemiology. Relatively few adequate surveys on exposed occupational populations have been reported. Almost all the studies undertaken failed to demonstrate an increased risk (*255, 256*). A marginal increase in incidence shown in one study (*257*) is not statistically significant (*26*).

A clearly significant threefold increase in the expected incidence of lung tumors reported among Cu smelters and concentrators is difficult to assess properly; the group was exposed to As, Cu, SO_2, and probably other potentially carcinogenic substances, as well as to Pb (*234*).

The well-established association of Pb with renal tumor induction in rats has focused attention on a possible similar relationship in humans. A comparison of 149 cases of Wilms' tumor (a renal tumor of children) with 149 matched nontumor controls showed that Pb-related occupations were significantly more prevalent among the fathers of Wilms' tumor cases (*258*). Although this study was considered inadequate by the IARC, several similar reports on the relationship between hydrocarbon-related occupations of fathers and childhood cancers have been quoted (*26*). More epidemiological evidence should be gathered on this issue.

Fishbein (*13*) reviewed the exposure levels to Pb in various environmental situations and concluded that they did not constitute a carcinogenic hazard for the general public. No relationship has been shown between Pb in drinking water and cancer of the stomach or any other site (*259*) or between Pb and cancer from trace elements in the human diet (*260*).

Conclusions. In view of so little firm epidemiological evidence for its carcinogenicity, lead is considered only as a possible carcinogenic hazard to humans. More detailed information is needed, particularly on the possible synergisms between Pb and other potentially carcinogenic chemicals.

Pb compounds are teratogenic and short-term assays show them to be genotoxic in a variety of in vivo and in vitro test systems. Besides demonstrating that chronic large exposures to Pb induce tumors in the kidney and probably at other sites, animal experiments also point to the possibility of a cocarcinogenic role for this metal.

Lithium. Li has proven useful in the treatment of manic depression and depressive illness and is now widely used for these purposes (*261*). It is also reported to relieve the neutropenia that results from certain cancer chemotherapies and other treatments (*262, 263*).

No firm evidence exists of Li carcinogenesis, although a few mutagenesis and clinical reports suggest a risk.

Li compounds caused chromosome damage in *Pisum* rootlets and in *Alium cepa* (*119*). Heck and Costa (*134*) reported that the carcinogenic potency of the relatively inactive amorphous NiS particles could be increased for Syrian hamster embryo cells in vitro by Li reduction. Clinical reports suggest that a Li induced side effect, leukocytosis, may be implicated in both the induction and reinduction of acute and chronic monocytic leukemia (*264–66*). Case–control studies should be conducted on the hazard of Li therapy (*267*) to determine whether the frequency of clinical reports of hematological malignancies is indeed greater than that attributable to chance (*264*). The leukemogenic effects, if any, of Li in experimental animal models should also be studied.

TIN. *Short-Term Assays.* Toxicity of Sn compounds is shown in Table VI. Ramel and Magnussen (*240*) showed nondisjunction of chromosomes in *Drosophila;* similarly Mitchell and Gerdes (*268*) showed mutagenesis in *Drosophila* with stannous fluoride; in this case fluoride ion toxicity can not be ruled out.

Significant single-strand breakage in human lymphocyte DNA by SN(II) but not Sn(IV) compounds was demonstrated (*111*). Sn compounds also suppressed DNA synthesis in mammalian cell systems (*269;* McLean and Swierenga, unpublished). However, Sn compounds were negative in the Rec assay (*33, 113, 114*) and only weakly positive in several plant toxicity assays (*34, 118*). Data for other assays are lacking.

Animal Experiments. Inorganic Sn did not affect tumor incidence in rodents when given in the drinking water over long periods (*246, 270, 271*). Similarly the intrathoracic injection of tin needles—of a comparable form and size to the asbestos needles that produce mesotheliomas and lung tumors—did not adversely affect mice (*272*). In a recent carcinogenesis bioassay by the U.S. National Institutes of Health (*273*), stannous chloride was judged not to be carcinogenic for the test animals, except for a possible increased incidence of C-cell tumors in the thyroid of male rats.

Epidemiology. No studies have indicated that tin in the workplace is an occupational cancer hazard, nor have any studies suggested that tin from the lining of cans constitutes a cancer risk (*8*). However, very few studies have been undertaken.

Conclusion. Although Sn has been judged to be noncarcinogenic on the basis of animal experiments, short-term assays indicate a considerable potential for DNA damage in animal and human cells. Thus, the possibility of carcinogenic risk cannot be excluded, and further studies on the toxicity of this element are needed.

ZINC. *Short-Term Assays.* Zn toxicity is shown in Table VI. Generally, Zn compounds have generally proved negative in cell-free DNA damage and microbial assays (*27, 33, 63, 111, 211, 274, 275*), but there have been a few exceptions. For example, Zn compounds were mutagenic in the Ames test (*25, 117, 276*) and in *Vicia faba* (*117*). Chromosome damage was reported in plant (*118*), rat bone marrow in vivo (*277*), and human cells (*277, 278*). Zn gave positive results in a Chinese hamster cell mutation assay (*124*) and negative results in the mouse lymphoma mutation assay (*123*). Cell transformation assay results have also been conflicting.

Animal Experiments. The production of teratomas by injecting $ZnCl_2$ into the testes of fowl by Michalowsky in 1926 has been cited as the first animal model of experimental carcinogenesis (*5*). This finding has been confirmed on numerous occasions with several different mammalian and avian species. Hormonal influence on these tumors, probably through the indirect stimulation of pituitary gonadotropin release, is also well established (*5, 279*). On the other hand, all attempts to induce tumors at other sites with Zn have proven negative (*270, 280*).

Zn was shown to have an anticarcinogenic effect in certain experimental systems. Its subcutaneous coinjection with Cd blocked the induction of interstitial cell tumors of the testis by the latter metal. Zn also inhibited the induction of sarcomas by Cd at the site of injection (*167, 169*). Interestingly, when these metals were injected intramuscularly into opposite legs, this response did not occur, therefore, the metal–metal inhibition must require local contact (*281*). Inhibition of organic chemical carcinogenesis with dietary Zn has also been indicated (*282*). The role and possible mechanisms involved in these interactions have been reviewed (*202*).

Epidemiology. Zn is an essential trace metal; it is a component of certain metalloenzymes and is involved in cell division via DNA polymerase. Epidemiological or clinical evidence has not associated this element with any increased incidence of industrial or environmental cancers in humans. The biological functions and toxicology of Zn have been reviewed (*283*).

Conclusion. Although Zn is classified in this chapter as a possible carcinogen, there is little or no evidence for considering it a potential primary carcinogen in humans. Some evidence suggests that this metal, particularly dietary Zn, may play an anticarcinogenic role; this possibility deserves further investigation in view of the chronic Zn insufficiencies among certain human population groups.

Other Inorganic Elements. A large number of miscellaneous inorganic elements have not been sufficiently tested or extensively reviewed for their potential carcinogenicity. One recent review is available (*284*). Some of these elements gave positive results in more or less isolated short-term assays (Table VII); others have occasionally been reported to be carcinogenic or to modify the incidence of tumors from other causes (Table VIII).

SHORT-TERM ASSAYS. Elements that were tested in several assays include Te, Mg, Mo, and Sb (Table VII). Te compounds caused hydrocephalus in offspring of rats exposed through contaminated drinking water; teratogenesis and transplacental transfer have been reviewed (*285*). These compounds were also positive in several microbial (*33, 113, 114*) and chromosome-damage (*69*) assays. Mo was positive in the Rec assay (*33, 113, 114*) and caused chromosome damage in *Euglena* (*286*). Mg was generally not genotoxic; however, it did cause malignant transformation with Syrian hamster embryo cells (*99*). Sb was positive in the enhanced virus transformation assay (*28*).

Sporadic reports of the genotoxicity of other elements not frequently tested, such as the rare earths, are also summarized in Table VII. The most common types of damage reported were chromosome aberrations in mammalian cells and toxicity for repair-deficient bacteria (Rec assay).

ANIMAL STUDIES. Table VIII summarizes the results of the available animal experimental and human statistical data on the carcinogenicity and teratogenicity of a number of trace elements. Traces of most of these elements may be found in human tissues. There is little evidence, with the possible exception of V, that any of these affect the incidence of cancers in humans. Reviews of the properties, metabolism, and toxicity—with some reference to mutagenicity, carcinogenicity, and teratology—of V, Ti, Te, In, and Ge may be found in the "Handbook of the Toxicology of Metals" (*287*). The effects of several of these elements on growth, survival, and the incidence of spontaneous tumors in mice and rats were studied by Schroeder et al. (*288–93*). These investigators designated these elements as "abnormal" trace elements and administered them in subtoxic doses in the drinking water throughout the lifetime of large groups of mice and rats. In addition to elements listed in Table VIII, these investigators also studied Sc, Zr, and Nb, none of which enhanced spontaneous tumor incidence in the strains studied (*290, 291*). Gd and Yb, when administered parenterally, have been associated with metastatic sarcomas in 10% of treated mice (*294*). However, these growths may have been in response to the smooth-surface foreign body effect of the metallic implants. Numerous spontaneous tumors were also recorded among the control mice in these experiments. The antitumor effect reported for Ge (*407*) was not significant in reducing the incidence of malignant lesions; however, it did significantly reduce the level for all tumors ($P < 0.05$).

Thallium has been considered as a potential carcinogen on theoretical grounds (*295*). For this reason, as well as others—(1) the increased incidence of lung carcinomas seen among workers in an antimony trioxide plant and (2) the significant concentrations of Sb and Tl present in some smelter dusts—animal inhalation studies should be undertaken on these elements (*296*).

The interaction of Mg and Pb in various dietary combinations was referred to in the section on Pb. The one study showed that an excess of Mg alone in the diet had no epithelial neoplastic action (0/284 rats) and no leukemogenic action (0/84

Table VII

Genotoxicity of Other Inorganic Elements: Short-Term Assays

Element	*In Vivo Exposure*[a]	*Cytotoxicity*	*Rec/Pol A Assays*[a]	*DNA Damage*[b]	*Mutation*		*Chromosome Aberrations*	*Mammalian Cell Transformation*[c]
					Bacteria	*Plant/Animal*		
Te	+ rat (*285*)		+ (*113, 114*) − (*33*)				+* (*69*)	
Mg			− (*33*)	− cell-free systems (*63, 211, 274*)		− mouse lymphoma (*123*)	− *Pisum* (*118*)	+ Syrian hamster (*99*) − enhanced virus trans. (*28*)
Mo			+ (*33, 113, 114*)		+ *E. coli* (*394*) − *E. coli* (*275*)		+ *Euglena* (*286*)	
Sb			+ (*113*) − (*33*)					+ enhanced virus trans. in hamster (*28*)
Hg	+* teratogenic in mice (*297*), placental transfer in humans (review, *298*), chromosome effects in humans (*299, 300*), and *Drosophila* (*240*)	+* human cervical carcinoma cells (*412*), plant cells (*34*)	− (*367*)	+ cell-free systems (*412*)	+ (*394*) − (*275*)	+ rice (*181*) +/− mouse lymphoma (*86*) − mouse mammary carcinoma (*122*)	+* human cervical carcinoma cells (*412*), *Pisum* (*118*), *Allium cepa* (*119*) −* human leukocytes (*69*)	+ enhanced virus trans. in hamster (*28*)

Ba	+ teratogenic in chick embryo (*370*)		− cell-free systems (33)		+ rice (*181*)		
B	+ teratogenic in chick embryo (*370*)						
Cs		+ (*114*)				+ *Pisum* (*118*)	
Cl		+ (*367*)					
Er						+ *Allium cepa* (*119*)	
F					+ *Drosophila* (*268*)		
Ge		+ (*414*)					
Ir		+ (*113, 114*)		− *Sal. typhimurium* (*309*)			
La						+ *Pisum* (*118*) *Allium cepa* (*119*)	
Nd						+ *Allium cepa* (*119*)	
Os		+ (*113, 114*)				+ *Pisum* (*118*)	
Pd						+ *Allium cepa* (*119*)	
Rh		+ (*113, 114*) − (*33*)		+ *Sal. typhimurium* (*309*)			
Rb			− cell-free system (*63*)				
Ru		− (*33*)		+ *Sal. typhimurium* (*309*)		+ *Allium cepa* (*119*)	
Sr					+ rice (*181*)	+ *Pisum* (*118*)	− (*68*)

continued on next page

Table VII Continued

Element	In Vivo Exposure[a]	Cytotoxicity	Rec/Pol A Assays[a]	DNA damage[b]	Mutation: Bacteria	Mutation: Plant/Animal	Chromosome Aberrations	Mammalian Cell Transformation[c]
Ta							+ *Pisum* (*118*) *Allium cepa* (*119*)	+ enhanced virus trans. (*28*)
Te			+ (*414*)					
Tl	+ teratogenic in chick embryo (*370*)						+ *Allium cepa* (*119*)	
Ti		+ chick hepatocytes (*391*)					+ *Pisum* (*118*)	− hamster (*66, 68*)
V		+ chick hepatocytes (*391*)	+ (*113, 114*)		+ *E. coli* (*394*)			
Yb							+ *Allium cepa* (*119*)	

Key: +, positive test result; −, negative test result; +/−, weakly positive test result; and *, includes data for human cells.
[a]Description of assays given in Table II footnotes.
[b]Includes biochemical assays.
[c]Includes enhanced virus transformation assay (*see* Table II).

Table VIII

Carcinogenic and Teratogenic Activities of Trace Elements

Element	*Species*	*Route*[a] *and Exposure*	*Activity*	*Ref.*
Ti	mouse	lifetime	negative	288
	rat	im, monthly × 6	fibrosarcoma	230
			lymphosarcoma	
V	mouse	lifetime	negative	407
	rat	lifetime	negative	289
	human	environmental	lung cancer	408
Ge	mouse	lifetime	antitumor	407
	rat	lifetime	negative	289
Te	mouse	lifetime	negative	292
	rat	lifetime	negative	293
	rat	day 9–15	hydrocephalus	409
Rh	mouse	lifetime	increased numbers of	291
Pd	mouse	lifetime	spontaneous tumors	
In	mouse	lifetime	negative	291
	hamster	iv, day 8	digital anomalies	410
	human	environmental	antitumor	411
Gd	mouse	sc, single	sarcomas (10%)	294
	mouse	lifetime	negative	291
Yb	mouse	sc, single	sarcomas (10%)	294
	mouse	lifetime	negative	291

[a]Route is oral unless indicated by im, intramuscular; iv, intravenous; or sc, subcutaneous. Route of human environmental exposure is undefined.

rats). An excess of both Mg and Pb enhanced the occurrence of renal tumors, and to a lesser extent, thyroid tumors and leukemias. Unfortunately, these and other interactions between Mg and Pb have not been reported in any detail (*252*).

MERCURY. *Short-Term Assays.* Hg compounds were positive in several short-term in vitro assays, such as the micronucleus test (*82*), and resulted in nondisjunction in *Drosophila* (*240*). They are teratogenic in mice (*297*); placental transfer has been shown for several species including humans (reviewed in Ref. 298).

Genotoxicity of Hg compounds in vitro is shown in Table VII. Positive results were reported for many of the assays in both lower and higher organisms, in particular, for the Rec assay (*33, 113, 114*), plant mutation assays (*34, 181*), and chromosome aberration tests (*118, 119, 299, 300*). In addition, Hg compounds were positive in a mammalian cell mutation assay (*86*) and the enhanced virus transformation assay (*28*).

Animal Studies. Conclusive evidence for Hg carcinogenicity was not demonstrated in the few animal studies reported. Lifetime exposure of mice to dimethylmercury showed no evidence of tumor activity (*301*). Druckrey et al. (*302*) reported the induction of sarcomas in rats after injections of liquid metallic Hg; however, this result may have been due to the smooth-surface foreign body effect of the solid mercury globules (*303*). Nixon et al. (*304*) reported an enhancing effect in rats for dimethylmercury on sodium nitrite plus ethylurea-induced transplacental schwannomas and ependymomas, but not on other neural tumors. In view of the broad spectrum of genotoxicity attributable to Hg in short-term assays and its reported role in enhancing the carcinogenicity of nitroso compounds, its possible role in chemical carcinogenesis deserves further investigation.

Noble Metals. SILVER, GOLD, AND PLATINUM. *Short-Term Assays.* Ag compounds have not been extensively tested in vitro. However, they were genotoxic in several assays (Table IX), such as fidelity of DNA synthesis (*27, 63*), a plant cytotoxicity assay (*34*), several mammalian cell mutation assays (*86, 124*), and the enhanced virus transformation assay (*28*). Generally, Ag compounds appeared to be negative in assays with the lower organisms. Au compounds induced chromosome aberrations in *Pisum* (*118*) and *Allium cepa* cells (*119*).

Pt coordination complexes form a new class of active anticancer agents. The most widely investigated compound, *cis*-diamminedichloroplatinum(II) (*cis*-DDP), is now in experimental clinical use as a chemotherapeutic agent. Recent evidence indicates that this compound may itself be carcinogenic.

In short-term tests, it is an extremely active genotoxic agent. Pt compounds are embryotoxic and teratogenic (reviewed in Ref. 305). The toxicity of Pt compounds in vitro is summarized in Table IX; except where otherwise stated, the compound tested was *cis*-DDP. Pt is strikingly positive in all test systems, including cell-free assays for DNA damage (*124, 306, 307*), mutation assays in microorganisms (*113, 114, 308–13*), and animal cell assays (*29, 123, 314–17*). Furthermore, Pt is an active chromosome-damaging agent; it causes aberrations (*118, 124, 316, 318, 319*) and sister chromatid exchanges (*316, 318*) in many species including humans. Pt causes mammalian cell transformation (*316*) and enhanced virus transformation (*28*).

Animal Experiments. cis-DDP increased the incidence of lung adenomas in A/Jax mice from 0.5–0.8% to 10–16% (*305*); it also appeared to act as an initiator of skin tumors in mice when applied in combination with the promoter croton oil; neither substance alone produced tumors. Subcutaneous injections of *cis*-DDP and DDP · *cis*-dichlorobis(pyrrolidine)platinum(II) induced sarcomas in rats (*305*).

Colloidal Ag, but not Au, administered subcutaneously and intravenously proved carcinogenic to rats (*320*). However, neither Ag nor Au intramuscular injections produced any tumors (*321*). A high occurrence of adverse reactions from Au therapy has been reported (*322*) that affected the lung, liver, blood, and skin; however, association with cancer has not been shown in humans.

Conclusions. The extensive positive data on *cis*-DDP in short-term assays and its reported activity as a primary carcinogen in rats and as a cofactor in mouse tumorigenesis emphasize that these antitumor complexes may pose a risk of further tumor induction with long-term treatment. In view of this uncertainty, further animal studies on the mechanism of *cis*-Pt tumorigenesis are required. Clear-cut evidence for carcinogenicity of Au and Ag compounds is lacking.

Foreign Body Carcinogenesis. Evgen'eva (*323*) induced tumors in the eyes of rats by introducing films of Pb into the eye chamber. Ag, Au, and Pt all induced sarcomas when implanted subcutaneously as smooth-surfaced discs in rats and mice (*324*). This response, which included sarcoma induction by nonmetallic discs of ivory and glass, was recognized as a relatively nonspecific foreign body carcinogenesis, and it has been confirmed in numerous experiments (*303, 325–27*).

The mixed results obtained with noble metals reflect the influences of differences in physical form of the implant (smooth vs. rough or solid vs. perforated), as well as the nature of the chemical compound and its solubility. These are aspects of the problem that do not seem to have been adequately addressed to date (*303*). The need to elucidate the mechanisms involved in foreign body carcinogenesis and to follow up the clinical use of metallic prosthetic devices (pins, plates, IUDs, etc.) would seem particularly pertinent at this time.

Several, predominantly veterinary, clinical reports of tumors in animals were associated with prosthetic implants (*223–25, 328*), It has also been shown experimentally that wear product particles from Co, Cr, and Mo alloy prostheses were carcinogenic to rats (*226, 227*). On the other hand, tests on seven alloys implanted as rods in rats failed to affect the tumor incidence or induce any sarcomas at site in rats (*329*).

As a 30–50-year latent period in man is not uncommon in metal carcinogenesis and in view of the increasingly early implantations of prosthetic devices, it would seem that further studies on alloy foreign body tumorigenesis are warranted.

Metal Cofactors in Carcinogenesis

Interactions of metals with each other or with organic chemical carcinogens have, in a number of instances, produced either anticarcinogenic or cocarcinogenic effects. Aside from directly affecting the incidence of malignant and nonmalignant tumors, these metals may alter tumor latency, dose–response, location, progression (rate of development), and frequency of metastases (*330*).

Anticarcinogenicity of metals has been reviewed by Sunderman (*77*); otherwise only sporadic reports, usually with specific metals, have appeared. These often conflicting reports on the synergisms and antagonisms of trace metals should receive further attention (*202*).

Several metals that do not seemingly act as primary carcinogens are discussed in this section in terms of their action either in enhancing or inhibiting the carcinogenic expression of other chemical carcinogens or in affecting spontaneous tumor incidence. Tables X and XI summarize these effects; short-term assay results for these compounds are shown in Table XII.

Aluminum. SHORT-TERM ASSAYS. Al was reported as inactive in a variety of short-term tests (Table XII). Al compounds did not decrease the fidelity of DNA synthesis (*27, 63*) or induce DNA damage in bacteria (*33*). They also failed to transform Syrian hamster embryo cells (*66*) and were negative in the enhanced virus transformation assay (*28*). Induction of chromosome aberrations was observed in vivo with mouse bone marrow cells (*331*) and in vitro with *Pisum* rootlets (*118*).

Table IX
Genotoxicity of Noble Metals: Short-Term Assays

Assay[a]		*Pt*[b]		*Ag*		*Au*
In vivo tests	+	embryotoxic and teratogenic (*305*), chromosome effects in *Drosophila* (*415*), rabbit (*416*), and mouse (*318*)				
	−	dominant lethal test (*417*)				
Cytotoxicity	+	Chinese hamster cells (*315*)	+	plant cells (*34*)		
DNA effects						
biochemical assays			+	(*27, 63*)		
Rec/Pol A assays	+	(*113, 114*)	−	(*33, 113, 114, 367*)		
DNA damage	+	mouse leukemia cells (*306*), Chinese hamster cells (*317*), plasmids (*307*)				
inhibition of DNA synthesis	+	mammalian cells (*418*)				
Chromosome aberrations	+*	human leukocytes (*318, 319*), Chinese hamster cells (*29, 316*), *Pisum* (*118*)			+	*Pisum* (*118*), *Allium cepa* (*119*)

Sister chromatid exchange	+*	human leukocytes (*318, 416*), Chinese hamster cells (*316*)		
Mutation				
bacteria	+	*E. coli* (*310*)		
	+	*Sal. typhimurium* (*308, 309, 311–13*)		
mammalian cells	+	Chinese hamster cells (*29, 124, 314–17*), mouse lymphoma cells (*123*)	+	Chinese hamster cells (*29*)
			+/−	mouse lymphoma cells (*86*)
Mammalian cell transformation	+	Chinese hamster cells (*316*)		
Enhanced virus transformation	+	(*28*)	+	(*28*)

Key: +, positive test result; −, negative test result; and +/−, weakly positive test result.
[a]Descriptions of assays are given in Table II footnotes.
[b]*cis*- and *trans*-Pt(II) and Pt salts.

Table X

Metals as Cofactors in Experimental Chemical Carcinogenesis: Tumor Inhibition

Metal	*Route*[a]	*Species*	*Tumor Model Affected*	*Ref.*
As	oral	mouse	topical MC skin tumors; various spontaneous tumors; mammary tumors in C3H strain	42 407 419
Al	sc	mouse	sc 4-nitroquinoline 1-oxide pulmonary adenomas	420 202
Co	ip	mouse	topical MC skin carcinoma, MC papilloma latency	219 202
Cu	oral	rat	ethionine hepatomas; methoxy dye hepatomas	233 421
Mn	im	rat	Ni_3S_2 or BP injection site sarcomas (on coinjection only)	77
Ni	oral	rat	dietary DMBA hepatomas	77
Se	oral	mouse	topical BP and DMBA skin tumors; spontaneous mammary tumors in the C_3H strain	353 419
	oral	rat	dimethylhydrazine and methyl-azoxymethanol colon carcinomas	423
Zn	sc	rat	Cd injection site sarcomas and interstitial cell (testes) tumors (on coinjection only)	202
	oral	mouse	topical MC skin tumors, DMBA salivary gland tumors; reduced growth	279 202

[a]im, intramuscular; ip, intraperitoneal; and sc, subcutaneous.

ANIMAL EXPERIMENTS. Only a few long-term tests on the potential carcinogenicity of Al have been reported (reviewed in Refs. 77 and 303). The most notable finding is that of a significant antitumor activity of Al compounds against the induction of lung tumors by 4-nitroquinoline 1-oxide in mice (*332*). This finding is particularly interesting in view of the ubiquitousness of aluminum oxide in the environment and its high concentration in human lung (*184*).

The only clearly positive report of tumorigenesis attributable to Al involves the induction of sarcomas in 9 out of 15 rats from implanted aluminum foil (*192*); the relevance of this report is obscured by the influence of solid-state and smooth-surface factors (*333*). Other investigations were essentially all negative. Al has not been included in the IARC lists of possible carcinogens (*23*).

Table XI

Metals as Cofactors in Experimental Chemical Carcinogenesis: Tumor Enhancement

Metal	*Route*[a]	*Species*	*Tumor Model Affected*	*Ref.*
As	it	rat	cocarcinogen for BP; synergism with $CuSO_4$ and Ca in synthetic Bordeaux mixture	46 47
Cr	it graft	rat	increased incidence of metastases with BP vs. BP only	424
Fe	it	hamster	cocarcinogen for BP for carcinoma of trachea and bronchi	425
	it	rat	cocarcinogen for BP for carcinoma of lung alveoli	426
	it	hamster	cocarcinogen for diethylnitrosamine	198
Pb	it	rat	synergism with BP for lung tumor induction, hepatoma development from 3-methyl-4-dimethylamino-azobenzene	254
Mg	oral	rat	Pb/Mg ratio influences on malignant lymphomas	252
Ti	it	hamster	cocarcinogen for BP for respiratory tract tumors	203

[a]it, intratracheal.

EPIDEMIOLOGY. There is little or no evidence available to suggest that specific Al compounds are carcinogenic. However, recent studies indicate that occupational exposure to the electrolytic refining of Al may constitute a cancer hazard by inducing, in particular, lung tumors and malignant lymphomas (*334, 335*). The risk, however, has been attributed to the release of tars in the "pot" rooms in smelter operations. The air in these rooms is known to contain carcinogenic polycyclic hydrocarbons, including benzo[*a*]pyrene with exposures lower than those experienced by coke oven workers in steel mills (*336*).

CONCLUSIONS. Epidemiological and experimental evidence does not indicate that Al is a primary carcinogen. However the possible role of Al as a cofactor in environmental carcinogenesis should be investigated further, particularly in regard to its anticarcinogenicity to organic chemical carcinogens.

Manganese. SHORT-TERM ASSAYS. Mn toxicity in short-term tests in vitro is shown in Table XII. Mn decreased fidelity of nucleic acid synthesis (*27, 63, 110, 211*) and was positive in several other test systems, including mutation assays in plant (*117,*

Table XII

Genotoxicity of Metal Cofactors: Short-Term Assays

Assay[a]		*Mn*		*Se*		*Al*
In vivo tests			+*	placental transfer in humans (*353*), teratogenic in chick embryos (*370*), and animals on pasture (*285*)	+	chromosome effects in mice (*331*)
			—*	no detectable teratogenesis in humans (*285*)		
Cytotoxicity	+/−	chick hepatocytes (*391*)				
DNA effects						
biochemical	+	(*27, 63, 110, 211, 274*)			−	(*63*)
Rec/Pol A assays	+	(*33*)	+	(*113, 114, 345, 430*)	−	(*33*)
	−	(*113, 114*)	−	(*33*)		
DNA damage	—*	strand breaks (*111*)	+*	human skin fibroblasts (*346*)		
Chromosome aberrations	+	mouse mammary carcinoma cells (*379*), *Vicia faba* (*117*), *Pisum* (*118*)	+*	human skin fibroblasts (*346*)	+	*Pisum* (*118*)
			—*	human leukocytes (*69*)		

Sister chromatid exchange			+*	human leukocytes (*347*)		
Mutation						
bacteria	+	*E. coli* (*427*)	+	*E. coli* (*394*)		
	+	phage (*428*)	+	*Sal. typhimurium* (*344*)		
	+	*Proteus mirabilis* (*429*)	+/−	*Sal. typhimurium* (*25, 345*)		
yeast/plants	+	*S. cerevisiae* (*337*), green algae (*338, 339*), *Vicia faba* (*117*)	+	barley (*431*)		
	−	rice (*181*)				
mammalian cells	+	Chinese hamster cells (*29, 65, 124*), mouse lymphoma cells (*86*)	−	Chinese hamster cells (*124*)		
	−	mouse mammary carcinoma cells (*122*)				
Mammalian cell transformation	+	Syrian hamster cells (*99*)			−	Syrian hamster cells (*66*)
Enhanced virus transformation	+	(*28*)			−	(*28*)

Key: +, positive test result; −, negative test result; and +/−, weakly positive test result.
[a]Description of assays given in Table II footnotes.

337–39) and animal (*29, 65, 86, 122, 124*) cells. Mn was positive in one cell transformation assay (*99*) and in the enhanced virus transformation assay (*28*).

Mn was also reported to have antimutagenic and anticarcinogenic activity (reviewed in Ref. 77). For example, Costa (*99*) showed inhibition of cell transformation by Ni_3S_2 in the presence of Mn.

ANIMAL EXPERIMENTS. Little or no evidence suggests that either malformations or malignancies are caused by the inhalation or ingestion of Mn (*340*). Manganous chloride has been implicated in shortening the latent period and enhancing the expectancy of lymphosarcoma in mice (*341*). In tests on 13 metal compounds injected into strain A mice, manganous sulfate was one of four metals that gave a significant increase in the incidence of lung adenomas in this strain (*342*).

Mn exerted a significant anticarcinogenic effect on Ni_3S_2 in rats. Both intramuscular and intrarenal injections of the metals were used, and the metal–metal interaction appeared dependent, as it did with Zn, on coinjection and local mixing (*343*). This finding, as well as inhibition by Mn dusts of hepatoma development induced by organic chemical carcinogens in rats, has been reviewed (*77*).

EPIDEMIOLOGY. No epidemiological evidence exists that cancer in humans may be caused by Mn. However, this metal, along with Mg, is a frequently interchangeable activator of a number of enzyme systems. It is also present in large quantities in melanin, although no relationship to melanoma induction is known (*184*).

Selenium. SHORT-TERM ASSAYS. Se compounds were teratogenic in several species, such as chickens, horses, cattle, and pigs; in some cases, exposure resulted from grazing on seleniferous range land (reviewed in Ref. 285). Although transplacental accumulation of selenium was shown for humans, the reviewer concluded that no detectable teratogenesis occurred.

In vitro assay results are shown in Table XII. Although several authors reported that Se compounds were active in the Ames test (*25, 344, 345*), only a few isolated reports of Se toxicity were found for mammalian cell assays, such as chromosome aberrations and DNA repair in human fibroblasts (*346*) and sister chromatid exchange in human lymphocytes (*347*). Se was negative in a Chinese hamster cell mutation assay (*124*); it was not tested in cell transformation assays.

Several authors have reported the antimutagenicity of Se compounds. This action has been reviewed by Shamberger (*348*), who concluded that antimutagenicity generally occurred at normal physiological levels, whereas mutagenicity was reported at 3–1000 times normal physiological levels.

ANIMAL EXPERIMENTS. Some evidence suggests that Se enhances the incidence of malignant tumors in rats and mice; however, whether it can act as a primary carcinogen is not clear despite a number of animal studies (*285*).

Diet, sex, age, strain, and various environmental factors, such as medication, appear to modify the pathotoxicological changes in animals that ingest Se; therefore its role in the onset of neoplasia is obscured (*349*). A high-protein diet reduced the incidence of several Se-related pathological changes in the rat, including neoplasia (*350*). Lifetime exposure of rats to drinking water that contained Se resulted in an increased tumor incidence over that in the controls

(*292*). Conversely, 5–15 ppm of Se as selenite significantly inhibited the incidence of mammary tumors in C3H mice; this anticancer effect was abolished by the addition of 200 ppm of $ZnCl_2$ to 5 ppm of Se (*351*).

Several studies affirm the role of Se (as sodium selenite) as a protective agent against a number of different organic chemical carcinogens; it reduced the incidence of DMBA- and BP-induced skin cancers in mice (*202*) and of dimethylhydrazine and methylazoxymethanol-induced colon cancers in mice and rats (*352*).

EPIDEMIOLOGY. No evidence exists for a causal relationship between a high-Se intake and an increased incidence of cancer in humans. A correlation has been shown, however, between a low-Se intake and an enhanced tumor incidence in humans (*260, 353*). The carcinogenic and anticarcinogenic effects of Se have been thoroughly reviewed (*354*).

CONCLUSION. The role of Se in carcinogenesis is equivocal. It appears to exert varying synergistic effects depending on the circumstances of its use. The evidence for its carcinogenicity in both animals and humans is, at best, tenuous. Recent reports on the antitumor activity of Se in animals and the inverse correlation of Se levels and tumor incidence in humans suggest that further studies are required.

Acknowledgment

The authors wish to thank Robert S. Stafford at the Environmental Mutagen Information Center at Oak Ridge for providing the in vitro test-related literature searches.

Literature Cited

1. Hammond, E.C. *Cancer* **1975**, *35*, 652.
2. Higginson, J. *Science (Washington, D.C.)* **1979**, *205*, 1363.
3. "IARC Monographs on the Evaluation of the Carcinogenic Risk of Chemicals to Man," Suppl. 1, 1979.
4. U.S. Department of Health and Human Services. Second Annual Report on Carcinogens, National Toxicology Program, Research Triangle Park, N.C., Dec. 1981.
5. Sunderman, F.W., Jr., in "Advances in Modern Toxicology," Vol. 2.; Goyer, R.A.; Mehlman, M.A., Eds.; Hemisphere Corp.: Washington, D.C., 1977; p. 257.
6. Kraybill, H.F. *Bull. N.Y. Acad. Sci.* **1978**, *54*, 413.
7. Hernberg, S. in "Cold Spring Harbor Conference on Cell Proliferation," Vol. 4; Hiatt, H.H.; Watson, J.D.; Winsten, J.A., Eds.; Cold Spring Harbor: Cold Spring Harbor, N.Y.: 1977, p. 147.
8. Furst, A. *Adv. in Modern Toxicol.* **1977**, *3*, 209.
9. Flessel, C.P.; Furst, A.; Radding, S.B. in "Metal ions in Biological Systems," Vol. 10; Sigel, H., Ed.; Marcel Dekker: New York, 1980; p. 23.
10. Hueper, W.C.; Conway, W.D. in "Chemical Carcinogenesis and Cancer"; Thomas Publishing Co: Springfield, 1964; p. 379.
11. Clayson, D.B. in "Chemical Carcinogenesis"; J. and A. Churchill Ltd.: London, 1962, p. 113.
12. Schinz, H.R.; Ühlinger, E. *Z. Krebsforsch.* **1942**, *52*, 425.

13. Fishbein, L. *J. Toxicol. Environ. Health* **1976**, *2*, 77.
14. Munroe, I.C. *Chem. Toxicol.* **1976**, *9*, 647.
15. Sunderman, F.W., Jr. *Fed. Proc.* **1978**, *37*, 40.
16. Bates, R.R. *EHP, Environ. Health Perspect.* **1979**, *28*, 303.
17. Tomatis, L. *Cancer Res.* **1978**, *38*, 887.
18. Saffiotti, U. in "Cold Spring Harbor Conference on Cell. Proliferation," Vol. 4; Hiatt, H.H.; Watson, J.D., Winston, J.A., Eds; Cold Spring Harbor: Cold Spring Harbor, N.Y., 1977; p. 1311.
19. Meyboom, R.H.B. in "Side Effects of Drugs Annual"; Dukes, M.N.G., Ed; Experta Medica: Amsterdam, 1977; p. 1985.
20. Lillenfield, A.M.; Pedersen, E.; David, J.E. in "Cancer Epidemiology, Methods of Study"; Lillenfield, A.M.; Gifford, A.J., Eds.; John Hopkins: Baltimore, 1967.
21. Norseth, T. in "Cold Spring Harbor Conference on Cell Proliferation," Vol. 4; Hiatt, H.H.; Watson, J.D.; Winston, J.A., Eds.; Cold Spring Harbor: Cold Spring Harbor, N.Y., 1977; p. 159.
22. National Institute of Occupational Safety and Health, U.S. Dept. of Health, Education and Welfare, Publ. No. 77–149, Washington, D.C., 1976.
23. Tomatis, L. in "Cold Spring Habor Conference on Cell Proliferation," Vol. 4; Hiatt, H.H.; Watson, J.D.; Winston, J.A., Eds; Cold Spring Harbor: Cold Spring Harbor, N.Y., 1977; p. 1339.
24. Stout, M.G.; Rawson, R.W. "Progress in Cancer Research Therapeutics," Vol. 17; Newell, G.R.; Ellison, N.M.; Eds.; Raven: New York, 1981; p. 243.
25. Hollstein, M.; McCann, J. *Mutat. Res.* **1979**, *65*, 133.
26. IARC Monographs on the Evaluation of the Carcinogenic Risk of Chemicals to Man, Vol. 23, 1980; p. 359.
27. Sirover, M.A.; Loeb, L.A. *Science (Washington, D.C.)* **1976**, *194*, 1434.
28. Casto, B.C.; Meyers, J.; DiPaolo, J.A. *Cancer Res.* **1979**, *39*, 193.
29. Hsie, A.W.; O'Neill, J.P.; San Sebastian, J.R.; Couch, D.B.; Brimer, P.A.; Sun, W.N.C.; Fuscoe, J.C.; Forbes, N.C.; Machanoff, R.; Riddle, J.C.; Hsie, M.H. in "The Fractionation and Analysis of Complex Environmental Mixtures"; Waters, M.D.; Nesnow, S.; Huisingh, J.L.; Sandhu, S.S.; Claxton, L., Eds.; Plenum: New York, 1979; p. 291.
30. DiPaolo, J.A.; Nelson, R.L.; Casto, B.C. *Br. J. Cancer* **1978**, *38*, 452.
31. "The OSHA Cancer Policy"; Occupational Health and Safety Letters, **1979**, *9*, 1.
32. Leonard, A.; Lauwerys, R.R. *Mutat. Res.* **1980**, *75*, 49.
33. Nishioka, H. *Mutat. Res.* **1975**, *31*, 185.
34. Oguni, I.; Suzuki-Nasu, K.; Masui, T. *Agric. Biol. Chem.* **1978**, *42*, 1425.
35. Bencko, V. *Environ. Health Perspect.* **1977**, *19*, 179.
36. Pelfrene, A. *J. Toxicol. Environ. Health* **1976**, *1*, 1003.
37. Leitch, A.; Kennaway, E.L. *Br. J. Med.* **1922**, *2*, 1107.
38. Fairhall, L.T.; Miller, J.W. *Public Health Rep.* **1941**, *56*, 1610.
39. Baroni, C.; van Esch, G.J.; Saffiotti, U. *Arch. Environ. Health* **1963**, *7*, 668.
40. Berteau, P.E.; Flom, J.; Dimmick, R.L.; Boyd, A.R. *Toxicol. Appl. Pharmacol.* **1978**, *45*, 323.
41. Boutwell, R.K. *J. Agric. Food Chem.* **1963**, *11*, 381.
42. Milner, J.E. *Arch. Environ. Health* **1969**, *18*, 7.
43. Kroes, R.; van Logten, J.; Berkvens, J.M.; De Vries, T.; van Esch, G.J. *Food Cosmet. Toxicol.* **1974**, *12*, 671.
44. Byron, W.R.; Bierbower, G.W.; Brouwer, J.B.; Hansen, W.H. *Toxicol. Appl. Pharmacol.* **1967**, *10*, 132.
45. Osswald, H.; Goerttler, K. *Verb. Dtsch. Geselisch. Pathol.* **1971**, *55*, 289.
46. Ishinishi, N.; Kodama, Y.;' Nobutomo, K.; Hisanaga, A. *EHP, Environ. Health Perspect.* **1977**, *19*, 191.

47. Ivankovic, S.; Eisenbrand, G.; Preussmann, R. *Int. J. Cancer* **1979**, *24*, 786.
48. Yeh, S. *Human Pathol.* **1973**, *4*, 469.
49. Milham, S., Jr.; Strong, T. *Environ. Res.* **1974**, *7*, 176.
50. Pershagen, G.; Elinder, C.G.; Bolander, A.M. *EHP, Environ. Health Perspect.* **1977**, *19*, 133.
51. Blot, W.J.; Fraumeni, J.F., Jr. *Lancet* **1975**, *2*, 142.
52. Osburn, H.S. *S. Afr. Med. J.* **1969**, *43*, 1307.
53. Lee, A.M.; Fraumeni, J.F., Jr. *JNCI, J. Natl. Cancer Inst.* **1969**, *42*, 1045.
54. Ott, M.; Holder, B.B.; Gordon, H.L. *Arch. Environ. Health* **1974**, *29*, 250.
55. Horiguchi, S.; Nakano, H.; Shinagawa, K.; Teramoto, K.; Kiyota, I. *Osaka City Med. J.* **1976**, *22*, 43.
56. Galy, P.; Touraine, R.; Brune, J.; Gallois, P.; Roudier, R.; Lorie, R.; Leheureux, P.; Wissendanger, T. *Lyon Med.* **1963**, *210*, 735.
57. Neubauer, O. *Br. J. Cancer* **1947**, *1*, 192.
58. Novey, H.S.; Martel, S.H. *J. Allergy* **1969**, *44*, 315.
59. Goldman, A.L. *Am. Rev. Resp. Dis.* **1973**, *108*, 1205.
60. Evans, S. *Br. J. Dermatol.* **1977**, *97*, 13.
61. Reymann, F.; Moller, R.; Nielsen, A. *Arch. Dermatol.* **1978**, *114*, 378.
62. Reeves, A.L. *Proc. Int. Congress Toxicol., Toronto* **1977**, p. 577.
63. Zakour, R.A.; Loeb, L.A.; Kunkel, T.A.; Koplitz, R.M. in "Trace Metals in Health and Disease"; Karasch, N., Ed.; Raven: New York, 1979; p. 135.
64. Luke, M.Z.; Hamilton, L.; Hollocher, T.C. *Biochem. Biophys. Res. Commun.* **1975**, *62*, 497.
65. Miyaki, M.; Akamatsu, N.; Ono, T.; Koyama, H. *Mutat. Res.* **1979**, *68*, 259.
66. DiPaolo, J.A.; Casto, B.C. *Cancer Res.* **1979**, *39*, 1008.
67. Pienta, R.J. in "Chemical Mutagens, Principles and Methods for their Dectection," Vol. 6; de Serres, F.J.; Hollaender, A., Eds; Plenum: New York, 1980; p. 175.
68. Casto, B.C.; Pieczynski, W.J.; Nelson, R.L.; DiPaolo, J.A. *Proc. Am. Assoc. Cancer Res.* **1976**, *17*, 12.
69. Paton, G.R.; Allison, A.C. *Mutat. Res.* **1972**, *16*, 332.
70. Talluri, M.V.; Guiggiani, V. *Caryologia* **1967**, *20*, 355.
71. Gardner, L.V.; Heslington, H.F. *Fed. Proc.* **1946**, *5*, 221.
72. Groth, D.H. *Environ. Res.* **1980**, *21*, 56.
73. Dutra, F.R.; Largent, E.J.; Roth, J. *AMA Arch. Pathol.* **1951**, *51*, 473.
74. Vorwald, A.J.; Pratt, P.C.; Urban, E.J. *Acta. Unio Int. Canc* **1955**, *11*, 735.
75. Groth, D.H.; MacKay, G.R. *Toxicol. Appl. Pharmacol.* **1971**, *19*, 392.
76. Sanders, C.L.; Cannon, W.C.; Powers, G.J. Health Phys. *1978*, *33*, 193.
77. Sunderman, F.W., Jr. in "Environmental Carcinogenesis"; Emmelot, P.; Krick, E., Eds.; Elsevier/North Holland: Amsterdam, 1979; p. 165.
78. Infante, P.F.; Wagoner, J.K.; Sprince, N.L. *Environ. Res.* **1980**, *21*, 35.
79. Wagoner, J.K.; Infante, P.F.; Bayliss, D.L. *Environ. Res.* **1980**, *21*, 15.
80. Mancuso, T.F. *Environ. Res.* **1980**, *21*, 48.
81. Griggs, K. *Science (Washington, D.C.)* **1973**, *181*, 842.
82. Jenssen, D.; Ramel, C. *Mutat. Res.* **1980**, *75*, 191.
83. Wild, D. *Mutat. Res.* **1978**, *56*, 319.
84. Bigaliev, A.B.; Elemesova, M.S.; Turebaev, M.N.; Bigalieva, R.K. *Zdravookhr. Kaz.* **1978**, *8*, 48.
85. Raffetto, G.; Parodi, S.; Parodi, C.; DeFerrari, M.; Troiano, R.; Brambilla, G. *Tumori,* **1977**, *63*, 503.
86. Oberly, T.J.; Piper, C.E. *Environ. Mutat.* **1980**, *2*, 281.
87. Leonard, A.; Lauwerys, R.R. *Mutat. Res.* **1980**, *76*, 227.
88. Hueper, W.C.; Payne, W.W. *Am. Ind. Hyg. Assoc. J.* **1959**, *20*, 274.

89. Laskin, S.; Kuschner, M.; Drew, R.T. in "Inhalation Carcinogenesis"; Hanna, M.G., Jr.; Nettesheim, P.; Gilbert, J.R., Eds; Atomic Energy Comm., Washington, D.C., 1970; p. 321.
90. Norseth, T. in "Trace Metals: Exposure and Health Effects"; DiFerrante, E., Ed.; Pergamon: London, 1979; p. 135.
91. Kuschner, M.; Laskin, S. *Am. J. Pathol.* **1971**, *64*, 183.
92. Nettesheim, P.; Hanna, M.G., Jr.; Doherty, D.G.; Newell, R.F.; Hellman, A. *JNCI, J. Natl. Cancer Inst.* **1971**, *47*, 1129.
93. Furst, A.; Schlauder, M.; Sasmore, D.P. *Cancer Res.* **1976**, *36*, 1779.
94. Baetjer, A.M.; Lowney, J.F.; Steffee, H.; Budacz, V. *Arch. Ind. Health* **1959**, *20*, 124.
95. Laskin, S. in "Research in Environmental Sciences"; Institute of Environmental Med., Washington, D.C., 1972; p. 92.
96. Levis, A.G.; Majone, F. *Br. J. Cancer* **1979**, *40*, 523.
97. Hueper, W.C. in "Recent Results in Cancer Research"; Springer Verlag: New York, 1966; p. 56.
98. Leonard, A. in "Trace Metals—Exposure and Health Effects"; DiFerranti, E., Ed.; Pergamon: New York, 1978; p. 199.
99. Costa, M. "Metal Carcinogenesis Testing—Principles and In Vitro Methods"; Humana: New Jersey; p. 27.
100. Royle, H. *Environ. Res.* **1975**, *10*, 39.
101. Langard, S.; Andersen, A.; Gylseth, B. *Br. J. Ind. Med.* **1980**, *37*, 114.
102. Enterline, P.E. *J. Occup. Med.* **1974**, *16*, 523.
103. Dalager, N.R.; Mason, T.J.; Fraumeni, J.F., Jr.; Hoover, R.; Payne, W.W. *J. Occup. Med.* **1980**, *22*, 25.
104. Blair, A. *J. Occup. Med.* **1980**, *22*, 158.
105. Blair, A.; Mason, T.J. *Arch. Environ. Health* **1980**, *35*, 92.
106. Poprovskaya, L.V.; Shabynina, N.K. *Gig. Tr. Prof. Zabol.* **1973**, *10*, 23.
107. Sunderman, F.W., Jr.; Allpass, P.R.; Mitchell, J.M.; Baselt, R.C.; Albert, D.M. Science (*Washington, D.C.)*, **1979**, *203*, 550.
108. Sunderman, F.W., Jr.; Shen, S.K.; Reid, M.C.; Allpass, P.R. in "Nickel Toxicology"; Brown, S.S.; Sunderman, F.W., Jr., Eds; Academic: New York, 1980; p. 113.
109. Sunderman, F.W., Jr. *EHP, Environ. Health Perspect.* **1981**, *40*, 131.
110. Miyaki, M.; Mutata, I.; Osabe, M.; Ono, T. *Biochem. Biophys. Res. Commun.* **1977**, *77*, 854.
111. McLean, J.R.; Williams, R.S.; Kaplan, J.G.; Birnbo, H.C. in "Progress in Mutation Research," Vol. 1; Elsevier/North Holland: Amsterdam, 1981; p. 828.
112. Hui, G.; Sunderman, F.W., Jr. *Carcinogenesis* **1980**, *1*, 297.
113. Kada, T.; Hirano, K.; Shirasu, Y. in "Chemical Mutagens Principles and Methods for their Detection," Vol. 6; de Serres, F.J.; Hollaender, A., Eds; Plenum: New York, 1980; p. 149.
114. Kanematsu, N.; Hara, M.; Kada, T. *Mutat. Res.* **1980**, *77*, 109.
115. LaVelle, J.M.; Witmer, C.M. *Environ. Mutagen.* **1981**, *3*, 320.
116. Swierenga, S.H.H.; Basrur, P.K. *Lab. Invest.* **1968**, *19*, 663.
117. Gläss, E. *Z. Bot.* **1956**, *44*, 1.
118. van Rosen, G. *Hereditas* **1954**, *40*, 258.
119. Levan, A. *Nature (London)* **1945**, *156*, 751.
120. Wulf, H.C. *Dan. Med. Bull.* **1980**, *27*, 40.
121. Saxholm, H.J.K.; Reith, A.; Brøgger, A. *Cancer Res.* **1981**, *41*, 4136.
122. Nishimura, M.; Umeda, M. *Mutat. Res.* **1978**, *54*, 246.
123. Amacher, D.E.; Paillet, S.C. *Mutat. Res.* **1980**, *78*, 279.
124. Hsie, A.W.; Johnson, N.P.; Couch, D.B.; San Sebastian, J.R.; O'Neill, J.P.; Hoeschele, J.D.; Rahn, R.O.; Forbes, N.L. in "Trace Metals in Health and Disease"; Karasch, N., Ed.; Raven: New York, 1979; p. 55.

125. Costa, M. in "Ultratrace Metal Analysis in Biological Sciences and Environment"; Risby, T.H., Ed.; ACS Advances in Chemistry Series No. 172; ACS: Washinton, D.C., 1979; p. 73.
126. Basrur, P.K.; Gilman, J.P.W. *Cancer Res.* **1967**, *27*, 1168.
127. Rivedal, E.; Sanner, T. *Cancer Res.* **1981**, *41*, 2950.
128. Webb, M.; Heath, J.C.; Hopkins, T. *Br. J. Cancer* **1972**, *26* 274.
129. Sutherland, R.B. "Report of the Division of Industrial Hygiene"; Ontario Dept. of Health, Toronto, 1959.
130. Gilman, J.P.W.; Ruckerbauer, G.M. *Cancer Res.* **1962**, *22*, 152.
131. Gilman, J.P.W. *Cancer Res.* **1962**, *22*, 158.
132. Gilman, J.P.W. Proc. 6th Can. Cancer Res. Conf., Pergamon: Toronto, 1966; p. 209.
133. Costa, M.; Simmons-Hansen, J.; Bedrossian, C.W.M.; Bonura, J.; Caprioli, R.M. *Cancer Res.* **1981**, *41*, 2868.
134. Heck, J.D.; Costa, M. *Cancer Lett.* **1982**, *15*, 19.
135. Hilderbrand, H.; Biserte, G. *Cancer* **1979**, *43*, 1358.
136. Hueper, W.C. *AMA Arch. Pathol.* **1958**, *65*, 600.
137. Sunderman, F.W.; Donnelly, A.J.; West, B.; Kincaid, J.F. *AMA Arch. Ind. Health* **1959**, *20*, 36.
138. Sunderman, F.W., Jr. *Ann. Clin. Lab. Sci.* **1977**, *7*, 377.
139. Ottolenghi, A.D.; Haseman, J.K.; Payne, W.W.; Falk, H.L.; McFarland, H.N. *JNCI, J. Natl. Cancer Inst.* **1975**, *54*, 1165.
140. Saknyn, A.V.; Blokhin, V.A. Vopr. Onkol. **1978**, *24*, 44.
141. Gilman, J.P.W. *Proc. Can. Fed. Biol. Soc.* **1980**, *23*, 121.
142. Yarita, T.; Nettesheim, P. *Cancer Res.* **1978**, *38*, 3140.
143. Kasprzak, K.S.; Marchow, L.; Breborowicz, J. *Res. Commun. Chem. Pathol. Pharmacol.* **1973**, *6*, 237.
144. Mukabo, K. *J. Nara Med. Assoc.* **1978**, *29*, 321.
145. Damjanov, I.; Sunderman, F.W., Jr.; Mitchell, J.M.; Allpass, P.R. *Cancer Res.* **1978**, *38*, 268.
146. Jasmin, G.; Solymoss, B. in "Inorganic and Nutritional Aspects of Cancer"; Schrauzer, G.N., Ed.; Plenum: New York, 1978; p. 69.
147. Roberts, R.S.; Julian, J.A.; Shannon, H.S.; Muir, D.C.F. in "Nickel Toxicology"; Braun, S.S.; Sunderman, F.W., Jr., Eds.; Academic: New York, 1980; p. 27.
148. Roberts, R.S.; Julian, T.A.; Muir, D.C.F. Internal Report, International Nickel Company Canada, June 1982.
149. NIOSH Criteria Document, U.S. Dept. of Health; Education & Welfare, Publication No. 77–164, May 1977.
150. Enterline, P.E.; Marsh, G.M. *JNCI, J. Natl. Cancer. Inst.* **1982**, *68*, 925.
151. Saknyn, A.V.; Shabynina, N.K. *Gig. Tr. Prof. Zabol.* **1973**, *17*, 25.
152. Pederson, E.; Høgetweit, A.C.; Andersen, A. *Int. J. Cancer* **1973**, *12*, 32.
153. Pederson, E.; Andersen, A.; Høgetweit, A.C. *Ann. Clin. Lab. Sci.* **1978**, *8*, 503.
154. Reed, D.; Lessard, R.; Maheux, B. *Am. J. Epidemiol.* **1978**, *108*, 233.
155. Torjussen, W. *Acta Otolaryngol.* **1979**, *88*, 279.
156. Nelen, J.M.B.; McEwan, J.D.; Thompson, D.W.; Walker, G.R.; Pearson, F.G. *Thoracic Cardiovasc. Surg.* **1979**, *77*, 522.
157. "IARC Monographs on the Evaluation of the Carcinogenic Risk of Chemicals to Man," Vol. 11, 1976.
158. Rohrer, S.R.; Shaw, S.M.; Van Sickle, D.C. in "Cadmium Toxicity"; Mennear, J.H., Ed.; Marcel Dekker: New York, 1979; p. 159.
159. Dhanze, J.R.; Jayaram, K.C. *Curr. Sci.* **1979**, *48*, 1008.
160. O'Riordan, M.L.; Hughes, E.G.; Evans, H.J. *Mutat. Res.* **1978**, *58*, 305.
161. Deaven, L.L.; Campbell, E.W. *J. Cell Biol.* **1978**, *79*, 131a.
162. Haddow, A.; Roe, F.J.C.; Dukes, C.E.; Mitchley, B.V.C. *Br. J. Cancer* **1964**, *18*, 667.

163. Kazantzi, G.; Hanbury, W.J. *Br. J. Cancer* **1966**, *20*, 190.
164. Heath, J.C.; Daniel, M.R. *Br. J. Cancer* **1964**, *18*, 124.
165. Furst, A. *Toxicol. Appl. Pharmacol.* **1978**, *45*, 305.
166. Roe, F.J.C.; Dukes, C.E.; Cameron, K.M.; Pugh, R.C.B.; Mitchley, B.C.V. *Br. J. Cancer* **1964**, *18*, 674.
167. Gunn, S.A.; Gould, T.C.; Anderson, W.A.D. *JNCI, J. Natl. Cancer Inst.* **1963**, *31*, 745.
168. Lucis, O.J.; Lucis, R.; Aterman, K. *Oncology* **1972**, *26*, 53.
169. Gunn, S.A.; Gould, T.C.; Anderson, W.A.D. *Proc. Soc. Exp. Biol. Med.* **1964**, *115*, 653.
170. Furst, A.; Cassetta, D.M.; Sasmore, O.P. *Proc. West. Pharmacol. Soc.* **1973**, *16*, 150.
171. Levy, L.S.; Roe, F.J.C.; Malcolm, D.; Kayantsis, G.; Clack, J.; Platt, H.S. *Ann. Occup. Hyg.* **1973**, *16*, 111.
172. Levy, L.S.; Clack, J. *Ann. Occup. Hyg.* **1975**, *17*, 205.
173. Scott, R.; Aughey, E. *Br. J. Urol.* **1978**, *50*, 25.
174. Lauwerys, R.R. in "Trace Metals, Exposure and Health Effects"; DiFerrante, E., Ed.; Pergamon Press: New York, 1978; p. 43.
175. Potts, C.L. *Ann. Occup. Hyg.* **1965**, *8*, 55.
176. Kipling, M.D.; Waterhouse, J.A.H. *Lancet* **1967**, *1*, 730.
177. Lemen, R.A.; Lee, J.S.; Wagoner, J.K.; Blejer, H.P. *Ann. N.Y. Acad. Sci*, **1976**, *271*, 273.
178. Kolonel, L.N. *Cancer* **1976**, *37*, 1782.
179. Whiting, R.F.; Stich, H.F.; Koropatnick, D.J. *Chem.-Biol. Interact.* **1979**, *26*, 267.
180. Brusick, D.B.; Gletten, F.; Japannath, D.; Weeker, U. *Mutat. Res.* **1976**, *38*, 386.
181. Reddy, T.P.; Vaidyanath, K. *Curr. Sci.* **1978**, *47*, 513.
182. Whiting, R.F.; Wei, L.; Stich, H.F. *Cancer Res.* **1981**, *41*, 1628.
183. Richmond, H.G. *Br. Med. J.* **1959**, *1*, 947.
184. Furst, A.; Haro, R.T. *Prog. Exp. Tumor Res.* **1969**, *12*, 102.
185. Fielding, J. *Scand. J. Haematol., Suppl.* **1977**, *32*, 100.
186. Haddow, A.; Horning, E.S. *JNCI, J. Natl. Cancer Inst.* **1960**, *24*, 109.
187. Hueper, W.C. *A.M.A. Arch. Pathol.* **1959**, *67*, 589.
188. Roe, F.J.C.; Haddow, A. *Br. J. Cancer* **1965**, *19*, 855.
189. Roe, F.J.C.; Carter, R.L. *Int. J. Cancer* **1967**, *2*, 370.
190. Langvad, E. *Int. J. Cancer* **1968**, *3*, 415.
191. Campbell, J.A. *Br. Med. J.* **1940**, *ii*, 275.
192. O'Gara, R.W.; Brown, J.M. *JNCI, J. Natl. Cancer Inst.* **1967**, *38*, 947.
193. Hueper, W.C.; Payne, W.W. *Arch. Environ. Health* **1962**, *5*, 445.
194. Saffiotti, U.; Cefis, F.; Shubik, P. *Proc. 3rd Quad. Int. Conf. Cancer* **1966**, 537.
195. Montesano, R.; Saffiotti, U.; Shubik, P. *Proc. Biol. Div. U.S. Atomic Energy Cancer Conf.* **1970**, 353.
196. Feron, V.J.; Emmelot, P.; Vossenaar, T. *Eur. J. Cancer* **1972**, *8*, 445.
197. Ho, W.; Furst, A. *Oncology* **1973**, *27*, 385.
198. Nettesheim, P.; Creasia, D.A.; Mitchell, T. *JNCI, J. Natl. Cancer Inst.* **1975**, *55*, 159.
199. Saffiotti, U.; Cefis, F.; Kolb, L.H. *Cancer Res.* **1968**, *28*, 104.
200. Creasia, D.A.; Nettesheim, P. in "Experimental Lung Cancer"; Karbe, E.; Park, J.F., Eds.; Springer-Verlag: Berlin, 1974; p. 234.
201. Fisher, G.L. in "Trace Metals in Health and Disease"; Karasch, N., Ed.; Raven Press: New York, 1979; p. 93.
202. Harris, C.L.; Smith, J.M.; Spora, M.B.; Saffiotti, U. *Proc. Am. Assoc. Cancer Res.* **1971**, *12*, 13.
203. Stenback, F.; Rowland, J. *Eur. J. Cancer* **1978**, *14*, 321.
204. Axelson, O.; Sjoberg, A. *J. Occup. Med.* **1979**, *21*, 419.
205. Anthoine, D.; Larny, P.; deRen, G.; Cervoni, P.; Petiet, G.; Schwartz, P.; Lamaze, R.; Zuck, P. *Ann. Méd. Nancy Est* **1979**, *18*, 461.

206. "IARC Monographs on the Evaluation of Carcinogenic Risk of Chemicals to Man," Vol. 1, Lyon, 1972.
207. Great Britain, Office of Population Census and Surveys. "Occupational Mortality 1970–1972," Registrar General's Diennial Supplement, England and Wales, 1978.
208. Egan, B.; Waxweiler, R.J.; Blade, L. *J. Environ. Pathol. Toxicol.* **1978**, *2*, 259.
209. Deconfle, P.; Wood, D.J. *Am. J. Epidemiol.* **1979**, *109*, 667.
210. Kraus, A.S.; Levin, M.L.; Gerhardt, P.R. *Am. J. Public Health* **1957**, *47*, 961.
211. Hoffmann, D.J.; Niyogi, S.K. *Science (Washington, D.C.)* **1977**, *198*, 513.
212. Vollmann, J. *Schweiz. Z. Allg. Pathol. Bakteriol.* **1938**, *1*, 440.
213. Thomas, J.A.; Thiery, J.P. *C.R. Acad. Sci.* **1953**, *236*, 1387.
214. Heath, J.C. *Nature (London)* **1954**, *173*, 822.
215. Morin, Y.; Daniel, P. *J. Can. Med. Assoc.* **1967**, *97*, 926.
216. Grice, H.C.; Goodman, T.; Munroe, I.C.; Wiberg, G.S.; Morrison, H.B. *Ann. N.Y. Acad. Sci.* **1969**, *156*, 189.
217. Saffiotti, U.; Cefis, F.; Kolb, L.H.; Grote, M.I. *Proc. Am. Assoc. Cancer Res.* **1963**, *4*, 59.
218. Wehner, A.P.; Busch, R.H.; Olson, R.J.; Craig, D.K. *Am. Ind. Hyg. Assoc. J.* **1977**, *38*, 338.
219. Kasirsky, G.; Gautieri, R.F.; Mann, D.E., Jr. *J. Pharm. Sci.* **1965**, *54*, 491.
220. Coates, E.O.; Watson, J.H.L. *Ann. Intern. Med.* **1971**, *75*, 709.
221. Hamilton, A. in "Industrial Toxicology"; Hardy, H.L., Ed.; Publ. Sci. Group Inc.: Acton, MA, 1973; p. 78.
222. Ferguson, A.B., Jr.; Akkahoshi, Y.; Laing, P.G.; Hodge, E.S. *J. Bone Jt. Surg.* **1962**, *44A*, 323.
223. Duke, V.E.; Fisher, D.E. *Cancer* **1972**, *30*, 1260.
224. Banks, W.C.; Morris, E.; Herron, M.R.; Green, R.W. *J. Am. Vet. Med. Assoc.* **1975**, *167*, 166.
225. Harrison, J.W.; McLain, D.L.; Hohn, R.B.; Wilson, G.P.; Cholman, J.A.; McGowan, K.N. *Clin. Orthop.* **1976**, *116*, 253.
226. Heath, J.C.; Freeman, M.A.; Swanson, S.A. *Lancet* **1971**, *1*, 564.
227. Swanson, S.A.V.; Freeman, M.A.R.; Heath, J.C. *J. Bone Jt. Surg.* **1973**, *55B*, 759.
228. Editorial *Lancet* **1976**, *2*, 2.
229. Herbert, V. in "The Pharmacological Basis of Therapeutics"; Goodman, A.G.; Gilman, A., Eds.; Macmillan: New York, 1975; p. 1320.
230. Furst, A. in "Environmental Geochemistry in Health and Disease"; Cannon, H.L.; Hopps, H.C., Eds.; Geol. Soc. Am.: Boulder, CO, 1971, p. 109.
231. Bresler, W.M. *Acta Unio Int. Cancrum* **1964**, *20*, 1501.
232. Pimental, J.C.; Marques, F. *Thorax* **1969**, *24*, 678.
233. Kamamoto, Y.; Makiura, S.; Sugihara, S.; Hiasa, Y.; Arai, M.; Ho, N. *Cancer Res.* **1973**, *33*, 1129.
234. Rencher, A.C.; Carter, M.W.; McKee, D.W. *J. Occup. Med.* **1977**, *19*, 754.
235. Kuratsune, M. *Jpn. J. Cancer Clin.* **1978**, *24*, 814.
236. Braun, W. *Dtsch. Med. Wochenschr.* **1958**, *83*, 870.
237. Latarget, R.; Galy, P.; Maret, G.; Gallois, P. *Mem. Acad. Chir.* **1964**, *90*, 384.
238. Pimental, J.C.; Menezes, A.P. *Gastroenterology* **1977**, *72*, 275.
239. Luthra, U.K.; Mitra, A.B.; Prabhakar, A.K.; Bhatnagar, P.; Agarwal, S.S. *Indian J. Med. Res.* **1978**, *68*, 78.
240. Ramel, C.; Magnussen, J. *Environ. Health. Perspect.* **1979**, *31*, 59.
241. Schwanitz, G.; Lehnert, G.; Gebhart, E. *Dtsch. Med. Wochenschr.* **1970**, *95*, 1636.
242. Kennedy, G.L.; Arnold, D.W. *Environ. Mut. Soc. Newsl.* **1971**, *5*, 37.
243. Zollinger, H.U. *Virchows. Arch. A: Pathol. Anat.* **1953**, *323*, 694.
244. Moore, M.R.; Meredith, P.A. *Arch. Toxicol.* **1979**, *42*, 87.
245. Van Esch, G.J.; Van Genderen, H.; Vink, H.H. *Br. J. Cancer* **1962**, *16*, 289.

246. Kanisawa, M.; Schroeder, H.A. *Cancer Res.* **1969**, *29*, 892.
247. Azar, A.: Trochmorvicz, H.J.; Maxfield, M.E. *Proc.—Int. Symp. Environ. Health Aspects Lead* 1973, Luxemburg, p. 199.
248. Van Esch, G.J.; Kroes, R. *Br. J. Cancer* **1969**, *23*, 765.
249. Zawirska, B.; Medras, K. *Arch. Immunol. Ther. Exp.* **1972**, *20*, 243.
250. Coogan, P.; Stern, L.; Hsu, G.; Hass, G. *Lab. Invest.* **1972**, *26*, 473.
251. Epstein, S.S.; Mantel, N. *Experientia* **1968**, *24*, 580.
252. McCreary, P.A.; Laing, G.H.; Coogan, P.S.; Hass, G.M. *Am. J. Pathol.* **1977**, *86*, 26A.
253. Kobayashi, N.; Okumoto, T. *JNCI, J. Natl. Cancer Inst.* **1974**, *52*, 1605.
254. Sagiura, K. *Nagoya-shiritsu Daigaku Igakkai Zasshi* **1972**, *23*, 332.
255. Malcolm, D. *Arch. Environ. Health* **1971**, *23*, 292.
256. Nelson, W.C.; Lykins, M.H.; MacKey, J.; Newell, V.A.; Findlea, J.T.; Hammer, D.T. *J. Chronic Dis.* **1973**, *26*, 105.
257. Cooper, W.C. *Ann. N.Y. Acad. Sci.* **1976**, *271*, 250.
258. Kantor, A.F.; Curnen, M.G.; Meigs, J.W.; Flannery, J.T. *J. Epidemiol. Community Health* **1979**, *33*, 253.
259. Elwood, P.C.; St. Leger, N.S.; Moore, F.; Morton, M. *Lancet* **1976**, *1*, 748.
260. Schrauzer, G.N.; White, D.A.; Schneider, C.J. *Bioinorg. Chem.* **1977**, *7*, 35.
261. Fieve, R.S. *Trends NeuroSci. (Pers. Ed.)* **1979**, *2*, 66.
262. Stein, R.S.; Flexner, J.M.; Graber, S.E. *Blood* **1979**, *54*, 636.
263. Stein, R.S. "Workshop on Effects of Lithium on Granulopoiesis and Immune Function"; Robinson, W.A., Rossof, A.H., Eds.; Plenum Press: New York, 1980.
264. Sethi, B.B.; Prakash, R.; Sethi, N. *Psychopharmacol. Bull.* **1981**, *4*, 5.
265. Orr, L.E.; McKennan, J.F. *Lancet* **1979**, *24*, 449.
266. Hammond, W.P.; Appelbaum, F. *N. Engl. J. Med.* **1980**, *302*, 808.
267. Leber, P. *Psychopharmacol. Bull.* **1981**, *2*, 10.
268. Mitchell, B.; Gerdes, R.A. *Fluoride* **1973**, *6*, 113.
269. McLean, J.R.; Kaplan, J.G. in "The Molecular Basis of Immune Cell Function"; Kaplan, J.G., Ed.; Elsevier/North-Holland: Amsterdam, 1981; p. 412.
270. Walters, M.; Roe, F.J.C. *Food Cosmet. Toxicol.* **1965**, *3*, 271.
271. Roe, F.J.C.; Boyland, E.; Millican, K. *Food Cosmet. Toxicol.* **1965**, *3*, 277.
272. Bischoff, F.; Bryson, G. *Res. Commun. Chem. Pathol. Pharmacol.* **1976**, *15*, 331.
273. National Toxicology Program; Technical Report Series No. 231; "Carcinogenesis Bioassay of Stannous Chloride"; U.S. Dept. of Health and Human Services, NIH, June 1982.
274. Murray, M.J.; Flessel, C.P. *Biochim. Biophys. Acta* **1976**, *425*, 256.
275. Venitt, S.; Levy, L.S. *Nature (London)* **1974**, *250*, 493.
276. Kalinina, L.M.; Polukhina, G.H. *Mutat. Res.* **1977**, *46*, 223.
277. Voroshilin, S.I.; Plotko, E.G.; Fink, T.V.; Nikifora, V.Y. *Tsitol. Genet.* **1978**, *12*, 241.
278. De Knudt, G.H. *Mutat. Res.* **1978**, *53*, 176.
279. Duncan, J.R.; Dreosti, I.E. *JNCI, J. Natl. Cancer. Inst.* **1975**, *55*, 195.
280. Heath, J.C.; Daniel, M.R.; Dingle, J.T.; Webb, M. *Nature (London)* **1962**, *193*, 592.
281. Furst, H.; Cassetta, D. *Proc. Am. Assoc. Cancer. Res.* **1972**, *13*, 62.
282. Mesrobian, A. *J. Dent. Res.* **1976**, *55*, B66.
283. Elinder, C.-G.; Piscator, M. in "Handbook on the Toxicology of Metals"; Friberg, L.; Nordberg, C.F.; Vouk, V.B., Eds.; Elsevier/North Holland: New York, 1979; p. 675.
284. Furst, A.; Radding, S.B. *Biol. Trace Element Res.* **1979**, *1*, 169.
285. Fishbein, L. in "Toxicology of Trace Elements"; Goyer, R.A.; Mehlman, M.A., Eds.; Hemisphere Publishing Corp.: Washington, D.C., 1977; p. 203.
286. Colmano, G. *Bull. Environ. Contam. Toxicol.* **1973**, *9*, 361.
287. "Handbook on the Toxicology of Metals"; Friberg, L.; Nordberg, G.F.; Vouk, V.B., Eds.; Elsevier/North Holland: Amsterdam, 1979.
288. Schroeder, H.A.; Balassa, J.J.; Vinton, W.H., Jr. *Nutrition (London)* **1964**, *83*, 239.

289. Schroeder, H.A.; Kanisawa, M.; Frost, D.V.; Mitchener, M. *J. Nutr.* 1968, *96*, 37.
290. Schroeder, H.A.; Mitchener, M.; Balassa, J.J.; Kanisawa, M.; Nason, A.P. *J. Nutr.* **1968**, *95*, 95.
291. Schroeder, H.A.; Mitchener, M. *J. Nutr.* **1971**, *101*, 1431.
292. Schroeder, H.A.; Mitchener, M. *J. Nutr.* **1971**, *101*, 1531.
293. Schroeder, H.A.; Mitchener, M. *Arch. Environ. Health* **1972**, *24*, 66.
294. Ball, R.A.; Van Gelder, G.; Green, J.W., Jr.; Reece, W.O. *Proc. Soc. Exp. Biol. Med.* **1970**, *135*, 426.
295. Groth, D.H. "Toxicology Research Projects Directory"; 1980, 05, #30109.
296. Groth, D.H. in "Effects and Dose Response Relationships of Toxic Metals"; Norberg, G.F., Ed.; Elsevier/North Holland: Amsterdam, 1976; p. 559.
297. Fuyuta, M.; Fujimoto, T.; Kiyofuji, E. *Acta Anat.* **1979**, *104*, 356.
298. Suzuki, T. in "Toxicology of Trace Elements"; Goyer, R.A.; Mehlman, M.A., Eds.; Hemisphere Publ. Co.: Washington, D.C., 1977; p. 6.
299. Popescu, H.I.; Negru, L.; Lancranjan, I. *Arch. Environ. Health* **1979**, *34*, 461.
300. Verschaeve, L.; Tassignon, J.-P.; Lefevre, M.; DeStoop, P.; Susanne, C. *Environ. Mutagenesis* **1979**, *1*, 259.
301. Schroeder, H.A.; Mitchener, M. *J. Nutr.* **1975**, *105*, 452.
302. Druckrey, H.; Hamperl, H.; Schmahl, D. *Z. Krebsforsch.* **1957**, *61*, 511.
303. Radding, S.B.; Furst, A. in "Molecular Basis of Environmental Toxicity"; Bhatnagar, R.S., Ed.; Ann Arbor Science Publ. Inc.: Ann Arbor, 1980; p. 359.
304. Nixon, J.E.; Koller, L.D.; Exon, J.H. *JNCI, J. Natl. Cancer Inst.* **1979**, *63*, 1057.
305. Leopold, W.R.; Miller, E.C.; Miller, J.A. *Cancer Res.* **1979**, *39*, 913.
306. Zwelling, L.A.; Anderson, T.; Kohn, K.W. *Cancer Res.* **1979**, *39*, 365.
307. Cohen, G.L.; Bauer, W.R.; Barton, J.K.; Lippard, S.J. *Science (Washington, D.C.)* **1979**, *203*, 1014.
308. Lecointe, P.; Macquet, J-P.; Butour, J-L.; Paoletti, C. *Mutat. Res.* **1977**, *48*, 139.
309. Monti-Bragadin, C.; Tomaro, C.M.; Banfi, E. *Chem.-Biol. Interact.* **1975**, *11*, 469.
310. Beck, D.J.; Brubaker, R.R. *Mutat. Res.* **1974**, *27*, 181.
311. Beck, D.J.; Fisch, J.E. *Mutat. Res.* **1980**, *77*, 45.
312. Suraikina, T.I.; Zakharova, I.A.; Mashkovsky, Y.S.; Fonshtein, L.M. *Tsitol. Genet.* **1979**, *13*, 486.
313. Andersen, K.S. *Mutat. Res.* **1979**, *67*, 209.
314. Taylor, R.T.; Happe, J.A.; Hanna, M.L.; Wu, R. *J. Environ. Sci. Health* **1979**, *A14*, 87.
315. Johnson, N.P.; Hoeschele, J.D.; Rahn, R.O.; Hsie, A.W. *Cancer Res.* **1980**, *40*, 1463.
316. Turnbull, D.; Popescu, N.C.; DiPaolo, J.A.; Myhr, B.C. *Mutat. Res.* **1979**, *66*, 267.
317. Zwelling, L.A.; Bradley, M.O.; Sharkey, N.A.; Anderson, T.; Kohn, K.W. *Mutat. Res.* **1979**, *67*, 271.
318. Wiencke, J.K.; Cervenka, J.; Paulus, H. *Mutat. Res.* **1979**, *68*, 69.
319. Meyne, J.; Lockhart, L.H.; Arrighi, F.E. *Mutat. Res.* **1979**, *63*, 201.
320. Schmaehl, D.; Steinhoff, D. *Z. Krebsforsch.* **1960**, *63*, 586.
321. Furst, A.; Schlauder, M.C. *J. Environ. Pathol. Toxicol.* **1977**, *1*, 51.
322. Schorn, D.; Anderson, I.F. *S. Afr. Med. J.* **1975**, *49*, 1505.
323. Evgen'eva, T.P. *Bull. Exp. Biol. Med. (Engl. Transl.)* **1972**, *74*, 1296.
324. Northdruft, H. *Naturwissenschaften*, **1955**, *42*, 75.
325. Oppenheimer, B.S.; Oppenheimer, E.T.; Danishefsky, I.; Stout, A.P. *Cancer Res.* **1956**, *16*, 439.
326. Northdurft, H. *Abh. Dtsch. Akad. Wiss. Berlin, Kl. Med.* **1960**, *3*, 80.
327. Northdruft, H. *Naturwissenschaften* **1962**, *49*, 18.
328. Sinibaldi, K.; Rosen, H.; Liu, S-K.; DeAngelis, M. *Clin. Orthop.* **1976**, *118*, 257.
329. Gaechter, A.; Alroy, J.; Anderson, G.B.J.; Galante, J.; Rostoker, W.; Schajowicz, F. *J. Bone Jt. Surg.* **1977**, *59*, 622.
330. Schmähl, D. *Oncology* **1976**, *2*, 73.

331. Manna, G.K.; Das, R.K. *Nucleus (Calcutta)* **1972**, *15*, 180.
332. Kobayashi, N.; Ide, G.; Katsuki, H.; Yamane, Y. *Gann* **1968**, *59*, 433.
333. Brand, K.G. in "Scientific Foundations of Oncology"; Symington, T.; Carter, R.L., Eds.; Wm. Heinmann: London, 1976; p. 490.
334. Milham, S., Jr. *J. Occup. Med.* **1979**, *21*, 475.
335. Gibbs, G.W.; Horowitz, I. *J. Occup. Med.* **1979**, *21*, 347.
336. Lloyd, J.W. *J. Occup. Med.* **1971**, *13*, 53.
337. Putrament, A.; Baronowska, H.; Ejchart, A.; Jachymczyk, W. *Mol. Gen. Genet.* **1977**, *151*, 69.
338. Singh, S.P.; Kashyap, A.K. *Environ. Exp. Bot.* **1978**, *18*, 47.
339. Sarma, T.A. *Indian J. Exp. Biol.* **1977**, *15*, 587.
340. Piscator, M. in "Handbook on the Toxicology of Metals"; Friberg, L.; Nordberg, G.F.; Vouk, V.B., Eds.; Elsevier/North Holland Press: Amsterdam, 1979; p. 485.
341. DiPaolo, J.A. *Fed. Proc.* **1964**, *23*, 393.
342. Stoner, G.D.; Shimkin, M.B.; Tronell, M.C.; Thompson, T.L.; Terry, L.S. *Cancer Res.* **1976**, *36*, 1744.
343. Sunderman, F.W., Jr.; Kasprzak, K.S.; Lan, T.J.; Minghetti, P.R.; Maenza, R.M.; Becker, N.; Onkelink, C.; Goldblatt, P.J. *Cancer Res.* **1976**, *36*, 1790.
344. Loefroth, G.; Ames, B.N. *Mutat. Res.* **1978**, *53*, 65.
345. Noda, M.; Takano, T.; Sakurai, H. *Mutat. Res.* **1979**, *66*, 175.
346. Lo, L.W.; Koropatnick, J.; Stich, H.F. *Mutat. Res.* **1978**, *49*, 305.
347. Ray, J.H.; Altenburg, L.C. *Mutat. Res.* **1978**, *54*, 343.
348. Shamberger, R.J. *Biol. Trace Element Res.* **1980**, *2*, 81.
349. Shapiro, J.R. *Ann. N.Y. Acad. Sci.* **1972**, *192*, 215.
350. Jaffe, W.G. *Arch. Latinoam. Nutr.* **1972**, *22*, 467.
351. Schrauzer, G.N.; White, D.A.; Schneider, C.J. *Bioinorg. Chem.* **1976**, *6*, 265.
352. Jacobs, M.M.; Jansson, B.; Griffin, C.A. *Cancer Lett.* **1977**, *2*, 133.
353. Shamberger, R.J.; Willis, C.E. *Clin. Lab. Sci.* **1971**, *2*, 211.
354. Glover, J.; Lavender, O.; Parizek, J.; Vouk, V. in "Handbook on the Toxicology of Metals"; Friberg, L.; Nordberg, G.F.; Vouk, V.B., Eds.; Elsevier/North Holland Press: Amsterdam, 1979; p. 555.
355. Tkeshelashvili, L.K.; Shearman, C.W.; Koplitz, R.M.; Zakour, R.A.; Loeb, L.A. *Proc. Am. Assoc. Cancer Res.* **1979**, *20*, 263.
356. Jung, E.G.; Trachsel, B.; Immich, H. *Germ. Med. Mth.* **1969**, *14*, 614.
357. Nakamuro, K.; Sayato, Y. *Mutat. Res.* **1981**, *88*, 73.
358. Oppenheim, J.P.; Fishbein, W.N. *Cancer Res.* **1965**, *25*, 980.
359. Wan, B.; Christian, R.T.; Soukup, S.W. *Environ. Mut.* **1982**, *4*, 493.
360. Röhr, G.; Bauchinger, M. *Mutat. Res.* **1976**, *40*, 125.
361. King, H.; Lunford, R.J. *J. Chem. Soc.* **1950**, *8*, 2086.
362. El-Sadek, L.M. *Egypt. J. Genet. Cytol.* **1972**, *1*, 218.
363. Rössner, P.; Cinatl, J.; Bencko, V. *Cesk. Hyg.* **1972**, *17*, 58.
364. Zanzoni, F.; Jung, E.G. *Arch. Dermatol. Res.* **1980**, *267*, 91.
365. Andersen, K.J.; Leighty, E.G.; Takahashi, M.T. *J. Agric. Food Chem.* **1972**, *20*, 649.
366. Simmon, V.F. *JNCI, J. Natl. Cancer Inst.* **1979**, *62*, 901.
367. Rosenkranz, H.S.; Leifer, Z. in "Chemical Mutagens, Principles and Methods for their Detection," Vol. 6; de Serres, F.J.; Hollaender, A., Eds.; Plenum Press: New York, 1980, p. 109.
368. Simmon, V.F.; Rosenkranz, H.S.; Zeiger, E.; Poirier, L.A. *JNCI, J. Natl. Cancer Inst.* **1979**, *62*, 911.
369. Maltoni, C. *Ann. N.Y. Acad. Sci,* **1976**, *271*, 444.
370. Ridgway, L.P.; Karnofsky, D.A. *Ann. N.Y. Acad. Sci.* **1952**, *55*, 203.
371. Nikiforov, Y.L.; Sakharova, M.N.; Beknazaryants, M.M.; Rapoport, I.A. *Dokl. Biol. Sci (Engl. Transl.)* **1970**, *194*, 520.

372. Nakamuro, K.; Yoshikawa, K.; Sayato, Y.; Kurata, H. *Mutat. Res.* **1978**, *58*, 175.
373. Tamino G. *Atti. Assoc. Genet. Ital.* **1977**, *22*, 69.
374. Majone, F. *Att. Assoc. Genet. Ital.* **1977**, *22*, 61.
375. Newbold, R.F.; Amos, J.; Connell, J.R. *Mutat. Res.* **1979**, *67*, 55.
376. Majone, F.; Levis, A.G. *Mutat. Res.* **1979**, *67*, 231.
377. Koshi, K. *Ind. Health* **1979**, *17*, 39.
378. Douglas, G.R.; Bell, R.D.L.; Grant, C.E.; Wytsma, J.M.; Bora, K.C. *Mutat. Res.* **1980**, *77*, 157.
379. Umeda, M.; Nishimura, M. *Mutat. Res.* **1979**, *67*, 221.
380. Tsuda, H.; Kato, K. *Mutat. Res.* **1977**, *46*, 87.
381. MacCrae, W.D.; Whiting, R.F.; Stich, H.F. *Chem.-Biol. Interact.* **1979**, *26*, 281.
382. Nestman, E.R.; Matula, T.; Douglas, G.R.; Bora, K.C.; Kowbel, D.J. *Mutat. Res.* **1979**, *66*, 357.
383. Tindall, K.R.; Warren, G.R.; Skaar, P.D. *Mutat. Res.* **1978**, *53*, 90.
384. Tomaro, M.; Banfi, E.; Venturini, S.; Monti-Bragadin, C. in "Proceedings of the 17th National Congress of the Italian Society for Microbiology," Padua, 1975; p. 411.
385. Petrilli, F.L.; De Flora, S. *Mutat. Res.* **1978**, *58*, 167.
386. Bonatti, S.; Meini, M.; Abbondanolo, A. *Mutat. Res.* **1975**, *38*, 147.
387. Tindall, K.R.; Hsie, A.W. *Environ. Mutagenesis* **1980**, *2*, 293.
388. Fradkin, A.; Janoff, A.; Lane, B.P.; Kuschner, M. *Cancer Res.* **1975**, *35*, 1058.
389. Jacquet, P.; Mayence, A. *Toxicol. Lett.* **1982**, *11*, 193.
390. Vasudev, V.; Krishnamurthy, N.B. *Curr. Sci.* **1979**, *48*, 1007.
391. Verne, J.; Fournier, E.; Aubert, M.; Hébert, S.; Richshoffer, N. *Rev. Int. Oceanogr. Méd.* **1974**, *XXXIII*, 147.
392. Mitra, R.S.; Bernstein, I.A. *J. Bacteriol.* **1978**, *133*, 75.
393. Shiraishi, Y.; Kurahashi, H.; Yosida, T.H. *Proc. Jpn. Acad.* **1972**, *48*, 133.
394. Yagi, T.; Nishioka, H. *Doshisha Daigaku Rikogaku Kenkyu Hokoku* **1977**, *18*, 63.
395. Mandel, R.; Ryser, J.P. *Environ. Mutagenesis* **1981**, *3*, 333.
396. Kury, G.; Crosby, R.J. *Toxicol. Appl. Pharmacol.* **1968**, *13*, 199.
397. Namba, M.; Nishitani, K.; Kimoto, T. *Jpn. J. Exp. Med.* **1978**, *48*, 303.
398. Varma, M.M.; Joshi, S.R.; Adeyemi, A.O. *Experientia* **1974**, *30*, 486.
399. Mukherji, S.; Maitra, P. *Indian. J. Exp. Biol.* **1976**, *14*, 519.
400. Bauchinger, M.; Schmid, E. *Mutat. Res.* **1972**, *14*, 95.
401. Beek, B.; Obe, G. *Experientia* **1974**, *30*, 1006.
402. Stella, M.; Rossi, R.; Martinucci, G.B.; Rossi, G.; Bonfante, A. *Biochem. Exp. Biol.* **1978**, *14*, 221.
403. Beek, B.; Obe, G. *Hum. Genet.* **1975**, *29*, 127.
404. Hessler, A. *Mutat. Res.* **1975**, *31*, 43.
405. Shargel, L.; Masnyj, J. *Toxicol. Appl. Pharmacol.* **1981**, *59*, 452.
406. Litton Bionetics, Inc. "Mutagenic Evaluation of Compound FDA 71–33, Stannous Chloride"; Natl. Technical Information Service, PB–245461, 1974.
407. Kanisawa, M.; Schroeder, H.A. *Cancer Res.* **1967**, *27*, 1192.
408. Stocks, P. *Br. J. Cancer* **1960**, *14*, 397.
409. Agnew, W.F. *Tetratology* **1972**, *6*, 331.
410. Ferm, V.H.; Carpenter, S.J. *Toxicol. Appl. Pharmacol.* **1970**, *16*, 166.
411. Hart, M.M.; Adamson, R.H. *Proc. Natl. Acad. Sci. (USA)* **1971**, *68*, 1623.
412. Umeda, M.; Saito, K.; Hirose, K.; Saito, M. *Jpn. J. Exp. Med.* **1969**, *39*, 47.
413. Gruenwedel, D.W.; Lu, D.S. *Biophys. Soc. Annu. Meet. Abstr.* 14th **1970**, 169A.
414. Kanematsu, K.; Kada, T. *Mutat. Res.* **1978**, *78*, 207.
415. Woodruff, R.C.; Valencia, R.; Lyman, R.F.; Earle, B.A.; Boyce, J.T. *Environ. Mutagenesis* **1980**, *2*, 133.
416. Morrison, W.D.; Huff, V.; Colyer, S.; Littlefield, G.; DuFrain, R. *Environ. Mutagenesis* **1980**, *2*, 298.

417. Arnold, D.W.; Kennedy, G.L., Jr.; Keplinger, M.L.; Calandra, J.C. *Genetics* **1975**, *80*, S10.
418. Harder, H.; Rosenberg, B. *Int. J. Cancer* **1970**, *6*, 207.
419. Schrauzer, G.N.; Ishmael, D. *Ann. Clin. Lab. Sci.* **1974**, *4*, 441.
420. Kobayashi, N.; Katsuki, H.; Yamane, Y. *Gann* **1970**, *61*, 239.
421. Fare, G.; Howell, J.S. *Cancer Res.* **1964**, *24*, 1279.
422. Shamberger, R.J. *JNCI, J. Natl. Cancer Inst.* **1970**, *44*, 931.
423. Jacobs, M.M. *Cancer* **1977**, *40*, 2557.
424. Lane, B.P.; Mass, M.J. *Cancer Res.* **1977**, *37*, 1476.
425. Saffiotti, U.; Montesano, R.; Sellakumar, R.R.; Kaufman, D.G. *JNCI, J. Natl. Cancer Inst.* **1972**, *49*, 1199.
426. Schreiber, H.; Martin, D.H.; Pazmino, M. *Cancer Res.* **1975**, *35*, 1654.
427. Demerec, M.; Janson, J. *Cold Spring Harbor Symp. Quant. Biol.* **1951**, *16*, 215.
428. Orgel, A.; Orgel, L.E. *J. Mol. Biol.* **1965**, *14*, 453.
429. Böhme, H. *Biol. Zentralbl.* **1961**, *80*, 5.
430. Nakamuro, K.; Yoshikawa, K.; Sayato, Y.; Kurata, H.; Tonormura, M.; Tonomura, A. *Mutat. Res.* **1976**, *40*, 177.
431. Walker, G.W.R.; Ting, K.P. *Can. J. Genet. Cytol.* **1967**, *9*, 314.
432. *Environ. Health Criter.* **1980**, *15*, 77.

11

Mineral Fiber Carcinogenesis

J. C. WAGNER

Pneumoconiosis Unit, Medical Research Council, Llandough Hospital, Penarth, Glamorgan, Wales

EVIDENCE STILL SUGGESTS A CARCINOGENIC ASSOCIATION for the various forms of asbestos, and recently, many other fibrous minerals have been recognized as potentially dangerous pollutants of the environment. The majority of these materials occur naturally, but some are synthetic. The natural fibers either are specifically exploited for commercial purposes or occur as atmospheric contaminants that are released during mining or tunnelling operations. Industry has been developing other mineral fibers as a cheap and reliable insulating substitute for asbestos. Minerals being exploited for a variety of purposes other than insulation and reinforcement are known to consist of fibers or elongated crystals, for example, some clays and some zeolites.

Although the biological effects of these mineral fibers have aroused considerable interest (*1–3*), information on many of the fibers is incomplete, and as yet their biological properties are largely unknown. For other fibers there is epidemiological evidence, or the results of experimental studies are known. Because some of these materials are of possible economic and environmental importance, it would be unwise to present preliminary information before full investigations are completed.

In this chapter, the fibrous minerals will be considered under the following headings: (1) asbestos minerals of commercial value; (2) asbestos minerals as potential environmental contaminants; (3) synthetic mineral fibers; (4) naturally occurring fibrous minerals of commercial value; and (5) naturally occurring fibrous minerals as potential environmental contaminants. Figures 1–4 are four types of fibers that are discussed; crocidolite (Figure 1), fine tremolite (Figure 2), and erionite (Figure 3) occur naturally, and rockwool (Figure 4) is synthetic.

Asbestos Minerals

Asbestos of Commercial Value. Practically all the present knowledge about the hazards associated with inhalation of fibrous mineral dusts has been obtained in studies of asbestos. Asbestos is now considered to consist of six naturally occurring minerals: chrysotile, crocidolite, amosite, anthophyllite, tremolite, and actinolite. Chrysotile is a member of a group of minerals referred to as the serpentines and is

0065-7719/84/0182-0631$06.00/1

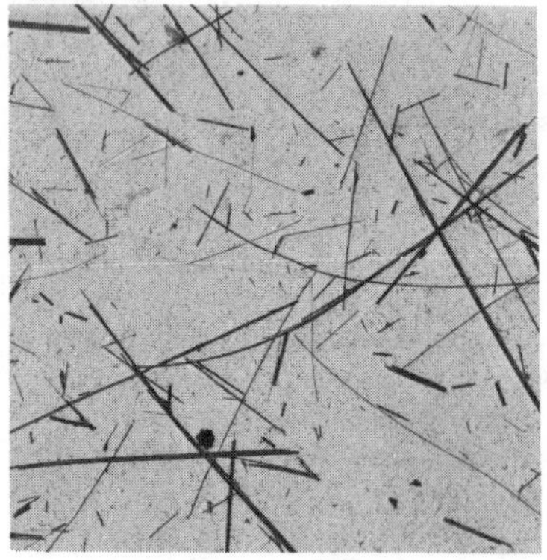

Figure 1. Crocidolite.

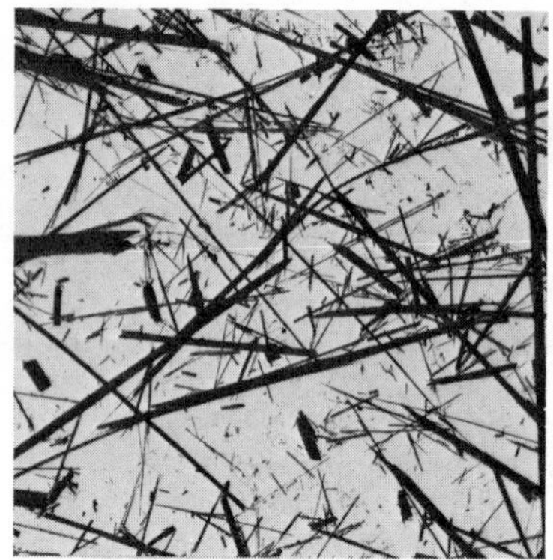

Figure 2. Fine tremolite (Korea).

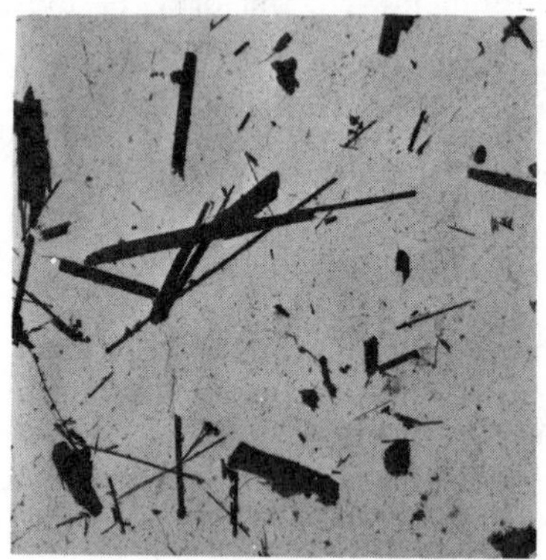

Figure 3. Erionite.

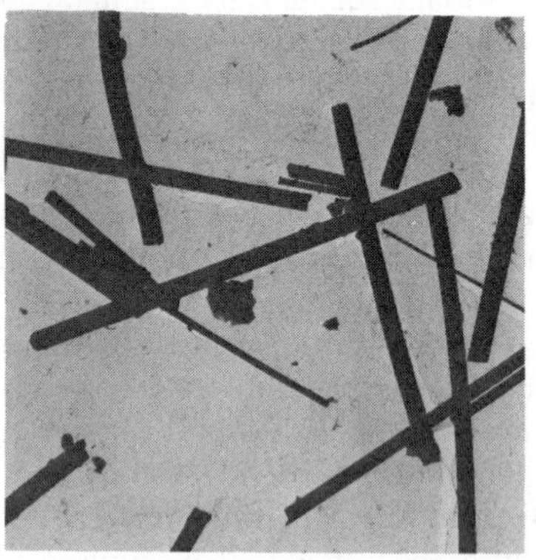

Figure 4. Rockwool (United States).

10 μm

composed almost exclusively of magnesium in combination with silica. Chrysotile has a sheet structure that curls to produce hollow tube-like fibers. The other five, members of the mineralogical group referred to as the amphiboles, are very similar in crystal structure, being chain silicates, but they vary in chemical composition. Crocidolite and amosite are iron-rich varieties, anthophyllite is a magnesium-rich mineral, and tremolite and actinolite contain a large amount of calcium together with magnesium.

The world production of asbestos in 1976 was 5×10^9 kg; 97% of this was chrysotile and the remainder was crocidolite and amosite. The commercial production of the other three amphiboles has been minimal in the past, but they are important as contaminants of other minerals and agricultural soil, as will be discussed later in this chapter. Chrysotile is widely distributed, with the largest commercial production from the Ural mountains in Russia, Quebec Province in Canada, Zimbabwe and Swaziland in Southern Africa, the Italian Alps, and Cyprus. Crocidolite now is mined almost exclusively in the Cape Province in

South Africa, and until recently in Western Australia. Amosite is exploited only in the Transvaal, but deposits have been discovered in Southern India.

Asbestos has over a thousand uses (*4*) so that the number of occupations in which exposure may have occurred is large. Crocidolite, because of its resistance to acids and sea water, was extensively used in naval insulation and fireproofing, as insulation for steam locomotive boilers, and later for soundproofing in passenger coaches. A significant amount was used in the insulation of buildings. The use of crocidolite and its importation into Britain has been severely limited since 1969 (*5*). Amosite has been used for thermal insulation, in floor tiles, and in the superstructure of ships. Chrysotile has been used for all other purposes, but particularly in asbestos cement products, insulation, fireproofing, and in the manufacture of friction materials such as brake linings and clutch plates. Chrysotile is still the main fiber used in textiles, but this is no longer a major section of the industry. The destruction or demolition of buildings, ships, and railway rolling stock is a source of environmental pollution.

Asbestos Minerals as Potential Environmental Contaminants. ASBESTIFORM MINERALS CONTAMINATING BANDED IRONSTONE. Although banded ironstone deposits frequently contain seams of fibrous silicates, most of which are small, occasionally large deposits occur. These large deposits are the source of the amphibole asbestos fibers that are exploited in the southern hemisphere. Other deposits are of no commercial value; for example, the taconite fibers in the Mesabi Range on the shores of Lake Superior. Although iron-ore mining in this region is causing contamination both of the atmosphere and the water of the lake, no evidence of a hazard to humans has been established. All the fibers are less than 5.0 μm long.

TREMOLITE AS A CONTAMINANT OF OTHER MINERAL DEPOSITS. Tremolite is an amphibole fiber; it is friable and of little economic importance, but has been used as an industrial talc. This fiber is a contaminant in talc and chrysotile deposits and is released when the materials are milled. It has been used as material for stuccoing of domestic dwellings in certain villages in Turkey (*6*), Cyprus, and elsewhere in the Eastern Mediterranean. In Turkey, villagers collect it from quarries that have been used for generations. In the vicinity of the chrysotile asbestos mine in Cyprus, tremolite is sometimes removed from the tailing dumps. In Korea there are mines producing tremolite for which a market is being sought.

POSSIBLE CONTAMINATION IN AGRICULTURE. Fibrous mineral contamination in agriculture has been appreciated only during the last few years, and may be shown to be of consequence. Evidence to date is still fragmentary. The only confirmed situation as far as asbestos is concerned is in Bulgaria, where the finding of pleural plaques in workers in the tobacco fields containing tremolite and anthophyllite in the soil has been reported (*7, 8*).

Synthetic Mineral Fibers

Synthetic mineral fibers can be divided into four groups: slag wools, rockwools, glass and ceramic wools, and filaments. The materials of each group consist of glassy mineral fibers. All man-made mineral fibers are formed from a liquid melt at temperatures of 1000–1500 °C, but the methods of producing the fibers vary.

All the man-made mineral fibers produced have glassy structures, and thus are not crystalline. Their length and diameter distributions differ considerably and are dependent on the method of production and the chemical composition. Usually, commercially produced fibers of man-made minerals are considerably coarser than asbestos fibers, although specialized samples have been produced with dimensions very similar to those of asbestos. These synthetic fibers fall into three broad categories of fiber size. The first is the continuous filament glass fibers that are used in textiles, and as a reinforcement for plastics and other materials; the products have fiber diameters greater than 8 μm. In the second category are insulation wools with fibers nominally 1–6 μm in diameter; however, there are ends that go down to 0.2 μm. The third category contains fibers smaller than 1.0 μm in diameter, which are used for specialized purposes such as scientific filter papers.

Man-made mineral fibers are usually coated with binding compounds to produce fabricated shapes and forms. In the past, insulation wool binders have included bitumen, urea, and phenol–formaldehyde resin compounds. Today, innovations in binding agents based on resin systems are continuously being made (*9*).

Naturally Occurring Fibrous Minerals

The naturally occurring fibrous minerals are a miscellaneous collection. The majority are silicates, but one metal, rutile (the fibrous form of titanium), is proving of interest because it has been recovered from the lungs of various industrial workers including slate-miners and processors. The two groups of fibrous silicates of particular current interest are the clays and the zeolites. Zeolites are a complex group of silicates formed by metamorphosis in deposits of volcanic ash. They are characterized by an open lattice structure useful for filtration, catalysis, and adsorption in the chemical industry and agriculture. Most of the commercially used zeolites are now synthesized and nonfibrous. Few of the natural materials are fibrous, but there are at least three—mordenite, clinoptilite, and erionite. These fibrous zeolites form hexagonal glassy rods that may occur singly or in strands and vary in diameter from deposit to deposit. Extremely fine erionite fibers have been found in a few deposits in Oregon in the United States and in central Turkey. The implications of erionite fibers will be explained later.

The absorbent clays have been used for various industrial purposes for many years, and recently there has been an increasing demand for these materials as cat litter. A chance discovery was that some of the material used for cat litter was fibrous in nature. Although these minerals appeared visually to consist of solid minerals, when finely group samples were examined under the transmission electron microscope, they were found to contain numerous short fine fibers. The fibers were particularly noticeable in minerals of the meerschaum ground including attapulgite, palygorscite, and sepiolite.

Sequelae of Exposure to Asbestos Dust

There have been numerous descriptions of the lesions resulting from exposure to asbestos dusts. Wagner (*10*) illustrated the lesions associated with the different types of fiber. The sequelae are as follows: (1) the presence of asbestos bodies in the sputum, (2) pleural plaques and diffuse pleural fibrosis, (3) interstitial pulmonary fibrosis (asbestosis), (4) carcinoma of the lung, (5) diffuse mesothelioma of pleura and peritoneum, and (6) an increased incidence of gastrointestinal tumors and possible increase in incidence of carcinoma of the larynx. On detailed investigation, each of these findings has provided problems that not only apply to asbestos exposure, but also have to be considered in the wider assessment of the other mineral fibers.

Asbestos Bodies and Fibers in the Sputum and Lung Tissue. Asbestos bodies consist of an iron–mucoprotein complex that surrounds the asbestos fibers after inhalation and retention in the lungs. These bodies usually have bulbous ends giving the appearance of drumsticks. Initially, the bodies were known as asbestosis bodies, suggesting that their presence was indicative of the presence of disease—asbestosis. It soon became clear that the presence of these coated fibers was at most indicative of occupational exposure to asbestos. Later, as more sensitive means of detection were developed (*11, 12*), it was realized that these bodies can be found in the lungs of practically everyone who has lived in an urban environment, and they are usually found around a core of amphibole fiber. Recently, these bodies have been identified in the lungs of animals exposed to glass fiber, and in humans, similar bodies have been seen surrounding erionite fibers (*13*). Under the transmission electron microscope, uncoated fibers are far more common in material extracted from macerated lung tissue; the ratio of fibers to asbestos bodies is greater than 1000:1. With the development of the more sophisticated techniques, it is obvious that a correct estimation of the number of fibers in either tissue or environmental samples can be obtained only by examination under a transmission electron microscope, otherwise the large number of fibers less than 0.5 μm in diameter will not be observed. The crucial question of the amount of fiber found in tissue that can be related to the diseases, which will be described later, cannot be stated with confidence at this stage. Also, the accuracy of result will depend on the type and size of fiber.

Pleural Plaques and Diffuse Pleural Fibrosis. Bilateral circumscribed areas of fibrous thickening on the lower portion of the chest wall below the mesothelium are characteristic of exposure to fibrous mineral dusts. These plaques are leaf-shaped, have an irregular embossed surface, and may be extensive. A frequent area for the development of these plaques is over the dome of the diaphragm.

Asbestosis. Asbestosis is a persistent slowly progressive interstitial fibrosis of the lung associated with the inhalation of asbestos dust, characterized by the finding of asbestos bodies and fibers in the tissue. The disease is fairly well established before there is recognition by radiological or physiological examination, the latter often being obscured by the effects of cigarette smoking. If exposure has been sufficient, then the disease will progress after the worker has left the industry. At present we are trying to establish how much fiber must be retained in lungs to cause asbestosis. In the cases of progressive fibrosis, the patients will eventually develop right heart failure.

Carcinoma of the Lung. Carcinoma of the lung in asbestos workers was first recognized in Britain in 1934, in the United States in 1935, and in Germany a few years later. In 1947, the Inspector of Factories in Britain reported that 15% of all death certificates for males that mentioned asbestosis attributed death to carcinoma of the lung (*14*). In 1955, this excessive risk was confirmed (*15*), by showing that those employed before 1930 in scheduled occupations in an asbestos textile factory had a death rate from lung cancer 10 times greater than that of the general population (*15*). In 1965, it was reported that 60% of the registered asbestos workers were dying of carcinoma of the lung (*16*).

The first demonstration of the joint action of cigarette smoking and occupational exposure to asbestos in producing lung cancer indicated that the two carcinogens acted multiplicatively (*17, 18*). More recently it was found that, relative to men who neither worked with asbestos nor smoked, the death rate for lung cancer was five times higher for men who worked with asbestos but did not smoke; it was 11 times higher for those who smoked but had not worked with asbestos; for those who both worked with asbestos and smoked, it was 53 times higher (*19*). Men and women working with asbestos have even more reason to give up smoking than smokers in the general population.

Diffuse Mesotheliomas of Pleura and Peritoneum. Diffuse mesotheliomas of both pleura and peritoneum are now accepted as being associated with exposure to asbestos dust. Occasional cases were recorded in the German literature in the 1940s, but the first series of cases was reported in 1960 from the crocidolite mining area in the Cape Province in South Africa (*20*). This association with exposure to asbestos dust now has been confirmed in most industrial countries throughout the world. In many of the cases, the exposure is for as little as 6 weeks, and there is no radiological or pathological evidence of pulmonary fibrosis. Recently, however, a dose relationship has been shown in the development of these tumors (*21*). Environmental exposure was a common finding in the cases of mesotheliomas from the Cape asbestos fields and in the vicinity of the mine in Western Australia, but not in the other asbestos mining areas. This type of tumor also has been observed in people living close to asbestos factories and has occurred in family situations when an asbestos worker has brought home fibers on clothing or hair, which has resulted in a tumor occurring in a relative. Cases have resulted from this type of exposure in early childhood. The average time between first exposure and diagnosis of the tumor is 40 yr, irrespective of the age at first exposure. The clinical aspects of mesothelioma have been described in a large series of cases (*22*). The possibility that the general public is at risk from asbestos in the ambient air has been raised on many occasions. There is no proof that this type of exposure has caused a mesothelioma.

The major controversy with regard to variety of asbestos concerns the mesotheliomas. Our original South African evidence indicated a clear association with crocidolite, and in South Africa this association is still valid (*23*). In Britain, as in other industrial countries, the majority of asbestos workers have been exposed to more than one type of fiber. Apart from actual mining areas, pure exposure is extremely rare. The South African experience with crocidolite is being repeated on a smaller scale at Wittenoom in Western Australia, where mesotheliomas are occurring both in those employed in the mines and in the environmentally exposed population. This has not occurred in any other mining situation. Gas-mask workers investigated by Jones et al. (*24*) appeared to have had a pure exposure to crocidolite, but Pooley's analysis of the lungs (*12*) confirmed the presence of a significant amount of chrysotile.

The technique developed by Pooley (*12*) for the identification of asbestos and other mineral fibers in lung tissue is the most useful method available for identifying individual exposures and emphasizing the complexity of the situation. The comparisons between the fibers in the lungs of the mesothelioma cases collected in Britain with those in the United States and Canada has shown that, in both countries, chrysotile fibers are found equally in cases and controls (*25*). In Britain it is crocidolite that is associated with mesothelioma, whereas in the United States it is usually amosite and, less frequently, crocidolite. One report (*26*) stated that mesotheliomas had occurred in factory workers who were exposed to amosite. Unfortunately, the fiber contents of these lungs have not been subjected to a detailed analysis. The Advisory Committee to the British Secretary of State for Employment (*27*) concluded that in the causation of mesotheliomas, crocidolite was more dangerous than chrysotile, and amosite may be intermediate between the two.

Other Cancers. A slight but significant increase in cancers of the gastrointestinal tract has been reported in studies in New York, Quebec, Belfast, and London (*28–31*). Although carcinoma of the larynx induced by mineral fibers has been reported (*32*), it has not been generally confirmed (*33*); the association seems to be more with heavy cigarette smoking.

Significance of Fiber Size

The importance of fiber size in the inhalation and retention of fibrous mineral dusts was first emphasized in a study (*34*) that showed that the fiber diameter is the most important factor in the deposition, and the length is only of minor significance. Later, in a study of the ultimate diameters of crocidolite and amosite fibers (*35*), the diameter was identified as a vital factor in assessing the probability of a fiber being associated with the development of a mesothelioma. Similar results were recorded from animal experiments in which asbestos and other mineral fibers were implanted into the pleural and peritoneal cavities of rats. The earlier results (*36–38*) were confirmed by Stanton's team (*39*). From all these investigations it now appears that the size of fiber responsible for mesotheliomas has a diameter of less than 0.25 μm, and probably a length greater than 5.0 μm. Fibers up to 3.0 μm in diameter inhaled and retained in the peripheral airways are associated with pulmonary fibrosis, and the effective length of at least 10 μm suggested by Timbrell in 1968 (*40*) has not been challenged. There is no agreement on the maximum length of fiber that would be hazardous. The most important finding in all these experiments was that mineral fibers other than asbestos having these diameters and lengths are capable of causing mesotheliomas. Whether this finding also applies to the development of pulmonary fibrosis is still under investigation. A significant factor in the fibrotic response may depend upon the ability of the material to survive in tissue. Studies on this aspect of the problem are being undertaken in many laboratories. The major producers of synthetic mineral fibers are investigating the production of significant quantities of fibers with specific length-to-diameter ratios for experimental studies. If durable fibers covering the suspected range of biological activity could be made available, it should be possible to test these hypotheses. Unfortunately, tremendous technical difficulties must be overcome before these fibers can be produced.

Effects of Other Fibers

In an attempt to clarify the significance of fibers in tissue, a detailed examination of a large series of cases is being undertaken (*24, 25, 41*). Included in this investigation are cases of mesothelioma from the United Kingdom, the United States, and Canada; fewer cases of mesotheliomas from Cyprus and central Turkey; cases of asbestosis from the United Kingdom and elsewhere; and a large number of lungs from adults with no evidence of industrial exposure.

Tremolite. IN VITRO STUDIES AND ANIMAL EXPERIMENTS. Three phases of tremolite have been studied experimentally (*42*): (a) a coarse flake-like fiber, (b) a fiber with a diameter of between 1.0 and 3.0 μm, and (c) a very fine fiber with a diameter less than 0.5 μm. In both the mammalian cell cytotoxicity tests and the pleural implantations, only the very fine tremolite fiber produced significant results with a marked cytotoxicity and a high incidence of mesotheliomas.

FINDINGS IN HUMANS. The flake-like tremolie used in the previous experiment was obtained from a talc mine in California. There is no evidence of disease among the miners and millers at this site. A coarse fibrous tremolite is found as a contaminant of the chrysotile deposits in Quebec Province in Canada. This fiber has been found in the lungs of workers from these mines (*43*), and is thought to be associated with pleural plaques and pulmonary fibrosis. In talc mines in the northern part of New York State, there is contamination by a coarse-fibered talc, and pulmonary fibrosis and carcinoma of the lung have been reported (*44*).

In an earlier section of this paper, the tremolite situation in the eastern Mediterranean was described. In eastern Turkey and Cyprus, where the tremolite is less than 0.5 μm in diameter, mesotheliomas have occurred. Elsewhere in Turkey, where the coarser fiber is used for stuccoing, large pleural plaques have been reported (*6*). The coarser tremolite and anthophyllite have been recorded in the lungs of agricultural workers in the tobacco growing areas in the Balkans, and these people develop massive calcified pleural plaques (*7, 45*).

Zeolites. ANIMAL EXPERIMENTS. Preliminary implantation experiments with very fine zeolite fibers (erionites) from Oregon and specific villages in central Turkey have produced a high incidence of mesotheliomas. This effect has not been seen with slightly coarser short-fibered erionite from New Zealand or mordenite from Japan. No reaction has been noted in animals exposed to nonfibrous synthetic zeolites.

STUDIES IN HUMANS. In central Turkey, a very high incidence of mesotheliomas has been reported from two widely separated villages. In both areas all the villagers use caves, which have been carved out of the volcanic tuff, for storage. The same material is used for building blocks and for surfacing the streets. It contains a variety of fibrous and nonfibrous zeolites, volcanic glass, and pumice. Although these materials are also present in all the surrounding villages, there is no evidence of mesotheliomas. The only significant difference is that, in certain caves in the affected villages, very fine erionite fibers are found and have been observed in lung tissue from several of the mesothelioma cases (*13*).

Synthetic Mineral Fibers. These materials are being intensively studied on both sides of the Atlantic. The investigations cover epidemiology, animal experimentation, and environmental and occupational studies of the dusts produced in industry. The results of all these studies were published in 1982 (*46*).

Fibrous Clays. These materials are being thoroughly investigated and it is expected that investigations will take several more years.

Discussion

The whole problem of the biological effects of mineral fibers still is under investigation. At this stage, the results of numerous current studies are necessary before definite conclusions can be reached. This statement may be optimistic. In spite of all the evidence accumulated during the last 20 years, the estimations of relative risks of exposure to the different types of asbestos still have not received universal acceptance.

The size of fiber appears to be a crucial factor in the production of mesotheliomas; apparently only relatively small amounts of material are necessary to produce these tumors providing the fibers are less than 0.2 μm in diameter. The length factor is not as clearly identified, but fibers of 1.0 μm are implicated; attaining more concrete evidence is dependent on the ability of the industry to produce fibers of specific size. Another factor that requires further study is the importance of the stability of the material in tissue. Is it important for the fibrous minerals to maintain an exact morphology for many years after retention in the tissues, or is only a short period essential? Many researchers believe that the fibers act as promoters in the development of the tumors, but no positive proof of this has been produced. Presumably as promoters, the substance would have to survive for a longer time than if they were initiators, but whether this could be measured in months or years is not known.

The actual mechanism of fine fiber carcinogenesis still remains unsolved. Numerous hypotheses have been suggested but none have been substantiated. Following the acceptance that crocidolite asbestos and possibly other types of this mineral, and finely fibered erionites are associated with mesotheliomas, it is essential that the whole situation be clarified as soon as possible. Fibrous minerals are of great economic importance and there will be an increasing need for acceptable forms for insulation, absorption, and filtration.

Literature Cited

1. "Biological Effects of Mineral Fibres"; Wagner, J. C., Ed.; IARC: Lyon, 1980; No. 30.
2. Wagner, J. C.; Berry, G.; Pooley, F. D. *Br. Med. Bull.* **1980**, *36*, 53–56.
3. Wagner, J. C.; Elmes, P. C. "Recent Advances in Occupational Health"; McDonald, J. C., Ed.; Churchill: London, 11, 1–13.
4. Hendry, N. W. *Ann. N. Y. Acad. Sci.* **1965**, *132*, 12–22.
5. "Asbestos—Health Precautions in Industry," Health & Safety Executive, 1970, Her Majesty's Stationery Office, London, No. 44.
6. Yazicioglu, S.; Ilcaytc, R.; Balci, B. S.; Sayli, B. S.; Yorulmaz, B. *Thorax* **1980**, *35*, 564–69.

7. Burilkov, T.; Michailova, L. *Environ. Res.* **1970**, *3*, 443–51.
8. Burilkov, T.; Michailova, L. *Int. Arch. Arbeitsmed.* **1972**, *29*, 95–101.
9. Wagner, J. C.; Berry, G.; Pooley, F. D. *Br. Med. Bull.* **1980**, *36*, 53–56.
10. Wagner, J. C. *Practitioner* **1979**, *223*, 28–33.
11. Thomson, J. G.; Kaschula, R. O. C.; MacDonald, R. R. *S. Afr. Med. J.* **1963**, *37*, 77–81.
12. Pooley, F. D. *Ann. Occup. Hyg.* **1975**, *18*, 181–86.
13. Sebastien, P.; Gaudichet, A.; Bignon, J.; Baris, Y. I. *Lab. Invest.* **1981**, *44*, 420–25.
14. "Annual Report of the Chief Inspector of Factories for the Year 1947 (CMD 7621)," Minister of Labour and National Service, Her Majesty's Stationery Office, London, 1949.
15. Doll, R. *Br. J. Ind. Med.* **1955**, *12*, 81–86.
16. Buchanan, W. D. *Ann. N. Y. Acad. Sci.* **1965**, *132*, 507–18.
17. Selikoff, I. J.; Hammond, E. C.; Churg, J. *JAMA, J. Am. Med. Assoc.* **1968**, *204*, 106–12.
18. Berry, G.; Newhouse, M. L.; Turok, M. *Lancet* **1972**, *2*, 476–79.
19. Selikoff, I. J.; Hammond, E. C. *JAMA, J. Am. Med. Assoc.* **1979**, *242*, 458–59.
20. Wagner, J. C.; Sleggs, C. A.; Marchand, P. *Br. J. Ind. Med.* **1960**, *17*, 260–71.
21. Newhouse, M. L.; Berry, G. *Br. J. Ind. Med.* **1976**, *33*, 147–51.
22. Elmes, P. C.; Simpson, M. J. C. *Q. J. Med.* **1976**, *45*, 427–49.
23. Webster, I. *S. Afr. Med. J.* **1973**, *47*, 165–71.
24. Jones, J. S. P.; Pooley, F. D.; Smith, P. G. "Environmental Pollution and Carcinogenic Risks"; Rosenfeld, C.; Davis, W., Eds.; IARC: Lyon, 1976; pp. 117–20, No. 13.
25. McDonald, A. D. "Biological Effects of Mineral Fibres"; Wagner, J. C., Ed.; IARC: Lyon, 1980, pp. 681–85, No. 30.
26. Selikoff, I. J.; Hammond, E. C.; Churg, J. *Arch. Environ. Health* **1972**, *25*, 183–86.
27. "Asbestos. Vol. 2: Papers Prepared for the Advisory Committee," Health and Safety Commission, 1979, Her Majesty's Stationery Office, London.
28. Hammond, E. C.; Selikoff, I. J.; Churg, J. *Ann. N. Y. Acad. Sci.* **1965**, *132*, 519–25.
29. McDonald, J. C.; McDonald, A. D.; Gibbs, G. W.; Siemsatycki, J.; Rossiter, C. E. *Arch. Environ. Health* **1971**, *22*, 677–86.
30. Elmes, P. C.; Simpson, M. J. C. *Br. J. Ind. Med.* **1971**, *28*, 226–36.
31. Newhouse, M. L. "Biological Effects of Asbestos"; Bogovski, P.; Gilson, J. C.; Timbrell, V.; Wagner, J. C., Eds.; World Health: Albany, NY, 1973; pp. 203–8.
32. Stell, P. M.; McGill, T. *Lancet* **1973**, *2*, 416–17.
33. Newhouse, M. L.; Gregory, M. M.; Shannon, H. "Biological Effects of Mineral Fibres"; Wagner, J. C., Ed.; IARC: Lyon, 1980; pp. 687–95, No. 30.
34. Timbrell, V. *Ann. N. Y. Acad. Sci.* **1965**, *132*, 255–73.
35. Timbrell, V.; Pooley, F. D.; Wagner, J. C. "Pneumoconiosis—Proceedings of the International Conference, Johannesburg"; Shapiro, H. A., Ed.; Oxford University Press: Cape Town, 1970; pp. 120–25.
36. Wagner, J. C. *Nature (London)* **1962**, *196*, 180–81.
37. Stanton, M. F.; Wrench, C. *JNCI, J. Natl. Cancer Inst.* **1972**, *48*, 797–821.
38. Pott, F.; Huth, F.; Friedrichs, K. H. *Zentralbl. Bakteriol. Parasitenkd. Infektionskr. Hyg., Abt. 1: Orig., Reihe B* **1972**, *155*, 463–69.
39. Stanton, M. F.; Layard, M. In "National Bureau of Standards Special Publication 506, Proceedings of the Workshop on Asbestos: Definitions and Measurement Methods"; NBS: Gaithersburg, MD, 1978; held July 18–20, 1977.
40. Timbrell, V.; Skidmore, J. W. "Internationale Konferenze der Biologische Wirkungen des Asbestes Dresden"; Holstein, E., Ed.; Dtsch. Zentralinst. Arbeitsmed: Berlin, 1968, pp. 52–56.

41. Wagner, J. C.; Pooley, F. D.; Berry, G.; Seal, R. M. E.; Munday, D. E.; Morgan, J.; Clark, N. J. BOHS Fifth International Symposium on Inhaled Particles, Cardiff, Wales; Walton, W. H., Ed.; 1980, Vol. 26, No. 1–4, pp. 423–31.
42. Wagner, J. C.; Chamberlain, M.; Brown, R. C.; Berry, G.; Pooley, F. D.; Davies, R.; Griffiths, D. M. *Br. J. Cancer* **1981**, *45*, 352.
43. Pooley, F. D. *Environ. Res.* **1976**, *12*, 281–98.
44. Kleinfeld, M.; Messite, J.; Kooyman. O.; Zaki, M. H. *Arch. Environ. Health* **1967**, *14*, 663–67.
45. Wagner, J. C. "Biological Effects of Mineral Fibres"; Wagner, J. C., Ed; IARC: Lyon, 1980; pp. 995–97, No. 30.
46. McConnell, E. E.; Wagner, J. C.; Skidmore, J. W.; Moore, J. A. in "Biological Effects of Man Made Fibres"; Report on IARC Meeting, Copenhagen, April 20–22, 1982 (Euro Reports and Studies 81) and Copenhagen WHO Reg. Office for Europe and IARC, 1983, 118–20.

AUTHOR INDEX

Bigger, C. Anita H., 41
Busby, Jr., William F., 945
Cartwright, R. A., 1
Clayson, D. B., 175
Connors, T. A., 1241
Cooke, M. A., 165
DiGiovanni, John, 1279
Dipple, Anthony, 41
Eisenbrand, G., 829
Evans, A. E. J., 277
Evans, I. A., 1171
Garner, R. C., 175
Gilman, John P. W., 577
Grasso, Paul, 1205
Greim, Helmut, 525
Kipling, M. D., 165
Kolar, G. F., 869
Lawley, P. D., 325
Martin, C. N., 175
Moschel, Robert C., 41
Osborne, M. R., 485
Parkes, H. G., 277
Preussmann, R., 643, 829
Schoental, R., 1137
Searle, C. E., 303
Slaga, Thomas J., 1279
Stewart, B. W., 643
Swierenga, Sabine H. H., 577
Wagner, J. C., 631
Weisburger, J. H., 1323
Williams, G. M., 1323
Wogan, Gerald N., 945
Wolff, Thomas, 525
Zedeck, Morris S., 915

INDEX

A

AAB—*See* Phenylazoacetanilide
AB—*See* Phenylazoaniline, aminoazobenzene
Acetaldehyde methylformylhydrazone, 920
6-Acetamidocoumarin, oncogenesis tests, 438*t*
Acetaminophen, liver necrosis, 187
Acetanilide
  metabolism, phenylhydroxylamine, 179
  modification of aromatic amine carcinogenesis, 262
Acetate esters, metabolic activation of aromatic amines, 184–87
Acetic acid, 1308*t*
N-Acetoxy-4-biphenylacetamide, carcinogenicity, 208*t*
2-Acetylaminofluorene—*See* 2-Fluorenylacetamide
N-Acetylation, enzymic, *N*-hydroxy compounds, 185
Acetylene tetrachloride, 540
Acetylene trichloride, 542
Acetylenic groups, in vivo conversion of drugs, 1265
N-Acetylethyleneimine, oncogenesis tests, 426–27*t*
Acid catalysis
  degradation and photolysis, dialkyltriazenes, 891
  reactions of monoalkyltriazenes, 885
Acidity
  effect on coupling of triazenes, 871
  urine, bladder carcinogenicity of aromatic amines, 183
Acrolein, 456
Acroosteolysis, 528
ACTH—*See* Adrenocorticotropin
Actinolite, 632
Actinomycin, 1079
  carcinogenicity, 1254
  tumor inhibition, 1297*t*
Action, 355
Activation steps, aromatic amines, 178
Activity, carcinogenic, chemical structure, 52
Acute aflatoxicosis, 969–70
Acute nonlymphocytic leukemias, 456
Acute toxicity, nitrosamines and nitrosamides, 652*t*
α-Acyloxynitrosamines, synthesis from α-nitrosamino ethers, 645
Additives, food, 1224–25
Adenine
  methylation, 365
  residues, benzo[*a*]pyrene modification, 124
Adenocarcinomas, induction, 916
Adenomas, lung, induced, benzo[*a*]pyrene derivatives, 103*t*
S-Adenosylmethionine, 366
Adrenocorticotropin, effect on AFB_1 carcinogenicity, 996*t*
Adrimycin, carcinogenicity, 1254
Adult animals, carcinogenicity, triazenes, 898
Aflatoxicosis
  acute, 969–70
  data, 979
Aflatoxin(s), 438, 945–1115, 1221
  alterations in RNA metabolism, 1078
  ammoniation, 965
  analogs, 1025–28
  animal feeds, 956–58
  beverages, eggs, and meat, 1112
  biochemical effects, 1076–93
  biological activity, 970–1028
  biological detoxification, 963–64
  carcinogenicity, 983–1004
  chemical inactivation, 964–66
  contamination
    food, 1222
    guidelines, 953
  control, 958–59
  dairy products, 1113–15
  detection in corn, 952
  detoxification, 958
  distribution, 1042
  elimination, 958
  excretion, 1029–76
  factors affecting metabolism, 1064–72
  factors affecting toxicity, 980–82
  formation, 958
  fruits, vegetables, and spices, 1110–11
  ginger root, 955
  grains, 1096–1100
  history, 946
  identification, 952
  inhibition of macromolecular synthesis, 1077–88
  interaction with mitochondria, 1089–91
  legumes, 1106–7
  liver cancer, 1222*t*
  lysomomal enzyme activities, 1092
  macromolecular binding
    adduct formation and removal, 1052
    characteristics, 1047–49
    to proteins, 1061
  metabolism, 1029–76
  metabolites, 1025–28
    factors affecting genotoxicity, 1027–28
  microorganisms, 971
  occurrence in agricultural commodities, 948–66

Aflatoxin(s)—*Continued*
oilseeds, 1104–7
particle-size effects, 955
peanut oil, destruction, 962
peanuts, 1101–3
physical elimination, 959
physical inactivation, 962–63
physical properties, 950–51*t*
pistachio nuts, 952
plants, 971
precursors, 1025–28
solubility, 947
solvent extraction, 960
sources, 1221
structure–activity relationships, 1093–94
teratogenicity, 1004–5
tissue distribution, 1029–76
toxicity, 971–83
tree nuts, 1108–9
Aflatoxin B_1, 945
as anticoagulant, 982
carcinogenicity in rats, 1221
detoxification, 1029, 1064
dihydrodiol, 1044
effect on cell cultures, 974
gene mutation effects, 1007–10*t*
genotoxicity, 1005–23
in vitro factors, 1030*t*, 1032*t*
hepatocarcinogenesis, 983–92
in vertebrates, 984–86*t*
hydrolysis products, HPLC, 1054
in vitro cell transformation, 1021*t*
liver cancer, 397
metabolic transformations, 1038–39*f*
metabolism, effects of sex, 1071
mouse, lethal dose, 1082
noncovalent binding, 1051
RNA synthesis
inhibition, 1079
selectivity, 1081
species susceptibility, 983
structure, 94, 947
teratogenic effects, 1005
treatment, protein, synthesis, and function, 1084–88
Aflatoxin B_1 dihydrodiol, DNA binding, 1050
Aflatoxin B_1-DNA adduct formation, 1059*t*
Aflatoxin B_1-guanyl modified DNA, hydrolytic pathways, 1060
Aflatoxin B_1-induced extrahepatic tumors, 992–94
Aflatoxin B_1-induced hepatocarcinogenesis, factors affecting, 995–99*t*
Aflatoxin B_1-modified DNA, hydrolysis products, 1057*f*, 1058*f*
Aflatoxin B_1 2,3-oxide, hydrolysis, 1069
Aflatoxin B_1-protein, binding mechanisms, 1062
Aflatoxin B_2
formation, 1045
reduction, 1046
structure, 947
Aflatoxin B_{2a}, 1040
in genotoxicity assays, 1024
Aflatoxin cogeners, 1000–4, 1023–25
Aflatoxin contamination, postharvest, control, 959
Aflatoxin D_1, isolation from peanut oil, 966
Aflatoxin exposure, and human disease, 966–70
Aflatoxin G_1
effects on rainbow trout, 980
structure, 947
Aflatoxin G_2, structure, 947
Aflatoxin–glutathione conjugate, 1045
excretion and distribution, 1042
Aflatoxin–guanine adduct, 1045
excretion and distribution, 1042
Aflatoxin H_1, 1044
Aflatoxin M_1, 1029, 1040, 1044
excretion and distribution, 1033*t*
Aflatoxin metabolites, 1000–4
Aflatoxin P_1, 1043–44
excretion and distribution, 1043*t*
Aflatoxin–protein conjugates, 1062
Aflatoxin Q_1, 979, 1044
Agaricus bisporus, 920
Agaritine, 920
Air balloons, nitrosamines, 847*t*
Albumin, aflatoxin B_1 inhibition, 1086
Alcohol, 21
feminization of males, 1159
incidence of esophageal cancer, 1141
ingestion of alkylating agents, 395
nitrosamine content, 1214*t*
testosterone synthesis, 1159
Aldrin
carcinogenicity in mice, 555, 556–57*t*
in humans, storage, 560
structure, 557
Alimentary toxic aleukia, 1142
Alkaline sucrose gradient analysis, *N*-nitroso carcinogens, 714
Alkanesulfonates, difunctional, oncogenesis tests, 457*t*
α-Alkoxynitrosamines, *N*-nitroso carcinogens, 645–48
Alkyl formates, oncogenesis tests, 420*t*
Alkyl halides
β-carbonyl substituted, 408, 409*t*
oncogenesis, 405*t*
Alkyl phosphates, 413
oncogenesis tests, 418–19*t*
Alkyl phosphotriesters, formation in DNA, 365
Alkyl sulfates, oncogenesis, 414–17*t*
Alkylaryltriazenes
biological effects, 896–904
chemistry and biological properties, 883–94
Alkylated bases, effect on template activity in vitro, 703
Alkylating agents
human cancer, 383–400
oncogenesis tests, chemical structure vs. reactivity, 404–60
tumor induction, 403
Alkylation
comparisons between experiments and humans, 466
DNA, in vivo dosimetry, 368
of nucleic acids, *N*-nitroso carcinogens, 698–704
triazenes, 887
Alkylation carcinogenesis, dose-response relationships, 378–83

Alkylation products, nitroso derived, in nucleic acids, 701
Alkylation repair, in mammalian cells, *N*-nitroso carcinogens, 722–28
S-Alkylcysteine, content determination, 378
O[6]-Alkyldeoxyguanosine triphosphate, induction of mutation, 361
Alkyldiarytriazenes, principal fragments in the mass spectrum, 880
Alkylguanine(s)
  isolation, 375
  repair removal, 360
  structures, 376
O[6]-Alkylguanine
  in DNA, biological role, related to *N*-nitroso carcinogens, 728
  elimination from mammalian DNA, 722
  persistence and tumorigenesis, 706–11
N-Alkylhistidines, content determination, 378
Alkyl-4-hydroxybutylnitrosamines, metabolic fate, 690
Alkylpurines, hydrolytic depurination, 455
Allium cepa roots, AFB_1 chromosome inductor, 1012*t*
Allyl chloride, 544
  oncogenesis, 406–7*t*
Allyl methanesulfonate, oncogenesis tests, 416–17*t*
Almonds, aflatoxins, 1108
Altered cells, multiplication, 1328
Ames test, bacterial screening tests, 1335
Amines
  aromatic, carcinogenicity, discussion, 175–83
  carcinogenic, analytical uses, 312
  deamination of primary, triazenes, 887
  nitrosation, in vivo conversion, 1262
  secondary, unusual formation, 648
Amino compounds, nitrosatable and nitrite, carcinogenesis, 672
Amino derivatives, five-membered heterocyclic ring compounds, 250
Amino groups, oxidation, in vivo conversion, 1258
Aminoacetonitrile, 934
  effect on *N*-nitroso carcinogenesis, 678*t*
2-Amino-9,10-anthracenedione, carcinogenicity, 259*t*
Aminoazo dyes
  metabolic activation, 190
  structure–activity relationship, 229
4-Aminobiphenyl
  See also 4-Biphenylamine
  and bladder cancer, 177
4-Aminodiphenylamine, carcinogenicity, 214*t*
1-Amino-2-methyl-9,10-anthracenedione, carcinogenicity, 259*t*
2-Amino-4-(5-nitro-2-furyl)thiazole, in vivo conversion, 1257
4-Amino-2-nitrophenol, carcinogenicity, 207*t*
4-Aminoquinoline 1-oxide, carcinogenic activity, 249*t*
Ammoniation, decontaminating oilseed meals, 965
Amosite, 632, 633
Amyl nitrile, 28
Analgesics, consumption related to cancer, 201
Analytical epidemiology, data, 14–16
Analytical methodology
  alkylation of nucleic acids, 699
  for *N*-nitroso compounds, 831–32
Analytical uses, carcinogenic amines, 312
Andrin, oncogenesis tests, 424*t*
Androgens, carcinogenicity, 1266
Anesthesiologists, cancer rate, 308
ANFT, in vivo conversion, 1257
Angelicalactone
  oncogenesis tests, 438*t*
  tumor inhibition, 2397*t*
Anguidine, carcinogenicity, 1249
Angular ring, unsubstituted, structure–activity relationships, 54
Aniles, metabolic activation, 187
Aniline(s), 278
  bladder cancer, 175
  carcinogenicity, 202*t*
    structure–activity relationship, 201
Aniline mustard
  oncogenesis tests, 450–51*t*
  structure, 374
Animal(s)
  metabolism, aromatic hydrocarbons, 71
  selection, carcinogenicity, evaluation, 1345
  small, tumors, bracken carcinogenicity, 1174
Animal feedstocks, toxin production, 956
Animal maintenance, bioassay of carcinogens, 1347
o-Anisidine, carcinogenicity, 203*t*
Ankylosing spondylitis, radiotherapy, 22, 22*t*
Antabuse, 377
  See also Disulfiram
Anthanthrene, carcinogenic activities, 140–41*t*
Anthopyllite, 632
Anthraanthracene, carcinogenic activities, 132*t*
Anthracene
  carcinogenic activities, 130*t*
  metabolic attack at the K region, 72
Anthracene derivatives, carcinogenic activities, 138–39*t*
Anthracene oil, 166
Anthramines, carcinogenic structure–activity relationship, 228
Anticancer agents, carcinogenicity, 1243–55
Antiinflammatory steroids, 1297
  effect on arachidonic acid metabolism, 1305*t*
  tumor inhibition, 1297*t*, 1298–1300, 1299*t*
Antimetabolites
  antitumor, carcinogenicity, 1251–53
  miscoding, 358
Antineoplastic drugs, carcinogenic reagants, 312
Antioxidants, 1282–86
  as inhibitors, 1306–7
  inhibition of chemical carcinogenesis, 1283*t*
Antipain, 1304
  carcinogenesis inhibitors, 1303*t*
Antituberculosis drug, 366
Antitumor antimetabolites, carcinogenicity, 1251–53
Antralin, epigenetic carcinogen, 1330*t*
AOM—*See* Azoxymethane
Apis mellifers, aflatoxins effect, 973

Arachidonic acid
  metabolism, inhibitors, 1304–6, 1305*t*
  tumor inhibition, 1298
Aralkyl halides, 408, 413
  oncogenesis tests, 411*t*
Aramite
  oncogenesis tests, 444–45*t*
  carcinogenicity in animals, 447
  structure, 395
Arecoline, structure, 395
Arene epoxides
  K region, synthesis, 110
  nomenclature, 46
  non-K region, synthesis, 112
  reactivity, 118
  transient metabolic intermediate, 68
Arenediazonium cations, carcinogenicity, 869
Aroclor, 1254
  effect on AFB_1 carcinogenicity, 997*t*
  inhibition of chemical carcinogenesis, 1291*t*
Aromatic amine(s)
  and bladder cancer, 287–90
  cancers, 277–98
  carcinogenicity, discussion, 175–272
  laboratory precautions, 315
  schools, 319
  toxicity, 277–78
Aromatic hydrocarbons, unsubstituted
  polycyclic, carcinogenic activities, 130–31*t*
  properties, 60–61*t*
Arsenic, 2
  carcinogenic action, 1267
  in food, 1224
  malignancy sites, 31*t*
Artemia salina, aflatoxins effect, 973
Arylamines, carcinogenic structure–activity relationship, 228
1-Aryl-3-methyltriazenes, decomposition products, 880
Asbestos, 33, 384
  composition, 631
  dust, exposure, 634–37
  epigenetic carcinogen, 1330*t*
  malignancy sites, 31*t*
  world production, 632
Asbestos bodies, composition, 635
Asbestos minerals, 631–33
Asbestosis, 635
Ascorbic acid
  effect on AFB_1 carcinogenicity, 996*t*
  effects on tumor promotion in mice, 1307*t*
Aspermia, 385
Aspirin, effect on arachidonic acid metabolism, 1305*t*
Assays, for neoplasm-promoting agents, 1338
Astragalin, bracken carcinogenicity, 1182, 1186
At-risk registers, 12
ATA—*See* Alimentary toxic aleukia
Ataxia telangiectasia, 19
  chromosomal instability, 396
Atmospheric pollution, sources, 1211
Audrosterone, role in protein synthesis inhibition, 1085
Auramine
  bladder cancer, 176
  carcinogenicity, 214*t*
Aurothioglucose, carcinogenicity, 1271
Azacytidine
  carcinogenicity, 1251, 1253
  structure, 367
Azathioprine, 399
  carcinogenicity, 1251, 1252
  epigenetic, 1330*t*
  structure, 399
Aziridine(s), 424
  oncogenesis tests, 426–27*t*
Azaridine ethanol, oncogenesis tests, 426–27*t*
Azo compounds, 915
Azo dyes
  benzidine-derived, metabolic activation, 191
  carcinogenicity in rodent liver, 1325
  structure–activity relationship, 229, 247
Azo group effect, *N,N*-dimethyl-*p*-phenylazoaniline, 234
Azo mustard, structure, 374
Azoxy compounds, 915
Azoxyethane, 919
Azoxymethane, oxidation to MAM, 933

B

B[*e*]P, role in tumor inhibition, 1295*t*
Baboon, aflatoxin B_1 toxicity, 978*t*
Baccharins, 1143
  structure, 1144
Bacillus, aflatoxins effect, 971
Bacillus megaterium
  aflatoxin B_1 chromosome inductor, 1011*t*
  aflatoxins effect, 971
Bacillus subtilis, gene mutation effects, 1007*t*, 1008*t*
Bacillus thuringiensis, aflatoxins effect, 971
Bacon
  DMN concentration, 1216
  frying, 833
  nitrosamine content, 1214*t*
Bacteria
  alkylation, *N*-nitroso carcinogens, 719–24
  mutagenesis, carcinogenicity, 1335
Barbiturates, enzyme-inducing agents, 258
Base damage
  See also Miscoding
  DNA damage produced by chemicals, 1335
Bathochromic shift, polynuclear compounds, 62
Bay region
  dihydrodiol epoxide, metabolic activation, 109
  structure, nomenclature systems, 44
BC—*See* Benzene hexachloride
BCNU—*See* Bis(chloroethyl)nitrosourea *and* *N*—Nitroso-*N,N'*-bis(2-chloroethyl)urea
Beans
  aflatoxins, 1106
  nitrosamine content, 1214*t*
Beef, polycyclic aromatic hydrocarbon content, 1210*t*
Beer
  malignancies caused, 21
  N-nitrosamines, 834–38
Beer brewing, aflatoxin destruction, 963
Benzacridines
  properties, 58*t*
  substituted, carcinogenic activities, 146–47*t*
Benzaldehyde pyridoxal, 858

Benzalpurine mustard, oncogenesis tests, 454*t*
Benzanthracene
  See also Benz[*a*]anthracene
  effect on aflatoxin B_1 carcinogenicity, 998*t*
Benzene
  carcinogenic activities, 130*t*
  malignancy sites, 31*t*
α-Benzene hexachloride, effect on aflatoxin B_1 carcinogenicity, 997*t*
Benzenediazonium cation, carcinogenicity, 869
Benzidine, 280–81
  carcinogenic reagents, 315
  carcinogenicity, 213*t*
    structure–activity relationship, 211
  metabolic activation, 189
  reactions with macromolecules, 197
  related to cancer in clinical chemists, 311
  role in bladder cancer, 175, 177, 281, 290
  structure, 280
Benzidine-derived azo dyes, metabolic activation, 191
3,3′-Benzidinedicarboxylic acid, carcinogenicity, 213*t*
Benzimidazole mustard, oncogenesis tests, 453*t*
Benzochrysenes, carcinogenic activities, 131*t*, 132*t*, 133*t*, 140–41*t*
Benzoflavone, 975, 1288
  influence on aflatoxin B_1 genotoxicity, 1030*t*
  inhibition of chemical carcinogenesis, 1287
  role in aflatoxin B_1 activation, 1068
Benzo[*b*]fluoranthene, structure, 166*f*
Benzo[*a*]naphthacene, carcinogenic activities, 130*t*
Benzo[*b*]pentaphene, carcinogenic activities, 132*t*
Benzo[*c*]pentaphene, carcinogenic activities, 132*t*
Benzo[*rst*]pentaphene, carcinogenic activities, 131*t*, 140–41*t*
Benzo[*ghi*]perylene, carcinogenic activities, 133*t*
Benzo[*c*]phenanthrene
  carcinogenic activities, 131*t*
  tumor-initiating activities of derivatives, 107*t*
Benzo[*c*]phenanthrene derivatives, carcinogenic activities, 138–39*t*
Benzo[*pqr*]picene, carcinogenic activities, 140–41*t*
Benzo[*a*]pyrene, 165
  carcinogenesis with *N*-nitroso compounds, 676*t*
  carcinogenic activities, 101*t*, 131*t*
  derivatives, carcinogenic activities, 101*t*
  genotoxic carcinogen, 1330*t*
  reactions with nucleic acids, 122–25
  structure, 166*f*
Benzo[*e*]pyrene
  carcinogenic activities, 130*t*
  tumor-initiating activities of derivatives, 106*t*
Benzo[*a*]pyrene derivatives
  lung adenomas induced, 103*t*
  tumor-initiating activity, 102*t*
Benzo[*a*]pyrene dihydrodiol epoxides, reactivity, 118
3,4-Benzphenanthrene—*See* Benzo[*c*]phenanthrene
Benzpyrene, nomenclature systems, 41
3,4-Benzpyrene—*See* Benzo[*a*]pyrene
Benzyl chloride, 529
  oncogenesis tests, 411*t*
  relative carcinogenicity, 382
Benz[*a*]anthracene, 73
  See also Benzanthracene
  carcinogenic activities, 131*t*
  derivatives, structure–activity relationships, 54
  early studies, carcinogenic activity, 50
  monosubstituted, carcinogenic activities, 134–35*t*
  reactions with nucleic acids, 122–25
  substituted, carcinogenic activities, 136–37*t*
  tumor-initiating activities of derivatives, 106–7*t*
Beta-hydroxylation, metabolism of *N*-nitroso carcinogens, 693
Beta-oxidized di-*n*-propylnitrosamines, metabolism, 691
Beta-oxidized nitrosamines, neighboring-group effect, 650
Betel, 25
Beverages
  aflatoxins, 1112
  N-nitrosamines, 834–38
BF—*See* Benzoflavone
BHA—*See* Butylated hydroxyanisole
BHT—*See* Butylated hydroxytoluene
Bis(chloromethyl) ether, 396
Bile acids, epigenetic carcinogen, 1330*t*
Bioassay
  aims, 1324
  history, 1324–26
  in vitro and in vivo tests, 1323–60
  requirements, 1324
Biochemical analysis, of tissue exposed to nitroso compounds, 704
Biochemical effects, aflatoxins, 1076–93
Biochemistry
  of O^6-methylguanine repair, *N*-nitroso carcinogens, 719–24
  polynuclear carcinogens, 66
Biological detoxification, aflatoxins, 963–54
Biological effects of alkylaryltriazenes, 896–904
Biomethylation
  anomalous, of DNA, 368
  DNA, 367
Biopolymers, interaction with triazenes, 906
Biotransformation
  of neoplasms, 1327
  N-nitroso carcinogens, 682–706
4-Biphenylacetamide
  carcinogenicity, 208*t*
  metabolic activation, 189
  reactions with macromolecules, 197
4-Biphenylacethydroxamic acid, carcinogenicity, 208*t*
Biphenylamine
  and bladder cancer, 177
  carcinogenic reagents, 315
  carcinogenic structure–activity relationship, 205
  carcinogenicity, 208*t*
  malignancy sites, 31*t*
  metabolic activation, 188
  modification of amine carcinogenesis, 260
  structure, 281*f*

Biphenyldimethylamine, carcinogenicity, 208*t*
Biphenylhydroxylamine, carcinogenicity, 208*t*
Birth control pills, liver tumors, 24
Bis(1-aziridinyl)morpholinophosphine sulfide, oncogenesis tests, 464–65*t*
Bis(2-chloroethyl) ether, 536
N-Bis(2-chloroethyl)-2-dimethoxyaniline, 369*t*
Bis(2-chloroethyl)methylamine, detoxification mechanism, 374
1,3-Bis(chloroethyl)-1-nitrosourea
  See also *N*-Nitroso-*N,N'*-bis(2-chloroethyl)urea
  oncogenesis tests, 450–51*t*
N,N-Bis(chloroethyl)triazene derivatives, medicinal applications, 872
Bis(2-chloroisopropyl) ether, 530
Bis(chloromethyl) ether, 439, 530
  DNA synthesis, inhibition, 402
  half-life, 396
  oncogenesis tests, 442–43*t*
  squamous carcinoma, 404
Bis(chloro-1-methylethyl) ether, 530
3,6-Bis(dimethylamino)acridine HCl, Acridine orange, carcinogenicity, 259*t*
Bis(3,4-epoxy-6-methylcyclohexylmethyl) adipate, oncogenesis tests, 463*t*
Bis(2,3-epoxy-2-methylpropyl) ether, oncogenesis tests, 463*t*
1'-Bis(2,3-epoxypropyl)-4,4'-bipiperidine, oncogenesis tests, 463*t*
1'-Bis(2,3-epoxypropyl)piperazine, oncogenesis tests, 463*t*
1'-Bis(ethyleneiminosulfonyl)propane, oncogenesis tests, 464–65*t*
1'-Bis(methanesulfonyloxy)propane, 459
Bisphenol diglycidyl ethers, oncogenesis tests, 461–62*t*
Black beans, aflatoxins, 1107
Black peppers, aflatoxins, 1111
Bladder cancer, 286–90
  anticancer drugs, 1246
  exposure to aromatic amines, 175
  industrial, 288–90
  N-nitroso carcinogens, 726
  United Kingdom, 10, 287, 288*t*
  worldwide variation, 5*t*
Bladder carcinogenesis
  naphthylamines, 224
  N-nitrosomethyl-*N*-alkylamines, 692
Bladder implantation, role in tumor induction, pellet, 256
Bladder neoplasms, malignant, in United Kingdom, 289*t*
Bladder tumors
  from aniline exposure, 278
  bracken carcinogenicity, 1175
  in sheep, *pteridium aquuilinum var esculentum*, 1180
Bleomycins, carcinogenicity, 1253
Blood glucose determinations, carcinogenic reagents, 311
Bloom's syndrome, chromosomal instability, 396
Blowing agents, use of triazene compounds, 872
Blue cheese, aflatoxins, 1114
Bond order, highest, related to carcinogenic activity, 59
Bone lesions, teratogenic effects, 1156
Bonito, polycyclic aromatic hydrocarbon content, 1210*t*
Botran, 559
Bovine enzootic hematuria, *pteridium aquuilinum var esculentum*, 1180
Bovolide, oncogenesis tests, 434–35*t*
Bowel cancer, 21
BP—*See* Benzo[*a*]pyrene, 1209
BPA—*See* Biphenylamine
BPAA—*See* 4-Biphenylacetamide
Bracken carcinogenicity, 1171–97, 1220
Breast cancer
  alkylating agent therapy, 398
  female, distribution, 6
  induction in female rats, 1343
Breast enlargement, precocious, 1156
Bromination, synthesis of arene epoxides and dihydrodiols, 112
9-Bromomethylanthracene, oncogenesis tests, 412*t*
7-Bromomethylbenz[*a*]anthracene, oncogenesis tests, 411*t*
7-Bromomethyl-12-methylbenz[*a*]anthracene, oncogenesis tests, 411*t*
3-Bromopropionic acidalbino, oncogenesis tests, 410*t*
Burkitt's lymphoma, 5
  Epstein–Barr virus presence, 27
Busulfan
  See also Myleran
  activity, 456
Butadiene dioxide, 401
  carcinogenicity, 369*t*
  oncogenesis tests, 461–62*t*
1-Butane sultone, 439
  oncogenesis tests, 440–41*t*
n-Butyl methanesulfonate, oncogenesis tests, 416–17*t*
n-Butyl stearate, oncogenesis tests, 420*t*
n-Butyl *p*-toluenesulfonate
  oncogenesis tests, 416–17*t*
  relative carcinogenicity, 382
Butylated hydroxyanisole, 935
  effects on hepatic microsomes, 1284–85
  effects on tumor promotion in mice, 1307*t*
  influence on aflatoxin B_1 genotoxicity, 1031*t*
  inhibition of chemical carcinogenesis, 1283*t*
Butylated hydroxytoluene
  effects on tumor promotion in mice, 1307*t*
  inhibition of chemical carcinogenesis, 1283*t*
  urethane tumorigenesis, 1286
Butyl-4-hydroxyanisoles, 1284
Butyrolactones, oncogenesis tests, 430–33*t*, 434–35*t*, 438*t*
N-Butyrylethyleneimine, oncogenesis tests, 426–27*t*

C

C-Nitroso compounds, carcinogenicity, 657*t*
Cadmium, malignancy sites, 31*t*
Calcium intake, effect on gastric cancer, 1194
Camembert, aflatoxins, 1114
cAMP, 1308*t*
Cancer
  as cause of death, 7
  causes, and social class, 7

Cancer—*Continued*
in England, 3
epidemiology, 1–34
defined, 1
gastric, bracken carcinogenicity, 1175
incidence, and age, 7*t*
mortality
males, occupation incidence, 14*t*
of chemists, 305*t*
natural history, 11–12
registeries, 11–12
sites, human, 21*t*
treatment, 10
Cancer theory, molecular level, 1207
Cantharadine, carcinogenicity, 1250
N-Caproylethyleneimine, oncogenesis tests, 426–27*t*
Captan
carcinogenicity in mice, 556–57*t*
structure, 557
Carbamate esters, metabolic activation of aromatic amines, 187
Carbamazepine, in vivo conversion, 1264
2-Carbazolylacetamide, carcinogenicity, 259*t*
3-Carbazolylacetamide, carcinogenicity, 259*t*
1-(4-Carboethoxyphenyl)-3,3-dimethyltriazene, principal target organs, 899*t*
Carbon black, exposure, 169
Carbon coupling, triazenes, 871
Carbon tetrachloride, 408, 537
aflatoxin B_1 carcinogenicity, 998*t*
effect on *N*-nitroso carcinogenesis, 678*t*
mechanisms, 562
oncogenesis, 406–7*t*
Carbonates, oncogenesis tests, 420*t*
β-Carbonyl-substituted alkyl halides, 408
oncogenesis, 409*t*
α-Carboxy-β-phenyl-β-propiolactone, oncogenesis tests, 430–33*t*
Carcinogen binding index, definition, 377
Carcinogenicity
in adult animals, triazenes, 898
correlation with mutagenicity, 369*t*
of 3,3-dialkyl-1-(3-pyridyl)triazenes to the rat fetus, 902*t*
evaluation, 1337, 1340, 1343
N-nitroso carcinogens, 653
structural requirements, 654–65
triazenes, 897
Carcinogenicity data, interpretation problems, 561
Carcinogenesis
diethylnitrosamine, median total dose and induction time, 666*t*
mechanisms, 1328
by *N*-nitroso compounds, mechanism, 697–728
steps, 18
transplacental, *N*-nitroso carcinogens, 671
Carcinogenic tars, early fluorescence studies, 50
Carcinogens, chemical, classes, 1329
Carcinomas
lung, in asbestos workers, 635–36
unsymmetrical *N*-nitrosamines, 659
Case, R. A. M., 290–93
Case-control studies, 16–17
Case fatality rate, definition, 15*t*
Cassava, aflatoxins, 1110
Castration, and rat aflatoxin B_1 metabolism, 1071
Cat, aflatoxin B_1 toxicity, 879*t*
Catecholamines, bracken carcinogenicity, 1182
Cattle, aflatoxin B_1 excretion, 1075
Cattle bracken poisoning, 1171
Causal connections, 1207
CBI—*See* Carcinogen binding index
CCNU—*See* (Chloroethyl)cyclohexylnitrosourea
Cell transformation
aflatoxin B_1 and in vitro, 1021*t*
evaluation of carcinogenicity, 1336
Cellular analysis of tissue responses, alkylation of DNA, 724
Ceramic wools, mineral fiber carcinogenesis, 633
Charge-transfer complex, carcinogenic activity, 60
Cheddar cheese, aflatoxins, 1115
Cheese
aflatoxins, 1114
nitrosamine content, 1214*t*
N-nitrosamines, 833
Cheilanthes sieberi, carcinogenicity, 1180
Chemical(s), purity, carcinogenicity evaluation, 1345
Chemical carcinogenesis
effects of protease inhibitors, 1303
effects of retinoids, 1301*t*
Chemical carcinogens
classes, 1329
definition, 1326
Chemical exposure
aflatoxin B_1 carcinogenicity, 1000–1
chemists, mortality rate, 304–8
chromosome studies, 310
Chemical inactivation, aflatoxins, 964–66
Chemical laboratories, carcinogen handling, 317
Chemical structure, carcinogenic activity, 52
Chemical studies, bracken carcinogenicity, 1181
Chemiluminescence detector, 829
Chemists
causes of death, 305*t*
epidemiological studies, 304–8
Swedish, causes of death, 307*t*
Chemotherapeutic agents, 24, 397–400
Chicken
aflatoxin B_1
excretion, 1076
toxicity, 978*t*
aflatoxin M_1, excretion, 1033*t*
embryos, aflatoxin B_1 chromosome inductor, 1015*t*
Childhood tumors, 8, 10
Chili peppers, aflatoxins, 1111
China, esophageal cancer, 1144
Chinese hamster
aflatoxin B_1 chromosome inductor, 1013*t*, 1014*t*
gene mutation effects of aflatoxin B_1, 1009*t*
Chlamydomonas reinhardii, gene mutation effects of AFB_1, 1008*t*
Chloral, 858
Chlorambucil
carcinogenicity, 1243, 1244
initiating agents, 401
oncogenesis tests, 450–51*t*
structure, 374

Chloramphenicol, in vivo conversion, 1257
Chlordane
carcinogenicity in mice, 555, 556–57*t*
structure, 557
Chlordecone
carcinogenicity, 547–51*t*
heptocellular carcinomas, 551
in humans, 560
mutagenicity tests, 553
structure, 550
use, 551
Chlordimeform
carcinogenicity in mice, 556–57*t*
structure, 558
Chlorinated hydrocarbons, role in tumor inhibition, 1293
Chlornaphazine, 24
carcinogenicity, 1246
structure, 398
Chloroacetaldehyde, 385
miscoding in polydeoxyribonucleotide templates, 357*t*
Chloroacetic acid, oncogenesis tests, 409*t*
Chloroacetone, oncogenesis tests, 409*t*
4-Chloro-4′-aminobiphenyl ether, carcinogenicity, 209*t*
p-Chloroaniline, carcinogenicity, 202*t*
Chlorobenzilate
carcinogenicity in mice, 556–57*t*
structure, 558
2-Chloro-4-biphenylamine, carcinogenicity, 208*t*
2-Chloro-1,3-butadiene, 526
1-Chloro-2-dinitrobenzene, carcinogenicity, 207*t*
1-Chloro-2-epoxypropane, 531
squamous carcinoma, 404
Chloroethers, malignancy sites, 31*t*
2-Chloroethyl derivatives of *N*-nitrosoureas, cytostatic properties, 681
N-(2-Chloroethyl)aminoazobenzene, oncogenesis tests, 444–45*t*
9-[2-(2-Chloroethylamino)ethylamino]-6-chloro-2-methoxycridine, oncogenesis tests, 444–45*t*
2-Chloroethylarylamines, 439
1-(Chloroethyl)cyclohexyl-1-nitrosourea, oncogenesis, 444–45*t*
Chloroethylene, 527
Chloroethylene oxide, 385
4-Chloro-6-ethyleneimino-2-phenylpyrimidine, oncogenesis tests, 426–27*t*
2-Chloroethyl-2-ethyl sulfide, miscoding, 365–66
2-3-(2-Chloroethylnitrosoureido)-D-glucopyranose, target organ, 786
N-(2-Chloroethyl)nitrosourethane, oncogenesis tests, 444–45*t*
2-Chloroethylphosphonic acid, structure, 447
2-Chloroethylsulfonic acid derivatives, 439
oncogenesis tests, 444–45*t*
2-Chloroethyltrimethylammonium chloride, 439
oncogenesis tests, 444–45*t*
Chloroform, 408, 537
mechanisms, 562
oncogenesis, 405*t*
Chloromethyl methyl ether, 396, 538
oncogenesis tests, 442–43*t*
9-Chloromethyl-*N*-anthracene, oncogenesis tests, 412*t*
9-Chloromethylbenz[*a*]anthracene, injections, 413
4-Chloromethylbiphenyl, 544
structure, 545
10-(Chloromethyl)-3-chloroanthracene, oncogenesis tests, 412*t*
10-(Chloromethyl)-3-methylanthracene, oncogenesis tests, 412*t*
7-Chloromethyl-12-methylbenz[*a*]anthracene, oncogenesis tests, 412*t*
4-Chloro-4′-nitrobiphenyl ether, carcinogenicity, 209*t*
α-Chloronitrosamines, synthesis of α-acyloxynitrosamines, 646
3-Chloroperbenzoic acid, 1050
1-(4-Chlorophenyl)-3,3-dimethyltriazene, principal target organs, 899*t*
Chlorophenylenediamines, carcinogenicity, 207*t*
Chloroprene, 526
administration, 527
malignancy sites, 31*t*
toxicology, 526
world production, 526
3-Chloropropene, 544
Chloropropham, 559
3-Chloropropionic acid, alkylating DNA, 353
Chloroquinone mustard, oncogenesis tests, 453*t*, 454*t*
α-Chlorotoluene, 529
Chlorotoluidines, carcinogenicity, 202*t*, 203*t*
Chlorpromazine
inhibition of chemical carcinogenesis, 1291*t*
tumor inhibition, 1297
Cholanthrene and derivatives, carcinogenic activities, 142–43*t*
Choline-deficient diet, 1083
Chromatin analysis, alkylation of nucleic acids by *N*-nitroso compounds, 711–14
Chromium
genotoxic carcinogen, 1330*t*
malignancy sites, 31*t*
Chromosomal damage, test for in vivo genotoxicity, 1340
Chromosome effects, in vitro assays, 1334
Chromosome studies, following chemical exposure, 310
Chromosome tests, evaluation of carcinogenicity, 1336
Chronic bioassay, experimental design, 1354
Chronic bioassay test systems, 1344
Chronic exposure, persistence of O^6-alkylguanine and tumorigenesis, 709
Chronic lymphocytic leukemia, alkylating agent therapy, 398
Chrysene
carcinogenic activities, 131*t*
tumor-initiating activity, 105
Chrysene derivatives
carcinogenic activities, 138–39*t*
tumor initiating activities, 106*t*
Chrysotile, 631–32, 633
Chymostatin, 1304
carcinogenesis inhibitors, 1303*t*

Cis-trans isomerism, 1,2,3-triazabutadienes, 895
triazene derivatives, 875
Cisplatin
carcinogenicity, 1243, 1248
oncogenesis tests, 452*t*
Citrinnin, effect on *N*-nitroso carcinogenesis, 678*t*
Citrus Red 2, 1224
Clavacin, oncogenesis tests, 434–35*t*
Clays, 634
Climatic conditions, bracken carcinogenicity, 1175
Clinical chemistry, carcinogenic reagents, 311
Clinoptilite, 634
Clofibrate, carcinogenicity, 1268
Clostridium, aflatoxins effect, 971
Clustering, definition, 10
Coal tar, 166
carcinogenic effect, 1267
creosote derivatives, 166
early investigations of carcinogenesis, 49
Coconut oils, polycyclic aromatic hydrocarbon content, 1210*t*
Coffee
aflatoxins, 1112
polycyclic aromatic hydrocarbon content, 1210*t*
Cohort studies, 17–18
Colon, aflatoxin B_1-induced tumors, 993
Colon cancer, fiber consumption, 924
Colon carcinogenesis, 918
experimental, 923–25
Colonic adenomatous polyps, induction, 916
Colpidium campylum, aflatoxin B_1 effect, 972
Combustion processes, PAH generation, 1294
Compensation, 294–95
Competitive risk, carcinogenic effect of two carcinogens, 675
Congeners, aflatoxin, 1023–25
Conjugation
and carcinogenic activity, 67
polynuclear compounds, related to carcinogenic activity, 62
Consumption, direct human, bracken fern, 1190
Conversion and recombination, by aflatoxin B_1, 1011*t*
Cooking, nitrosamine formation, 1215
Copra, aflatoxins, 1105
Corn, aflatoxins, 1096
detection, 952
Corticosteroids
treatment, bracken carcinogenicity, 1173
effect on aflatoxin B_1 carcinogenicity, 996*t*
Cortisol, tumor inhibition, 1299*t*
Cortisone, tumor inhibition, 1297*t*
Cosmetics, nitrosamines, 842–45
Cottage cheese, aflatoxins, 1115
Cottonseed, aflatoxins, 1104
Coumarins, highly substituted—*See also* Aflatoxins
oncogenesis tests, 438*t*
tumor inhibition, 1297*t*, 1298
N-Coupling, triazenes, 871
Cow, excretion of aflatoxin M_1, 1035*t*
CPFA—*See* Cyclopropenoid fatty acids
Creosote derivatives, of coal tar, 166
Cresidine, carcinogenicity, 203*t*
Crocidolite, 632, 633
Crop contamination, atmospheric pollution, 1211
Cross-linkage, DNA damage produced, 1335
Crotocin, lethal dose, 1139*t*
Crude incidence rate, definition, 15*t*
Cultured cells, aflatoxin potency, 973–76
Cumulative incidence rate, definition, 15*t*
Cutaneous application, administration of test chemicals, 1349
Cutting oils, 170
Cyanogenesis, bracken carcinogenicity, 1182
Cycasin, 915–38, 1219
carbohydrate moiety, 915
carcinogenesis, 918
neurotoxicity, 932
occurrence, 915
Cyclamate, 1225
Cyclamate–saccharin combination, 1225
Cyclic nitrosamines
metabolism, 693
structure–activity relationships, 661
target organ, 763–77
Cyclic sulfides, 439
oncogenesis tests, 440–41*t*
N-Cycloethyleneureidoazobenzene, oncogenesis tests, 426–27*t*
Cyclohexane dimethane sulfonates, reactions and metabolism, 458
Cycloheximide, 982
Cyclopenta[*a*]phenanthrene and derivatives, carcinogenic activities, 142–43*t*
Cyclophosphamide, 24
carcinogenicity, 1243, 1245
DNA alkylation, 370–71*t*
metabolism, 456
Cyclopropenoid fatty acids
effect on aflatoxin B_1 carcinogenicity, 997*t*, 998*t*
tumor induction by aflatoxin B_1, 1000–1
Cyclops fuscus, aflatoxins effect, 973
Cyproheptadine, in vivo conversion, 1264
Cysteamines
protection from aflatoxin B_1, 981
tumor inhibition, 1297*t*
Cysteine
influence on aflatoxin B_1 genotoxicity, 1030*t*
protection from aflatoxin B_1, 981
[3H]-Cytidine triphosphate incorporation, inhibition by aflatoxin B_1, 1079
Cytochrome P-448 complexation, inhibition by flavones, 1068
Cytochrome P-450, and carcinogenic activity, 66
Cytomegalus virus, immune suppression, 28
Cytosine arabinoside, carcinogenicity, 1251, 1253
Cytostatic properties, 2-chloroethyl derivatives of *N*-nitrosoureas, 681
Cytotoxic therapy, with Myleran, 460
Cytotoxin, mode of action, 1330*t*
Cytoxan, oncogenesis tests, 453*t*

D

DAB—*See* Dimethyl-*p*-phenylazoaniline
Dacarbazine, 1243
carcinogenicity, 1248
DACPM—*See* Methylenebis(2-chloroaniline)

Dairy products
  aflatoxins, 1113–15
  bracken carcinogenicity, 1191
  N-nitrosamines, 833
Damage, fixation, 1328
DAMPM—*See* Methylenebis(2-methylaniline)
DAPM—*See* Methylenedianiline
Dates, aflatoxins, 1110
Db[a,c]A, role in tumor inhibition, 1295*t*
DDT—*See* Dichlorodiphenyltrichloroethane
15-Deacetyl, structure, 1148*t*
4-Deacetyl neosolaniol, structure 1148*t*
Deacetylation, metabolic detoxification of aromatic amines, 193
Deamination of primary amines, triazenes, 887
Death(s)
  causes, chemists, 305*t*
  in U.S., 396
    common causes, 3*t*
Decane oxide, influence on aflatoxin B_1 genotoxicity, 1030*t*
Decarbazine, oxidative demethylation, 377
Decision point approach
  results, 1358*t*
  systematic approach to evaluate carcinogenicity, 1332
Dediazoniation, dialkylaryltriazenes, 894
Definition, chemical carcinogens, 1326
Degradation
  acid-catalyzed, and photolysis, dialkyltriazenes, 891
  reactions of monoalkyltriazenes, 885–87
Dehydroacetic acid, 395
  oncogenesis tests, 437*t*
Dehydrogenation, selective, synthesis of arene epoxides and dihydrodiols, 112
Dehydroxylation, metabolic detoxification of aromatic amines, 193
DEN—*See* Diethylnitrosamine
Deoxyguanosine, reactions with styrene oxides, 425
2-Deoxy-2-(*N*-methyl-*N*-nitrosoureido)-D-glucopyranose, target organ, 781
Deoxyribonucleic acid—*See* DNA
3-(β-D-2-Deoxytribosyl)-7,8-dihydropyrimido[2,1-*i*]purine-9-one, 353
DES—*See* Diethylstilbestrol
Descriptive epidemiology, 13–14
Desmethyl trichlorphon, as genotoxic agents, 393
Detoxification
  aflatoxin B_1, 1064
  mechanisms, aromatic amines, 191
  pathway with phenobarbital, 1066
Dexamethasone, tumor inhibition, 1297–98, 1297*t*, 1299*t*
DFMO, two-stage promotion, inhibition, 1309
Diacetoxyscirpenol, 1147
Diacetylbenzidine, carcinogenicity, 213*t*
Diacetylhydrazine, 937
Diacetylscirpenol, lethal dose, 1139*t*
Dialkylaryltriazenes, chemistry and biological properties, 889
3,3-Dialkyl-1-(3-pyridyl)triazenes, toxicity, to the rat fetus, 902*t*
Dialkyltriazenes, reactions of, 891–94
Diallate
  carcinogenicity in mice, 556–57*t*
  structure, 558
2,4-Diaminoanisole, carcinogenicity, 206*t*
3,3′-Diaminobenzidine, carcinogenicity, 213
4′-Diamino-3′-dichlorobiphenyl, 530
4′-Diamino-3′-dichlorodiphenylmethane, structure, 544
4′-Diaminodiphenylmethane—*See* 4,4′-Methylenedianiline
4′-Diaminophenyl—*See* Benzidine
Dianhydrogalacticol, carcinogenicity, 1249
o,o′-Dianisidine, carcinogenicity, 213*t*
Diastereomers, nomenclature, 45
Diazepam, in vivo conversion, 1261
N-Diazo coupling
  acid-catalyzed reversal, dialkylaryltriazenes, 892
  preparation of dialkylaryltriazenes, 889
  preparation of monoalkylaryltriazenes, 884, 888
Dibenzamine, carcinogen, 1250
Dibenz[*a*]anthracene
  carcinogenic activity, 131*t*, 140–41*t*
  carcinogenic activity, early studies, 50
  tumor-initiating activity, 105
    of derivatives, 106*t*, 107*t*
Dibenzo[*a,h*]anthracene, structure, 166*f*
Dibenzo[*b*]chrysene, carcinogenic activities, 132*t*
Dibenzo[*b,def*]chrysene
  carcinogenic activities, 131*t*, 140–41*t*
Dibenzo[*def,no*]chrysene
  See also Dibenzopyrene
  carcinogenic activities, 132*t*
Dibenzodioxins, 533–34
  halogenated, 532
Dibenzofurans, 533–34
  halogenated, structure–activity relationship, 534
  structures, 534
3-Dibenzofuranylacetamide, carcinogenicity, 259*t*
3-Dibenzofuranylamine, carcinogenicity, 259*t*
Dibenzo[*a*]naphthacene, carcinogenic activities, 132*t*, 133*t*
Dibenzo[*de,gr*]napthacene, carcinogenic activities, 132*t*
Dibenzo[*fg,op*]napthacene, carcinogenic activities, 132*t*
Dibenzo[*b,g*]phenanthrene, carcinogenic activities, 132*t*
Dibenzo[*c,g*]phenanthrene, carcinogenic activities, 133*t*
Dibenzopyrene
  See also Naphtho[1,2,3,4-*def*]chrysene *and* Dibenzo[*b,def*]chrysene
  carcinogenic activities, 133*t*
  structure, 166*f*
Dibenzothiophenylacetamides, carcinogenicity, 259*t*
N,N-Dibenzyl-2-chloroethylamine, carcinogenicity, 1250
Dibromoacetophenone, effect on arachidonic acid metabolism, 1305*t*
1-Dibromo-3-chloropropane, 385, 553–54
  carcinogenicity, 547–51*t*

1-Dibromo-3-chloropropane—*Continued*
mutagenicity effects, 554
sterility effects, 554
Dibromodulcitol, oncogenesis tests, 450–51*t*
Dibromoethane, 538, 539
1,2-Dibromoethane, DNA alkylation, 370–71*t*
Dibromomannitol, oncogenesis tests, 450–51*t*
Di-*n*-butyl sulfate
oncogenesis tests, 414–15*t*
relative carcinogenicity, 382
1,1-Di-*n*-butylhydrazine, 923
Dibutylnitrosamine, metabolism, 688
Dichlone, 559
3,3′-Dichlorobenzidine, 283, 530–31, 544
carcinogenic reagents, 315
carcinogenicity, 213*t*
interaction with polyribonucleotides, 531
structure, 283, 544
1,4-Dichloro-2-butene, 526
Dichlorodiphenyldichloroethane
carcinogenicity in mice, 556–57*t*
structure, 558
Dichlorodiphenyldichloroethylene
carcinogenicity in mice, 556–57*t*
in humans, storage, 560
structure, 559
Dichlorodiphenyltrichloroethane
carcinogenicity in mice, 556–57*t*
in humans, storage, 560
inhibition of chemical carcinogenesis, 1291*t*
structure, 558
1,2-Dichloroethane, 539
Dichloroethylenes, 528, 529
Di(2-chloroethyl)methylamine, oncogenesis tests, 448–49*t*
Dichloromethane, 538
commercial importance, 538
α,α-Dichloromethyl ether, oncogenesis tests, 442–43*t*
2-(2,4-Dichlorophenoxy)propionic acid, 559
Dichlorvos
DNA methylation, 393
as genotoxic agents, 393
oncogenesis tests, 418–19*t*
structures, 559
Dicryl, 559
Dicyclohexylnitrosamines, structure–activity relationship, 657
Dieldrin, 424
carcinogenicity in mice, 555, 556–57*t*
effect on aflatoxin B_1 carcinogenicity, 997*t*
in humans, storage, 560
oncogenesis tests, 424*t*
structure, 396, 558
1,2,3,4-Diepoxycyclohexane, oncogenesis tests, 463*t*
1,2,5,6-Diepoxycyclooctane, oncogenesis tests, 463*t*
1,2,6,7-Diepoxyheptane, oncogenesis tests, 461–62*t*
1,2,5,6-Diepoxyhexane, oncogenesis tests, 461–62*t*
1,2,7,8-Diepoxyoctane, oncogenesis tests, 461–62*t*
1,2,4,5-Diepoxypentane, oncogenesis tests, 461–62*t*
9,10,12,13-Diepoxystearic acid, oncogenesis tests, 463*t*
Dietary factors, 27, 1227–32
and aflatoxin B_1 carcinogenicity, 994
aflatoxin B_1 metabolism, 1070–72
observations in animals, 1230–32
Dietary protein, effect on hepatotoxicity, 980
Diethanolamine, 845
Diethyl carbonate, oncogenesis tests, 420*t*
Diethyl epoxysuccinate, structure, 395
Diethyl maleate, 1069
tumor inhibition, 1297*t*
Diethyl sulfate
oncogenesis tests, 414–15*t*
relative carcinogenicity, 382
N-Diethylacetylethyleneimine, oncogenesis tests, 426–27*t*
Diethylamine, lowest effective carcinogenic doses, 670*t*
Diethyl-2-chlorovinyl phosphate, oncogenesis tests, 418–19*t*
Diethyldithiocarbamate, 1285
Diethyl-*S*-ethylmercaptoethanol thiophosphate, oncogenesis tests, 418–19*t*
Diethyl-*S*-[ethylthioethyl]phosphorodithioate, oncogenesis tests, 418–19*t*
1,2-Diethylhydrazine, carcinogenesis, 919
Diethyl-*p*-nitrophenyl thiophosphate, oncogenesis tests, 418–19*t*
Diethylnitrosamine, 1216
combination effects in carcinogenesis, 676*t*
dose–response relationships, 667*f*
effects
on aflatoxin B_1 carcinogenicity, 997*t*
of xenobiotics on carcinogenesis, 678*t*
Diethylnitrosamine carcinogenesis, median total dose and induction time, 666*t*
Diethyl-1-phenyltriazene
principal target organs, 899*t*
transplacental carcinogenesis in rats, 900*t*
3,3-Diethyl-1-(3-pyridyl)triazene
principal target organs, 899*t*
transplacental carcinogenesis in rats, 900*t*
Diethylstilbestrol, 24
causes, 1205
epigenetic carcinogen, 1330*t*
structure, 1155
Diffuse pleural fibrosis, as indication of fibrous mineral exposure, 635
1,1-Difluoroethylene, 529
α-Difluoromethylornithine, stage-specific inhibitors, 1309*t*
Difunctional alkylating agents, 396
Difunctional epoxides, 460
Difunctional ethyleneimines, 460
Difunctional sulfonates, 456
Diglycidyl ether, oncogenesis tests, 461–62*t*
Dihalomethanes, 538
16,17-Dihydro-15*H*-cyclopenta]*a*]phenanthrene and derivatives, carcinogenic activities, 142–43*t*
trans-1,2-Dihydro-1,2-dihydroxynaphthalene, breakdown of sulfates, 72*f*
Dihydrodiol
activity of benzo[*a*]pyrene derivative, 101*t*
formation, catalysis, 1069

Dihydrodiol—*Continued*
lung adenomas induced by benzo[*a*]pyrene derivative, 103*t*
non-K region, synthesis, 112
tumorigenic activity of benzo[*a*]pyrene derivative, 102*t*
Dihydrodiol epoxides
activity of benzo[*a*]pyrene derivative, 101*t*
lung adenomas induced by benzo[*a*]pyrene derivative, 103*t*
nomenclature, 44
tumorigenic activity of benzo[*a*]pyrene derivative, 102*t*
vicinal, reactivity, 118
Dihydrodiol route, metabolic, aromatic hydrocarbons, 73
Dihydro-2,3-hydroxy aflatoxin B_1—*See* Aflatoxin B_1 dihydrodiol
5,6-Dihydroretinoic acid, 1302*t*
3,3′-Dihydroxybenzidine, carcinogenicity, 213*t*
3,3′-Diindolymethane, inhibition of chemical carcinogenesis, 1291*t*
Diiodomethane, 538
Diisopropyl fluorophosphate, oncogenesis tests, 418–19*t*
Diisopropyl sulfate, 413
oncogenesis tests, 414–15*t*
Diketene, oncogenesis tests, 438*t*
Dimethane sulfonates
SN_1 elimination reactions, 459
structure, 398
Dimethanesulfonoxyhexanes, oncogenesis tests, 457*t*
2,4-Dimethoxyaniline, carcinogenicity, 203*t*
3,3′-Dimethoxybenzidine-3-(*o*-dianisidine), carcinogenic reagents, 315
Dimethyl carbamoylchloride, squamous carcinoma, 404
Dimethyl dithiophosphate of diethyl mercaptosuccinate, oncogenesis, 418–19*t*
Dimethyl hydroxy-2,2,2-trichloroethyl phosphonate, oncogenesis tests, 418–19*t*
α,β-Dimethyl maleic anhydride, oncogenesis tests, 434–35*t*
Dimethyl selenide, exposure, 1145
Dimethyl sulfate, 384
DNA alkylation, 370–71*t*, 373*t*
miscoding in polydeoxyribonucleotide templates, 357*t*
oncogenesis tests, 414–15
relative carcinogenicity, 382
squamous carcinoma, 404
Dimethylamine, lowest effective carcinogenic doses, 670*t*
Dimethylamine salts, of phenoxyalkanoic acid, 845
4-Dimethylaminoazobenzene
See also Dimethyl-4-phenylazoaniline
carcinogenesis with *N*-nitroso compounds, 676*t*
4-Dimethylaminostilbene, carcinogenesis with *N*-nitroso compounds, 676*t*
Dimethylbenz[*a*]anthracene(s), 168
carcinogenic activities, 136–37*t*
tumor-initiating activity, derivatives, 108*t*
Dimethylbenz[*a*]anthracene derivatives, carcinogenic activities, 136–37*t*
Dimethylbenz[*a*]anthracene tumor, inhibition by TCDD, 1292*f*
3,3′-Dimethylbenzidine, carcinogenic reagents, 315
Dimethylbiphenylamines, carcinogenicity, 209*t*
Dimethylcarbamoyl chloride, 531
Dimethyl-2,2-chlorovinyl phosphate, oncogenesis tests, 418–19*t*
1,7-Dimethylchrysene, structure, 169*f*
2,5-Dimethyl-1,2,5,6-diepoxyhex-3-yne, oncogenesis tests, 461–62*t*
Dimethylformamide, structure, 352
Dimethylhydrazine, 922
alkylation of nucleic acids, 927
carcinogenesis, 918
conversion in liver, 937
tumor induction, genetic variation, 925
1,2-Dimethylhydrazine, metabolism to methylazoxymethanol, 917
Dimethyl-1-(2-methylphenyl)triazene, principal target organs, 899*t*
Dimethyl-1-(4-nitrophenyl)triazene, principal target organs, 899*t*
Dimethylnitrosamine
combination effects in carcinogenesis, 676*t*
effects of xenobiotics on carcinogenesis, 678*t*
in frankfurters, 1216
genotoxic carcinogen, 1330*t*
3,3′-Dimethyl-2-oxetanone, oncogenesis tests, 430–33*t*
N-Dimethyl-4-phenylazoaniline
derivatives, structure–activity relationship, 233
liver carcinogenicity, 235–36*t*
reactions with macromolecules, 196
substituent effect, 234*t*
3-Dimethyl-1-phenyltriazene
mass spectrometry data, 879
mutagenicity, 901
principal target organs, 899*t*
transplacental carcinogenesis in rats, 900*t*
Dimethyl-1-(3-pyridyl-*N*-oxide)triazene, principal target organs, 899*t*
Dimethyl-1-(3-pyridyl)triazene, principal target organs, 899*t*
Dimethyltriazene conformation, triazenes, 873
N,N-Dimethyltriazene, medicinal applications, 872
5-(3,3-Dimethyltriazeno)imidazole-4-carboxamide, oxidative demethylation, 377
β,β-Dimethyltrimethylene oxide, oncogenesis tests, 430–33*t*
2,6-Dinitroaniline, 845
Dinitroaniline derivatives, 845
N,N′-Dinitroso-*N,N′*-diethylethylenediamine, target organ, 761
N,N′-Dinitroso-*N,N′*-dimethylethylenediamine, target organ, 761
N,N′-Dinitroso-*N,N′*-dimethyloxamide, target organ, 797
N,N′-Dinitroso-*N,N′*-dimethylphthalamide, target organ, 798
N,N′-Dinitroso-2,5-dimethylpiperazine, target organ, 774

N,N′-Dinitroso-*N,N′*-dimethyl-1,3-propanediamine, target organ, 761
N,N′-Dinitrosohomopiperazine, target organ, 774
N,4-Dinitroso-*N*-methylaniline, target organ, 761
N,N′-Dinitroso-2-methylpiperazine, target organ, 773
N,N′-Dinitrosopentamethylenetetramine, target organ, 775
N,N′-Dinitrosoperhydropyrimidine, target organ, 775
N,N′-Dinitrosopiperazine, target organ, 773
N,N′-Dinitroso-2,3,5,6-tetramethylpiperazine, target organ, 774
2,4-Dinitrotoluene, carcinogenicity, 206*t*
Diol–epoxide metabolites, 394
Diphenylamine, 284
  structure, 285*f*
Diphenylhydantoin, in vivo conversion, 1264
Diphenylnitrosamine, structure–activity relationship, 658
α,α-Diphenyl-β-propiolactone, oncogenesis tests, 430–33*t*
Dipole movements, triazene compounds, 875
Di-*n*-propylnitrosamines, metabolism of β-oxidized, 691
Direct-acting carcinogen, mode of action, 1330*t*
Dishwashing compounds, nitrosamines, 850
7,12-Disubstituted benz[*a*]anthracenes, carcinogenic activities, 136–37*t*
1,1-Disubstituted hydrazines, 929
Disulfiram, 377, 1285
  effects
    N-nitroso carcinogenesis, 678*t*
    tumor promotion in mice, 1307*t*
  inhibition of chemical carcinogenesis, 1283*t*
Dithiocarbamates, 855, 1227
Dithranol, carcinogenicity, 1272
DMBA—*See* Dimethylbenz[*a*]anthracene
DMH—*See* 1,2-dimethylhydrazine
DNA
  alkylation, 353, 367
    extent after carcinogen doses, 370–71*t*
    in vivo dosimetry, 368
  alkylation repair, *N*-nitroso carcinogens, 722–28
  bases, miscoding, 356*f*
  β-propiolactone reactions, 353
  binding
    aflatoxins, 1049
    polynuclear aromatics, 122–25
    vs. protein binding, 1062
  biomethylation, 368
    cytotoxic action, 367
  carcinogen binding index, methyl methanesulfonate, 372
  carcinogens that interact with and alter, 1329
  damage
    alkylating agents, 1243
    antimetabolites, 1251
    in vitro assays, 1334
    indicators, 365
    measurement discussion, 1335
  damage and repair, aflatoxin B_1-induced, 1017–20*t*
  deficient biomethylation, 367

DNA—*Continued*
  fragmentation, test for in vivo genotoxicity, 1340
  hypomethylation, 367
  in vivo, stability of alkylated components, 705
  in vivo alkylation, 372
    by epoxides
  methylation by dichlorvos, 385
  nitroso compounds as alkylating agents, 698
  O-alkylation, bases, 354
  reactions
    with aromatic amines, 193–201
    with 4-nitroquinoline, 247
  repair
    error-prone, 365
    mechanisms, 365
  repair-induced structural change, *N*-nitroso carcinogens, 714–16
  replication, 354
  role of O^6-alkylguanine in *N*-nitroso carcinogens, 728
  single-strand scission, 1254
  synthesis
    inhibition, 1077
    MAM effects, 927
    partial hepatectomy stimulation, 1077
  transformation, 351
DNA-adduct formation, 1053
DNA–aflatoxin B_1 adduct formation, 1059
Doctors, cancer rate, 308
Dodecane, carcinogenic enhancement, 168
Dog, aflatoxin B_1 toxicity, 978*t*
Domestic soots, 165
Dominant lethal test, test for in vivo genotoxicity, 1340
Dose dependence, equation, 379
Dose–response studies
  alkylation carcinogenesis, 378–83
  N-nitroso carcinogens, 665–71
Dose selection, rationale, 1350
Double bonds
  epoxidation, conversion of drugs, 1263
  reactive, related to carcinogenic activity, 57
Drinking water, arsenic, 1224
Drosophila melanogaster
  aflatoxin B_1 chromosome inductor, 1012*t*
  aflatoxins effect, 973
  gene mutation effects of aflatoxin B_1, 1010*t*
  somatic eye-color mutations, 351
Drugs
  anticancer, carcinogenicity, 1241–55
  converted to carcinogens in vivo, 1255–66
  iatrogenic cancer, 24–25
  naturally occurring, carcinogenicity, 1253–55
  nitrosamines, 845
DTIC—*See* Decarbazine
Duck(s)
  aflatoxin B_1 hepatocarcinogenicity, 984*t*
  aflatoxin B_1 toxicity, 978*t*
  excretion of aflatoxin M_1, 1033*t*
  susceptibility to aflatoxin B_1, 992
Dyes
  azo, structure–activity relationship, 247

Dyes—*Continued*
phenylazonaphthol, structure–activity relationship, 240
use of triazene compounds, 972

E

Edam cheese, aflatoxins, 1114
Eggs, aflatoxins, 1112
5,8,11,14-Eicosatetraynoic acid
effect on arachidonic acid metabolism, 1305*t*
tumor inhibition, 1297*t*
Elaiomycin, structure, 920
Elastatinal, 1304
carcinogenesis inhibitors, 1303*t*
Electrochemical oxidation, triazenes, 892
Electron(s)
pi, density distributions, related to carcinogenic activities, 57
properties related to carcinogenic activity, 60
Electron transport, in vitro inhibition by aflatoxin B_1, 1090
Electronic structure, related to carcinogenic activity, 58
Electrophilic character, reactive carcinogenic organic compounds, 869
Embryotoxicity, *N*-nitroso carcinogens, 653
α-Emitters, 22
Enantiomer(s)
nomenclature, 45
tumorigenic activity of benzo[*a*]pyrene derivative, 102
Endogenous modification, aromatic amine carcinogenesis, 263
Endogenous nitrosation, availability of nitrosating agents, 858
Endogenous synthesis, sources, 1211
Endoplasmic reticulum, activation of aromatic amines, 180
Endosulfan, 559
Endrin, 424
Environmental carcinogens, 829
Environmental factors, data support, 1141
Environmental *N*-nitrosamines, preformed, 832–33
Environmental pollution, 26
sources, 633
Enzymatic activation, dialkylaryltriazenes, 904
Enzymatic repair, of alkylated DNA, 467
Enzyme(s)
acetylation, *N*-hydroxy compounds, 185
action, metabolic detoxification of aromatic amines, 192
bioactivation of nitrosamines, 685
conversions, activation of aromatic amines, 180
in vivo assays, 1339
inhibition of chemical carcinogenesis, 1291*t*
involved in metabolism, polynuclear carcinogens, 66
microsomal, 1065–67
modification of aromatic amine carcinogenesis, 258
reduction, activation of aromatic amines, 183
role in tumor inhibition, 1290
Epibromohydrin, oncogenesis tests, 424*t*
Epichlorohydrin, 531
administration, 531
carcinogenicity, 368
Epichlorohydrin—*Continued*
as initiator, 421
mutagenicity, 368
oncogenesis tests, 422–23*t*, 424*t*
squamous carcinoma, 404
structure, 352
Epidemiologic studies, bracken carcinogenicity, 1193
Epidemiologist, role, 277
Epidemiology
advantages and disadvantages, 1–2
defined, 1
descriptive, 13–14
founder, 11
history, 2–3
methods, 13–18
role of chemists, 304–8
Epidermal superoxide dismutase, decreasing levels, 1306
Epigenetic carcinogen(s), 1329
mode of action, 1330*t*
vs. genotoxic, 525
Epigenetic mechanisms, 525
Epodyl, oncogenesis tests, 461–62*t*
Epoxide(s)
activity of benzo[*a*]pyrene derivative, 101*t*
arene
nomenclature, 46
reactivity, 118
carcinogenicity, 1249
difunctional
inactive, oncogenesis tests, 463*t*
oncogenesis tests, 461–62*t*
dihydrodiol, nomenclature, 44
hydrocarbon, first synthesis, 68
in vivo alkylation of DNA, 421
K-region arene, synthesis, 110
lung adenomas induced by benzo[*a*]pyrene derivative, 103*t*
monofunctional
inactive, 424*t*
oncogenesis tests, 422–23*t*
non-K-region arene, synthesis, 112
tumorigenic activity of benzo[*a*]pyrene derivative, 102*t*
vicinal dihydrodiol, reactivity, 118
Epoxide hydrase inhibitors, 1069
Epoxide hydrolase, and carcinogenic activity, 67
1,2-Epoxybutane, oncogenesis tests, 422–23*t*, 424*t*
1,2-Epoxybut-3-ene, 421
oncogenesis tests, 422–23*t*
Epoxycyclohexane, oncogenesis tests, 424*t*
Epoxycyclooctane, oncogenesis tests, 424*t*
1,2-Epoxydodecane, oncogenesis tests, 424*t*
1,2-Epoxyhexadecane, oncogenesis tests, 422–23*t*
4,5-Epoxy-3-hydroxyvaleric acid β-lactone, oncogenesis tests, 430–33*t*, 438*t*
3,4-Epoxymethylcyclohexylmethyl-3,4-epoxy-6-methylcyclohexanecarboxylate, oncogenesis, 461–62*t*
2,3-Epoxy-2-methylpropyl acrylate, oncogenesis tests, 424*t*

5,6-Epoxyretinoic acid, 1302t
9,10-Epoxystearic acid, oncogenesis tests, 424t
Erionite, 634
  structure, 632
Error-prone repair, DNA, 365
Escherichia coli
  aflatoxin B_1 chromosome inductor, 1011t
  bacterial screening tests, 1335
  differential repair, 1017t
  gene mutation effects of aflatoxin B_1, 1008t
  induced phage reactivation, 1017t
Escherichia coli-arginine, gene mutation effects of aflatoxin B_1, 1007t
Esophageal cancer, 21, 1141–46
  bracken carcinogenicity, 1194
  in China, 1144
  N-methyl-*N*-nitrosoaniline, 869
  nutrition effects, 1229
  role of selenium, 1142–46
  worldwide variation, 6t
Ester(s), 413
  fatty acids, 413, 421
  metabolic activation of aromatic amines, 184–87
  oncogenesis tests, 420t
  synthesis from α-nitrosamino ethers, 645
Ester trichothecenes, 1149
Esterification, activation of aromatic amines, 183
Estradiol
  epigenetic carcinogen, 1330t
  role in protein synthesis inhibition, 1085
  structure, 1155
Estrogen(s)
  anabolic action, 1155–57
  bone lesions, inductions, 1156
  carcinogenicity, 1266
  in vivo conversion to carcinogens, 1265
Estrogenic agents, 1151–59
  sources, 1155
Ethanol pretreatment, toxic effects, enhancement, 982
Ethenoadenine, miscoding and efficiency, 357t
Ethenocytosine, miscoding and efficiency, 357t
O^6,O^7-Ethenoguanine, structure, 355f
α-Ethers of nitrosamines, *N*-nitroso carcinogens, 645–48
Ethionamide, carcinogenicity, 1272
Ethionine, DNA alkylation, 370–71t
Ethoglucid, carcinogenicity, 1249
p-Ethoxyacetanilide, carcinogenicity, 203t
Ethoxyquin, inhibition of chemical carcinogenesis, 1283t
Ethyl acrylate, oncogenesis tests, 420t
Ethyl alcohol, effect on *N*-nitroso carcinogenesis, 678t
Ethyl bromoacetate, oncogenesis tests, 409t
Ethyl chloroacetate, oncogenesis tests, 409t
Ethyl formate, oncogenesis tests, 420t
Ethyl methanesulfonate
  alkylation of nucleic acids, 699
  classification, 359
  distinguishing, 361
  DNA alkylation, 370–71t, 373t
  lung adenomas induction, 383
  oncogenesis tests, 416–17t
  somatic eye-color mutations, 351
Ethyl *p*-toluenesulfonate
  oncogenesis tests, 416–17t
  relative carcinogenicity, 382
Ethylene chlorohydrin, oncogenesis, 406–7t
Ethylene dibromide, 539–40
  DNA alkylation, 370–71t
  in vivo alkylating agents, 385
  incidence of malignant neoplasms, 379
  oncogenesis, 406–7t
  synergistic effects, 376–77
Ethylene dichloride, 539
  inhalation administration, 408
  oncogenesis, 406–7t
Ethylene glycol bis(2,3-epoxy-2-methylpropyl)ether, oncogenesis tests, 463t
Ethylene oxide
  alkylation of cysteine, 378
  hystidine alkylation, 378
  oncogenesis tests, 422–23t
  skin painting, 421
Ethylene sulfide
  carcinogenic index, 439
  oncogenesis tests, 440–41t
  relative carcinogenicity, 382
1,1′-Ethylenebis[3-(2-chloroethyl)-3′-nitrosourea], target organ, 785
Ethyleneimines
  difunctional, 460
  genotoxic carcinogen, 1330t
  monofunctional, 424, 428
    oncogenesis tests, 426–27t
  polyfunctional, 460
    oncogenesis tests, 464–65t
Ethyleneiminosulfonylpentane, oncogenesis tests, 426–27t
Ethyleneiminosulfonylpropane, oncogenesis tests, 426–27t
Ethyleneoxycyclohexane, oncogenesis tests, 424t
1-Ethyleneoxy-3,4-epoxycyclohexane, oncogenesis tests, 461–62t
Ethylenethiourea, 1227
2-Ethylhexyldiphenyl phosphate, oncogenesis tests, 418–19t
N-Ethylmaleimide, oncogenesis tests, 438t
N-Ethyl-*N*-nitrosoureas
  carcinogenicity, 368
  DNA alkylation, 370–71t, 373t
  genotoxic carcinogen, 1330t
  mutagenicity, 368
Etiologic agents, classifications, 19–29
ETU—*See* Ethylenethiourea
ETYA—*See* 5,8,11,14-Eicosatetraynoic acid
Evaluation, final, results obtained in chronic bioassays, 1355
Excitation energies, polynuclear compounds, carcinogenic activity, 62
Exogenous
  exposure, *N*-nitroso compounds, 829–31
  modification of aromatic amine carcinogenesis, 263
Exposure, time to appearance of cancer, 1140
Extended anilines, metabolic activation, 188
Extraheptic tumors, aflatoxin B_1-induced, 992–94
Eye tumor—*See* Retinoblastoma

F

F—*See* Fluocinolone
FA—*See* Fluocinolone acetonide
FAA—*See* 2-Fluorenylacetamide
Factories, nitrosamines, 856
Fanconi's anemia, chromosomal instability, 396
Farm livestock, tumors, bracken carcinogenicity, 1177
Farr, William, 11
Fat, effect on aflatoxin B_1 carcinogenicity, 995*t*
Fatty acids, esters, 413, 421
FCA—*See* Fluclorolone acetonide
Fecal occult blood, detection, carcinogenic reagents, 311
Feedstuff components, effect on aflatoxin B_1 carcinogenicity, 996*t*
Females, cancer deaths, secular trends, 9*f*
Fern, bracken, carcinogenicity, 1171–97
Ferret, aflatoxin B_1 hepatocarcinogenicity, 985*t*
Fiber size, significance in mineral fiber carcinogenesis, 637
Fibrinogen, aflatoxin B_1 inhibition, 1086
Fibrous clays, 639
Figs, aflatoxins, 1110
Filaments, mineral fiber carcinogenesis, 633
Filberts, aflatoxins, 1109
Fire retardants, 534–36
Fisetin, 976
Fish
  aflatoxins, 1112
  N-nitrosamines, 833
  nitrosamine contamination, 1215
  nitrosamine content, 1214*t*
  polycyclic aromatic hydrocarbon content, 1210*t*
  susceptibility to aflatoxin B_1, 983
Fish meal, nitrosamines, 850
Five-membered rings, 428
  oncogenesis tests, 434–35*t*
Flavones
  inhibition of chemical carcinogenesis, 1287
  inhibition of cytochrome P-448 complexation, 1068
  as tumor inhibitors, 1286–90
Flavonoids, bracken carcinogenicity, 1186–90
Fluclorolone acetonide, 1299*t*
  epidermal DNA synthesis inhibition, 1299
  tumor inhibition, 1299*t*
Fluocinolone, tumor inhibition, 1299*t*
Fluocinolone acetonide, 1299
  epidermal DNA synthesis, inhibition, 1299
  stage-specific inhibitors, 1309*t*
  tumor inhibition, 1299*t*
Fluocinonide, 1299*t*
Fluoranthene, role in tumor inhibition, 1295*t*
2-Fluorenylacetamide, 1206
  activation of aromatic amines, 180
  carcinogenic structure–activity relationship, 218
  metabolic activation, 190
  modification of aromatic amine carcinogenesis, 260
  reactions with macromolecules, 193
Fluorescence, carcinogenic materials, 49
Fluorobiphenylamine, carcinogenicity, 208*t*, 209*t*
Fluorbiprofen, tumor inhibition, 1297*t*
5-Fluorouracil, carcinogenicity, 1251, 1253
Foam rubbers, synthetic, use of triazene compounds, 872
Foci induction in rodent liver, altered, 1341
Folpet, 559
Food
  aflatoxin contamination, 1222
  carcinogens, 1205–33
  N-nitrosamines, 832–33
  polycyclic aromatic hydrocarbons, 1209–13
Food additives, 1224–25
Food carcinogens
  fungal sources, 1220–23
  metals, 1223–24
  plant sources, 1219–20
Food dyes, structure–activity relationship, 240
Foodstuffs
  nitrosamine content, 1214*t*
  polycyclic aromatic hydrocarbon content, 1210*t*
Formaldehyde, 397, 858
  in vivo conversion to carcinogens, 1260
Formamide, structural requirements for carcinogenicity, 655*t*
Formylhydrazine, tumorigenicity, 920
Four-membered rings, 428
  oncogenesis tests, 430–33*t*
Frankfurters, DMN concentration, 1216
Free radicals, triazenyl, electronic configurations, 874
Free valence number, related to carcinogenic activity, 59
Freon, oncogenesis, 406–7*t*
Fruits, aflatoxins, 1110–11
Frying, effects on NDMA, 832
Frying oils, 1224–25
Fucinolone, epidermal DNA synthesis inhibition, 1299
Fumaric acid, bracken carcinogenicity, 1182
Fungal sources, of food carcinogens, 1220–23
Fungicide captan, structure, 395
Furazolidone, toxicity, 1256*t*
Furium, toxicity, 1256*t*
Furosemide, in vivo conversion to carcinogens, 1264
Fursarenon-X, influence on aflatoxin B_1 genotoxicity, 1031*t*
Fusaria, secondary metabolites, 1138
Fusarial mycotoxins, 1137–64
  epidemiological considerations, 1140–41
Fusarial toxins, protection, 1159–61
Fusarium microfungi, 1138
Fused-ring amines
  carcinogenic structure–activity relationship, 218
  metabolic activation, 190

G

Gamma-ray emission, 23
Garlic, aflatoxins, 1110
Gas chromatography, detection of zearalenone, 1152
Gastric cancer
  bracken carcinogenicity, 1175, 1193
  effect of calcium intake, 1194
Gastrointestinal tract, dietary effects, 1140

Gavage, administration of test chemicals, 1348
Gene expression, by aflatoxin B_1, 1016*t*
Genetic factors, 1206–7
Genite R-99, 559
Genitourinary tract disease, abnormal tryptophan metabolism, 257
Genotoxic carcinogen, 525, 1329
  mode of action, 1330*t*
Genotoxicity
  aflatoxin B_1, 1005–23
    in vitro factors, 1030*t*
    in vivo factors, 1032*t*
  vs. epigeneticity, 525
Genotoxicity evaluation, decision point 1, 1337
Geographical effects, bracken carcinogenicity, 1175
GH—*See* Insulin
Ginger root, aflatoxins, 955
Glass wools, mineral fiber carcinogenesis, 633
Gloves, nitrosamines, 847*t*
Glucose determinations, blood, carcinogenic reagents, 311
Glucuronides, metabolic activation of aromatic amines, 187
Glutathione
  binding to aflatoxins, 1069
  influence on aflatoxin B_1 genotoxicity, 1031*t*
Glutathione epoxide, influence on aflatoxin B_1 genotoxicity, 1031*t*
Glutathione peroxidase, selenium as cofactor, 1285
Glutathione transferase, 374
  and carcinogenic activity, 67
Glycidal ester of dodecanoic acid, oncogenesis tests, 422–23*t*
Glycidal ester of dodecanoic stearic acid, oncogenesis tests, 422–23*t*
Glycidal ester of hexanoic acid, oncogenesis tests, 422–23*t*
Glycidaldehyde, 421
  carcinogenicity, 368
  mutagenicity, 368
  oncogenesis tests, 422–23*t*
Glycidol, oncogenesis tests, 422–23*t*, 424*t*
Glycidyl ester of stearic acid, oncogenesis tests, 424*t*
Glycol sulfate, oncogenesis tests, 414–15*t*
Glycopeptides, carcinogenicity, 1253
Glycosides, bracken carcinogenicity, 1186
Goat, excretion of aflatoxin M_1, 1036*t*
Gossypol 3-methylcoumarin, polymerized corn oil, effect on aflatoxin B_1 carcinogenicity, 996*t*
Grade, definition, 3
Gradient analysis, alkaline sucrose, *N*-nitroso carcinogens, 714
Grain
  aflatoxins, 1096–1100
  polycyclic aromatic hydrocarbon content, 1210*t*
Gramine, structure, 838
Granuloma pouch assay, test for in vivo genotoxicity, 1340
Great Britain, esophageal cancer, 1144
Grignard method, preparation of monoalkylaryltriazeness, 883
Grignard reagent, preparation of trialkyltriazenes, 894
Groundnuts, aflatoxins, 1101
Growth hormone, effect on aflatoxin B_1 carcinogenicity, 996*t*
GSHP—*See* Glutathione peroxidase
Guanine, nitroso compound as alkylating agent, 698
Guinea pig
  aflatoxin B_1 toxicity, 978*t*
  excretion of aflatoxin M_1, 1035*t*
Guppy, aflatoxin B_1 hepatocarcinogenicity, 984*t*

H

Haloalkyl ether, 439
  oncogenesis tests, 442–43*t*
Halogenated dibenzodioxins, 532
Halogenated dibenzofurans, structure–activity relationship, 534
Halogenated hydrocarbons
  inhibition of chemical carcinogenesis, 1291*t*
  role in tumor inhibition, 1290
Halothane, effect on *N*-nitroso carcinogenesis, 678*t*
Ham, polycyclic aromatic hydrocarbon content, 1210*t*
Hamster(s)
  aflatoxin B_1 toxicity, 978*t*
  dichlorodiphenyltrichloroethane, 555
  golden syrian, aflatoxin B_1 chromosome inductor, 1014*t*
  syrian, aflatoxin B_1 hepatocarcinogenicity, 984*t*
HAQO—*See* Hydroxylaminoquinoline 1-oxide
Harderian glands, aflatoxin B_1-induced tumors, 993
Hazards, laboratory, carcinogens, 303–20
HBV—*See* Hepatitis B virus
HC—*See* Corticosteroids
HCC—*See* Hepatocellular carcinoma
Health risk assessment, carcinogens and promoters, 1357
Healthy worker effect, 29
HeLa cells, RNA synthesis, inhibition, 1080
Helical polysome formation, 1087
Heliothis zea, aflatoxins effect, 973
Hemangioendothelioma, 918
Hematuria, bovine enzootic, *pteridium aquuilinum var esculentum*, 1180
Hemisulfur mustard, DNA alkylation, 370–71*t*
Hemoglobin, in vivo alkylation, detection, 394
Hemorrhagic bracken poisoning, sheep, 1179
Hepatectomy, partial, stimulation of DNA synthesis, 1077
Hepatic cancer, causes, 1205
Hepatic hyperplastic nodules, induction, 916
Hepatic tumors, causes, 1205
Hepatitis B virus, human liver cancer, 968
Hepatitis B virus infection, as cocarcinogen, 394
Hepatocarcinogenicity, AFB_1 in vertebrates, 984–86*t*
Hepatocellular carcinoma, 968
  induction, 366, 916
Hepatotoxicity
  effect of dietary protein, 980
  4,4′-methylenedianiline, 283

Heptabromobiphenyl, mixtures, 534
Heptachlor, 553
  carcinogenicity, 547–51*t*
  structure, 550
Heptachlor epoxide
  carcinogenicity, 547–51*t*
  hepatocarcinoma, 552
  in humans, storage, 560
  structure, 550
Heptachlor–heptachlor epoxide mixture, mutagenicity, 553
Heritable germline effects, by aflatoxin B_1, 1014*t*
Heritable translocation, test for in vivo genotoxicity, 1340
Heterocarbon metabolites and derivatives, nomenclature systems, 42
Heterocyclic amines
  metabolic activation, 191
  reactions with macromolecules, 200
Heterocyclic compounds
  aromatic, nomenclature systems, 41
  carcinogenic, activities, 144–45*t*
  structure–activity relationship, 247–59
Heterolytic and enzymatic activation, dialkylaryltriazenes, 904
Hexabromobiphenyl, mixtures, 534
Hexachlorobenzene, 546
  carcinogenicity, 547–51*t*
  in humans, storage, 560
  swiss mice, administration, 552
Hexachlorobutadiene, 532
  carcinogenicity, 548–51*t*
Hexachloroethane, 540
Hexacyclic aromatic hydrocarbon derivatives, carcinogenic activities, 140–41*t*
Hexaepoxysqualene, oncogenesis tests, 463*t*
Hexachlorobutadiene, target organ, 532
Hexakis(1-aziridinyl)-2,2,4,4,6,6-hexahydrotriazatriphosphorine, oncogenesis, 464–65*t*
1,1′-Hexamethylenebis[3-(2-chloroethyl)-3′-nitrosourea], target organ, 785
Hexamethylenetetramine, in vivo conversion to carcinogens, 1260
Hexamethylphophoramide, 397
Hexylbis(1,6-methylnitroso)nitroguanidine, target organ, 794
High-fat diet(s)
  and aflatoxin metabolism, 1071
  effect on aflatoxin B_1 carcinogenicity, 995*t*
High-pressure liquid chromatography
  analysis, nucleic acids, alkylation, 700
  detection of zearalenone, 1152
  separation of AFB_1 hydrolysis products, 1054
Highest bond order, related to carcinogenic activity, 59
Histiocytic lymphoma, causes, 399
Histiocytomas, with chlordane, 555
Histopathology, definition, 3
Hodgkin's disease
  alkylating agent therapy, 398
  distribution, 6
Hordenine, structure, 838
Hormonal effects, on aflatoxin B_1 carcinogenicity, 1000
Hormonal status, effects on aflatoxin B_1 metabolism, 1071
Hormone(s)
  mode of action, 1330*t*
  modification of aromatic amine carcinogenesis, 263
Hospital personnel, chemical exposure related to cancer rate, 308–12
Host-mediated mutagenicity, test for in vivo genotoxicity, 1340
HPLC—*See* High-pressure liquid chromatography
HT-2 toxin, structure, 1148*t*
Human(s)
  and aflatoxin exposure, 966–70
  cancer
    and alkylating agents, 383–400
    two-stage process, 379
  cancer sites, 21*t*
  consumption of bracken fern, 1190
  foods, aflatoxins, 949–56
  inactivation, INH, 938
  indirect, consumption, bracken fern, 1190
  liver cancer, aflatoxins, 967–69, 967*t*
  lung fibroblasts, aflatoxin B_1 effects, 1022*t*
  nitrosamine synthesis, 1218
  variability, 19
Human cells
  DNA fragmentation, 1020*t*
  unscheduled DNA synthesis, 1018*t*
Human leukocytes, aflatoxin B_1 chromosome inductor, 1013*t*
Human lymphoblasts, gene mutation effects of aflatoxin B_1, 1009*t*
Human lymphocytes, aflatoxin B_1 chromosome inductor, 1014*t*
Human skin fibroblasts, aflatoxin B_1 chromosome inductor, 1013*t*
Hycanthone, carcinogenicity, 1269
Hydralazine, 932
Hydrazides, carcinogenicity, 1269
Hydrazine(s), 366, 919
  1,1-disubstituted, 929
  metabolism, 937
  mushroom-derived, 919–20
  structural requirements for carcinogenicity, 655*t*
  structure, 919
Hydrazine derivatives, 915–38
  mutagenicity, 931–38
Hydrazobenzene, carcinogenicity, 213*t*
Hydrazodicarboxybis(methylnitrosamide), target organ, 782
Hydrocarbon(s)
  carcinogenesis, foundations for scientific study, 49
  derivatives
    with five-membered rings, activities, 142–43*t*
    tumor-initiating activities, 106–8*t*
  unsubstituted polycyclics, activities, 130–31*t*
  various sites, metabolic reactions, 67
Hydrocarbon dihydrodiols, nomenclature, 44
Hydrocarbon epoxides, first synthesis, 68
Hydrocarbon–nucleoside interaction products, 122–25

Hydrocortisone 8, effect on aflatoxin B_1 carcinogenicity, 996*t*
Hydrogen bond, intramolecular, effect on hydrolytic reactivity of dihydrodiol epoxides, 121
Hydrolysis, vicinal dihydrodiol epoxides, 120
α-Hydroperoxynitrosamines, synthesis, 647
Hydroquinone mustard, oncogenesis tests, 450–51*t*
N-Hydroxy derivatives, activation of aromatic amines, 178
3-Hydroxy-2,2-dimethylbutyric acid β-lactone, oncogenesis, 438*t*
N-Hydroxy-*p*-ethoxyacetanilide, carcinogenicity, 203*t*
3-(2-Hydroxyethyl)-3-methyl-1-phenyltriazene, principal target organs, 899*t*
4-Hydroxyhexenoic acid lactones, oncogenesis tests, 434–35*t*, 438*t*
4-Hydroxylaminopyridine 1-oxide, carcinogenic activity, 249*t*
Hydroxylaminoquinoline 1-oxide(s)
  carcinogenic activity, 249*t*
  reaction with DNA, RNA, and protein, 247
  substituted, structure–activity relationship, 248*t*
o-Hydroxylation, detoxification pathway for aromatic amines, 191
α-Hydroxylation, metabolic activation of nitrosamines, 657
β-Hydroxylation, metabolism of *N*-nitroso carcinogens, 693
3-Hydroxymethyl-1-phenyltriazene, principal target organs, 899*t*
α-Hydroxynitrosamines, chemistry, 647
α-Hydroxy-*N*-nitrosamines, *N*-nitroso carcinogens, 644–48
Hydroxypurine derivatives, carcinogenicity, 251*t*
3-Hydroxy-2,2,4-trimethylheptanoic acid β-lactone, oncogenesis tets, 438*t*
Hyoscine, carcinogenicity, 1250
Hypolipidemic drugs, carcinogenicity, 1268
Hypomethylation of DNA, causes, 367
Hypophysectomy, 981
  in male rats, 1083

I

Iatrogenic cancer and drugs, 24–25
Ice cream, aflatoxins, 1115
Immunosuppressants, 24, 310
  mode of action, 1330*t*
In vitro effects, of alkylated bases on template activity, 703
In vitro tests, 1323–60
In vitro transformation, 350
In vivo, DNA, stability of alkylated components, 705
In vivo alkylation
  by nitroso compounds, 701
  detection and quantification, 375
In vivo dosimetry, 368–78
In vivo nitrosation, 857–60
Incidence density, definition, 15*t*
Indan epoxide, oncogenesis tests, 424*t*
Independent additive risk, carcinogenic effect of two carcinogens, 675
Indole, structure–activity relationship, 255
Indole-3-acetonitrile, inhibition of chemical carcinogenesis, 1291*t*
Indole-3-carbinol, inhibition of chemical carcinogenesis, 1291*t*
Indomethacin, 1305
  effect on arachidonic acid metabolism, 1305*t*
  tumor inhibition, 1297*t*
Industry
  exposure to chemicals, 383–97
  incidence of bladder cancer, 288–90
Inflammation, malignancy development, 25
INH—*See* Isoniazid *and* Isonicotinic acid hydrazide
Inhalation studies, 466
Inhibition, 1279–1311
  effect of two carcinogens, 675
  of tumor initiation, 1282–98
  of tumor promotion, 1298–1310
Inhibitors, 1297
Initiation, definition, 18
Initiators, tumor, characteristics, 1281
Injection molding, occupational exposure to *N*-nitrosamines, 853*t*
Inorganic carcinogen, mode of action, 1330*t*
Insulin, effect on aflatoxin B_1 carcinogenicity, 996*t*
Intragastric intubation, administration of test chemicals, 1348
Intramolecular hydrogen bond, effect on hydrolytic reactivity of dihydrodiol epoxides, 121
Intraperitoneal injection, administration of test chemicals, 1350
Intravenous injection, administration of test chemicals, 1350
Invertebrates, aflatoxins effect, 972–73
Iodacetamide, alkylating DNA, 353
Iodoacetic acid, oncogenesis tests, 409*t*
7-Iodomethyl-12-methylbenz[*a*]anthracene, oncogenesis tests, 412*t*
3-Iodopropionic acid
  alkylating DNA, 353
  oncogenesis tests, 410*t*
Ionization potentials, and carcinogenic activity, 61
IR absorption, triazenes, 876
Irradiation, 21
  background dose, 22
  low doses, 22
  risk estimates, 22*t*
Isomerization, 1,2-naphthalene epoxide to naphthol, mechanism, 71*f*
Isoniazid
  See also Isonicotinic acid hydrazide
  metabolism, 922
    mechanism, 1270
Isonicotinic acid hydrazide, structure, 366
Isophosphamide
  carcinogenicity, 1246
  oncogenesis tests, 454*t*
Isopropyl alcohol, maligancy sites, 31*t*
Isopropyl-α-(2-methylhydrazino)-*p*-toluamide (HCl)—*See* Procarbazine

Isoquercitrin, bracken carcinogenicity, 1182, 1186
IUPAC nomenclature and classification, triazenes, 870

J

Japanese food, nitrosamines, 840*t*
Japanese quail, susceptibility to dietary aflatoxin, 977

K

K region, 62–63*t*
  arene epoxides, synthesis, 110
  aromatic hydrocarbons, metabolic attack, 72
  indices, related to carcinogenic activity, 59
  unsubstituted aromatic hydrocarbons, 60–61*t*
K-region dihydrodiols, synthesis, 112
Kadlubar's suggestion, for miscoding, 356, 358
Kaempferol, bracken carcinogenicity, 1186
Kanechlor, inhibition of chemical carcinogenesis, 1291*t*
Kanechlor 500, 545–46
  hepatic tumors, 1293
Kenya, liver cancer incidence, 1222*t*
  aflatoxin exposure, 967*t*
Kepone
  carcinogenicity, 547–51*t*
  structure, 550
  use, 551

L

L region
  unreactive, related to carcinogenic activity, 59
  unsubstituted aromatic hydrocarbons, 60–61*t*
Laboratory hazards, carcinogens, 303–20
Laboratory use, potent carcinogens, 315
Laburnum, 1220
Lactones, 428
  carcinogenicity, 395
  oncogenesis tests, 430–38*t*
  reactions with cysteine, 436
Lasiocarpine, effect on aflatoxin B_1 carcinogenicity, 997*t*
Laurylamine, 845
N-Laurylethyleneimine, oncogenesis tests, 426–27*t*
Lead, inhibition of chemical carcinogenesis, 1291*t*
Leather particles, malignancy sites, 31*t*
Leather-tanning industry, nitrosamines, 856
Legal liability in Britain, 295–96
Legislation, 297–98
  influence on manufacturers, 297
Legumes, aflatoxins, 1106–7
Lesions, asbestos dust exposure, 634–35
Leukemia
  acute nonlymphocytic, 456
  irradiation risks, 22*t*
Leukocyte myeloperoxidase, carcinogenic reagents, 312
Leupeptin, 1304
  carcinogenesis inhibitors, 1303*t*
Lewis acids, acid-catalyzed degradation of monoalkyltriazenes, 887
Life table rate, definition, 15*t*
Lime, tobacco mixture, 25
Limonene dioxide, oncogenesis tests, 463*t*
Limonene monoxide, oncogenesis tests, 424*t*
Lindane
  carcinogenicity, 548–51*t*
  in humans, storage, 560
Lipid synthesis, aflatoxins, 1091–92
Lipotrope-deficient diet, effect on aflatoxin B_1 carcinogenicity, 995*t*
Liver
  cancer, nutrition effects, 1229
  in rodent, altered Foci induction, 1341
Liver cancer, 21
  N,N-dimethyl-*p*-phenylazoanilines, 235–36*t*
  human
    aflatoxins, 967–69, 967*t*
    hepatitis B virus, 968
  polybrominated biphenyls, 535
Liver carcinogenesis, test for promoting activity, 1339
Liver cell tumor(s)
  primary, 5
    worldwide variation, 6*t*
  uses, 363
Liver DNA, methylation, 363
Liver enzyme-inducing agents, 261
Liver tumor(s), 918
  birth control pills, 25
  induction, 917
    by *N*-nitroso carcinogens, 658
Livestock, tumors, bracken carcinogenicity, 1177
Local carcinogenic action, 466
Lomustine, oncogenesis tests, 444–45*t*
Loveless hypothesis, on miscoding, 355
Lubricating oils, 170
Lung(s), aflatoxin B_1induced tumors, 993
Lung adenoma, induction and correlations, 369
Lung cancer, 2
  alkylating agent therapy, 398
  and asbestos workers, 635–36
  causes, 1205
  worldwide variation, 5*t*
Lung tissue, asbestos presence, 635
Luteoskyrin, 1222–23
Lymphoblastic leukemia, age occurrence, 10
Lymphosarcoma, alkylating agent therapy, 398
Lysogeny, induction in *E. coli*, 352
Lysomomal enzyme activities, aflatoxins, 1092

M

MAB—*See* Methylaminoazobenzene
Mackerel, polycyclic aromatic hydrocarbon content, 1210*t*
Macromolecular binding
  aflatoxins, 1046–64
    adduct formation and removal, 1052
    characteristics, 1049–52
    to proteins, 1061
Macromolecular synthesis, inhibition, aflatoxins, 1077
Macromolecules, reactions with aromatic amines, 193–201
Macrozamin, 915
  carbohydrate moiety, 915
Magenta, related to bladder cancer, 176

Maleic acid hydrazide, 845
Maleic anhydride, oncogenesis tests, 434–35*t*
Maleic hydrazide, 922
in vivo alkylation, 438
oncogenesis tests, 437*t*
structure, 395
Males, cancer deaths, secular trends, 9*f*
Malignancies, increasing, 8
Malignant, and DNA repair, *N*-nitroso carcinogens, 714
Malondialdehyde, 858
Malt
direct-fire kilned, 834
NDMA formation, heating, 836*t*
NDMA reduction, 837*f*
MAM—*See* Methylazoxymethanol
Mammalian cells, alkylation repair, *N*-nitroso carcinogens, 722–28
Mammalian cytogenetics, by aflatoxin B_1, 1012*t*
Mammary adenocarcinoma, causes, 1205
Man-made mineral fibers, 634
Mannitol myleran
carcinogenicity, 369*t*
mutagenicity, 369*t*
oncogenesis tests, 457*t*
Mannomustine
carcinogenicity, 1249
oncogenesis tests, 450–51*t*
Margarine, polycyclic aromatic hydrocarbon content, 1210*t*
Marmoset, aflatoxin B_1 hepatocarcinogenicity, 985*t*
Mass spectrometry, triazenes, 879
Maximum tolerated dose, determination, 1353
Mayonnaise, polycyclic aromatic hydrocarbon content, 1210*t*
Meat
aflatoxins, 1112
nitrosamine content, 1214*t*
polycyclic aromatic hydrocarbon content, 1210*t*
Mechanism(s), chemical carcinogenesis, 51
Mechanism of action, dialkylaryltriazenes, 904
Medicines, 1241–73
Melphalan, 369*t*, 1243, 1244
mutagenicity, 369*t*
oncogenesis tests, 450–51*t*
Membrane transport, 1092
Menadione, effect on aflatoxin B_1 toxicity, 981
Mercaptopurine, 1251, 1252
epigenetic carcinogen, 1330*t*
Mesothelioma, 33
Metabolic activation
aromatic amines, 179*f*
dialkylaryltriazenes, 904
nitrosamines, α-hydroxylation, 657
N-nitroso carcinogens, 682
polynuclear aromatic carcinogens, 126
Metabolic breakdown, sulfates or glucosiduronates, 72*f*
Metabolic intermediate, transient, arene epoxides, 68
Metabolic pathways
in vivo conversion of medicines to carcinogens, 1255
primary, naphthalene, 73
Metabolic reactions, various sites on hydrocarbons, 67
Metabolism
abnormal tryptophan, genitourinary tract disease, 257
aromatic hydrocarbons, in animals, 71
cyclophosphamide, mechanism, 1245
dibutylnitrosamine, 688
enzymes involved, polynuclear carcinogens, 66
isoniazid, mechanism, 1270
methylamino groups, in vivo conversion, 1260
microsomal, mechanism, naphthalene, 69*f*
N-nitrosomethyl-*n*-alkylamines, 692
oxidized di-*n*-propylnitrosamines, 691
structure relationships, 1334
Metabolites
secondary, microfungi, 1138
tryptophan, 256
Metal, as food carcinogens, 1223–24
Metal foils, epigenetic carcinogen, 1330*t*
Metal-working industries, nitrosamines, 856
α-Metallated nitrosamines, synthesis of α-acyloxynitrosamines, 646
Methanesulfonic acid 2-chloroethyl ester, oncogenesis tests, 444–45*t*
Methapyrilene, in vivo conversion to carcinogens, 1260
Methapyrilene hydrochloride, in vivo conversion, 1261
Methenamine, in vivo conversion, 1260
Methoscopolamine bromide, carcinogenicity, 1250
Methotrexate, carcinogenicity, 1251
2-Methoxy-3-benzofuranylamine, carcinogenicity, 259*t*
3-Methoxy-4-biphenylamine, carcinogenicity, 209*t*
Methoxychlor, 554
carcinogenicity, 547–51*t*
structure, 551
Methoxy(octenyl-ONN-azoxy)-2-butanol
See also Elaiomycin
structure, 920
4-[(*p*-Methoxyphenyl)azo]-*o*-anisidine, carcinogenicity, 231*t*
Methyl bromide, 408
oncogenesis, 405*t*
Methyl CCNU—*See* *N*-Nitroso-*N*-(2-chloroethyl)-*N*′-(4-methylcyclohexyl)urea
Methyl chloride, 408
Methyl iodide
oncogenesis, 405*t*
relative carcinogenicity, 382
Methyl iodine, 408
Methyl malvalatete, effect on aflatoxin B_1 carcinogenicity, 998*t*
Methyl methanesulfonate
alkylation
of cysteine, 378
of guanine, 378
of nucleic acids, 699
carcinogen binding index to DNA, 372
DNA alkylation, 370–71*t*, 373*t*
half-life, 374
hystidine alkylation, 378
oncogenesis tests, 414–15*t*

Methyl methanesulfonate—*Continued*
relative carcinogenicity, 382
thymoma yield, 403
Methyl protoanemonin, oncogenesis tests, 434–35*t*
N-Methyl resonances, triazenes, 878
Methyl sterculate, effect on aflatoxin B_1 carcinogenicity, 998*t*
Methyl substituent, effect on carcinogenic activity, 54
Methyl *p*-toluenesulfonate, oncogenesis tests, 416–17*t*
Methylacetoxymethylnitrosamine, effects of xenobiotics on carcinogenesis, 678*t*
Methyladenine, 364
excretion, 377
Methylamine, destruction of aflatoxins, 964
Methylamino groups, metabolism, in vivo conversion, 1260
N-Methylaminoazobenzene, metabolic activation, 190
Methylating agents, precautions in laboratory use, 317
Methylazoxymethanol, 915–38
carcinogenesis, 918
cell-transforming activity, 932
degradation, 934
effect on DNA synthesis, 927
inhibition of protein synthesis, 928
metabolism from 1,2-dimethylhydrazine, 917
tumors induced, 916
Methylazoxymethanol β-D-glucoside—*See* Cycasin
7-Methylbenz[*a*]anthracene, tumor-initiating activities of derivatives, 107*t*
8-Methylbenz[*a*]anthracene, tumor-initiating activities of derivatives, 108*t*
10-Methylbenz[*a*]anthracene, 168
7-Methylbenz[*a*]anthracene derivatives, carcinogenic activities, 136–37*t*
Methylbenzo[*a*]fluorene, structure, 169*f*
Methylbenzylamine, 857
4′-Methyl-4-biphenylacetamide, carcinogenicity, 209*t*
2-Methyl-4-biphenylamine(s), carcinogenicity, 209*t*
Methyl-2-butylhydrazine, 923
Methylchloroform, 541
3-Methylcholanthrene, 351
carcinogenesis with *N*-nitroso compounds, 676*t*
inhibition of chemical carcinogenesis, 1291*t*
modification of aromatic amine carcinogenesis, 260
tumor-initiating activities of derivatives, 107*t*
5-Methylchrysene, tumor-initiating activities of derivatives, 108*t*
4-Methylcoumarin, inhibition of chemical carcinogenesis, 1291*t*
2-Methyldiacetylbenzidine, carcinogenicity, 213*t*
Methylene chloride, in vivo alkylating agents, 385
Methylene dichloride, 408
oncogenesis, 405*t*
Methylene disulfonates, 397
4,4′-Methylenebis(2-carbomethoxyaniline), carcinogenicity, 214*t*
4,4′-Methylenebis(2-chloroaniline), 283–84
carcinogenicity, 214*t*
structure, 283, 544
4,4′-Methylenebis(2-methylaniline), carcinogenicity, 214*t*
4,4′-Methylenedianiline, 282–83
carcinogenicity, 214*t*
structure, 282
structure–activity relationship, 211
N-Methyl-*N*-formylhydrazine, 919
Methylguanine, 364
*O*⁶-Methylguanine
mechanism of repair, 468
miscoding and efficiency, 357*t*
promutagenic effect, repair pathways, 362*f*
repair, biochemistry, *N*-nitroso carcinogens, 719–24
Methylhydrazine, tumor induction, 920
2-Methylnitro-9,10-anthracenedione, carcinogenicity, 259*t*
6-[(1-Methyl-4-nitroimidazol-5-yl)thio]purine, azathioprine, 259*t*
Methylnitronitrosoguanidine, body penetration, 372
N-Methyl-*N*′-nitro-*N*-nitrosoguanidine
carcinogenicity, 368
distinguishing, 361
DNA alkylation, 370–71*t*, 373*t*
mutagenicity, 368
relative carcinogenicity, 382
structure, 360
4-(*N*-Methyl-*N*-nitrosamine)-1-(3-pyridyl)-1-butanone
concentrations, 843*t*
metabolism, 696
precursor, 842
N-Methyl-*N*-nitroso compounds, activation, 360
N-Methyl-*N*-nitrosoaniline, esophageal carcinogenicity, 869
N-Methyl-*N*-nitrosocarbamoyl)-L-ornithine, target organ, 780
N-Methyl-*N*-nitrosourea
carcinogenicity, 368
combination effects in carcinogenesis, 676*t*
DNA alkylation, 370–71*t*, 373*t*
effects of xenobiotics on carcinogenesis, 678*t*
liver protein exhaustion, 364
miscoding in polydeoxyribonucleotide templates, 357*t*
mutagenicity, 368
structure, 360
thymoma yield, 403
1-(4-Methyloxyphenyl)-3,3-dimethyltriazene, principal target organs, 899*t*
Methylphenylnitrosamine, effects of xenobiotics on carcinogenesis, 678*t*
3-Methyl-1-phenyl-3-(2-sulfoethyl)triazene, principal target organs, 899*t*
Methylpurines, removal from DNA, 363*t*
4-Methylpyrene, structure, 169*f*
α-Methyltetronic acid, oncogenesis tests, 434–35*t*
*O*⁴-Methylthymine, 361
miscoding and efficiency, 357*t*

Methyl-*p*-toluenesulfonate, relative carcinogenicity, 382
Metronidazole, in vivo conversion, 1257
Mice—*See* Mouse
Microfungi, secondary metabolites, 1138
Microorganisms, aflatoxins, 971
Microsomal, triazenes, 906
Microsomal enzyme inducers, 1065–67
Milk
  aflatoxins, 1113
  bracken carcinogenicity, 1191
Milk substitutes, 955
Millet, aflatoxins, 1100
Mineral fiber(s)
  carcinogenesis, 631–39
    significance of fiber size, 637
  synthetic, 639
Mineral oil(s), 2
  induced cancer, 170
  isolated compounds, 168
Mink, aflatoxin B_1 excretion, 1076
Mirex
  carcinogenicity, 547–51*t*
  mutagenicity tests, 553
  structure, 551
  use, 551
Miscoding, 357–60
  alkylating agents, 358–59
  antimetabolites, 358
  carcinogenic action, 355
  DNA, 353–54
  DNA bases, 356*f*
  N^2-guaninyl derivatives, 356, 358
  Kadlubar's suggestion, 356, 358
  Loveless' hypothesis, 355
  mutagens, distinguishing, 361
Misonidazole, 1257
Mitochondrial function, aflatoxins, 1089–91
Mitomycin c
  DNA damage, 374
  oncogenesis tests, 464–65*t*
Mixed-function oxidase system, and carcinogenic activity, 66
MNNG—*See* *N*-Methyl-*N*′-nitro-*N*-nitrosoguanidine
MOCA—*See* Methylenebis(2-chloroaniline)
Models, for statistical approaches, 1208
Modification, aromatic amine carcinogenesis, 258–63
Mold growth, influences, 948
Molecular geometry and triazene structure, 873
Molecular orbital energies, various triazene groups, 874
Molecular structure, triazenes, 872
Monkey
  AFB_1 excretion, 1072–73
  AFB_1 hepatocarcinogenicity, 986*t*
  AFB_1 toxicity, 978*t*
  excretion of AFM_1, 1037*t*
Monkey cells
  DNA fragmentation, 1019*t*
  unscheduled DNA synthesis, 1018*t*
Monoalkylaryltriazenes, chemistry and biological properties, 883–89
Monochloroacetaldehyde diethyl acetal, oncogenesis tests, 442–43*t*
Monocrotaline, effect on aflatoxin B_1 carcinogenicity, 997*t*
Monofunctional alkyl sulfates, 413
Monofunctional epoxides, 421, 424
Monofunctional ethyleneimines, 424, 428
Monomethyl sulfate, relative carcinogenicity, 382
Monomethylbenz[*a*]anthracenes, properties, 62–63*t*
Monosubstituted benz[*a*]anthracenes, carcinogenic activities, 134–35*t*
Moolgavkar equation, 379
Mordenite, 634
Morpholine, 858
  derivatives, 845
    nitrosamine contamination, 844*t*
  tumor induction by *N*-nitroso derivatives, 661
Mortality data, 12
  chemists, and cancer, 304–8
Mortality surveillance system, 11
Mouse
  AFB_1 chromosome inductor, 1014*t*, 1015*t*
  AFB_1 excretion, 1074–75
  AFB_1 hepatocarcinogenicity, 984*t*
  AFB_1 toxicity, 978*t*
  aflatoxin congener and metabolites, 1004
  bracken carcinogenicity, 1175
  excretion of AFM_1, 1034*t*
  kidney, AFB_1 treatment, 1082
  PB treatment, 1065
  susceptibility to AFB_1, 1082
  swiss, AFB_1 chromosome inductor, 1014*t*
Mouse skin
  carcinogenesis process, 51
  painting, 1325
Mozambique, liver cancer incidence, aflatoxin exposure, 967t
MTD—*See* Maximum tolerated dose
Mucinous adenocarcinomas, induction, 916
Mule Spinning Regulations of 1952, 172
Multigeneration experiments, *N*-nitroso carcinogens, 670
Multiple dose, persistence of O^6-alkylguanine and tumorigenesis, 709
Multistage model, 1280
Mung beans, 1106
Murine leukemia virus, induction, 351
Mussels, polycyclic aromatic hydrocarbon content, 1210*t*
Mustard(s), two-stage carcinogenesis, 455
Mustard gas, 384
  causes, 1205
  cytotoxic action, 365–67
  malignancy sites, 32*t*
  oncogenesis tests, 448–49*t*
Mutagenesis, 467
  bacterial, evaluation of carcinogenicity, 1335
  in vitro assays, 1334
Mutagenicity
  aflatoxins, 1005–30
  correlation with carcinogenicity, 369*t*
  effects of ring-substituted triazenes, 903
  N-nitroso carcinogens, 677–81
  shikimic acid, 1186
  triazenes, 901

Mutation
  demonstration of the nature, 463
  induction in DNA, 361
Mycology, aflatoxins, 948
Mycotoxins, 945, 1138
  fusarial, 1137–64
    epidemiological considerations, 1140–41
Myeloperoxidase determination, carcinogenic reagents, 312
Myleran
  activity, 456
  alkylation mechanism, contraindication, 459
  carcinogenicity, 1243, 1247
  cytotoxic, 458
  DNA alkylation, 370–71*t*
  oncogenesis tests, 457*t*
  reactions and metabolism, 458
  structure, 458
N-Myristoyethyleneimine, oncogenesis tests, 426–27*t*
  Mytomycin C, carcinogenicity, 1254

N

Naphthacene, carcinogenic activities, 130*t*
Naphthalene
  mechanism for microsomal metabolism, 69*f*
  metabolic attack at the K region, 72
1,2-Naphthalene epoxide
  mechanism for isomerization to naphthol, 71*f*
  transient metabolic intermediate, 70
2′,3′-Naphtho-1,2-anthracene—*See* Pentaphene
2′,2′-Naphtho-2,3-phenanthrene—*See* Benzo[*a*]naphthacene
Naphtho[1,2,3,4-*def*]chrysene
  See also Dibenzopyrene
  carcinogenic activities, 133*t*, 140–41*t*
Napthoflavone, inhibition of cytochrome P-448 complexation, 1068
Naphtho[8,1,2-*cde*]naphthacene
  See also Naphtho[2,3-*a*]pyrene
  carcinogenic activities, 133*t*
Naphtho[2,3-*a*]pyrene
  See also Naphtho[8,1,2-*cde*]naphthacene
  carcinogenic activities, 133*t*
Naphtho[1,2-*b*]triphenylene, carcinogenic activities, 132*t*
Naphthylamine(s), 278, 279, 280, 354
  and bladder cancer, 175, 290
  carcinogenic reagents, 315
  carcinogenic structure–activity relationship, 224
  causes, 1205
  genotoxic carcinogen, 1330*t*
  malignancy sites, 31*t*
  metabolic activation, 190
  metabolites, 356
  reaction with macromolecules, 195
  structure, 279, 280
Naphthylamine mustard
  and bladder cancer, 177
  carcinogenicity, 369*t*
  mutagenicity, 369*t*
  oncogenesis tests, 450–51*t*
  structure, 398
Naphthylthiourea, 278–80
  and bladder cancer, 177
  structure, 279
Nasopharyngeal carcinoma, 5
  worldwide variation, 6*t*
NAT—*See* *N*-Nitrosoanatabine
Natural products, with anticancer activity, carcinogenicity, 1253–55
NDBA—*See* *N*-Nitrosodi-*n*-butylamine
NDEA—*See* *N*-Nitrosodiethylamine
NDEIA—*See* *N*-Nitrosodiethanolamine
NDMA—*See* *N*-Nitrosodimethylamine
NDPA—*See* *N*-Nitrosodi-*n*-propylamine
NDPhA—*See* *N*-Nitrosodiphenylamine
Negative-ion MS, 952
Neoplasia, 3
  See also Tumor induction
  deaths in United Kingdom, 8*f*
Neoplasm(s)
  common, in U.S., 4*t*
  common sites, 4*t*
  interaction with receptors, 1327
  skin, induction in mice, 1342
Neoplasm-promoting agents, assays for, 1338
Neoplastic conversion, 1327
Neoplastic development and progression, 1328
  sequence of events, 1327
Neosolaniol, structure, 1148*t*
Neurospora crassa, gene mutation effects of AFB_1, 1008*t*
Neutron emission, 23
Newborns, 993
Nickel
  genotoxic carcinogen, 1330*t*
  malignancy sites, 31*t*
Nicotine, 842
Nifuradene, toxicity, 1256*t*
Nifuroxime, toxicity, 1256*t*
Nigerian foods, aflatoxins, 954
Nipples, nitrosamines, accelerator effects, 850
Nitramine, structural requirements for carcinogenicity, 655*t*
Nitrate-treated products, 832
Nitrilotriacetic acid, epigenetic carcinogen, 1330*t*
Nitrite, 858–59
Nitrite amino compounds, combined administration, 672
Nitrite and nitrosatable amino compounds, combined administration, 672
Nitrite-treated products, 832
Nitro compounds, laboratory precautions, 315
Nitro derivatives
  five-membered heterocyclic ring compounds, 250
  potential carcinogenicity, 1257
Nitro groups, in vivo conversion, 1255
3-Nitro-*p*-acetophenetidine, carcinogenicity, 207*t*
9-Nitroacridine 9-oxide, carcinogenic activity, 249*t*
5-Nitro-*o*-anisidine, carcinogenicity, 206*t*
4-Nitroanthranilic acid, carcinogenicity, 203*t*
4-Nitrobiphenyl
  carcinogenic reagents, 315
  carcinogenicity, 208*t*
  malignancy sites, 32*t*
2-Nitrochlorobenzene, carcinogenicity, 203*t*

Nitrofuran(s)
metabolic activation, 191
used as medicines, toxicity, 1256*t*
Nitrofuran compounds, reduction of a nitro group, 182
Nitrofurantoin, toxicity, 1256*t*
Nitrofurazone, toxicity, 1256*t*
2-Nitrofuryl compounds, tumor induction, 253–54*t*
N-[4-(5-Nitro-2-furyl)-2-thiazolyl]formamide, 1257
conversion to carcinogens, 1257
metabolism, inhibition, 1306
Nitrogen-centered free radicals, triazenes, 874
Nitrogen mustard, 439, 447, 455–56
carcinogenicity, 1243
detoxification mechanism, 374
difunctional, oncogenesis tests, 450–51*t*
DNA alkylation, 370–71*t*
monofunctional, oncogenesis tess, 444–45*t*
oncogenesis tests, 448–49*t*, 453*t*
tumor rate effects, 401
Nitrogen mustard hydrochloride, carcinogenicity, 1244
Nitroimidazoles, in vivo conversion, 1256
Nitromide, 1257
2-Nitro-*p*-phenylenediamine, carcinogenicity, 207*t*
4-Nitro-*o*-phenylenediamine, carcinogenicity, 207*t*
4-Nitropyridine 1-oxide, carcinogenic activity, 249*t*
4-Nitroquinoline 1-oxide
metabolic activation, 191
structure–activity relationship, 182
substituted, structure–activity relationship, 248*t*
Nitrosamides, mutagenicity, 677–81
N-Nitrosamides, transplacental carcinogenesis, 671
N-Nitrosamides and derivatives, target organ, 778–801
Nitrosamine(s), 1213–19
activation and detoxification pathways, 683–88
average daily intake, 838
contamination, in rubber chemicals, 844*t*
cyclic, target organ, 763–77
food, 832–33
formation
in vivo, 1217–19
inhibition, 858
in intestine, 1218
metabolism, 688
migration, 848*t*
natural occurrence, 1216–17
occupational exposure, 851–57
preformed environmental, 832–33
in rubber articles, 847*t*
structural requirements for carcinogenicity, 655*t*
structures, 849
synthesis in humans, 1218
tobacco, 839
tobacco smoke, 839–42
tobacco specific, 840
unusual formation, 648
N-Nitrosamine(s)
mutagenicity, 677–81
neighboring-group effect, 650
pharmacokinetics, 682
structure–activity relationships, 657–65
subacute toxicity, 651
symmetrical, target organ, 732–47
unsymmetrical, target organ, 748–62
Nitrosamino ethers, synthesis of α-acyloxynitrosamines, 645
Nitrosatable amino compounds, carcinogenesis by combined administration, 672
Nitrosation
amines, in vivo conversion, 1262
catalysis, 858
drugs, 845
endogenous, availability of nitrosating agents, 858
in vivo, 857–60
reactions, 857
N-Nitroso carcinogens
discussion, 643–801
in the environment, 829–60
N-Nitroso compounds
determination, 831
endogenous exposure, 830
exogenous exposure, 829–31
formation in tobacco smoke, 829
Nitroso-derived alkylation products, identification in nucleic acids, 701
N-Nitroso-(1-acetoxybutyl)-3-carbomethoxypropylamine, target organ, 747
N-Nitroso-1-acetoxydi-*n*-butylamine, target organ, 747
N-Nitroso-*N*-(acetoxymethyl)-*n*-butylamine, target organ, 751
N-Nitrosoacetoxymethyl-*tert*-butylamine, target organ, 752
N-Nitroso-*N*-(1-acetoxymethyl)ethylamine, target organ, 748
N-Nitroso-*N*-(acetoxymethyl)isobutylamine, target organ, 762
N-Nitrosoacetoxymethylphenylamine, target organ, 762
Nitroso(acetoxymethyl)-*n*-propylamine, target organ, 750
N-Nitroso-*N'*,*O*-acetyl-3,5-dimethylpiperazine, target organ, 772
N-Nitrosoaldicarb, target organ, 797
N-Nitroso-*N*-alkyl-*N'*-nitrosoguanidines, 664
N-Nitroso-*N*-allyl(2-hydroxyethyl)amine, target organ, 759
N-Nitroso-*N*-allyl(2-hydroxypropyl)amine, target organ, 759
N-Nitroso-*N*-allylurea, target organ, 787
Nitrosoamino acids, synthesis of α-acyloxynitrosamines, 646
N-Nitrosoanatabine
concentrations, 843*t*
target organ, 768
Nitrosoazetidine, target organ, 763
N-Nitrosobaygon, target organ, 796
N-Nitroso-*N'*-benzoyl-3,5-dimethylpiperazine, target organ, 773
N-Nitroso-*N*-benzylurea, target organ, 789

N-Nitroso(2-bisacetoxyethyl)amine, target organ, 737
N-Nitroso(2-bisacetyoxypropyl)amine, target organ, 740
N-Nitroso-N,N'-bis(2-chloroethyl)urea, target organ, 785
N-Nitroso(2-bischloropropyl)amine, target organ, 741
N-Nitroso[2-bis(diethoxy)ethyl]amine, target organ, 737
N-Nitroso(2-bisethoxyethyl)amine, target organ, 736
N-Nitrosobis(2-hydroxyethyl)amine, dose–response studies, 668
N-Nitrosobis(2-hydroxyethyl)amine, target organ, 736
N-Nitrosobis(2-hydroxypropyl)amine, target organ, 739
N-Nitrosobis(2-methoxyethyl)amine, target organ, 736
N-Nitrosobis(2-oxopropyl)amine, target organ, 740
N-Nitrosobis(4,4,4-trifluorobutyl)amine, target organ, 745
N-Nitroso-di-n-butylamine, bladder tumor induction, 658
N-Nitroso-N-n-butyl-tert-butylamine, target organ, 746
N-Nitroso-N-n-butylbutyramide, target organ, 801
N-Nitroso-N-n-butyl-N'-n-butylurea, target organ, 788
N-Nitroso-N-n-butylethylsuccinamate, target organ, 801
N-Nitroso-N-n-butyl-N-(3-carboxypropyl)amine, target organ, 745
N-Nitroso-N-n-butyl(3-hydroxybutyl)amine, target organ, 743, 744
N-Nitroso-N-n-butyl-N'-nitroguanidine, target organ, 793
N-Nitroso-N-n-butyl(2-oxobutyl)amine, 744
N-Nitroso-N-n-butyl-n-pentylamine, target organ, 760
N-Nitroso-4-tert-butylpiperidine, target organ, 768
N-Nitroso-N-n-butylurea, target organ, 787
N-Nitroso-sec-N-butylurea, target organ, 788
N-Nitroso-N-n-butylurethane, target organ, 795
N-Nitrosobuxten, target organ, 796
N-Nitrosocarbaryl, target organ, 796
N-Nitroso-N'-carboethyoxypiperazine, target organ, 773
N-Nitrosocarbofurane, target organ, 797
N-Nitroso-N-carboxymethylurea, target organ, 799
N-Nitrosochlorodiazepoxide, target organ, 758
N-Nitroso-N-(2-chloroethyl)-N',N'-diethylurea, target organ, 786
N-Nitroso-N-(2-chloroethyl)-N',N'-dimethylurea, target organ, 786
N-Nitroso-N-(2-chloroethyl)-N',N'-morpholinourea, target organ, 786
N-Nitroso-N-(2-chloroethyl)-N'-(2-hydroxyethyl)urea, target organ, 785
N-Nitroso-N-(2-chloroethyl)-N'-(2-methanesulfonyloxyethyl)urea, target organ, 785
N-Nitroso-N-(2-chloroethyl)-N'-(4-methylcyclohexyl)urea, target organ, 785
N-Nitroso-N-(2-chloroethyl)urea, target organ, 785
N-Nitroso-N-(2-chloroethyl)urethane, target organ, 795
N-Nitroso-3-chloropiperidine, target organ, 766
N-Nitroso-4-chloropiperidine, target organ, 766
N-Nitrosocimelidin, target organ, 800
N-Nitroso-4-cyclohexylpiperidine, target organ, 776
N-Nitroso-N-cyclohexylurea, target organ, 789
N-Nitrosodecamethyleneamine, target organ, 770
N-Nitrosodialkylamines, metabolites, 356
N-Nitrosodiallylamine, target organ, 742
N-Nitrosodibenzylamine, target organ, 746
N-Nitroso-3,4-dibromopiperidine, target organ, 766
N-Nitrosodibutylamine, metabolic fate, 689
N-Nitrosodi-sec-butylamine, target organ, 658, 745
N-Nitrosodi-n-butylamine, target organ, 742
N-Nitroso-3,4-dichloropiperidine, target organ, 766
N-Nitroso-3,4-dichloropyrrolidine, target organ, 763
N-Nitrosodicyclohexylamine, target organ, 746
N-Nitrosodiethylamine
  See also Diethylnitrosamine
  target organ, 734
Nitroso-5,6-dihydrouracil, target organ, 791
N-Nitroso-N-(2,3-dihydroxypropyl)(2-hydroxypropyl)amine, target organ, 741
N-Nitroso-N-(2,3-dihydroxypropyl)(2-oxopropyl)amine, target organ, 741
N-Nitrosodiisobutylamine, target organ, 745
N-Nitrosodiisopropylamine, target organ, 742
Nitrosodimethylamine, carcinogenic activity, 643
N-Nitrosodimethylamine(s), 363, 829, 845
  activation, 360
  acute toxicity, 360
  in air, 851t
  in beer, 834, 835t
  carcinogen binding index, 376
  liver protein exhaustion, 364
  liver toxicity, 651
  in malt, 836t, 837t
  precursors, 837
  structure, 360, 838
  target organ, 732
N-Nitroso-2,6-dimethylmorpholine
  target organ, 770, 771
N-Nitroso-2,6-dimethylpiperidine, target organ, 768
N-Nitroso-3,5-dimethylpiperidine, target organ, 768, 772
N-Nitroso-2,5-dimethylpyrrolidine, target organ, 763
N-Nitroso-N,N'-dimethylurea, target organ, 780
N-Nitrosodi-n-octylamine, target organ, 746
N-Nitrosodi-n-pentylamine, target organ, 746

N-Nitrosodiphenylamine(s), 855
target organ, 746
N-Nitrosodi-*n*-propylamine, target organ, 738
N-Nitrosododecamethylamine, target organ, 770
N-Nitrosoephedrine, target organ, 755
N-Nitroso-3,4-epoxypiperidine, target organ, 766
N-Nitroso-*N*-ethylbenzylamine, target organ, 760
N-Nitroso-*N*-ethylbiuret, target organ, 784
N-Nitroso-*N*-ethyl-*n*-butylamine, target organ, 759
N-Nitroso-*N*-ethyl-*tert*-butylamine, target organ, 759
N-Nitroso-*N*-ethyl(3-carboxypropyl)amine, target organ, 759
N-Nitroso-*N*-ethyl-*N'*,*N'*-diethylurea, target organ, 784
N-Nitrosoethylenethiourea, target organ, 790
N-Nitrosoethylisopropylamine
structure–activity relationship, 657
target organ, 758
N-Nitroso-*N*-ethyl(2-hydroxyethyl)amine, target organ, 736, 758
N-Nitroso-*N*-ethyl(4-hydroxybutyl)amine, target organ, 759
N-Nitroso-*N*-ethyl-(1-methoxyethyl)amine, target organ, 737
N-Nitroso-*N*-ethyl(d_5)-*N'*-nitroguanidine, target organ, 800
N-Nitroso-*N*-ethyl-*N'*-nitroguanidine, target organ, 793
N-Nitrosoethyl-4-picolylamine, target organ, 760
N-Nitroso-*N*-ethyl(2,2,2-trifluoroethyl)amine, target organ, 736
N-Nitroso-*N*-ethylurea, target organ, 782
N-Nitroso-*N*-ethyl(d_2)urea, target organ, 799
N-Nitroso-*N*-ethylurethane, target organ, 795
N-Nitroso-*N*-ethyl(d_5)urethane, target organ, 800
N-Nitroso-*N*-ethylvinylamine, target organ, 737
N-Nitroso-*N*-(2-fluoroethyl)urea, target organ, 785
N-Nitrosofolic acid, target organ, 760
N-Nitrosoguvacoline, target organ, 767
N-Nitrosoheptamethyleneamine, target organ, 769
N-Nitrosoheptamethylenimine, target organ, 776
N-Nitroso-*N*-*n*-heptylurea, target organ, 789
N-Nitroso-*N*-*n*-hexyl-*N'*-nitroguanidine, target organ, 794
N-Nitroso-*N*-*n*-hexylurea, target organ, 789
N-Nitrosohydantoin, target organ, 790
N-Nitrosohydrazines, carcinogenicity, 657*t*
N-Nitroso-1-hydroperoxydi-*n*-butylamine, target organ, 747
N-Nitroso-*N*-(4-hydroxybutyl)pentylamine, target organ, 760
N-Nitroso-*N*-(2-hydroxyethyl-*n*-butylamine), target organ, 759
N-Nitroso-(2-hydroxyethyl)(2,3-dihydroxypropyl)amine, target organ, 762
N-Nitroso-(2-hydroxyethyl)(2-hydroxypropyl)amine, target organ, 762
N-Nitroso-*N*-(2-hydroxyethyl)isopropylamine, target organ, 758
N-Nitroso-*N*-(2-hydroxyethyl)urea, target organ, 784
N-Nitrosohydroxylamines, carcinogenicity, 657*t*
N-Nitroso-α-hydroxymethyl-*n*-butylamine, synthesis, 647
N-Nitroso-3'-hydroxynornicotine, target organ, 764
N-Nitroso-4-hydroxypiperidine, target organ, 765
N-Nitroso-3-hydroxypiperidine, target organ, 765
N-Nitrosohydroxyproline, target organ, 763
N-Nitroso-*N*-(3-hydroxypropyl)butylamine, target organ, 760
N-Nitroso-*N*-(2-hydroxypropyl)(2-oxopropyl)amine, target organ, 740
N-Nitroso-2-hydroxypropylurea, target organ, 799
N-Nitroso-3-hydroxypyrrolidine, 833
target organ, 763
N-Nitrosoimidazolidone, target organ, 790
N-Nitrosoiminodiacetic acid, target organ, 737
N-Nitrosoiminodiacetonitrile, target organ, 737
N-Nitrosoiminodipropionitrile, target organ, 741
N-Nitrosoindoline, target organ, 775
N-Nitroso-*N*-isobutyl-*N'*-nitroguanidine, target organ, 794
N-Nitroso-*N*-isobutylurea, target organ, 788
N-Nitrosoisonipecotic acid, target organ, 767
N-Nitroso-*N*-isopropylurea, target organ, 787
N-Nitrosolandrin, target organ, 796
N-Nitrosomethomyl, target organ, 797
N-Nitroso-2-methoxy-2,6-dimethylmorpholine, target organ, 776
N-Nitrosomethylacetamide, target organ, 797
N-Nitrosomethylacetoxymethylamine, target organ, 733, 734
N-Nitroso-*N*-methyl-*N'*-acetylurea, target organ, 781
N-Nitrosomethyl-*n*-alkylamines with long alkyl chains, metabolism, 692
N-Nitrosomethylallylamine, target organ, 750
N,N-Nitrosomethylaminoacetonitrile, target organ, 749
N-Nitroso-*N*-methyl-4-aminoazobenzene, target organ, 757
N-Nitroso-*N*-methyl-4-aminobenzaldehyde, target organ, 757
N-Nitrosomethylaminobenzylideneindene, target organ, 757
N-Nitroso-*N*-methylaminopyridine, target organ, 757
4-(*N*-Nitroso-4-methylamino)-4-(3-pyridyl)butanal, target organ, 755
N-Nitrosomethylamino-1-(3-pyridyl)-1-butanone, target organ, 755
N,N-Nitrosomethylaminosulfolane, target organ, 756
N-Nitrosomethylbenzamide, target organ, 798
N-Nitroso-*N*-methyl-*N'*-(2-benzothiazolyl)urea, target organ, 781
N-Nitrosomethylbenzylamine, 845
O^6-MeG in esophageal DNA, 708
target organ, 754
N-Nitroso-*N*-methyl-*N'*,*N'*-bis(2-chloroethyl)urea, target organ, 782

N-Nitrosomethylbiuret, target organ, 782
N-Nitroso-N-methyl(n-butyl-d_2)amine, target organ, 750, 751
N-Nitroso-N-methyl-n-butylamine, target organ, 751
N-Nitroso-tert-methylbutylamine, target organ, 751
N-Nitroso-N-methyl(butyroxymethyl)amine, target organ, 734
N-Nitroso-N-methyl-N′-carboxymethylurea, target organ, 780
N-Nitroso-N-methyl-3-carboxypropylamine, target organ, 761
N-Nitroso-N-methyl(2-chloroethyl)amine, target organ, 749
N-Nitrosomethylcyanamide, target organ, 798
N-Nitrosomethylcyclohexylamine
  structure–activity relationship, 657
  target organ, 755
N-Nitroso-N-methyl-n-decylamine, target organ, 753
N-Nitroso-1-N-methyl-deoxy-D-galactidole, target organ, 756
N-Nitroso-N-methyldeoxy-D-glucitole, target organ, 756
N-Nitroso-N-methyl-N′,N′-diethylurea, target organ, 782
N-Nitroso-N-methyl-2,3-dihydroxypropylamine, target organ, 761
N-Nitroso-N-methyl(dimethylbenzyl)amine, target organ, 754
N-Nitroso-N-methyl(dimethylbutan-3-one)amine, target organ, 752
N-Nitroso-N-methyl-N′,N′-dimethylurea, target organ, 782
N-Nitroso-N-methyl-n-dodecylamine, target organ, 753, 845
N-Nitroso-N-methylethylamine, target organ, 748, 761
N-Nitroso-N-methyl-β-D-galactosylamine, target organ, 756
N-Nitroso-N-methyl-β-D-glucosylamine, target organ, 755
N-Nitroso-N-methyl-n-heptylamine, target organ, 752
N-Nitroso-N-methyl-n-hexylamine, target organ, 752
N-Nitroso-N-methyl(4-hydroxy-n-butyl)amine, target organ, 751
N-Nitrosomethylmethoxymethylamine, 733
N-Nitroso-N-methyl(methylbenzyl)amine, target organ, 754
N-Nitroso-2-methyl-2-morpholine, target organ, 770
N-Nitroso-N-methyl-N′-nitroguanidine, target organ, 791, 799
N-Nitroso-N-methyl-n-nonylamine, target organ, 753
N-Nitroso-N-methyl-n-octylamine, target organ, 753
N-Nitroso-2-methyloxazolidine, target organ, 775
N-Nitroso-5-methyloxazolidine, target organ, 764, 801
N-Nitroso-N-methyl(2-oxopropyl)amine, target organ, 750
N-Nitroso-N-methyl-n-pentylamine, target organ, 752
N-Nitrosomethylphenidate, target organ, 769
N-Nitrosomethylphenylamine, target organ, 756
N-Nitroso-N-methyl(2-phenylethyl)amine, target organ, 754, 762
N-Nitroso-N-methyl-N′-phenylurea, target organ, 781
N-Nitroso-N′-methylpiperazine, target organ, 772
N-Nitroso-2-methylpiperidine, target organ, 767
N-Nitroso-3-methylpiperidine, target organ, 767
N-Nitroso-4-methylpiperidine, target organ, 768
N-Nitroso-3-methylpiperid-4-one, target organ, 767
N-Nitrosomethylpropionamide, target organ, 797
N-Nitroso-n-methylpropylamine, target organ, 749
N-Nitroso-5-methylpyrrolidone, target organ, 798
N-Nitrosomethylstearylamine, 845
4-(4-N-Nitrosomethylstyryl)quinoline, target organ, 757
N-Nitroso-n-methyltetradecylamine, target organ, 753
Nitrosomethyltoluenesulfonamide, target organ, 798
N-Nitroso-n-methyl(2,2,2-trifluoroethyl)amine, target organ, 749
Nitroso-n-methylundecylamine, target organ, 753
Nitrosomethylurea
  multigeneration experiment, 672t
  target organ, 778, 799
N-Nitrosomethylurethane, target organ, 794, 800
N-Nitroso-N-methylvinylamine, target organ, 749
N-Nitrosomorpholine
  carcinogenesis with N-nitroso compounds, 676t
  target organ, 770
N-Nitrosonornicotine
  metabolism, 693, 695
  target organ, 763
N-Nitrosonornicotine N-oxide, target organ, 764
N-Nitrosooctamethyleneamine, target organ, 769
N-Nitroso-N-n-octylurea, target organ, 789
N-Nitrosooxazolidine, target organ, 764, 801
N-Nitroso-N-(2-oxopropyl)butylamine, target organ, 760
N-Nitroso-2-oxopropyl-(2-oxobutyl)amine, target organ, 760
N-Nitroso-N-n-pentyl-N′-nitroguanidine, target organ, 794
N-Nitroso-N-n-pentylurea, target organ, 788
N-Nitroso-N-n-pentylurethane, target organ, 796
N-Nitroso-N-phenylbenzylamine, target organ, 760
N-Nitroso-N-phenyl-N′,N′-dimethylurea, target organ, 790
N-Nitroso-N-(2-phenylethyl)urea, target organ, 790
N-Nitroso-4-phenylpiperidine, target organ, 768

N-Nitroso-N-phenylurea, target organ, 790
N-Nitrosopipecolic acid, target organ, 767
N-Nitrosopiperazine, target organ, 772
N-Nitrosopiperidine
  metabolism, 693
  target organ, 764
N-Nitroso-4-piperidone, target organ, 765
N-Nitrosoproline, target organ, 763
N-Nitrosoproline ethyl ester, target organ, 763
N-Nitroso-N-n-propyl-(1-acetoxypropyl)amine, target organ, 742
N-Nitroso-N-n-propyl(4-hydroxybutyl)amine, target organ, 759
N-Nitroso-N-n-propyl(2-hydroxypropyl)amine, target organ, 738
N-Nitroso-N-n-propyl(1-methoxypropyl)amine, target organ, 742
N-Nitroso-N-n-propyl-N'-nitroguanidine, target organ, 793
N-Nitroso-N-n-propyl(2-oxopropyl)amine, target organ, 738
N-Nitroso-N-n-propylpropionamide, target organ, 797
N-Nitroso-N-n-propylurea, target organ, 786
N-Nitroso-N-n-propylurethane, target organ, 795
N-Nitrosopyrrolidine
  metabolism, 694
  target organ, 763
N-Nitrosopyrrolidone, target organ, 798
N-Nitrososarcosine, target organ, 749
N-Nitrososarcosine ethyl ester, target organ, 749
N-Nitrosotetrahydro-1,3-oxazine
  target organ, 771, 776
N-Nitroso-1,2,3,4-tetrahydropyridine, target organ, 766
N-Nitroso-1,2,3,6-tetrahydropyridine, target organ, 766
N-Nitroso-2,2,6,6-tetramethylpiperidine, target organ, 766
N-Nitroso-2,2,6,6-tetramethylpiperidine, target organ, 768
N-Nitrosothiomorpholine, target organ, 771
N-Nitroso-N-tridecylurea, target organ, 789
N-Nitrosotrimethylpiperazine, target organ, 772
N-Nitroso-N,N',N'-tris(2-chloroethyl)urea, target organ, 786
N-Nitroso-N-undecylurea, target organ, 789
N-Nitrosourea
  carcinogenicity, 1249
  2-chloroethyl derivatives, 681
Nitrothiazoles, in vivo conversion, 1256
5-Nitro-o-toluidine, carcinogenicity, 206t
Nitrovin, toxicity, 1256t
4-Nitrozuinoline 1-oxide, structure-activity relationship, 247
NMNG—*See* N-Nitroso-N-methyl-N'-nitroguanidine
NMOR—*See* N-Nitrosomorpholine
NMR data, triazenes, 875, 878
NNK—*See* 4-(N-Methyl-N-nitrosamino)1-(3-pyridyl)-1-butanone
NNN—*See* N-Nitrosonornicotine
Nobiletin, 976
Nocardia, aflatoxins effect, 971
Nomenclature, polynuclear compounds, 41
Non K-region arene expoxides, synthesis, 112
Non K-region dihydrodiols, synthesis, 112
N-Nonanoylethyleneimine, oncogenesis tests, 426–27t
Nonbonding molecular orbital coefficient, 64
Nonionizing radiation, 23
Nonlymphocytic leukemia, secondary acute, 398
NPIP—*See* N-Nitrosopiperidine
NPRO—*See* N-Nitrosoproline
NPYR—*See* N-Nitrosopyrrolidine
NQO—*See* 4-Nitroquinoline 1-oxide
NSAR*See* N-Nitrososarcosine
Nucleic acids
  alkylation, N-nitroso carcinogens, 698–704
  macromolecular binding of aflatoxins, 1046–61
    characteristics, 1047–49
  reactions with polynuclear aromatics, 122–25
  nitroso-derived alkylation products, 701
Nucleophilic properties, monoalkyltriazenes, 888
Nucleophilicities, polynuclear compounds, related to carcinogenic activity, 62
Nucleoside–hydrocarbon interaction products, 122–25
Nurses, cancer rate, 308
Nursing-bottle tests, nitrosamines, 847t

O

Oats, aflatoxins, 1099
Occult blood, fecal, detection, carcinogenic reagents, 311
Occupation
  as cancer cause, 29–34
  as source of hazards, 30
Occupational cancer, causes, 165–73
Occupational hazards and malignancy, 31t
Octachlorodi-n-propyl ether, oncogenesis tests, 442–43t
ODC—*See* Ornithine decarboxylase
Oil(s)
  as cause of occupational cancer, 165–73
  frying, 1224-25
Oil-soluble derivatives, 1-phenylazo-2-naphthol, 241
Oilseeds, in aflatoxins, 1104–7
Olefinic double bonds, epoxidation and in vivo conversion, 1263
N-Oleyethyleneimine, oncogenesis tests, 426–27t
Onc gene, 351
Oncogenesis tests
  with aklylating agents, 400–4
    chemical structure vs. reactivity, 404–60
Oncopeltus fasciatus, aflatoxins effect, 973
Onions, aflatoxins, 1110
Oral intake, administration of test chemicals, 1348
Organ-specific effects, N-nitrosamines, 688
Organ specificity
  N-nitroso carcinogens, 665
  symmetrical dialkylnitrosamines, 658
Organochlorine pesticides, 546–53, 1226
Organochlorines, 553
Organotropic effects, N-nitroso carcinogens, 697
Ornithine dicarboxylase, activity, 1307

Osborne-Mendel rats, toxaphene effects, 553
OSHA standards, 297
Ostrimia nubilalis, aflatoxins effect, 973
Ouabain systems, functional enzyme, need, 361
Ovariectomy, and rat liver microsomal activity, 1071
Ovary cancer, alkylating agent therapy, 398
Ovex, 559
Oxetanes, 428
  oncogenesis tests, 430–33*t*
Oxidation
  activation of aromatic amines, 179
  amino groups, in vivo conversion, 1258
  dialkylaryltriazenes, 892
Oxidative decarboxylation of nitrosoamino acids, synthesis of α-acyloxynitrosamines, 646
Oxidative phosphorylation, 1089
Oxime, structural requirements for carcinogenicity, 655*t*
7-(2-Oxoethyl)guanine, structure, 355*f*
5-Oxomethyl ester, bracken carcinogenicity, 1197
S-Oxydibenzothiophenyl-2-acetamide, carcinogenicity, 259*t*
Oysters, polycyclic aromatic hydrocarbon content, 1210*t*
Ozonization, destruction of aflatoxins, 964

P

PAA—*See* Phenanthrenylacetamide
Pacifiers, nitrosamines, 846, 847*t*
PAH—*See* Polycyclic aromatic hydrocarbons
Pancreas cancer
  deaths, 8
  derivatives of di-*n*-propylnitrosamine, 691
Panfuran, toxicity, 1256*t*
Panmyelotoxicoses, 1142
Papilloma induction, kinetics, 381
Papillomas, unsymmetrical *N*-nitrosamines, 659
Paprkia, aflatoxins, 1111
Paracetamol, major metabolite of phenacetin, 1259
4-Parahydroxyanisole, effects on tumor promotion in mice, 1307*t*
Parasorbic acid, oncogenesis tests, 437*t*
Partial hepatectomy, effect on aflatoxin B_1 carcinogenicity, 998*t*
Patulin, oncogenesis tests, 434–35*t*
PB—*See* Phenobarbital
PCB—*See* Polychlorinated biphenyl(s)
Peanut(s), 1221
  in aflatoxins, 1101–3
Peanut butter, aflatoxins, 1103
Peanut candies, aflatoxins, 1103
Peanut meal, aflatoxin contamination, 958
Peanut oil
  aflatoxin destruction, 962
  unrefined, aflatoxin decontamination, 961
Peas, aflatoxins, 1107
Pecans, aflatoxins, 1108
Pellet, bladder implantation, role in tumor induction, 256
Penicillin
  injection-site sarcomas, 428
  possible reactions, 429
Penicillin G, oncogenesis tests, 430–33*t*
Penicillinic acid, 428
  oncogenesis tests, 434–35*t*
  possible reactions, 429
Pentacene, carcinogenic activities, 130*t*
Pentacholoromethane, 540
Pentacyclic aromatic hydrocarbon derivatives, 140–141*t*
Pentalin, 540
Pentamethyleneiminedithiocarbamate, piperidine salt, nitrosamine contamination, 844*t*
Pentaphene, carcinogenic activities, 130*t*, 140–41*t*
Pepper, aflatoxins, 1111
Pepstatin, 1304
  carcinogenesis inhibitors, 1303*t*
Peracid epoxidation, synthesis of vicinal dihydrodiol epoxides, 112
Perchlorobutadiene, 532
Perchloroethane, 540
  See also Hexachloroethane
Perchloroethylene, 541
  mechanisms, 562
Periplaneta americana, aflatoxins effect, 973
Peritoneum, diffuse mesotheliomas, 636
Perylene, carcinogenic activities, 130*t*, 140–41*t*
Pesticides, 546–61, 1226
  exposure, 383–97
  in humans, 560
  nitrosamines, 845–46
  organochlorine, 546–53
Petroleum oils, 167–68
Phage induction by aflatoxin B_1, 1011*t*
Pharmacokinetics, *N*-nitroso carcinogens, 682
Pharmacological properties, use of triazene compounds, 872
Phenacetin, 24, 1258
  abuse, 24
Phenanthramines, carcinogenic structure–activity relationship, 228
Phenanthrene
  carcinogenic activities, 130*t*
  derivatives
    carcinogenic activities, 138–39*t*
    tumor-initiating activity, 106*t*
  metabolic attack at the K region, 72
  role in tumor inhibition, 1295*t*
  tumor-initiating activity, 105
Phenathrene dihydrodiol, tumor-initiating activity, 105
2-Phenanthrylacetamide, reactions with macromolecules, 196
Phenazopyridine, in vivo conversion, 1260
Phenelzine, carcinogenicity, 1269
Phenidone, effect on arachidonic acid metabolism, 1305*t*
Phenobarbital
  AFB_1 carcinogenicity, 998*t*
  effect on AFB_1 measurements, 1066
  modification of aromatic amine carcinogenesis, 261
  in *N*-nitroso carcinogenesis, 678*t*
  stimulation of aflatoxin B_1 metabolism, 1065
Phenol(s)
  epigenetic carcinogen, 1330*t*
  metabolic intermediates in the enzymic formation, 70

Phenothiazines, inhibition of chemical carcinogenesis, 1291*t*
Phenoxybenzamine, carcinogenicity, 1247
4-Phenylazoaniline derivatives, structure–activity relationship, 229
4-(Phenylazo)-*o*-anisidine, carcinogenicity, 231*t*
4-(Phenylazo)acetanilide, carcinogenicity, 231*t*
4-(Phenylazo)diacetanilide, carcinogenicity, 231*t*
4-(Phenylazo)-*N*-phenylacethydroxamic acid, carcinogenicity, 231*t*
1-Phenylazo-2-naphthol, oil-soluble derivatives, 241
Phenylazonaphthol dyes, structure–activity relationship, 240
Phenylazonaphthols, structure–activity relationship, 243
4-(Phenylazo)-*N*-phenyldroxylamine, carcinogenicity, 231*t*
N-Phenylbenzeneamine—*See* Diphenylamine
Phenylenediamine(s), carcinogenicity, 206*t*
Phenylhydroxylamine, acetanilide metabolism, 179
N-Phenyl-2-naphthylamine, 285
  structure, 285
N-Phenylphenylenediamine, carcinogenicity, 207*t*
Phenytoin, in vivo conversion, 1264
Phorbol ester(s), 381
  epigenetic carcinogen, 1330*t*
Phorbol myristyl acetate, 526
Phosphate esters, metabolic activation of aromatic amines, 187
Phosphodiesterase, 1308*t*
Phosphonates, 413
  oncogenesis tests, 418–19*t*
Phosphoric acid triester, 393
Photodynamic action, polynuclear compounds, carcinogenic activity, 62
Photolysis
  and acid-catalyzed degradation, dialkyltriazenes, 891
  dialkyltriazenes, 892
Physical elimination, aflatoxins, 959
Physical inactivation, aflatoxins, 962–63
Pi bonding, and carcinogenic activity, 65
Pi electron(s)
  density distributions, related to carcinogenic activities, 57
  distribution, effect on carcinogenetic activity, 56
Picene, carcinogenic activities, 130*t*, 140–41*t*
Pig
  AFB_1 excretion, 1075
  AFB_1 toxicity, 978*t*
  AFM_1 excretion, 1036*t*
Piperazine, 858
  predominant sites of tumor induction by *N*-nitroso derivatives, 661
Piperidine
  lowest effective carcinogenic doses, 670*t*
  predominant sites of tumor induction by *N*-nitroso derivatives, 661
Pistachio nuts
  aflatoxins, 1109
  detection of aflatoxins, 952
Pitch, exposure, 170
Plant(s)
  aflatoxins, 971
  food carcinogens, 1219–20
Plant cytogenetics, by aflatoxin B_1, 1012*t*
Plant flavonoids, 976
  influence on aflatoxin B_1 genotoxicity, 1030*t*
Platinum diammines, 455
Pleura, diffuse mesotheliomas, 636
Pleural fibrosis, diffuse, as indication of fibrous mineral exposure, 635
Pleural plaques, as indication of fibrous mineral exposure, 635
Podophylline toxin, carcinogenicity, 1250
Poisoning
  cattle bracken, 1171
  hemorrhagic bracken, sheep, 1179
Polyamine synthesis, 1308*t*
Polybrominated biphenyl(s), 534–35
Polycholorinated biphenyl(s), 545–46, 1292
  accumulation, 545
  effect on AFB_1 carcinogenicity, 997*t*
Polychlorinated camphene(s), carcinogenicity, 547–51*t*
Polychlorinated hydrocarbons, epigenetic carcinogen, 1330*t*
Polychloroprene, 527
Polycyclic aromatic hydrocarbons
  botanical sources, 1210–12
  enzyme-inducing agents, 258
  exposure to laboratory personnel, 316
  in food, 1209–13
  role in tumor inhibition, 1293–97, 1295*t*
  two-stage initiation–promotion, 1294
  unsubstituted, carcinogenic activities, 130–31*t*
Polycyclic hydrocarbons, malignancy sites, 31*t*
Polyfunctional ethyleneimines, 460
Polyinosinicpolycytidylic acid, tumor inhibition, 1297*t*
Polymer foils, epigenetic carcinogen, 1330*t*
Polymorphism, bracken carcinogenicity, 1175
Polynuclear carcinogens
  nomenclature, 41
  related to structure, 55
Polysome disaggregation, 1086
Polysome formation, helical, 1087
Polytetrafluoroethylene, 527
Polyvinyl bromide, 536
Polyvinylidene fluoride, 529
Postharvest aflatoxin contamination, control, 959
Potency, carcinogenic reagents, 314
Pott, Percivall, 1324
Precocious breast enlargement, 1156
Pregnancy, diethylstibestrol use, 24
Prevalence rate, definition, 15*t*
Primary amines, deamination, triazenes, 887
Primary liver cell tumors, 5
Primary metabolic routes, naphthalene, 73
Primates, susceptibility to aflatoxin B_1, 991
Procarbazine, 921, 1243
  carcinogenicity, 1249
  metabolism, 921
  structure, 921
Progestins
  carcinogenicity, 1266
  in vivo conversion, 1265

Proline, bracken carcinogenicity, 1197
Prometalol hydrochloride, carcinogenicity, 1272
Promoter(s), 18
  mode of action, 1330*t*
  tumor, characteristics, 1281
Promutagenic base(s), removal, 362, 364
Promutagens
  3-methyladenine, 364
  7-methylguanine, 354
1,3-Propane sultone
  carcinogenic index, 439
  carcinogenicity, 368
    relative, 382
  DNA synthesis, inhibition, 402
  mutagenicity, 368
  oncogenesis tests, 440–41*t*
Propargyl methanesulfonate, oncogenesis tests, 416–17*t*
Propazine, 559
β-Propiolactone
  alkylating DNA, 353
  carcinogenic index, 428
  carcinogenicity, 368
  DNA synthesis, inhibition, 402
  induction of skin tumors, 402
  initiating agents, 401
  mutagenicity, 368
  oncogenesis tests, 401, 430–33*t*
  reactions with DNA, 353
  relative carcinogenicity, 382
  structure, 352
Propyl gallate, influence on aflatoxin B_1 genotoxicity, 1031*t*
n-Propyldiazonium ion, 467
Propylene glycol, 1224
Propylene oxide, oncogenesis tests, 422–23*t*
1,2-Propyleneimine, oncogenesis tests, 426–27*t*
Prostaglandin synthetase inhibitors, tumor inhibition, 1298
Prostate cancer, worldwide variation, 5*t*
Protease inhibitors, 1302–4
  chemical and radiation carcinogenesis, 1303
Protein, 980
  effect on aflatoxin B_1 carcinogenicity, 996*t*
  macromolecular binding by aflatoxins, 1061
  reaction with 4-nitroquinoline, 247
  synthesis and function, aflatoxin B_1 treatment, 1084–88
Protein binding, vs. DNA binding, 1062
Protein synthesis
  in monkeys, inhibition, 1085
  inhibition, 928
Protein undernutrition, in rats, 1231
Protolysis
  dialkyltriazenes, 891
  reactions of monoalkyltriazenes, 885–87
Prototypes, molecular, triazenes, 872
Protozoa, aflatoxin B_1 effect, 972
Psoralens, carcinogenicity, 1250, 1268
Ptaquiloside, bracken carcinogenicity, 1197
Pteraquilin, bracken carcinogenicity, 1182
Pteridium aquuilinum—See Bracken carcinogenicity
Purine oxides, structure-activity relationship, 250
Purines, role in aflatoxin B_1-nucleic acid interactions, 1051
PyAB—*See* 4-*N*-Pyrrolidinylazobenzene
Pyrene
  carcinogenic activities, 130*t*
  inactive derivatives, carcinogenic activities, 138–39*t*
  role in tumor inhibition, 1295*t*
Pyrimethamine, carcinogenicity, 1272
Pyrolysis, dialkylaryltriazenes, 893
Pyrrole, derivatives, structure-activity relationship, 250
Pyrrolidine
  lowest effective carcinogenic doses, 670*t*
  predominant sites of tumor induction by *N*-nitroso derivatives, 661
4-*N*-Pyrrolidinylazobenzene, structure-activity relationship, 238
Pyrrolizidine alkaloid(s), 1219
  effect on AFB_1 carcinogenicity, 997*t*

Q

Quail, Japanese, susceptibility to dietary aflatoxin, 977
Quaternary ammonium compounds, 845
Quercetin, 976, 1196
  bracken carcinogenicity, 1186–90
  inhibition of chemical carcinogenesis, 1287
Quercetin pentamethyl ether, inhibition of chemical carcinogenesis, 1287
Quinacrine ethyl half-mustard, oncogenesis tests, 444–45*t*
Quinacrine ethyl mustard, oncogenesis tests, 453*t*
Quinoline 1-oxide, carcinogenic activity, 249*t*
Quinones, enzyme-inducing agents, 258
Quintozene, 559

R

RA—*See* Retinoic acid
Rabbit, aflatoxin B_1 toxicity, 978*t*
Radiation carcinogenesis
  effects of protease inhibitors, 1303
  effects of retinoids, 1301*t*
Radioimmunoassay, alkylation of nucleic acids, 700
Radon, 2
Rainbow trout
  AFB_1 hepatocarcinogenicity, 984*t*
  AFB_1 toxicity, 978*t*
  AFG_1 effects on, 980
  aflatoxin congener and metabolites, 1002
  embryos, for aflatoxin carcinogenicity, 987
Raisins, aflatoxins, 1110
Rapidogen dyeing process, use of triazene compounds, 872
Rat(s)
  AFB_1 excretion, 1073–74
  AFB_1 toxicity, 978*t*
  aflatoxin congener and metabolites, 1001–2
  excretion of aflatoxin M_1, 1033*t*
  lethal dose of selenium, 1145
  PB treatment, 1065
  protein undernutrition, 1231
  Sprague-Dawley, aflatoxin B_1 chromosome inductor, 1014*t*
  susceptibility to aflatoxin B_1, 988

Rat liver cells, AFB_1 effects, 1021*t*
γ-Ray emission, 23
Reactive double bond, related to carcinogenic activity, 57
Reagents
  carcinogenic, clinicial chemistry, 311
  possible carcinogenicity, 313
Reduction, activation of aromatic amines, 182
Repair-induced structural change in DNA, *N*-nitroso carcinogens, 714–16
Repair mechanism, O_6-methylguanine, 468
Repair process, cell division, 362
Repair system, 361–62
Reproductive factors, 28
Reserpine, carcinogenicity, 1271
Resonance theory, and carcinogenic activity, 65
Resorcinoldiglycidyl ether, oncogenesis tests, 463*t*
Resorptive carcinogenic action, triazenes, 906
Respiration, in vitro inhibition by AFB_1, 1090
Retinal, 1302*t*
  effect on carcinogenesis, 1301*t*
Retinoblastoma, in children, 9–10
Retinoic acid, 1302*t*
  effect on carcinogenesis, 1301–t
Retinoids, as inhibitors, 1300–2
Retinol, 1302*t*
  effect on carcinogenesis, 1301*t*
  influence on AFB_1 genotoxicity, 1031*t*
Retinyl acetate, 1302*t*
  effect on carcinogenesis, 1301*t*
Retinyl methyl ether, effect on carcinogenesis, 1301*t*
Retinyl palmitate, 1302*t*
Retinylidene dimedone, effect on carcinogenesis, 1301*t*
Retonioic acid, stage-specific inhibitors, 1309*t*
Riboflavin
  effect on aflatoxin B_1 carcinogenicity, 995*t*
  tumor inhibition, 1297*t*
Ribs, polycyclic aromatic hydrocarbon content, 1210*t*
Rice, aflatoxins, 1098
Rifampycine, carcinogenicity, 1271
RNA, reaction with 4-nitroquinoline, 247
RNA metabolism, alterations, aflatoxins, 1078
RNA synthesis
  in vitro nucleolar, 1080–81
  inhibition by AFB_1, 1079
  selectivity of AFB_1, 1081
Rock fern, carcinogenicity, 1180
Rockwool
  mineral fiber carcinogenesis, 633
  structure, 632
Rodent cells
  DNA fragmentation, 1019*t*, 1020*t*
  unscheduled DNA synthesis, 1018*t*
Romadur, aflatoxins, 1114
Roridin A, 1143
  lethal dose, 1139*t*
Rosenkranz, bacterial screening tests, 1335
Rubber articles, nitrosamines, 847*t*
Rubber chemicals, nitrosamine contamination, 844*t*
Rubber factories, and bladder cancer, 177
Rubber industry
  N-nitrosamines, occupational exposure, 853*t*
  nitrosamine exposure, 851–56
Rubber products, nitrosamines, 846
Rubber toys, nitrosamines, 847*t*
Rubratoxin, toxic effects, enhancement, 982
Rutile, 634

S

SA—*See* Stilbenamine
SAA—*See* Stilbenylacetamide
Saccharin, 1225
  epigenetic carcinogen, 1330*t*
Saccharin-cyclamate combination, 1225
Saccharomyces cerevisiae, AFB_1 chromosome inductor, 1011*t*, 1012*t*
Safe dose, definition, 1207–8
Safrole, 1220
Saguinus oedipomidas, aflatoxin B_1 hepatocarcinogenicity, 985*t*
Salmo gaidneri—*See* Trout
Salmon, aflatoxin B_1 hepatocarcinogenicity, 984*t*
Salmonella
  aflatoxicol mutagenicity, 1041
  aflatoxins effect, 972
  gene mutation effects of AFB_1, 1007*t*
Salmonella typhimurium
  AFB_1
    binding, 1055
    gene mutation effects, 1007*t*, 1008*t*
  bacterial screening tests, 1335
  gene mutation effects of aflatoxin B_1, 1008*t*
Salt bath curing, *N*-nitrosamines, occupational exposure, 853*t*
Sarkomycin, oncogenesis tests, 434–35*t*
Sausage, polycyclic aromatic hydrocarbon content, 1210*t*
Schools, aromatic amines, 319
Science education, carcinogens, 319
Scopolamine, carcinogenicity, 1250
Screening, 294
Scrotal cancer, 170–72
  chimney sweeps, 2
  first related to soot exposure, 49
  prognosis and prevention, 172
Sebaceous gland suppression, test for in vivo genotoxicity, 1340
Secondary amines, nitrosation, 648
Selenium, 1223
  effects on tumor promotion in mice, 1307*t*
  inhibition
    of chemical carcinogenesis, 1283*t*
    of tumor formation, 1285
  lethal dose in rats, 1145
  role in esophageal cancer, 1142–46
  toxicity, 1144
  tumorigenicity role, 924
Selenium compounds, photosensitivity, 1144
Septic angina, 1142
Sesame seeds, aflatoxins, 1105
Sex, effects on AFB_1 metabolism, 1071
Sex organs, abnormalities, 1157
Shale oil, 167
Sheep
  AFB_1 excretion, 1075
  AFB_1 toxicity, 978*t*
  AFM_1 excretion, 1037*t*

Shikimic acid, bracken carcinogenicity, 1182–86
Short-term tests, in vitro, 1334
Shrimp, aflatoxins, 1112
Sigma bonding, and carcinogenic activity, 65
Simazine, 559
Single-dose carcinogenicity, *N*-nitroso carcinogens, 669
Single-dose studies, persistence of O^6-alkylguanine in DNA, 706–11
Sister chromatid exchange, by AFB_1, 1014*t*
Six-membered rings, 429
  oncogenesis tests, 437*t*
Skin cancer
  AFB_1-induced, 993
  worldwide variation, 5*t*
Skin neoplasm induction in mice, 1342
Skin tumors
  induction, 402
  protein binding, 401
Slag wools, mineral fiber carcinogenesis, 633
Small animals, tumors, bracken carcinogenicity, 1174
Smoking, 20–21
  related to chemical exposure and cancer rate, 310–11
SOD—*See* Superoxide dismutase
Sodium cyanate, tumor inhibition, 1297*t*
Sodium saccharin, effect on *N*-nitroso carcinogenesis, 678*t*
Soil contamination, sources, 1211
Solid-state carcinogen, mode of action, 1330*t*
Solvent(s), 536–43
Solvent extraction, aflatoxins, 960
Solvent pollution, exposure, related to cancer rate, 309
Soot, 49, 169–70
  as cause of occupational cancer, 165–73
  domestic, 165
Sorbic acid, 395, 429
  oncogenesis tests, 437*t*
Sorghum, aflatoxins, 1099
Soybean(s), aflatoxins, 1106
Soybean oil, nitrosamine content, 1214*t*
Specialized registries, 12
Species responses to carcinogens, 1206
Specific locust test, test for in vivo genotoxicity, 1340
Spectroscopy, triazenes, 872, 875–83
Sperm abnormality, test for in vivo genotoxicity, 1340
Spices, aflatoxin, 1110–11
Spironolactone, carcinogenicity, 1272
Spodoptera frugiperda, aflatoxins effect, 973
Spores, bracken carcinogenicity, 1197
Sputum, asbestos presence, 635
Squamous neoplasms, bracken carcinogenicity, 1176
Stability of alkylated components, DNA in vivo, 705
Stage-specific inhibitors of two-stage promotion, 1309–10
Staggers, bracken, 1171
Standardized mortality ratio, definition, 15*t*
Statistical approach, 1207–9
Steak, polycyclic aromatic hydrocarbon content, 1210*t*
N-Stearoylethyleneimine, oncogenesis tests, 426–27*t*
Stem cells, types, 380
Stereoisomers, nomenclature, 45
Stereoselective synthesis, synthesis of vicinal dihydrodiol epoxides, 112
Sterility, shikimic acid, 1186
Steroid(s)
  antiinflammatory, 1297
    tumor inhibition, 1297*t*, 1298–1300, 1299*t*
  carcinogenicity, 126
  enzyme-inducing agents, 258
  modification of aromatic amine carcinogenesis, 263
Steroid hormone mechanisms, alterations, 1088–89
Steroid structure, related to polynuclear carcinogens, 54
Stilbenamines, carcinogenic structure–activity relationship, 215
4-Stilbenylacetamide
  metabolic activation, 189
  reactions with macromolecules, 197
Stomach, AFB_1-induced tumors, 994
Stomach cancer
  bracken carcinogenicity, 1193
  nutrition effects, 1229
  protective factors, 1194
  worldwide variation, 5*t*
Strand breakage, types of DNA damage produced by chemicals, 1335
Streptomyces, aflatoxins effect, 971
Strobane, carcinogenicity in mice, 556–57*t*
Structural change in DNA, repair-induced, *N*-nitroso carcinogens, 714–16
Structural requirements for carcinogenicity, *N*-nitroso carcinogens, 654–65
Structure, chemical, carcinogenic activity, 52, 1333
Structure–activity relationship(s)
  aflatoxins, 1093–94
  carcinogenic potential of aromatic amines, 201–65
  N-nitrosamines, 657–65
  triazenes, 896
Styrene epoxide, effect in microsomal metabolism of naphthalene, 70
Styrene oxide, 421
  influence on AFB_1 genotoxicity, 1030*t*
  oncogenesis tests, 422–23*t*
  reactions with deoxyguanosine, 425
  structure, 394
Subcutaneous injection, 1325
  administration of test chemicals, 1349
Substituent effect, *N,N*-dimethyl-*p*-phenylazoaniline, 234*t*
Substituted benzacridines, carcinogenic activities, 146–47*t*
Substituted benzo[*a*]pyrene derivatives, carcinogenic activities, 140–41*t*
Substituted benz[*a*]anthracenes, carcinogenic activities, 136–37*t*
Substituted dibenz[*a,h*]anthracene derivatives, carcinogenic activities, 140–41*t*
Succinic acid, bracken carcinogenicity, 1182
Succinic anhydrides, oncogenesis tests, 434–35*t*

Sulfate esters, metabolic activation of aromatic amines, 185–87
Sulfhydryl compounds, binding to aflatoxins, 1069
Sulfonates, 413
  oncogenesis, 414–17*t*
Sulfur mustard(s), 447, 455–56
  oncogenesis tests, 448–49*t*
  tumor inhibition, 1297*t*
Sultones, 439
  oncogenesis tests, 440–41*t*
Sunflower seeds, aflatoxins, 1105
Superoxide dismutase, epidermal, decreasing levels, 1306
Survival rate, definition, 15*t*
Swaziland, liver cancer incidence, aflatoxin exposure, 967*t*
Sweden, cancer mortality rate for chemists, 306
Sweeteners, 1225–26
Symmetrical *N*-nitrosamines, target organ, 732–47
Symmetrical nitrosamines, structure–activity relationship, 658
Synergistic effect, carcinogenic effect of two carcinogens, 675
Synthetic foam rubbers, use of triazene compounds, 872
Syrian hamster(s)
  embryo cells, AFB_1 effects, 1021*t*
  kidney cells, AFB_1 effects, 1022*t*
  susceptibility to AFB_1, 992

T

T-2 tetraol, structure, 1148*t*
T-2 toxin, 1146
  deacylation, 1148
  effects on the immune system, 1149–50
  in vitro tests, 1147
  influence on AFB_1 genotoxicity, 1031*t*
  isolation, 1146
  lethal dose, 1139*t*
  metabolism, 1148–49
  structure, 1148
TAME—*See* Tosylalanyl methyl ester
Tangeretin, 976
Tar, exposure, 170
Target organ(s)
  bracken carcinogenicity, 1179
  cyclic nitrosamines, 763–77
  dialkylaryltriazenes in rats, 899
  N-nitrosamides, 778–801
  symmetrical dialkylnitrosamines, 658
  symmetrical *N*-nistroamines, 732–47
  unsymmetrical *N*-nitrosamines, 748–62
Tars
  as cause of occupational cancer, 165–73
  carcinogenic, early fluorescence studies, 50
TCB—*See* 3,3′,4,4′-Tetrachlorobiphenyl
TCDD—*See* 2,3,7,8-Tetrachlorodibenzo-*p*-dioxin
TCP—*See* 2,4,6-Trichlorophenol
Tea, polycylic aromatic hydrocarbon content, 1210*t*
Teats, nursing-bottle, nitrosamines, 847*t*
Telodrin, 559
TEM—*See* Triethylenemelamine
Template activity in vitro, effect of alkylated bases, 703
Teratogenicity
  aflatoxins, 1004–5
  3,3-dialkyl-1-(3-pyridyl)triazenes, 902*t*
  N-nitroso carcinogens, 653
  shikimic acid, 1186
  triazenes, 901
Test chemicals, administration, bioassay of carcinogens, 1347
Testicular DNA synthesis inhibition, test for in vivo genotoxicity, 1340
Testosterone
  role in protein synthesis inhibition, 1085
  synthesis by alcohol, 1159
3,3′,4,4′-Tetrachlorbiphenyl, inhibition of chemical carcinogenesis, 1291*t*
2,3,7,8-Tetrachlordibenzo-*p*-dioxin, 532–33, 1290
  genetic regulation of AFB_1 metabolism, 1067
  inhibition of chemical carcinogenesis, 1291*t*
  structure, 532
  tumor inhibition, 1292*f*
Tetrachlorethylene, 541
1,1,2,2-Tetrachloroethane, 540
Tetrachloromethane, 537
2,3,5,6-Tetrachloro-4-nitroanisole, carcinogenicity, 203*t*
Tetrachlorvinphos
  carcinogenicity in mice, 556–57*t*
  structure, 559
Tetracyclic aromatic hydrocarbon derivatives, carcinogenic activities, 138–39*t*
12-*O*-Tetradecanoylphorbol-13-acetate, 1280
  tumor promotion, retinoid, inhibition, 1301*t*
Tetraethylthiuram disulfide, nitrosamine contamination, 844*t*
Tetrafidon, 559
Tetrafluoroethylene, 527
Tetrafluoro-*m*-phenylenediamine, carcinogenicity, 206*t*
Tetrahydrocortisol, tumor inhibition, 1299*t*
1,3,5,7-Tetramethylanthracene, structure, 169*f*
2′,3,4′,6′-Tetramethylbiphenylamine, carcinogenicity, 209*t*
1,3,6,8-Tetramethylcarbazole, structure, 169*f*
1,2,7,8-Tetramethyldibenzothiophene, structure, 169*f*
Tetramethylthiuram disulfide, nitrosamine contamination, 844*t*
Thailand
  liver cancer incidence, 1222*t*
    aflatoxin exposure, 967*t*
Thermostability, bracken carcinogenicity, 1175
Thiaminase, bracken carcinogenicity, 1172
Thin-layer chromatography
  detection of zearalenone, 1152
  of trichothecenes, 1150
4,4′-Thiodianiline, carcinogenicity, 213*t*
Thionitrosamine, structural requirements for carcinogenicity, 655*t*
Thiophene, derivatives, structure–activity relationship, 250
Thiophosphates, oncogenesis tests, 418–19*t*
Thiophosphonates, 413
Thiotriethylenephosphoramide, carcinogenicity, 1249

Thiourea, 1220
Thiuram sulfides, 855
Thorotrast, carcinogenicity, 1271
Three-ring hydrocarbons, 168
Thymic lymphoma, kinetics of induction, 381
Thymime, nitroso compounds as alkylating agents, 699
Tilsit, aflatoxins, 1114
Time dependence, equation, 379
Time experiments, dose effect and dose induction, *N*-nitroso carcinogens, 665
Tire industry
  N-nitrosamines, occupational exposure, 853*t*
  nitrosamine levels, 852
Tissue, exposure to nitroso compounds, biochemical analysis, 704
Tissue responses, cellular analysis, *N*-nitroso carcinogens, 724
Titanium, fibrous form, 634
TLC—*See* Thin-layer chromatography
TLCK—*See* Tosyllysyl chloromethyl ketone
Tobacco, 20–21
  lime mixture, 25
  nitrosamines, 839
  nitrosodiethanolamine, 844*t*
Tobacco smoke
  N-nitroso compounds, 829
  N-nitrosodiethanolamine, 844*t*
  nitrosamines, 839–42
  volatile *N*-nitrosamines, 841*t*
Tobacco-specific nitrosamines, 840
α-Tocopherol
  effect on AFB_1 toxicity, 981
  effects on tumor promotion in mice, 1307*t*
o,o'-Tolidine, carcinogenicity, 213*t*
o-Tolidine, related to cancer in clinical chemists, 311
Toluenediamine(s), carcinogenicity, 206*t*
Toluidine(s), 285–86
  carcinogenicity, 202*t*
  structure, 286
p-Toluidine mustard, oncogenesis tests, 450–51*t*
4-(*m*-Tolylazo)aniline, carcinogenicity, 231*t*
o-Tolylazo-*m*-toluene, structure–activity relationship, 240
2-(*o*-Tolylazo)-*p*-toluidine(s), carcinogenicity, 231*t*
Tosylalanyl methyl ester, 1302*t*
Tosyllysyl chloromethyl ketone, 1302
  carcinogenesis inhibitors, 1303*t*
  stage-specific inhibitors, 1309*t*
Tosylphenylalanyl chloromethyl ketone, 1302
  carcinogenesis inhibitors, 1303*t*
Toxaphene, 551
  carcinogenicity, 547–51*t*
  in vivo metabolism, 553
  technical grade, 552–53
Toxicity
  acute and chronic, triazenes, 896
  aflatoxins, 971–83
  3,3-dialkyl-1-(3-pyridyl)triazenes to the rat fetus, 902*t*
  N-nitroso carcinogens, 651
  ring-substituted triazenes, 903
Toxicology
  of chloroprene, 526
  preliminary, carcinogenicity evaluation, 1350
Toxin production in animal feedstocks, 956
TPA—*See* 12-*O*-Tetradecanoylphorbol-13-acetate
TPCK—*See* Tosylphenylalanyl chloromethyl ketone
Transformation
  cell, evaluation of carcinogenicity, 1336
  in vitro, 350
Transplacental carcinogenesis
  N-nitroso carcinogens, 671
  triazenes, principal target organs, 899*t*
Trauma, malignancy development, 25
Tree nuts, in aflatoxins, 1108–9
Tree shrew, aflatoxin B_1 hepatocarcinogenicity, 985*t*
Tremolite, 632
  as contaminant, 633
  fine, structure, 632
  human studies, 638
  in vitro studies, 638
Trenimon
  carcinogenicity, 1249
  oncogenesis tests, 464–65*t*
Treosulfan, carcinogenicity, 1248
Triafur, toxicity, 1256*t*
Trialkyltriazenes, preparation, 894
1,2,3-Triazabutadienes, preparation, 895
Triazenium salts, preparation, 894
Triazines, carcinogenic potential, 869–907
Tributyrin, oncogenesis tests, 420*t*
Tricaprylin, oncogenesis tests, 420*t*
Trichloroaniline, carcinogenicity, 203*t*
Trichloroethane(s), 541, 542
Trichloroethylene, 542–43
Trichloromethane, 537
Trichlorophenol(s), 554
  carcinogenicity, 547–51*t*
Trichlorophenoxyacetic acid, 559
Trichloropropane 2,3-oxide, influence on AFB_1 genotoxicity, 1031*t*
Trichlorphon, 413, 560
  as genotoxic agents, 393
  oncogenesis tests, 418–19*t*
  structure, 385
Trichodermin, lethal dose, 1139*t*
Trichothecenes, 1139*t*
  detection, 1150–51
  determination, biological methods, 1150
  effects on the immune system, 1149–50
  ester, 1149
  oxidation, 1143
  structure, 1139
  thin-layer chromatography, 1150
Trichothecin, lethal dose, 1139*t*
Trichothecolones, structure, 1139
Tricothecenes, carcinogenicity, 1249
Tricyclic aromatic hydrocarbon derivatives, carcinogenic activities, 138–39*t*
Triepoxydecane, oncogenesis tests, 461–62*t*
Triethanolamine, 845
Triethylene glycol, oncogenesis tests, 461–62*t*
Triethylenemelamine(s)
  carcinogen binding index, 376
  carcinogenicity, 369*t*, 1249
  DNA alkylation, 370–71*t*
  initiating agents, 401
  mutagenicity, 369*t*
  oncogenesis tests, 464–65*t*
  relative carcinogenicity, 382

13-Trifluoromethyl, 1302*t*
Trifluraline, 846
3,4,5-Trihydroxycyclohexane-1-carboxylic acid—*See* Shikimic acid
Trimethyl phosphate, oncogenesis tests, 418–19*t*
Trimethylaniline(s), carcinogenicity, 202*t*
2′,3,5′-Trimethyl-4-biphenylamine, carcinogenicity, 209*t*
Trimethylene oxide, 428
  See also Oxetanes
  carcinogenic index, 428
  oncogenesis tests, 430–33*t*
  relative carcinogenicity, 382
2,2,4-Trimethyl-3-hydroxy-3-penenoic acid β-lactone, oncogenesis 438*t*
2,3,6-Trimethylnaphthalene, structure, 169*f*
1,2,8-Trimethylphenantrene, structure, 169*f*
N,N′,N′-Trinitrosohexahydro-1,3,5-triazine, target organ, 775
Triphenylene, carcinogenic activities, 130*t*
Tris(1-aziridinyl)phosphine oxide, oncogenesis tests, 464–65*t*
Tris(1-aziridinyl)phosphine sulfide, oncogenesis tests, 464–65*t*
Tris(2-chloroethyl)amine, oncogenesis tests, 448–49*t*
Tris(2,3-dibromo)phosphate
  oncogenesis tests, 418–19*t*
  structure, 393, 535
Trivial nomenclature, polynuclear aromatic carcinogens, 48
Trout, rainbow—*See* Rainbow trout
Trp-P-1—*See* 3-Amino-1,4-dimethyl-5*H*-pyrido[4,3-*b*]indole
Trp-P-2—*See* 3-Amino-1-methyl-5*H*-pyrido[4,3-*b*]indole
Trypan blue, structure–activity relationship, 243
Tryptophan, structure–activity relationship, 255
Tryptophan pyrrolase, aflatoxin B_1 inhibition, 1086
Trytophan metabolites, epigenetic carcinogen, 1330*t*
Tumors
  bladder, bracken carcinogenicity, 1175
  in farm livestock, bracken carcinogenicity, 1177
  mouse, bracken carcinogenicity, 1175
  in sheep, *pteridium aquuilinum var esculentum*, 1180
  in small animals, bracken carcinogenicity, 1174
  stage, 3–4
  treatment, 10
Tumor induction, 3, 467
  See also Neoplasia
  aniline and its derivatives, 202–3*t*
  benzidine and its derivatives, 213*t*
  benzo[*a*]pyrene derivatives, 102*t*
  biphenylamine(s) and its derivatives, 208–9*t*
  bladder, role of implanted pellet, 256
  derivatives of 4-phenylazoaniline, 231–32*t*
  dialkylaryltriazenes, 904
  factors involved, 52*f*
  fluorenamine(s) and related compounds, 220–22*t*
  fused-ring amines, 225–26*t*
  inhibition, 1282–98
Tumor induction—*Continued*
  methylenedianiline and related compounds, 214*t*
  nitrofuryl compounds, 253–54*t*
  nitroquinoline 1-oxide analogs, 249*t*
  phenylenediamines and related substances, 206–7*t*
  stilbenamines and related compounds, 216–17*t*
Tumor initiators, characteristics, 1281
Tumor promoters, characteristics, 1281
Tumor promotion
  in mouse skin
    effects of retinoids, 1302*t*
    inhibitors, 1308*t*
  in vitro tests, 1338
  in vivo assays, 1339
  inhibition, 1298–1310
Tumor transplantation, 926
Tumorigenesis, persistence of O^6-alkylguanine, 706–11
Tupala glis, aflatoxin B_1 hepatocarcinogenicity, 985*t*
Two-stage carcinogenesis, 1280*f*
  bladder, *N*-nitroso carcinogens, 726
  model, 380
Two-stage promotion
  in mouse skin, stage-specific inhibitors, 1309*t*
  stage-specific inhibitors, 1309–10
Type-C virus, biologic promotion in DNA, 350

U

Ubiquinone, effect on aflatoxin B_1 toxicity, 981
Uganda, liver cancer incidence, 1222*t*
United Kingdom
  bladder cancer, 287, 288*t*
  cancer mortality rate for chemists, 307
United States, cancer mortality rate for chemists, 304
Unreactive L region, related to carcinogenic activity, 59
Unrefined peanut oil, aflatoxin decontamination, 961
α,β-Unsaturated γ-lactones, 428
Unsubstituted angular ring, structure–activity relationships, 54
Unsubstituted aromatic hydrocarbons, properties, 60–61*t*
Unsubstituted polycyclic aromatic hydrocarbons, carcinogenic activities, 130–31*t*
Unsymmetrical nitrosamines
  structure–activity relationship, 659–61
  target organ, 748–62
Uracil mustard
  carcinogenicity, 369*t*
  mutagenicity, 369*t*
  oncogenesis tests, 453*t*
Urethane
  DNA synthesis, inhibition, 402
  structure, 375
Urethane(ethyl carbamate), DNA alkylation, 370–71*t*
Urinary metabolism
  aromatic hydrocarbons, 72
  dialkylaryltriazenes, 905
  dialkylnitrosamines, 690

Urine acidity, bladder carcinogenicity of aromatic amines, 183
Uterine cytosol receptor, aflatoxin M_1 effects, 1088
UV absorption, triazenes, 876
UV light, 23
UV radiation, malignancy sites, 31*t*

V

Vaginal cancer, causes, 1205
Valence number, free, related to carcinogenic activity, 59
Vegetables
  aflatoxins, 1110–11
  nitrosamine content, 1214*t*
  polycyclic aromatic hydrocarbon content, 1210*t*
Verrucarin A, 1143
  lethal dose, 1139*t*
Vertebrates, aflatoxin toxicity, 976
Vesical cancer, causes, 1205
Vicinal dihydrodiol epoxides, 115
  reactivity, 118
Vicinal *trans*-dihydrodiols, nomenclature, 46
Vinblastine, carcinogenicity, 1253
Vincristine, carcinogenicity, 1253
Vinyl bromide, 536
Vinyl chloride, 527
  carcinogen binding index, 376
  causes, 1205
  DNA alkylation, 370–71*t*
  genotoxic carcinogen, 1330*t*
  malignancy sites, 31*t*
  metabolites, 356
    miscoding, 354
  mutagenicity, 528
  oncogenesis, 406–7*t*
  relevant metabolites, 385
  target cells, 376
Vinyl trichloride, 542
Vinylcyclohexene dioxide, oncogenesis tests, 461–62*t*
Vinylene carbonate, 429
  oncogenesis tests, 434–35*t*
1-Vinyl-3,4-epoxycyclohexane, oncogenesis tests, 424*t*
Vinylidene chloride, 528
  oncogenesis, 406–7*t*
Vinylidene chloride carcinogenicity, 529
Vinylidene fluoride, 529
Virtually safe dose, definition, 1207–8
Viruses, role in human malignancy, 27–28
Vitamin A
  deficiency, effect on AFB_1 carcinogenicity, 995*t*
  effect on carcinogenesis, 1301*t*
Vitamin A palmitate, effect on carcinogenesis, 1301*t*
Vitamin C
  effect on AFB_1 carcinogenicity, 996*t*
  inhibition of chemical carcinogenesis, 1283*t*
Vitamin content, effects on aflatoxin toxicity, 980
Vitamin E, inhibition of chemical carcinogenesis, 1283*t*
Vitamin K1, effect on aflatoxin B_1 toxicity, 981
Volatility, carcinogenic reagents, 314

W

Walnuts, aflatoxins, 1109
Water
  nitrosamine content, 1214*t*
  nitrosamines, 848
Water hose production, *N*-nitrosamines, occupational exposure, 853*t*
Wheat, aflatoxins, 1098
Wine, aflatoxins, 1112
Wood particles, malignancy sites, 31*t*

X

X-rays
  malignancy sites, 31*t*
  pregnancy, hazards, 22
Xanthine oxides, structure–activity relationship, 250
Xenobiotics, modifying effects on *N*-nitroso carcinogenesis, 678*t*
Xenylamine—*See* 4-Biphenylamine
Xeroderma pigmentes, 19
Xeroderma pigmentosum, 365
  DNA alkylation repair, *N*-nitroso carcinogens, 723
Xylidine(s), carcinogenicity, 202*t*

Y

Yogurt, aflatoxins, 1115

Z

Z—*See* Zearalenone
Zearalenol, structure, 1153
Zearalenone, 1151
  biological action, 1152–57
  biosynthesis from acetate, 1151
  destruction, 1159
  detection methods, 1152
  effects
    on animals, 1154
    in sheep, 1151
  hydrolysis, 1158
  maternal and fetal effects, 1156
  metabolism, 1157–59
  occurrence, 1153
  production, 1153
  teratogenic effects, 1156
Zearelenol, 1152
Zeolites, 634
  human studies, 638
Zeranol, 1152
  structure, 1153
Zinc dibutyldithiocarbamate, nitrosamine contamination, 844*t*
Zinc diethyldithiocarbamate, nitrosamine contamination, 844*t*
Zinc pentamethyleneiminedithiocarbamate, nitrosamine contamination, 844*t*
Zoxazolamine hydroxylase, aflatoxin B_1 inhibition, 1086